Infectious Diseases: In Context

SECOND EDITION

Infectious Diseases: In Context

SECOND EDITION

VOLUME 2

Macrophage Activation Syndrome to Zoonoses

Thomas Riggs, Editor

GALE
A Cengage Company

Farmington Hills, Mich • San Francisco • New York • Waterville, Maine
Meriden, Conn • Mason, Ohio • Chicago

GALE
A Cengage Company

Infectious Diseases: In Context, Second Edition

Thomas Riggs, Editor

Project Editor: Tracie Moy

Acquisitions Editor: Jessica Bomarito

Editorial Staff: Mike Tyrkus

Rights Acquisition and Management: Ashley M. Maynard and Carissa Poweleit

Imaging: John L. Watkins

Product Design: Kristine A. Julien

Composition: Amy Darga

Manufacturing: Rita Wimberley

For product information and technology assistance, contact us at **Gale Customer Support, 1-800-877-4253.**
For permission to use material from this text or product, submit all requests online at **www.cengage.com/permissions.**
Further permissions questions can be emailed to **permissionrequest@cengage.com**

Cover photographs: 3D rendering influenza virus, Rost9/Shutterstock.com; Vaccinating a child, CNKO2/Shutterstock.com; Tick crawling on human skin, Henrik Larsson/Shutterstock.com; Vaccine containers, Paula Bronstein/Getty Images; Hand in glove collects water sample, PRESSLAB/Shutterstock.com; Hands of old woman suffering from leprosy, NikomMaelao Production/Shutterstock.com; Fumigation machine to kill mosquitoes carrying Zika, BOONJAEM/Shutterstock.com.

Inside art: 3D rendering Influenza Virus H1N1, Rost9/Shutterstock.com.

LIBRARY OF CONGRESS CATALOGING-IN-PUBLICATION DATA

Names: Riggs, Thomas J., editor.
Title: Infectious diseases : in context / Thomas J. Riggs, editor.
Description: Second edition. | Farmington Hills, Mich : Gale, A Cengage Company, [2018] | Includes bibliographical references and index.
Identifiers: LCCN 2018002810 | ISBN 9781410381286 (set : alk. paper) | ISBN 9781410381293 (vol. 1 : alk. paper) | ISBN 9781410381309 (vol. 2 : alk. paper) | ISBN 9781410381316 (ebook)
Subjects: MESH: Communicable Diseases | Encyclopedias
Classification: LCC RC111 | NLM WC 13 | DDC 616.003—dc23
LC record available at https://lccn.loc.gov/2018002810

Gale
27500 Drake Rd.
Farmington Hills, MI 48331-3535

978-1-4103-8128-6 (set)
978-1-4103-8129-3 (vol. 1)
978-1-4103-8130-9 (vol. 2)

This title is also available as an e-book.
978-1-4103-8131-6

Contact your Gale sales representative for ordering information.

Printed in the United States
1 2 3 4 5 6 7 22 21 20 19 18

Contents

Advisors and Contributors xv

Introduction xvii

About the *In Context* Series xxi

About This Book xxiii

Using Primary Sources xxvii

Glossary xxxi

Chronology lxi

VOLUME 1

African Sleeping Sickness 1

AIDS 7

AIDS: Origin of the Modern Pandemic 17

Airborne Precautions 21

Alveolar Echinococcosis 24

Amebiasis 27

Anellovirus 30

Angiostrongyliasis 35

Animal Importation 39

Anisakiasis 43

Anthrax 47

Anti-Cytokine Antibody Syndrome 53

Antibacterial Drugs 56

Antibiotic Resistance 61

Antimicrobial Soaps 66

Antiviral Drugs 70
Arthropod-borne Disease 74
Ascariasis 78
Asilomar Conference 81
Aspergillosis 84
Avian Influenza 87
B Virus (Cercopithecine herpesvirus 1) Infection 91
*Babesiosis (*Babesia *Infection)* 95
Bacterial Disease 99
Balantidiasis 102
Baylisascaris *Infection* 105
Biological Weapons Convention 109
Bioterrorism 113
Blastomycosis 121
Blood Supply and Infectious Disease 125
Bloodborne Pathogens 129
Botulism 133
Bovine Spongiform Encephalopathy (Mad Cow Disease) 136
Brucellosis 140
Burkholderia 144
Buruli (Bairnsdale) Ulcer 147
Campylobacter *Infection* 151
Cancer and Infectious Disease 154
Candidiasis 157
Cat Scratch Disease 161
CDC (Centers for Disease Control and Prevention) 164
Chagas Disease 171
Chickenpox (Varicella) 175
Chikungunya 180
Childhood-Associated Infectious Diseases, Immunization Impacts 184
Chlamydia *Infection* 189
Chlamydia Pneumoniae 193
Cholera 197

Climate Change and Infectious Disease 203
Clostridium difficile *Infection* 209
CMV (Cytomegalovirus) Infection 214
Coccidioidomycosis 218
Cohorted Communities and Infectious Disease 223
Cold Sores 226
Colds (Rhinitis) 228
Contact Lenses and Fusarium *Keratitis* 232
Contact Precautions 235
Creutzfeldt-Jakob Disease 239
Crimean-Congo Hemorrhagic Fever 243
Cryptococcus neoformans *Infection* 247
Cryptosporidiosis 251
Culture and Sensitivity 254
Cyclosporiasis 258
Demographics and Infectious Disease 261
Dengue and Dengue Hemorrhagic Fever 266
Developing Nations and Drug Delivery 270
Diphtheria 274
Disinfection 280
Dracunculiasis 283
Droplet Precautions 286
Dysentery 289
Ear Infection (Otitis Media) 293
Eastern Equine Encephalitis 296
Ebola 300
Economic Development and Infectious Disease 306
Emerging Infectious Diseases 311
Encephalitis 315
Endemnicity 320
Enterovirus 71 infection 324
Epidemiology 328
Epstein-Barr Virus 335

Escherichia coli *O157:H7* 338
Exposed: Scientists Who Risked Disease for Discovery 342
Fifth Disease 347
Filariasis 350
Food-Borne Disease and Food Safety 354
Gastroenteritis (Common Causes) 358
Genetic Identification of Microorganisms 362
Genital Herpes 365
Germ Theory of Disease 366
Giardiasis 371
GIDEON 375
Glanders (Melioidosis) 378
Globalization and Infectious Disease 383
Gonorrhea 387
H5N1 391
Haemophilus Influenzae 394
Hand, Foot, and Mouth Disease 397
Handwashing 400
Hantavirus 404
Helicobacter pylori 409
Helminth Disease 414
Hemorrhaghic Fevers 418
Hepatitis A 422
Hepatitis B 426
Hepatitis C 430
Hepatitis D 434
Hepatitis E 437
Herpes Simplex 1 Virus 440
Herpes Simplex 2 Virus 444
Histoplasmosis 448
HIV 453
Hookworm (Ancylostoma) *Infection* 457
Host and Vector 461

Hot Tub Rash (Pseudomonas aeruginosa *Dermatitis*) 465
HPV (Human Papillomavirus) Infection 468
Immigration and Infectious Disease 472
Immune Response to Infection 476
Impetigo 480
Infection Control and Asepesis 483
Influenza 488
Influenza Pandemic of 1918 493
Influenza Pandemic of 1957 499
Influenza, Tracking Seasonal Influences and Virus Mutation 503
Isolation and Quarantine 508
Japanese Encephalitis 511
Kawasaki Disease 515
Koch's Postulates 519
Kuru 522
Lassa Fever 526
Legionnaires' Disease (Legionellosis) 529
Legislation, International Law, and Infectious Diseases 533
Leishmaniasis 538
Leprosy (Hansen's Disease) 543
Leptospirosis 548
Lice Infestation (Pediculosis) 552
Listeriosis 556
Liver Fluke Infection 560
Lung Fluke (Paragonimus) Infection 565
Lyme Disease 569

VOLUME 2

Macrophage Activation Syndrome 575
Malaria 578
Marburg Hemorrhagic Fever 585
Marine Toxins 589
Measles (Rubeola) 593

Médicins Sans Frontièrs (Doctors without Borders) 599
Meningitis, Bacterial 604
Meningitis, Viral 607
Microbial Evolution 611
Microorganisms 615
Microscope and Microscopy 618
Microsporidiosis 622
Monkeypox 626
Mononucleosis 630
Mosquito-Borne Diseases 636
MRSA 640
Mumps 644
Mycotic Disease 649
National Institute of Allergy and Infectious Diseases 653
Necrotizing Fasciitis 657
Nipah Virus Encephalitis 662
Nocardiosis 666
Norovirus Infection 669
Nosocomial (Healthcare–Associated) Infections 673
Notifiable Diseases 678
Opportunistic Infection 682
Outbreaks: Field-Level Response 685
Pandemic Preparedness 690
Parasitic Diseases 694
Personal Protective Equipment 699
Pink Eye (Conjunctivitis) 702
Pinworm (Enterobius vermicularis) *Infection* 705
Plague, Early History 709
Plague, Modern History 715
Pneumocystis jirovecii *Pneumonia* 721
Pneumonia 725
Polio Eradication Campaign 732
Polio (Poliomyelitis) 736

Powassan Virus 741

President's (Obama Adminstration) Initiative on Combating Antibiotic Resistance 744

Prion Disease 748

ProMED 751

Protozoan diseases 753

Psittacosis 759

Public Health and Infectious Disease 762

Puerperal Fever 767

Q Fever 771

Rabies 775

Rapid Diagnostic Tests for Infectious Diseases 781

Rat-Bite Fever 785

Re-emerging Infectious Diseases 789

Relapsing Fever 795

Resistant Organisms 799

Retroviruses 805

Rickettsial Disease 809

Rift Valley Fever 813

Ringworm 817

River Blindness (Onchocerciasis) 820

Rocky Mountain Spotted Fever 824

Rotavirus Infection 828

RSV (Respiratory Syncytial Virus Infection) Infection 832

Rubella 836

Salmonella *Infection (Salmonellosis)* 840

Sanitation 844

SARS (Severe Acute Respiratory Syndrome) 847

Scabies 852

Scarlet Fever 856

Schistosomiasis (Bilharzia) 860

Scrofula: The King's Evil 865

Sepsis as a WHO Priority 868

Severe Fever With Thrombocytopenia Syndrome 871
Sexually Transmitted Infections 875
Shigellosis 880
Shingles (Herpes Zoster) Infection 885
Smallpox 890
Smallpox Eradication and Storage 896
Sporotrichosis 901
St. Louis Encephalitis 905
Standard Precautions 908
Staphylococcus aureus *Infection* 911
Sterilization 914
Strep Throat 917
Streptococcal Infections, Group A 920
Streptococcal Infections, Group B 924
Strongyloidiasis 928
Swimmer's Ear and Swimmer's Itch (Cercarial Dermatitis) 931
Syphilis 934
*Taeniasis (*Taenia *Infection)* 940
Talaromycosis 944
Tapeworm Infection 948
Tetanus 952
Tick-Borne Diseases 956
Toxic Shock 961
*Toxoplasmosis (*Toxoplasma *Infection)* 964
Trachoma 967
Travel and Infectious Disease 970
Trichinellosis 972
Trichomoniasis 975
Tropical Infectious Diseases 979
Tuberculosis 983
Tularemia 989
Typhoid Fever 993
Typhus 997

UNICEF ... 1003
United Nations Millennium Goals and Infectious Disease ... 1007
Urinary Tract Infection ... 1012
USAMRIID (United States Army Medical Research Institute of Infectious Diseases) ... 1015
Vaccines and Vaccine Development ... 1020
Vancomycin-Resistant Enterococci ... 1025
Vector-Borne Disease ... 1029
Venezuelan Equine Encephalitis Virus ... 1033
Viral Disease ... 1037
Virus Hunters ... 1043
War and Infectious Disease ... 1047
Water-Borne Disease ... 1053
West Nile Virus ... 1057
Whipworm (Trichuriasis) ... 1062
Whooping Cough (Pertussis) ... 1066
Women and Infectious Disease ... 1071
World Health Organization (WHO) ... 1076
World Trade and Infectious Disease ... 1081
Yaws ... 1087
Yellow Fever ... 1092
Yersiniosis ... 1096
Zika Virus ... 1100
Zoonoses ... 1105

Sources Consulted ... 1111
General Index ... 1203

Advisors and Contributors

While compiling this volume, the editors relied on the expertise and contributions of the following scientists, scholars, and researchers, who served as advisors, academic reviewers, or contributors for *Infectious Diseases: In Context.*

Susan Aldridge, Ph.D.
Independent scholar and writer
London, United Kingdom

William Arthur Atkins, M.S.
Independent scholar and writer
Pekin, Illinois

Stephen A. Berger, M.D.
Founder and Medical Advisor
Tel Aviv Medical Center
Tel Aviv, Israel

Agnieszka Caruso, PhD
Canon Biomedical
Rockville, Maryland

Laura J. Cataldo, PhD
Independent Scholar
Myersville, Maryland

L. S. Clements, MD, PhD
Assistant Professor of Pediatrics
University of South Alabama College of Medicine
Mobile, Alabama

Bryan Davies, LLB
Writer and Journalist
Ontario, Canada

Paul Davies, PhD
Director
Science Research Institute
Adjunct Professor
Paris-Sorbonne
Paris, France

Larry Gilman, PhD
Independent Scholar and Journalist
Sharon, Vermont

Tony Hawas, MA
Writer and Journalist
Brisbane, Australia

Brian D. Hoyle, PhD
Microbiologist
Nova Scotia, Canada

Kenneth T. LaPensee, PhD, MPH
Epidemiologist and Medical Policy Specialist
Hampton, New Jersey

Adrienne Wilmoth Lerner, JD
Independent Scholar
Jacksonville, Florida

Ted McDermott, MFA
Writer and Journalist
Butte, Montana

Caryn Neumann, PhD
Senior Lecturer, Interdisciplinary and Communication Studies
Miami University
Oxford, Ohio

James Overholtzer, MA
Independent Scholar
Seattle, Washington

Anna Marie Roos, PhD
Reader and Programme Leader, School of History & Heritage
University of Lincoln
Lincoln, United Kingdom

Kausalya Santhanam, PhD
Founder
SciVista IP & Scientific Communication
India

Claire Skinner, MFA
Writer and Editor
Tucson, Arizona

Constance K. Stein, PhD
Director of Cytogenetics and Associate Professor
SUNY Upstate Medical University
Syracuse, New York

Samuel D. Uretsky, PharmD
Independent Researcher and Writer
New York, New York

Malini Vashishta, PhD
Independent Scholar and Medical Writer
Windsor, California

Jack Woodall, PhD
Former Director, Nucleus for the Investigation of Emerging Infectious Diseases
Institute of Medical Biochemistry,
Center for Health Sciences
Federal University of Rio de Janeiro
Rio de Janeiro, Brazil

Melanie Barton Zoltán, MS
Independent Scholar
Amherst, Massachusetts

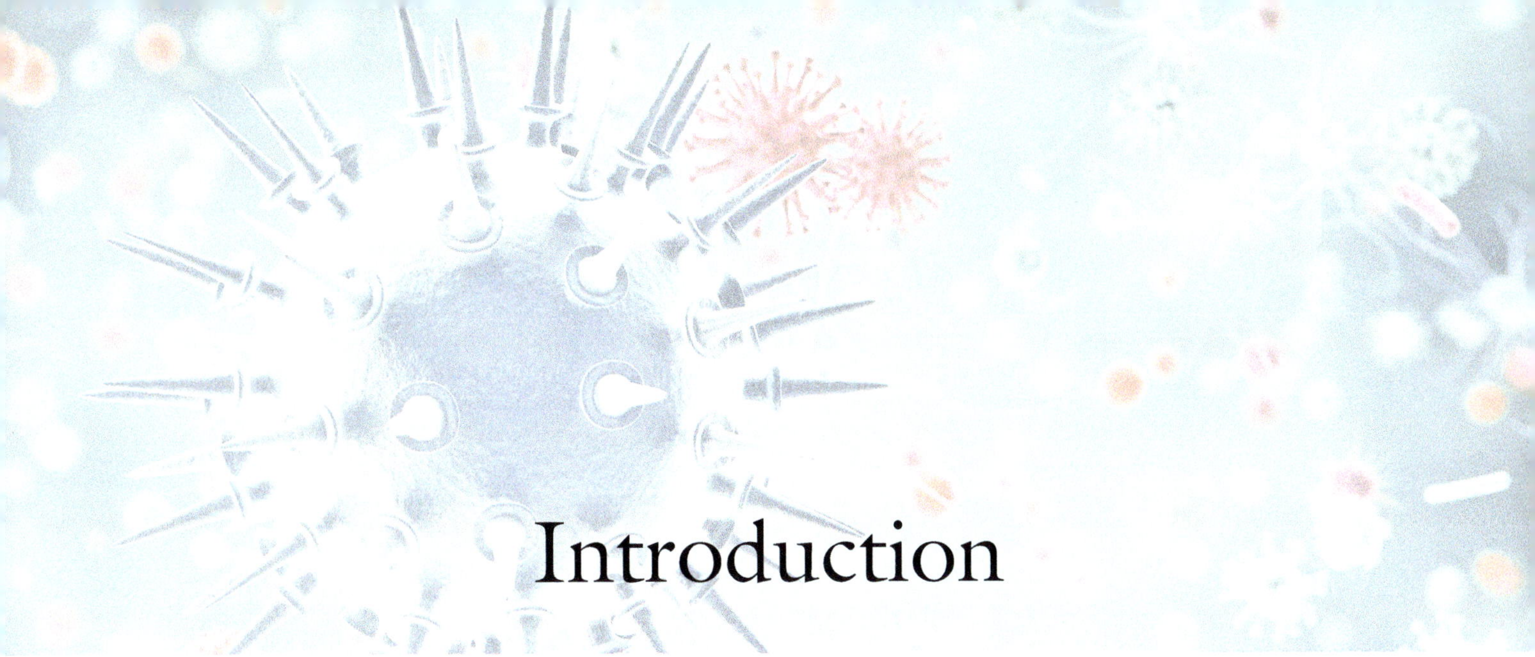

Introduction

Ever since humankind's ancestors first descended from the trees and adopted a bipedal lifestyle in the East African savanna, our species has been victim to two major biothreats: large carnivores and seemingly invisible microbial pathogens. Competing large carnivores were dispatched relatively quickly by *Homo sapiens*, which literally means "wise man," but microorganisms remained invisible and completely unknown to early humans. Yet our species needed to develop a sophisticated innate and adaptive immune system to defend against these microorganisms. Throughout history our forbearers must have fallen prey to a multitude of endemic and epidemic microbial diseases, and infections have taken a terrible toll on human populations.

When the first modern humans appeared in Africa about 170,000 years ago, they lived a predatory existence as scattered bands of hunter-gatherers. However, humans lacked the speed, agility, size, strength, and endowment of traditional weapons featured by most large carnivores such as fangs, thick hides, large claws, and powerful jaws. Our species had to learn to become predators by deploying their relatively few but ultimately decisive assets. Humans possessed three major advantages over their carnivorous competitors: 1) unusually large brains to cooperate and learn through their communication skills; 2) apposable thumbs for tool making; and 3) knowledge of the many uses of fire to survive. Remarkably, the capacity to maintain and control fire was passed down from our closest primate ancestor, *Homo erectus*, which acquired the skill over 1 million years earlier. In addition to providing light, warmth, and some protection against large predators, fire presented an opportunity to limit intestinal parasites by cooking meat before eating it. Helminthic intestinal parasites slowly sap the strength and vitality of their human hosts. Living a life relatively free from parasitism provided humans with a major advantage over other mammals.

Becoming predators had its advantages, but frequent nicks and scratches and intermittent bleeding episodes must have inevitably accompanied this lifestyle. Our thin skins and the lack of decent footwear likely made minor injuries commonplace when chasing prey. Those fortunate enough to possess rapid clotting capacity and an early and intense innate immune response following injury enjoyed an evolutionary advantage over bleeders and poor wound-healers. Regrettably, what were considered survival traits for our ancestors are a liability in modern times. We are now plagued by an excessive risk of clotting tendencies (including deep venous thrombosis, strokes, and myocardial infarction). Likewise, our overly reactive immune responses and propensity to overcompensate from inflammatory stimuli contribute to accelerating incidence of localized and systemic inflammatory states such as sepsis, asthma, multiple sclerosis, and inflammatory bowel disease.

Humans spread out over time from East Africa about 35,000 years ago to populate much of the world's tropical and temperate climates. Yet the entire human population expanded very little for tens of thousands of years. Our collective fate as a species was forever altered about 8,000 years ago with the first successful human efforts to domesticate plants. This seminal event in human history first took place along the Fertile Crescent in the Middle East and was later copied elsewhere, when feasible. Manipulating the environment to maintain favored plant life for human consumption greatly accelerated the yields from a given parcel of land compared to searching for scattered edible plants in the environment. These first agrarian societies were later joined by domesticated animals that could be employed to carry heavy loads, as a source of animal milk, and as animal meat for slaughter. Horses and oxen could also be harnessed to plows to till the soil and further improve crop yields. Jump on a horse's back and later add wheel-and-axel-fitted chariots or wagons, and you have the essential elements of a transportation system that existed for thousands of years.

Putting aside our wandering, predatory ways to settle down as farmers had an immediate and profound impact on humankind. The first effect was food security and a reduced fear of starvation. Second, high crop yields provided women of childbearing age ready access to food, resulting in increased fertility and fecundity rates. Third, a steady source of nutrition freed up at least some members of a farm community to perform more specialized labor. Individuals with a penchant for tool making could become full-time tool makers, good weavers could become permanent weavers, people with a talent for pottery making became full-time pottery makers, and so on. Food could now be provided by someone else in a specialized workforce.

The agrarian lifestyle necessitated human habitation living within fixed dwellings near the fields. Gone were the days of small, nomadic bands of humans scattered over the land hunting for food. People now became close-knit members of towns crowded together in proximity to each other and their animals. This living arrangement created a novel risk for humankind. Some of the deadliest epidemics in history are zoonotic infections, which are infectious diseases found in animals that spread and adapt to replicate in human hosts. Domesticated farm animals serve as unrecognized and unwanted reservoirs for zoonotic infections. These animals have gradually acquired some form of immune defense or tolerance to the manifest disease produced by these microorganisms. When the infections "jump" species and infect their human overseers, massive and potentially lethal epidemics can occur.

This has occurred numerous times in the past and continues in the early 21st century in such diseases as the H7N9 bird flu strain passed from chickens to humans and the Middle Eastern Respiratory Syndrome–associated coronavirus infections spread from camels to humans. Many other examples of zoonotic epidemic diseases are recorded in history. For example, the smallpox virus in humans was likely derived from the camel pox virus and is probably the single greatest killer of humankind throughout history. The black plague in 14th-century Europe was likely derived from city-dwelling, peri-domestic rats. When the bacterial pathogen *Yersinia pestis* first jumped species to humans it caused infection of the lymph glands (bubonic plague) and then via the respiratory tract (pneumonic plague). This disease killed millions over a five-year period in Europe, tearing at the very fabric of Western civilization. Bovine tuberculosis from infected, unpasteurized cow's milk was likely the origin of the first human cases of tuberculosis. Tuberculosis has become a common cause of death ever since. This single chronic lung infection has killed, and continues to kill, over a million patients worldwide each year.

Increasingly our forefathers migrated to crowded population centers, and the human population exploded. This trend continues in the 21st century. We are still on the ascending limb of an exponential expansion of human population. Evidence indicates that it took tens of thousands of years for our species to reach our first billion around 1830 CE. It took about 100 years to reach the second billion in 1930. Yet it took only 12 years to go from 6 billion (1999) to 7 billion people (2011), and it will be an estimated 13 years until we reach 8 billion people. For the first time in history, the majority of people now reside in cities. Many megacities (defined as greater than 10 million inhabitants) are bursting at the seams with overstretched needs for clean water, sufficient goods and services, adequate sewage disposal, and enough living space to handle the expanding population needs.

Living in densely populated spaces facilitates the spread of microbial pathogens by the respiratory tract by sharing a common airspace in poorly ventilated rooms. Food preparation and distribution into large cities under suboptimal sanitary conditions and inadequate sewage disposal puts city dwellers at great risk of foodborne illness and waterborne outbreaks. Even urban mosquito-borne outbreaks are an increasing risk in megacities in developing countries due to poor water drainage systems and standing water sources from old tires and other debris from human activities. As cities get larger and people accumulate under confined spaces, the risk of contagion rises. With ready access to international flights, we are increasingly susceptible to a major epidemic event. A newly reassorted influenza virus strain or a similar respiratory virus will most likely be the cause of the next pandemic. This is one reason why so much effort is going into finding a universal vaccine option to protect people from this potentially deadly virus. Deliberate release of a genetically enhanced hybrid virus as a weapon of bioterrorism is also a possibility. A pan-resistant, highly transmissible bacterial pathogen that has evolved resistance to all major antibiotics is also a possibility.

Remarkably, the existence of pathogenic microorganisms was entirely unknown until 1683, when Dutch microscopist Antoni van Leeuwenhoek (1632–1723) peered down his glass lens magnifier to first identify bacteria. It took almost 200 years to confirm their pathogenic significance by the establishment of the germ theory of disease by Louis Pasteur (1822–1895), Robert Koch (1843–1910), and many others. At least 1,500 known species of microbial pathogens have been identified that can harm humans. To be a pathogen, the microorganism must possess the ability to evade host barrier defenses and immune clearance mechanisms. Further, it must be able to replicate faster that the innate and acquired clearance capacity to remove pathogens from the patient. The struggle continues between the human host and microbial pathogens even in the 21st century.

Consider that, as of 2018, up to one-third of the entire human population was latently infected with tuberculosis. This mycobacterial organism can reawaken and spread within the host if his or her immune defenses fail them. Reactivation of tuberculosis can spread to unsuspecting people living close to the infected patient at any time. The upper airways of up to 60 percent of children in day care centers are colonized with the common respiratory pathogen *Streptococcus pneumoniae*. *Staphylococcus aureus* is found in the nose of least one-third of humans, and 5 to 10 percent are colonized by *Neisseria meningitidis*. These constant microbial treats are countered by a continuously acting array of innate and acquired host defenses that hold back potential invaders. Patients born with primary immune deficiencies do not have to wait long to be recognized because of the usual onslaught of opportunistic pathogens to which we are all exposed, but they are more susceptible. In addition to endemic infectious disease risks, epidemic diseases continue to plague us on a regular basis. Despite concerted vaccine-induced mitigation strategies, annual influenza epidemics exact a toll on human populations. As of 2018 Brazil was experiencing an entirely newly recognized epidemic of microcephaly and Guillain-Barré syndrome from a previously unknown mosquito-borne flavivirus known as Zika virus. At the same time, the ancient scourge of Yellow Fever, which is caused by a similar, but highly lethal flavivirus, has reappeared and become epidemic in regions of Brazil.

The detailed study of pathogenic microbiology teaches us that, while we are controlling some pathogens, many others are not under our thumb and can still cause us harm. Smallpox and possibly polio have likely been eliminated by concerted control efforts featuring vaccine eradication strategies. We have been less effective eliminating pathogens with antimicrobial chemotherapy. The promise of precision medicine with ready access to molecular biology tools to eradicate pathogens remains an attractive but not as yet unproven method to vanquish our microbial adversaries. We still need new ideas in our continuing efforts to control microorganisms.

This book describes in some detail the nature of essentially all the common microbial pathogens known to infect humans. Content experts who prepared each chapter use a templated format, which provides a succinct yet thorough and up-to-date summary of each pathogen and its clinical infectious disease manifestations. The book provides a detailed and ready access reference text of pathogenic microbiology.

Steven Opal, M.D.
Professor of Medicine, Infectious Disease Division,
Alpert Medical School of Brown University

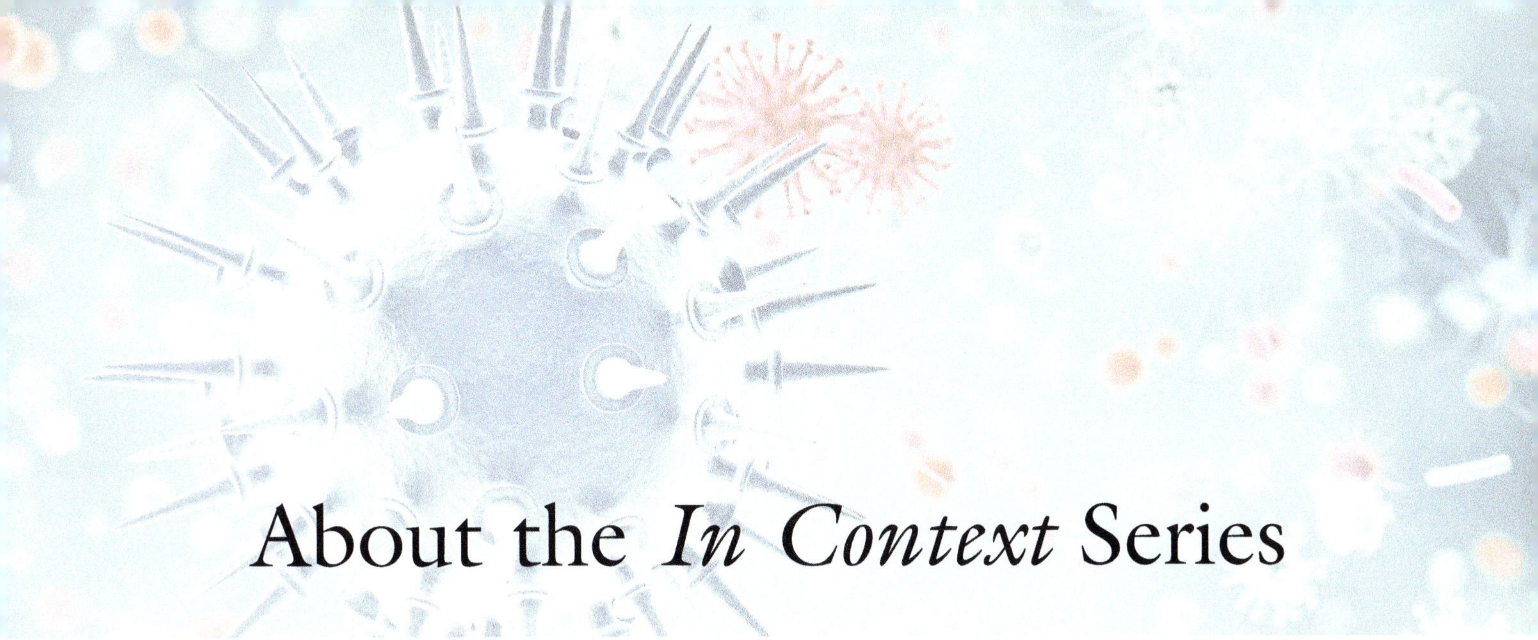

About the *In Context* Series

Written by subject matter experts and aimed primarily at high school students and an interested general readership, the *In Context* series serves as an authoritative reference guide to essential concepts of science, the impacts of recent changes in scientific consensus, and the effects of science on social, political, and legal issues.

In Context books align with, and support, national science standards and high school science curriculums. Cross-curricular in nature, the series addresses the intersections of science and the humanities, and facilitates higher-level thinking that is critical to student achievement. Original essays written by subject matter experts and supplemental primary source documents serve the requirements of high school and international baccalaureate programs. Entries are designed to present foundational concepts, provide insights on leading social issues, and spur critical thinking about connections between science and society.

In Context books also give special coverage to the impact of science on daily life, commerce, travel, and the future of industrialized and impoverished nations. Entries include Words to Know sidebars designed to facilitate understanding and increase reading retention without overwhelming readers with scientific terminology.

Entries include standardized subheads tailored to the subject matter of each book. To facilitate further research, each entry includes a listing of resources (books, periodicals, and websites) and references to related entries.

In addition to maps, charts, tables and graphs, each *In Context* title has approximately 250 topic-related images that visually enrich the content. Each *In Context* title includes a chronology of major events related to the topic, a topic-specific glossary, a bibliography, and an index especially prepared to coordinate with the volume topic.

Disclaimer: This information is not a tool for self-diagnosis or a substitute for professional care.

About This Book

The goal of *Infectious Diseases: In Context* is to help high school and early college-age students understand the essential facts and deeper cultural connections of topics and issues related to the scientific study of infectious disease.

The relationship of science to complex ethical and social considerations is evident, for example, when considering the general rise of infectious diseases that sometimes occurs as an unintended side effect of the otherwise beneficial use of medications. Approximately one-quarter of the world's population is infected with tuberculosis (TB). Although for most people the infection is inactive, the organism causing some new cases of TB is evolving toward a greater resistance to the antibiotics that were once effective in treating TB. These statistics take on a social dimension given that TB disproportionately affects social groups such as the elderly, minorities, and people infected with human immunodeficiency virus (HIV). In 2017 TB was a leading cause of death for individuals infected with HIV.

To encourage the reader to explore the relationship between science and culture, as space allows, we have included primary sources that enhance the content of *In Context* entries. Drawn from popular media, accessible scholarly journals, and historical sources, these documents include firsthand accounts from patients and medical professionals, in-depth case studies, foundational works of scientific thought, and government documents that shed light on the topics under study. In keeping with the philosophy that much of the benefit from using primary sources derives from the reader's own process of inquiry, the contextual material introducing each primary source provides an unobtrusive introduction and springboard to critical thought.

General Structure

Infectious Diseases: In Context, Second Edition is a collection of more than 260 entries that provide insight into increasingly important and urgent topics associated with the study of infectious disease.

The articles in the book are meant to be understandable by anyone with a curiosity about topics related to infectious disease, and the second edition of *Infectious Diseases: In Context* has been designed with ready reference in mind:

- Entries are arranged alphabetically rather than by chronology or scientific subfield.
- The **chronology** (timeline) includes many of the most significant events in the history of infectious disease and advances of science. Where appropriate, related scientific advances are included to offer additional context.

- An extensive glossary provides readers with a ready reference for content-related terminology. In addition to defining terms within the text, specific Words to Know sidebars are placed within each entry.
- A bibliography section (citations of books, periodicals, and websites) offers additional resources to those resources cited within each entry.
- A **comprehensive general index** guides the reader to topics and people mentioned in the book.

Entry Structure

In Context entries are designed so that readers may navigate entries with ease. Toward that goal, entries are divided into easy-to-access sections:

- **Introduction**: An opening section designed to clearly identify the topic.
- **Words to Know** sidebar: Essential terms that enhance readability and critical understanding of entry content.
- Established but flexible **rubrics** customize content presentation and identify each section, enabling the reader to navigate entries with ease. Inside *Infectious Diseases: In Context* entries, readers will find two key schemes of organization. Most entries contain internal discussions of **Disease History, Characteristics, and Transmission**, followed by **Scope and Distribution**, then a summary of **Treatment and Prevention**. General social or science topics may have a simpler structure discussing, for example, **History and Scientific Foundations**. Regardless, the goal of *In Context* entries is a consistent, content-appropriate, and easy-to-follow presentation.
- **Impacts and Issues**: Key scientific, political, or social considerations related to the entry topic.
- **Bibliography**: Citations of books, periodicals, and websites used in preparation of the entry or that provide a stepping stone to further study.
- **"See also" references** clearly identify other content-related entries.

Infectious Diseases: In Context Special Style Notes

Please note the following regarding topics and entries included in *Infectious Diseases: In Context*:

- Primary source selection and the composition of sidebars are not attributed to authors of signed entries to which the sidebars may be associated. In all cases the sources for sidebars containing external content (e.g., a CDC policy position or medical recommendation) are clearly indicated.
- The Centers for Disease Control and Prevention (CDC) includes parasitic diseases with infectious diseases, and the editors have adopted this scheme.
- A detailed understanding of biology and chemistry is neither assumed nor required for *Infectious Diseases: In Context*. Accordingly, students and other readers should not be intimidated or deterred by the sometimes complex names of chemical molecules or biological classification. Where necessary, sufficient information regarding chemical structure or species classification is provided. If desired, more information can easily be obtained from any basic chemistry or biology reference.

Bibliography Citation Formats (How to Cite Articles and Sources)

In Context titles adopt the following citation format:

BIBLIOGRAPHY

Books

Magill, Gerard, ed. *Genetics and Ethics: An Interdisciplinary Study.* New York: Fordham University Press, 2003.

Verlinsky, Yury, and Anver Kuliev. *Practical Preimplantation Genetic Diagnosis.* New York: Springer, 2005.

Periodicals

Byrd, Allyson L., and Julia A. Segre. "Adapting Koch's Postulates." *Science* 351, no. 6270 (January 15, 2016): 224–226. This article can also be found online at http://science.sciencemag.org/content/351/6270/224 (accessed January 16, 2018).

Eldin, Carole, et al. "From Q Fever to *Coxiella burnetii* Infection: A Paradigm Change." *Clinical Microbiology Reviews* 30, no. 1 (January 2017): 115–190.

Websites

ADEAR. Alzheimer's Disease Education and Referral Center. National Institute on Aging. http://www.alzheimers.org/generalinfo.htm (accessed January 23, 2018).

"Discussion by the Genetics and Public Policy Center." PGD: Preimplantation Genetic Diagnosis. http://dnapolicy.org/downloads/pdfs/policy_pgd.pdf (accessed January 23, 2006).

Genetics and Public Policy Center. http://dnapolicy.org/index.jhtml.html (accessed January 23, 2018).

There are, however, alternative citation formats that may be useful to readers and examples of how to cite articles in often used alternative formats are shown below.

APA Style

Books

Kübler-Ross, Elizabeth. (1969) *On Death and Dying.* New York: Macmillan. Excerpted in K. Lee Lerner and Brenda Wilmoth Lerner, eds. (2006) *Medicine, Health, and Bioethics: Essential Primary Sources*, Farmington Hills, Mich.: Thomson Gale.

Periodicals

Venter, J. Craig, et al. (2001, February 16). "The Sequence of the Human Genome." *Science*, vol. 291, no. 5507, pp. 1304–51. Excerpted in K. Lee Lerner and Brenda Wilmoth Lerner, eds. (2006) *Medicine, Health, and Bioethics: Essential Primary Sources*, Farmington Hills, Mich.: Thomson Gale.

Websites

Johns Hopkins Hospital and Health System. "Patient Rights and Responsibilities." Retrieved January 14, 2006 from http://www.hopkinsmedicine.org/patients/JHH/patient_rights.html. Excerpted in K. Lee Lerner and Brenda Wilmoth Lerner, eds. (2006) *Medicine, Health, and Bioethics: Essential Primary Sources*, Farmington Hills, Mich.: Thomson Gale.

Chicago Style

Books

Kübler-Ross, Elizabeth. *On Death and Dying.* New York: Macmillan, 1969. Excerpted in K. Lee Lerner and Brenda Wilmoth Lerner, eds. *Medicine, Health, and Bioethics: Essential Primary Sources*, Farmington Hills, MI: Thomson Gale, 2006.

Periodicals

Venter, J. Craig, et al. "The Sequence of the Human Genome." *Science* (2001): 291, 5507, 1304–1351. Excerpted in K. Lee Lerner and Brenda Wilmoth Lerner, eds. *Medicine, Health, and Bioethics: Essential Primary Sources*, Farmington Hills, MI: Thomson Gale, 2006.

Websites

Johns Hopkins Hospital and Health System. "Patient Rights and Responsibilities." http://www.hopkinsmedicine.org/patients/JHH/patient_rights.html (accessed January 14, 2006). Excerpted in K. Lee Lerner and Brenda Wilmoth Lerner, eds. *Medicine, Health, and Bioethics: Essential Primary Sources*, Farmington Hills, MI: Thomson Gale, 2006.

MLA Style

Books

Kübler-Ross, Elizabeth. *On Death and Dying*, New York: Macmillan, 1969. Excerpted in K. Lee Lerner and Brenda Wilmoth Lerner, eds. *Medicine, Health, and Bioethics: Essential Primary Sources*, Farmington Hills, Mich.: Thomson Gale, 2006.

Periodicals

Venter, J. Craig, et al. "The Sequence of the Human Genome." *Science*, 291 (16 February 2001): 5507, 1304–51. Excerpted in K. Lee Lerner and Brenda Wilmoth Lerner, eds. *Terrorism: Essential Primary Sources*, Farmington Hills, Mich.: Thomson Gale, 2006.

Web Sites

"Patient's Rights and Responsibilities." Johns Hopkins Hospital and Health System. 14 January 2006. http://www.hopkinsmedicine.org/patients/JHH/patient_rights.html. Excerpted in K. Lee Lerner and Brenda Wilmoth Lerner, eds. *Terrorism: Essential Primary Sources*, Farmington Hills, Mich.: Thomson Gale, 2006.

Style (Natural and Social Sciences)

Books

Kübler-Ross, Elizabeth. *On Death and Dying*, (New York: Macmillan, 1969). Excerpted in K. Lee Lerner and Brenda Wilmoth Lerner, eds. *Medicine, Health, and Bioethics: Essential Primary Sources*, (Farmington Hills, Mich.: Thomson Gale, 2006).

Periodicals

Venter, J. Craig, et al. "The Sequence of the Human Genome." *Science*, 291 (16 February 2001): 5507, 1304–1351. Excerpted in K. Lee Lerner and Brenda Wilmoth Lerner, eds. *Medicine, Health, and Bioethics: Essential Primary Sources*, (Farmington Hills, Mich.: Thomson Gale, 2006).

Websites

Johns Hopkins Hospital and Health System. "Patient's Rights and Responsibilities." available from http://www.hopkinsmedicine.org/patients/JHH/patient_rights.html; accessed14 January 2006. Excerpted in K. Lee Lerner and Brenda Wilmoth Lerner, eds. *Medicine, Health, and Bioethics: Essential Primary Sources*, (Farmington Hills, Mich.: Thomson Gale, 2006).

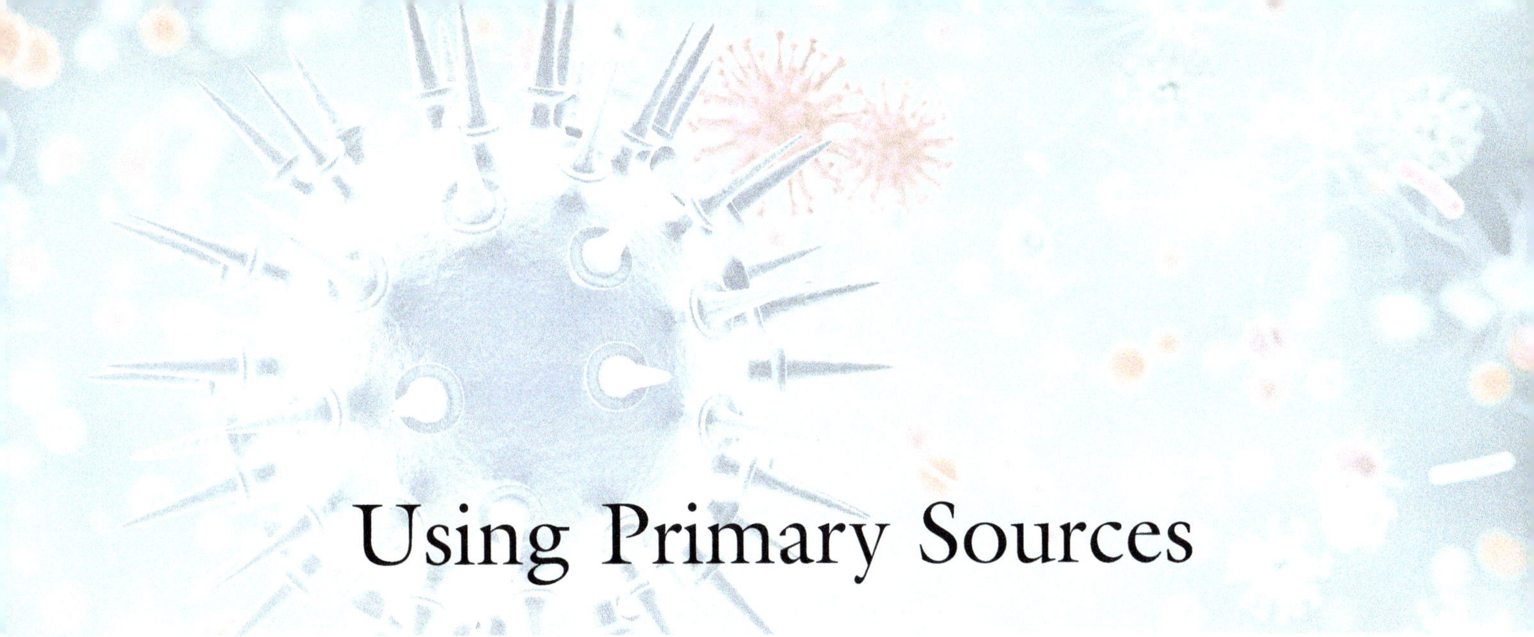

Using Primary Sources

The definition of what constitutes a primary source is often the subject of scholarly debate and interpretation. Although primary sources come from a wide spectrum of resources, they are united by the fact that they individually provide insight into the historical *milieu* (context and environment) during which they were produced.

Primary sources include materials such as newspaper articles, press dispatches, autobiographies, essays, letters, diaries, speeches, song lyrics, posters, works of art—and in the 21st century, Web logs (blogs)—that offer direct, first-hand insight or witness to events of their day.

Categories of primary sources include:

- Documents containing firsthand accounts of historic events by witnesses and participants. This category includes diary or journal entries, letters, email, newspaper articles, interviews, memoirs, and testimony in legal proceedings.
- Documents or works representing the official views of both government leaders and leaders of other organizations. These include primary sources such as policy statements, speeches, interviews, press releases, government reports, research studies, and legislation.
- Works of art, including (but certainly not limited to) photographs, poems, and songs, including advertisements and reviews of those works that help establish an understanding of the cultural environment with regard to attitudes and perceptions of events.
- Secondary sources. In some cases, secondary sources or tertiary sources may be treated as primary sources. For example, if an entry written many years after an event, or to summarize an event, includes quotes, recollections, or retrospectives (accounts of the past) written by participants in the earlier event, the source can be considered a primary source.

Analysis of Primary Sources

The primary material collected in this volume is not intended to provide a comprehensive or balanced overview of a topic or event. Rather, the primary sources are intended to generate interest and lay a foundation for further inquiry and study.

In order to properly analyze a primary source, readers should remain skeptical and develop probing questions about the source. Using historical documents requires that readers analyze them carefully and extract specific information. However, readers must also read "beyond the text" to garner larger clues about the social impact of the primary source.

In addition to providing information about their topics, primary sources may also supply a wealth of insight into their creator's viewpoint. For example, when reading a news article about an outbreak of disease, consider whether the reporter's words also indicate something about his or her origin, bias (an irrational disposition in favor of someone or something), prejudices (an irrational disposition against someone or something), or intended audience.

Students should remember that primary sources often contain information later proven to be false, or contain viewpoints and terms unacceptable to future generations. It is important to view the primary source within the historical and social context existing at its creation. If, for example, a newspaper article is written within hours or days of an event, later developments may reveal some assertions in the original article as false or misleading.

Test New Conclusions and Ideas

Whatever opinion or working hypothesis readers form, it is critical that they then test that hypothesis against other facts and sources related to the incident. For example, it might be wrong to conclude that factual mistakes are deliberate unless evidence can be produced of a pattern and practice of such mistakes with an intent to promote a false idea.

The difference between sound reasoning and preposterous conspiracy theories (or the birth of urban legends) lies in the willingness to test new ideas against other sources, rather than rest on one piece of evidence such as a single primary source that may contain errors. Sound reasoning requires that arguments and assertions guard against argument fallacies that utilize the following:

- false dilemmas (only two choices are given when in fact there are three or more options);
- arguments from ignorance (*argumentum ad ignorantiam*; because something is not known to be true, it is assumed to be false);
- possibilist fallacies (a favorite among conspiracy theorists who attempt to demonstrate that a factual statement is true or false by establishing the possibility of its truth or falsity. An argument where "it could be" is usually followed by an unearned "therefore, it is.");
- slippery slope arguments or fallacies (a series of increasingly dramatic consequences is drawn from an initial fact or idea);
- begging the question (the truth of the conclusion is assumed by the premises);
- straw man arguments (the arguer mischaracterizes an argument or theory and then attacks the merits of their own false representations);
- appeals to pity or force (the argument attempts to persuade people to agree by sympathy or force);
- prejudicial language (values or moral goodness, good and bad, are attached to certain arguments or facts);
- personal attacks (*ad hominem*; an attack on a person's character or circumstances);
- anecdotal or testimonial evidence (stories that are unsupported by impartial observation or data that is not reproducible);
- *post hoc* (after the fact) fallacies (because one thing follows another, it is held to cause the other);
- the fallacy of the appeal to authority (the argument rests upon the credentials of a person, not the evidence).

Despite the fact that some primary sources can contain false information or lead readers to false conclusions based on the information presented, they remain an invaluable resource regarding past events. Primary sources allow readers and researchers to come as close as possible to understanding the perceptions and context of events and thus to more fully appreciate how and why misconceptions occur.

Glossary

A

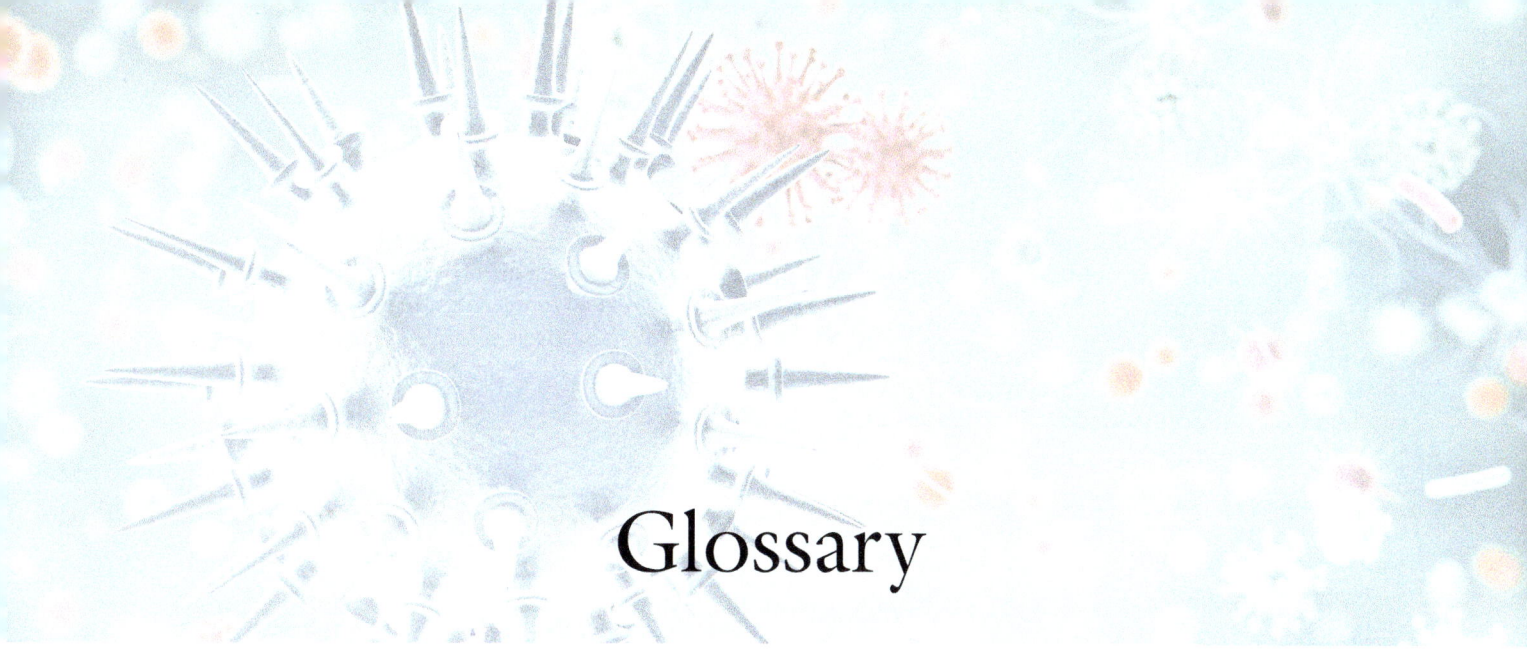

ABIOGENESIS: Also known as spontaneous generation. The incorrect theory that living things can be generated from nonliving things.

ABIOTIC: The portion of an ecosystem that is not living, such as water or soil.

ABSCESS: A pus-filled sore, usually caused by a bacterial infection. It results from the body's defensive reaction to foreign material. Abscesses are often found in the soft tissue under the skin in areas such as the armpit or the groin. However, they may develop in any organ, and they are commonly found in the breast and gums. If they are located in deep organs such as the lung, liver, or brain, abscesses are far more serious and call for more specific treatment.

ACARACIDES: Chemicals that kill mites and ticks.

ACQUIRED (ADAPTIVE) IMMUNITY: The ability to resist infection that develops according to circumstances and is targeted to a specific pathogen. There are two types of acquired immunity, known as active and passive. Active immunity is either humoral, involving production of antibody molecules against a bacterium or virus, or cell-mediated, where T-cells are mobilized against infected cells. Infection and immunization can both induce acquired immunity. Passive immunity is induced by injection of the serum of a person who is already immune to a particular infection.

ACQUIRED IMMUNODEFICIENCY SYNDROME (AIDS):A disease of the immune system caused by the human immunodeficiency virus (HIV). It is characterized by the destruction of a particular type of white blood cell and increased susceptibility to infection and other diseases.

ACTIVE INFECTION: An infection that is currently producing symptoms or in which the infective agent is multiplying rapidly. In contrast, a latent infection is one in which the infective agent is present but not causing symptoms or damage to the body or reproducing at a significant rate.

ACUTE INFECTION: An infection of rapid onset and of short duration that either resolves or becomes chronic.

ADAPTIVE IMMUNITY: Another term for acquired immunity, referring to the resistance to infection that develops through life and is targeted to a specific pathogen. There are two types of adaptive immunity, known as active and passive. Active immunity is either humoral, involving production of antibody molecules against a bacterium or virus, or cell-mediated, in which T cells are mobilized against infected cells. Infection and immunization can both induce acquired immunity. Passive immunity is induced by injection of the serum of a person who is already immune to a particular infection.

ADHESION: Physical attraction between different types of molecules.

AEROBES: Aerobic microorganisms require the presence of oxygen for growth. Molecular oxygen functions in the respiratory pathway of the microbes to produce the energy necessary for life. Bacteria, yeasts, fungi, and algae are capable of aerobic growth.

AEROSOL: Particles of liquid or solid dispersed as a suspension in gas.

AGGREGATIONS: When blood clots (becomes solid, usually in response to injury), cells called platelets form clumps called aggregations. An instrument called an aggregometer measures the degree of platelet aggregation in blood.

AIDS (ACQUIRED IMMUNODEFICIENCY SYNDROME): A disease of the immune system caused by the human immunodeficiency virus (HIV). It is characterized by the destruction of a particular type of white blood cell and increased susceptibility to infection and other diseases.

AIRBORNE PRECAUTIONS: Procedures designed to reduce the chance that certain disease-causing (pathogenic) microorganisms will be transmitted through the air.

AIRBORNE TRANSMISSION: The ability of a disease-causing (pathogenic) microorganism to be spread through the air by droplets expelled during sneezing or coughing.

ALLELE: Any of two or more alternative forms of a gene that occupy the same location on a chromosome.

ALLERGY: An excessive or hypersensitive response of the immune system to substances (allergens) in the environment. Instead of fighting off a disease-causing foreign substance, the immune system launches a complex series of actions against the particular irritating allergen. The immune response may be accompanied by a number of stressful symptoms, ranging from mild to life threatening. In rare cases an allergic reaction leads to anaphylactic shock—a condition characterized by a sudden drop in blood pressure, difficulty in breathing, skin irritation, collapse, and possible death.

ALPHAVIRUS: A genus of small, spherical RNA viruses. The genus contains some of the most important human and animal pathogens, such as chikungunya virus; Sindbis virus; Semliki Forest virus; Western, Eastern, and Venezuelan equine encephalitis viruses; and the Ross River virus. Alphaviruses are transmitted by arthropods, in particular mosquitoes.

ALVEOLUS: A tiny air sac located within the lungs. The exchange of oxygen and carbon dioxide takes place within these sacs.

AMEBIC DYSENTERY: An inflammation of the intestine caused by the parasite *Entamoeba histolytica.* The severe form of the malady is characterized by the formation of localized lesions (ulcers) in the intestine, especially in the region known as the colon; abscesses in the liver and the brain; vomiting; severe diarrhea with fluid loss leading to dehydration; and abdominal pain. Also referred to as amebiasis or amoebiasis.

AMERICAN TYPE CULTURE COLLECTION (ATCC): A not-for-profit bioscience organization that maintains the world's largest and most diverse collection of microbiological life. Many laboratories and institutions maintain their own stockpile of microorganisms, usually those that are in frequent use in the facility. Some large culture collections are housed and maintained by universities or private enterprises, but none of these rivals the ATCC in terms of size.

AMPLIFICATION: A process by which something is made larger or the quantity of something is increased.

ANADROMOUS: Fish that migrate from ocean (salt) water to fresh water, such as salmon.

ANAEROBIC BACTERIA: Bacteria that grow without oxygen; also called anaerobic bacteria or anaerobes. Anaerobic bacteria can infect deep wounds, deep tissues, and internal organs where there is little oxygen. These infections are characterized by abscess formation, foul-smelling pus, and tissue destruction.

ANTHELMINTIC: Medicines that rid the body of parasitic worms.

ANTHRAX: A disease that is caused by the bacterium *Bacillus anthracis.* The bacterium can enter the body via a wound in the skin (cutaneous anthrax), via contaminated food or liquid (gastrointestinal anthrax), or via inhalation (inhalation anthrax).

ANTIBACTERIAL: A substance that reduces or kills germs (bacteria and other microorganisms but not viruses). Also often a term used to describe a drug used to treat bacterial infections.

ANTIBIOTIC: A drug, such as penicillin, used to fight infections caused by bacteria. Antibiotics act only on bacteria and are not effective against viruses.

ANTIBIOTIC RESISTANCE: The ability of bacteria to resist the actions of antibiotic drugs.

ANTIBIOTIC SENSITIVITY: The susceptibility of a bacterium to an antibiotic. Each type of bacteria can be killed by some types of antibiotics and not be affected by other types. Different types of bacteria exhibit different patterns of antibiotic sensitivity.

ANTIBODIES: Proteins found in the blood that help fight against foreign substances called antigens. Antigens, which are usually proteins or polysaccharides, stimulate the immune system to produce antibodies, or Y-shaped immunoglobulins. The antibodies inactivate the antigen and help remove it from the body. While antigens can be the source of infections from pathogenic bacteria and viruses, organic molecules detrimental to the body from internal or environmental sources also act as antigens. Genetic engineering and the use of various mutational mechanisms allow the construction of a vast array of antibodies (each with a unique genetic sequence).

ANTIBODY-ANTIGEN BINDING: Antibodies are produced by the immune system in response to antigens (material perceived as foreign). The antibody response to a particular antigen is highly specific and often involves a physical association between the two molecules. Biochemical and molecular forces govern this association.

ANTIBODY RESPONSE: The specific immune response that utilizes B cells to kill certain kinds of antigens.

ANTIFUNGAL: Antifungals (also called antifungal drugs) are medicines used to fight fungal infections. They are of two kinds, systemic and topical. Systemic antifungal drugs are medicines taken by mouth or by injection to treat infections caused by a fungus. Topical antifungal drugs are medicines applied to the skin to treat skin infections caused by a fungus.

ANTIGEN: A substance, usually a protein or polysaccharide, that stimulates the immune system to produce antibodies. While antigens can be the source of infections from pathogenic bacteria and viruses, organic molecules detrimental to the body from internal or environmental sources also act as antigens.

ANTIGENIC DRIFT: The gradual accumulation of mutations in genes, such as in gene coding for surface proteins, over a given period.

ANTIGENIC SHIFT: An abrupt and major genetic change, such as in gene coding for surface proteins of a virus.

ANTIMICROBIAL: Slows the growth of bacteria or is able to kill bacteria. Antimicrobial materials include antibiotics (which can be used inside the body) and disinfectants (which can only be used outside the body).

ANTIRETROVIRAL (ARV) DRUGS: Drugs that prevent the reproduction of a type of virus called a retrovirus. The human immunodeficiency virus (HIV), which causes acquired immunodeficiency syndrome (AIDS), is a retrovirus. These ARV drugs are therefore used to treat HIV infections. These medicines cannot prevent or cure HIV infection, but they help to keep the virus in check.

ANTIRETROVIRAL (ARV) THERAPY: A form of drug therapy that prevents the reproduction of a type of virus called a retrovirus. Human immunodeficiency virus (HIV), which causes acquired immunodeficiency syndrome (AIDS), is a retrovirus. ARV drugs are used to treat HIV infections and keep the virus in check, but they cannot prevent or cure the infection.

ANTISENSE DRUG: A drug that binds to messenger RNA (mRNA), thereby blocking gene activity. Some viruses have mRNA as their genetic material, so an antisense drug can inhibit their replication.

ANTISEPTIC: A substance that prevents or stops the growth and multiplication of microorganisms in or on living tissue.

ANTITOXIN: An antidote to a toxin that neutralizes the toxin's poisonous effects.

ANTIVIRAL DRUGS: Compounds that are used to prevent or treat viral infections, via the disruption of an infectious mechanism used by the virus, or to treat the symptoms of an infection.

ARACHNID: An arthropod that belongs to class Arachnida, such as a spider or scorpion. Arachnids have eight legs, which differentiates them from six-legged insects.

ARBOVIRUS: A virus that is typically spread by blood-sucking insects, most commonly mosquitoes. Over 100 types of arboviruses cause disease in humans. Yellow fever and dengue fever are two examples.

ARENAVIRUS: A virus that belongs in a viral family known as Arenaviridae. The name arenavirus derives from the appearance of the spherical virus particles when cut into thin sections and viewed using a transmission electron microscope. The interior of the particles is grainy or sandy in appearance, due to the presence of ribosomes that have been acquired from the host cell. The Latin designation *arena* means "sandy."

ARTHROPOD: A member of the largest single animal phylum, consisting of organisms with segmented bodies, jointed legs or wings, and exoskeletons.

ARTHROPOD-BORNE DISEASE: A disease caused by one of a phylum of organisms characterized by exoskeletons and segmented bodies.

ARTHROPOD-BORNE VIRUS: A virus caused by one of a phylum of organisms characterized by exoskeletons and segmented bodies.

ASEPSIS: Without germs, more specifically without microorganisms.

ASPIRATION: The drawing out of fluid from a part of the body; it can cause pneumonia when stomach contents are transferred to the lungs through vomiting.

ASSAY: A determination of an amount of a particular compound in a sample (e.g., to make chemical tests to determine the relative amount of a particular substance in a sample). A method used to quantify a biological compound.

ASYMPTOMATIC: A state in which an individual does not exhibit or experience symptoms of a disease.

ATAXIA: An unsteadiness in walking or standing that is associated with brain diseases such as kuru or Creutzfeldt-Jakob disease.

ATOPY: An inherited tendency toward hypersensitivity toward immunoglobulin E, a key component of the immune system, which plays an important role in asthma, eczema, and hay fever.

ATROPHY: Decreasing in size or wasting-away of a body part or tissue.

ATTENUATED STRAIN: A bacterium or virus that has been weakened. Often used as the basis of a vaccine against the specific disease caused by the bacterium or virus.

AUTOCLAVE: A device designed to kill microorganisms on solid items and in liquids by exposure to steam at a high pressure.

AUTOIMMUNE DISEASE: A disease in which the body's defense system attacks its own tissues and organs.

AUTOIMMUNITY: A condition in which the immune system attacks the body's cells, causing tissue destruction. Autoimmune diseases are classified as either general, in which the autoimmune reaction takes place simultaneously in a number of tissues, or organ specific, in which the autoimmune reaction targets a single organ. Autoimmunity is accepted as the cause of a wide range of disorders and is suspected to be responsible for many more. Among the most common diseases attributed to autoimmune disorders are rheumatoid arthritis, systemic lupus erythematosus (lupus), multiple sclerosis, myasthenia gravis, pernicious anemia, and scleroderma.

AUTOINFECTION: The reinfection of the body by a disease organism already in the body, such as eggs left by a parasitic worm.

B

B CELL: Also known as B lymphocyte; a kind of cell produced in bone marrow that secretes antibodies.

BABESIOSIS: An infection of the red blood cells caused by *Babesia microti*, a form of parasite (parasitic sporozoan).

BACILLUS ANTHRACIS: The bacterium that causes anthrax.

BACTEREMIA: This condition occurs when bacteria enter the bloodstream through, for example, a wound or an infection or through a surgical procedure or injection. Bacteremia may cause no symptoms and resolve without treatment, or it may produce fever and other symptoms of infection. In some cases, bacteremia leads to septic shock, a potentially life-threatening condition.

BACTERIA: Single-celled microorganisms that live in soil, water, plants, and animals and whose activities range from the development of disease to fermentation. They play a key role in the decay of organic matter and the cycling of nutrients. Bacteria exist in various shapes, including spherical, rod-shaped, and spiral. Some bacteria are agents of disease. Different types of bacteria cause many sexually transmitted infections, including syphilis, gonorrhea, and chlamydia. Bacteria also cause diseases such as typhoid, dysentery, and tetanus. Bacterium is the singular form of bacteria.

BACTERIOCIDAL: The treatment of a bacterium such that the organism is killed. A bactericidal treatment is always lethal and is also referred to as sterilization.

BACTERIOLOGICAL STRAIN: A bacterial subclass of a particular tribe and genus.

BACTERIOPHAGE: A virus that infects bacteria. When a bacteriophage that carries the diphtheria toxin gene infects diphtheria bacteria, the bacteria produce diphtheria toxin.

BACTERIOSTATIC: Refers to a treatment that restricts the ability of the bacterium to grow.

BASIDIOSPORE: A fungal spore of Basidiomycetes. Basidiomycetes are classified under the Fungi kingdom as belonging to the phylum Mycota (i.e., Basidiomycota), class Mycetes (i.e., Basidiomycetes). Fungi are frequently parasites that decompose organic material from their hosts, such as the parasites that grow on rotten wood, although some may cause serious plant diseases such as smuts (Ustomycetes) and rusts (Teliomycetes). Some live in a symbiotic relationship with plant roots (Mycorrhizae). A cell type termed *basidium* is responsible for sexual spore formation in Basidiomycetes, through nuclear fusion followed by meiosis, thus forming haploid basidiospores.

BED NET: A type of netting that provides protection from diseases caused by insects such as flies and mosquitoes. It is often used when sleeping to allow air to flow through its mesh structure while preventing insects from biting.

BIFURCATED NEEDLE: A bifurcated needle is a needle that has two prongs with a wire suspended between them. The wire is designed to hold a certain amount of vaccine. Development of the bifurcated needle was a major advance in vaccination against smallpox.

BIOINDICATOR: A living organism whose status in an ecosystem offers an idea of the health of its environment.

BIOFILM: A population of microorganisms that forms following the adhesion of bacteria, algae, yeast, or fungi to a surface. These surface growths can be found in natural settings, such as on rocks in streams, and in infections, such as those that occur on catheters. Microorganisms can colonize living and inert natural and synthetic surfaces.

BIOINFORMATICS: The development of new database methods to store genomic information (information related to genes and the genetic sequence), computational software programs, and methods to extract, process, and evaluate this information. Also known as computational biology, bioinformatics also refers to the refinement of existing techniques to acquire the genomic data. Finding genes and determining their function, predicting the structure of proteins and sequence of ribonucleic acid (RNA) from the available sequence of deoxyribonucleic acid (DNA), and determining the evolutionary relationship of proteins and DNA sequences are aspects of bioinformatics.

BIOLOGICAL WARFARE: As defined by the United Nations, the use of any living organism, such as a bacterium or virus, or an infective component, such as a toxin, to cause disease or death in humans, animals, or plants. In contrast to bioterrorism, biological warfare is the state-sanctioned use of biological weapons on an opposing military force or civilian population.

BIOLOGICAL WEAPON: A weapon that contains or disperses a biological toxin, disease-causing microorganism, or other biological agent intended to harm or kill plants, animals, or humans.

BIOMAGNIFICATION: The increasing concentration of compounds at a higher trophic level or the tendency of organisms to accumulate certain chemicals to a concentration larger than that occurring in their inorganic, nonliving environment, such as soil or water, or, in the case of animals, larger than in their food.

BIOMODULATOR: Short for biologic response modulator. An agent that modifies some characteristic of the immune system, which may help in the fight against infection.

BIOSAFETY LABORATORY: A laboratory that deals with all aspects of potentially infectious agents or biohazards.

BIOSAFETY LEVEL 4 FACILITY: A specialized biosafety laboratory that deals with dangerous or exotic infectious agents or biohazards that are considered high risks for spreading life-threatening diseases, either because the disease is spread through aerosols or because there is no therapy or vaccine to counter the disease.

BIOSHIELD PROJECT: A joint effort between the US Department of Homeland Security and the Department of Health and Human Services. The program was tasked with improving treatment of diseases caused by biological, chemical, and radiological weapons.

BIOSPHERE: The sum of all life-forms on Earth and the interaction among those life-forms.

BIOTECHNOLOGY: Use of biological organisms, systems, or processes to make or modify products.

BIOWEAPON: A weapon that uses bacteria, viruses, or poisonous substances made by bacteria or viruses.

BLOOD-BORNE PATHOGENS: Disease-causing agents carried or transported in the blood. Blood-borne infections are those in which the infectious agent is transmitted from one person to another via contaminated blood.

BLOODBORNE: Via the blood. For example, bloodborne pathogens are pathogens (disease-causing agents) carried or transported in the blood. Bloodborne infections are those in which the infectious agent is transmitted from one person to another via contaminated blood. Infections of the blood can occur as a result of the spread of an ongoing infection caused by bacteria such as *Yersinia pestis*, *Haemophilus influenzae*, or *Staphylococcus aureus*.

BOTULINUM TOXIN: One of the most poisonous substances known. The toxin, which can be ingested or inhaled, and which disrupts transmission of nerve impulses to muscles, is naturally produced by the bacterium *Clostridium botulinum*. Certain strains of *C. baratii* and *C. butyricum* can also produce the toxin.

BOTULISM: An illness produced by a toxin that is released by the soil bacterium *Clostridium botulinum*.

One type of toxin is also produced by *Clostridium baratii*. The toxins affect nerves and can produce paralysis. The paralysis can affect the functioning of organs and tissues that are vital to life.

BROAD SPECTRUM: A series of objects or ideas with great variety between them. In medicine the term is often applied to drugs that act on a large number of different disease-causing agents.

BROAD-SPECTRUM ANTIBIOTICS: Drugs that kill a wide range of bacteria rather than just those from a specific family. For example, Amoxicillin is a broad-spectrum antibiotic that is used against many common illnesses such as ear infections.

BRONCHIOLITIS: An inflammation (-itis) of the bronchioles, the small air passages in the lungs that enter the alveoli (air sacs).

BUBO: A swollen lymph gland, usually in the groin or armpit, characteristic of infection with bubonic plague.

BUSHMEAT: The meat of terrestrial wild and exotic animals, typically those that live in parts of Africa, Asia, and the Americas; also known as wild meat.

C

CADAVER: The body of a deceased human, especially one designated for scientific dissection or other research.

CAMPYLOBACTERIOSIS: Campylobacteriosis is a bacterial infection of the intestinal tract of humans. The infection, which typically results in diarrhea, is caused by members of the genus *Campylobacter*. In particular, *Campylobacter jejuni* is the most common cause of bacterial diarrhea in the United States, with more occurrences than salmonella (another prominent disease-causing bacteria associated with food poisoning). Worldwide, approximately 5 to 14 percent of all diarrhea may be the result of campylobacteriosis.

CAPSID: The protein shell surrounding a virus particle.

CARBOLIC ACID: An acidic compound that, when diluted with water, is used as an antiseptic and a disinfectant.

CARCINOGEN: Any biological, chemical, or physical substance or agent that can cause cancer. There are more than 100 different types of cancer, which can be distinguished by the type of cell or organ that is affected, the treatment plan employed, and the cause of the cancer. Most of the carcinogens that are commonly discussed come from chemical sources artificially produced by humans. Some of the better-known carcinogens are the pesticide DDT (dichlorodiphenyltrichloroethane), asbestos, and the carcinogens produced when tobacco is smoked.

CASE FATALITY RATE: The rate of patients suffering disease or injury that die as a result of that disease or injury during a specific period of time.

CASE FATALITY RATIO: A ratio indicating the amount of people who die as a result of a particular disease, usually expressed as a percentage or as the number of deaths per 1,000 cases.

CATALYST: Substance that speeds up a chemical process without actually changing the products of reaction.

CD4+ T CELLS: A type of T cell found in the immune system that are characterized by the presence of a CD4 antigen protein on their surface. These are the cells most often destroyed as a result of HIV infection.

CELL CYCLE AND CELL DIVISION: The series of stages that a cell undergoes while progressing to division is known as cell cycle. For an organism to grow and develop, the organism's cells must be able to duplicate themselves. Three basic events must take place to achieve this duplication: the deoxyribonucleic acid (DNA), which makes up the individual chromosomes within the cell's nucleus must be duplicated; the two sets of DNA must be packaged into two separate nuclei; and the cell's cytoplasm must divide itself to create two separate cells, each complete with its own nucleus. The two new cells —products of the single original cell—are known as daughter cells.

CELL MEMBRANE: The cell is bound by an outer membrane that, as described by a membrane model termed the fluid mosaic model, is composed of a phospholipid lipid bilayer with proteins—molecules that also act as receptor sites—interspersed within the phospholipid bilayer. Varieties of channels exist within the membrane. In eukaryotes (cells with a true nucleus) there are a number of internal cellular membranes that can partition regions within the cells' interior. Some of these membranes ultimately become continuous with the nuclear membrane. Bacteria and viruses do not have inner membranes.

CENTERS FOR DISEASE CONTROL AND PREVENTION (CDC): One of the primary public health institutions in the world. The CDC is headquartered in Atlanta,

Georgia, with facilities at nine other sites in the United States. The centers are the focus of US government efforts to develop and implement prevention and control strategies for diseases, including those of microbiological origin.

CESTODE: A class of worms characterized by flat, segmented bodies, commonly known as tapeworms.

CHAGAS DISEASE: A human infection that is caused by a microorganism that establishes a parasitic relationship with a human host as part of its life cycle. The disease is named for the Brazilian physician Carlos Chagas, who in 1909 described the involvement of the flagellated protozoan known as *Trypanosoma cruzi* in a prevalent disease in South America.

CHAIN OF TRANSMISSION: The route by which an infection is spread from its source to a susceptible host. An example of a chain of transmission is the spread of malaria from an infected animal to humans via mosquitoes.

CHANCRE: A sore that occurs in the first stage of syphilis at the place where the infection entered the body.

CHEMILUMINESCENT SIGNAL: The production of light from a chemical reaction. A variety of tests to detect infectious organisms or target components of the organisms relies on the binding of a chemical-containing probe to the target and the subsequent development of light following the addition of a reactive compound.

CHEMOTHERAPY: The treatment of a disease, infection, or condition with chemicals that have a specific effect on its cause, such as a microorganism or cancer cell. The first modern therapeutic chemical was derived from a synthetic dye. Sulfonamide drugs developed in the 1930s, penicillin and other antibiotics of the 1940s, hormones developed in the 1950s, and later drugs that interfere with cancer cell metabolism and reproduction have all been part of the chemotherapeutic arsenal.

CHICKENPOX: Chickenpox (also called varicella disease and sometimes spelled chicken pox) is a common and extremely infectious childhood disease that can also affect adults. It produces an itchy, blistery rash that typically lasts about a week and is sometimes accompanied by a fever.

CHILDBED FEVER: A bacterial infection occurring in women following childbirth, causing fever and, in some cases, blood poisoning and possible death.

CHLORINATION: A chemical process that is used primarily to disinfect drinking water and spills of microorganisms. The active agent in chlorination is the element chlorine, or a derivative of chlorine (e .g., chlorine dioxide). Chlorination is a swift and economical means of destroying many, but not all, microorganisms that are a health threat in fluids such as drinking water.

CHRONIC: Chronic infections persist for prolonged periods of time—months or even years—in the host. This lengthy persistence is due to a number of factors, which can include masking of the disease-causing agent (e.g., bacteria) from the immune system, invasion of host cells, and the establishment of an infection that is resistant to antibacterial agents.

CHRONIC FATIGUE SYNDROME (CFS): A condition that causes extreme tiredness. People with CFS have debilitating fatigue that lasts for six months or longer. They also have many other symptoms. Some of these symptoms are pain in the joints and muscles, headache, and sore throat. CFS appears to result from a combination of factors.

CILIA: Specialized arrangements of microtubules that have two general functions. They propel certain unicellular organisms, such as paramecium, through the water. In multicellular organisms, if cilia extend from stationary cells that are part of a tissue layer, they move fluid over the surface of the tissue.

CIRRHOSIS: A chronic, degenerative, irreversible liver disease in which normal liver cells are damaged and are then replaced by scar tissue. Cirrhosis changes the structure of the liver and the blood vessels that nourish it. The disease reduces the liver's ability to manufacture proteins and process hormones, nutrients, medications, and poisons.

CLINICAL TRIALS: According to the National Institutes of Health, a clinical trial is "a research study to answer specific questions about vaccines or new therapies or new ways of using known treatments." These studies allow researchers to determine whether new drugs or treatments are safe and effective. When conducted carefully, clinical trials can provide fast and safe answers to these questions.

CLOACA: The cavity into which the intestinal, genital, and urinary tracts open in vertebrates such as fish, reptiles, birds, and some primitive mammals.

CLUSTER: A grouping of individuals contracting an infectious disease or foodborne illness very close in time or place.

COCCIDIUM: Any single-celled animal (protozoan) belonging to the subclass Coccidia. Some coccidia species can infest the digestive tract, causing coccidiosis.

COHORT: A group of people (or any species) sharing a common characteristic. Cohorts are identified and grouped in cohort studies to determine the frequency of diseases or the kinds of disease outcomes over time.

COHORTING: The practice of grouping people with similar infections or symptoms together to reduce transmission to others.

COLONIZATION: The process of occupation and increase in number of microorganisms at a specific site.

COLONIZE: To persist and grow at a given location.

COMMUNITY-ACQUIRED INFECTION: An infection that develops outside of a hospital, in the general community. It differs from hospital-acquired infections in that those who are infected are typically in better health than hospitalized people.

CONGENITAL: Existing at the time of birth.

CONJUNCTIVITIS: An inflammation or redness of the lining of the white part of the eye and the underside of the eyelid (conjunctiva) that can be caused by infection, allergic reaction, or physical agents such as infrared or ultraviolet light. Conjunctivitis (also called pink eye) is one of the most common eye infections in children and adults in the United States. Luckily, it is also one of the most treatable infections. Because it is so common in the United States and around the world and is often not reported to health organizations, accurate statistics are not available for conjunctivitis.

CONTACT PRECAUTIONS: Actions developed to minimize the transfer of microorganisms directly by physical contact and indirectly by touching a contaminated surface.

CONTAGIOUS: A disease that is easily spread among a population, usually by casual person-to-person contact.

CONTAMINATION: The unwanted presence of a microorganism or compound in a particular environment. That environment can be in the laboratory setting, for example, in a medium being used for the growth of a species of bacteria during an experiment. Another environment can be the human body, where contamination by bacteria can produce an infection. Contamination by bacteria and viruses can occur on several levels and their presence can adversely influence the results of experiments. Outside the laboratory, bacteria and viruses can contaminate drinking water supplies, foodstuffs, and products, thus causing illness.

COWPOX: A disease that is caused by the cowpox or catpox virus. The virus is a member of the orthopoxvirus family. Other viruses in this family include the smallpox and vaccinia viruses. Cowpox is a rare disease and is mostly noteworthy as the basis of the formulation, over 200 years ago, of an injection by Edward Jenner that proved successful in curing smallpox.

CREPITANT: A crackling sound that accompanies breathing, a common symptom of pneumonia or other diseases of the lungs.

CREUTZFELDT-JAKOB DISEASE (CJD): A transmissible, rapidly progressing, fatal neurodegenerative disorder related to bovine spongiform encephalopathy (BSE), commonly called mad cow disease.

CULL: The selection, often for destruction, of a part of an animal population. Often done just to reduce numbers, a widespread cull was carried out during the epidemic of bovine spongiform encephalopathy (BSE or mad cow disease) in the United Kingdom during the 1980s.

CULTURE: A single species of microorganism that is isolated and grown under controlled conditions. The German bacteriologist Robert Koch first developed culturing techniques in the late 1870s. Following Koch's initial discovery, medical scientists quickly sought to identify other pathogens. In the 21st century bacteria cultures are used as basic tools in microbiology and medicine.

CULTURE AND SENSITIVITY: Laboratory tests that are used to identify the type of microorganism causing an infection and the compounds to which the identified organism is sensitive and resistant. In the case of bacteria, this approach permits the selection of antibiotics that will be most effective in dealing with the infection.

CUTANEOUS: Pertaining to the skin.

CYST: A closed cavity or sac or the dormant stage of life of some parasites when they live inside an enclosed area, covered by a tough outer shell.

CYTOKINE: One of a family of small proteins that mediate an organism's response to injury or infection. Cytokines operate by transmitting signals between cells in an organism. Minute quantities of cytokines are secreted, each by a single cell type, to regulate functions in other cells by binding with specific receptors. Their interactions with the receptors produce secondary signals that inhibit or enhance the action of certain genes within the cell. Unlike endocrine hormones, which can act throughout the body, most cytokines act locally near the cells that produced them.

CYTOTOXIC: Able to kill cells. Cytotoxic drugs kill cancer cells but may also have applications in killing bacteria.

D

DEBRIDEMENT: The medical process of removing dead, damaged, or infected tissue from pressure ulcers, burns, and other wounds to speed healing of the surrounding healthy tissue.

DEFINITIVE HOST: The organism in which a parasite reaches reproductive maturity.

DEGRADATION (CELLULAR): The destruction of host cell components, such as DNA, by infective agents such as bacteria and viruses.

DEHYDRATION: The loss of water and salts essential for normal bodily function. It occurs when the body loses more fluid than it takes in. Water is important to the human body because it makes up about 70 percent of the muscles, around 75 percent of the brain, and approximately 92 percent of the blood. A person who weighs about 150 pounds (68 kilograms) will contain about 80 quarts (just over 75 liters) of water. About 2 cups of water are lost each day just from regular breathing. If the body sweats more and breathes more heavily than normal, the human body loses even more water. Dehydration occurs when that lost water is not replenished.

DEMENTIA: From the Latin word dement, meaning "away mind," a progressive deterioration and eventual loss of mental ability that is severe enough to interfere with normal activities of daily living. Dementia lasts more than six months, has not been present since birth, and is not associated with a loss or alteration of consciousness. It is a group of symptoms caused by gradual death of brain cells. Dementia is usually caused by degeneration in the cerebral cortex, the part of the brain responsible for thoughts, memories, actions, and personality. Death of brain cells in this region leads to the cognitive impairment that characterizes dementia.

DEMOGRAPHICS: The characteristics of human populations or specific parts of human populations, most often reported through statistics.

DEOXYRIBONUCLEIC ACID (DNA): A double-stranded, helical molecule that forms the molecular basis for heredity in most organisms.

DERMATOPHYTE: A parasitic fungus that feeds off keratin, a protein that is abundant in skin, nails, and hair and therefore often causes infection of these body parts.

DIAGNOSIS: Identification of a disease or disorder.

DIARRHEA: To most individuals, diarrhea means an increased frequency or decreased consistency of bowel movements; however, the medical definition is more exact than this explanation. In many developed countries, the average number of bowel movements is three per day. However, researchers have found that diarrhea, which is not a disease, best correlates with an increase in stool weight; a stool weight above 10.5 ounces (300 grams) per day generally indicates diarrhea. This is mainly due to excess water, which normally makes up 60 to 85 percent of fecal matter. In this way, true diarrhea is distinguished from diseases that cause only an increase in the number of bowel movements (hyperdefecation) or incontinence (involuntary loss of bowel contents). Diarrhea is also classified by physicians into acute, which lasts one to two weeks, and chronic, which continues for longer than four weeks. Viral and bacterial infections are the most common causes of acute diarrhea.

DIATOM: Algae are a diverse group of simple, nucleated, plantlike aquatic organisms that are primary producers. Primary producers are able to utilize photosynthesis to create organic molecules from sunlight, water, and carbon dioxide. Ecologically vital, algae account for roughly half of the photosynthetic production of organic material on Earth in both freshwater and marine environments. Algae exist either as single cells or as multicellular organizations. Diatoms are microscopic, single-celled algae that have intricate glass-like outer cell walls partially composed of silicon. Different species of diatom can be identified based on the structure of these walls. Many diatom species are planktonic, suspended in the water column moving at the mercy of water currents. Others remain attached to submerged surfaces. One bucketful of water may contain millions of diatoms. Their abundance makes them important food sources in aquatic ecosystems.

DIMORPHIC: The occurrence of two different shapes or color forms within the species, usually occurring as sexual dimorphism between males and females.

DINOFLAGELLATE: Microorganisms that are regarded as algae. Their wide array of exotic shapes and, sometimes, armored appearance, is distinct from other algae. The closest microorganisms in appearance are the diatoms.

DIPHTHERIA: A potentially fatal, contagious bacterial disease that usually involves the nose, throat, and air passages but may also infect the skin. Its most striking feature is the formation of a grayish membrane covering the tonsils and upper part of the throat.

DISINFECTANT: Disinfection and the use of chemical disinfectants is one key strategy of infection control. Disinfectants reduce the number of living microorganisms, usually to a level that is considered safe for the particular environment. Typically, this entails the destruction of those microbes that are capable of causing disease.

DISSEMINATED: The previous distribution of a disease-causing microorganism over a larger area.

DISSEMINATION: The spreading of a disease in a population or over a large geographic area or the spreading of disease organisms in the body.

DISTAL: From the same root word as distant, the medical word for distant from some agreed-on point of reference. For example, the hand is at the distal end of the arm from the trunk.

DNA: Deoxyribonucleic acid, a double-stranded, helical molecule that is found in almost all living cells and that determines the characteristics of each organism.

DNA FINGERPRINTING: A range of techniques used to show similarities and dissimilarities between the deoxyribonucleic acid (DNA) present in different individuals or organisms.

DNA PROBES: Substances or agents that bind directly to a predefined specific sequence of nucleic acids in deoxyribonucleic acid (DNA).

DORMANT: Inactive but still alive. A resting, nonactive state.

DROPLET: A drop of water or other fluid that is fewer than 5 microns (a millionth of a meter) in diameter.

DROPLET TRANSMISSION: The spread of microorganisms from one space to another (including from person to person) via droplets that are larger than 5 microns in diameter. Droplets are typically expelled into the air by coughing and sneezing.

DRUG RESISTANCE: Develops when an infective agent, such as a bacterium, fungus, or virus, develops a lack of sensitivity to a drug that would normally be able to control or even kill it. This tends to occur with overuse of anti-infective agents, which selects out populations of microbes most able to resist them, while killing off those organisms that are most sensitive. The next time the anti-infective agent is used, it will be less effective, leading to the eventual development of resistance.

DYSENTERY: An infectious disease that has ravaged armies, refugee camps, and prisoner-of-war camps throughout history. The disease is still a major problem in developing countries with primitive sanitary facilities.

DYSPLASIA: Abnormal changes in tissue or cell development.

E

ECOLOGY: The study of the relationships among communities of living things.

ECTOPARASITES: Parasites that cling to the outside of their host rather than their host's intestines. Common points of attachment are the gills, fins, or skin of fish.

ELBOW BUMP: A personal greeting that involves two people touching elbows instead of shaking hands. It is recommended by the World Health Organization for use by researchers handling highly infectious organisms such as Ebola virus.

ELECTROLYTES: Compounds that ionize in a solution. Electrolytes dissolved in the blood play an important role in maintaining the proper functioning of the body.

ELECTRON: A fundamental particle of matter carrying a single unit of negative electrical charge.

EMBRYONATED: When an embryo has been implanted in a female animal.

EMERGING INFECTIOUS DISEASE: A new infectious disease such as severe acute respiratory syndrome (SARS) or West Nile virus, as well as a previously known disease such as malaria, tuberculosis, or bacterial pneumonia that is appearing in a new form that is resistant to drug treatments.

ENCEPHALITIS: A type of acute brain inflammation, most often due to infection by a virus.

ENCEPHALOMYELITIS: Simultaneous inflammation of the brain and spinal cord.

ENCEPHALOPATHY: Any abnormality in the structure or function of the brain.

ENCYSTED LARVAE: Larvae that are not actively growing and dividing and are more resistant to environmental conditions.

ENDEMIC: Present in a particular area or among a particular group of people.

ENDOCYTOSIS: A process by which host cells allow the entry of outside substances, including viruses, through their cell membranes.

ENTERIC: Involving the intestinal tract or relating to the intestines.

ENTEROBACTERIAL: Infections Infections caused by a group of bacteria that dwell in the intestinal tract of humans and other warm-blooded animals. The bacteria are all Gram-negative and rod-shaped. As a group they are termed Enterobacteriaceae. A prominent member of this group is Escherichia coli. Other members are the various species in the genera Salmonella, Shigella, Klebsiella, Enterobacter, Serratia, Proteus, and Yersinia.

ENTEROPATHOGEN: A virus or pathogen that invades the large or small intestine, causing disease.

ENTEROTOXIN: A class of toxin produced by bacteria. Unlike exotoxins, which are released by bacteria, enterotoxins reside with the bacterial cells.

ENTEROVIRUS: A group of viruses that contain ribonucleic acid as their genetic material. They are members of the picornavirus family. The various types of enteroviruses that infect humans are referred to as serotypes, in recognition of their different antigenic patterns. The different immune response is important, as infection with one type of enterovirus does not necessarily confer protection to infection by a different type of enterovirus. There are 64 different enterovirus serotypes. The serotypes include polio viruses, coxsackie A and B viruses, echoviruses, and a large number of what are referred to as non-polio enteroviruses.

ENZOOTIC: Affecting animals, naturally present in an environment, and occurring at regular intervals.

ENZYMES: Molecules that act as critical catalysts in biological systems. Catalysts are substances that increase the rate of chemical reactions without being consumed in the reaction. Without enzymes, many reactions would require higher levels of energy and higher temperatures than exist in biological systems. Enzymes are proteins that possess specific binding sites for other molecules (substrates). A series of weak binding interactions allows enzymes to accelerate reaction rates. Enzyme kinetics is the study of enzymatic reactions and mechanisms. Enzyme inhibitor studies have allowed researchers to develop therapies for the treatment of diseases, including AIDS.

ENZYME-LINKED IMMUNOSORBENT ASSAY (ELISA): A technique used to detect antibodies or infectious agents in a sample. The procedure involves interactions via serial binding to a solid surface, usually a polystyrene multiwell plate. The result is a colored product that correlates to the amount of analyte present in the original sample.

EPIDEMIC: From the Greek epidemic, meaning "prevalent among the people," it is most commonly used to describe an outbreak of an illness or a disease in which the number of individual cases significantly exceeds the usual or expected number of cases in any given population.

EPIDEMIOLOGIST: One who studies the various factors that influence the occurrence, distribution, prevention, and control of disease, injury, and other health-related events in a defined human population. By the application of various analytical techniques, including mathematical analysis of the data, the probable cause of an infectious outbreak can be pinpointed.

EPIDEMIOLOGY: The study of the various factors that influence the occurrence, distribution, prevention, and control of disease, injury, and other health-related events in a defined human population. By the application of various analytical techniques, including mathematical analysis of the data, the probable cause of an infectious outbreak can be pinpointed.

EPIZOOTIC: The abnormally high occurrence of a specific disease in animals in a particular area, similar to a human epidemic.

EPSTEIN-BARR VIRUS (EBV): Part of the family of human herpes viruses. Infectious mononucleosis (IM) is the most common disease manifestation of this virus, which, once established in the host, can never be completely eradicated. Little can be done to treat EBV; most methods can only alleviate resultant symptoms.

EQUID: A mammal of the horse family, such as a horse, donkey, mule, or zebra.

ERADICATE: To get rid of; the permanent reduction to zero of global incidence of a particular infection.

ERADICATION: The process of destroying or eliminating a microorganism or disease.

ERYTHEMA: Skin redness due to excess blood in capillaries (small blood vessels) in the skin.

ESCHAR: Any scab or crust forming on the skin as a result of a burn or disease. Scabs from cuts or scrapes are not eschars.

ETIOLOGY: The study of the cause or origin of a disease or disorder.

EX SITU: A Latin term meaning "from the place" or removed from its original place.

EXECUTIVE: Order Presidential orders that implement or interpret a federal statute, administrative policy, or treaty.

EXOTOXIN: A toxic protein produced during bacterial growth and metabolism and released into the environment.

EYE DROPS: Saline-containing fluid that is added to the eye to cleanse the eye or as the solution used to administer antibiotics or other medication.

F

FASCIA: A type of connective tissue made up of a network of fibers. It is best thought of as being the packing material of the body. Fascia surrounds muscles, bones, and joints and lies between the layers of skin. It functions to hold these structures together, protecting them and defining the shape of the body. When surrounding a muscle, fascia helps prevent a contracting muscle from catching or causing excessive friction on neighboring muscles.

FEBRILE: Pertaining to a fever.

FECAL-ORAL ROUTE: The spread of disease through the transmission of minute particles of fecal material from one organism to the mouth of another. This can occur by drinking contaminated water; eating food exposed to animal or human feces, such as food from plants watered with unclean water; or preparing food without practicing proper hygiene.

FECES: Solid waste excreted from a living body.

FIBROBLAST: A cell type that gives rise to connective tissue.

FILOVIRUS ANY: RNA virus that belongs to the family Filoviridae. Filoviruses infect primates. Marburg virus and Ebola virus are filoviruses.

FLAGELLUM: A hairlike structure in a cell that serves as an organ of locomotion.

FLAVIVIRUS: A single genus of ribonucleic acid (RNA) viruses that belong to the family Flaviviridae. Flaviviruses are found in arthropods but can infect humans and animals. Examples are dengue, yellow fever, West Nile, Japanese encephalitis, and Zika.

FLEA: Any parasitic insect of the order Siphonaptera. Fleas can infest many mammals, including humans, and can act as carriers (vectors) of disease.

FLORA: In microbiology, the collective microorganisms that normally inhabit an organism or system. Human intestines, for example, contain bacteria that aid in digestion and are considered normal flora.

FOCUS: In medicine, a primary center of some disease process (for example, a cluster of abnormal cells). Foci is plural for focus (more than one focus).

FOMITE: An object or a surface to which infectious microorganisms such as bacteria or viruses can adhere and be transmitted. Papers, clothing, dishes, and other objects can all act as fomites. Transmission is often by touch.

FOOD PRESERVATION: Any one of a number of techniques used to prevent food from spoiling, such as canning, pickling, drying or freeze-drying, irradiation, pasteurization, smoking, and the addition of chemical additives. Food preservation has become an increasingly important component of the food industry as fewer people eat foods produced on their own lands and as consumers expect to purchase and consume foods that are out of season.

FULMINANT INFECTION: An infection that appears suddenly and whose symptoms are immediately severe.

G

GAMETOCYTE: A germ cell with the ability to divide for the purpose of producing gametes, either male gametes called spermatocytes or female gametes called oocytes.

GAMMA GLOBULIN: A group of soluble proteins in the blood, most of which are antibodies that can mount a direct attack on pathogens and can be used to treat various infections.

GANGRENE: The destruction of body tissue by a bacteria called Clostridium perfringens or a combination of Streptococci and Staphylococci bacteria. C. perfringens is widespread; it is found in soil and the intestinal tracts of humans and animals. It becomes dangerous only when its spores germinate, producing toxins and destructive enzymes, and germination occurs only in an anaerobic environment (one almost totally devoid of oxygen). While gangrene can develop in any part of the body, it is most common in fingers, toes, hands, feet, arms, and legs, the parts of the body most susceptible to restricted blood flow. Even a slight injury in such an area is at high risk of causing gangrene. Early treatment with antibiotics, such as penicillin, and surgery to remove the dead tissue will often reduce the need for amputation. If left untreated, gangrene results in amputation or death.

GASTROENTERITIS: An inflammation of the stomach and the intestines. Commonly called the stomach flu.

GENE: The fundamental physical and functional unit of heredity. Whether in a microorganism or in a human cell, a gene is an individual element of an organism's genome and determines a trait or characteristic by regulating biochemical structure or metabolic process.

GENE THERAPY: The treatment of inherited diseases by corrective genetic engineering of the dysfunctional genes. It is part of a broader field called genetic medicine, which involves the screening, diagnosis, prevention, and treatment of hereditary conditions in humans. The results of genetic screening can pinpoint a potential problem to which gene therapy can sometimes offer a solution. Genetic defects are significant in the total field of medicine, with up to 15 out of every 100 newborn infants having a hereditary disorder of greater or lesser severity. More than 2,000 genetically distinct inherited defects have been classified as of 2018, including diabetes, cystic fibrosis, hemophilia, sickle cell anemia, phenylketonuria, Down syndrome, and cancer.

GENETIC ENGINEERING: The altering of the genetic material of living cells to make them capable of producing new substances or performing new functions. When the genetic material within the living cells (i.e., genes) is working properly, the human body can develop and function smoothly. However, should a single gene (even a tiny segment of a gene) go awry, the effect can be dramatic deformities, disease, and even death are possible.

GENOME: All of the genetic information for a cell or organism. The complete sequence of genes within a cell or virus.

GENOTYPE: The genetic information that a living thing inherits from its parents that affects its makeup, appearance, and function.

GEOGRAPHIC FOCALITY: The physical location of a disease pattern, epidemic, or outbreak; the characteristics of a location created by interconnections with other places.

GEOGRAPHIC INFORMATION SYSTEM (GIS): A system for archiving, retrieving, and manipulating data that has been stored and indexed according to the geographic coordinates of its elements. The system generally can utilize a variety of data types, such as imagery, maps, tables, etc.

GEOGRAPHIC MEDICINE: Also called geomedicine, the study of how human health is affected by climate and environment.

GERM THEORY OF DISEASE: A fundamental tenet of medicine that states that microorganisms, which are too small to be seen without the aid of a microscope, can invade the body and cause disease.

GLOBAL OUTBREAK ALERT AND RESPONSE NETWORK (GOARN): A collaboration of resources for the rapid identification, confirmation, and response to outbreaks of international importance.

GLOBALIZATION: The integration of national and local systems into a global economy through increased trade, manufacturing, communications, and migration.

GLOMERULONEPHRITIS: Inflammation of the kidneys. Mostly it affects the glomeruli, the small capsules in the kidney where blood flowing through capillaries transfers body wastes to urine.

GLYCOPROTEIN: A protein that contains a short chain of sugar as part of its structure.

GRAM-NEGATIVE BACTERIA: Bacteria whose cell walls are composed of an inner and outer membrane that are separated from one another by a region called the periplasm. The periplasm also contains a thin but rigid layer called the peptidoglycan.

GRANULOCYTE: Any cell containing granules (small, grain-like objects). The term is often used to refer to a type of white blood cell (leukocyte).

GROUP A STREPTOCOCCUS (GAS): A type (specifically a serotype) of the Streptococcus bacteria, based on the antigen contained in the cell wall.

GUILLAIN-BARRÉ SYNDROME: A rare condition in which the body's immune system attacks the nerves. It can cause muscle weakness, nerve tingling, and paralysis and may be triggered by an infection.

H

HARM-REDUCTION STRATEGY: In public health, a public policy scheme for reducing the amount of harm caused by a substance such as alcohol or tobacco. The phrase may refer to any medical strategy directed at reducing the harm caused by a disease, substance, or toxic medication.

HELMINTH: A representative of various phyla of wormlike animals.

HELMINTHIC DISEASE: An infection by parasitic worms such as hookworms or flatworms, known as helminths. A synonym for helminthic is verminous.

HELSINKI DECLARATION: A set of ethical principles governing medical and scientific experimentation on human subjects. It was drafted by the World Medical Association and was originally adopted in 1964.

HEMAGGLUTININ: Often abbreviated as HA, hemagglutinin is a glycoprotein, a protein that contains a short chain of sugar as part of its structure.

HEMOLYSIS: The destruction of blood cells, an abnormal rate of which may lead to lowered levels of these cells. For example, hemolytic anemia is caused by destruction of red blood cells at a rate faster than they can be produced.

HEMORRHAGE: Very severe, massive bleeding that is difficult to control.

HEMORRHAGIC FEVER: A high fever caused by viral infection that features a high volume of bleeding. The bleeding is caused by the formation of tiny blood clots throughout the bloodstream. These blood clots, also called microthrombi, deplete platelets and fibrinogen in the bloodstream. When bleeding begins, the factors needed for the clotting of the blood are scarce. Thus, uncontrolled bleeding (hemorrhage) ensues.

HEPA (HIGH-EFFICIENCY PARTICULATE AIR) FILTER: A filter that is designed to nearly totally remove airborne particles that are 0.3 microns (millionth of a meter) in diameter or larger. Such small particles can penetrate deeply into the lungs if inhaled.

HEPADNAVIRIDAE: A family of hepadnaviruses composed of two genera, Avihepadnavirus and Orthohepadnavirus. Hepadnaviruses have partially double-stranded DNA, and they replicate their genome in the host cells using an enzyme called reverse transcriptase. Because of this, they are also termed retroviruses. The viruses invade liver cells (hepatocytes) of vertebrates. When hepadna retroviruses invade a cell, a complete viral double-stranded (ds) DNA is made before it randomly inserts in one of the host's chromosomes. Once part of the chromosomal DNA, the viral DNA is then transcribed into an intermediate messenger RNA (mRNA) in the hosts' nucleus. The viral mRNA then leaves the nucleus and undergoes reverse transcription, which is mediated by the viral reverse transcriptase.

HEPATITIS AND HEPATITIS VIRUSES: Hepatitis is an inflammation of the liver, a potentially life-threatening disease most frequently caused by viral infections but that may also result from liver damage caused by toxic substances such as alcohol and certain drugs. There are five major types of hepatitis viruses: hepatitis A (HAV), hepatitis B (HBV), hepatitis C (HCV), hepatitis D (HDV), and hepatitis E (HEV).

HERD IMMUNITY: A resistance to disease that occurs in a population when a proportion of them have been immunized against it. The theory is that it is less likely that an infectious disease will spread in a group where some individuals are unlikely to contract it.

HERPESVIRUS: A family of viruses, many of which cause disease in humans. The herpes simplex 1 and herpes simplex 2 viruses cause infection in the mouth or on the genitals. Other common types of herpesvirus include chickenpox, Epstein-Barr virus, and cytomegalovirus. Herpesvirus is notable for its ability to remain latent, or inactive, in nerve cells near the area of infection, and to reactivate long after the initial infection. Herpes simplex 1 and 2, along with chicken pox, cause familiar skin sores. Epstein-Barr virus causes mononucleosis. Cytomegalovirus also causes a flu-like infection but can be dangerous to the elderly, infants, and those with weakened immune systems.

HETEROPHILE ANTIBODY: An antibody found in the blood of someone with infectious mononucleosis, also known as glandular fever.

HIGH-LEVEL DISINFECTION: A process that uses a chemical solution to kill all bacteria, viruses, and other disease-causing agents except for bacterial endospores and prions. High-level disinfection should be distinguished from sterilization, which removes endospores (a bacterial structure that is resistant to radiation, drying, lack of food, and other conditions potentially lethal to the bacteria) and prions (misshapen proteins that can cause disease) as well.

HIGHLY ACTIVE ANTIRETROVIRAL THERAPY (HAART): The name given to the combination of drugs given to people with human immunodeficiency virus (HIV) infection to slow or stop the progression of their condition to AIDS (acquired immunodeficiency syndrome). HIV is a retrovirus, and the various components of HAART block its replication by different mechanisms.

HISTAMINE: A hormone that is chemically similar to the hormones serotonin, epinephrine, and norepinephrine. A hormone is generally defined as a chemical produced by a certain cell or tissue that causes a specific biological change or activity to occur in another cell or tissue located elsewhere in the body. Specifically, histamine plays a role in localized immune responses and in allergic reactions.

HISTOCOMPATIBILITY: The histocompatibility molecules (proteins) on the cell surfaces of one individual of a species are unique. Thus, if the cell is transplanted into another person, the cell will be recognized by the immune system as being foreign. The histocompatibility molecules act as antigens in the recipient and so can also be called histocompatibility antigens or transplantation antigens. This is the basis of the rejection of transplanted material.

HISTOPATHOLOGY: The study of diseased tissues. A synonym for histopathology is pathologic histology.

HIV (HUMAN IMMUNODEFICIENCY VIRUS): The virus that causes acquired immunodeficiency syndrome (AIDS).

HOMOZYGOUS: A condition in which two alleles for a given gene are the same.

HORIZONTAL GENE TRANSFER: A major mechanism by which antibiotic resistance genes get passed between bacteria. It accounts for many hospital-acquired infections.

HORIZONTAL TRANSMISSION: The transmission of a disease-causing microorganism from one person to another, unrelated person by direct or indirect contact.

HOST: An organism that serves as the habitat for a parasite or possibly for a symbiont. A host may provide nutrition to the parasite or symbiont, or it may simply provide a place in which to live.

HOST FOCALITY: The tendency of some animal hosts, such as rodents carrying hantavirus and other viruses, to exist in groups in specific geographical locations and act as a local reservoir of infection.

HUMAN GROWTH HORMONE: A protein that is made and released from the pituitary gland, which increases growth and manufacture of new cells.

HUMAN IMMUNODEFICIENCY VIRUS (HIV): A class of viruses known as the retroviruses. These viruses are known as RNA viruses because they have RNA (ribonucleic acid) as their basic genetic material instead of DNA (deoxyribonucleic acid).

HUMAN T-CELL LEUKEMIA VIRUS (HTLV): Also known as human T-cell lymphotropic viruses, human T-cell leukemia viruses are divided into two known types: HTLV-1 and HTLV-2. HTLV-1 is often carried by people with no obvious symptoms, though it can cause a number of maladies, such as abnormalities of the T cells and B cells, a chronic infection of the myelin covering of nerves that causes degeneration of the nervous system, sores on the skin, and inflammation of the inside of the eye. HTLV-2 infection usually does not produce any symptoms. However, in some people a cancer of the blood known as hairy cell leukemia can develop.

HYBRIDIZATION: The process of combining two or more different molecules or organisms to create a new molecule or organism. Often called a hybrid organism.

HYGIENE: Health practices that minimize the spread of infectious microorganisms between people or between other living things and people. Inanimate objects and surfaces such as contaminated cutlery or a cutting board may be a secondary part of this process.

HYPERENDEMIC: Endemic (commonly present) in all age groups of a population. A related term is holoendemic, meaning a disease that is present more in children than in adults.

HYPERINFECTION: An infection that is caused by a very high number of disease-causing microorganisms. The infection results from an abnormality in the immune system that allows the infecting cells to grow and divide more easily than would normally be the case.

I

IATROGENIC: Any infection, injury, or other disease condition caused by medical treatment.

IMMUNITY HUMORAL REGULATION: One way in which the immune system responds to pathogens is by producing soluble proteins called antibodies. This is known as the humoral response and involves the activation of a special set of cells known as the B lymphocytes, because they originate in the bone marrow. The humoral immune response helps in the control and removal of pathogens such as bacteria, viruses, fungi, and parasites before they enter host cells. The antibodies produced by the B cells are the mediators of this response.

IMMIGRATION: The relocation of people to a different region or country from their native lands. Also, the movement of organisms into an area where they were previously absent.

IMMUNE GLOBULIN: A type of protein found in blood. The immune globulins (also called immunoglobulins) are Y-shaped globulins that act as antibodies, attaching themselves to invasive cells or materials in the body so that they can be identified and attacked by the immune system. There are five immune globulins, designated IgM, IgG, IgA, IgD, and IgE.

IMMUNE RESPONSE: The body's production of antibodies or some types of white blood cells in response to foreign substances.

IMMUNE SYNAPSE: Before they can help other immune cells respond to a foreign protein or pathogenic organism, helper T cells must first become activated. This process occurs when an antigen-presenting cell submits a fragment of a foreign protein, bound to a Class II MHC molecule (virus-derived fragments are bound to Class I MHC molecules), to the helper T cell. Antigen-presenting cells are derived from bone marrow and include both dendritic cells and Langerhans cells, as well as other specialized cells. Because T cell responses depend on direct contact with their target cells, their antigen receptors, unlike antibodies made by B cells, exist bound to the membrane only. In the intercellular gap between the T cell and the antigen-presenting cell, a special pattern of various receptors and complementary ligands forms that is several microns in size.

IMMUNE SYSTEM: The body's natural defense system that guards against foreign invaders and that includes lymphocytes and antibodies.

IMMUNO-BASED TEST: A medical technology that tests for the presence of a disease by looking for a reaction between disease organisms that may be present in a tissue or fluid sample and antibodies contained in the test kit.

IMMUNOCOMPROMISED: Having an immune system with reduced ability to recognize and respond to the presence of foreign material.

IMMUNODEFICIENCY: When part of the body's immune system is missing or defective, thus impairing the body's ability to fight infections. As a result, the person with an immunodeficiency disorder will have frequent infections that are generally more severe and last longer than usual.

IMMUNOGENICITY: The capacity of a host to produce an immune response to protect itself against infectious disease.

IMMUNOLOGY: The study of how the body responds to foreign substances and fights off infection and other disease. Immunologists study the molecules, cells, and organs of the human body that participate in this response.

IMMUNOSUPPRESSION: A reduction of the ability of the immune system to recognize and respond to the presence of foreign material.

IMPETIGO: A very localized bacterial infection of the skin. It tends to afflict primarily children but can occur in people of any age. Impetigo caused by the bacteria Staphylococcus aureus (or staph) affects children of all ages, while impetigo caused by the bacteria called group A streptococci (Streptococcus pyogenes or strep) is most common in children ages two to five years.

IMPORTED CASE OF DISEASE: An instance of disease in which an infected person who is not yet showing symptoms travels from his or her home country to another country and develops symptoms of the disease there.

IN SITU: A Latin term meaning "in place" or in the body or natural system.

INACTIVATED VACCINE: A vaccine that is made from disease-causing microorganisms that have been killed or made incapable of causing the infection. The immune system can still respond to the presence of the microorganisms.

INACTIVATED VIRUS: A virus that is incapable of causing disease but still stimulates the immune system to respond by forming antibodies.

INCIDENCE: The number of new cases of a disease or an injury that occur in a population during a specified period of time.

INCUBATION PERIOD: The time between exposure to a disease-causing virus or bacterium and the appearance of symptoms of the infection. Depending on the microorganism, the incubation time can range from a few hours, such as with food poisoning due to Salmonella, to a decade or more, such as with acquired immunodeficiency syndrome (AIDS).

INFECTION CONTROL: Policies and procedures used to minimize the risk of spreading infections, especially in hospitals and health care facilities.

INFECTION CONTROL PROFESSIONAL (ICP): A nurse, doctor, laboratory worker, microbiologist, public health official, or other specialist in the prevention and control of infectious disease. ICPs develop methods to control infection and instruct others in their use. These methods include proper handwashing; correct wearing of protective masks, eye guards, gloves, and other specialized clothing; vaccination; monitoring for infection; and investigating ways to treat and prevent infection. Courses and certifications are available for those wishing to become ICPs.

INFORMED CONSENT: An ethical and informational process in which a person learns about a procedure or clinical trial, including potential risks or benefits, before deciding to voluntarily participate in a study or undergo a particular procedure.

INNATE IMMUNITY: Resistance against disease that an individual is born with, as distinct from acquired immunity, which develops with exposure to infectious agents.

INOCULUM: A substance such as a virus, bacterial toxin, or viral or bacterial component that is added to the body to stimulate the immune system, which then provides protection from an infection by the particular microorganism.

INPATIENT: A patient who is admitted to a hospital or clinic for treatment, typically requiring the patient to stay overnight.

INSECTICIDE: A chemical substance used to kill insects.

INTERMEDIATE HOST: An organism infected by a parasite while the parasite is in a developmental, not sexually mature form.

INTERMEDIATE-LEVEL DISINFECTION: A form of disinfection that kills bacteria, most viruses, and mycobacteria.

INTERNATIONAL HEALTH REGULATIONS: Regulations introduced by the World Health Organization (WHO) that aim to control, monitor, prevent, protect against, and respond to the spread of disease across national borders while avoiding unnecessary interference with international movement and trade.

INTERTRIGO: A skin rash, often occurring in obese people on parts of the body symmetrically opposite each other. Sometimes called eczema intertrigo, it is caused by irritation of skin trapped under hanging folds of flesh such as pendulous breasts.

INTRAVENOUS: In the vein. For example, the insertion of a hypodermic needle into a vein to instill a fluid, withdraw or transfuse blood, or start an intravenous feeding.

IONIZING RADIATION: Any electromagnetic or particulate radiation capable of direct or indirect ion production in its passage through matter. In general use: Radiation that can cause tissue damage or death.

IRRADIATION: A method of preservation that treats food with low doses of radiation to deactivate enzymes and to kill microorganisms and insects.

ISOLATION: Within the health community, precautions taken in the hospital to prevent the spread of an infectious agent from an infected or colonized patient to susceptible people. Isolation practices are designed to minimize the transmission of infection.

ISOLATION AND QUARANTINE: Public health authorities rely on isolation and quarantine as two important tools among the many they use to fight disease outbreaks. Isolation is the practice of keeping a disease victim away from other people, sometimes by treating them in their homes or by the use of elaborate isolation systems in hospitals. Quarantine separates people who have been exposed to a disease but have not yet developed symptoms from the general population. Both isolation and quarantine can be entered voluntarily by patients when public health authorities request it, or it can be compelled by state governments or by the federal Centers for Disease Control and Prevention.

J

JAUNDICE: A condition in which a person's skin and the whites of the eyes are discolored a shade of yellow due to an increased level of bile pigments in the blood as a result of liver disease. Jaundice is sometimes called icterus, from a Greek word for the condition.

K

KERITITIS: Sometimes called corneal ulcers, an inflammation of the cornea, the transparent membrane that covers the colored part of the eye (iris) and pupil of the eye.

KOCH'S POSTULATES: A series of conditions that must be met for a microorganism to be considered the cause of a disease. German microbiologist Robert Koch (1843–1910) proposed the postulates in 1890.

KOPLIK SPOTS: Red spots with a small blue-white speck in the center found on the tongue and the insides of the cheeks during the early stages of measles. Also called Koplik's sign, they are named after American pediatrician Henry Koplik (1858–1927).

L

LARVAE: Immature forms (wormlike in insects; fishlike in amphibians) of an organism capable of surviving on its own. Larvae do not resemble the parent and must go through metamorphosis, or change, to reach the adult stage.

LATENT: Potential or dormant, as in a condition that is not yet manifest or active.

LATENT INFECTION: An infection already established in the body but not yet causing symptoms or having ceased to cause symptoms after an active period.

LATENT VIRUS: Viruses that can incorporate their genetic material into the genetic material of the infected host cell. Because the viral genetic material can then be replicated along with the host material, the virus becomes effectively "silent" with respect to detection by the host. Latent viruses usually contain the information necessary to reverse the latent state. The viral genetic material can leave the host genome to begin the manufacture of new virus particles.

LEGIONNAIRES' DISEASE: A type of pneumonia caused by Legionella bacteria. The bacterial species responsible for Legionnaires' disease is L. pneumophila. Major symptoms include fever, chills, muscle aches, and a cough that is initially nonproductive. Definitive diagnosis relies on specific laboratory tests for the bacteria, bacterial antigens, or antibodies produced by the body's immune system. As with other types of pneumonia, Legionnaires' disease poses the greatest threat to people who are elderly, ill, or immunocompromised.

LENS: An almost clear, biconvex structure in the eye that, along with the cornea, helps to focus light onto the retina. It can become infected, causing inflammation, for example, when contact lenses are improperly used.

LEPTOSPIRE: Also called a leptospira, any bacterial species of the genus Leptospira. Infection with leptospires causes leptospirosis.

LESION: The tissue disruption or the loss of function caused by a particular disease process.

LIPOPOLYSACCHARIDE (LPS): A molecule that is a constituent of the outer membrane of gram-negative bacteria. LPS is also be referred to as endotoxin. It helps protect the bacterium from host defenses and can contribute to illness in the host.

LIVE VACCINE: A virus or bacteria that has been weakened (attenuated) to cause an immune response in the body without causing disease. Live vaccines are preferred to killed vaccines, which use a dead virus or bacteria, because they cause a stronger and longer-lasting immune response.

LOW-LEVEL DISINFECTION: A form of disinfection that is capable of killing some viruses and some bacteria.

LYMPHADENOPATHY: Any disease of the lymph nodes, or the glandlike bodies that filter the clear intercellular fluid called lymph to remove impurities..

LYMPHATIC SYSTEM: The body's network of organs, ducts, and tissues that filters harmful substances out of the fluid that surrounds body tissues. Lymphatic organs include the bone marrow, thymus, spleen, appendix, tonsils, adenoids, lymph nodes, and Peyer's patches (in the small intestine). The thymus and bone marrow are called primary lymphatic organs, because lymphocytes are produced in them. The other lymphatic organs are called secondary lymphatic organs. The lymphatic system is a complex network of thin vessels, capillaries, valves, ducts, nodes, and organs that runs throughout the body, helping protect and maintain the internal fluids system of the entire body by both producing and filtering lymph and by producing various blood cells. The three main purposes of the lymphatic system are to drain fluid back into the bloodstream from the tissues, to filter lymph, and to fight infections.

LYMPHOCYTE: A type of white blood cell, such as a B or T lymphocyte, that functions as part of the lymphatic and immune systems by stimulating antibody formation to attack specific invading substances.

M

M PROTEIN: An antibody found in unusually large amounts in the blood or urine of patients with multiple myeloma, a form of cancer that arises in the white blood cells that produce antibodies.

MACAQUE: Any short-tailed monkey of the genus Macaca. Macaques, including rhesus monkeys, are often used as subjects in medical research because they are relatively affordable and resemble humans in many ways.

MACULOPAPULAR: A macule is any discolored skin spot that is flush or level with the surrounding skin surface; a papule is a small, solid bump on the skin. A maculopapular skin disturbance is one that combines macules and papules.

MAJOR HISTOCOMPATIBILITY COMPLEX (MHC): The proteins that protrude from the surface of a cell that identify the cell as "self." In humans, the proteins coded by the genes of the major histocompatibility complex (MHC) include human leukocyte antigens (HLA), as well as other proteins. HLA proteins are present on the surface of most of the body's cells and are important in helping the immune system distinguish "self" from "non-self" molecules, cells, and other objects.

MALAISE: A general or nonspecific feeling of unease or discomfort, often the first sign of disease infection.

MALIGNANT: A general term for cells that can dislodge from the original tumor and invade and destroy other tissues and organs.

MATERIEL: A French-derived word for equipment, supplies, or hardware.

MEASLES: An infectious disease caused by a virus of the paramyxovirus group. It infects only humans, and the infection results in life-long immunity to the disease. It is one of several exanthematous (rash-producing) diseases of childhood, the others being rubella (German measles), chickenpox, and scarlet fever. The disease is particularly common in both preschool and young school children.

MENINGITIS: An inflammation of the meninges, the three layers of protective membranes that line the spinal cord and the brain. Meningitis can occur when there is an infection near the brain or spinal cord, such as a respiratory infection in the sinuses, the mastoids, or the cavities around the ear. Disease organisms can also travel to the meninges through the bloodstream. The first signs may be a severe headache and neck stiffness followed by fever, vomiting, a rash, and, then, convulsions leading to loss of consciousness. Meningitis generally involves two types: nonbacterial meningitis, or aseptic meningitis, and bacterial meningitis, or purulent meningitis.

MENINGITIS BELT: The Meningitis Belt is an area of Africa south of the Sahara Desert, stretching from the Atlantic to the Pacific coast, where meningococcal meningitis is common.

MEROZOITE: The motile, infective stage of malaria responsible for disease symptoms.

MESSENGER RIBONUCLEIC ACID (MRNA): A molecule of RNA that carries the genetic information for producing one or more proteins; mRNA is produced by copying one strand of DNA, but in eukaryotes it is able to move from the nucleus to the cytoplasm (where protein synthesis takes place).

MICROBICIDE: A compound that kills microorganisms such as bacteria, fungi, and protozoa.

MICROCEPHALY: A rare neurological condition in which the head of a baby is significantly smaller than that of other children of the same age and sex. This can cause developmental delays, intellectual disability, and movement and coordination difficulties. When detected at birth, it results from abnormal growth in the womb.

MICROFILIAE: Live offspring produced by adult nematodes within the host's body.

MICROORGANISM: With only a single currently known exception (i.e., Epulopiscium fishelsonia, a bacterium that is billions of times larger than the bacteria in the human intestine and is large enough to view without a microscope), microorganisms are minute organisms that require microscopic magnification to view. To be seen, they must be magnified by an optical or electron microscope. The most common types of microorganisms are viruses, bacteria, blue-green bacteria, some algae, some fungi, yeasts, and protozoans.

MIGRATION: In medicine, the movement of a disease symptom from one part of the body to another, apparently without cause.

MIMICKED: In biology, mimicry is the imitation of another organism, often for evolutionary advantage. A disease that resembles another (for whatever reason) is sometimes said to have mimicked the other. Pathomimicry is the faking of symptoms by a patient, also called malingering.

MINIMAL INHIBITORY CONCENTRATION (MIC): The lowest level of an antibiotic that prevents growth of the particular type of bacteria in a liquid food source after a certain amount of time. Growth is detected by clouding of the food source. The MIC is the lowest concentration of the antibiotic at which the no cloudiness occurs.

MITE: A tiny arthropod (insect-like creature) of the order Acarina. Mites may inhabit the surface of the body without causing harm or may cause various skin ailments by burrowing under the skin. The droppings of mites living in house dust are a common source of allergic reactions.

MMR (MEASLES, MUMPS, RUBELLA) VACCINE: A vaccine given to protect someone from measles, mumps, and rubella. The vaccine is made up of viruses that cause the three diseases. The viruses are incapable of causing the diseases but can still stimulate the immune system.

MONO SPOT TEST: A blood test used to check for infection with the Epstein-Barr virus, which causes mononucleosis.

MONOCLONAL ANTIBODIES: Antibodies produced from a single cell line that are used in medical testing and, increasingly, in the treatment of some cancers.

MONONUCLEAR LEUKOCYTE: A type of white blood cell active in the immune system.

MONOVALENT VACCINE: A vaccine that is active against just one strain of a virus, such as the one that is in common use against the poliovirus.

MORBIDITY: From the Latin morbus, "sick," it refers to both the state of being ill and the severity of the illness. A serious disease is said to have high morbidity.

MORPHOLOGY: The study of form and structure of animals and plants. Also, the outward physical form possessed by an organism.

MORTALITY: The condition of being susceptible to death. The term mortality comes from the Latin word mors, which means death. Mortality can also refer to the rate of deaths caused by an illness or injury (e.g., "Rabies has a high mortality rate").

MOSQUITO COILS: Spirals of inflammable paste that, when burned, steadily release insect repellent into the air. They are often used in Asia, where many coils release octachlorodipropyl ether, which can cause lung cancer.

MOSQUITO NETTING: Fine meshes or nets hung around occupied spaces, especially beds, to keep out disease-carrying mosquitoes. Mosquito netting is a cost-effective way of preventing malaria.

MRSA (METHICILLIN-RESISTANT STAPHYLOCOCCUS AUREUS): Bacteria resistant to most penicillin-type antibiotics, including methicillin.

MUCOCUTANEOUS: A region of the body in which mucosa (mucous membrane) transitions to skin. Mucocutaneous zones occur in animals, at the body orifices. In humans mucocutaneous zones are found at the lips, nostrils, conjunctivae, urethra, vagina (in females), foreskin (in males), and anus.

MULTIBACILLARY: The more severe form of leprosy (Hansen's disease). It is defined as the presence of more than five skin lesions on the patient with a positive skin-smear test. The less severe form of leprosy is called paucibacillary leprosy.

MULTIDRUG RESISTANCE: A phenomenon that occurs when an infective agent loses its sensitivity against two or more of the drugs that are used against it.

MULTIDRUG THERAPY: The use of a combination of drugs against infection, each of which attacks the infective agent in a different way. This strategy can help overcome resistance to anti-infective drugs.

MUTABLE VIRUS: A virus whose DNA changes rapidly so that drugs and vaccines against it may not be effective.

MUTATION: A change in an organism's deoxyribonucleic acid (DNA) that occurs over time and may render it less sensitive to the drugs that are used against it.

MYALGIA: Muscular aches and pain.

MYCOBACTERIA: A genus of bacteria that contains the bacteria causing leprosy and tuberculosis. The bacteria have unusual cell walls that are harder to dissolve than the cell walls of other bacteria.

MYCOTIC: Having to do with or caused by a fungus. Any medical condition caused by a fungus is a mycotic condition, also called a mycosis.

MYCOTIC DISEASE: A disease caused by fungal infection.

N

NATIONAL ELECTRONIC TELECOMMUNICATIONS SYSTEM FOR SURVEILLANCE (NETSS): A computerized public health surveillance information system that provides the US Centers for Disease Control and Prevention (CDC) with weekly data regarding cases of nationally notifiable diseases.

NECROPSY: A medical examination of a dead body; also called an autopsy.

NECROTIC TISSUE: Dead tissue in an otherwise living body. Tissue death is called necrosis.

NEEDLESTICK INJURY (NSI): Any accidental breakage or puncture of the skin by an unsterilized medical needle (syringe) is a needlestick injury. Health care providers are at particular risk for needlestick injuries, which may transmit disease, because of the large number of needles they handle.

NEGLECTED TROPICAL DISEASE: Many tropical diseases are considered to be neglected because, despite their prevalence in less-developed areas, new vaccines and treatments are not being developed for them. Malaria was once considered to be a neglected tropical disease, but recently a great deal of research and money have been devoted to its treatment and cure.

NEMATODE: Also known as a roundworm; a type of helminth characterized by a long, cylindrical body.

NEURAMINIDASE (NA): A glycoprotein, which is a protein that contains a short chain of sugar as part of its structure.

NEUROTOXIN: A poison that interferes with nerve function, usually by affecting the flow of ions through the cell membrane.

NEUTROPHIL: A type of white blood cell that phagocytizes foreign microorganisms, releasing a bacteria-killing chemical known as lysozyme. Neutrophils are prominent in the inflammatory response.

NOBEL PEACE PRIZE: An annual prize bequeathed by Swedish inventor Alfred Nobel (1833–1896) and awarded by the Norwegian Nobel Committee to an individual or organization that has "done the most or the best work for fraternity between the nations, for the abolition or reduction of standing armies and for the holding and promotion of peace congresses."

NODULE: A small, roundish lump on the surface of the skin or of an internal organ.

NONGOVERNMENTAL ORGANIZATION (NGO): A voluntary organization that is not part of any government; often organized to address a specific issue or perform a humanitarian function.

NORMAL FLORA: The bacteria that normally inhabit some part of the body, such as the mouth or intestines. Normal flora are essential to health.

NOROVIRUS: A type of virus that contains ribonucleic acid as the genetic material and causes an intestinal infection known as gastroenteritis. A well-known example is Norwalk-like virus.

NOSOCOMIAL INFECTION: An infection that is acquired in a hospital. More precisely, the US Centers for Disease Control and Prevention (CDC) in Atlanta, Georgia, defines a nosocomial infection as a localized infection or an infection that is widely spread throughout the body that results from an adverse reaction to an infectious microorganism or toxin that was not present at the time of admission to the hospital.

NOTIFIABLE DISEASE: A disease that the law requires be reported to health officials when diagnosed. Also called a reportable disease.

NUCLEOTIDE: The basic unit of a nucleic acid. It consists of a simple sugar, a phosphate group, and a nitrogen-containing base.

NUCLEOTIDE SEQUENCE: A particular ordering of the chain structure of nucleic acid that provides the necessary information for a specific amino acid.

NUCLEUS, CELL: Membrane-enclosed structure within a cell that contains the cell's genetic material and controls its growth and reproduction. (Plural: nuclei.)

NUTRITIONAL SUPPLEMENTS: Substances necessary to health, such as calcium or protein, that are taken in concentrated form to compensate for dietary insufficiency, poor absorption, unusually high demand for that nutrient, or other reasons.

NYMPH: In aquatic insects, the larval stage.

O

ONCOGENIC VIRUS: A virus capable of changing the cells it infects so that the cells begin to grow and divide uncontrollably.

OOCYST: A spore phase of certain infectious organisms that can survive for a long time outside the organism and therefore continue to cause infection and resist treatment.

OOPHORITIS: An inflammation of the ovary, which happens in certain sexually transmitted diseases.

OPPORTUNISTIC INFECTION: An infection that occurs in people whose immune systems are diminished or are not functioning normally. Such infections are opportunistic insofar as the infectious agents take advantage of their hosts' compromised immune systems and invade to cause disease.

OPTIC SOLUTION: Any liquid solution of a medication that can be applied directly to the eye.

ORAL REHYDRATION THERAPY: Restoring body water levels by giving the patient fluids through the mouth (orally). Often, a special mixture of water, glucose, and electrolytes called oral rehydration solution is given.

ORCHITIS: Inflammation of one or both testicles. Swelling and pain are typical symptoms. Orchitis may be caused by various sexually transmitted diseases or escape of sperm cells into the tissues of the testicle.

OUTBREAK: The appearance of new cases of a disease in numbers greater than the established incidence rate or the appearance of even one case of an emergent or rare disease in an area.

OUTPATIENT: A person who receives health care services without being admitted to a hospital or clinic for an overnight stay.

OVA: Mature female sex cells produced in the ovaries. (Singular: ovum.)

OVIPOSITION: Ovum is Latin for "egg." To oviposition is to position or lay eggs, especially when done by an insect.

P

PANCREATITIS: An inflammation of the pancreas, an organ that is important in digestion. Pancreatitis can be acute (beginning suddenly, usually with the patient recovering fully) or chronic (progressing slowly with continued, permanent injury to the pancreas).

PANDEMIC: An epidemic that occurs in more than one country or population simultaneously. Pandemic means "all the people."

PAPULAR: A small, solid bump on the skin; papular means pertaining to or resembling a papule.

PAPULE: A small, solid bump on the skin.

PARAMYXOVIRUS: A type of virus that contains ribonucleic acid as the genetic material and has proteins on its surface that clump red blood cells and assist in the release of newly made viruses from the infected cells. Measles virus and mumps virus are two types of paramyxoviruses.

PARASITE: An organism that lives in or on a host organism and that gets its nourishment from that host. The parasite usually gains all the benefits of this relationship, while the host may suffer from various diseases and discomforts or show no signs of the infection. The life cycle of a typical parasite usually includes several developmental stages and morphological changes as the parasite lives and moves through the environment and one or more hosts. Parasites that remain on a host's body surface to feed are called ectoparasites, while those that live inside a host's body are called endoparasites. Parasitism is a highly successful biological adaptation. There are more known parasitic species than nonparasitic ones, and parasites affect just about every form of life, including most all animals, plants, and even bacteria.

PAROTITIS: Inflammation of the parotid gland. There are two parotid glands, one on each side of the jaw, at the back. Their function is to secret saliva into the mouth.

PAROXYSM: In medicine, a fit, convulsion, or seizure. Paroxysm may also be a sudden worsening or recurrence of disease symptoms.

PASTEURIZATION: Pasteurization is a process in which fluids such as wine and milk are heated for a predetermined time at a temperature that is below the boiling point of the liquid. The treatment kills any microorganisms that are in the fluid but does not alter the taste, appearance, or nutritive value of the fluid.

PATHOGEN: A disease-causing agent, such as a bacterium, a virus, a fungus, or another microorganism.

PATHOGENIC: Causing or capable of causing disease.

PAUCIBACILLARY: An infectious condition, such as a certain form of leprosy, characterized by few, rather than many, bacilli, which are a rod-shaped type of bacterium.

PCR (POLYMERASE CHAIN REACTION): A widely used technique in molecular biology involving the amplification of specific sequences of genomic DNA.

PERMETHRIN: A synthetic chemical used as insecticide. It is commonly used for insect control and can be found on food, crops, livestock, pets, and clothing. It affects the nervous system of the insects, resulting in death if consumed or touched by them. Humans and pets are more resistant to the effects but should still avoid consuming food covered with it, touching it, or breathing it.

PERSISTENCE: The length of time a disease remains in a patient. Disease persistence can vary from a few days to life-long.

PESTICIDE: A substance used to reduce the abundance of pests or any living thing that causes injury or disease to crops.

PHAGOCYTOSIS: The process by which certain cells engulf and digest microorganisms and consume debris and foreign bodies in the blood.

PHENOTYPE: The visible characteristics or physical shape produced by a living thing's genotype.

PLAGUE: A contagious disease that spreads rapidly through a population and results in a high rate of death.

PLASMID: A circular piece of DNA that exists outside of the bacterial chromosome and copies itself independently. Scientists often use bacterial plasmids in genetic engineering to carry genes into other organisms.

PLEURAL CAVITY: The lungs are surrounded by two membranous coverings, the pleura. One of the pleura is attached to the lung, the other to the ribcage. The space between the two pleura, the pleural cavity, is normally filled with a clear lubricating fluid called pleural fluid.

PNEUMONIA: Inflammation of the lung accompanied by filling of some air sacs with fluid (consolidation). Pneumonia can be caused by a number of infectious agents, including bacteria, viruses, and fungi.

POSTEXPOSURE PROPHYLAXIS: Treatment with drugs immediately after exposure to an infectious microorganism. The aim of this approach is to prevent an infection from becoming established.

POSTHERPETIC NEURALGIA: Neuralgia is pain arising in a nerve that is not the result of any injury. Postherpetic neuralgia is neuralgia experienced after infection with a herpesvirus, namely Herpes simplex or Herpes zoster.

POTABLE: Water that is clean enough to drink safely.

PREVALENCE: The actual number of cases of disease or injury that exists in a population.

PRIMARY HOST: An organism that provides food and shelter for a parasite while allowing it to become sexually mature. A secondary host is one occupied by a parasite during the larval or asexual stages of its life cycle.

PRIONS: Proteins that are infectious. Indeed, the name prion is derived from "proteinaceous infectious particles." The discovery of prions and confirmation of their infectious nature overturned a central dogma that infections were caused only by intact organisms, particularly microorganisms such as bacteria, fungi, parasites, or viruses. Because prions lack genetic material, the prevailing attitude was that a protein could not cause disease.

PRODROMAL SYMPTOMS: The earliest symptoms of a disease.

PRODROME: A symptom indicating the disease's onset; it may also be called a prodroma. For example, painful swallowing is often a prodrome of infection with a cold virus.

PROPHYLAXIS: Pre-exposure treatment (e.g., immunizations) to prevent the onset or recurrence of a disease.

PROSTRATION: A condition marked by nausea, disorientation, dizziness, and weakness caused by dehydration and prolonged exposure to high temperatures; also called heat exhaustion or hyperthermia.

PROTOZOA: Single-celled, animal-like microscopic organisms that live by taking in food rather than making it by photosynthesis and must live in the presence of water. (Singular: protozoan.) Protozoa are a diverse group of single-celled organisms, with more than 50,000 different types represented. The vast majority are microscopic, many measuring less than 5 one-thousandth of an inch (0.005 millimeters), but some, such as the freshwater Spirostomun, may reach 0.17 inches (3 millimeters) in length, large enough to enable it to be seen with the naked eye.

PRURITIS: The medical term for itchiness.

PRURULENT: Containing, discharging, or producing pus.

PUERPERAL: An interval of time around childbirth, from the onset of labor through the immediate recovery period after delivery.

PUERPERAL FEVER: A bacterial infection present in the blood (septicemia) that follows childbirth. The Latin word puer, meaning "boy" or "child," is the root of this term. Puerperal fever was much more common before the advent of modern aseptic practices, but infections still occur. Louis Pasteur showed that puerperal fever is most often caused by Streptococcus bacteria, which is now treated with antibiotics.

PULMONARY: Having to do with the lungs or respiratory system. The pulmonary circulatory system delivers deoxygenated blood from the right ventricle of the heart to the lungs and returns oxygenated blood from the lungs to the left atrium of the heart. At its most minute level, the alveolar capillary bed, the pulmonary circulatory system is the principle point of gas exchange between blood and air that moves in and out of the lungs during respiration.

PURULENT: Any part of the body that contains or releases pus. Pus is a fluid produced by inflamed, infected tissues and is made up of white blood cells, fragments of dead cells, and a liquid containing various proteins.

PUSTULE: A reservoir of pus visible just beneath the skin. It is usually sore to the touch and surrounded by inflamed tissue.

PYELONEPHRITIS: Inflammation caused by bacterial infection of the kidney and associated blood vessels.

PYROGENIC: A substance that causes fever. The word pyrogenic comes from the Greek word pyr, meaning fire.

Q

QUANTITATED: An act of determining the quantity of something, such as the number or concentration of bacteria in an infectious disease.

QUARANTINE: The practice of separating from the general population people who have been exposed to an infectious agent but have not yet developed symptoms. In the United States, this can be done voluntarily or involuntarily by the authority of states and the federal Centers for Disease Control and Prevention.

R

RALES: French term for a rattling sound in the throat or chest.

RASH: A change in appearance or texture of the skin. A rash is the popular term for a group of spots or red, inflamed skin that is usually a symptom of an underlying condition or disorder. Often temporary, a rash is only rarely a sign of a serious problem.

REASSORTMENT: A condition resulting when two or more different types of viruses exchange genetic material to form a new, genetically different virus.

RECEPTOR: Protein molecules on a cell's surface that act as a "signal receiver" and allow communication between cells.

RECOMBINANT DNA: DNA that is cut using specific enzymes so that a gene or DNA sequence can be inserted.

RECOMBINATION: A process during which genetic material is shuffled during reproduction to form new combinations. This mixing is important from an evolutionary standpoint because it allows the expression of different traits between generations. The process involves a physical exchange of nucleotides between duplicate strands of deoxyribonucleic acid (DNA).

RED TIDE: Red tides are a marine phenomenon in which water is stained a red, brown, or yellowish color because of the temporary abundance of a particular species of pigmented dinoflagellate (these events are known as blooms). Also called phytoplankton, or planktonic algae, these single-celled organisms of the class Dinophyceae move using a taillike structure called a flagellum. They also photosynthesize, and it is their photosynthetic pigments that can tint the water during blooms. Dinoflagellates are common and widespread. Under appropriate environmental conditions, various species can grow very rapidly, causing red tides. Red tides occur in all marine regions with a temperate or warmer climate.

REEMERGING DISEASE: Many diseases once thought to be controlled are reappearing to infect humans again. These are known as reemerging diseases because they have not been common for a long period of time and are starting to appear again among large population groups.

REEMERGING INFECTIOUS DISEASE: Illnesses such as malaria, diphtheria, tuberculosis, and polio that were once nearly absent from the world but are starting to cause greater numbers of infections once again. These illnesses are reappearing for many reasons. Malaria and other mosquito-borne illnesses increase when mosquito-control measures decrease. Other diseases are spreading because people have stopped being vaccinated, as happened with diphtheria after the collapse of the Soviet Union. A few diseases are reemerging because drugs to treat them have become less available or drug-resistant strains have developed.

REHYDRATION: Dehydration is excessive loss of water from the body; rehydration is the restoration of water after dehydration.

REITER'S SYNDROME: Named after German doctor Hans Reiter (1881–1969), a form of arthritis (joint inflammation) that appears in response to bacterial infection in some other part of the body. Also called Reiter syndrome, Reiter disease, or reactive arthritis.

RELAPSE: A return of symptoms after the patient has apparently recovered from a disease.

REPLICATE: To duplicate something or make a copy of it. All reproduction of living things depends on the replication of DNA molecules or, in a few cases, RNA molecules. Replication may be used to refer to the reproduction of entire viruses and other microorganisms.

REPLICATION: A process of reproducing, duplicating, copying, or repeating something, such as the duplication of DNA or the recreation of characteristics of an infectious disease in a laboratory setting.

REPORTABLE DISEASE: By law, occurrences of some diseases must be reported to government authorities when observed by health care professionals. Such diseases are called reportable diseases or notifiable diseases. Cholera and yellow fever are examples of reportable diseases.

RESERVOIR: The animal or organism in which a virus or parasite normally resides.

RESISTANCE: Immunity developed within a species (especially bacteria) via evolution to an antibiotic or other drug. For example, bacteria may acquire of genetic mutations that render them invulnerable to the action of antibiotics.

RESISTANT BACTERIA: Microbes that have lost their sensitivity to one or more antibiotic drugs through mutation.

RESISTANT ORGANISM: An organism that has developed the ability to counter something trying to harm it. Within infectious diseases, the organism, such as a bacterium, has developed a resistance to drugs, such as antibiotics.

RESPIRATOR: Any device that assists a patient in breathing or takes over breathing entirely for them.

RESTRICTION ENZYME: A special type of protein that can recognize certain DNA sequences and cut DNA to isolate specific genes. These DNA fragments may be joined together to create new stretches of DNA.

RETROVIRUS: Viruses in which the genetic material consists of ribonucleic acid (RNA) instead of the usual deoxyribonucleic acid (DNA). Retroviruses produce an enzyme known as reverse transcriptase that can transform RNA into DNA, which can then be permanently integrated into the DNA of the infected host cells.

REVERSE TRANSCRIPTASE: An enzyme that makes it possible for a retrovirus to produce deoxyribonucleic acid (DNA) from ribonucleic acid (RNA).

RHINITIS: An inflammation of the mucous lining of the nose. A nonspecific term that covers infections, allergies, and other disorders whose common feature is the location of their symptoms. These symptoms include infected or irritated mucous membranes, producing a discharge, congestion, and swelling of the tissues of the nasal passages. The most widespread form of infectious rhinitis is the common cold.

RIBONUCLEIC ACID (RNA): Any of a group of nucleic acids that carry out several important tasks in the synthesis of proteins. Unlike DNA (deoxyribonucleic acid), it has only a single strand. Nucleic acids are complex molecules that contain a cell's genetic information and the instructions for carrying out cellular processes. In eukaryotic cells, the two nucleic acids, ribonucleic acid (RNA) and deoxyribonucleic acid (DNA), work together to direct protein synthesis. Although it is DNA that contains the instructions for directing the synthesis of specific structural and enzymatic proteins, several types of RNA actually carry out the processes required to produce these proteins. These include messenger RNA (mRNA), ribosomal RNA (rRNA), and transfer RNA (tRNA). Further processing of the various RNAs is carried out by another type of RNA called small nuclear RNA (snRNA). The structure of RNA is similar to that of DNA, however, instead of the base thymine, RNA contains the base uracil in its place.

RING VACCINATION: The vaccination of all susceptible people in an area surrounding a case of an infectious disease. Because vaccination makes people immune to the disease, the hope is that the disease will not spread from the known case to other people. Ring vaccination was used in eliminating the smallpox virus.

RNA VIRUS: A virus whose genetic material consists of either single- or double-stranded ribonucleic acid (RNA) rather than deoxyribonucleic acid (DNA).

ROUNDWORM: Also known as nematodes, a type of helminth characterized by long, cylindrical bodies. Roundworm infections are diseases of the digestive tract and other organ systems that are caused by roundworms. Roundworm infections are widespread throughout the world, and humans acquire most types of roundworm infection from contaminated food or by touching the mouth with unwashed hands that have come into contact with the parasite larva. The severity of infection varies considerably from person to person. Children are more likely to have heavy infestations and are also more likely to suffer from malabsorption and malnutrition than adults.

ROUS SARCOMA VIRUS: Named after American doctor Francis Peyton Rous (1879–1970), a virus that can cause cancer in some birds, including chickens. It was the first known virus capable of causing cancer.

RUMINANTS: Cud-chewing animals with a four-chambered stomachs and even-toed hooves.

S

SANITATION: The use of hygienic recycling and disposal measures that prevent disease and promote health through sewage disposal, solid waste disposal, waste material recycling, and food processing and preparation.

SCHISTOSOMES: Blood flukes.

SEIZURE: A sudden disruption of the brain's normal electrical activity accompanied by altered consciousness or other neurological and behavioral abnormalities. Epilepsy is a condition characterized by recurrent seizures that may include repetitive muscle jerking called convulsions. Seizures are traditionally divided into two major categories: generalized seizures and focal seizures. Within each major category, however, there are many different types of seizures. Generalized seizures come about due to abnormal neuronal activity on both sides of the brain, whereas focal seizures, also named partial seizures, occur in only one part of the brain.

SELECTION: A process that favors one feature of organisms in a population over another feature found in the population. This occurs through differential reproduction—those with the favored feature produce more offspring than those with the other feature, such that they become a greater percentage of the population in the next generation.

SELECTION PRESSURE: The influence of various factors on the evolution of an organism. An example is the overuse of antibiotics, which provides a selection pressure for the development of antibiotic resistance in bacteria.

SELECTIVE PRESSURE: The tendency of an organism that has a certain characteristic to be eliminated from an environment or to increase in number. An example is the increased prevalence of bacteria resistant to multiple kinds of antibiotics.

SENTINEL: An epidemiological method in which a subset of the population is surveyed for the presence of communicable diseases. Also, an animal used to indicate the presence of disease within an area.

SENTINEL SURVEILLANCE: A method in epidemiology where a subset of the population is surveyed for the presence of communicable diseases. Also, a sentinel is an animal used to indicate the presence of disease within an area.

SEPSIS: A bacterial infection in the bloodstream or body tissues. Sepsis is a very broad term covering the presence of many types of microscopic disease-causing organisms. It is also called bacteremia. Closely related terms include septicemia and septic syndrome.

SEPTIC: Infected with bacteria, particularly in the bloodstream.

SEPTICEMIA: Prolonged fever, chills, anorexia, and anemia in conjunction with tissue lesions.

SEQUENCING: Finding the order of chemical bases in a section of DNA.

SEROCONVERSION: The development in the blood of antibodies to an infectious organism or agent. Typically, seroconversion is associated with infections caused by bacteria, viruses, and protozoans. But seroconversion also occurs after the deliberate inoculation with an antigen in the process of vaccination. In the case of infections, the development of detectable levels of antibodies can occur quickly, in the case of an active infection, or can be prolonged, in the case of a latent infection. Seroconversion typically heralds the development of the symptoms of the particular infection.

SEROLOGIC TEST: A test of the blood or other body fluid, such as spinal fluid, in which serum or the body fluids collected are used to look for antibodies.

SEROTYPE: Also known as a serovar, a class of microorganism based on the types of antigens (molecules that elicit an immune response) presented on the surface of the microorganism. A single species may have thousands of serotypes with medically distinct behaviors.

SEXUALLY TRANSMITTED INFECTION (STI): STIs vary in their susceptibility to treatment, their signs and symptoms, and the consequences if they are left untreated. Some are caused by bacteria. These usually can be treated and cured. Others are caused by viruses and can typically be treated but not cured.

SHED: To cast off or release. In medicine, the release of eggs or live organisms from an individual infected with parasites is often referred to as shedding.

SHOCK: A medical emergency in which the organs and tissues of the body are not receiving an adequate flow of blood. This condition deprives the organs and tissues of oxygen (carried in the blood) and allows the buildup of waste products. Shock can result in serious damage or even death.

SOCIOECONOMIC: Concerning both social and economic factors.

SOUTHERN BLOT ANALYSIS: An electrophoresis technique in which pieces of deoxyribonucleic acid (DNA) that have resulted from enzyme digestion are separated from one another on the basis of size, followed by the transfer of the DNA fragments to a flexible membrane. The membrane can then be exposed to various probes to identify target regions of the genetic material.

SPECIAL PATHOGENS BRANCH: A group within the US Centers for Disease Control and Prevention (CDC) whose goal is to study highly infectious viruses that produce diseases within humans.

SPIROCHETE: A bacterium shaped like a spiral. Spiral-shaped bacteria live in contaminated water, sewage, soil, and decaying organic matter, as well as inside humans and animals.

SPONGIFORM: The clinical name for the appearance of brain tissue affected by prion diseases, such as Creutzfeldt-Jakob disease or bovine spongiform encephalopathy (mad cow disease). The disease process leads to the formation of tiny holes in brain tissue, giving it a spongy appearance.

SPONTANEOUS: Generation Also known as abiogenesis, the incorrect and discarded assumption that living things can be generated from nonliving things.

SPORE: A dormant form assumed by some bacteria, such as anthrax, that enables the bacterium to survive high temperatures, dryness, and lack of nourishment for long periods of time. Under proper conditions, the spore may revert to the actively multiplying form of the bacteria.

SPOROZOAN: The fifth phylum of the kingdom Protista, known as Apicomplexa, comprises several species of obligate intracellular protozoan parasites classified as sporozoa or sporozoans, because they form reproductive cells known as spores. Many sporozoans are parasitic and pathogenic species, such as Plasmodium falciparum, Plasmodium malariae, Plasmodium vivax, Toxoplasma gondii, Pneumocystis carinii, Cryptosporidium parvum and Cryptosporidium muris, The sporozoa reproduction cycle has both asexual and sexual phases. The asexual phase is schizogony (from the Greek, meaning "generation through division"), in which merozoites (daughter cells) are produced through multiple nuclear fissions. The sexual phase is sporogony (i.e., generation of spores) and is followed by gametogony, or the production of sexually reproductive cells termed gamonts.

SPOROZOITE: Developmental stage of a protozoan (e.g., a malaria protozoan), during which it is transferred from vector (with malaria, a mosquito) to a human host.

STAINING: The use of chemicals to identify target components of microorganisms.

STANDARD PRECAUTIONS: The safety measures taken to prevent the transmission of disease-causing bacteria. These measures include proper handwashing; wearing gloves, goggles, and other protective clothing; proper handling of needles; and sterilization of equipment.

STERILIZATION: The complete killing or elimination of living organisms in the sample being treated. Sterilization is absolute. After the treatment, the sample is either devoid of life or the possibility of life (as from the subsequent germination and growth of bacterial spores), or living organisms are still present or could grow if they were present.

STRAIN: A subclass or a specific genetic variation of an organism.

STREP THROAT: An infection caused by group A Streptococcus bacteria. The main target of the infection is the mucous membranes lining the pharynx. Sometimes the tonsils are also infected (tonsillitis). If left untreated, the infection can develop into rheumatic fever or other serious conditions.

STREPTOCOCCUS: A genus of bacteria that includes species such as Streptococci pyogenes, a species of bacteria that causes strep throat.

SUPERINFECTION: A new infection that occurs in a patient who already has some other infection. For example, a bacterial infection appearing in a person who already had viral pneumonia would be a superinfection.

SURVEILLANCE: The systematic analysis, collection, evaluation, interpretation, and dissemination of data. Public health surveillance assists in the identification of health threats and the planning, implementation, and evaluation of responses to those threats.

SYLVATIC: Meaning "pertaining to the woods," the term refers to diseases such as plague that are spread by animals including ground squirrels and other wild rodents.

SYSTEMIC: Any medical condition that affects the whole body (i.e., the whole system) is systemic.

T

T CELL: An immune-system white blood cell that enables antibody production, suppresses antibody production, or kills other cells. When a vertebrate encounters substances capable of causing it harm, a protective system known as the immune system comes into play. This system is a network of many different organs that work together to recognize foreign substances and destroy them. The immune system can respond to the presence of a disease-causing agent (pathogen) in two ways. Immune cells called the B cells can produce soluble proteins (antibodies) that can accurately target and kill the pathogen. This branch of immunity is called humoral immunity. In cell-mediated immunity, immune cells known as the T cells produce special chemicals that can specifically isolate the pathogen and destroy it.

TAPEWORM: Parasitic flatworms of class Cestoidea, phylum Platyhelminthes, that live inside the intestine. Tapeworms have no digestive system but absorb predigested nutrients directly from their surroundings.

T CELL VACCINE: A vaccine that relies on eliciting cellular immunity, rather than humoral antibody-based immunity, against infection. T cell vaccines are being developed against the human immunodeficiency virus (HIV) and hepatitis C.

TICK: Any blood-sucking parasitic insect of suborder Ixodides, superfamily Ixodoidea. Ticks can transmit a number of diseases, including Lyme disease and Rocky Mountain spotted fever.

TOGAVIRUS: is a single-stranded ribonucleic acid (RNA) virus.

TOPICAL: Any medication that is applied directly to a particular part of the body's surface(e.g., a topical ointment).

TOXIC: Something that is poisonous and that can cause illness or death.

TOXIN: A poison produced by a living organism.

TOXOID: A bacterial toxin that has been altered chemically to make it incapable of causing damage but still capable of stimulating an immune response. Toxoids are used to stimulate antibody production, which is protective in the event of exposure to the active toxin.

TRANSFUSION-TRANSMISSIBLE INFECTIONS: Any infection that can be transmitted to a person by a blood transfusion (addition of stored whole blood or blood fractions to a person's own blood). Some diseases that can be transmitted in this way are acquired immunodeficiency syndrome (AIDS), hepatitis B, hepatitis C, syphilis, malaria, and Chagas disease.

TRANSMISSION: Microorganisms that cause disease in humans and other species are known as pathogens. The transmission of pathogens to a human or other host can occur in a number of ways, depending on the microorganism.

TREMATODES: Also called flukes, a type of parasitic flatworm. In humans flukes can infest the liver, lung, and other tissues.

TRICLOSAN: A chemical that kills bacteria.

TRISMUS: The medical term for lockjaw, a condition often associated with tetanus, which is an infection by the Clostridium tetani bacillus. In trismus or lockjaw, the major muscles of the jaw contract involuntarily.

TROPHOZOITE: The amoeboid, vegetative stage of the malaria protozoa.

TYPHUS: A disease caused by various species of Rickettsia, characterized by fever, rash, and delirium. Insects such as lice and chiggers transmit typhus. Two forms of typhus, epidemic typhus and scrub typhus, are fatal if untreated.

U

ULCER: An open sore on the inside or outside of the body that is accompanied by disintegration or necrosis of the surrounding tissue.

ULCERATIVE STI: Any kind of sexually transmitted infection (STI) that results in genital ulcers. This includes herpes, syphilis, chancroid, and gonorrhea. Herpes is the most common.

UNIVERSAL PRECAUTION: An infection-control strategy in which all human blood and other material is assumed to be potentially infectious, specifically with organisms such as human immunodeficiency virus (HIV) and hepatitis B virus. The precautions are aimed at preventing contact with blood or the other materials.

V

VACCINATION: The inoculation, or use of vaccines, to prevent specific diseases within humans and animals by producing immunity to such diseases. It is the introduction of weakened or dead viruses or microorganisms into the body to create immunity by the production of specific antibodies.

VACCINE: A substance that is introduced to stimulate antibody production and thus provide immunity to a particular disease.

VACCINIA VIRUS: A usually harmless virus that is closely related to the virus that causes smallpox, a dangerous disease. Infection with the vaccinia virus confers immunity against smallpox, so vaccinia virus has been used as a vaccine against smallpox.

VARICELLA ZOSTER IMMUNE GLOBULIN (VZIG): A preparation that can give people temporary protection against chickenpox after exposure to the Varicella virus. It is used for children and adults who are at risk of complications of the disease or who are susceptible to infection because they have weakened immunity.

VARICELLA ZOSTER VIRUS (VZV): A member of the alpha herpes virus group and is the cause of both chickenpox (also known as varicella) and shingles (herpes zoster).

VARIOLA VIRUS: The virus that causes smallpox. It is one of the members of the poxvirus group (family Poxviridae). The virus particle is brick shaped and contains a double strand of deoxyribonucleic acid (DNA). The variola virus is among the most dangerous of all the potential biological weapons.

VARIOLATION: The premodern practice of deliberately infecting a person with smallpox to make them immune to a more serious form of the disease. It was dangerous but did confer immunity on survivors.

VECTOR: Any agent that carries and transmits parasites and diseases. Also, an organism or a chemical used to transport a gene into a new host cell.

VECTOR-BORNE DISEASE: One in which the pathogenic microorganism is transmitted from an infected individual to another individual by an arthropod or other agent, sometimes with other animals serving as intermediary hosts. The transmission depends on the attributes and requirements of at least three different living organisms: the pathologic agent, either a virus, protozoa, bacteria, or helminth (worm); the vector, commonly arthropods such as ticks or mosquitoes; and the human host.

VENEREAL DISEASE: Diseases that are transmitted by sexual contact. They are named after Venus, the Roman goddess of female sexuality.

VESICLE: A membrane-bound sphere that contains a variety of substances in cells.

VIRAL SHEDDING: The movement of the herpes virus from the nerves to the surface of the skin. During shedding the virus can be passed on through skin-to-skin contact.

VIRION: A mature virus particle consisting of a core of ribonucleic acid (RNA) or deoxyribonucleic acid (DNA) surrounded by a protein coat. This is the form in which a virus exists outside of its host cell.

VIRULENCE: The ability of a disease organism to cause disease. A more virulent organism is more infective and liable to produce more serious disease.

VIRUS: Essentially nonliving repositories of nucleic acid that require the presence of a living prokaryotic or eukaryotic cell for the replication of the nucleic acid. There are a number of different viruses that challenge the human immune system and that may produce disease in humans. A virus is a small, infectious agent that consists of a core of genetic material—either deoxyribonucleic acid (DNA) or ribonucleic acid (RNA)—surrounded by a shell of protein. Very simple microorganisms, viruses are much smaller than bacteria that enter and multiply within cells. Viruses often exchange or transfer their genetic material (DNA or RNA) to cells and can cause diseases such as chickenpox, hepatitis, measles, and mumps.

VISCERAL: Pertaining to the viscera. The viscera are the large organs contained in the main cavities of the body, especially the thorax and abdomen—for example, the lungs, stomach, intestines, kidneys, or liver.

W

WATERBORNE DISEASE: Diseases that are caused by exposure to contaminated water. The exposure can occur by drinking the water or having the water come in contact with the body. Examples of waterborne diseases are cholera and typhoid fever.

WAVELENGTH: A distance of one cycle of a wave; for instance, the distance between the peaks on adjoining waves that have the same phase.

WEAPONIZATION: The use of any bacterium, virus, or other disease-causing organism as a weapon of war. Among other terms, it is also called germ warfare, biological weaponry, and biological warfare.

WEIL'S DISEASE: Named after German doctor Adolf Weil (1848–1916), a severe form of leptospirosis or seven-day fever, which is a disease caused by infection with the corkscrew-shaped bacillus Leptospira interrogans.

WILD VIRUS: A genetic description referring to the original form of a virus, first observed in nature. It may remain the most common form in existence, but mutated forms develop over time and sometimes become the new wild virus.

Z

ZOONOSES: Diseases of microbiological origin that can be transmitted from animals to people. The causes of the diseases can be bacteria, viruses, parasites, or fungi.

ZOONOTIC: A disease that can be transmitted between animals and humans. Examples of zoonotic diseases are anthrax, plague, and Q fever.

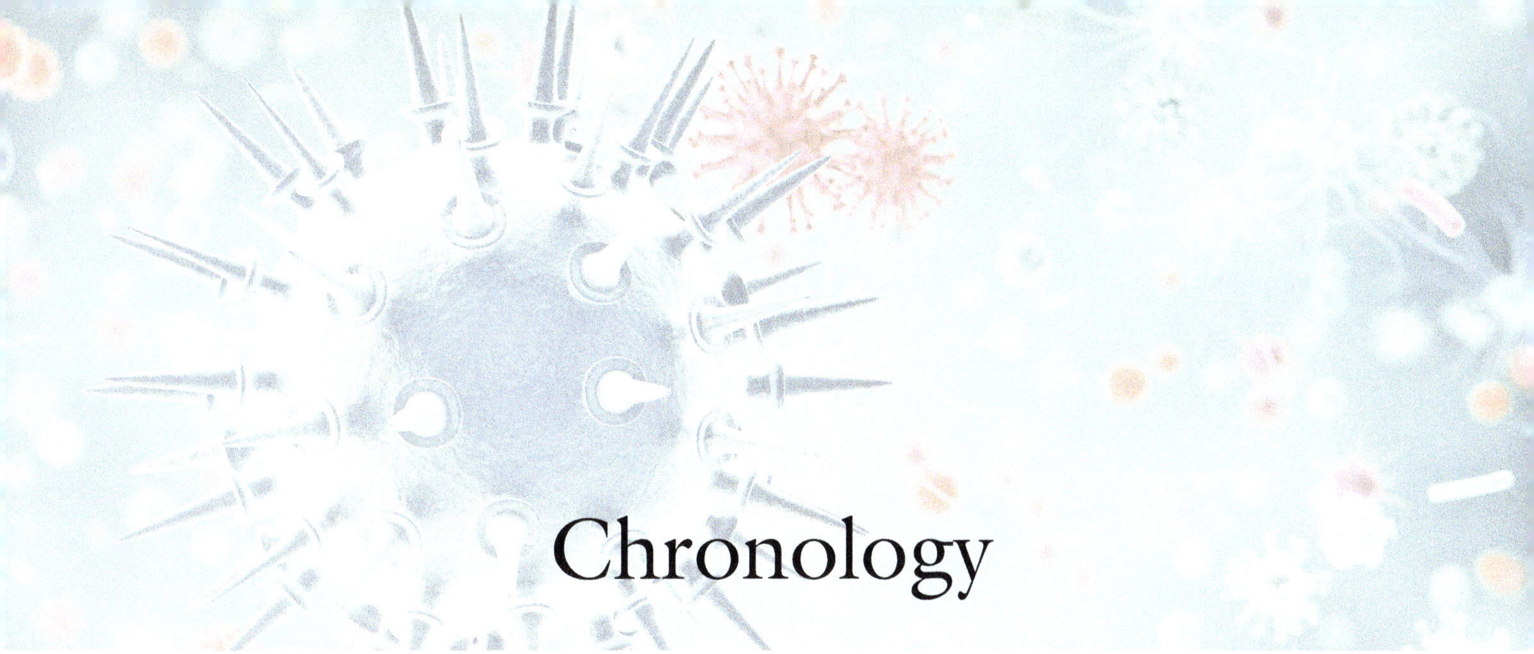

Chronology

BC

c. 2500 The characteristic symptoms of malaria are first described in Chinese medical writings.

c. 1000 Hindu physicians exhibit broad clinical knowledge of tuberculosis. In India, the Laws of Manu consider it to be an unclean, incurable disease and an impediment to marriage.

c. 430 Plague of Athens caused by unknown infectious agent. One-third of the population (increased by those fleeing the Spartan army) die.

c. 400 Hippocrates (460–370 BCE), Greek physician, and his disciples establish their medical practice based on reason and experiment. They attribute disease to natural causes and use diet and medication to restore the body's balance of humors.

c. 400 Hippocratic texts recommend irrigation with fresh water as a treatment for septic wounds.

c. 300 A medical school is set up in Alexandria, where the first accurate anatomical observations using dissection are made. The principal exponents of the school are Greek physician Herophilus (c. 335 BCE–c. 280 BCE) and Greek physician Erasistratus (c. 304 BCE–c. 250 BCE).

c. 300 Herophilus, Greek anatomist, establishes himself as the first systemic anatomist and the first to perform human dissections.

91 Greek scientific medicine takes hold in Rome when the physician Asclepiades (c. 130 BCE–40 BCE) of Bithynia settles in the West.

AD

c. 30 Aulus Cornelius Celsus, Roman encyclopedist, writes his influential book *De Re Medicina*. The work contains descriptions of many conditions and operations and is probably drawn mostly from the collection of writings of the school of Hippocrates. It is rediscovered during the 15th century and becomes highly influential.

c. 75 Dioscorides (c. 40–c. 90), Greek physician, writes the first systematic pharmacopoeia. His *De Materia Medica* in five volumes provides accurate botanical and pharmacological information. It is preserved by the Arabs and, when translated into Latin and printed in 1478, becomes a standard botanical reference.

150 Claudius Galen (129–c. 210), Greek physician, says that pus formation is required for wound healing. This proves to be incorrect and hinders the treatment of wounds for centuries.

c. 160 Bubonic plague (termed "barbarian boils") sweeps China.

c. 160 Galen, in his *De Usu Partium*, describes the pineal gland as a secretory organ that is important to thinking. He names it the pineal because it resembles a pine cone.

c. 166 Plague in Rome (possibly smallpox or bubonic plague) eventually kills millions throughout the weakening Roman empire.

167 Stabiae, a popular health resort for tuberculosis sufferers, is established near Naples, Italy. It is believed that the fumes from nearby Mt. Vesuvius are beneficial for lung ulcers.

170 Galen first describes gonorrhea.

c. 200 Galen describes internal inflammations as caused by personal factors.

c. 370 Basil of Caesarea (330–379) founds and organizes a large hospital at Caesarea (near Palestine).

c. 400 Fabiola, a Christian noblewoman, founds the first nosocomium, or hospital, in Western Europe. After establishing the first hospital in Rome, she establishes a hospice for pilgrims in Porto, Italy.

430 Earliest recorded plague in Europe is an epidemic that breaks out in Athens, Greece.

c. 500 During this century the "plague of Justinian" kills about 1 million people.

529 Benedict of Nursia founds the monastery at Monte Cassino in central Italy. It becomes, if not an actual medical school, at least an important center of scholarship in which medicine played a great part. It also acquires great fame throughout the West, and its medical teachings are spread by the Benedictines to their monasteries scattered all over Europe.

610 In China Ch'ao Yuan-fang (550–630) writes a treatise on the causes and symptoms of diseases. Medical knowledge spreads from China to Japan via the Korean peninsula.

644 Rotharus, King of Lombardy (c. 606–652; also called Rothari), issues his edict ordering the segregation of all lepers.

c. 700 Benedictus Crispus, archbishop of Milan from 681 to about 730, writes his *Commentarium Medicinale*, an elementary practical manual in verse. It describes the use of medicinal plants for curing illnesses.

c. 850 Christian physician Sabur ibn Sahl of Jundishapur compiles a 22-volume work on antidotes that dominates Islamic pharmacopeia for the next 400 years.

c. 850 Islamic philosopher Al-Kindi (813–873) writes his *De Medicinarum Compositarum Gradibus*, which attempts to base dosages of medicine on mathematical measurements.

c. 875 Bertharius (c. 810–883), the abbot of Montcasino from 857 to 884, writes two treatises, *De Innumeris Remediorum Utilitatibus* and *De Innumeris Morbis*, that give insight into the kind of medicine practiced in the monasteries.

896 Abu Bakr al-Razi (c. 845–c. 930; also known as Rhazes), Persian physician and alchemist, distinguishes between the specific characteristics of measles and smallpox. He is also believed to be the first to classify all substances into the great classification of animal, vegetable, and mineral.

c. 900 First medical books written in Anglo-Saxon appear, including *Lacnunga* and *Leech Book of Bald*.

c. 955 Jewish "prince of medicine," Isaac Israeli (c.855–955), dies. He writes classic works on fever and uroscopy, as well as *Guide of the Physicians*.

c. 980 Abu al-Qasim Al-Zahrawi (936–1013), known as Abucasis, creates a system and method of human dissection along with the first formal specific surgical techniques.

c. 1000 Ibn Sina (c. 980–1037), or Avicenna, publishes *Al-Quanun*, or Canon of Medicine, where he held that medicines could be discovered and tried by experiment or by reasoning.

1137 St. Bartholomew's hospital is founded in London.

1140 Bologna, Italy, begins to develop as a major European medical center. In the next century, the Italian physician Taddeo Alderotti (c. 1233–1303) opens a school of medicine there.

1200 Physicians in Italy begin to write case histories that describe symptoms and observable pathology of diseases.

c. 1267 Roger Bacon (1214–1292), English philosopher and scientist, asserts that natural phenomena should be studied empirically.

1302 First formally recorded postmortem or judicial autopsy is performed in Bologna, Italy, by Italian physician Bartolomeo da Varignana. A postmortem is ordered by the court in a case of suspected poisoning.

1333 Public botanical garden is established in Venice, Italy, to grow herbs that have medical uses.

1345 First apothecary shop or drug store opens in London.

1348 The beginning of a three-year epidemic caused by *Yersinia pestis* kills almost one-third of the population of urban Europe. In the aftermath of the epidemic, measures are introduced by the Italian government to improve public sanitation, marking the origin of public health.

1374 As the plague spreads, the Republic of Ragusa places the first quarantines on crews of ships thought to be infected.

1388 Richard II (1367–1400), king of England, establishes the first sanitary laws in England.

1489 Typhus is first brought to Europe by soldiers who had been fighting in Cyprus.

1491 First anatomical book to contain printed illustrations is German physician Johannes de Ketham's *Fasciculus Medicinae*.

1492 Venereal diseases, smallpox, and influenza are brought by the Columbus expedition (and subsequent European explorers) to the New World. Millions of native peoples eventually die from these diseases because of a lack of prior exposure to stimulate immunity. In some regions whole villages succumb, and across broader regions up to 95 percent of the native population dies.

1525 Gonzalo Hernandez de Oviedo y Valdes (1478–1557) of Spain publishes the first systematic description of the medicinal plants of Central America.

1525 Paracelsus (1493–1541), Swiss physician and alchemist, begins the use of mineral substances as medicines.

1527 Paracelsus publicly burns the writings of Galen in Basel, Switzerland. He rejects the traditional medical methods as irrational, and he founds iatrochemistry, asserting that the body is linked in some way to the laws of chemistry.

1528 Italian physician Girolamo Fracastoro (c. 1478–1553), also known as Fracastorius, describes an epidemic of typhus among French troops invading Naples.

1530 Fracastorius writes his poem called "Syphilis" (*Syphilis sive Morbus Gallici*), which gives the definitive name to the sexually transmitted infection that is spreading throughout Europe.

1536 Paracelsus publishes his surgical treatise, *Chirurgia Magna*.

1543 Andreas Vesalius (1514–1564), Dutch anatomist, publishes his *De Corporis Humani Corporis Fabrica*, the first accurate book on human anatomy. Its illustrations are of the highest level of both realism and art, and the result revolutionizes biology.

1546 Fracastorius writes his *De Contagione et Contagiosis Morbis*, which contains new ideas on the transmission of contagious diseases and is considered the scientific beginning of that study.

1567 A book on miner's tuberculosis by Paracelsus is posthumously published.

1602 Felix Platter (1536–1614), Swiss anatomist, publishes his *Praxis Medica*, which is the first modern attempt at the classification of diseases.

1621 Johannes Baptista van Helmont (1577–1635), Dutch physician and alchemist, writes his *Ortus Medicinae* in which he becomes one of the founders of modern pathology. He studies the anatomical changes that occur in disease.

1624 Adriaan van den Spigelius (1578–1625), Dutch anatomist, publishes the first account of malaria.

1640 Juan del Vigo introduces cinchona into Spain. Native to the Andes, the bark of this tree is processed to obtain quinine, used in the treatment of malaria.

1642 First treatise on the use of cinchona bark (quinine powder) for treating malaria is written by Spanish physician Pedro Barba (1608–1671).

1648 René Descartes (1596–1650), French philosopher and mathematician, writes *De Homine*, the first European textbook on physiology. He considers the body to be a material machine and offers his mechanist theory of life.

1648 Willem Piso (1611–1678), Dutch physician and botanist (also called Le Pois), points out the effectiveness of ipecac against dysentery in his book *De Medicina Brasiliensi*. He is among the first to become acquainted with tropical diseases, and he distinguishes between yaws and syphilis.

1660 The Royal Society of London is founded in England with Henry Oldenburg (c. 1618–1677) as secretary and Robert Hooke (1635–1702) as curator of experiments. Two years later, in 1662, King Charles II (1630–1685) grants it a royal charter, and it becomes known as the "Royal Society of London for the Promotion of Natural Knowledge."

1665 Bubonic plague epidemic in London kills 75,000 people. It is during this scourge that English scientist and mathematician Isaac Newton (1642–1727) leaves school in London and stays at his mother's farm in the country. There he formulates his laws of motion.

1665 First drawing of the cell is made by Robert Hooke (1635–1703), English physicist. While observing a sliver of cork under a microscope, Hooke notices it is composed of a pattern of tiny rectangular holes he calls "cells" because each looks like a small, empty room. Although he does not observe living cells, the name is retained.

1665 Hooke publishes his landmark book on microscopy, *Micrographia*. Containing some of the most beautiful drawings of microscopic observations ever made, his book led to many discoveries in related fields.

1666 Robert Boyle (1627–1691), English physicist and chemist, publishes *The Origine of Formes and Qualities* in which he begins to explain all chemical reactions and physical properties through the existence of small, indivisible particles or atoms.

1668 Francesco Redi (1626–1697), Italian physician, conducts experiments to disprove spontaneous generation. He shows that maggots are not born spontaneously but come from eggs laid by flies. He publishes his *Esperienze Intorno all Generazione degli Insetti*.

1671 Michael Ettmüller (1644–1683), German physician, attributes the contagiousness of tuberculosis to sputum.

1672 French physician Le Gras introduces ipecac into Europe. The root of the Brazilian plant ipecacuanha is used to cure dysentery.

1674 Antoni van Leeuwenhoek (1632–1723), Dutch biologist and microscopist, observes "animacules" in lake water viewed through a ground glass lens. This observation of what will eventually be known as bacteria represents the start of the formal study of microbiology.

1675 John Josselyn, English botanist, publishes an account of the plants and animals he encounters while living in America and indicates that tuberculosis existed among Native Americans before the arrival of Europeans.

1677 Antoni van Leeuwenhoek (1632–1723), Dutch biologist and microscopist, discovers spermatozoa and describes them in a letter he publishes in *Philosophical Transactions* in 1679. That year Johan Ham also sees them microscopically, but the semen he observes comes from a patient suffering from gonorrhea, and Ham concludes that spermatozoa are a consequence of the disease.

1700 Bernardino Ramazzini (1633–1714), Italian physician, publishes the first systematic treatment on occupational diseases. His book, *De Morbis Artificum*, opens an entirely new department of modern medicine—diseases of trade or occupation and industrial hygiene.

1721 The word *antiseptic* first appears in print.

1730 British physician George Martine (1702–1743) performs the first tracheostomy on a patient with diphtheria.

1735 Botulism first described.

1748 British physician John Fothergill (1712–1780) describes diphtheria in "Account of the Putrid Sore Throat."

1762 Marcus Anton von Plenciz Sr. (1705–1786), Austrian physician, expresses the idea that all infectious diseases are caused by living organisms and that there is a specific organism for each disease.

1767 William Heberden (1710–1801), English physician, demonstrates that chickenpox is not a mild form of smallpox but a different disease.

1780 George Adams (1750–1795), English engineer, devises the first microtome. This mechanical instrument cuts thin slices for examination under a microscope, thus replacing the imprecise procedure of cutting by handheld razor.

1789 Polio is first described by English physician Michael Underwood (1736–1820) in England.

1796 Edward Jenner (1749–1823) uses cowpox virus to develop a smallpox vaccine. By modern standards, this was human experimentation, as Jenner injected healthy eight-year-old James Phillips with cowpox and then after a period of months with smallpox.

1798 Government legislation is passed to establish hospitals in the United States devoted to the care of ill mariners. This initiative leads to the establishment of a Hygienic Laboratory that eventually grows to become the National Institutes of Health (NIH).

1800 Marie-François-Xavier Bichat (1771–1802) publishes his first major work, *Treatise on Tissues*, which establishes histology as a new scientific discipline. Bichat distinguishes 21 kinds of tissue and relates particular diseases to particular tissues.

1801 A hospital is established in London to treat the victims of typhus.

1802 English chemist John Dalton (1766–1844) introduces modern atomic theory into the science of chemistry.

1814 The Royal Hospital for Diseases of the Chest is founded in London in an attempt to keep consumptive patients (people with tuberculosis) segregated.

1816 The stethoscope, which is an important tool for diagnosing pneumonia, is introduced by René Laënnec (1781–1826).

1817 Start of first cholera pandemic, which spreads from Bengal to China in the east and to Egypt in the west.

1818 William Charles Wells (1757–1817), Scottish American physician, suggests the theory of natural selection in an essay dealing with human color variations. He notes that dark-skinned people seem more resistant to tropical diseases than lighter-skinned people. Wells also calls attention to selection carried out by animal breeders. Jerome Lawrence, James Cowles Prichard (1786–1848), and others make similar suggestions but do not develop their ideas into a coherent and convincing theory of evolution.

1818 Xavier Bichat (1771–1802), French physician, publishes his first major work, *Trait, des membranes en general*, in which he propounds the notion of tissues. This work also founds histology, distinguishing 21 kinds of tissue and relating disease to them.

1820 First United States *Pharmacopoeia* is published.

1824 Start of second cholera pandemic, which penetrates as far as Russia and also reaches England, North America, the Caribbean, and Latin America.

1826 Pierre Bretonneau (1778–1862), French physician, describes and names diphtheria in his specification of diseases.

1829 Salicin, the precursor of aspirin, is purified from the bark of the willow tree.

1831 Charles Darwin (1809–1882), English naturalist, begins his historic voyage on the HMS *Beagle* (1831–1836). His observations during the voyage lead to his theory of evolution by means of natural selection.

1835 Jacob Bigelow (1787–1879), American physician, publishes his book *On Self-Limited Diseases*, in which he states the commonsense idea that some diseases will simply run their course and subside without the benefit of any treatment from a physician.

1836 Theodor Schwann (1810–1882), German physiologist, carries out experiments that refute the theory of the spontaneous generation. He also demonstrates that alcoholic fermentation depends on the action of living yeast cells. The same conclusion is reached independently by French physicist Charles Cagniard de la Tour (1777–1859).

1837 Pierre-François-Olive Rayer (1793–1867), French physician, is the first to describe the disease glanders as found in humans and to prove that it is not a form of tuberculosis.

1838 Angelo Dubini (1813–1902), Italian physician, discovers *Ankylostoma duodenale*, the cause of hookworm disease, in the intestinal tract.

1838 Matthias Jakob Schleiden (1804–1881) notes that the nucleus first described by Scottish botanist Robert Brown (1773–1858) is a characteristic of all plant cells. Schleiden describes plants as a community of cells and cell products. He helps establish cell theory and stimulates Theodor Schwann's recognition that animals are also composed of cells and cell products.

1839 Third cholera pandemic begins with entry of British troops in Afghanistan and travels to Persia, Central Asia, Europe, and the Americas.

1841 Friedrich Gustav Jacob Henle (1809–1885), German pathologist and anatomist, publishes his *Allegemeine Anatomie*, which becomes the first systematic textbook of histology (the study of minute tissue structure and includes the first statement of the germ theory of communicable disease).

1842 Edwin Chadwick (1800–1890), a pioneer in sanitary reform, reports that deaths from typhus in 1838 and 1839 in England exceeded those from smallpox.

1842 Oliver Wendell Holmes (1809–1894), American physician, recommends that surgeons wash their hands using calcium chloride to prevent spread of infection from corpses to patients.

1843 First outbreak of polio in the United States occurs.

1843 Gabriel Andral (1797–1876), French physician, is the first to urge that blood be examined in cases of disease.

1846 American Medical Association establishes a code of ethics for physicians that declares their obligation to treat victims of epidemic diseases even at a risk to their own lives.

1847 A series of yellow fever epidemics sweeps the American Southern states. The epidemics recur for more than 30 years.

1847 The first sexually transmitted infection clinic is opened at the London Docks Hospital.

1849 John Snow (1813–1858), English physician, first states the theory that cholera is a waterborne disease. During a cholera epidemic in London in 1854, Snow breaks the handle of the Broad Street Pump, thereby shutting down the main source of disease transmission during the outbreak.

1849 Snow publishes the groundbreaking paper "On the Transmission of Cholera."

1855 Third, or modern, pandemic of plague probably begins in Yunan province, China.

1857 Louis Pasteur demonstrates that lactic acid fermentation is caused by a living organism. Between 1857 and 1880, he performs a series of experiments that refute the doctrine of spontaneous generation. He also introduces vaccines for fowl cholera, anthrax, and rabies, based on attenuated strains of viruses and bacteria.

1858 Rudolf Ludwig Carl Virchow (1821–1902), German physician, publishes his landmark paper "Cellular Pathology" and establishes the field of cellular pathology.

Virchow asserts that all cells arise from preexisting cells (*Omnis cellula e cellula*). He argues that the cell is the ultimate locus of all disease.

1859 Darwin publishes his landmark book *On the Origin of Species by Means of Natural Selection.*

1861 Carl Gegenbaur (1826–1903), German anatomist, confirms Theodor Schwann's suggestion that all vertebrate eggs are single cells.

1862 First demonstration of pasteurization.

1864 Fourth cholera pandemic starts and revisits locations of previous pandemics.

1865 An epidemic of rinderpest kills 500,000 cattle in Great Britain. Government inquiries into the outbreak pave the way for the development of contemporary theories of epidemiology and the germ theory of disease.

1865 French physiologist Claude Bernard (1813–1878) publishes *Introduction to the Study of Human Experimentation*, which advocates, "Never perform an experiment which might be harmful to the patient even if advantageous to science."

1866 Austrian botanist and monk Johann Gregor Mendel (1822–1884) discovers the laws of heredity and writes the first of a series of papers on heredity (1866–1869). The papers formulate the laws of hybridization. Mendel's work is disregarded until 1900, when Dutch botanist Hugo de Vries (1848–1935) rediscovers it. Unbeknownst to both Darwin and Mendel, Mendelian laws provide the scientific framework for the concepts of gradual evolution and continuous variation.

1867 British surgeon Joseph Lister (1827–1912) publishes a study that implicates microorganisms with infection. Based on this, his use of early disinfectants during surgery markedly reduces postoperative infections and death.

1867 Robert Koch (1843–1910), German bacteriologist, establishes the role of bacteria in anthrax, providing the final piece of evidence in support of the germ theory of disease. Koch goes on to formulate postulates that, when fulfilled, confirm bacteria or viruses as the cause of an infection.

1868 Carl August Wunderlich (1815–1877), German physician, publishes his major work on the relation of animal heat or fever to disease. He is the first to recognize that fever is not itself a disease but rather a symptom.

1869 Johann Friedrich Miescher (1844–1895), Swiss physician, discovers nuclein, a new chemical isolated from the nuclei of pus cells. Two years later he isolates nuclein from salmon sperm. This material comes to be known as nucleic acid.

1871 German biologist Ferdinand Julius Cohn (1828–1898) coins the term *bacterium.*

1871 First US city to use a filter on its public water supply is Poughkeepsie, New York. The evidence mounts that much disease is spread by contaminated drinking water.

1873 Franz Anton Schneider describes cell division in detail. His drawings include both the nucleus and chromosomal strands.

1875 Cohn publishes a classification of bacteria in which the genus name *Bacillus* is used for the first time.

1875 Koch's postulates used for the first time to demonstrate that anthrax is caused by *Bacillus anthracis*, validating the germ theory of disease.

1877 Louis Pasteur first distinguishes between aerobic and anaerobic bacteria.

1877 Paul Ehrlich (1854–1915), German bacteriologist, recognizes the existence of the mast cells of the immune system.

1877 Koch describes new techniques for fixing, staining, and photographing bacteria.

1877 Wilhelm Friedrich Kühne (1837–1900), German physiologist, proposes the term *enzyme* (meaning "in yeast"). Kühne establishes the critical distinction between enzymes, or "ferments," and the microorganisms that produce them.

1878 Lister publishes a paper describing the role of a bacterium he names *Bacterium lactis* in the souring of milk.

1878 Koch publishes his landmark findings on the etiology or cause of infectious disease.

Koch's postulates state that the causative microorganism must be located in a diseased animal and that, after it is cultured or grown, it must then be capable of causing disease in a healthy animal. Finally, the newly infected animal must yield the same bacteria as those found in the original animal.

1878 Thomas Burrill (1839–1916), American botanist, demonstrates that a plant disease (pear blight) is caused by a bacterium (*Micrococcus amylophorous*).

1879 Albert Neisser (1855–1916), German physician, identifies the bacterium *Neiserria gonorrhoeoe* as the cause of gonorrhea.

1880 C. L. Alphonse Laveran (1845–1922), French physician, isolates malarial parasites in erythrocytes of infected people and demonstrates that the organism can replicate in the cells.

1880 The first issue of the journal *Science* is published by the American Association for the Advancement of Science.

1881 Fifth cholera pandemic begins and is widespread in China and Japan in the Far East, as well as Germany and Russia in Europe, although the disease does not spread in North America.

1881 *Streptococcus pneumoniae*, a major cause of bacterial pneumonia, is discovered independently by Pasteur and US Army physician George Sternberg (1838–1915).

1882 Angelina Fanny Hesse (1850–1934) and Walther Hesse (1846–1911) in Koch's laboratory develop agar as a solid grow medium for microorganisms. Agar replaces gelatin as the solid growth medium of choice in microbiology.

1882 Friedrich August Johannes Loffler (1852–1915), German bacteriologist, and F. Schulze discover the bacterium causing glanders, a contagious and destructive disease of animals, especially horses, that can be transmitted to humans.

1883 German-Swiss pathologist Edwin Klebs (1834–1913) and German bacteriologist Friedrich Loeffler (1852–1915) independently discover *Corynebacterium diphtheriae*, the bacterium that causes diphtheria.

1883 Koch discovers *V. cholerae* as the causative agent of cholera in Egypt.

1883 Surgical gowns and headgear begin to be used by surgeons.

1884 Élie Metchnikoff (1845–1916), Russian microbiologist, discovers the antibacterial activity of white blood cells, which he calls phagocytes, and formulates the theory of phagocytosis. He also develops the cellular theory of vaccination.

1884 Danish bacteriologist Hans Christian Gram (1853–1938) develops the Gram stain, a method of categorizing bacteria into one of two groups (Gram positive and Gram negative) based on the chemical reaction of the bacteria cell walls to a staining procedure.

1884 Pasteur and coworkers publish a paper titled *A New Communication on Rabies.* Pasteur proves that the causal agent of rabies can be attenuated and that the weakened virus can be used as a vaccine to prevent the disease. This work serves as the basis of future work on virus attenuation, vaccine development, and the concept that variation is an inherent characteristic of viruses.

1885 Francis Galton (1822–1911) devises a new statistical tool, the correlation table.

1885 Pasteur inoculates a boy, Joseph Meister, against rabies. Meister had been bitten by a dog infected with rabies, and the treatment saved his life. This is the first time Pasteur uses an attenuated (weakened) germ on a human being.

1885 Russian hematologist Antonin Filatov makes the first formal description of mononucleosis.

1885 Theodor Escherich (1857–1911), German-Austrian pediatrician, identifies a bacterium inhabiting the human intestinal tract that he names *Bacterium coli* and shows that the bacterium causes infant diarrhea and gastroenteritis. The bacterium is subsequently named *Escherichia coli.*

1886 Italian physician Camillo Golgi (c. 1843–1926) describes two forms of malaria, with fever occurring every two and every three days, respectively.

1887 Julius Richard Petri (1852–1921), German microbiologist, develops a culture dish that has a lid to exclude airborne contaminants. The innovation is subsequently termed the Petri dish.

1888 Galton publishes *Natural Inheritance*, considered a landmark in the establishment of biometry and statistical studies of variation. Galton also proposes the Law of Ancestral Inheritance, a statistical description of the relative contributions to heredity made by previous generations.

1888 Martinus Wilhelm Beijerinck (1851–1931), Dutch botanist, uses a growth medium enriched with certain nutrients to isolate the bacteria *Rhizobium*, demonstrating that nutritionally tailored growth media are useful in bacterial isolation.

1888 The diphtheria toxin is discovered by French physician Émile Roux (1853–1933) and French bacteriologist Alexandre Yersin (1863–1943).

1888 The Institute Pasteur is formed in France.

1890 Emil von Behring (1854–1917), German bacteriologist, uses his new discovery of antitoxins to develop an antitoxin for diphtheria—a disease that usually brought death to the children it attacked.

1891 First child is treated with the diphtheria antitoxin.

1891 Ehrlich discovers that methyl blue dye immobilizes malaria bacterium and begins searching for other, more potent microbial dyes.

1891 Ehrlich proposes that antibodies are responsible for immunity.

1891 Prussian State dictates that even jailed prisoners must give consent prior to treatment (for tuberculosis).

1891 Koch proposes the concept of delayed type hypersensitivity.

1892 Dmitry Ivanovsky (1864–1920), Russian microbiologist, demonstrates that filterable material causes tobacco mosaic disease. The infectious agent is subsequently showed to be the tobacco mosaic virus. Ivanovsky's discovery heralds the field of virology.

1892 First vaccine for diphtheria becomes available.

1892 Neisser, the discoverer of gonorrhea bacteria, injects human subjects with syphilis, prompting debate and leading to regulations on human experimentation.

1892 German physician Richard Pfeiffer (1858–1945) discovers *Haemophilius influenzae*, a cause of both pneumonia and influenza.

1894 Yersin isolates *Yersinia (Pasteurella) pestis*, the bacterium responsible for bubonic plague.

1894 German physicist Wilhelm Conrad Röntgen, 1845–1923) discovers X-rays.

1895 German chemist Heinrich Dreser (1860–1924), working for the Bayer Company in Germany, produces a drug he thought to be as effective an analgesic as morphine, but without its harmful side effects. Bayer begins mass production of diacetylmorphine and in 1898 markets the new drug under the brand name "heroin" as a cough sedative.

1896 Edmund Beecher Wilson (1856–1939), American zoologist, publishes the first edition of his highly influential treatise *The Cell in Development and Heredity*. Wilson calls attention to the relationship between chromosomes and sex determination.

1896 William Joseph Dibdin (1850–1925), English engineer, and his colleague improve the sewage disposal systems in England with the introduction of a bacterial system of water purification. These improvements greatly reduce the number of waterborne diseases such as cholera and typhoid fever.

1897 American physician William Welch describes and names *Plasmodium falciparum*, a protozoan parasite and cause of malaria.

1898 First state-run sanatorium for tuberculosis in the United States opens in Massachusetts.

1898 Loeffler and German bacteriologist Paul Frosch (1860–1928) publish their *Report on Foot-and-Mouth Disease*. They prove that this animal disease is caused by a filterable virus and suggest that similar agents might cause other diseases.

1898 Beijerinck discovers and names the causative agent of the tobacco mosaic disease. He describes it as a new type of microscopically visible organism that eventually comes to be known as a virus.

1898 The First International Congress of Genetics is held in London.

1898 The transmission of plague by flea-infested rodents is shown by French bacteriologist Paul-Louis Simond (1858–1947).

1899 A meeting to organize the Society of American Bacteriologists is held at Yale University. The society will later become the American Society for Microbiology.

1899 George Henry Falkiner Nuttall (1862–1937), American biologist, first summarizes the role of insects, arachnids, and myriapods as transmitters of bacterial and parasitic diseases.

1899 Start of the sixth cholera pandemic, which affects the Far East, apart from sporadic outbreaks in parts of Europe.

1900 Austrian biologist Karl Landsteiner (1868–1943) discovers the blood-agglutination phenomenon and the four major blood types in humans.

1900 Pandemic plague becomes widely disseminated throughout the world, reaching Europe, North and South America, India, the Middle East, Africa, and Australia.

1900 Ehrlich proposes the theory concerning the formation of antibodies by the immune system.

1900 Walter Reed (1851–1902), American surgeon, discovers that the yellow fever virus is transmitted to humans by a mosquito. This is the first demonstration of a viral cause of a human disease.

1901 Joseph Everett Dutton (1874–1905), English physician, and his colleague J. L. Todd discover the parasite *Trypanosoma gambiense* that is responsible for African sleeping sickness.

1902 Ronald Ross (1857–1932), a British officer with the Indian Medical Service, receives the Nobel Prize for identifying mosquitoes as the transmitter of malaria.

1904 Ehrlich discovers a microbial dye called trypan red that helps destroy the trypanosomes that cause such diseases as sleeping sickness. This is the first such active agent against trypanosomes (parasitic protozoa).

1905 Fritz Richard Schaudinn (1871–1906), German zoologist, discovers *Treponema pallidum*, the organism or parasite causing syphilis. His discovery of this almost invisible parasite is due to his consummate technique and staining methods.

1905 Jules Bordet (1870–1961), Belgian bacteriologist, and his colleague, Octave Gengou (1875–1957), discover the bacillus of whooping cough (*B. pertussis*). Bordet goes on to discover a method of immunization against this dreaded childhood disease.

1906 Charles Nicolle (1866–1936) of the Pasteur Institute in Paris shows a link between typhus and lice.

1906 The Pure Food and Drugs Act is passed in the United States, beginning the organization that would become the Food and Drug Administration (FDA).

1906 Viennese physician Clemens von Pirquet (1874–1929) coins the term *allergy* to describe the immune reaction to certain compounds.

1907 Laveran identifies malaria parasites (protozoa) in blood.

1907 Charles Franklin Craig (1872–1950), American physician, and Percy Moreau Ashburn (1872–1940), American surgeon, work in the Philippines and are the first to prove that dengue fever (also called breakbone fever) is caused by a virus.

1907 Clemens Peter Pirquet von Cesenatico (1874–1929), Austrian physician, first introduces the cutaneous, or skin, reaction test for the diagnosis of tuberculosis.

1907 English biologist William Bateson (1861–1926) urges his colleagues to adopt the term *genetics* to indicate the importance of the new science of heredity.

1909 Sigurd Orla-Jensen (1870–1949) proposes that the physiological reactions of bacteria are primarily important in their classification.

1909 American zoologist and geneticist Thomas Hunt Morgan (1866–1945) selects the fruit fly *Drosophila* as a model system for the study of genetics. Morgan and his coworkers confirm the chromosome theory of heredity and realize the significance of the fact that certain genes tend to be transmitted together. Morgan postulates the mechanism of "crossing over." His associate, Alfred Henry Sturtevant (1891–1970) demonstrates the relationship between crossing over and the rearrangement of genes in 1913.

1909 Walter Reed General Hospital opens in Washington, D.C.

1909 Danish botanist Wilhelm Johannsen (1857–1927) argues the necessity of distinguishing between the appearance of an organism and its genetic constitution. He invents the terms *gene* (carrier of heredity), *genotype* (an organism's genetic constitution), and *phenotype* (the appearance of the actual organism).

1910 Howard Taylor Ricketts (1871–1910), discoverer of the *Rickettsia* genus of bacteria, dies of the *Rickettsia*-caused disease typhus while investigating an outbreak in Mexico City.

1910 Ehrlich announces his discovery of an effective treatment for syphilis. He names this new drug Salvarsan (now arsphenamine). His discovery marks the first chemotherapeutic agent for a bacterial disease.

1911 The first known retrovirus, Rous sarcoma virus, is discovered by Peyton Rous (1879–1970), who also showed that the virus could induce cancer.

1912 The United States Public Health Service is established.

1913 Béla Schick (18771967) designs a skin test that determines immunity to diphtheria.

1914 Frederick William Twort (1877–1950), English bacteriologist, and Felix H. D'Herelle (1873–1949), Canadian-Russian physician, independently discover bacteriophage, viruses that destroy bacteria.

1915 A typhus epidemic in Serbia causes 150,000 deaths.

1915 Stanislaus von Prowazek (1875–1915), Czech parasitologist, dies of typhus when investigating an outbreak in a Russian prisoner of war camp, having identified *R. prowazekii*, the causative agent.

1915 US Public Health Office allows induction of pellagra in Mississippi prisoners.

1916 D'Herelle carries out further studies of the agent that destroys bacterial colonies and gives it the name bacteriophage (bacteria-eating agent). D'Herelle and others unsuccessfully attempt to use bacteriophages as bactericidal therapeutic agents.

1917 D'Arcy Wentworth Thompson (1860–1948) publishes *On Growth and Form*, which suggests that the evolution of one species into another occurs as a series of transformations involving the entire organism rather than a succession of minor changes in parts of the body.

1918 Global influenza pandemic kills more people than numbers of soldiers who died fighting during World War I (1914–1918). By the end of 1918, more than 25 million people die from virulent strain of Spanish influenza.

1918 American geneticist Thomas Hunt Morgan (1866–1945) and coworkers publish *The Physical Basis of Heredity*, a survey of the remarkable development of the new science of genetics.

1919 James Brown uses blood agar to study the destruction of blood cells by the bacterium *Streptococcus.* He observes three reactions that he designates alpha, beta, and gamma.

1919 The Health Organization of the League of Nations was established for the prevention and control of disease around the world.

1920 Data on diphtheria is gathered for the first time in the United States, showing approximately 13,000 deaths per year.

1920 Sprunt and Evans coined the term *infectious mononucleosis*, as they described the abnormal mononuclear leukocytes observed in patients with the condition.

1921 Otto Loewi (1873–1961), German American physiologist, discovers that acetylcholine functions as a neurotransmitter. It is the first such brain chemical to be so identified.

1922 British parasitologist John Stephens (1865–1946) describes *P. ovale.*

1924 Albert Jan Kluyver (1888–1956), Dutch microbiologist and biochemist, publishes *Unity and Diversity in the Metabolism of Microorganisms.* He demonstrates that different microorganisms have common metabolic pathways of oxidation, fermentation, and synthesis of certain compounds. Kluyver also states that life on Earth depends on microbial activity.

1924 The last urban epidemic of plague in the United States begins in Los Angeles.

1926 American chemist James B. Sumner (1887–1955) publishes a report on the isolation of the enzyme urease and his proof that the enzyme is a protein. This idea is controversial until 1930 when American biochemist John Howard Northrop (1891– 1987) confirms Sumner's ideas by crystallizing pepsin. Sumner, Northrop, and Wendell Meredith Stanley (1904–1971) ultimately share the Nobel Prize in Chemistry in 1946.

1927 Thomas Rivers (1888–1962), American bacteriologist and virologist, publishes a paper that differentiates bacteria from viruses, establishing virology as a field of study that is distinct from bacteriology.

1928 British bacteriologist Frederick Griffith (1877–1941) discovers that certain strains of pneumococci could undergo some kind of transmutation of type. After injecting mice with living R type pneumococci and heat-killed S type, Griffith is able to isolate living virulent bacteria from the infected mice. Griffith suggests that some unknown "principle" had transformed the harmless R strain of the pneumococcus to the virulent S strain.

1928 Philip (1894–1972) and Cecil Drinker (1887–1958) of Harvard School of Public Health introduce the "iron lung" for treatment of paralytic polio.

1928 Scottish biochemist Alexander Fleming (1881–1955) discovers penicillin. In his published report (1929), Fleming observes that the mold *Penicillium notatum* inhibits the growth of some bacteria. This is the first antibacterial, and it opens a new era of "wonder drugs."

1929 Fleming publishes his account of the bacteriolytic power of penicillin.

1929 Scientist Francis O. Holmes introduces the technique of "local lesion" as a means of measuring the concentration of tobacco mosaic virus. The method becomes extremely important in virus purification.

1929 Willard Myron Allen (1904–1993), American physician, and George Washington Corner (1889–1981), American anatomist, discover progesterone. They demonstrate that it is necessary for the maintenance of pregnancy.

1930 Max Theiler (1899–1972), South African–born American virologist, demonstrates the advantages of using mice as experimental animals for research on animal viruses. Theiler uses mice in his studies of the yellow fever virus.

1930 British geneticist Ronald A. Fisher (1890–1962) publishes *Genetical Theory of Natural Selection*, a formal analysis of the mathematics of selection.

1930 United States Food, Drug, and Insecticide Administration is renamed the Food and Drug Administration (FDA).

1932 At Tuskegee, Alabama, African American sharecroppers become unknowing and unwilling subjects of experimentation on the untreated natural course of syphilis. Even after penicillin came into use in the 1940s, the men remained untreated.

1932 William J. Elford (1900–1952) and Christopher H. Andrewes (1896–1988) develop methods of estimating the sizes of viruses by using a series of membranes as filters. Later studies prove that the viral sizes obtained by this method were comparable to those obtained by electron microscopy.

1933 "Regulation on New Therapy and Experimentation" decreed in Germany.

1934 Discovery of chloroquine is announced by scientist Hans Andersag (1902–1955) at Bayer in Germany.

1934 J. B. S. Haldane (1892–1964), British geneticist, presents the first calculations of the spontaneous mutation frequency of a human gene.

1934 John Marrack (1886–1976) begins a series of studies that leads to the formation of the hypothesis governing the association between an antigen and the corresponding antibody.

1935 Wendall Meredith Stanley (1904–1971), American biochemist, discovers that viruses are partly protein-based. By purifying and crystallizing viruses, he enables scientists to identify the precise molecular structure and propagation modes of several viruses.

1936 George P. Berry (1898–1986) and Helen M. Dedrick report that the Shope virus could be "transformed" into myxomatosis/Sanarelli virus. This virological curiosity was variously referred to as "transformation," "recombination," and "multiplicity of reactivation." Subsequent research suggests that it is the first example of genetic interaction between animal viruses, but some scientists warn that the phenomenon might indicate the danger of reactivation of virus particles in vaccines and in cancer research.

1937 American researcher H. R. Cox (1907–1986) cultures *Rickettsiae* in the yolks of fertilized hens' eggs, opening the door to research into a vaccine.

1938 American biochemist Emory L. Ellis (1906–2003) and German American biophysicist Max Delbrück (1906–1981) perform studies on phage replication that mark the beginning of modern phage work. They introduce the "one-step growth" experiment, which demonstrates that, after bacteriophages attack bacteria, replication of the virus occurs within the bacterial host during a "latent period," after which viral progeny are released in a "burst."

1939 Ernest Chain (1906–1979), German-born British biochemist, and Howard Florey (1898–1968), Australian pathologist and pharmacologist, refine the purification of penicillin, allowing the mass production of the antibiotic.

1939 Swiss chemist Paul Müller (1899–1965) discovers the insecticidal properties of DDT.

1939 American virologist Richard E. Shope (1901–1966) reports that the swine influenza virus survived between epidemics in an intermediate host. This discovery is an important step in revealing the role of intermediate hosts in perpetuating specific diseases.

1941 American scientists George W. Beadle (1903–1989) and Edward L. Tatum (1909–1975) publish their classic study on the biochemical genetics titled *Genetic Control of Biochemical Reactions in Neurospora*. Beadle and Tatum irradiate red bread mold *Neurospora* and prove that genes produce their effects by regulating particular enzymes. This work leads to the one-gene-one-enzyme theory.

1941 Norman M. Gregg (1892–1966) of Australia discovers that rubella (German measles) during pregnancy can cause congenital abnormalities. Children of mothers who had rubella during their pregnancy are found to suffer from blindness, deafness, and heart disease.

1941 The term *antibiotic* is coined by Russian American microbiologist Selman Waksman (1888–1973).

1942 Jules Freund (1890–1960) and Katherine McDermott identify adjuvants (e.g., paraffin oil) that act to boost antibody production.

1942 Italian microbiologist Salvador E. Luria (1912–1991) and Delbrück demonstrate statistically that inheritance of genetic characteristics in bacteria follows the principles of genetic inheritance proposed by Darwin. For their work, the two, along with American bacteriologist Alfred Day Hershey (1908–1997), are awarded the 1969 Nobel Prize in Medicine or Physiology.

1942 Neil Hamilton Fairley (1891–1966), Australian physician, wins a Fellowship to the Royal Society for work on anemia caused by the rupture of red blood cells in malaria.

1943 At University of Cincinnati Hospital, experiments are performed using mentally disabled patients.

1943 Penicillin starts to become available as a therapy for Allied troops.

1944 Oswald T. Avery (1877–1955), Colin M. MacLeod (1909–1972), and Maclyn McCarty (1911–2005) publish a landmark paper on the pneumococcus transforming principle. The paper is titled "Studies on the Chemical Nature of the Substance Inducing Transformation of Pneumococcal Types." Avery suggests that the transforming principle seems to be deoxyribonucleic acid (DNA), but contemporary ideas about the structure of nucleic acids suggest that DNA does not possess the biological specificity of the hypothetical genetic material.

1944 Waksman introduces streptomycin.

1944 To combat battle fatigue during World War II (1939–1945), nearly 200 million amphetamine tablets are issued to American soldiers stationed in Great Britain during the war.

1944 The United States Public Health Service Act is passed.

1944 University of Chicago Medical School professor Alf Alving conducts malaria experiments on more than 400 Illinois prisoners.

1945 Joshua Lederberg (1925–2008) and Tatum demonstrate genetic recombination in bacteria.

1946 Physicists Felix Bloch (1905–1983) and Edward Mills Purcell (1912–1997) develop nuclear magnetic resonance (NMR) as a viable tool for observation and analysis.

1946 American geneticist Hermann J. Muller (1890–1967) is awarded the Nobel Prize in Medicine or Physiology for his contributions to radiation genetics.

1946 Delbrück and W. T. Bailey Jr. publish a paper titled "Induced Mutations in Bacterial Viruses." Despite some confusion about the nature of the phenomenon in question, this paper establishes the fact that genetic recombinations occur during mixed infections with bacterial viruses. Hershey and American scientist R. Rotman make the discovery of genetic recombination in bacteriophage simultaneously and independently. Hershey and his colleagues prove that this phenomenon can be used for genetic analyses. They construct a genetic map of phage particles and show that phage genes can be arranged in a linear fashion.

1946 Nazi physicians and scientists are tried by international court at Nuremberg, Germany.

1947 Four years after the mass production and use of penicillin, microbial resistance is detected.

1947 Nuremberg Code is issued regarding voluntary consent of human subjects.

1948 American scientist Barbara McClintock (1902–1992) publishes her research on transposable regulatory elements ("jumping genes") in maize. Her work was not appreciated until similar phenomena were discovered in bacteria and fruit flies in the 1960s and 1970s. McClintock was awarded the Nobel Prize in Physiology or Medicine in 1983.

1948 Chloramphenicol and tetracycline are shown to be effective treatments for typhus.

1948 James V. Neel (1915–2000), American geneticist, reports evidence that the sickle-cell disease is inherited as a simple Mendelian autosomal recessive trait.

1948 The World Health Organization (WHO) is formed. WHO subsequently becomes the principle international organization managing public health–related issues on a global scale. Headquartered in Geneva, Switzerland, by 2002 WHO becomes an organization of more than 190 member countries. It contributes to international public health in areas including disease prevention and control, promotion of good health, addressing disease outbreaks, initiatives to eliminate diseases (e.g., vaccination programs), and development of treatment and prevention standards.

1949 John F. Enders (1897–1985), Thomas H. Weller (1915–2008), and Frederick C.

Robbins (1916–2003) publish "Cultivation of Polio Viruses in Cultures of Human Embryonic Tissues." The report by is a landmark in establishing techniques for the cultivation of poliovirus in cultures on non-neural tissue and for further virus research. The technique leads to the polio vaccine and other advances in virology.

1949 Macfarlane Burnet (1899–1985), Australian virologist, and his colleagues begin studies that lead to the immunological tolerance hypothesis and the clonal selection theory. Burnet receives the 1960 Nobel Prize in Physiology or Medicine for this research.

1950 Dr. Joseph Stokes of the University of Pennsylvania infects 200 women prisoners with viral hepatitis.

1950 American microbial ecologist Robert Hungate (1906–2004) develops the roll-tube culture technique, which is the first technique that allows anaerobic bacteria to be grown in culture.

1951 Esther M. Lederberg (1922–2006), American microbiologist, discovers a lysogenic strain of *Escherichia coli* K12 and isolates a new bacteriophage called lambda.

1951 Rosalind Franklin (1920–1958), English chemist, obtains sharp X-ray diffraction photographs of deoxyribonucleic acid (DNA).

1951 The eradication of malaria from the United States is announced.

1951 University of Pennsylvania under contract with US Army conducts psychopharmacological experiments on hundreds of Pennsylvania prisoners.

1952 Hershey and American biologist Martha Chase (1927–2003) publish their landmark paper "Independent Functions of Viral Protein and Nucleic Acid in Growth of Bacteriophage." The famous "blender experiment" suggests that DNA is the genetic material.

1952 James T. Park and Jack L. Strominger (1925–) demonstrate that penicillin blocks the synthesis of the peptidoglycan of bacteria. This represents the first demonstration of the action of a natural antibiotic.

1952 Karl Maramorosch (1915–2016), Austrian-born American virologist, demonstrates that some viruses can multiply in both plants and insects. This work leads to new questions about the origins of viruses.

1952 Joshua and Esther Lederberg develop the replica plating method that allows for the rapid screening of large numbers of genetic markers. They use the technique to demonstrate that resistance to antibacterial agents such as antibiotics and viruses is not induced by the presence of the antibacterial agent.

1952 Polio peaks in the United States, with 57,268 cases recorded.

1952 Italian American virologist Renato Dulbecco (1914–2012) develops a practical method for studying animal viruses in cell cultures. His so-called plaque method is comparable to that used in studies of bacterial viruses, and the method proves to be important in genetic studies of viruses. These methods are described in his paper "Production of Plaques in Monolayer Tissue Cultures by Single Particles of an Animal Virus."

1952 Franklin completes a series of X-ray crystallography studies of two forms of DNA. Her colleague, Maurice Wilkins (1916–2004), gives information about her work to James Watson (1928–).

1952 Waksmanis awarded the Nobel Prize in Physiology or Medicine for his discovery of streptomycin, the first antibiotic effective against tuberculosis.

1952 William G. Gochenour demonstrates that pretibial fever (also called Fort Bragg Fever) is not caused by a virus but rather is an infection caused by a microorganism called *Leptospira*.

1952 William Hayes isolates a strain of *E. coli* that produces recombinants thousands of times more frequently than previously observed. The new strain of K12 is named Hfr (high-frequency recombination) by Hayes.

1953 Watson and British molecular biologist Francis Crick (1916–2004) publish two landmark papers in the journal *Nature*: "Molecular Structure of Nucleic Acids: A Structure for Deoxyribonucleic Acid," and "Genetical Implications of the Structure of Deoxyribonucleic Acid." Watson and Crick propose a double helical model for DNA and call attention to the genetic implications of their model. Their model is based, in part, on the X-ray crystallographic work of Franklin and the biochemical work of Erwin Chargaff (1905–2002). Their model explains how the genetic material is transmitted.

1953 Jonas Salk (1914–1995), American virologist, begins testing a polio vaccine composed of a mixture of killed viruses.

1954 Enders, Weller, and Robbins receive the Nobel Prize in Physiology or Medicine for their work on poliovirus

1954 Enders and Thomas Peebles (1921–2010), American pediatrician, develop the first vaccine for measles. A truly practical and successful vaccine requires more time.

1954 Salk produces the first successful anti-poliomyelitis vaccine, which prevents paralytic polio. It is soon (1955) followed by the development of the first oral vaccine by Polish American virologist Albert Bruce Sabin (1906–1993).

1954 Weller isolated the varicella zoster virus from chickenpox lesions.

1955 Fred L. Schaffer and Carlton E. Schwerdt report on their successful crystallization of the polio virus. Their achievement is the first successful crystallization of an animal virus.

1955 Salk's inactivated polio vaccine is approved for use.

1955 National Institutes of Health organizes a Division of Biologics Control within the FDA following death from faulty polio vaccine.

1956 Alfred Gierer and Gerhard Schramm demonstrate that naked RNA from tobacco mosaic virus is infectious. Subsequently, infectious RNA preparations are obtained for certain animal viruses.

1956 Niels Kaj Jerne (1911–1994), Danish-English immunologist, proposes the clonal selection theory of antibody selection to explain how white blood cells are able to produce a large range of antibodies.

1956 Researchers start hepatitis experiments on mentally disabled children at the Willowbrook State School.

1957 Alick Isaacs (1921–1967), Scottish virologist, demonstrates that antibodies act only against bacteria. This means that antibodies are not one of the body's natural forms of defense against viruses. This knowledge eventually leads to the discovery of interferon this same year by Isaacs and his colleague Jean Lindenmann (1924–2015) of Switzerland. They find that the generation of a small amount of protein is the body's first line of defense against a virus.

1957 Isaacs and Lindenmann publish their pioneering report on the drug interferon, a protein produced by interaction between a virus and an infected cell that can interfere with the multiplication of viruses.

1957 French biologist François Jacob (1920–2013) and French microbial geneticist Élie Wollman (1917–2008) demonstrate that the single linkage group of *Escherichia coli* is circular and suggest that the different linkage groups found in different Hfr strains result from the insertion at different points of a factor in the circular linkage group that determines the rupture of the circle.

1957 The World Health Organization advances the oral polio vaccine developed by Sabin as a safer alternative to the Salk vaccine.

1958 Beadle, Tatum, and Joshua Lederberg are awarded the Nobel Prize in Physiology or Medicine. Beadle and Tatum were honored for the work in *Neurospora* that led to the one-gene-one-enzyme theory. Lederberg was honored for discoveries concerning genetic recombination and the organization of the genetic material of bacteria.

1958 American geneticist and molecular biologists Matthew Meselson (1930–) and

Franklin Stahl (1929–) publish their landmark paper "The Replication of DNA in *Escherichia coli*," which demonstrated that the replication of DNA follow the semiconservative model.

1959 Sabin announces successful results from testing live attenuated polio vaccine. His vaccine eventually is preferred over the Salk vaccine, because it can be administered orally and offers protection with a single dose.

1959 English biochemist Rodney Porter (1917–1985) begins studies that lead to the discovery of the structure of antibodies. Porter receives the 1972 Nobel Prize in Physiology or Medicine for this research.

1959 American biologist Robert L. Sinsheimer reports that bacteriophage ÛX174, which infects *Escherichia coli*, contains a single-stranded DNA molecule rather than the expected double-stranded DNA. This provides the first example of a single-stranded DNA genome.

1959 Sydney Brenner (1927–) and Robert W. Horne publish a paper titled "A Negative Staining Method for High Resolution Electron Microscopy of Viruses." The two researchers develop a method for studying the architecture of viruses at the molecular level using the electron microscope.

1961 Crick, Brenner, and others propose that a molecule called transfer RNA uses a three-base code in the manufacture of proteins.

1961 French pathologist Jacques Miller (1931–) discovers the role of the thymus in cellular immunity.

1961 Jewish American biochemist and geneticist Marshall Warren Nirenberg (1927–2010) synthesizes a polypeptide using an artificial messenger RNA (a synthetic RNA containing only the base uracil) in a cell-free protein-synthesizing system. The resulting polypeptide only contains the amino acid phenylalanine, indicating that UUU was the codon for phenylalanine. This important step in deciphering the genetic code is described in the landmark paper by Nirenberg and German biochemist J. Heinrich Matthaei (1929–), "The Dependence of Cell-Free Synthesis in *E. coli* upon Naturally Occurring or Synthetic Polyribonucleotides." This work establishes the messenger concept and a system that could be used to work out the relationship between the sequence of nucleotides in the genetic material and amino acids in the gene product.

1961 Noel Warner establishes the physiological distinction between the cellular and humoral immune responses.

1962 Watson, Crick, and Wilkins are awarded the Nobel Prize in Physiology or Medicine for their work in elucidating the structure of DNA.

1962 United States Congress passes Kefauver-Harris Drug Amendments that shift the burden of proof of clinical safety to drug manufacturers. For the first time drug manufacturers had to prove their products were safe and effective before they could be sold.

1963 Sabin's live polio vaccine is approved for use.

1964 British pathologist Michael Epstein (1921–) and Irish virologist Yvonne Barr (1921–2016) discover the Epstein-Barr virus that is the cause of mononucleosis.

1964 Retrovir is developed as a cancer treatment. While not useful for cancer, the drug subsequently becomes the first drug approved for the treatment of acquired immunodeficiency syndrome (AIDS).

1964 World Medical Association adopts Helsinki Declaration.

1965 Anthrax vaccine adsorbed (AVA) is approved for use in the United States.

1965 Jacob, André Lwoff (1902–1994), and Jacques Monod (1910–1976) are awarded the Nobel Prize in Physiology or Medicine for their discoveries concerning genetic control of enzymes and virus synthesis.

1966 Bruce Ames (1928–), American biochemist, develops a test to screen for compounds that cause mutations, including those that are cancer causing. The so-called Ames test utilizes the bacterium *Salmonella typhimurium*.

1966 Daniel Carleton Gajdusek (1923–2008), American pediatrician, transfers for the first time a viral disease of the central nervous system from humans to another species. The viral disease kuru is found in New Guinea and is spread by the ritual eating of the deceased's brains.

1966 FDA and National Academy of Sciences begin investigation of effectiveness of drugs previously approved because they were thought safe.

1966 Nirenberg and Har Gobind Khorana (1922–2011) lead teams that decipher the genetic code. All of the 64 possible triplet combinations of the four bases (the codons) and their associated amino acids are determined and described.

1966 Merck, Sharp, and Dohme Laboratories began research into a varicella-zoster vaccine.

1966 *New England Journal of Medicine* article exposes unethical Tuskegee syphilis study.

1966 NIH Office for Protection of Research Subjects ("OPRR") is created.

1966 Paul D. Parman and Harry M. Myer Jr. develop a live-virus rubella vaccine.

1967 A hemorrhagic fever outbreak in Marburg, Germany, occurs. The virus responsible is subsequently named the marburg virus, and the disease is called marburg hemorrhagic fever.

1967 British physician Maurice Henry Pappworth (1910–1994) publishes "Human Guinea Pigs," advising that "no doctor has the right to choose martyrs for science or for the general good."

1968 FDA administratively moves to Public Health Service.

1968 American molecular biologist Mark Ptashne (1940–) and biochemist Walter Gilbert (1932–) independently identify the bacteriophage genes that are the repressors of the lac operon.

1968 Robert W. Holley (1922–1993), Khorana, and Nirenberg are awarded the Nobel Prize in Physiology or Medicine for their interpretation of the genetic code and its function in protein synthesis.

1968 Werner Arber (1929–), Swiss microbiologist, discovers that bacteria defend themselves against viruses by producing DNA-cutting enzymes. These enzymes quickly become important tools for molecular biologists.

1969 By Executive Order, the United States renounces first use of biological weapons and restricts future weapons research programs to issues concerning defensive responses (e.g., immunization, detection, etc.).

1969 Jonathan R. Beckwith (1935–), American molecular biologist, and colleagues isolate a single gene.

1969 Delbrück, Hershey, and Luria are awarded the Nobel Prize in Physiology or Medicine for their discoveries concerning the replication mechanism and the genetic structure of viruses.

1969 US Surgeon General William Stewart (1921–2008) announces, "The time has come to close the book on infectious diseases."

1970 First outbreak of drug-resistant tuberculosis recorded in the United States.

1970 American geneticist Howard Martin Temin (1934–1994) and American biologist David Baltimore (1938–) independently discover reverse transcriptase in viruses. Reverse transcriptase is an enzyme that catalyzes the transcription of RNA into DNA.

1972 Biological and Toxin Weapons Convention (BWC) is signed. BWC prohibits the offensive weaponization of biological agents (e.g., anthrax spores). It also prohibits the transformation of biological agents with established legitimate and sanctioned purposes into agents of a nature and quality that could be used to effectively induce illness or death.

1972 Introduction of amoxicillin, a drug related to penicillin, which is a treatment of choice for bacterial pneumonia.

1972 Michiaka Takahashi (1928–2013), Japanese virologist, isolates the varicella virus from a three-year-old patient and named it

Oka, after the patient's name. The isolated virus is later used by Merck to develop a vaccine.

1972 Paul Berg (1926–) and researcher Herbert Boyer (1936–) produce the first recombinant DNA molecules.

1972 Recombinant technology emerges as one of the most powerful techniques of molecular biology. Scientists can splice together pieces of DNA to form recombinant genes. As the potential uses, therapeutic and industrial, became increasingly clear, scientists and venture capitalists establish biotechnology companies.

1973 Concerns about the possible hazards posed by recombinant DNA technologies, especially work with tumor viruses, leads to the establishment of a meeting at Asilomar, California. The proceedings of this meeting are subsequently published by the Cold Spring Harbor Laboratory as a book titled *Biohazards in Biological Research.*

1973 Boyer and Stanley Cohen (1922–) create recombinant genes by cutting DNA molecules with restriction enzymes. These experiments mark the beginning of genetic engineering.

1974 National Research Act establishes "The Common Rule" for protection of human subjects.

1974 Peter C. Doherty (1940–) and Rolf Zinkernagel (1944–) discover the basis of immune determination of self and nonself.

1975 César Milstein (1927–2002), Argentinian biochemist, and Georges J. F. Köhler (1946–1995), German immunologist, create monoclonal antibodies.

1975 Baltimore, Dulbecco, and Temin share the Nobel Prize in Physiology or Medicine for their discoveries concerning the interaction between tumor viruses and the genetic material of the cell and the discovery of reverse transcriptase.

1975 HHS promulgates Title 45 of Federal Regulations titled "Protection of Human Subjects," requiring appointment and utilization of Institutional Review Board (IRB).

1976 First outbreak of Ebola virus observed in Zaire, resulting in more than 300 cases with a 90 percent death rate.

1976 Swine flu outbreaks identified in soldiers stationed in New Jersey. Virus identified as H1N1 virus causes concern due to its similarities to H1N1 responsible for Spanish Flu pandemic. President Gerald Ford (1913–2006) calls for emergency vaccination program. More than 20 deaths result from Guillain-Barre syndrome related to the vaccine.

1977 Carl R. Woese (1928–2012) and George E. Fox (1945–) publish an account of the discovery of a third major branch of living beings, the Archaea. Woese suggests that an rRNA database could be used to generate phylogenetic trees.

1977 Earliest known AIDS victims in the United States are two homosexual men in New York who are diagnosed as suffering from Kaposi's sarcoma.

1977 Frederick Sanger (1918–2013), British biochemist, develops the chain termination (dideoxy) method for sequencing DNA and uses the method to sequence the genome of a microorganism.

1977 The first known human fatality from H5N1 avian flu occurs in Hong Kong.

1977 The last reported smallpox case is recorded. Ultimately, WHO declares the disease eradicated.

1979 National Commission issues Belmont Report.

1979 The last case of wild poliovirus infection is recorded in the United States.

1980 Congress passes the Bayh-Dole Act. The act is amended by the Technology Transfer Act in 1986.

1980 In *Diamond v. Chakrabarty*, the US Supreme Court rules that a genetically modified bacterium can be patented.

1980 Researchers successfully introduce a human gene, which codes for the protein interferon, into a bacterium.

1980 The FDA promulgates 21 CFR 50.44, prohibiting the use of prisoners as subjects in clinical trials.

1981 AIDS is officially recognized by the US Centers for Disease Control and Prevention (CDC), and the first clinical description of this disease is made. It soon becomes recognized that AIDS is an infectious disease caused by a virus that spreads virtually exclusively by infected blood or body fluids.

1981 First disease-causing human retrovirus, human T-cell leukemia virus, is discovered.

1981 The first cases of AIDS are reported among previously healthy young men in Los Angeles and New York presenting with *Pneumocystis carinii* pneumonia and Kaposi's sarcoma.

1982 FDA approves the first genetically engineered drug, a form of human insulin produced by bacteria.

1983 *Escherichia coli* O157:H7 is identified as a human pathogen.

1983 Luc Montagnier (1932–), French virologist, and Robert Gallo (1937–), American biomedical researcher, discover the human immunodeficiency virus (HIV) that causes AIDS.

1984 Jerne, Kohler, and Milstein are awarded the Nobel Prize in Physiology or Medicine for theories concerning the specificity in development and control of the immune system and the discovery of the principle for production of monoclonal antibodies.

1984 WHO begins a program to control trypanosomiasis.

1985 British geneticist Alec Jeffreys (1950–) develops "genetic fingerprinting," a method of using DNA polymorphisms (unique sequences of DNA) to identify individuals. The method, which has been used in paternity, immigration, and murder cases, is generally referred to as "DNA fingerprinting."

1985 First vaccine for *H. influenzae* type B is licensed for use.

1985 Japanese molecular biologist Susumu Tonegawa (1939–) discovers the genes that code for immunoglobulins. He receives the 1986 Nobel Prize in Physiology or Medicine for this discovery.

1985 American biochemist Kary Mullis (1944–), while working at Cetus Corporation, develops the polymerase chain reaction (PCR), a new method of amplifying DNA. This technique quickly becomes one of the most powerful tools of molecular biology. Cetus patents PCR and sells the patent to Hoffman-LaRoche Inc. in 1991.

1986 Congress passes the National Childhood Vaccine Injury Act, requiring patient information on vaccines and reporting of adverse events after vaccination.

1986 First genetically engineered vaccine approved for human use is the hepatitis B vaccine. The FDA gives its approval.

1986 First license to market a living organism that was produced by genetic engineering is granted by the US Department of Agriculture. It allows Biologics Corporation to sell a virus that is used as a vaccine against a herpes disease in pigs.

1986 International Committee on the Taxonomy of Viruses officially names the AIDS virus as HIV.

1987 An illness outbreak in Prince Edward Island, Canada, which sickens over 100 people and kills 3, leads to the first isolation and identification of domoic acid.

1987 Maynard Olson (1943–) creates and names yeast artificial chromosomes (YACs), which provides a technique to clone long segments of DNA.

1987 US Congress charters a Department of Energy (DOE) advisory committee, the Health and Environmental Research Advisory Committee (HERAC), which recommends a 15-year, multidisciplinary, scientific, and technological undertaking to map and sequence the human genome. DOE designates multidisciplinary human genome centers. National Institute of General Medical Sciences at the National Institutes of Health (NIH NIGMS) begins funding genome projects.

1988 First report of vancomycin-resistant enterococci, a type of *Streptococcus* that is resistant to almost all antibiotics.

1988 The Human Genome Organization (HUGO) is established by scientists to coordinate international efforts to sequence the human genome. The Human Genome Project officially adopts the goal of determining the entire sequence of DNA comprising the human chromosomes.

1988 WHO and its partners announce the Global Polio Eradication Initiative.

1989 Ebola-Reston virus is the source of an outbreak at an animal facility in Virginia. The outbreak becomes the basis for the best-selling book *The Hot Zone.*

1989 Sidney Altman (1939–) and Thomas R. Cech (1947–) are awarded the Nobel Prize in Chemistry for their discovery of ribozymes (RNA molecules with catalytic activity). Cech proves that RNA can function as a biocatalyst as well as an information carrier.

1990 Only 24 cases of diphtheria reported in the United States during preceding 10-year period.

1991 Cholera returns to the Western Hemisphere when an outbreak in Peru spreads to other Latin American countries.

1991 WHO announces CIOMS Guidelines (the International Ethical Guidelines for Biomedical Research Involving Human Subjects).

1992 American biochemist J. Craig Venter (1946–) establishes the Institute for Genomic Research (TIGR) in Rockville, Maryland. TIGR later sequences the genome of *Haemophilus influenzae* and many other bacterial genomes.

1993 An international research team, led by Daniel Cohen of the Center for the Study of Human Polymorphisms in Paris, produces a rough map of all 23 pairs of human chromosomes.

1993 Beginning in April, a five-week contamination of the drinking water supply of Milwaukee, Wisconsin, by *Cryptosporidium parvum* sickens 400,000 people and kills an estimated 104 people.

1993 Hanta virus emerges in the United States in a 1993 outbreak on a Native American reservation in the Four Corners area (corners of Utah, Colorado, New Mexico, and Arizona). The resulting Hanta pulmonary syndrome (HPS) has a 43 percent mortality rate.

1993 Outbreaks in Moscow and St. Petersburg mark the return of epidemic diphtheria to the Western world.

1994 AZT (zidovudine) is approved by the FDA for use in reducing maternal-fetal HIV transmission.

1994 DOE announces the establishment of the Microbial Genome Project as a spin-off of the Human Genome Project.

1994 Ebola-Ivory Coast virus is discovered.

1994 Geneticists determine that DNA repair enzymes perform several vital functions, including preserving genetic information and protecting the cell from cancer.

1994 WHO declares the Americas free of polio.

1994 WHO reports the start of epidemics of plague in Malawi, Mozambique, and India after a 15-year absence.

1995 Edward B. Lewis (1918–2004), Christiane Nüsslein-Volhard (1942–), and Eric F. Wieschaus (1947–), developmental biologists, share the Nobel Prize in Physiology or Medicine to cover discrimination based on genetic information related to illness, disease, or other conditions.

1995 Peter Funch and Reinhardt Kristensen (1948–) create a new phylum, Cycliophora, for a novel invertebrate called *Symbion pandora*, which is found living in the mouths of Norwegian lobsters.

1995 Public awareness of the potential use of chemical or biological weapons by a terrorist group increases following an attack by Aum Shinrikyo, a Japanese cult, which releases sarin gas in a Tokyo subway, killing a dozen people and sending thousands to the hospital.

1995 FDA approves the varicella-zoster vaccine developed by Merck for vaccinations of people 12 months and older.

1995 The Programme Against African Trypanosomiasis (PAAT) is created.

1995 The sequence of *Mycoplasma genitalium* is completed. *M. genitalium*, regarded as the smallest known bacterium, is considered a model of the minimum number of genes needed for independent existence.

1996 H5N1 avian flu virus is identified in Guangdong, China.

1996 International participants in the genome project meet in Bermuda and agree to formalize the conditions of data access. The agreement, known as the "Bermuda Principles," calls for the release of sequence data into public databases within 24 hours.

1996 Scientists report further evidence that individuals with two mutant copies of the CC-CLR-5 gene are generally resistant to HIV infection.

1996 William R. Bishai and coworkers report that SigF, a gene in the tuberculosis bacterium, enables the bacterium to enter a dormant stage.

1997 The DNA sequence of *Escherichia coli* is completed.

1997 William Jacobs Jr. (1955–) and Barry Bloom create a biological entity that combines the characteristics of a bacterial virus and a plasmid (a DNA structure that functions and replicates independently of the chromosomes). This entity is capable of triggering mutations in *Mycobacterium tuberculosis.*

1997 Outbreaks of highly pathogenic H5N1 influenza are reported in poultry at farms and live animal markets in Hong Kong.

1998 A live, orally administered rotavirus vaccine is approved for use in the United States. Use was discontinued in 1999 due to complications in some vaccinated children.

1998 Venter forms a company (later named Celera) and predicts that the company would decode the entire human genome within three years. Celera plans to use a "whole genome shotgun" method, which would assemble the genome without using maps. Venter says that his company would not follow the Bermuda Principles concerning data release.

1998 DOE (Office of Science) funds bacterial artificial chromosome and sequencing projects.

1998 Scientists find that an adult human's brain can, with certain stimuli, replace cells. This discovery heralds potential breakthroughs in neurology.

1998 World Health Organization reports a resurgence in tuberculosis (TB) cases worldwide. TB is killing more people than at any other point in history. Recommends Directly Observed Therapy (DOT) treatment, which is 95 percent effective in curing patients, even in developing nations.

1999 Pharmaceutical research in Japan leads to the discovery of donepezil (Aricept), the first drug intended to help ward off memory loss in Alzheimer's disease and other age-related dementias.

1999 Scientists announce the complete sequencing of the DNA making up human chromosome 22. The first complete human chromosome sequence is published in December 1999.

1999 NIH and the Office for Protection from Research Risks (OPRR) require researchers conducting or overseeing human subjects to ethics training.

1999 The public genome project responds to Venter's challenge with plans to produce a draft genome sequence by 2000. Most of the sequencing is done in five centers, known as the "G5": the Whitehead Institute for Biomedical Research in Cambridge, Massachusetts; the Sanger Centre near Cambridge, England; Baylor College of Medicine in Houston; Washington University in St. Louis; and the DOE's Joint Genome Institute (JGI) in Walnut Creek, California.

2000 On June 26, 2000, leaders of the public genome project and Celera announce the completion of a working draft of the entire human genome sequence. Ari Patrinos of the DOE helps mediate disputes between the two groups so that a fairly amicable joint announcement could be presented at the White House in Washington, D.C.

2000 Office for Protection from Research Risks (OPRR) becomes part of the Department of Health and Human Services, Office of Human Research Protection (OHRP).

2000 The federal government approves irradiation of raw meat, the only technology known to kill *E. coli* O157 bacteria while preserving the integrity of the meat.

2000 The first volume of Annual Review of *Genomics and Human Genetics* is published. Genomics is defined as the new science dealing with the identification and characterization of genes and their arrangement in chromosomes and human genetics as the science devoted to understanding the origin and expression of human individual uniqueness.

2000 The municipal water supply of Walkerton, Ontario, Canada, is contaminated in the summertime by a strain of the bacterium *Escherichia coli* O157:H7, sickening 2,000 people and killing 7.

2000 WHO declares the Western Pacific region, including China, free of polio.

2001 In February the complete draft sequence of the human genome is published. The public sequence data is published in the British journal *Nature*, and the Celera sequence is published in the American journal *Science*. Increased knowledge of the human genome allows greater specificity in pharmacological research and drug interaction studies.

2001 Microbiologists reveal that bacteria possess an internal protein structure similar to that of human cells.

2001 Researchers at Eli Lilly in Minneapolis sequence the genome of *Streptococcus pneumoniae*.

2001 Letters containing a powdered form of *Bacillus anthracis*, the bacteria that causes anthrax, are mailed to government representatives, members of the news media, and others in the United States. More than 20 cases and 5 deaths eventually result. As of August 2007, the case remains open and unsolved.

2001 The Chemical and Biological Incident Response Force (CBIRF) sends a 100-member initial response team into the Dirksen Senate Office Building in Washington alongside Environmental Protection Agency (EPA) specialists to detect and remove anthrax. A similar mission was undertaken at the Longworth House Office Building in October, when samples were collected from more than 200 office spaces.

2001 The Pan African Trypanosomiasis and Tsetse Eradication campaign (PATTEC) begins operation.

2002 Following September 11, 2001, terrorist attacks on the United States, the Public Health Security and Bioterrorism Preparedness and Response Act of 2002 is passed to improve the ability to prevent and respond to public health emergencies.

2002 In June 2002 traces of biological and chemical weapon agents are found in Uzbekistan on a military base used by US troops fighting in Afghanistan. Early analysis dates and attributes the source of the contamination to former Soviet Union biological and chemical weapons programs that used the base.

2002 In the aftermath of the September 11, 2001, terrorist attacks on the United States, the US government dramatically increases funding to stockpile drugs and other agents that could be used to counter a bioterrorist attack.

2002 Scientists determine that stockpiled smallpox vaccine doses can be effective if diluted to one-tenth their original concentration, greatly enhancing the number of doses available to respond to an emergency.

2002 Severe acute respiratory syndrome (SARS) virus is found in patients in China, Hong Kong, and other Asian countries. The newly discovered coronavirus is not identified until early 2003. The spread of the virus reaches epidemic proportions in Asia and expands to the rest of the world.

2002 The Best Pharmaceuticals for Children Act passed to improve safety and efficacy of patented and off-patent medicines for children.

2002 The Defense Advanced Research Projects Agency (DARPA) initiates the Biosensor Technologies program in 2002 to develop fast, sensitive, automatic technologies for the detection and identification of biological warfare agents.

2002 The Pathogen Genomic Sequencing program is initiated by the Defense Advanced Research Project Agency (DARPA) to focus on characterizing the genetic components of pathogens to develop novel diagnostics, treatments, and therapies for the diseases they cause.

2002 The planned destruction of stocks of the smallpox-causing Variola virus at the two remaining depositories in the United States and Russia is delayed over fears that large-scale production of the vaccine might be needed in the event of a bioterrorist action.

2002 WHO declares the 51 countries of its European region free of polio.

2003 Almost 500,000 civic and health care workers at strategic hospitals, governmental facilities, and research centers across the United States are slated to receive smallpox immunizations as part of a strategic plan for ready response to a biological attack using the smallpox virus.

2003 An international research team funded by NINR found that filters made from old cotton saris cut the number of cholera cases in rural Bangladesh villages almost in half. Other inexpensive cloth should work just as well in other parts of the world where cholera is endemic. This simple preventive measure has the potential to make a significant impact on a global health problem.

2003 By early May WHO officials have confirmed reports of more than 3,000 cases of SARS from 18 different countries with 111 deaths attributed to the disease. United States health officials reported 193 cases with no deaths. Significantly, all but 20 of the US cases are linked to travel to infected areas, and the other 20 cases are accounted for by secondary transmission from infected patients to family members and health care workers. Health authorities assert that the emergent virus responsible for SARS will remain endemic (part of the natural array of viruses) in many regions of China well after the current outbreak is resolved.

2003 Canadian scientists at the British Columbia Cancer Agency in Vancouver announce the sequence of the genome of the coronavirus most likely to be the cause of SARS. Within days scientists at the CDC in Atlanta, Georgia, offer a genomic map that confirms more than 99 percent of the Canadian findings.

2003 Differences in outbreaks in Hong Kong between 1997 and 2003 cause investigators to conclude that the H5N1 virus has mutated.

2003 Following approximately five deaths by heart attack correlated to individuals receiving the new smallpox vaccine, US health officials at the CDC announce a suspension of administration of the vaccine to patients with a history of heart disease until the matter can be fully investigated.

2003 Preliminary trials for a malaria vaccine are scheduled to begin in malaria-endemic African areas, where approximately 3,000 children die from the disease every day.

2003 SARS cases in Hanoi reach 22, as a simultaneous outbreak of the same disease occurs in Hong Kong. WHO issues a global alert about a new infectious disease of unknown origin in both Vietnam and Hong Kong.

2003 SARS is added to the list of quarantinable diseases in the United States.

2003 Studies indicate that women with a history of some sexually transmitted infections, including the human papillomavirus, are at increased risk for developing cervical cancer.

2003 Studies show no correlation between immunization schedules and sudden infant death syndrome (SIDS) occurrences.

2003 The first case of an unusually severe pneumonia occurs in Hanoi, Vietnam, and is identified two days later as severe acute respiratory syndrome (SARS) by Italian physician and epidemiologist Carlo Urbani (1956–2003), who formally identifies

SARS as a unique disease and names it. Urbani dies of SARS later that year.

2003 The first case of bovine spongiform encephalopathy (BSE, mad cow disease) in the United States is found in a cow in Washington state. Investigations later reveal that the cow was imported from a Canadian herd, which included North America's first "homegrown" case of BSE six months earlier.

2003 WHO takes the unusual step of issuing a travel warning that describes SARS as a worldwide health threat. WHO officials announce that SARS cases, and potential cases, have been tracked from China to Singapore, Thailand, Vietnam, Indonesia, Philippines, and Canada.

2003 the United States invades Iraq and finds chemical, biological, and nuclear weapons programs, but no actual weapons.

2003 WHO Global Influenza Surveillance Network intensifies work on development of a H5N1 vaccine for humans.

2004 A 35-year-old television producer in the Guangdong province of China is the first person to become ill with SARS since the end of May 2003, the initial outbreak of the newly identified disease. Within two weeks three other people are suspected of having SARS in the region, and teams from WHO return to investigate possible human-to-human, animal-to-human, and environmental sources of transmission of the disease.

2004 Chinese health officials in the Guangdong province of China launch a mass slaughter of civet cats, a cousin of the mongoose considered a delicacy and thought to be a vector of SARS, in an attempt to control the spread of the disease.

2004 Project BioShield Act of 2004 authorizes US government agencies to expedite procedures related to rapid distribution of treatments as countermeasures to chemical, biological, and nuclear attack.

2005 H5N1 virus, responsible for avian flu, moves from Asia to Europe. WHO attempts to coordinate multinational disaster and containment plans. Some nations begin to stockpile antiviral drugs.

2005 WHO reports outbreaks of plague in the Democratic Republic of the Congo.

2005 FDA Drug Safety Board is founded.

2005 US president George W. Bush (1946–) addresses the issue of HIV/AIDS in black women in the United States, acknowledging it as a public health crisis.

2006 European Union bans the importation of avian feathers (non-treated feathers) from countries neighboring or close to Turkey.

2006 Mad cow disease confirmed in an Alabama cow as third reported case in the United States.

2006 More than a dozen people are diagnosed with avian flu in Turkey, but United Nations (UN) health experts assure the public that human-to-human transmission is still rare and only suspected in a few cases in Asia.

2006 Researchers begin human trials for vaginal microbicide gels.

2007 Texas governor Rick Perry (1950–) adds the HPV vaccine to the list of required vaccines for school-age girls.

2007 Four people are hospitalized with botulism poisoning in the United States after more than 90 potentially contaminated meat products, including canned chili, were removed from grocery shelves across the country.

2007 The CDC issues a rare order for isolation when a New Jersey man infected with a resistant strain of tuberculosis flies on multiple trans-Atlantic commercial flights.

2008 The CDC issues a health advisory after a widespread outbreak of measles in the United States.

2008 An outbreak of salmonellosis linked to peppers imported from Mexico causes more than 1,400 to become ill in the United States between April and August.

2008 A case of Marburg Hemorrhagic Fever is diagnosed in the Netherlands. The patient, a Dutch woman, had recently returned from Uganda, where she contracted the virus. WHO calls on Uganda's Ministry of

Health to advise all tourists against entering caves where bats might be present.

2008 WHO reports that there is an outbreak of the H5N1 virus, often called the "bird flu," in Indonesia. Of the 139 confirmed cases of the virus, 113 have people died.

2009 The 2009 flu pandemic is caused by the H1N1 virus, also known as the "swine flu." CDC estimates place the global death toll between 151,700 and 575,000 during the 2008–2009 flu season.2010 Following a destructive earthquake, a cholera outbreak begins in Haiti and the Dominican Republic, affecting more than 800,000 people and killing nearly 10,000 by May 2017.

2010 WHO releases first report on neglected tropical diseases (NTDs) to highlight challenges and draw attention to eradication efforts.

2010 The Affordable Care Act (ACA) is signed into law in the United States. Purposes of the law included making health insurance more affordable and expanding insurance coverage.

2011 WHO Strategic Technical Advisory Group for Neglected Tropical Diseases adopts a roadmap for controlling, eliminating, and eradicating NTDs by 2020.

2011 An outbreak of haemolytic uremic syndrome, a rare condition linked to *Escherichia coli* bacteria, sickens 276 people in Germany.

2011 A measles outbreak in Europe affects 33 countries, with more than 6,500 people contracting the virus. In response, WHO issues new vaccination and travel recommendations for adults and children.

2012 United Nations Foundation launches the Shot@Life program to provide vaccines for children around the globe.

2012 An outbreak of pertussis (whooping cough) sickens 48,277 people in the United States. This is the largest number of cases since 1955.

2012 Contamination at a Massachusetts compounding pharmacy leads to an outbreak of fungal meningitis in the United States. Roughly 800 people become ill, and 76 die.

2012 The first case of Middle East Respiratory Syndrome Coronavirus (MERS-CoV, initially known as "novel virus") is identified in Saudi Arabia. By 2017 more than 2,000 cases have been reported.

2012 Pre-exposure prophylaxis (PrEP) goes on the market. The medication, which is recommended to people with high risk of contracting HIV, lowers the risk of acquiring the disease. 2013 Polio reemerges in Syria as a consequence of civil war. WHO responds with an immunization drive.

2013 First local transmission of chikungunya occurs in the Americas. Mosquitoes in the Caribbean are found to be spreading the virus to humans.

2013 An Ebola outbreak begins in Guinea in December.

2014 The Ebola virus spreads throughout Guinea and to Liberia and Sierra Leone, becoming widespread in both. Cases are reported in other West African nations, and travelers and returning aid workers introduce cases to the United States, Spain, the United Kingdom, and Italy.

2014 WHO releases its first report on antimicrobial resistance.

2014 WHO declares the South-East Asia Region (comprising Bangladesh, Bhutan, Democratic People's Republic of Korea, India, Indonesia, Maldives, Myanmar, Nepal, Sri Lanka, Thailand, and Timor-Leste) free of polio.

2014 The WHO director-general declares the spread of wild poliovirus a Public Health Emergency of International Concern.

2014 FDA announces the approval of a vaccine (Trumenba) for Group B meningococcal disease.

2014 An outbreak of polio in Pakistan results in more than 300 reported cases and new efforts to eradicate the virus in the country. Immunization efforts lead to a reduction in the number of reported cases to five in 2017.

2014 President Barack Obama (1961–) signs Executive Order 13676: Combating Antibiotic-Resistant Bacteria. The order directs federal agencies to address the problem of bacteria that are becoming resistant to the antibiotics commonly used to treat them.

2015 The Pan American Health Organization declare the Americas free of the endemic transmission of rubella.

2015 Chikungunya becomes a notifiable disease in the United States.

2015 A measles outbreak in the United States affects 189 people in 24 states. Most cases occur in individuals who have not received the measles vaccine.

2015 The US government releases the National Action Plan for Combating Multidrug-Resistant Tuberculosis in response to the growing threat of multidrug-resistant ad extensively drug-resistant tuberculosis.

2016 An outbreak of Rift Valley Fever (RVF) in Niger kills 33 people. This is the largest number of RVF fatalities since the 2005–2007 epidemic in Kenya.

2016 WHO declares a public health emergency due to the Zika virus, which is spreading rapidly in the Americas and causing miscarriage, stillbirth, and birth defects, including microcephaly.

2017 A cholera epidemic begins in Yemen in April. By January 2018 WHO estimates that 1 million have contracted the disease and more than 2,000 have died.

2017 An outbreak of norovirus in Yolo County, California, schools causes more than 2,800 people to become ill.

2017 A large outbreak of plague begins in Madagascar in August, causing 2,119 confirmed and suspected cases by early November, when the Madagascar Ministry of Health declares the outbreak contained. During the outbreak WHO advises against any travel or trade restrictions, citing the low risk of international transmission.

2017 An outbreak of Seoul virus in the United States causes 17 people to become ill. Infected rats are found in Colorado, Georgia, Illinois, Iowa, Minnesota, Missouri, Pennsylvania, South Carolina, Tennessee, Utah, and Wisconsin.

2017 A monkeypox outbreak occurs in Nigeria, with 172 suspected and 61 confirmed cases between September and December.

2017 The WHO Strategic Technical Advisory Group for Neglected Tropical Diseases adds chromoblastomycosis and other deep mycoses, scabies and other ectoparasites, and snakebite envenoming to the list of neglected tropical diseases.

2017 WHO declares that the Zika virus is no longer a public health emergency. The disease remains a risk for pregnant women who live in areas where Zika transmission occurs.

2017 The CDC reports that rates of Hepatitis C are rising in the United States as a result of the opioid drug epidemic. Hepatitis C can be transmitted between people who share injection drug paraphernalia.

2017 A listeriosis outbreak linked to contaminated deli meats sickens 1,000 people in South Africa and becomes the largest recorded listeria outbreak.

2018 An outbreak of Lassa fever in Nigeria becomes the largest recorded. WHO reports 317 confirmed cases, 764 suspected cases, and 72 deaths in January and February, more than in all of 2016.

2018 An outbreak of the vaccine-preventable disease yellow fever occurs in Brazil. WHO records 723 confirmed cases and 237 deaths.

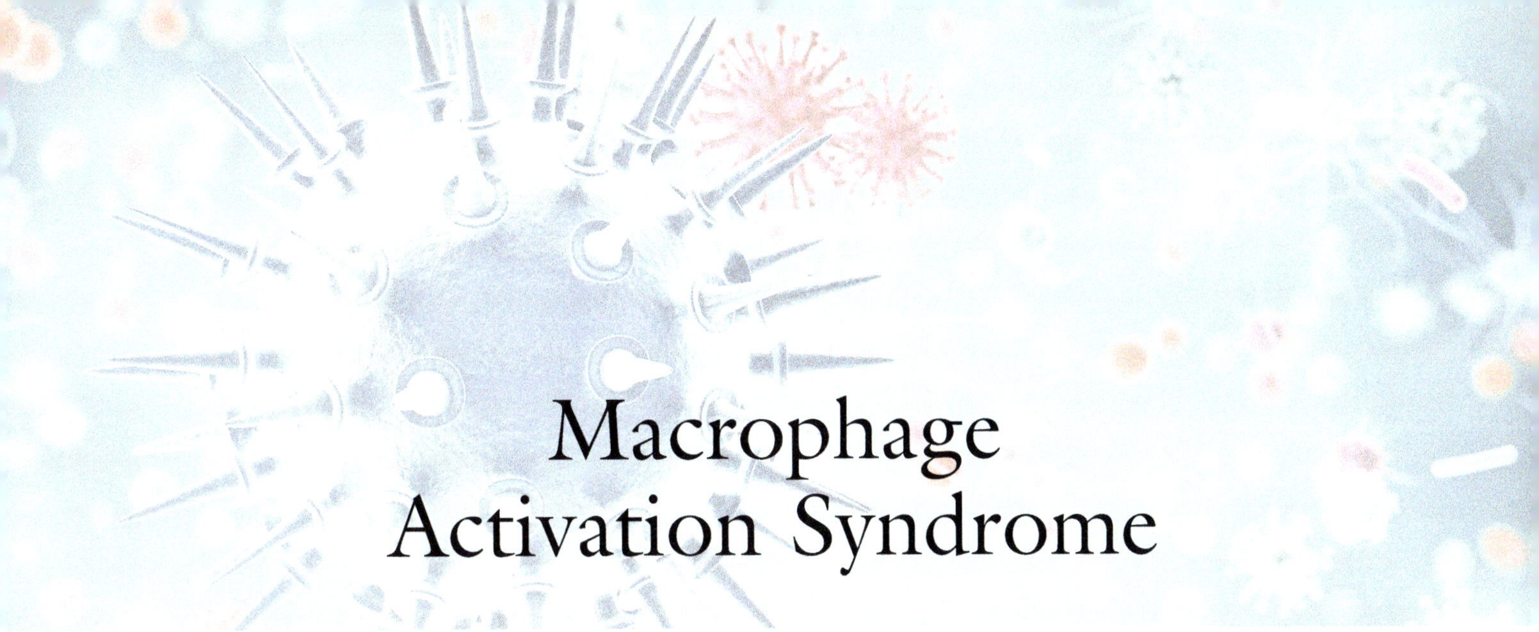

Macrophage Activation Syndrome

Introduction

Macrophage activation syndrome (MAS) is a potentially fatal complication of rheumatic diseases. It occurs when white blood cells called macrophages attack the body. It is characterized by high fever, lymph node abnormalities, and liver and spleen enlargement. It can ultimately lead to multiple organ failure. MAS usually occurs in the context of Still's disease in adults or a rheumatic disease such as systemic juvenile idiopathic arthritis (SJIA). More rarely it occurs in patients with systemic lupus erythematosus (SLE) and Kawasaki disease.

Disease Characteristics and Clinical Findings

MAS is considered a subset of diseases known as hemophagocytic lymphohistiocytosis (HLH). HLH is a general term that describes a spectrum of diseases characterized by accumulations of activated macrophages. It is an aggressive and life-threatening syndrome that causes an overactivation of the immune system. It is most common in infants and young children but can affect people of any age.

Unlike predominant forms of HLH that are inherited, MAS is a disease that occurs in a heterogeneous group of diseases, ranging from infections to tumors to rheumatologic disorders. The term *macrophage activation syndrome* was first coined to describe patients with SJIA in 1985.

Among children MAS is most commonly seen in patients with SJIA. About 10 percent of patients with SJIA develop MAS, whereas mild, "subclinical" MAS may be seen in as many as one-third of patients with SJIA. In adults MAS is most frequently associated with adult-onset Still's disease, SLE, and various vasculitis (blood vessel inflammation) syndromes, according to limited epidemiologic studies. Although the reason for development of MAS in some people with SJIA is not known, infection has been identified as a likely trigger in nearly one-third of patients.

The clinical findings in MAS are often dramatic and evolve rapidly. Typically, patients become acutely ill, with persistent fever, changes to mental status, and abnormalities in the lymph nodes. In addition, the liver and spleen are enlarged, and there is liver dysfunction.

In a multicenter study of 362 patients with MAS conducted by Francesca Minoia and coauthors published in *Arthritis & Rheumatology*, almost all of the patients with MAS presented with fever. A large proportion had enlargement of the liver and spleen. A smaller proportion of patients showed lymph node abnormalities. The central nervous system was affected in nearly one-third of patients. Symptoms included seizures, lethargy, irritability, headache, and coma. About 20 percent of the patients had skin, mucosal, and gastrointestinal bleeding.

A hemorrhagic syndrome with widespread intravascular blood clotting is a prominent feature of MAS. These clinical symptoms are associated with a sudden fall in at least two of three blood cell counts (leukocytes, erythrocytes, and platelets). The fall in platelet count is also usually an early finding. Such reduction in blood counts may be due to increased destruction of the cells by phagocytosis, the process by which certain cells engulf and digest microorganisms and consume debris and foreign bodies in the blood.

WORDS TO KNOW

IMMUNE SYSTEM The body's natural defense system that guards against foreign invaders and that includes lymphocytes and antibodies.

PHAGOCYTOSIS The process by which certain cells engulf and digest microorganisms and consume debris and foreign bodies in the blood.

MACROPHAGES AND THE IMMUNE SYSTEM

Macrophages (big eaters) are a type of white blood cell that engulfs and digests cellular debris, foreign substances, microbes, cancer cells, and anything else that has foreign proteins on its surface. This process is called phagocytosis (cell eating). Macrophages are found in essentially all tissues, where they patrol for potential foreign organisms. They move by changing their shape and can take various forms throughout the body. Depending on their location, they may be called histiocytes, Kupffer cells, alveolar macrophages, microglia, or another name. Besides phagocytosis, they play a critical role in initiating specific defense mechanisms by recruiting other immune cells such as lymphocytes. In humans dysfunctional macrophages cause severe diseases such as chronic granulomatous disease, which can result in frequent infections as well as MAS.

In a 2009 article in *Arthritis & Rheumatism*, Allesandro Parodi and coauthors offered preliminary guidelines for diagnosis of MAS as a complication of juvenile SLE, including simultaneous finding of at least one clinical criterion and two laboratory criteria. Clinical criteria include fever, enlargement of liver and spleen, bleeding disorder, and central nervous system dysfunction. Laboratory criteria for MAS include reduction in blood cell counts or platelet counts, increased levels of the enzymes aspartate transaminase and lactate dehydrogenase, increased levels of triglycerides (fat) and ferratin (iron), and decreased levels of the clotting protein fibrinogen. The elevation of ferritin is particularly marked (above 10,000 ng/mL) in most patients and appears to parallel the degree of macrophage activation.

In 2016 the classification criteria for MAS complicating SJIA were slightly amended, as reported by Angello Ravelli and colleagues in *Annals of the Rheumatic Diseases.* Diagnosis of MAS was contingent on the patient presenting fever with high ferritin levels and any two of low platelet counts, high aspartate transaminase and triglyceride levels, and decreased fibrinogen levels.

MAS is a life-threatening condition associated with high mortality rates. Therefore, early recognition of this syndrome and immediate therapeutic intervention to produce a rapid response are critical. Most clinicians start with intravenous corticosteroid therapy, mostly methylprednisolone (30 milligrams per kilogram for three consecutive days) followed by oral prednisolone (2 to 3 milligrams per kilogram per day in four divided doses). If MAS does not improve with corticosteroids, several drugs are used, including the immunosuppressants cyclosporine A and cyclophosphamide.

■ Issues and Impacts

Although mortality rates of MAS can reach 20 percent, MAS is diagnosed relatively early, and outcomes are improving due to increasing awareness. Validated diagnostic criteria are making early diagnosis easier. A substantial proportion of MAS patients experience recurrent episodes, and these patients may require closer monitoring.

There have been no long-term studies regarding which treatments are the most effective for MAS. Treatment of the disease has involved trial and error. Immunosuppressant drugs designed to treat rheumatoid arthritis called interleukin-1 (IL-1) inhibitors may be helpful in treating MAS, taken in conjunction with steroidal drugs.

SEE ALSO *Childhood-Associated Infectious Diseases, Immunization Impacts; Demographics and Infectious Disease; Immune Response to Infection; Kawasaki Disease*

BIBLIOGRAPHY

Books

Cimaz, Rolando, and Thomas Lehman, eds. *Pediatrics in Systemic Autoimmune Diseases.* 2nd ed. Oxford, UK: Elsevier, 2016.

Periodicals

Bracaglia, Claudia, Giusi Prencipe, and Fabrizio F. Benedetti. "Macrophage Activation Syndrome: Different Mechanisms Leading to One Clinical Syndrome." *Pediatric Rheumatology* 15 (January 2017): 5–12. This article can also be found online at https://ped-rheum.biomedcentral.com/articles/10.1186/s12969-016-0130-4 (accessed March 12, 2018).

Hadchouel, Michelle, Anne-Marie Prieur, and Claude Griscelli. "Acute Hemorrhagic, Hepatic and Neurologic Manifestations in Juvenile Rheumatoid Arthritis: Possible Relationship to Drugs or Infection." *Journal of Pediatrics* 106 (1985): 561–566.

Minoia, Francesca, et al. "Clinical Features, Treatment, and Outcome of Macrophage Activation Syndrome Complicating Systemic Juvenile Idiopathic Arthritis." *Arthritis & Rheumatology* 66 (2014): 3160–3169. This article can also be found online at http://onlinelibrary.wiley.com/doi/10.1002/art.38802/full (accessed March 12, 2018).

Parodi, Allesandro, et al. "Macrophage Activation Syndrome in Juvenile Systemic Lupus Erythematosus: A Multinational Multicenter Study of Thirty-Eight Patients." *Arthritis & Rheumatism* 60, no. 11 (2009): 3388–3399. This article can also be found online at http://onlinelibrary.wiley.com/doi/10.1002/art.24883/pdf (accessed March 12, 2018).

Ravelli, Angello, et al. "2016 Classification Criteria for Macrophage Activation Syndrome Complicating Systemic Juvenile Idiopathic Arthritis." *Annals of the Rheumatic Diseases* 75, no. 3 (2016): 481–489. This article can also be found online at http://ard.bmj.com/content/75/3/481.info (accessed March 12, 2018).

Sawhney, S., P. Woo, and K. J. Murray. "Macrophage Activation Syndrome: A Potentially Fatal Complication of Rheumatic Disorders." *Archives of Disease in Childhood* 85 (June 2001): 421–426. This article can also be found online at http://adc.bmj.com/content/archdischild/85/5/421.full.pdf (accessed March 12, 2018).

Websites

Saldana, José Ignacio. "Macrophages." British Society for Immunology. https://www.immunology.org/public-information/bitesized-immunology/cells/macrophages (accessed March 12, 2018).

Malini Vashishtha

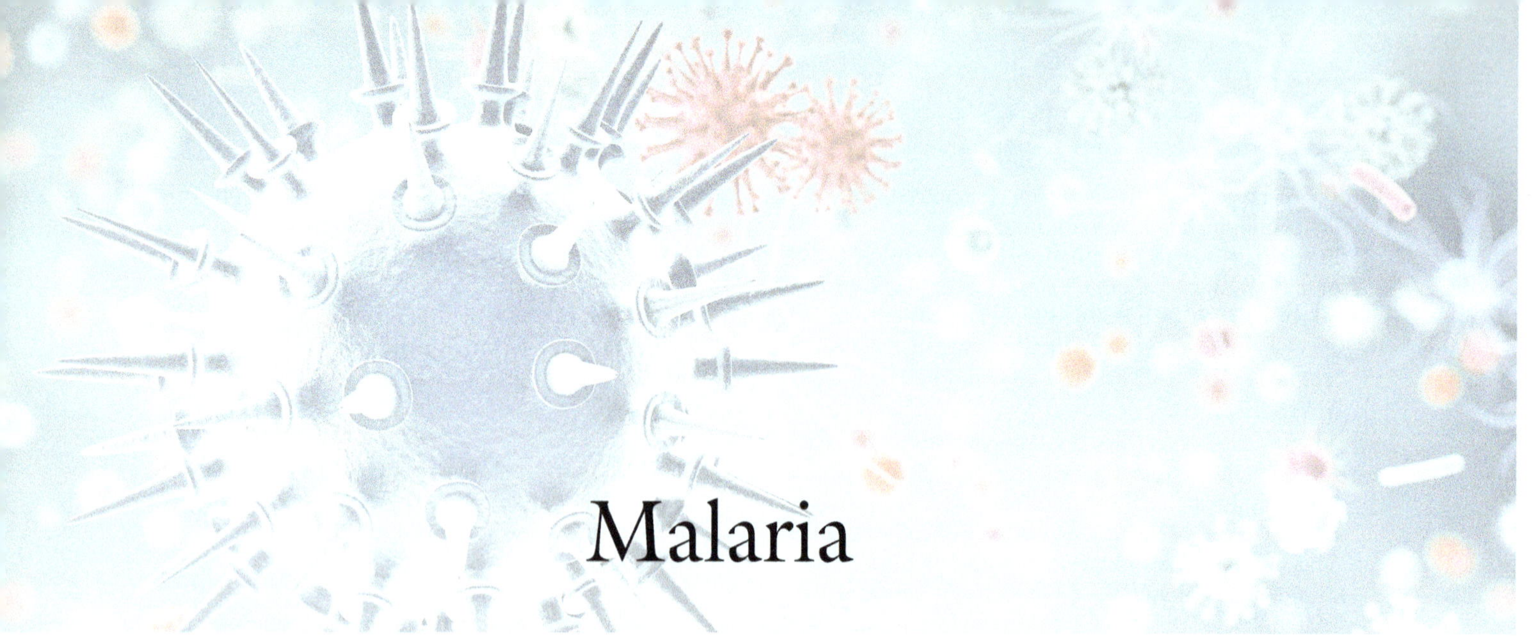

Malaria

Introduction

Malaria is the leading cause of death worldwide from parasitic infection. According to the World Health Organization (WHO), there were more than 216 million cases of malaria each year in tropical and subtropical regions of the world as of 2016. That year there were 1 to 2 million deaths, most of which occur in sub-Saharan Africa, with children being disproportionately affected.

The word *malaria* means "bad air," which used to be considered the cause of the disease. In the 19th century, it was established that malaria is caused by *Plasmodia*, which are single-celled parasites carried by mosquitoes belonging to the *Anopheles* genus. Five species of *Plasmodia* are involved in malaria: *P. falciparum*, *P. vivax*, *P. ovale*, *P. malariae*, and, to a lesser extent, *P. knowlesi*, which generally only affects animals but sometimes humans too. Malaria caused by *P. falciparum* is by far the most serious and the cause of most fatalities.

There are several drugs that can be used for both treatment and prevention of malaria. However, parasites have

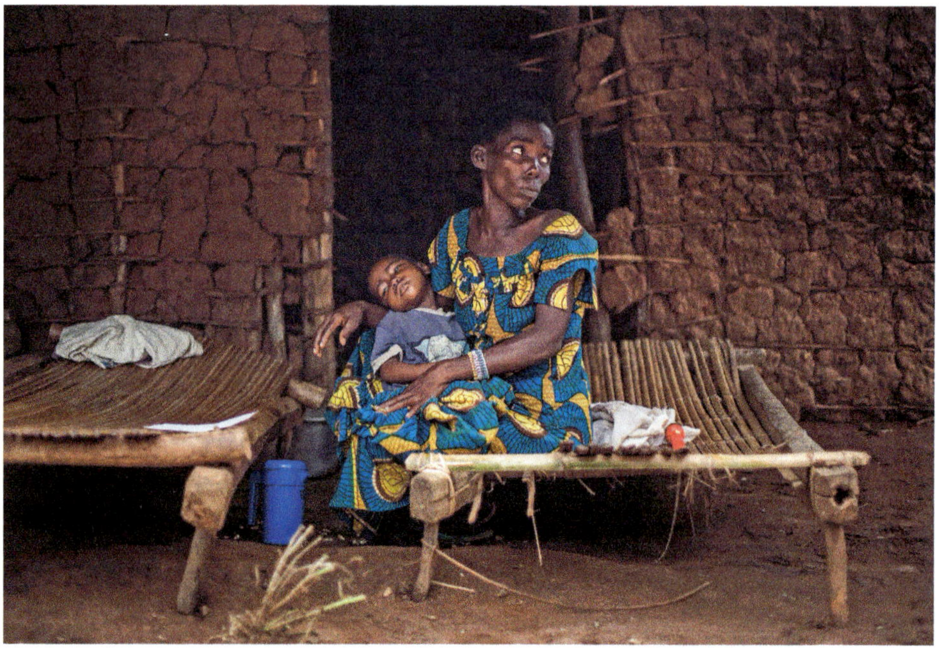

A mother and child await treatment for malaria, a deadly parasitic infection characterized by cycles between fever and chills, at a health center in the Democratic Republic of the Congo during a 2017 outbreak. © JOHN WESSELS/AFP/Getty Images

WORDS TO KNOW

ENDEMIC Present in a particular area or among a particular group of people.

GAMETOCYTE A germ cell with the ability to divide for the purpose of producing gametes, either male gametes called spermatocytes or female ones called oocytes.

MEROZOITE The motile, infective stage of malaria responsible for disease symptoms.

MORBIDITY From the Latin *morbus*, "sick," it refers to both the state of being ill and the severity of the illness. A serious disease is said to have high morbidity.

PARASITE An organism that lives in or on a host organism and that gets its nourishment from that host. The parasite usually gains all the benefits of this relationship, whereas the host may suffer from various diseases and discomforts or show no signs of the infection. The life cycle of a typical parasite includes several developmental stages and morphological changes as the parasite lives and moves through the environment and one or more hosts. Parasites that remain on a host's body surface to feed are called ectoparasites, whereas those that live inside a host's body are called endoparasites. Parasitism is a highly successful biological adaptation. There are more known parasitic species than nonparasitic ones, and parasites affect just about every form of life, including most all animals, plants, and even bacteria.

PROPHYLAXIS Pre-exposure treatment (e.g., immunizations) to prevent the onset or recurrence of a disease.

REEMERGING DISEASE Many diseases once thought to be controlled are reappearing to infect humans again. These are known as reemerging diseases because they have not been common for a long period of time and are starting to appear again among large population groups.

SPOROZOITE Developmental stage of a protozoan (e.g., a malaria protozoan), during which it is transferred from vector (with malaria, a mosquito) to a human host.

evolved resistance to one of the main ones, chloroquine, in certain areas. A vaccine for malaria has been developed, and pilot programs to test the efficacy and safety of the vaccine were ongoing as of 2018.

Disease History, Characteristics, and Transmission

What historical accounts of war call "marsh fever," "intermittent fever," or "remittent fever" match current descriptions of malaria. One of the earliest recorded casualties of malaria may have been the great military campaigner of ancient Greece, Alexander the Great (356 BCE–323 BCE), who died of a fever. Malaria and dysentery also caused sickness during the Crusades (1095–c.1300). It was a major cause of disease among European armies on campaigns in tropical regions up to the 1820s, when quinine extracted from cinchona bark was found to be useful in both treating and preventing the disease.

However, quinine proved to be only a partial solution to malaria among the military, for it continued to be a problem during World War I (1914–1918) in some locations in Eastern Europe, the Middle East, and North Africa. In 1918 a large number of British and French troops in Macedonia contracted malaria despite the use of quinine. In World War II (1939–1945), quinine supplies were limited, and military commanders had lost their faith in it. Many of the Allies turned to the synthetic drug mepacrine instead. This was shown to have a dramatic effect in reducing the rate of malaria among Australian troops in New Guinea and among Allied troops in Burma. The insecticide DDT was introduced in 1944 and was sprayed from the air to protect troops operating in marshy malarial areas of Myanmar (then Burma) and Italy.

The malaria parasite enters the body through the bite of an infected female *Anopheles* mosquito and travels through the blood to the liver and then back to the blood, undergoing a complex life cycle. The incubation time of malaria is typically between 7 and 30 days and sometimes longer. For travelers returning from areas where malaria is endemic, symptoms may, therefore, not start until well after their return home. Sometimes people are infected with two or more species of *Plasmodium.*

People who live in areas where malaria is hyperendemic generally acquire immunity to the disease. The authors of a 2009 study published in *Clinical Microbiology Reviews* noted that such immunity "provides solid protection against severe morbidity and mortality." In fact, most people who live in hyperendemic areas generally do not become sick from malaria, despite the fact that they are continuously infected with the *Plasmodium.*

The specific pattern of symptoms experienced in a bout of malaria depends on which of the four species of *Plasmodium* is responsible for the disease. High fever with chills, headache, aching limbs, nausea, and diarrhea are common symptoms, however. Often the patient will experience a cycle of shivering and chills followed by flushing, fever, and profuse sweating. This bout of symptoms tends to spike every day or so and is related to the parasites bursting out of the red blood cells they have infected.

In severe malaria, there may be swollen liver, pallor (paleness), jaundice (yellowing of the skin and eyes), anemia (reduced ability of blood to transport oxygen), and respiratory distress. Complications are most common among babies, children, pregnant women, people with weak immune systems, and travelers and are usually caused by *P. falciparum* malaria. Cerebral malaria is the most serious complication of malaria and is associated with high mortality rates. The other *Plasmodium* species do not cause cerebral malaria. The symptoms of cerebral malaria include seizures, stupor, and coma. However, a full recovery is possible, with or without malaria-associated morbidity, including movement problems and blindness.

Other complications of *P. falciparum* malaria include a swollen spleen, kidney failure, and low blood sugar. The latter occurs because the parasites consume glucose much faster than red blood cells do, therefore depleting the body's supplies. Death from a ruptured spleen has been reported in *P. vivax* malaria.

The risk of relapse depends on the type of malaria the patient has. *P. falciparum* malaria, although responsible for most fatalities, does not actually lead to long-term relapse. However, survivors may suffer flare-ups over the year after the first attack. *P. vivax* causes a relapsing form of the disease, lasting up to five years, because of dormant parasites residing in the liver. *P. ovale* causes a similar condition, although it is far less common. *P. malariae* may produce long-term kidney disease called nephrotic syndrome if a person is infected with *P. malariae* continually or chronically.

The process by which *Plasmodia* parasites are transmitted begins with the bite of the infected female *Anopheles* mosquito, which takes a blood meal from the host. The infectious sporozoite form of the parasite is injected into the skin through the mosquito's salivary glands and travels through the bloodstream to the liver. They then reproduce asexually within liver cells. This process takes one to two weeks. During this period the patient will not have any symptoms.

The infected liver cells rupture, releasing parasite forms called merozoites, which enter red blood cells, maturing and multiplying. This process takes about 48 hours. The parasites then rupture the red blood cell, releasing more merozoites, which go on to infect further red blood cells. The release of the merozoites causes inflammation and a release of toxins, which causes a spike of fever. This stage can cause a massive increase in the number of parasites, particularly in *P. falciparum*, because this species infects all types of red blood cells. It is possible for more than 5 percent of all the red blood cells in the body to contain *P. falciparum* parasites.

In a further twist to this complex life cycle, some *Plasmodium* merozoites develop within the red blood cells into sexual forms, known as gametocytes. If another mosquito bites, it may take up these parasites in the blood meal. The parasites can mate sexually inside the mosquito to form more sporozoites, ready to complete the cycle from the beginning with the next bite of the same, or another, host.

P. vivax and *P. ovale* have a hepatic form that lies dormant for several weeks, giving rise to relapse symptoms when they are released into the blood. *P. malariae* may be transmitted from person to person through blood and organ donations from people who are already infected with the parasite, even though they may not have symptoms. Each stage in the life cycle of each species of *Plasmodium* has a specific morphology, which allows for accurate diagnosis in expert hands.

Scope and Distribution

According to WHO, there are around 216 million symptomatic cases of malaria every year in 91 countries. In 2016 there were 445,000 reported deaths caused by the disease. Also that year 90 percent of the malaria cases and 91 percent of deaths from malaria occurred in Africa. The majority of deaths were children.

In the United States there are approximately 1,700 cases of malaria each year, mainly occurring in travelers returning from endemic areas. Around 12 people die in the United States each year from malaria. Most people in the United States who have malaria contracted it while visiting malarial areas without taking prophylactic steps to prevent the illness.

Malaria is endemic in some tropical and subtropical regions, including areas of sub-Saharan Africa, Southeast Asia, the Western Pacific, Haiti, and parts of South America. The parasites require a temperature of at least 68°F (20°C) to complete their life cycle. Besides temperature, humidity and rainfall are factors affecting the transmission of malaria. The disease is endemic in more than 106 countries, with almost half of the world's population at risk.

Malaria has been known for more than 4,000 years. The disease used to be even more widespread than it is in the 21st century. Endemic malaria has been eliminated from almost 29 countries as of 2016. (Elimination is considered to have occurred when a country has been free of indigenous malaria for three years.) In 2016 some 44 countries that had not eliminated malaria had 10,000 malaria cases or fewer. This was an improvement from 2010, when only 37 countries with malaria could report the same. Some Pacific islands do not have malaria, despite favorable climatic factors, because *Anopheles* mosquitoes do not live there. *Plasmodium* parasites have differing geographical distributions. *P. falciparum* has the widest spread and is found in tropical areas, especially sub-Saharan Africa. *P. vivax* occurs in Asia, Central and South America, and some locations in Africa. *P. ovale* primarily occurs in west sub-Saharan Africa but is also found in the Western Pacific. *P. malariae* is found throughout the world. *P. knowlesi* occurs in Southeast Asia, especially Malaysia. It is primarily a disease of macaques, a species of monkey, but it can occasionally infect humans. There are about 430 species in the *Anopheles* genus, and only 30 to 40 transmit malaria. Some prefer to bite nonhuman animals, whereas others are active inside rather than outside. Therefore, risk of contracting malaria depends on the nature of the local mosquito population.

Returning travelers are especially at risk of malaria, as are pregnant women. Malaria should always be suspected if someone develops fevers and chills up to one year after return from a malarial area. Malaria in a pregnant woman can cause fetal death or low birth weight. The disease can also be passed on during childbirth and will cause severe anemia in the newborn.

Malaria has often accompanied military campaigns throughout the course of human history because the disease is encouraged by the conditions of war. The movement of troops or refugees leads to the spread of many kinds of parasites, including *Plasmodia*, and those without immunity are at risk when they travel to areas where the disease is endemic. Moreover, war may damage drainage and irrigation systems, which encourages the breeding of mosquitoes.

■ Treatment and Prevention

Treatment for malaria depends on a number of factors, including where the malarial infection was obtained, which *Plasmodium* species is causing the disease, and which antimalarial drugs the *Plasmodium* species is resistant to, if any. The health and age of the patient also plays a role in determining treatment. Pregnant women, for example, will need a different treatment protocol than the rest of the population. Each country has its own treatment guidelines for malaria.

Several drugs can be used for the treatment and prevention of malaria. In most cases of uncomplicated malaria, WHO recommends treatment with artemisinin-based combination therapies (ACTs). ACTs combine artemisinin with another antimalarial drug. Drug resistance has begun to emerge in some areas, with chloroquine-resistant *P. falciparum* being a problem in Africa and elsewhere, and chloroquine-resistant *P. vivax* in Southeast Asia.

Unlike WHO, the Centers for Disease Control and Prevention (CDC) does not recommend ACTs for treatment of malaria in the United States. Artemisinin is only available by request from the CDC and only in severe cases of malaria. There is concern among US health care professionals that artemisinin is harmful to the heart and should be used only when other treatment approaches are not working or if there are extenuating circumstances. The CDC recommends treating most cases of malaria in the United States with the antimalarial drugs chloroquine, Malarone® (a combination of atovaquone and proguanil), Coartem® (a combination of artemether and lumefantrine), quinine sulfate in combination with an antibiotic such as doxycycline, and mefloquine.

Patients with malaria need close medical attention as well as medication. Often this means supervision in a hospital setting. It is especially important that fluid balance and glucose levels are maintained.

Prevention of malaria involves taking prophylactic medication before, during, and after travel to malarial areas. Chloroquine, doxycycline, mefloquine, Malarone®, and primaquine are often prescribed for malaria prophylaxis (prevention). Would-be travelers should take advice from the CDC or their national equivalent on the specific protection they need. Pregnant women, in particular, need prophylaxis. Only doxycycline is not recommended for use during pregnancy.

The other key to prevention is avoiding the bite of the *Anopheles* mosquito. This can be challenging, as it is smaller and less conspicuous than some other mosquito species, and a bite could go unnoticed. *Anopheles* mosquitoes bite primarily between dusk and dawn. Wearing clothes of thick, woven material, such as cotton, that cover most of the body and sleeping under bed nets impregnated with permethrin insecticide are helpful, along with the use of an insect repellent containing DEET on exposed areas of skin and inside the home. Malaria sometimes occurs despite preventive measures, including medication, so those who are at risk should still be on the lookout for telltale symptoms such as fever.

Some people in endemic areas develop a natural immunity to malaria over time. If they leave the endemic area, their immunity wanes and then disappears over the course of a few years.

■ Impacts and Issues

An effective vaccine would be an enormous advance in the global fight against malaria. As of 2018 there was no vaccine that completely immunized people against the disease. However, the vaccine RTS,S/AS01, also known as Mosquirix®, was available for children in three countries in Africa: Ghana, Kenya, and Malawi. Mosquirix® partially immunized children to malaria from the *P. falciparum* parasite. Studies from 2009 to 2014 showed that vaccination with Mosquirix® prevented 4 of 10 cases of *P. falciparum*–caused cases of uncomplicated malaria in children who were given the vaccine between 5 and 17 months. WHO states that the vaccine should not replace antimalarial practices, such as sleeping under mosquito nets that have been treated with insecticide at night.

There have been many needless deaths because of wrong or delayed diagnosis of malaria. Many doctors in countries (often temperate ones) that do not have many malaria cases are unfamiliar with malaria and may not realize that gastrointestinal symptoms are often prominent in the disease. Fever may not be the only symptom. Returning travelers may assume that, if they have taken prophylactic medication, then protection is assured. Symptoms setting in several weeks or even months after return from a malarial area may wrongly be assumed to be severe influenza.

The correct diagnosis of malaria depends on identifying the parasites in a blood smear, often treated with Giemsa stain. Both thin and thick smears are usually examined. The thin smear preserves the morphology of the parasites so that the species involved can be identified. The thick smear contains more parasites and allows for more rapid diagnosis. When levels of parasites in the blood fall between bouts of fever, the smear may appear negative, even if the person has the disease. Three negative smears, taken at intervals, are required to definitively exclude the disease.

Malaria continues to be a global health problem. People who live in areas where the disease is endemic need greater access to treatment for malaria, and more people need insecticide-treated mosquito nets for sleeping and insecticide-treated homes. Moreover, increased movements by travelers and migrants on a global scale are likely to add to the risk of reintroducing malaria to countries where it had previously been eradicated. As most scientists agree that Earth's temperature is rising, it is likely that more areas of the world will become habitats for the *Anopheles* mosquito and its parasites. Therefore, the search for a vaccine and new antimalarial drugs has never been more urgent.

PRIMARY SOURCE

Forward to *World Malaria Report 2017* by Dr. Tedros Adhanom Ghebreyesus, Director-General, World Health Organization

SOURCE: *"World Malaria Report 2017." World Health Organization, 2017. http://apps.who.int/iris/bitstream/10665/259492/1/9789241565523-eng.pdf?ua=1 (accessed February 23, 2018).*

INTRODUCTION: *In the foreword to the World Health Organization's (WHO)* World Malaria Report *2017, WHO director-general Tedros Adhanom Ghebreyesus (1965–) summarizes the state of malaria across the globe in 2017. He noted that cases of malaria increased by 5 million from 2015 to 2016, a troubling sign. He also expressed concern that the burden of the disease rests primarily on poor people who live in sub-Saharan Africa. Many of these people do not have access to mosquito nets. Moreover, their homes often are not sprayed with insecticide to kill malaria-spreading mosquitoes. Many people who need prompt diagnosis and treatment of malaria do not receive adequate care. Further, there has not been enough monetary investment by the global community or by affected countries to fully eradicate the disease.*

For many years, the global response to malaria was considered one of the world's great public health achievements. WHO reported time and again on the massive roll-out of effective disease cutting tools, and on impressive reductions in cases and deaths.

Last December, we noted a troubling shift in the trajectory of this disease. The data showed that less than half of countries with ongoing transmission were on track to reach critical targets for reductions in the death and disease caused by malaria. Progress appeared to have stalled.

The *World Malaria Report 2017* shows that this worrying trend continues. Although there are some bright spots in the data, the overall decline in the global malaria burden has unquestionably leveled off. And, in some countries and regions, we are beginning to see reversals in the gains achieved.

Global disease burden and trends

In 2016, 91 countries reported a total of 216 million cases of malaria, an increase of 5 million cases over the previous year. The global tally of malaria deaths reached 445 000 deaths, about the same number reported in 2015.

Although malaria case incidence has fallen globally since 2010, the rate of decline has stalled and even reversed in some regions since 2014. Mortality rates have followed a similar pattern.

The WHO African Region continues to account for about 90% of malaria cases and deaths worldwide. Fifteen countries—all but one in sub-Saharan Africa—carry 80% of the global malaria burden. Clearly, if we are to get the global malaria response back on track, supporting the most heavily affected countries in this region must be our primary focus.

Extending health care to all

As WHO Director-General, achieving universal health coverage is my top priority. This is based on the moral conviction that all people should be guaranteed access to the health services they need, when and where they need them, regardless of where they live or their financial status.

To this end, how have countries fared in delivering services that prevent, diagnose and treat malaria for all in need? While we have made important headway, the pace of progress must be greatly accelerated if we are to reach our global malaria targets for 2020 and beyond.

In 2016, just over half (54%) of people at risk of malaria in sub-Saharan Africa were sleeping under an insecticide-treated mosquito net—the primary prevention method. This level of coverage represents a considerable increase since 2010 but is far from the goal of universal access.

Spraying the inside walls of homes with insecticides (indoor residual spraying, IRS) is another important prevention measure. The report documents a precipitous drop in IRS coverage in the WHO African Region since 2010, as well as declines in all other WHO regions over this same period.

Prompt diagnosis and treatment is the most effective means of preventing a mild case of malaria from developing into severe disease and death. In the WHO African Region, most people who seek treatment for malaria in the public health system receive an accurate diagnosis and effective medicines.

However, access to the public health system remains far too low. National-level surveys in the WHO African Region show that only about one third (34%) of children with a fever are taken to a medical provider in this sector.

Inadequate investment

A minimum investment of US$ 6.5 billion will be required annually by 2020 in order to meet the 2030 targets of the WHO global malaria strategy. The US$2.7 billion invested in 2016 represents less than half of that amount. Of particular concern is that, since 2014, investments in malaria control have, on average, declined in many high-burden countries.

Malaria response at a cross-roads

The choice before us is clear. If we continue with a "business as usual" approach—employing the same level of resources and the same interventions—we will face near-certain increases in malaria cases and deaths.

It is our hope that countries and the global health community choose another approach, resulting in a boost in funding for malaria programmes, expanded access to effective interventions and greater investment in the research and development of new tools.

As I have said before, countries must be in the driver's seat; they alone are ultimately responsible for the health of their citizens. Universal health coverage is indeed a political choice—one that takes courage, compassion and long-term vision.

After spending many years fighting the scourge of malaria in Ethiopia, I know that we are up against a tough adversary. But I am also convinced that this is a winnable battle. With robust financial resources and political leadership, we can—and will—swing the pendulum back towards a malaria-free world.

SEE ALSO *Climate Change and Infectious Disease; Travel and Infectious Disease; Tropical Infectious Diseases; Vector-Borne Disease*

BIBLIOGRAPHY

Books

Staines, Henry M., and Sanjeev Krishna, eds. *Treatment and Prevention of Malaria: Antimalarial Drug Chemistry, Action and Use.* Basel, Switzerland: Springer Basel, 2012.

Periodicals

Doolan, Denise L., Carlota Dobaño, and J. Kevin Baird. "Acquired Immunity to Malaria." *Clinical Microbiology Reviews* 22, no. 1 (2009): 13–36. This article can also be found online at https://www.ncbi.nlm.nih.gov/pmc/articles/PMC2620631/ (accessed February 23, 2018).

Khuu, Diana, et al. "Malaria-Related Hospitalizations in the United States, 2000–2014." *American Journal of Tropical Medicine and Hygiene* 97, no. 1 (July 2017): 213–221. This article can also be found online at https://www.ajtmh.org/content/journals/10.4269/ajtmh.17-0101 (accessed February 23, 2018).

Websites

"Eliminating Malaria." World Health Organization, 2016. http://apps.who.int/iris/bitstream/10665/205565/1/WHO_HTM_GMP_2016.3_eng.pdf (accessed February 23, 2018).

"Guidelines for the Treatment of Malaria, 3rd ed." World Health Organization, 2015. http://apps.who.int/iris/bitstream/10665/162441/1/9789241549127_eng.pdf?ua=1&ua=1 (accessed February 26, 2018).

Hotez, Peter, and Jennifer Herricks. "One Million Deaths by Parasites." PLOS Speaking of Medicine Community Blog, January 16, 2015. http://blogs.plos.org/speakingofmedicine/2015/01/16/one-million-deaths-parasites/ (accessed February 23, 2018).

"Malaria." Centers for Disease Control and Prevention, January 26, 2018. http://www.cdc.gov/malaria (accessed February 21, 2018).

"Malaria." World Health Organization. http://www.who.int/topics/malaria/en (accessed February 21, 2018).

"World Malaria Report 2017." World Health Organization, 2017. http://apps.who.int/iris/bitstream/10665/259492/1/9789241565523-eng.pdf?ua=1 (accessed February 23, 2018).

Susan Aldridge
Claire Skinner

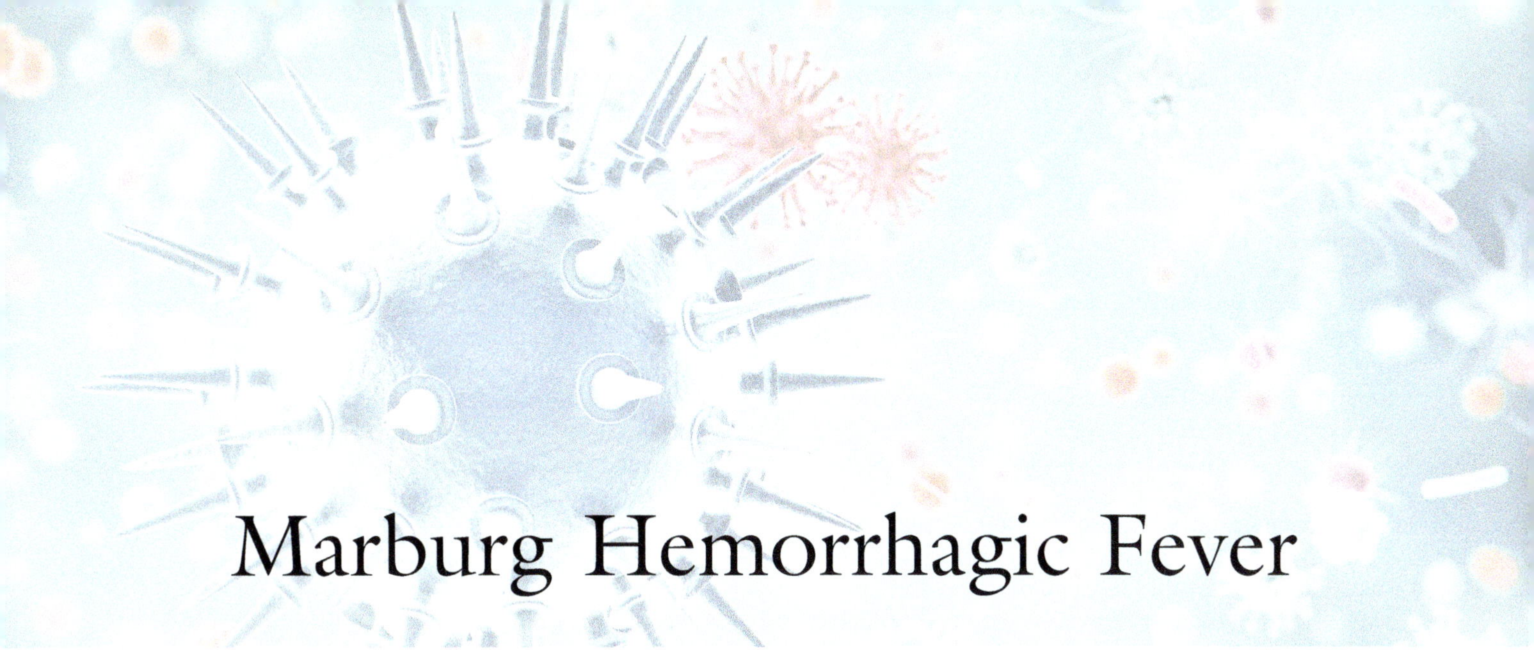

Marburg Hemorrhagic Fever

■ Introduction

Marburg hemorrhagic fever is one of a group of severe infections known as hemorrhagic fevers. The term *hemorrhagic* denotes the ability of these viral diseases to cause massive bleeding (hemorrhaging).

Marburg hemorrhagic fever is caused by a type of virus called a filovirus. The virus contains ribonucleic acid (RNA) as its genetic material. The discovery of the agent of Marburg hemorrhagic fever led to the creation of the filovirus viral group. Other filoviruses that have been identified include the four strains (types) of Ebola virus.

■ Disease History, Characteristics, and Transmission

Both Marburg fever and Marburg virus were discovered in 1967. At that time outbreaks of the fever occurred in three laboratories where scientists were studying the virus. One of these labs was located in the German city of Marburg, from which the names of the disease and the virus were taken.

More than 30 people became ill during this initial outbreak. The source of the virus was found to be African green monkey tissues that had been imported to the lab from Uganda as part of an effort to develop a polio vaccine. Victims included not only laboratory staff who were directly exposed to the virus but also family members and caregivers who contracted the illness from a staff member with the disease. This pattern of transmission helped establish the contagious nature of the virus.

The next reported case occurred in 1975 and was determined to have been acquired in Zimbabwe. Another case was reported in 1980, this time in western Kenya. Cases reported in 1987 and 1998 also originated in other African countries. An outbreak in 2004–2005 in Angola sickened 252 people and killed 227, a 90 percent mortality rate. Since then, according to statistics from the World Health Organization (WHO), only about 22 cases were reported prior to 2015.

The exact mechanism of transmission of the virus to humans is thought to be through fruit bats, which are likely the natural host of the virus. Once someone is infected, human-to-human transmission can occur by direct contact or contact with blood or other body fluids of the infected person. Other methods of transmission include handling medical equipment or touching surfaces that are contaminated with fluids infected with the virus. Even con-

WORDS TO KNOW

ENDEMIC Present in a particular area or among a particular group of people.

FILOVIRUS Any RNA virus that belongs to the family *Filoviridae*. Filoviruses infect primates. Examples include Marburg virus and Ebola virus.

HEMORRHAGIC FEVER A high fever caused by viral infection that features a high volume of bleeding. The bleeding is caused by the formation of tiny blood clots throughout the bloodstream. These blood clots, also called microthrombi, deplete platelets and fibrinogen in the bloodstream. When bleeding begins, the factors needed for the clotting of the blood are scarce. Thus, uncontrolled bleeding (hemorrhage) ensues.

HOST An organism that serves as the habitat for a parasite or a symbiont. A host may provide nutrition to the parasite or symbiont, or it may simply provide a place in which to live.

RESERVOIR An animal or organism in which a virus or parasite normally resides.

tact with a dead body can pass on the infection if the virus remains in the blood of the recently deceased person.

Symptoms appear suddenly between 2 and 21 days after infection. Presumably, during this incubation period, the virus is commandeering host cell replication machinery so that deoxyribonucleic acid (DNA) can be synthesized from the viral RNA. The DNA then is used to produce the necessary components for new viruses.

The symptoms of Marburg hemorrhagic fever include fever, chills, and headache. Initial symptoms may be mistaken for influenza. Approximately five days later, a rash appears mainly on the chest, stomach, and back. Nausea with vomiting, chest and abdominal pain, and diarrhea can develop. Subsequently, more severe symptoms may appear, including liver dysfunction with jaundice, pancreas inflammation, rapid weight loss, liver failure, and hemorrhaging. At this stage organ failure often leads to a rapid death.

According to WHO, the overall death rate from Marburg hemorrhagic fever is about 50 percent. During an outbreak the death rate ranges from 24 to 90 percent. Those who recover may display a number of recurring diseases, such as hepatitis.

Scope and Distribution

Marburg hemorrhagic fever is endemic in Africa. As of 2017 it had not been discovered to be indigenous to any other continent. The fruit bat is a natural reservoir of the infection.

Treatment and Prevention

As of 2017 there was no cure or specific treatment for Marburg hemorrhagic fever. There was also no vaccine, although the development of an Ebola vaccine has offered hope that a Marburg vaccine could be developed. Rather, combating the infection involves standard precautions by attending physicians and other caregivers, such as handwashing and changing surgical garb before examining or tending to another patient. In addition, precautions to prevent the spread of the virus include wearing protective gowns, caps, foot covers, and masks equipped with face shields to guard against a spill or spray of blood. Treatment has largely been a catch-up effort designed to keep a patient stabilized and, in the worst cases, alive by the maintenance of blood pressure, fluid levels, and the proper concentrations of electrolytes. Also, ensuring that the blood remains capable of clotting can help reduce loss of blood during hemorrhaging.

Even diagnosing the disease is challenging. In its early stages the disease displays symptoms that are similar to influenza, malaria, and typhoid fever. In addition, once symptoms appear, the disease can swiftly worsen.

The presence of the viral genetic material can be detected using a number of molecular techniques. This can confirm the presence of the virus just a few days after infection. However, because there have been so few cases and because Marburg hemorrhagic fever is not a disease that is easily studied in the laboratory, the diagnostic significance of these molecular advances is unclear.

Impacts and Issues

Outbreaks of Marburg hemorrhagic fever are sporadic. This limits the number of people who are affected by the disease. However, this does not diminish the severity of the illness. The rapid onset of the disease and its high death rate can cause panic in the communities affected.

Despite the rarity of Marburg hemorrhagic fever, outbreaks can occur. The most recent large-scale example is the outbreak that occurred in 2005 in Uige,

Known Marburg Hemorrhagic Fever Infections (1967–2014)

Year	Country	Probable Origin	Human Cases	Reported Deaths	Mortality Rate
1967	Germany and Yugoslavia	Uganda	31	7	23%
1975	South Africa	Zimbabwe	3	1	33%
1980	Kenya	Kenya	2	1	50%
1987	Kenya	Kenya	1	1	100%
1990	Russia	Russia	1	1	100%
1998–2000	Democratic Republic of the Congo (DRC)	DRC	154	128	83%
2004–2005	Angola	Angola	252	227	90%
2007	Uganda	Uganda	4	1	25%
2008	United States	Uganda	1	0	0%
2008	Netherlands	Uganda	1	1	100%
2012	Uganda	Uganda	15	4	27%
2014	Uganda	Uganda	1	1	100%

SOURCE: Adapted from "Chronology of Marburg Hemorrhagic Fever Outbreaks." US Centers for Disease Control and Prevention. 2014. Available from: https://www.cdc.gov/vhf/marburg/resources/outbreak-table.html

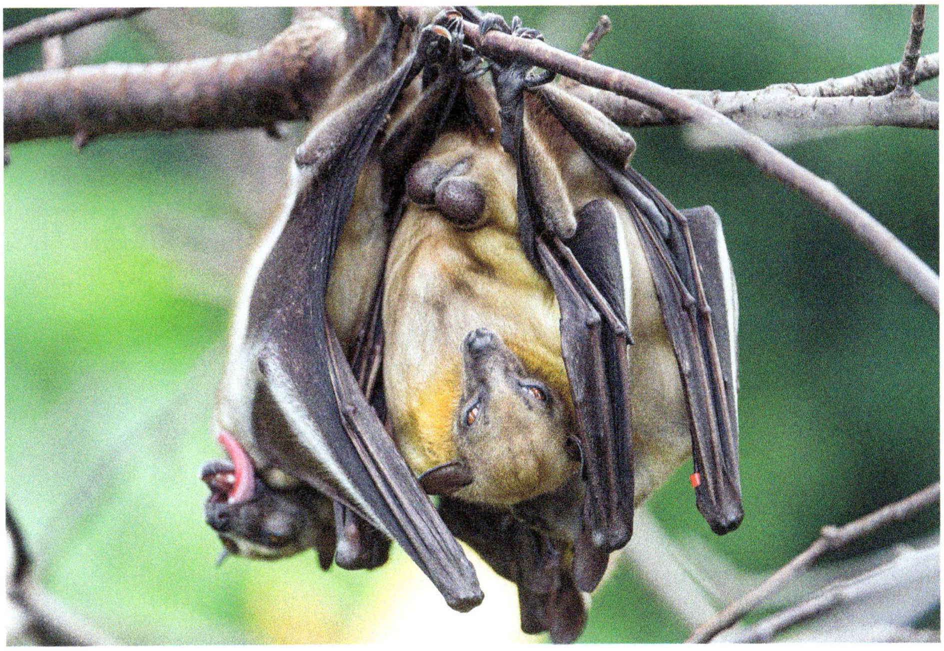

Rousettus aegyptiacus, the African fruit bat, is thought to be the natural host of the Marburg virus. Although Marburg fever is a deadly disease in humans, infected fruit bats do not exhibit symptoms of illness. © *Picture by Tambako the Jaguar/Getty Images*

Angola, where at least 252 were confirmed to have become infected. Of these, 227 died.

Investigations of the 2005 Angolan outbreak determined that one cause was the unsafe use of needles to deliver injections in homes, medical clinics, and a pediatric ward. Reuse of the needles, which were intended to be used once and disposed of, facilitated the spread of the virus. In the aftermath of the outbreak, WHO instituted a safe injection campaign, which was still active in 2017 and which has helped reduce the reuse of contaminated needles in the region.

The isolated nature of the Angolan regions affected contributed to the spread of the disease. Medical care was rudimentary, and clinics were not always adequately supplied to cope with the infection. Cultural practices, such as the open viewing and touching of the deceased prior to burial, also likely contributed to the spread of the virus. WHO has worked to increase awareness of the disease, especially in rural areas. Increased understanding of the disease and its spread, as well as alterations in behavior and cultural practices, may help reduce the potential for future outbreaks.

Despite efforts following the Angolan outbreak, small outbreaks of Marburg hemorrhagic fever have continued, particularly in Uganda. In 2012 15 people in Uganda contracted the virus, and 4 died. In 2017 there was another outbreak in Kween District in eastern Uganda. As of November 2017, two people in the region were confirmed to have the disease, and a third was suspected to have had it. All three died. In response to the outbreak, additional efforts were made to educate the region's residents about disease treatment and safe burial practices. Community leaders spoke on local radio stations to explain the disease and precautions necessary to halt its spread.

Perhaps the greatest impact of the disease has been as an example of how diseases spread from their natural, nonhuman hosts to humans. Identification of the natural host of a disease and the regions in which the natural host exists in greatest numbers is vital if the disease is to be eradicated. In the case of Marburg hemorrhagic fever, the natural host is thought to be a primate.

Avoiding contact with primates in the wild, including consuming their meat as food, reduces the risk of contracting the disease.

The study of Marburg hemorrhagic fever requires a high-containment facility called a biosafety level 4 laboratory, where airflow into and out of the laboratory is controlled and stringent precautions regarding the wearing of protective clothing and decontamination following work with the virus are enforced. These steps help ensure that the virus does not escape the laboratory and that researchers are protected from infection. Efforts to educate the medical community about Marburg symptomology are also important because the virus can quickly infect health care workers and has the potential to rapidly spread into the community. This potential for rapid person-to-person spread combined with the ferocity of the disease has heightened concerns that the Marburg virus could be used as an agent of bioterrorism.

SEE ALSO *Ebola; Emerging Infectious Diseases; Hemorrhagic Fevers*

BIBLIOGRAPHY

Books

Barrett, Ron, and George J. Armelagos. *An Unnatural History of Emerging Infections*. Oxford, UK: Oxford University Press, 2013.

Johnson, Nicholas, ed. *The Role of Animals in Emerging Viral Diseases*. Boston: Elsevier/AP, 2014.

Periodicals

Henry, Ronnie, and Frederick A. Murphy. "Etymologia: Marburg Virus." *Emerging Infectious Diseases* 23, no. 10 (October 2017): 1689.

Reynolds, Pierce, and Andrea Marzi. "Ebola and Marburg Virus Vaccines." *Virus Genes* 53, no. 4 (August 2017): 501–515.

Websites

"Health Workers Urged to Work with Communities to Stop Marburg." World Health Organization, November 4, 2017. http://www.afro.who.int/news/health-workers-urged-work-communities-stop-marburg (accessed November 29, 2017).

"Marburg Hemorrhagic Fever." Centers for Disease Control and Prevention, December 1, 2014. https://www.cdc.gov/vhf/marburg/index.html (accessed November 20, 2017).

"Marburg Virus Disease." World Health Organization, October 2017. http://www.who.int/mediacentre/factsheets/fs_marburg/en/ (accessed November 20, 2017).

Brian Hoyle

Marine Toxins

Introduction

Marine toxins are naturally occurring compounds that can contaminate some types of seafood. The seafood may not show any signs of contamination but, if eaten, can cause various human illnesses.

Disease History, Characteristics, and Transmission

Marine toxins have probably existed for thousands of years. Biblical accounts of illnesses match the symptoms of paralytic shellfish poisoning, and the Red Sea may have been named "red" because of the frequent explosive growth of certain algae. Accounts of the consequences of marine toxins date back centuries. For example, a June 17, 1793, entry in a diary kept by the ship's surgeon during an expedition led by Captain George Vancouver (1757–1789) off the West Coast of North America describes the death of a shipmate that is consistent with the effects of eating contaminated mussels.

In the coastal regions of the United States, the illnesses most frequently caused by marine toxins are scombrotoxic fish poisoning, ciguatera poisoning, paralytic shellfish poisoning, neurotoxic shellfish poisoning, and amnesic shellfish poisoning.

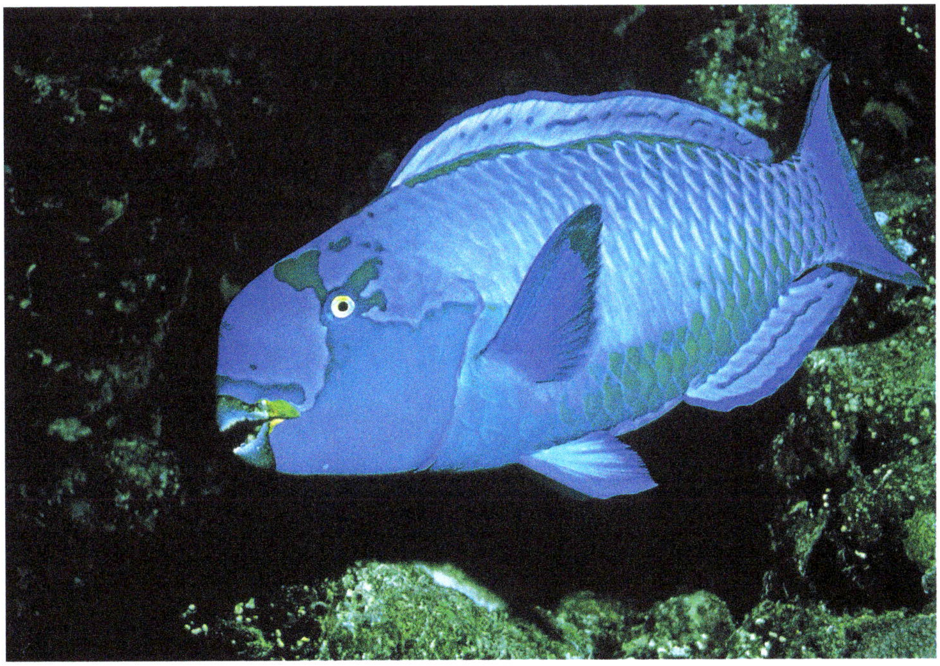

Chlorurus gibbus, also known as the heavybeak parrotfish or steephead parrotfish. Consuming this fish is known to carry risks of ciguatera poisoning. © Peter Scoones/Science Source

WORDS TO KNOW

BIOMAGNIFICATION The increasing concentration of compounds at higher trophic level or the tendency of organisms to accumulate certain chemicals to a concentration larger than that occurring in their inorganic, non-living environment, such as soil or water, or in the case of animals, larger than in their food.

DEGRADATION (CELLULAR) Means breakdown and refers to the destruction of host cell components, such as DNA, by infective agents such as bacteria and viruses.

DIATOM Algae are a diverse group of simple, nucleated, plantlike aquatic organisms that are primary producers. Primary producers are able to utilize photosynthesis to create organic molecules from sunlight, water, and carbon dioxide. Ecologically vital, algae account for roughly half of photosynthetic production of organic material on Earth in both freshwater and marine environments. Algae exist either as single cells or as multicellular organizations. Diatoms are microscopic, single-celled algae that have intricate glass-like outer cell walls partially composed of silicon. Different species of diatom can be identified based upon the structure of these walls. Many diatom species are planktonic, suspended in the water column moving at the mercy of water currents. Others remain attached to submerged surfaces. One bucketful of water may contain millions of diatoms. Their abundance makes them important food sources in aquatic ecosystems.

DINOFLAGELLATE Microorganisms that are regarded as algae. Their wide array of exotic shapes and, sometimes, armored appearance is distinct from other algae. The closest microorganisms in appearance are the diatoms.

HISTAMINE A hormone that is chemically similar to the hormones serotonine, epinephrine, and norepinephrine. A hormone is generally defined as a chemical produced by a certain cell or tissue that causes a specific biological change or activity to occur in another cell or tissue located elsewhere in the body. Specifically, histamine plays a role in localized immune responses and in allergic reactions.

RED TIDE A marine phenomenon in which water is stained a red, brown, or yellowish color because of the temporary abundance of a particular species of pigmented dinoflagellate (these events are known as blooms). Also called phytoplankton, or planktonic algae, these single-celled organisms of the class Dinophyceae move using a tail-like structure called a flagellum. They also photosynthesize, and it is their photosynthetic pigments that can tint the water during blooms. Dinoflagellates are common and widespread. Under appropriate environmental conditions, various species can grow very rapidly, causing red tides. Red tides occur in all marine regions with a temperate or warmer climate.

Scombrotoxic fish poisoning is a bacterial illness caused by the degradation of fish (mainly tuna and bonito). The bacteria degrade fish proteins, and a by-product of the protein decomposition is a group of compounds called histamines. When the spoiled fish is eaten, the high histamine level causes poisoning. Symptoms may begin only a few minutes after eating the seafood or several hours later. They include the development of a rash, flushing of the skin, sweating, and headache. As the body tries to expel the poison, abdominal pain, vomiting, and diarrhea also can occur. Some people also experience a burning or metallic sensation in the mouth.

The symptoms of scombrotoxic fish poisoning are temporary and tend to fade after a few hours. Usually no treatment is necessary, although some people benefit from antihistamines, which counteract the effects produced by the excess histamines, as well as from the drug epinephrine. Symptoms can be more severe in those who are taking some medications that slow the breakdown of histamine.

The second most common type of illness caused by marine toxins in the United States is ciguatera poisoning. This type of poisoning is due to the contamination of tropical reef fish by tiny marine plants called dinoflagellates. The illness is an example of what is termed *biological magnification* or *biomagnification.* In this case, the dinoflagellates are present in fish species that are food for a larger species. That species in turn becomes food for a larger marine animal. This pattern continues, with the concentration of the poison increasing from creature to creature. The animal at the top of this food chain (with ciguatera poisoning, it is often the barracuda) may have a high concentration of the poison. The person who eats that animal ingests the accumulated load of toxin. In addition to the barracuda, other fishes may contain high levels of the dinoflagellate toxin, including grouper, sea bass, snapper, and mullet. These popular sport fishes are found in tropical waters off of Hawaii, the Virgin Islands, Puerto Rico, and islands in the South Pacific.

MARINE MICROORGANISMS

Marine microorganisms often inhabit a harsh environment. Ocean temperatures are generally very cold—approximately 37.4° F (about 3° C) on average—and this temperature tends to remain this cold except in shallow areas. About 75 percent of the oceans of the world are below 3,300 feet (1000 meters) in depth. The pressure on objects like bacteria at increasing depths is enormous.

Some marine bacteria have adapted to the pressure of the ocean depths and require the presence of the extreme pressure to function. Such bacteria are barophilic if their requirement for pressure is absolute or barotrophic if they can tolerate both extreme and near-atmospheric pressures. Similarly, many marine bacteria have adapted to the cold growth temperatures. Those that tolerate the temperatures are described as psychrotrophic, while those bacteria that require the cold temperatures are termed *psychrophilic* ("cold loving").

Marine microbiology has become the subject of much commercial interest. Compounds with commercial potential as nutritional additives and antimicrobials are being discovered from marine bacteria, actinomycetes, and fungi. For example, the burgeoning marine nutraceuticals market for products such as omega 3 fatty acid represents billions of dollars annually. As relatively little is still known of the marine microbial world, as compared to terrestrial microbiology, many more commercial and medically relevant compounds undoubtedly remain undiscovered.

In coastal regions of the United States, Canada, and other maritime countries, government agencies monitor ocean catches and aquaculture facilities for the presence of the various toxic species. Detection of these toxic species can lead to the closure of a region to fishing and the sale of commercially raised seafood until the problem is resolved.

The health risk posed by marine toxins has been balanced somewhat by the discovery that some marine toxins can act as anticancer drugs. A 2006 University of Wisconsin study reported that marine toxins can bind to a cell component called actin and that this interaction can disable rapidly growing cells, including cancer cells.

Symptoms of ciguatera poisoning usually appear within minutes of eating a contaminated fish. They include nausea with vomiting, abdominal cramps, diarrhea, sweating, headache, muscle aches, dizziness, itchy skin, and general weakness. More unusual symptoms are possible, such as alterations in taste and temperature sensations, and nightmares and hallucinations may occur. The symptoms tend to fade in one to four weeks.

Paralytic shellfish poisoning is caused by another dinoflagellate that can explode in numbers during an event called a red tide. The name refers to the appearance of the water, which becomes discolored by the presence of vast numbers of the reddish-brown dinoflagellates. The affected marine creatures are often filter-feeders—those that feed by straining sea water to remove tiny nutrients. The toxin-laden dinoflagellates accumulate in mussels, clams, oysters, crabs, and scallops. Lobsters also can become contaminated.

Symptoms of paralytic shellfish poisoning begin within several minutes to several hours of eating contaminated seafood. Initially, the symptoms are mild and include numbness of the face, arms, and legs; more severe symptoms follow, including dizziness, nausea, and loss of coordination. Some people become paralyzed and can die when they become unable to breathe.

Neurotoxic shellfish poisoning is another illness that is caused by a dinoflagellate. Shellfish are involved; they concentrate the toxin during filter-feeding. As with the other illnesses caused by marine toxins, symptoms tend to occur soon after consuming the contaminated seafood. Symptoms include dizziness; numbness; a tingling sensation in the mouth, arms, and legs; and loss of coordination. Recovery occurs within several days.

Finally, amnesic shellfish poisoning is a rare event that is caused by a microscopic plant (diatom) called Nitzchia pungens. Concentration of the diatom in shellfish, such as mussels, also concentrates a component of the diatom known as domoic acid. When contaminated mussels are eaten, the domoic acid causes an intestinal upset, dizziness, headache, and loss of orientation. In severe cases, there can be brain damage when domoic acid attaches to chemical receptors in brain cells, disrupting cell function. Permanent loss of memory, paralysis, and death can result.

■ Scope and Distribution

Marine toxins are found in coastal regions in almost all parts of the globe, except at the higher latitudes of the Arctic and Antarctic. Different illnesses often have different distributions. For example, neurotoxic shellfish poisoning tends to occur in the Gulf of Mexico and along the southern Atlantic Coast of the United States. However, the 2015 finding of the neurotoxin in mussels off the coast of Alaska indicates that the range of the dinoflaggellate is increasing. Some researchers believe the warming global climate may be the reason.

Illnesses caused by marine toxins occur in greater numbers in more equatorial regions because the warmer waters encourage the growth of the microorganisms that produce the toxins. However, outbreaks occur during the warmer months in other regions.

There is no evidence that gender or race influences a person's susceptibility to marine toxins. The elderly and those with a less efficient immune system may be more at risk.

Treatment and Prevention

Treatment typically involves making the patient as comfortable as possible and waiting for the illness to pass. Scombrotoxic fish poisoning can be treated with drugs aimed at neutralizing the effects of the excess histamine.

There are no vaccines that provide protection against poisoning by marine toxins. The best prevention strategy is to use caution when eating seafood. For example, eating raw shellfish is risky and should be avoided. Warnings about algal blooms and reports of seafood-related illnesses should be taken seriously. Seafood from the affected region should be avoided until public health officials have determined that the danger is over.

Impacts and Issues

In the United States about 30 people are poisoned by the toxins in seafood each year. The consequences of this poisoning can range from a short-term and inconvenient illness to permanent damage, memory loss, and death.

Because coastal areas often attract tourists and tourists often want to sample the local seafood, an outbreak of poisoning by a marine toxin can affect the local economy. For example, in 1987 there was an outbreak of amnesic shellfish poisoning on Prince Edward Island, Canada, which sickened more than 100 people and caused several deaths. In the years following the outbreak, fear over consumption of seafood and a lingering perception that the coast of the province was dangerous caused a marked drop in visitors. This adversely affected the island's economy, which relies heavily on summer tourism.

Periodic outbreaks involving larger numbers of people also occur. In fact, studies by the Woods Hole Oceanographic Institution and the US National Oceanographic and Atmospheric Administration indicate that the frequency of algal blooms has been increasing along the coasts of the United States and other countries since the 1970s. While the cause of the increased number of blooms is not absolutely certain, a general consensus among scientists is that the documented warming of the coastal oceans has made conditions more favorable for algal growth. If so, a consequence of global warming could be more algal blooms and more cases of marine toxin–related illness.

SEE ALSO *Water-Borne Disease*

BIBLIOGRAPHY

Books

Botana, Luis M., and Natalia Vilariño, eds. *Climate Change and Marine and Freshwater Toxins.* Berlin: Walter de Gruyter GmbH, 2015.

Periodicals

McPartlin, Daniel A., et al. "Biosensors for the Monitoring of Harmful Algal Blooms." *Current Opinion in Biotechnology* 45 (June 2017): 164–169.

Websites

"Marine Environments." Centers for Disease Control and Prevention. https://www.cdc.gov/habs/illness-symptoms-marine.html (accessed November 20, 2017).

McColl, Karen. "High Levels of Paralytic Shellfish Poisoning Found off Haines, Alaska." CBC News, December 23, 2015. http://www.cbc.ca/news/canada/north/psp-levels-high-along-haines-coast-says-report-1.3371953 (accessed November 20, 2017).

Brian Hoyle

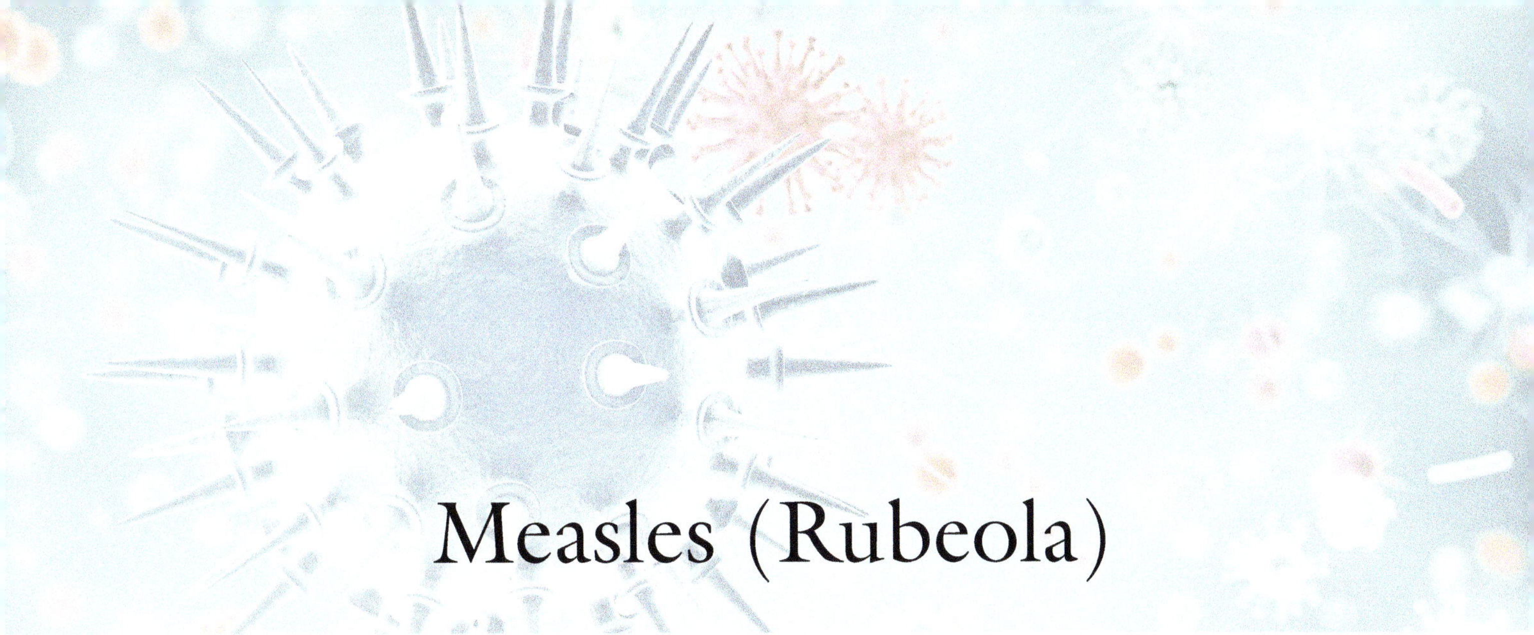

Measles (Rubeola)

Introduction

Measles is an acute viral illness that was once one of the most common diseases of childhood. The clinical name for measles is rubeola, which comes from the Latin word *ruber*, meaning "red," and is a reference to the pinkish-red rash that is characteristic of the disease.

Measles is a highly infectious disease that is spread by coughs, sneezes, and person-to-person contact. It will occasionally lead to serious and even potentially fatal complications, such as pneumonia and encephalitis. Once someone has had measles, they are usually immune for life.

Vaccination was introduced in the 1960s in the Western world and has led to a dramatic reduction in the number of children contracting measles. For example, according to the World Health Organization (WHO), the number of global deaths from measles decreased by 84 percent from 2000 to 2016. However, the disease is still present in human populations and causes thousands of deaths each year.

Because humans are the only hosts for the measles virus, it should be possible to eradicate measles through universal vaccination. This requires a global effort to bring the vaccine to children in all areas of the world.

Disease History, Characteristics, and Transmission

Measles is caused by a virus from the Paramyxoviridae family, which also includes the influenza and mumps viruses. It is a single-stranded, enveloped, ribonucleic acid (RNA) virus, which means that its genetic material is RNA rather than deoxyribonucleic acid (DNA).

The incubation time of the measles virus is one to two weeks. The virus first infects the epithelial cells lining the upper respiratory tract and then spreads to the rest of the body. In what is called typical or natural measles, the early symptoms are like those of a common cold and include coughing, sneezing, sore throat, and fever. Within a few days, characteristic small white spots called Koplik spots develop inside the mouth. A day or so later, a rash appears, starting behind the ears and spreading to the face and down the body and lasting for three or four days. The appearance of a rash may coincide with a spike in fever, sometimes to more than 104°F (40°C).

Up to 30 percent of measles patients experience complications, with most occuring in individuals under five years or over 20 years. Complications include pneumonia, diarrhea, and otitis media, a middle ear infection that can lead to deafness. Encephalitis, an inflammation of the brain, is a complication in an estimated 1 out of 1,000 cases of measles. Mortality from measles complications is highest among infants under two years old and in adults. For every 1,000 children who contract measles, around one or two will die.

There is also a modified form of measles that occurs among those who have been incompletely vaccinated.

WORDS TO KNOW

AEROSOL Particles of liquid or solid dispersed as a suspension in gas.

KOPLIK SPOTS Red spots with a small blue-white speck in the center found on the tongue and the insides of the cheeks during the early stages of measles. Also called Koplik's sign, they are named after American pediatrician Henry Koplik (1858–1927).

MORTALITY The condition of being susceptible to death. The term *mortality* comes from the Latin word *mors*, which means death. Mortality can also refer to the rate of deaths caused by an illness or injury (e.g., "Rabies has a high mortality rate").

Modified measles is less severe than typical measles and Koplik spots may be absent. However, the risk of complications is the same. Rarely, a form of the disease called atypical measles may occur, usually among those who received the vaccine in the 1960s. Atypical measles is characterized by sudden onset of fever, muscle pain, abdominal pain, and headache. Koplik spots are rarely present, and pneumonia is a common complication. Subacute sclerosing panencephalitis is an extremely rare degenerative disease of the brain and nervous system that is thought to arise from persistent measles infection in the brain. It occurs at a rate of around 5 to 10 per 1 million cases and develops anywhere from one month to seven years after measles exposure.

Measles is spread through the aerosol route—that is, through coughs and sneezes—and also by person-to-person contact. It is a very infectious diseases with around 90 percent of those being exposed becoming infected. A person is infectious for four days before the rash appears and four days after the rash fades.

Measles in the mother can affect pregnancy by causing miscarriage, preterm birth, and other issues.

■ Scope and Distribution

Almost all children developed measles before the introduction of the measles vaccine in 1963. The disease was most common in the winter and early spring.

Before the introduction of the vaccine, there were around 500,000 cases of measles a year in the United States that were reported to the Centers for Disease Control and Prevention (CDC), although the CDC notes that the number of cases was underreported and is likely somewhere between 3 and 4 million. Of the approximately 500,000 measles cases reported to the CDC each year, some 48,000 people were hospitalized, 1,000 experienced encephalitis, and 400 to 500 died.

There was a sharp decline in measles cases following mass vaccination programs. But there was resurgence beginning in 1983 among those who had not been vaccinated and among previously vaccinated teenagers. By 1989 there were 19,000 reported cases. A revised vaccination strategy that called for two doses instead of one brought measles under control again. By 1993 cases were down to fewer than 1,000 annually in the United States, where it has remained despite occasional outbreaks. The United States declared in 2000 that measles was eliminated from the country.

Since 2000 there have been cases of measles in the United States, and there have been a number of outbreaks. Some have been caused by a person contracting measles in another country and then returning to the United States. This occurred in 2014 when unvaccinated Amish travelers caught measles in the Philippines and brought the disease with them back to Ohio. (Some Amish do not vaccinate their children.)

Measles is a worldwide disease. There are about 19 cases of measles per 1 million people, according to the CDC. WHO reported 89,780 deaths from measles in 2016. This was the first time in modern history that there

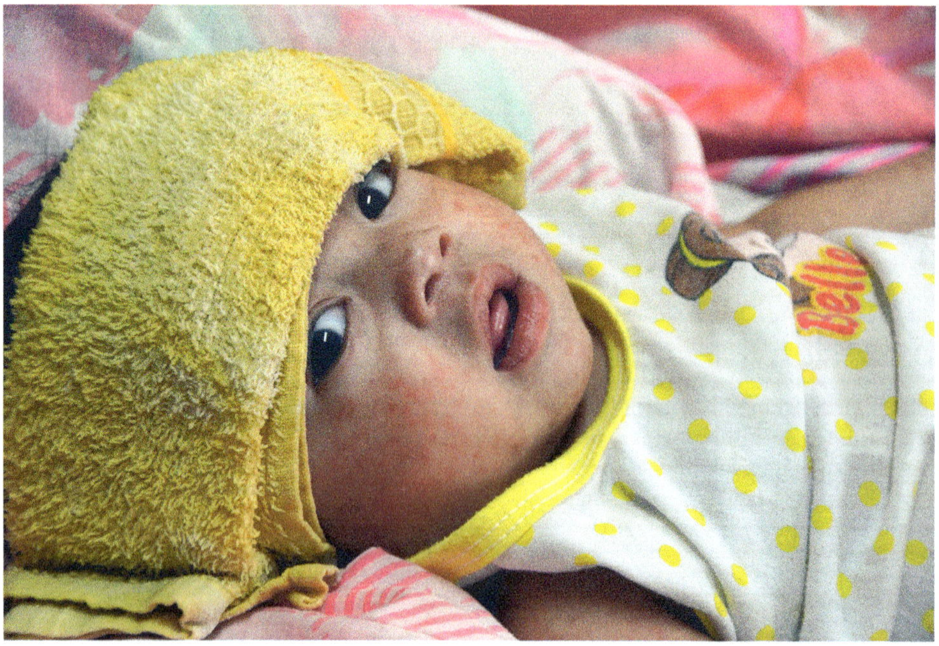

A baby in Manilla, Philippines, exhibiting a rash caused by the infectious respiratory disease measles. © *CDC/Jim Goodson/Science Source*

were less than 100,000 deaths in a year from the disease. Most deaths from measles occur in developing countries where vaccines may not be readily available.

Measles is a leading cause of death among children. The death rate from measles in developing countries is higher than in developed countries. People who are malnourished, who lack appropriate amounts of vitamin A, and who do not have access to adequate health care are particularly at risk of dying from the disease. According to WHO, about 3 to 6 percent of these cases result in death. For displaced people, such as those living in refugee camps, the mortality rate can be as high as 30 percent. Patients with weakened immunity, including those with human immunodeficiency virus (HIV) or acquired immunodeficiency syndrome (AIDS), are at risk of complications from measles.

Treatment and Prevention

Treatment of measles is often unnecessary, although antibiotics may be given for secondary bacterial infections. Vitamin A may be useful in very severe cases and in countries where this vitamin deficiency is common. The antiviral drug ribavirin may be used in very severe cases also, as well as in patients with weakened immunity.

The spread of measles can be prevented by good hygiene, including handwashing. People with measles should isolate themselves while they are infectious and not attend school, day care, or work.

The best way to prevent measles is by vaccination. A killed (inactive) vaccine was introduced in 1963, followed by a live (active) vaccine from the late 1960s. In the early 21st century, it is typical to give a combined measles, mumps, and rubella (MMR) vaccine—one dose between 12 and 15 months and a second at four to six years old. Most people can receive MMR, but it is not usually recommended for people with weakened immunity or for pregnant women.

According to WHO, 85 percent of children were vaccinated against measles in 2016. This was up 13 percent from the year 2000, when only 72 percent of children were vaccinated.

Impacts and Issues

The Measles Initiative was established by the American Red Cross, the CDC, the United Nations Children's Fund (UNICEF), and WHO in 2001. In 2012 the Measles Initiative was renamed the Measles & Rubella Initiative (M & R Initiative), and it expanded its focus to include elimination of the disease rubella. The goal of the M & R Initiative is to eliminate deaths from measles and to prevent congenital rubella syndrome through mass vaccination programs. The M & R Initiative hopes to accomplish this goal by the year 2020.

SOCIAL AND PERSONAL RESPONSIBILITY

Have you been near someone with measles? Or do think you have? If so, the Centers for Disease Control and Prevention (CDC) suggest that you:

"Immediately call your doctor and let him or her know that you have been exposed to someone who has measles. Your doctor can

- determine if you are immune to measles based on your vaccination record, age, or laboratory evidence, and
- make special arrangements to evaluate you, if needed, without putting other patients and medical office staff at risk.

If you are not immune to measles, MMR [measles, mumps, and rubella] vaccine or a medicine called immune globulin may help reduce your risk developing measles. Your doctor can help to advise you, and monitor you for signs and symptoms of measles.

If you do not get MMR or immune globulin, you should stay away from settings where there are susceptible people (such as school, hospital, or childcare) until your doctor says it's okay to return. This will help ensure that you do not spread it to others."

Recent measles outbreaks in the United States have occurred in part because some parents choose not to vaccinate their children. These individuals either do not believe that vaccines are effective, because they do not believe measles is a serious disease or because they are afraid of the side effects of vaccines. This is a problem from a public health perspective: recent outbreaks of measles have occurred in places with a significantly large number of unvaccinated children. In December 2014, for example, an international tourist infected with measles visited Disney theme parks in Orange County, California, and inadvertently spread the disease. The outbreak spread from California to other states, as well as to Canada and Mexico, ultimately infecting 147 people. The majority of people who caught the disease were either unvaccinated or had an unknown vaccination status. Unvaccinated people who caught the disease at the Disney parks were either too young to receive the vaccination (11 months old or younger) or were not vaccinated due to personal beliefs.

The authors of a 2016 article for the *Journal of the American Medical Association* showed that US citizens who are unvaccinated are more likely to contract measles than their vaccinated counterparts. "A substantial proportion of the US measles cases in the era after elimination were intentionally unvaccinated," they stated. Moreover, the authors observed that "the phenomenon of vaccine refusal was associated with an increased risk for measles among people who refuse vaccines and among fully vaccinated individuals."

Although two doses of the MMR vaccine are about 97 percent effective, a very small percentage of people who have been vaccinated against measles and are exposed to measles will get sick. For these people, the vaccine did not elicit the appropriate immunological response and they did not develop enough or effective enough antibodies to be immune to measles. Although the people for whom the vaccine is not fully effective may get measles when exposed to the virus, they are more likely than their unvaccinated counterparts to get less sick from the disease, and they are less likely to spread to the disease to others.

PRIMARY SOURCE

Anti-Vaccine Activists Spark a State's Worst Measles Outbreak in Decades

SOURCE: *Sun, Lena H. "Anti-Vaccine Activists Spark a State's Worst Measles Outbreak in Decades."* Washington Post *(May 5, 2017). This article can also be found online at https://www.washingtonpost.com/national/health-science/anti-vaccine-activists-spark-a-states-worst-measles-outbreak-in-decades/2017/05/04/a1fac952-2f39-11e7-9dec-764dc781686f_story.html?utm_term=.fbe17e5ac742 (accessed February 13, 2018).*

INTRODUCTION: *The following article describes the reasons why some members of the Somali American community in Minneapolis, Minnesota, refused to vaccinate their children against measles and how this caused the 2017 measles outbreak there. The author of the article writes that some Somali Americans refuse vaccinations for their children because they fear that vaccines cause autism and are unsafe. Since 2008 the Somali American community has been targeted by anti-vaccine activists who encouraged them not to vaccinate their children.*

MINNEAPOLIS—The young mother started getting advice early on from friends in the close-knit Somali immigrant community here. Don't let your children get the vaccine for measles, mumps and rubella—it causes autism, they said.

Suaado Salah listened. And this spring, her 3-year-old boy and 18-month-old girl contracted measles in Minnesota's largest outbreak of the highly infectious and potentially deadly disease in nearly three decades. Her daughter, who had a rash, high fever and cough, was hospitalized for four nights and needed intravenous fluids and oxygen.

"I thought: 'I'm in America. I thought I'm in a safe place and my kids will never get sick in that disease,'" said Salah, 26, who has lived in Minnesota for more than a decade. Growing up in Somalia, she'd had measles as a child. A sister died of the disease at age 3.

Salah no longer believes that the MMR vaccine triggers autism, a discredited theory that spread rapidly through the local Somali community, fanned by meetings organized by anti-vaccine groups. The activists repeatedly invited Andrew Wakefield, the founder of the modern anti-vaccine movement, to talk to worried parents.

Immunization rates plummeted, and last month the first cases of measles appeared. Soon there was a full-blown outbreak, one of the starkest consequences of an intensifying anti-vaccine movement in the United States and around the world that has gained traction in part by targeting specific communities.

"It's remarkable to come in and talk to a population that's vulnerable and marginalized and who doesn't necessarily have the capacity for advocacy for themselves, and to take advantage of that," said Siman Nuurali, a Somali American clinician who coordinates the care of medically complex patients at Children's Hospitals and Clinics of Minnesota. "It's abhorrent."

Although extensive research has disproved any relationship between vaccines and autism, the fear has become entrenched in the community. "I don't know if we will be able to dig out on our own," Nuurali said.

Anti-vaccine activists defend their position and their role, saying they merely provided information to parents.

"The Somalis had decided themselves that they were particularly concerned," Wakefield said last week. "I was responding to that."

He maintained that he bears no fault for what is happening within the community. "I don't feel responsible at all," he said.

MMR vaccination rates among U.S.-born children of Somali descent used to be higher than among other children in Minnesota. But the rates plummeted from 92 percent in 2004 to 42 percent in 2014, state health department data shows, well below the threshold of 92 to 94 percent needed to protect a community against measles.

Wakefield, a British activist who now lives in Texas, visited Minneapolis at least three times in 2010 and 2011 to meet privately with Somali parents of autistic children, according to local anti-vaccine activists. Wakefield's prominence stems from a 1998 study he authored that claimed to show a link between the vaccine and autism. The study was later identified as fraudulent and was retracted by the medical journal that published it, and his medical license was revoked.

The current outbreak was identified in early April. As of Friday, there were 44 cases, all but two occurring in people who were not vaccinated and all but one in children

10 or younger. Nearly all have been from the Somali American community in Hennepin County. A fourth of the patients have been hospitalized. Because of the dangerously low vaccination rates and the disease's extreme infectiousness, more cases are expected in the weeks ahead.

Measles, which remains endemic in many parts of the world, was eliminated in the United States at the start of this century. It reappeared several years ago as more people —many wealthier, more educated and white—began refusing to vaccinate their children or delaying those shots.

The ramifications already have been significant. A 2014–2015 measles outbreak infected 147 people in seven states and spread to Mexico and Canada. In California, high school students were sent home because of infected classmates. One patient who was unknowingly infectious visited a hospital and exposed dozens of pregnant women and babies, including those in the neonatal intensive care unit. Another adult patient was hospitalized and on a breathing machine for three weeks.

Federal guidelines typically recommend that children get the first vaccine dose at 12 to 15 months of age and the second when they are 4 to 6 years old. The combination is 97 percent effective in preventing the viral disease, which can cause pneumonia, brain swelling, deafness and, in rare instances, death. State health officials are now recommending doses for babies as young as 6 months if there is concern for ongoing measles exposure.

Minnesota's Somali community is the largest in the country. The roots of the outbreak there date to 2008, when parents raised concerns that their children were disproportionately affected by autism spectrum disorder. A limited survey by the state health department the following year found an unexpectedly high number of Somali children in a preschool autism program. But a University of Minnesota study found that Somali children were about as likely as white children to be identified with autism, although they were more likely to have intellectual disabilities.

Around that time, health-care providers began receiving reports of parents refusing the MMR vaccine.

As parents sought to learn more about the disorder, they came across websites of anti-vaccine groups. And activists from those groups started showing up at community health meetings and distributing pamphlets, recalled Lynn Bahta, a longtime state health department nurse who has worked with Somali nurses to counter MMR vaccine resistance within the community.

At one 2011 gathering featuring Wakefield, Bahta recalled, an armed guard barred her, other public health officials and reporters from attending.

Fear of autism runs so deep in the Somali community that parents whose children have recently come down with measles insist that measles is preferable to risking autism. One father, who did not want his family identified to protect its privacy, sat helplessly by his daughter's bed at Children's Minnesota hospital last week as she struggled to breathe during coughing fits.

The 23-month-old was on an IV for fluids and had repeatedly pulled out the oxygen tube in her nose. Her older brother, almost 4, endured a milder bout. Neither had received the MMR vaccine.

The children now have antibodies to protect against measles, but they still need the vaccine to prevent mumps and rubella. Their father, who is 33 and studying mechanical engineering while working as a mechanic, wants to wait. His worry: autism. A colleague has a son "who is mute."

"I would hold off until she's 3 ... or until she fluently starts talking," he said.

His wife no longer harbors doubts, however. As soon as both children are well, she said, "they are going to get the shot."

The pervasive mistrust was evident Sunday night during a meeting, sponsored by several anti-vaccine groups, that drew a mostly Somali crowd of 90 to a Somali-owned restaurant here. Patti Carroll, a member of the Vaccine Safety Council of Minnesota, described its goal as giving parents more information, including about their right to refuse to vaccinate. People have been "bullied big-time" by doctors and public health officials, she said.

The presentation by anti-vaccine activist Mark Blaxill drew cheers and applause. Blaxill, a Boston businessman whose adult daughter has autism, played down the threat of measles and played up local autism rates.

"When you hear people from the state public health department saying there is no risk, that [vaccines] are safe, this is the sort of thing that should cause you to be skeptical," Blaxill said.

Two pediatricians in the audience stepped up to a microphone to denounce the claims.

"I am very concerned, especially in the midst of a measles outbreak, to have folks come into a community impacted by this disease and start talking about links between MMR and autism," said Andrew Kiragu, interim chief of pediatrics at Hennepin Medical Center in Minneapolis. "This is a travesty."

He and the other doctors were interrupted by boos and yelling.

"For God's sake, I want to know if vaccines are safe!" Sahra Osman shouted. She has a nearly adult son who received an autism diagnosis when he was 3. "My people are suffering! We're not ignorant. I read a lot. I know a lot. I educate myself. . . You don't know what you are talking about."

While scores of studies from around the world have shown conclusively that vaccines do not cause autism, that is often not a satisfactory answer for Somali American parents. They say that if science can explain that vaccines do not cause autism, science should be able to say what *does.*

But researchers don't really know. A growing body of evidence suggests that brain differences associated with autism may be found early in infancy—well before children receive most vaccines. Other studies have found that alterations in brain-cell development related to autism may occur before birth. There are some genetic risk factors for autism, and advanced parental age has been associated with the condition.

Meanwhile, the ongoing spread of the anti-vaccine message is making it harder to control the burgeoning number of measles cases.

The groups continue advising parents, "in the middle of their crisis," on how to opt out of vaccines, said pediatric nurse practitioner Patsy Stinchfield, an infection-control expert leading the outbreak response at Children's Minnesota. That message is "exactly the opposite of what clinicians and public health officials are urging, which is to get vaccinated as soon as possible."

Staffers at her hospital have been working round-the-clock to vaccinate hundreds of people who may have been exposed; an MMR dose given within 72 hours of exposure can prevent measles.

When their two sick children are well, Suaado Salah and her husband, Tahlil Wehlie, plan to talk to friends and acquaintances to spread the word that the anti-vaccine groups are wrong and that all youngsters should get immunized. "Because when the kids get sick, it's going to affect everybody. It's not going to affect only the family who have the sick kid," she said. "They make sick for everybody. That's when you wake up and say, 'Okay, what happened?'"

But she understands the apprehension that fed the outbreak. With a parent whose child has autism, she said, "it's something that you're looking for an answer for how it happened and what happened to your kid."

See Also *Childhood Infectious Diseases, Immunization Impacts; Mumps; Rubella*

BIBLIOGRAPHY

Books

Bennett, John E., Raphael Dolin, and Martin J. Blaser. *Mandell, Douglas, and Bennett's Principles and Practice of Infectious Diseases.* 8th ed. Philadelphia: Elsevier/Saunders, 2015.

Periodicals

Brown, Katrina F., et al. "Factors Underlying Parental Decisions about Combination Childhood Vaccinations Including MMR: A Systematic Review." *Vaccine* 28, no. 26 (June 11, 2010): 4235–4248. This article can also be found online at https://www.sciencedirect.com/science/article/pii/S0264410X10005761 (accessed February 15, 2018).

Majumder, Maimuna S., et al. "Substandard Vaccination Compliance and the 2015 Measles Outbreak." *JAMA Pediatrics* 169, no. 5 (May 2015): 494–495. This article can also be found online at https://jamanetwork.com/journals/jamapediatrics/fullarticle/2203906 (accessed February 15, 2018).

Phadke, Varun K., Robert A. Bednarczyk, and Daniel A. Salmon. "Association between Vaccine Refusal and Vaccine-Preventable Diseases in the United States: A Review of Measles and Pertussis." *JAMA* 315, no. 11 (2016): 1149–1158. This article can also be found online at https://jamanetwork.com/journals/jama/article-abstract/2503179?tab=cme&redirect=true (accessed February 13, 2018).

Zipprich, Jennifer, et al. "Measles Outbreak—California, December 2014–February 2015." *Morbidity and Mortality Weekly Report* 64, no. 6 (February 15, 2018): 153–154. This article can also be found online at https://www.cdc.gov/mmwr/preview/mmwrhtml/mm6406a5.htm?s_cid=mm6406a5_w (accessed February 15, 2018).

Websites

Doucleff, Michaeleen. "Why Mumps and Measles Can Spread Even When We're Vaccinated." NPR, April 18, 2014. https://www.npr.org/sections/health-shots/2014/04/18/304155213/why-mumps-and-measles-can-spread-even-when-were-vaccinated (accessed February 15, 2018).

"Measles." World Health Organization, January 2018. http://www.who.int/mediacentre/factsheets/fs286/en/ (accessed February 13, 2018).

"Measles (Rubeola)." Centers for Disease Control and Prevention, February 5, 2018. https://www.cdc.gov/measles/index.html (accessed February 13, 2018).

"Year in Review: Measles Linked to Disneyland." Centers for Disease Control and Prevention, December 2, 2015. https://blogs.cdc.gov/publichealthmatters/2015/12/year-in-review-measles-linked-to-disneyland/ (accessed February 15, 2018).

Susan Aldridge
Claire Skinner

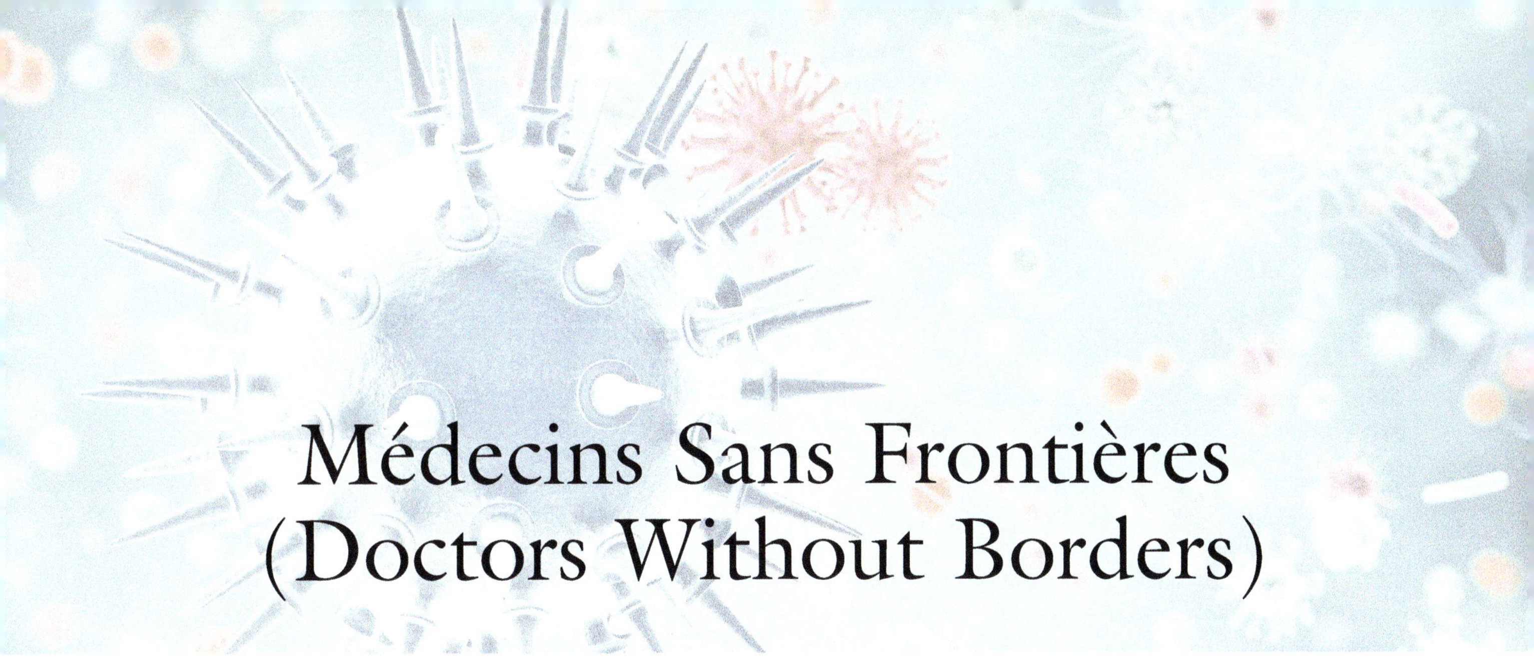

Médecins Sans Frontières (Doctors Without Borders)

Introduction

Médecins Sans Frontières (MSF), known in English as Doctors Without Borders, is an international, independent humanitarian organization designed to provide assistance in emergency situations caused by war or armed conflict, drought, famine, epidemics, disasters (either natural or humanmade), or lack of available health care. It was established in 1971. Among the characteristics that distinguish MSF from other charitable organizations are its independence from government funding (roughly 89 percent of its funding comes from private donations) and its ability and willingness to make public opinion statements. In February 2018 MSF had branches in 28 countries around the world.

Médecins Sans Frontières was awarded the Nobel Peace Prize in 1999 "in recognition of the organization's pioneering humanitarian work on several continents." The organization was thrust into the spotlight again during the 2014–2016 Ebola virus outbreak in West Africa. MSF led the initial medical efforts to treat people infected with Ebola and to contain the outbreak. The organization was sharply critical of the global public health community's response, which it found slow and tepid.

History and Scientific Foundations

Because MSF is an independent international organization, it has no political ties or limitations to prevent it from responding to any situation thought likely to benefit from its assistance. It was not designed to become involved in international governmental affairs. For those involved in the local response of MSF, the effort is a humanitarian one. Traveling staff are primarily volunteers (although their personal expenses are paid, and they may receive a small stipend) who are willing to make themselves available with little notice; they are typically deployed in an area for 6 to 12 months. Assigned locations may be remote and dangerous. MSF hires local staff and provides them with training and materials, and all personnel (MSF core and local staff) work in cooperation with other local and international emergency and relief organizations.

MSF is staffed by physicians, nurses, health care providers, logisticians, technicians, technical and nonmedical personnel, sanitation and water experts, and administrative workers. There is a small core of paid staff, a large number of volunteer workers, and a significant number of local

WORDS TO KNOW

EPIDEMIOLOGY The study of the various factors that influence the occurrence, distribution, prevention, and control of disease, injury, and other health-related events in a defined human population. By the application of various analytical techniques, including mathematical analysis of the data, the probable cause of an infectious outbreak can be pinpointed.

NOBEL PEACE PRIZE An annual prize bequeathed by Swedish inventor Alfred Nobel (1833–1896) and awarded by the Norwegian Nobel Committee to an individual or organization that has "done the most or the best work for fraternity between the nations, for the abolition or reduction of standing armies and for the holding and promotion of peace congresses."

NONGOVERNMENTAL ORGANIZATION (NGO) A voluntary organization that is not part of any government; often organized to address a specific issue or perform a humanitarian function.

POTABLE Water that is clean enough to drink safely.

staffers hired at each major site. MSF had 468 projects in 71 countries in 2016, not including search-and-rescue operations.

Applications and Research

MSF's primary tasks are the provision of basic and emergency physical and mental health care on-site at hospitals and clinics (either existent or created locally by MSF staff), the performance of surgery, the provision of vaccinations and immunizations, the delivering of babies, and the allocation of ready-to-use therapeutic food (RUTF) to malnourished children. MSF also employs experts who are able to dig and construct wells or bring in potable (safe to drink) water to establish a means of supplying clean drinking water. When necessary, MSF also assists in creating temporary shelters and can supply blankets and plastic sheeting materials.

In addition to its emergency operations, MSF operates longer-term projects to treat infectious and communicable diseases such as human immunodeficiency virus (HIV) and acquired immunodeficiency syndrome (AIDS), tuberculosis, and sleeping sickness (a widespread tropical disease spread by the bite of an infected tsetse fly), and to provide physical and mental health treatment for marginalized groups, including drug users, sex workers, street children, incarcerated people, and migrants and other displaced people. MSF also has an expert epidemiology section, which has been used around the world to diagnose, treat, monitor, and contain epidemics of cholera, meningitis, and measles, among other diseases.

By traveling in small teams and enlisting local resources, MSF teams have penetrated war zones and reached refugee groups and epidemic epicenters. Because of its size, well-trained staff, and ability to hire significant numbers of local people to meet personnel needs, MSF is generally able to respond quickly to emergencies. Its teams use highly specialized kits and equipment packs that enable them to carry all needed supplies with them when they mobilize, so they are literally able to "hit the ground running" with no delay before they can begin emergency operations.

Their field kits are tailored to be an exact match for the type of emergency situation, geographic conditions, terrain, environmental conditions, and estimated patient population size. They can set up portable operating theatres, clinics, and hospitals immediately upon arrival in an affected area. They have created myriad treatment and response protocols that are customized to fit any necessary situation; their kits and protocols have been adopted by emergency and relief organizations worldwide.

Impacts and Issues

One of the unique aspects of MSF, in contrast to nearly all other relief and aid organizations, is its commitment to combining humanitarian medical care with outspoken opinion on the causes of worldwide suffering. It is equally vocal on perceived impediments to the provision of effective medical care. For example, MSF has spoken publicly against pharmaceutical companies that refuse to manufacture pediatric dosages of AIDS-related drugs or to provide affordable and appropriate medica-

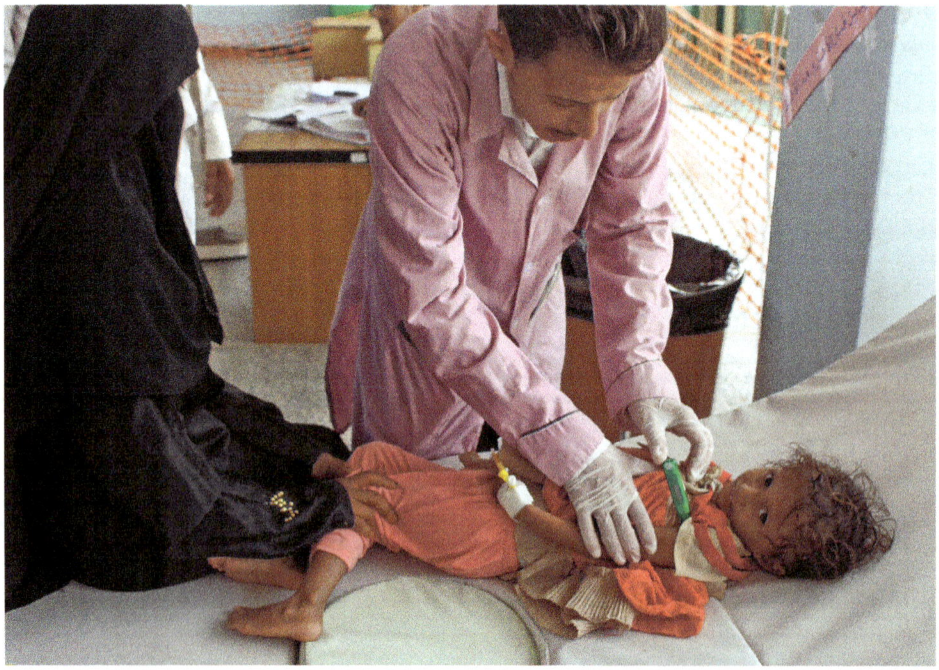

A doctor with Médicins Sans Frontièrs (Doctors Without Borders) cares for a Yemeni child believed to be infected with cholera in 2017. *© AFP Contributor/Getty Images*

tions to African countries hardest hit by the AIDS pandemic. MSF has sought (and received) audiences with the United Nations (UN), various international and governmental organizations, and the worldwide media in an effort to communicate the needs of its various patient groups and to educate the world on violations of international humanitarian doctrines that its teams have witnessed or that they argue have been perpetrated across the globe. Researchers, academics, and scientists associated with MSF publish scholarly articles, create media campaigns, engage in public education programs, and offer presentations and exhibits at local and international conferences in an effort to create public awareness of medical and living conditions in underserved, impoverished, and war-torn areas of the world. MSF has launched a major initiative called the Campaign for Access to Essential Medicines, through which it is trying to help underserved or marginalized populations obtain safe, effective, affordable treatments for such diseases as HIV/AIDS, tuberculosis, and malaria.

MSF led the global response to the Ebola virus outbreak that began in March 2014 in Guinea and spread throughout Guinea, Liberia, and Sierra Leone. MSF personnel were the first to identify in spring 2014 that the mysterious and deadly illness was Ebola and not another viral hemorrhagic fever. By June 2014 MSF publicly stated that the Ebola outbreak was out of control, that it no longer had the resources to fight it on its own, and that governments and other international actors needed to join the effort. The outbreak of the dangerous tropical disease took more than 11,000 lives before it was officially declared over by the World Health Organization (WHO) in January 2016. (MSF, however, argued that the outbreak officially ended in June 2016 after the last flare-up in Liberia.)

According to a report published by MSF in 2015, the international community did not respond to its June 2014 plea for assistance. MSF wrote that the governments of Guinea and Sierra Leone refused to acknowledge the epidemic and that WHO in Guinea and Sierra Leone were slow to act, waiting months before mobilizing emergency teams. Slow response from governments and WHO, MSF contended, meant that some MSF-staffed Ebola treatment centers were extremely understaffed and underprepared. In Monrovia, Liberia, for instance, the MSF center ELWA 3 was at full capacity and was forced to turn away most people with the disease. People died waiting in line to receive care. MSF noted that fear of the Ebola virus—its high mortality rate and disturbing physical symptoms—deterred the international community from investing in the outbreak's containment. MSF argued in its report that it was not until two people with Ebola arrived in the developed world in August and September 2014 (one in Spain and one in the United States) that the international community fully mobilized to respond.

In September 2014 MSF addressed the UN Security Council and called on UN members to assist in the Ebola response by dispatching their biohazard and disaster response teams to Ebola-affected areas. In its 2015 report, MSF wrote, "Helpful pledges of equipment and logistical support came in September, yet sufficient deployment of qualified and trained medical staff to treat patients on the ground did not." This meant that local health care workers and international groups, like MSF, were the ones on the frontlines, not governments.

The work of MSF on the ground in West Africa during the Ebola outbreak, as well as its work alerting the world at large to the Ebola outbreak and its demands for action, positioned MSF as an outspoken advocate of accessible medical care for all people (not just those living in developed countries) and a vocal critic of public and private health organizations that respond poorly to health care emergencies.

PRIMARY SOURCE

Doctors Without Borders Has Mixed Feelings about Award for Ebola Work

SOURCE: *Kelto, Anders. "Doctors Without Borders Has Mixed Feelings about Award for Ebola Work." NPR, September 18, 2015. https://www.npr.org/sections/goatsandsoda/2015/09/18/441417614/americas-nobel-goes-to-doctors-without-borders (accessed February 27, 2018).*

INTRODUCTION: *Médecins Sans Frontières (MSF), or Doctors Without Borders, is an international humanitarian organization that provides emergency medical assistance in more than 70 nations. MSF's mission is to provide medical care in to the world's neediest populations, often those touched by war, conflict, epidemic disease, natural disaster, and famine. In the following interview, the head of MSF's United States board of directors, Deane Marchbein, talks to National Public Radio (NPR) correspondent Anders Kelto about the organization's work in West Africa during the Ebola virus outbreak there in 2014 and 2015 and the prestigious award MSF won for its efforts. Marchbein admits she has some ambivalence about MSF receiving an award. She then describes MSF's on-the-ground work in West Africa, her concern that the world is not prepared for another Ebola outbreak, and her hope for better tools for quickly diagnosing Ebola, among other topics.*

The Lasker Award, given for outstanding contributions to medicine and medical research, is sometimes referred to as "America's Nobel Prize." Since the award was established in 1945, more than 80 laureates have gone on to win the Nobel.

The medical aid group Medicins Sans Frontieres (Doctors Without Borders) is one of four recipients this year, accepting the award for its contributions to the fight against Ebola. I spoke with the president of the U.S. Board of Directors, Dr. Deane Marchbein, who was in New York for the presentation.

First of all, congratulations on winning the Lasker.

Thank you. But this award is for our colleagues in the field who were on the front lines of the Ebola outbreak since the beginning. So many of them suffered so much and worked so hard to help people. They put in extremely long hours in very hot and dangerous conditions, having to wear hazmat suits inside tents filled with sick patients and with huge lines of people waiting to get in. The hazmat suits you have to put on so carefully and take off even more carefully so that you don't contaminate yourself. It's incredibly dangerous and exhausting work. And many health care workers from local communities died in disproportional numbers. The numbers are just staggering.

I think a lot of people picture Doctors Without Borders as a mostly Western organization, with American and European doctors parachuting into Africa. But that's not exactly the case.

No. First of all, for every foreign doctor there are roughly 10 locally hired staff, most of them health care workers. These are the people who were leading the fight against Ebola and providing so much of the most important and dangerous care. Without good local staff, we would not have been able to do much of anything. The international staff come and go, so the local staff provide the institutional memory. I learn more from the local staff members than I do from anyone else, especially about how to communicate with patients.

Secondly, our international staff is global. Many of the doctors who were traveling to West Africa to fight Ebola were from other parts of Africa. Some were from Asia and Australia. And also Europe and North America. It's an incredibly interesting group of people.

Give us a sense of MSF's involvement in the early days of the Ebola outbreak.

We were in Guinea when the first case was identified, and we helped identify the first case. We were involved in direct patient care. We set up treatment centers; we had people on the front lines treating patients. In previous epidemics, there would typically be one case in a remote area, so we would set up a treatment center in that area and the outbreak would be contained. This Ebola outbreak was different because it appeared in many places at once. Unfortunately, our initial effort to get national leaders and the World Health Organization to recognize that this was bigger and different and catastrophic fell on deaf ears.

A lot has been written about the failed international response to Ebola. Do you think the world is now better prepared for the next big outbreak, whether Ebola or something else?

I'm not sure. I know there's a big focus on global health security right now, with the U.S. and other nations investing lots of money in epidemiological responses—tracking the spread of diseases. That's good. But I'm not seeing a focus on who is going to do direct patient care. There's a lot more to an epidemic than just the epidemiology. Research and development needs to step up their game. We need better diagnostic tools. Can you imagine if we had a good point-of-care diagnostic test for Ebola? Then we could instantly determine who to admit and who to discharge. If we had really effective treatments, that would also be a game changer. Vaccine developments are starting to look promising. MSF is now vaccinating its front-line health care workers, and we hope to have more good data on effectiveness soon. But I'm concerned that these vaccines might be stockpiled in wealthy nations and won't make it to poor and middle-income countries. So overall, if you ask if I'm optimistic, I'd say I'm not.

Where do things stand with Ebola now?

The numbers have decreased dramatically. Over the last couple weeks, there have only been one or two new cases per week. We are still following nearly 300 contacts in Sierra Leone and Guinea. We need to get to zero. The tail end of an epidemic is long and difficult. For example, right now what's disturbing is that we're still seeing new cases not related to the contacts we're following. We're still seeing unsafe burials, which says to me we still have a long way to go. We need to focus on education so that people know how to stay safe.

And the long-term effects of Ebola are frightening. So many health care workers died during the outbreak—doctors, nurses, ambulance drivers, midwives. And these are countries that already had fragile medical infrastructures. So, for example, the Ebola outbreak has taken a lot of progress that's been made in maternal mortality and pushed it back 20 years.

What do you see as MSF's role in international health care going forward?

We're used to being the guys on the ground who just do it. We're not used to being the guys in the meeting who establish policy. Ebola and the Lasker Award have now given us visibility that, to be honest, we're not comfortable with. Ebola has pushed us to be visible in ways that we've never had to be before. Going forward, we now have a responsibility to share with others. It's important that we collaborate with other actors. Are we in a position to dictate the international response to medical crises? Absolutely not. But we do have on-the-ground experience that's important. And we have to share that. The Lasker award has given us the forum to engage with others in the global health community in a meaningful way.

This year, NPR won a Peabody Award for its coverage of the Ebola outbreak. I felt conflicted about this. There's something strange about celebrating an award that's grounded in unspeakable suffering. Do you have the same feeling with the Lasker?

Absolutely. We're excited about the recognition. We're deeply appreciative. And, again, this is about the people in the field who were doing the hardest, most dangerous work. But there's also a real feeling of guilt that our success and our fame is a direct result of other people's extreme misery.

SEE ALSO *CDC (Centers for Disease Control and Prevention); Developing Nations and Drug Delivery; United Nations Millennium Goals and Infectious Disease; World Health Organization (WHO)*

BIBLIOGRAPHY

Books

Fox, Renée C. *Doctors Without Borders: Humanitarian Quests, Impossible Dreams of Médecins Sans Frontières.* Baltimore, MD: Johns Hopkins University Press, 2014.

Redfield, Peter. *Life in Crisis: The Ethical Journey of Doctors Without Borders.* Berkeley: University of California Press, 2013.

Periodicals

O'Carroll, Lisa. "Ebola Crisis Brutally Exposed Failures of the Aid System, Says MSF." *Guardian* (March 23, 2014). This article can also be found online at https://www.theguardian.com/global-development/2015/mar/23/ebola-crisis-response-aid-who-msf-report-sierra-leone-guinea (accessed February 27, 2018).

Torjesen, Ingrid. "World Leaders Are Ignoring Worldwide Threat of Ebola, Says MSF." *BMJ* 349 (September 5, 2014). This article can also be found online at http://www.bmj.com/content/349/bmj.g5496 (accessed February 27, 2018).

Websites

"Founding of MSF." Doctors Without Borders/Médecins Sans Frontières. http://www.doctorswithoutborders.org/founding-msf (accessed February 27, 2018).

"The Nobel Peace Prize 1999: Médecins Sans Frontières." Nobelprize.org. http://nobelprize.org/peace/laureates/1999/index.html (accessed February 26, 2018).

"Pushed to the Limit and Beyond: A Year into the Largest Ever Ebola Outbreak." Doctors Without Borders/Médecins Sans Frontières, March 19, 2015. https://www.msf.org.uk/sites/uk/files/ebola_-_pushed_to_the_limit_and_beyond.pdf (accessed February 27, 2018).

Paul Davies
Claire Skinner

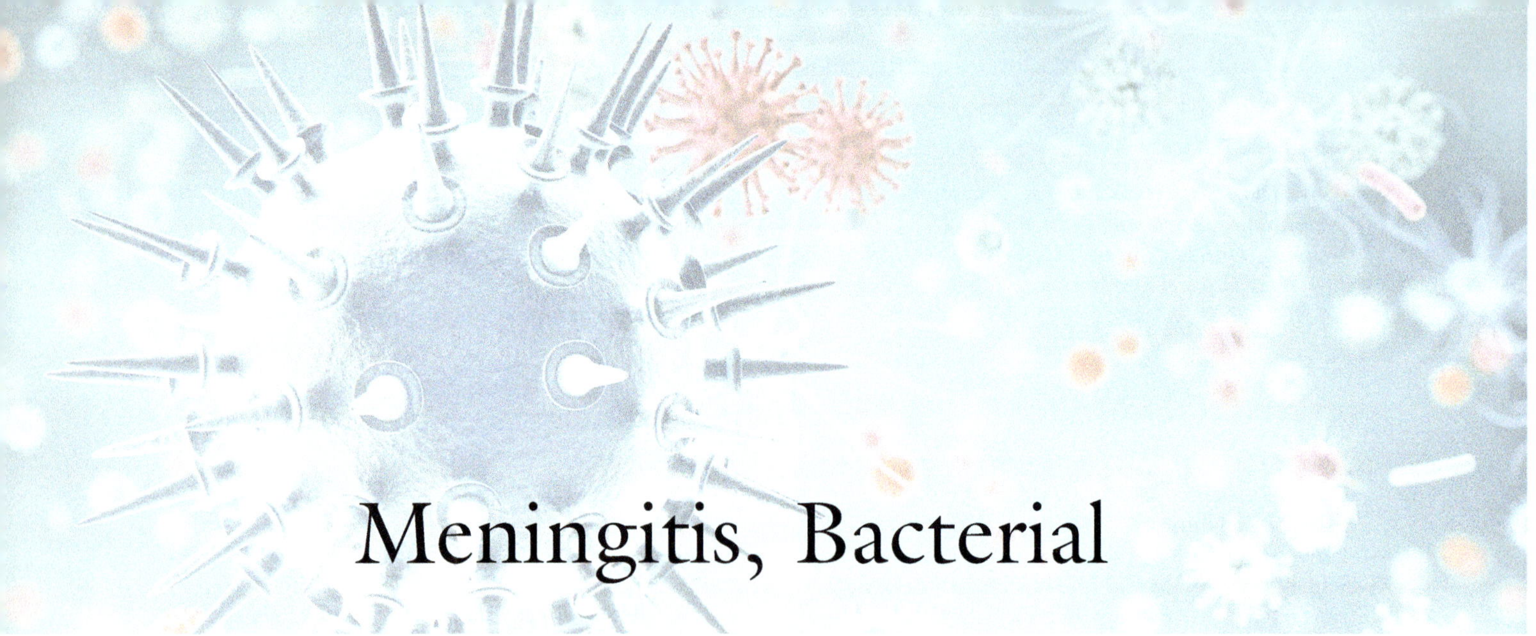

Meningitis, Bacterial

Introduction

Bacterial meningitis refers to an acute disease caused by several different types of bacteria. The disease causes the meninges, the membrane that surrounds the brain and the spinal cord, to become inflamed. Inflammation-related swelling of the membrane can cause serious problems, including septicemia, brain damage, coma, and death.

Bacterial meningitis results from a bacterial infection of the blood that spreads to the cerebrospinal fluid, which is the fluid that flows around the meninges. The illness is serious. If not treated, the death rate is high. Those who survive may be left with lifelong disabilities including impaired hearing due to damage to the hair cells of the ear responsible for converting sound waves to the electrical signals that the brain can interpret. Longer-term problems also include paralysis, mental dysfunction, and paralysis.

WORDS TO KNOW

BIOFILM A population of microorganisms that forms following the adhesion of bacteria, algae, yeast, or fungi to a surface. These surface growths can be found in natural settings such as on rocks in streams or in infections such as can occur on catheters. Microorganisms can colonize living or inert, natural or synthetic surfaces.

INTRAVENOUS In the vein. For example, the insertion of a hypodermic needle into a vein to instill a fluid, withdraw or transfuse blood, or start an intravenous feeding.

MENINGITIS BELT An area of Africa, south of the Sahara Desert, stretching from the Atlantic to the Pacific coasts, where meningococcal meningitis is common.

SEPTICEMIA Blood poisoning characterized by prolonged fever, chills, anorexia, and anemia in conjunction with tissue lesions.

STRAIN A subclass or a specific genetic variation of an organism.

Disease History, Characteristics, and Transmission

Like other bacterial diseases, such as plague and anthrax, bacterial meningitis has likely been occurring for thousands of years. Comparison of the genetic material of the bacteria that cause meningitis with other bacteria indicates that bacterial meningitis is ancient in its origin. Documented descriptions of the disease date back to 1805, when an outbreak was described in Geneva, Switzerland. In the 19th century meningitis also decimated the ruling family in Japan.

Bacterial meningitis can be caused by a number of different strains of bacteria. The bacteria that are the most common causes are *Neisseria meningitidis* (also known as meningococcus), *Streptococcus pneumoniae* (also known as pneumococcus), and *Listeria monocytogenes.* Less commonly, *Pseudomonas aeruginosa*, *Staphylococcus aureus*, *Streptococcus agalactiae*, and *Haemophilus influenzae* type b (also known as Hib) can cause meningitis. In addition, *Mycobacterium tuberculosis* can be a problem in developing countries.

The less common bacteria are often not a health concern. But, in someone whose immune system is inefficiently functioning due to age, illness, or deliberate immunosuppression (as occurs following organ transplantation to avoid rejection of the transplant), the bacteria are capable of causing meningitis infection.

The source of the infection is sometimes never determined. It is known that bacteria can spread from an ear infection to the meninges. The most common source is the spread of bacteria into the bloodstream from an infection in the heart (endocarditis). In endocarditis the infecting bacteria can adhere to tissues and produce a colony of bacteria that is enclosed in a slime-like overlay. The organized structure, which is called a biofilm, can then slough off bacteria into the bloodstream.

Infection of the meninges by bacteria usually produces a fever, a headache, sensitivity to light, and mental disorientation. In addition, when the spinal cord is involved, a person can experience pain in the neck and the legs that becomes progressively worse. These symptoms also occur in the type of meningitis that is caused by viruses. Distinction between the two types of meningitis usually requires obtaining the bacteria from the cerebrospinal fluid. The bacteria are detected when the cerebrospinal fluid is added to a culture (a source of nutrients for the bacteria). With time the bacteria grow and divide repeatedly to form a visible mound of cells, called a colony.

Bacteria can also be detected by a staining procedure called a Gram stain. Depending on which of two stains the bacteria retain, they may be distinguished as Gram-positive (bacteria with a single membrane) or Gram-negative (bacteria with two membranes). This distinction is important for determining the most effective antibiotic to use. *Streptococcus pneumoniae* is an example of a Gram-positive bacterium that can cause meningitis. *Neisseria meningitidis* is an example of a Gram-negative bacterium that causes meningitis.

In the meningitis caused by *Neisseria meningitidis*, the first symptom to appear is often a rash that appears as small, reddish or purple spots. The rash can spread quickly over the middle part of the body, legs, the conjunctiva in the eyes, and parts of the hands and feet.

Scope and Distribution

Bacterial meningitis occurs all over the world. In areas such as sub-Saharan Africa, the disease is especially prevalent.

The main reason for the global distribution of bacterial meningitis is the equally wide distribution of the bacteria. Some of the bacteria capable of causing meningitis are normally found in the mouth. These can be spread from person to person by coughing or kissing.

In developed countries, including the United States, meningitis is rare and occurs as isolated cases. More widespread epidemics still occur in other parts of the world, especially in northern Africa.

Treatment and Prevention

Bacterial meningitis is treated with antibiotics. The choice of the antibiotic depends on the bacterium causing the infection. When treating an infection suspected of being meningitis, several antibiotics effective against the widest variety of bacteria are often used even before

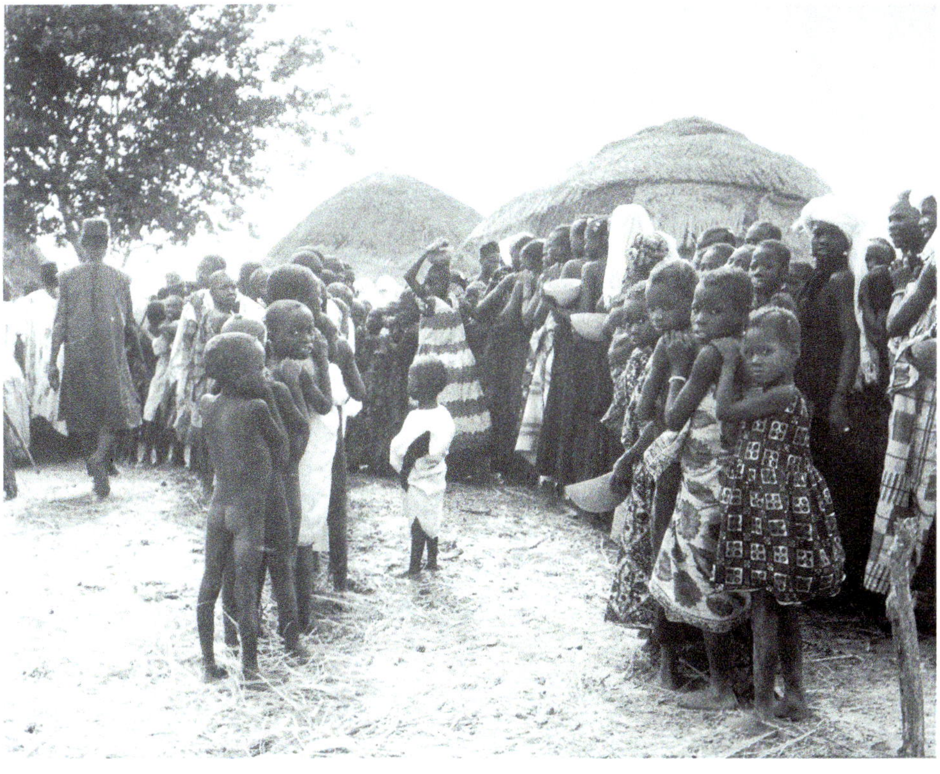

Villagers in Africa's "meningitis belt" are particularly at risk of contracting the disease. © Bettmann/Getty Images

ASEPTIC AND BACTERIAL MENINGITIS

The meninges are a series of three membranes covering the brain and spinal cord that act to protect and partition the central nervous system (CNS). The membranes comprising the meninges are the dura mater, arachnoid layer, and pia mater.

Meningitis is an inflammation of the meninges that can occur when there is an infection near the brain or spinal cord, such as a respiratory infection in the sinuses, mastoids, or cavities around the ear. Disease organisms can also travel to the meninges through the bloodstream. The first signs may be a severe headache and neck stiffness followed by fever, vomiting, and a rash and then convulsions leading to loss of consciousness.

Meningitis generally involves two types: nonbacterial meningitis, which is often called aseptic meningitis, and bacterial meningitis, which is referred to as purulent meningitis. Nonbacterial meningitis may be caused by viruses, drug reactions, or central nervous syndrome disorders.

the cause of the infection has been identified. This is done because rapid treatment is important in minimizing the danger of the infection. Once the cause of the infection has been determined, the antibiotic therapy can be adjusted to target the particular bacterium.

Antibiotics are usually given intravenously. This produces a high level of the antibiotic throughout the body. Because the antibiotic can be continuously supplied, the dose can remain consistent during the several weeks of treatment usually required.

Vaccines directed toward *Neisseria* and *Haemophilus* have lessened childhood meningitis dramatically. As of 2017 these included three meningococcal A conjugate vaccines (which protect against two or more pathogens) and a vaccine directed against the outer layer (capsule) of the bacteria. In addition, both newborns and the elderly benefit from vaccines against *Streptococcus pneumoniae*. The American Association of Pediatrics recommends vaccinating newborns against pneumococcal meningitis as early as six weeks after birth. The US Centers for Disease Control and Prevention (CDC) recommends vaccination for everyone over the age of 65.

As of 2017 research efforts focused on group A vaccines. Group A meningococcus still caused large epidemics in Africa, as well as India, Pakistan, Nepal, and China. Group A outbreaks had not occurred in North America since the 1950s.

■ Impacts and Issues

Bacterial meningitis continues to be a significant health concern, especially in some underdeveloped regions of the world. As of June 2015, more than 220 million people under 29 years of age had been vaccinated in 15 nations in Africa. In both underdeveloped and developed countries, the disease is a serious health concern for infants less than a year old. The high fever that can accompany bacterial meningitis can cause seizures. Because bacterial meningitis is contagious, infants in day care facilities are at increased risk for the disease.

Despite the ongoing problem of bacterial meningitis, the introduction of vaccines has greatly reduced the prevalence of the infection. For survivors of a bacterial meningitis infection, hearing loss can be a consequence. Artificial implants in an area of the ear called the cochlea can sometimes restore hearing to a level that allows normal function. However, to be fully effective, the implant must be installed within weeks of the end of an infection. This is because the fluid that has accumulated in the ear changes consistency over time and becomes almost jellylike, making installation of an implant impossible.

SEE ALSO *Bacterial Disease; Childhood Infectious Diseases, Immunization Impacts; Meningitis, Viral*

BIBLIOGRAPHY

Books

Preux, Pierre-Marie, and Michel Dumas. *Neuroepidemiology in Tropical Health.* New York: Academic Press, 2017.

Periodicals

Costerus, Joost M., et al. "Community-Acquired Bacterial Meningitis." *Current Opinion in Infectious Diseases* 30, no. 1 (February 2017): 135–141.

Websites

"Meningitis." Centers for Disease Control and Prevention, April 10, 2017. https://www.cdc.gov/meningitis/index.html (accessed November 20, 2017).

"Meningococcal Meningitis." World Health Organization, December 2017. http://www.who.int/mediacentre/factsheets/fs141/en/ (accessed November 29, 2017).

"Meningococcal Vaccination: What Everyone Should Know." Centers for Disease Control and Prevention, May 19, 2017. https://www.cdc.gov/vaccines/vpd/mening/public/index.html (accessed November 20, 2017).

Brian Hoyle

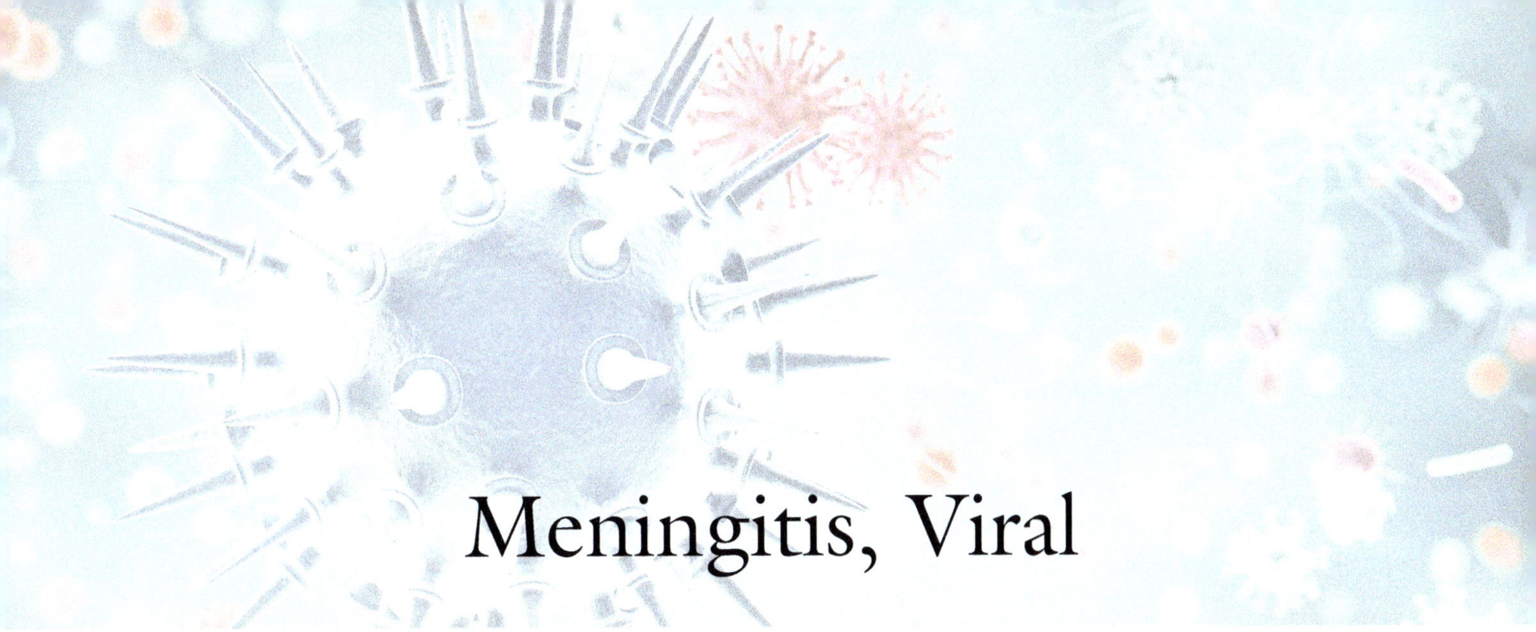

Meningitis, Viral

Introduction

Meningitis is an inflammation of the meninges, which are the tissues covering the brain and spinal cord. In 2015 approximately 380,000 people died from meningitis, according to the Meningitis Research Foundation. Of the more than 1 million that survived, many live with physical and mental problems such as permanent scars, arthritis, and brain injuries caused by the malady.

There are two types of meningitis: bacterial meningitis and aseptic meningitis. Bacterial meningitis, such as meningococcal meningitis, is a bacterial infection. Aseptic meningitis is caused by viral, fungal, or other infection. It also may have a noninfectious cause such as an underlying illness. Some types of aseptic meningitis respond to antibiotic treatment, but viral meningitis does not. Aseptic meningitis causes tens of thousands of hospital admissions per year in the United States alone. Sometimes viral meningitis is referred to as aseptic meningitis, probably because viruses are most commonly the cause of aseptic meningitis.

Viral meningitis is less serious than bacterial meningitis. Most people who contract viral meningitis recover without treatment, but sometimes treatment is necessary, especially to some of the most vulnerable humans: babies and young children. In addition, viral meningitis is difficult to differentiate between the other types of meningitis so it is prudent to visit a medical professional when the symptoms common to meningitis occur.

The symptoms of meningitis vary, but severe headache, neck stiffness, and an aversion to light are common. Accurate diagnosis of the cause of meningitis, through examination of the cerebrospinal fluid, is important because treatment for bacterial meningitis needs to begin as soon as possible. Viral meningitis is rarely fatal but may occasionally cause permanent disability.

Disease History, Characteristics, and Transmission

More than 80 percent of cases of aseptic meningitis are caused by viruses. These include arboviruses, enteroviruses (ribonucleic acid [RNA] viruses within the family *Picornaviridae*), herpesviruses, human immunodeficiency virus (HIV), influenza (flu) virus, measles, mumps, and the rodent-borne virus lymphocytic choriomeningitis (LCM).

The enteroviruses, such as Enterovirus 71, account for around 90 percent of cases of viral meningitis. These viruses live in the human intestine. They are also a common cause of colds, sore throats, stomach upsets, and diarrhea. Until the introduction of the MMR (measles, mumps, and rubella) vaccine, the mumps virus was the most common cause of viral meningitis among children under five years of age.

Although viral meningitis is usually considered a mild illness, it often requires physician care or hospitalization for treatment, especially for those at higher risk than most people, including children younger than five (even more so for babies younger than one month) and people with weakened immune systems. Some symptoms of viral meningitis are caused by pressure on the brain from inflamed meninges and include a severe headache and stiffness of the neck.

Viruses Associated with Meningitis

Arboviruses (viruses borne by mosquitoes and ticks, such as West Nile virus and La Crosse virus)

Enteroviruses (ribonucleic acid [RNA] viruses within the family *Picornaviridae*)

Herpesviruses (including varicella-zoster virus, which causes chickenpox and shingles, and herpes simplex viruses)

Human immunodeficiency virus (HIV) (causes acquired immunodeficiency syndrome [AIDS])

Influenza (flu) virus

Lymphocytic choriomeningitis (LCM) virus (a rodent-borne virus that is a member of the family *Arenaviridae*)

Measles

Mumps

WORDS TO KNOW

ARBOVIRUS A virus typically spread by blood-sucking insects, most commonly mosquitoes. More than 100 types of arboviruses cause disease in humans. Yellow fever and dengue are two examples.

ARTHROPOD A member of the largest single animal phylum, consisting of organisms with segmented bodies, jointed legs or wings, and exoskeletons.

BACTERIA Single-celled microorganisms that live in soil, water, plants, and animals and whose activities range from the development of disease to fermentation. They play a key role in the decay of organic matter and the cycling of nutrients. Bacteria exist in various shapes, including spherical, rod-shaped, and spiral. Some bacteria are agents of disease. Different types of bacteria cause many sexually transmitted diseases, including syphilis, gonorrhea, and chlamydia. Bacteria also cause diseases such as typhoid, dysentery, and tetanus. Bacterium is the singular form of bacteria.

DNA Deoxyribonucleic acid, a double-stranded, helical molecule that is found in almost all living cells and that determines the characteristics of each organism.

ENTEROVIRUS A group of viruses that contain ribonucleic acid as their genetic material. They are members of the picornavirus family. The various types of enteroviruses that infect humans are referred to as serotypes, in recognition of their different antigenic patterns. The different immune response is important, as infection with one type of enterovirus does not necessarily confer protection to infection by a different type of enterovirus. There are 64 different enterovirus serotypes. The serotypes include polio viruses, coxsackie A and B viruses, echoviruses, and a large number of what are referred to as non-polio enteroviruses.

HERPESVIRUS A family of viruses, many of which cause disease in humans. The herpes simplex 1 and herpes simplex 2 viruses cause infection in the mouth or on the genitals. Other common types of herpesvirus include chickenpox, Epstein-Barr virus, and cytomegalovirus. Herpesvirus is notable for its ability to remain latent, or inactive, in nerve cells near the area of infection, and to reactivate long after the initial infection. Herpes simplex 1 and 2, along with chickenpox, cause familiar skin sores. Epstein-Barr virus causes mononucleosis. Cytomegalovirus also causes a flu-like infection but can be dangerous to the elderly, infants, and those with weakened immune systems.

VIRUS Essentially nonliving repositories of nucleic acid that require the presence of a living prokaryotic or eukaryotic cell for the replication of the nucleic acid. There are a number of different viruses that challenge the human immune system and that may produce disease in humans. A virus is a small, infectious agent that consists of a core of genetic material—either deoxyribonucleic acid (DNA) or ribonucleic acid (RNA)—surrounded by a shell of protein. Very simple microorganisms, viruses are much smaller than bacteria that enter and multiply within cells. Viruses often exchange or transfer their genetic material (DNA or RNA) to cells and can cause diseases such as chickenpox, hepatitis, measles, and mumps.

A high fever and photophobia (aversion to light) are also common side effects of enterovirus-associated meningitis. Patients may have a strong desire to be in a quiet, dark room. Additional symptoms in infants include a low desire to eat, irritability, and sleepiness or trouble waking up from sleep. Other symptoms in adults include sleepiness or trouble waking up from sleep, nausea, vomiting, loss of appetite, and lack of energy.

Many people with viral meningitis experience nonspecific symptoms such as vomiting, cough, diarrhea, loss of appetite, and rash. Many such cases are mistaken as the flu. Where symptoms are severe, bacterial meningitis might be suspected, and immediate hospital admission is appropriate. Occasionally, the virus affects the brain itself, causing encephalitis, an inflammation that can lead to lasting brain damage.

The symptoms of viral meningitis have a rapid onset, usually within 3 to 10 days after exposure. Other causes of aseptic meningitis may produce disease following a slower course. In the early stages, it can be difficult to distinguish aseptic and bacterial meningitis. One clue is that the person with aseptic meningitis usually remains alert. Confusion and disorientation may occur with bacterial meningitis, along with neurological abnormalities such as deafness or visual disturbances; such symptoms are uncommon in viral meningitis.

It is more difficult to identify the symptoms of viral meningitis in infants. Fever, fretfulness and irritability, difficulty in waking up, or refusal to eat may be noted.

An individual with possible meningitis symptoms should seek prompt medical attention. Though viral meningitis is generally less severe, early symptoms of viral and

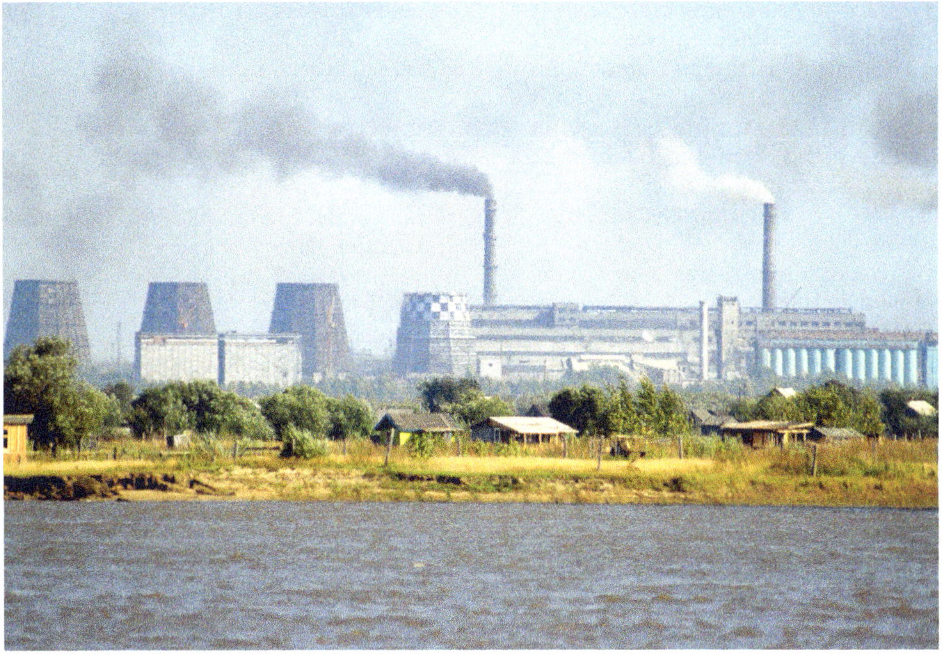

Summer outbreaks of viral meningitis are common in Khabarovsk, Russia. Swimmers in the Amur River are at risk of contracting the disease. © *Wolfgang Kaehler/LightRocket/Getty Images*

bacterial meningitis may be difficult to distinguish without medical testing. Bacterial meningitis requires antibiotic treatment and can cause permanent disability or death if left untreated.

Diagnosis involves an examination of the cerebrospinal fluid (CSF), the watery fluid that bathes and protects the brain and spinal cord. A sample of CSF is removed from around the spinal cord in a procedure called a lumbar puncture (sometimes called a spinal tap). Bacteria can usually be cultured from this in cases of bacterial meningitis.

In addition, diagnosis can involve the use of PCR tests, where PCR stands for polymerase chain reaction, a technique used to analyze deoxyribonucleic acid (DNA). In such tests the results can correctly diagnosis viral meningitis with an estimated sensitivity of more than 95 percent. Other diagnostic tools include collecting samples by swabbing the nose and throat for further testing in a laboratory. Stool and urine samples are sometimes also taken for diagnostic testing.

Most people make a full recovery from viral meningitis, with no lasting effects. Sometimes recovery is slow, with patients experiencing headache, tiredness, fatigue, depression, and loss of concentration for many months.

Transmission of meningitis depends on the underlying viral cause. Enteroviruses, the most common cause, are spread through direct contact with the saliva, mucus, or nasal mucous of an infected person. Person-to-person transmission through exposure to coughs and sneezes, shaking hands, or touching something previously handled by a sufferer is possible, although unusual.

Enteroviruses are also shed into the feces of people who are infected. Children who are not yet toilet trained may spread the virus in this way. Adults changing the diaper of an infected infant may therefore be at risk. The infectious period lasts from about 3 days after a person has been infected until 10 days after they develop the symptoms of viral meningitis.

Scope and Distribution

Viral meningitis is far more common than bacterial meningitis. It is found mainly among babies, children, and adolescents. There are an estimated 300,000 cases per year in the United States. Because many mild cases are not reported to a physician, the true number of cases is unknown. Moreover, as the main purpose of hospital investigations is to rule out bacterial meningitis, the specific virus involved in an aseptic case is often not detected.

There are seasonal variations in viral meningitis, depending on the virus involved. Viruses borne by arthropods, such as mosquitoes and ticks, cause disease most often in late summer and early fall. Enteroviruses follow a similar seasonal pattern. Mumps virus tends to cause meningitis most often in late winter and early spring, whereas herpes meningitis does not have a seasonal pattern.

Treatment and Prevention

There is no general antiviral treatment for viral meningitis, although the antiviral drug acyclovir (ACV) might be used if the cause is found to be herpes simplex. Accurate diagnosis is needed to be sure the cause really is viral. Bacterial meningitis and some types of aseptic meningitis respond to antibiotic therapy. Sometimes antibiotics will be started straight away if a person is admitted to hospital with any form of meningitis, but these will be discontinued if the cause is found to be viral. Bedrest, fluids, and medication to relieve pain and fever are the best approach to alleviating the symptoms associated with viral meningitis.

It is difficult to prescribe a specific way of preventing viral meningitis because there are so many different causes of the disease. The MMR vaccine will prevent meningitis caused by the measles and mumps virus. Because the majority of cases are caused by enteroviruses, which are spread by infected saliva and other bodily secretions, good personal hygiene stems transmission. Regular and thorough handwashing can stop enteroviruses from spreading. Potentially contaminated surfaces should be cleaned with soap and water or diluted bleach. These precautions are especially important in institutions such as child care centers, schools, public bathing facilities, and dormitories.

■ Impacts and Issues

Viral meningitis is a serious condition. Though viral meningitis may be alleviated without treatment, individuals who suspect that they have meningitis should seek medical care. Viral meningitis rarely has serious long-term health consequences in otherwise healthy individuals. Bacterial meningitis, however, can be life threatening. Because early symptoms of viral and bacterial meningitis are similar, prompt and accurate diagnosis is necessary to distinguish between the two forms of meningitis.

In August 2006 an outbreak of viral meningitis was reported from the region of Khabarovsk, on the Russia–China border, affecting more than 800 children. It is thought they contracted the infection through either swimming in the Amur River or from drinking its waters. There had been ongoing summer outbreaks of viral meningitis in this area for some time, arising usually from fecal contamination of the Amur's waters. Swimming is therefore prohibited in the summer months. During the 2006 outbreaks, public health doctors tried to stem the outbreak by asking parents to keep their children away from social activities, as the meningitis could be spread by infected air droplets.

The Meningitis Research Foundation, a nonprofit organization in the United Kingdom, aims to more accurately and quickly identify the causes of individual cases of meningitis so that improved drugs and vaccines can be developed to better counteract the disease. As such, in 2015 it coordinated a study to determine if new genomic techniques could be developed and used to increase the accuracy and speed of diagnosing meningitis in children, while at the same time reducing the costs for diagnosis and treatment. The research study began on May 14, 2015, and was still active as of February 2018.

See Also *Enterovirus 71 Infection; Herpes Simplex 1 Virus; Herpes Simplex 2 Virus; HIV; Influenza; Measles (Rubeola); Mumps*

BIBLIOGRAPHY

Books

Christodoulides, Myron, ed. *Meningitis: Cellular and Molecular Basis.* Wallingford, UK: CAB International, 2013.

Ferri, Fred F. *Ferri's Clinical Advisor 2018.* Philadelphia: Elsevier, 2018.

Myers, James W., and Jonathan P. Moorman. *Gantz's Manual of Clinical Problems in Infectious Disease.* Philadelphia: Wolters Kluwer, 2015.

Shrader, Anthony L., ed. *Meningitis: Symptoms, Management and Potential Complications.* Hauppage, NY: Nova Biomedical, 2014.

Periodicals

McGill, F., M. J. Griffiths, and T. Solomon. "Viral Meningitis: Current Issues in Diagnosis and Treatment." *Current Opinion in Infectious Diseases* 30, no. 2 (April 2017): 248–256. This article can also be found online at https://www.ncbi.nlm.nih.gov/pubmed/28118219 (accessed February 22, 2018).

Websites

"Meningitis and You—the Facts." Meningitis Now. https://www.meningitisnow.org/fight-for-now/wtf-meningitis/identifying-disease/meningitis-and-you-facts/ (accessed February 16, 2018).

Pollard, Andrew, et al. "Using New Genomic Techniques to Identify the Causes of Meningitis in UK Children." Meningitis Research Foundation, May 14, 2015. https://www.meningitis.org/research-projects/genomic-techniques-identify-causes-of-meningitis (accessed February 16, 2018).

"Viral Meningitis." Centers for Disease Control and Prevention, April 15, 2016 https://www.cdc.gov/meningitis/viral.html (accessed February 16, 2018).

"Viral Meningitis." Meningitis Now. https://www.meningitisnow.org/meningitis-explained/what-is-meningitis/types-and-causes/viral-meningitis/ (accessed February 16, 2018).

"Viral Meningitis." Meningitis Research Foundation. https://www.meningitis.org/meningitis/what-is-meningitis/viral-meningitis (accessed February 16, 2018).

Wan, Cordia. "Viral Meningitis." Medscape, August 22, 2017. https://emedicine.medscape.com/article/1168529-overview (accessed February 16, 2018).

Susan Aldridge
William Arthur Atkins

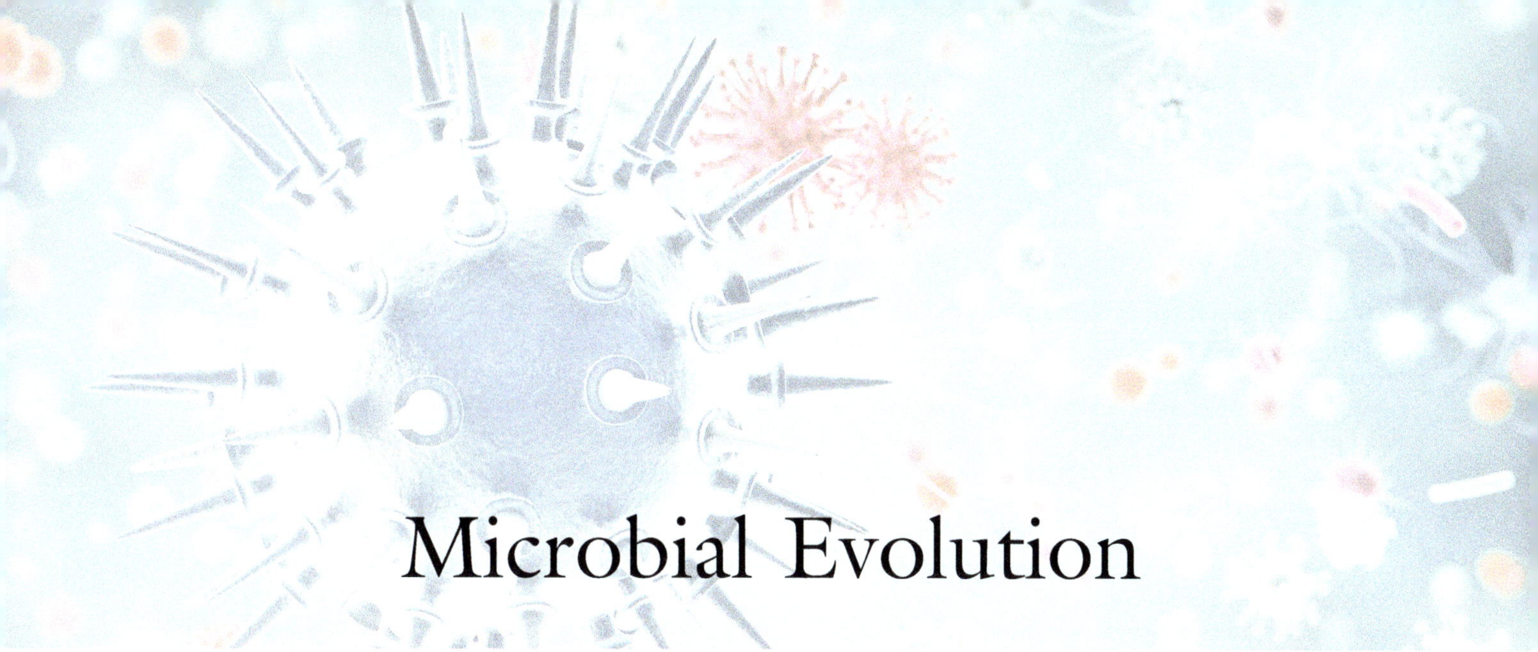

Microbial Evolution

Introduction

Microbial evolution refers to the genetically driven changes that occur in microorganisms and that are retained over time. Some microbial changes can be in response to a selective pressure. The best examples of this are the various changes that can occur in bacteria in response to the presence of antibiotics. These changes can make an individual bacterium less susceptible or completely resistant to the killing action of one or more antibiotics.

Other microbial changes can occur randomly in the absence of any selective pressure. These changes, which often are due to a change in the sequence of the units (nucleotides) that comprise an organism's genetic material, can confer an advantage to the organism, as compared to unaltered organisms. In the classic scenario of evolution, such an advantageous trait will be retained and can be passed on to future generations of the organism.

Gene transfer between bacteria can occur even between species that are not related to one another. This so-called horizontal gene transfer is an important form of microbial evolution that occurs in nature, and it can be important in infectious disease—for example, in the acquisition of a gene that determines antibiotic resistance.

In contrast to Darwinian evolution, which takes place over millions of years, microbial evolution can occur within hours. This is because some bacteria can grow and divide in about 20 minutes under ideal growth conditions. A bacterium containing an altered gene that confers a survival advantage can, over 24 hours, give rise to thousands of progeny that carry the same gene. Each new bacterium can in turn give rise to thousands of progeny by the next day. Thus, a mutation can rapidly spread in a bacterial population and, because the trait is capable of being transferred to unrelated bacteria, to other bacterial populations as well.

Human-imposed selective pressures, such as the overuse or misuse of antibiotics; factory-farm types of agriculture that crowd animals in a small space; and the encroachment of humans on previously undisturbed territory are influencing microbial evolution and the emergence or re-emergence of infectious diseases.

WORDS TO KNOW

ANTIBIOTIC RESISTANCE The ability of bacteria to resist the actions of antibiotic drugs.

BACTERIOPHAGE A virus that infects bacteria. When a bacteriophage that carries the diphtheria toxin gene infects diphtheria bacteria, the bacteria produce diphtheria toxin.

HORIZONTAL GENE TRANSFER A major mechanism by which antibiotic resistance genes get passed between bacteria. It accounts for many hospital-acquired infections.

MUTATION A change in an organism's DNA that occurs over time and may render it less sensitive to drugs that are used against it.

PLASMID A circular piece of DNA that exists outside of the bacterial chromosome and copies itself independently. Scientists often use bacterial plasmids in genetic engineering to carry genes into other organisms.

SELECTIVE PRESSURE The tendency of an organism that has a certain characteristic to be eliminated from an environment or to increase in numbers. An example is the increased prevalence of bacteria resistant to multiple kinds of antibiotics.

■ History and Scientific Foundations

Darwinian evolution can be depicted as a tree, with the original organism at the base of the trunk and the myriad evolutionary changes that occur over time generating the branches and even smaller twigs at their tips. Put another way, this route of evolution is vertical, with genetic changes transferred from one generation of a species to succeeding generations.

In contrast, evidence that has been accumulating since the 1970s has firmly established that microbial evolution occurs differently. The tree analogy is inaccurate when describing microbial evolution. Rather, microbial evolution is considered more like a web or a net, with the transfer of genetic information occurring between many different species simultaneously rather than between succeeding generations of one type of microbe.

This wider, interspecies transfer is called horizontal transfer. It is one route by which a bacterium can become resistant to one or more antibiotics. A bacterium that carries the genetic determinants for resistance to an antibiotic may be able to transfer the gene to another, unrelated bacterium, which then also becomes resistant to the antibiotic.

The transfer of genes between bacteria can occur in several ways. A gene that resides in the deoxyribonucleic acid (DNA) of a donor bacterium can be transferred to the recipient bacterium through a tube that transiently connects the two cells. Once inside the recipient, the inserted DNA can become part of the recipient's genome (its hereditary information encoded in its DNA) and express its encoded product.

Bacterial genes can also reside on more mobile genetic elements known as plasmids. Plasmids are more easily transferable between bacteria. Genes that code for products that render a cell resistant to particular antibiotics can be located on plasmids. If a bacterium that possesses an antibiotic-resistance gene is adjacent to another bacterium (not necessarily the same type of bacterium), a copy of the plasmid can move to the recipient bacterium, which then becomes resistant to the antibiotic(s).

A third genetic mechanism of bacterial evolution involves bacteriophages—viruses that specifically infect a type of bacteria (for example, various types of coliphages infect various strains of *Escherichia coli*). When a bacteriophage infects a bacterium, the viral genetic material can insert into the host's genetic material. When the viral material is excised, some of the host's genetic material can be removed as well, to become part of the genome of the bacteriophage. A subsequent infection by the bacteriophage of another bacterium can transfer genes from the first bacterium to the second bacterial host. If the new gene confers an advantage to the second bacterium, it will be retained and passed on to subsequent generations of that bacterium.

The processes described above are directed in the sense that a genetic trait that changes an organism is transferred from one organism to another. In contrast, a final mechanism of microbial evolution—mutation—can occur

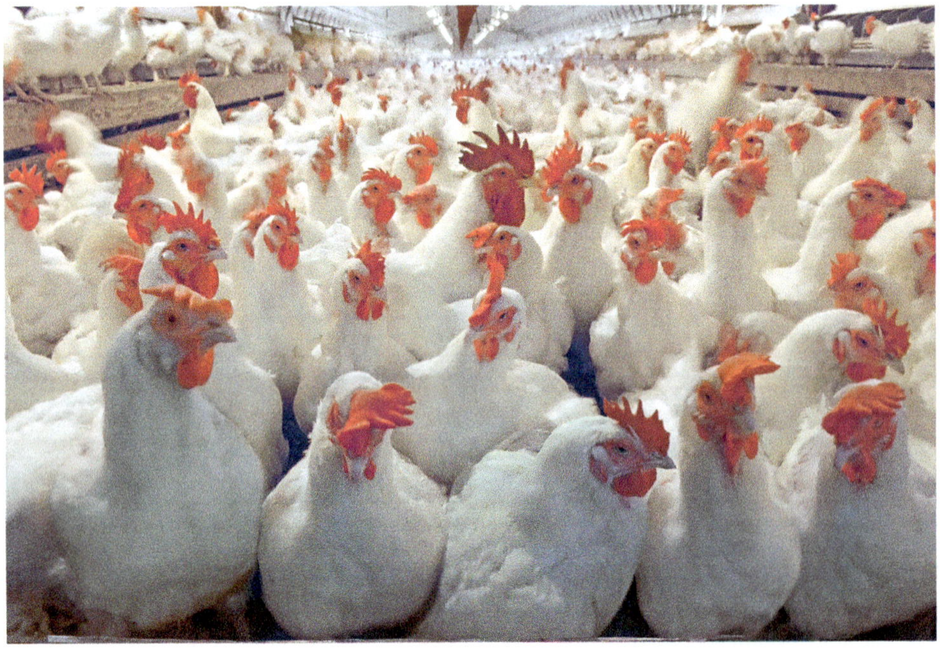

Crowded poultry farms created the perfect conditions for the evolution of avian influenza. © *Lester Lefkowitz/Getty Images*

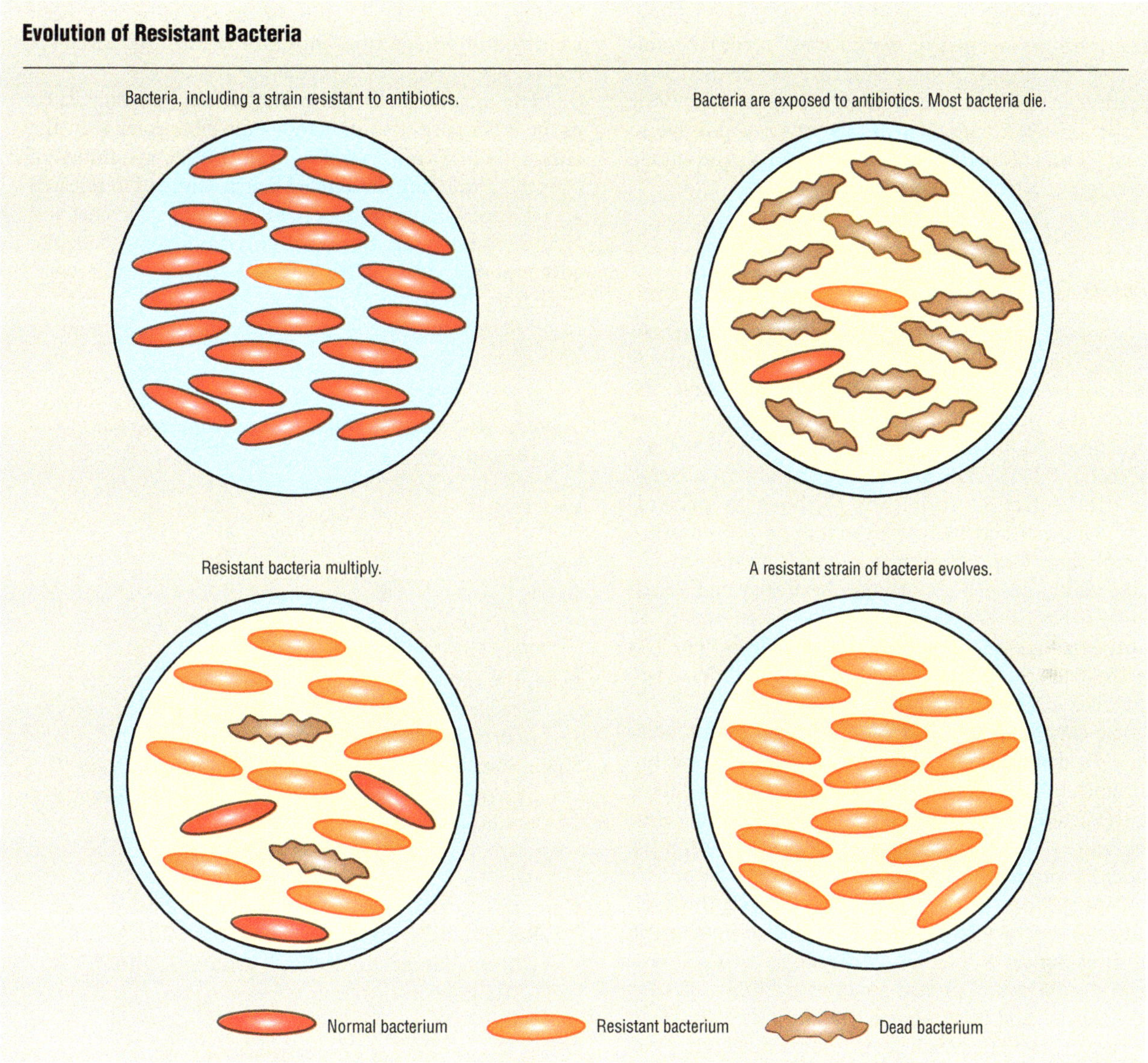

randomly. A change in the arrangement of nucleotides that makes up a gene can occur by chance during the replication of the DNA. For example, one nucleotide can be substituted for another. Alternatively, additional nucleotides may be accidentally inserted or may be deleted. If the genetic change is not drastic enough to completely disable the gene's action, then the protein produced will be different. Sometimes this difference can be advantageous to the microbe. For example, the altered protein may produce enhanced activity of an enzyme that degrades antibiotics, or it may produce a membrane protein that adopts a different three-dimensional configuration that makes the microbial surface more resistant to antimicrobial compounds. Once again, such an advantageous mutation will be retained and can be passed to subsequent generations.

Applications and Research

The ability of bacteria to evolve via horizontal gene transfer has been exploited in genetic engineering that involves the deliberate insertion of a certain gene into a recipient bacterium and the expression of the gene product by the recipient. Indeed, this aspect of biotechnology is essentially a faster version of the natural pace of microbial evolution.

The acquisition of a gene by a microorganism can be tracked. Similar genes can be isolated from various organisms, and the sequence of nucleotides that makes up the gene can be deduced. By comparing the gene sequences, researchers can determine how precisely the sequences match. Sequences from different organisms that match exactly provide strong evidence that the gene arose in a single organism and was passed on to another organism. Because changes in a genetic sequence will occur randomly over time, the degree of gene difference can be used as an indication of how recently a gene was acquired by one microbe, relative to another. In this way, it is possible to generate a sort of map of the movement of a gene among microbes over a long period of time.

■ Impacts and Issues

The ability of disease-causing microorganisms, particularly bacteria and viruses, to evolve is a fundamentally important factor in infectious diseases. For example, the horizontal acquisition of a gene that encodes for the production of a potent and destructive toxin created *Escherichia coli* O157:H7, which can cause a serious and even lethal infection in humans. Without the gene, *E. coli* is a normal and harmless resident of the intestinal tract of warm-blooded creatures, including humans. In another example, genetic changes have spawned a variety of *Mycobacterium tuberculosis* that is resistant to all antibacterial agents used to treat tuberculosis. The fact that the bacterium is also easily passed from person to person is a cause for concern.

The emergence of avian influenza (caused by an influenza virus designated H5N1) is one example of how human agricultural practices can influence microbial evolution. The tremendous crowding-together of poultry that is done to optimize the income generated by a poultry farm made it easier for viral disease to spread in a flock. Then, the ability of many viruses to rapidly mutate allowed the avian influenza virus to spread—first from bird to human and later from human to human. While the latter is still rare, sporadic outbreaks of human-transmitted H5N1 infection have occurred, and the geographic range of the virus seems to be expanding. The possibility that this serious and sometimes fatal disease will develop into a global epidemic is real and has spurred efforts by agencies, including the World Health Organization (WHO) and the US Centers for Disease Control and Prevention (CDC), to monitor the disease and participate in efforts to develop a vaccine.

As of 2017 other emerging microbial diseases include Zika virus encephalopathy, H1N1 virus responsible for swine influenza ("swine flu"), chikungunya virus infection, and various bacterial infections that are resistant to multiple antibiotics. For example, the chikungunya virus has expanded its range from Africa, Asia, and Europe prior to 2013 to the Caribbean, North America, and South America. As of 2017 illnesses due to the virus have been identified in 45 countries in the Americas, with over 1.7 million suspected cases, according to the CDC.

The fact that microbial evolution can be manipulated in the laboratory has implications for bioterrorism. In the aftermath of World War II (1939–1945), a number of countries, including the United States, engaged in research aimed at designing more potently infectious bacterial and viral diseases. While this research was discontinued, the advent of molecular biology in the 1970s has created legitimate fears that rogue nations, organizations, or individuals could design and deploy a deadly version of a contagious microorganism.

SEE ALSO *Antibiotic Resistance; Emerging Infectious Diseases*

BIBLIOGRAPHY

Books

Bayry, Jagadeesh, ed. *Emerging and Re-emerging Infectious Diseases of Livestock.* New York: Springer, 2017.

Pulcini, Céline, et al, eds. *Antimicrobial Stewardship, Volume 2: Developments in Emerging and Existing Infectious Diseases.* London: Elsevier, 2017.

Shah, Sonia. *Pandemic: Tracking Contagions, from Cholera to Ebola and Beyond.* New York: Sarah Crichton, 2016.

Periodicals

Collier, Beth-Ann, et al. "Clinical Development of a Recombinant Ebola Vaccine in the Midst of an Unprecedented Epidemic." *Vaccine* 35, no. 35 (2017): 4465–4469.

Websites

"Final Trial Results Confirm Ebola Vaccine Provides High Protection against Disease." World Health Organization. http://www.who.int/mediacentre/news/releases/2016/ebola-vaccine-results/en/ (accessed November 15, 2017).

"NIAID Emerging Infectious Diseases/Pathogens." National Institute of Allergy and Infectious Diseases. https://www.niaid.nih.gov/research/emerging-infectious-diseases-pathogens (accessed November 15, 2017).

Brian Hoyle

Microorganisms

■ Introduction

Microorganisms, also called microbes, are life forms that are too small to be seen with the naked eye but that play an important role in human health and disease. The main types of microorganisms are bacteria, fungi, protozoa, and viruses. The first three are unicellular organisms, of which only bacteria have a nucleus. Viruses, however, need to be inside a host cell to survive.

Microbes occupy a wide range of ecological niches. Some live inside the human intestine or on the skin; others are found in soil, on the ocean floor, or even in the Arctic ice cap. Microbes have potential for both benefit and harm, and accordingly they may be nonpathogenic or pathogenic. Gut flora, for example, keep the digestive system healthy by breaking down and metabolizing indigestible food products. On the other hand, pathogenic microbes cause a wide range of diseases, ranging from cold and flu to tuberculosis, acquired immunodeficiency syndrome (AIDS), and cholera. In addition, commensal microorganisms are present on body surfaces such as the skin, mucosa, respiratory tract, and vagina.

■ History and Scientific Foundations

Microbes were first observed in 1674 by Dutch biologist Antoni van Leeuwenhoek (1632–1723) using a primitive microscope he had invented. He observed what he called "animalcules" of all shapes and sizes in samples from many sources. The origin and function of these life forms was widely discussed over the next two centuries, but it was not until the 19th century that Louis Pasteur (1822–1895) and Robert Koch (1843–1910) finally laid down the scientific foundations of microbiology.

Pasteur's work in the 1870s and 1880s showed that putrefaction depended on the action of microbes. He later developed pasteurization, a technique of gentle heating that stops food and drink from spoiling by decreasing their levels of microbial contamination. Meanwhile, Koch isolated the anthrax bacillus in 1876 and the tuberculosis bacillus in 1882. By the end of the century, the microbes responsible for plague, meningitis, gonorrhea, typhoid, tetanus, diphtheria, dysentery, and pneumonia had been discovered and characterized.

Koch pushed forward the germ theory of disease, which rested on his four postulates. First, the microorganism had to be present in all cases of the disease. Second, one had to be able to isolate the responsible microorgan-

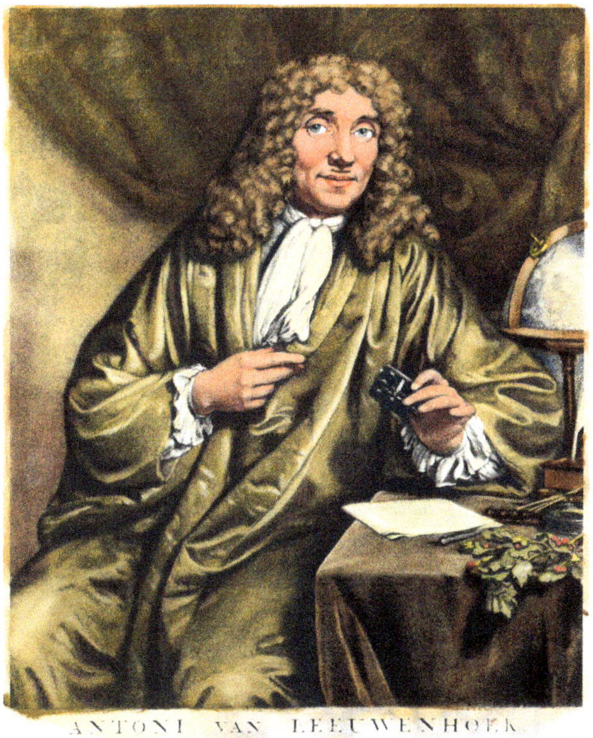

Dutch biologist Antoni van Leeuwenhoek. With the help of his new invention, the microscope, Leeuwenhoek discovered microorganisms in 1674. © Bettmann/Getty Images

WORDS TO KNOW

COLONIZATION The process of occupation and increase in number of microorganisms at a specific site.

COMMENSALISM A relationship wherein two different organisms share the same area/region but neither benefit each other or cause harm to each other.

IMMUNOCOMPROMISED Having an immune system with reduced ability to recognize and respond to the presence of foreign material.

PATHOGEN A disease-causing agent, such as a bacterium, a virus, a fungus, or another microorganism.

PUTREFACTION The process of decay or decomposition by which organic matter is broken down.

ism and then cultivate and identify it in the laboratory. Finally, on reinjection to other lab animals, the disease had to be reproduced and remain the same as the original pathogen.

Bacteria are single-celled organisms of 2 micrometers average length and 0.5 micrometers average diameter. They occur in a range of characteristic shapes from which their names are sometimes derived: for instance, rods (bacilli), spheres or ovals (cocci), and spirals (spirochaetes). Bacteria do not have a nucleus, and their genetic material (deoxyribonucleic acid [DNA]) lies free in the cell or on tiny circular structures called plasmids. They cause a range of infections, including sore throats, pneumonia, and food poisoning, as well as serious diseases such as tuberculosis (caused by mycobacterium species).

Fungi and protozoa have a cell structure that is more like that of a human cell, with the nucleus carrying their DNA. Protozoa are single-celled microbes, including diverse types of organisms such as plasmodia and trypanosomes, which often have complex life cycles and interactions with their human hosts. They cause some serious tropical diseases, including malaria.

The fungi group includes yeasts, molds, and mushrooms. They play an important role in decomposing biological material, such as dead plants, and in the food and drink industry. Some fungi cause diseases of the skin or hair, such as athlete's foot. Some fungi remain as common flora in healthy individuals but may become pathogenic in immunocompromised hosts (for example, the Candida species, which causes thrush, yeast infections, and more). Viruses were first discovered in the late 1880s when it was realized that some disease agents could pass through filters that would usually hold back the smallest bacteria. These filtrates were implicated in diseases such as yellow fever and foot-and-mouth disease (a disease of animals). Unlike other microbes, viruses need a living cell to thrive and replicate. Without a host, they die. Viruses are responsible for a range of human diseases, including hepatitis, AIDS, the common cold, influenza, and some forms of pneumonia and meningitis.

REAL-WORLD USE OF MICROBES

- Polymerase chain reaction (popularly known as PCR) is a technique widely used in molecular biology to amplify a single copy of a segment of deoxyribonucleic acid (DNA) into thousands of copies.
- PCR is used in clinical and research laboratories for a broad array of applications, such as research involving DNA cloning and sequencing, diagnostics, forensic science, and other genetic manipulations.
- Kary Mullis (1944–) developed PCR for Cetus Corporation in 1983. It revolutionized molecular biology and earned him the Nobel Prize in Chemistry in 1993.

■ Applications and Research

Understanding microbiology leads to a better appreciation of many diseases, which can allow for more accurate diagnosis and effective treatment. Sometimes one microorganism can cause many different diseases, such as the bacterium *Staphylococcus aureus*, which causes strep throat, scarlet fever, and toxic shock syndrome. On the other hand, one disease can often be caused by many different microorganisms. For instance, pneumonia can be caused by adenovirus, respiratory syncytial virus, influenza virus, parainfluenza virus, and cytomegalovirus. Among bacteria the following are known to cause pneumonia: *Streptococcus pneumoniae*, *Chlamydia pneumoniae*, *Haemophilus influenzae*, *Klebsiella pneumonia*, and *Pseudomonas aeruginosa*. The disease can also be caused by mycoplasma, which are organisms that have some of the characteristics of both bacteria and viruses.

Most microorganisms are actually harmless to human health. There are two kinds of pathogens: strict pathogens and opportunistic pathogens. A strict pathogen is always associated with disease; these include *Mycobacterium tuberculosis*, which causes tuberculosis (TB) and rabies virus. However, most human infections are caused by opportunistic pathogens, which normally live on the skin or in the nose or mouth or in the surroundings without causing any problems. However, if they enter unprotected sites like the blood, they may cause disease. Among the most common of the opportunistic pathogens are *Pneumocystis carinii*, *Candida albicans*, and cytomegalovirus, which often cause complications among those with HIV/AIDS.

Impacts and Issues

Infectious diseases, including HIV/AIDS, malaria, and tuberculosis, continue to claim millions of lives each year. There are also emerging infections, such as severe acute respiratory syndrome (SARS), Zika virus, and bird flu, that have the potential to cause pandemics. However, science has shown that infections can be defeated: smallpox has been eradicated, and polio and measles are nearly eradicated.

Antibiotics (which are active against bacteria and fungi but not viruses) have been the major weapon against infection. Starting with the introduction of penicillin in the 1940s, doctors now have a wide range of drugs against infections such as TB. Antiviral drugs are also making AIDS a chronic disease rather than a death sentence. However, microorganisms are developing resistance against these pharmaceutical weapons, so it is vital that scientists continue to extend their understanding of microbial physiology so new drugs against infection can be developed.

Vaccines are the other major tool against microbial disease. They generally contain either a killed or weakened version of the microbe or a part of the organism, such as a protein borne on its surface, which can elicit an immune response. There is an urgent need for the development of vaccines against malaria, AIDS, and hepatitis C.

A new and more detailed level of understanding of microbiology may come from genetics. The genomes of several medically significant microbes have now been sequenced. The genomics approach means a better understanding of how microorganisms cause human illnesses and new opportunities for developing more effective antibiotics, antivirals, and vaccines.

See Also *Antibiotic Resistance; Germ Theory of Disease; Koch's Postulates; Microbial Evolution; Microscope and Microscopy*

BIBLIOGRAPHY

Books

Lock, Stephen, Stephen Last, and George M. Dunea, eds. *The Oxford Illustrated Companion to Medicine*. Oxford, UK: Oxford University Press, 2001.

Murray, Patrick, Ken S. Rosenthal, and Michael A. Pfaller. *Medical Microbiology*. Philadelphia: Elsevier, 2016.

Periodicals

Benedict, Kaitlin, et al. "Emerging Issues, Challenges, and Changing Epidemiology of Fungal Disease Outbreaks." *Lancet Infectious Diseases* 17, no. 12 (December 2017): e403–e411.

Yates, Tom A., et al. "The Transmission of *Mycobacterium tuberculosis* in High Burden Settings." *Lancet* 16, no. 2 (February 2016): 227–238.

Websites

"Antibiotic/Antimicrobial Resistance." Centers for Disease Control and Prevention, January 8, 2018. https://www.cdc.gov/drugresistance/index.html (accessed January 29, 2018).

"Basic Concepts in Microscopy." Zeiss. https://www.zeiss.com/microscopy/us/solutions/reference/basic-microscopy.html (accessed January 29, 2018).

"The Nobel Prize in Chemistry 2014." Nobelprize.org. http://www.nobelprize.org/nobel_prizes/chemistry/laureates/2014/ (accessed January 29, 2018).

"Polymerase Chain Reaction (PCR)." National Center for Biotechnology Information (NCBI). https://www.ncbi.nlm.nih.gov/probe/docs/techpcr/ (accessed February 5, 2018).

Susan Aldridge
Kausalya Santhanam

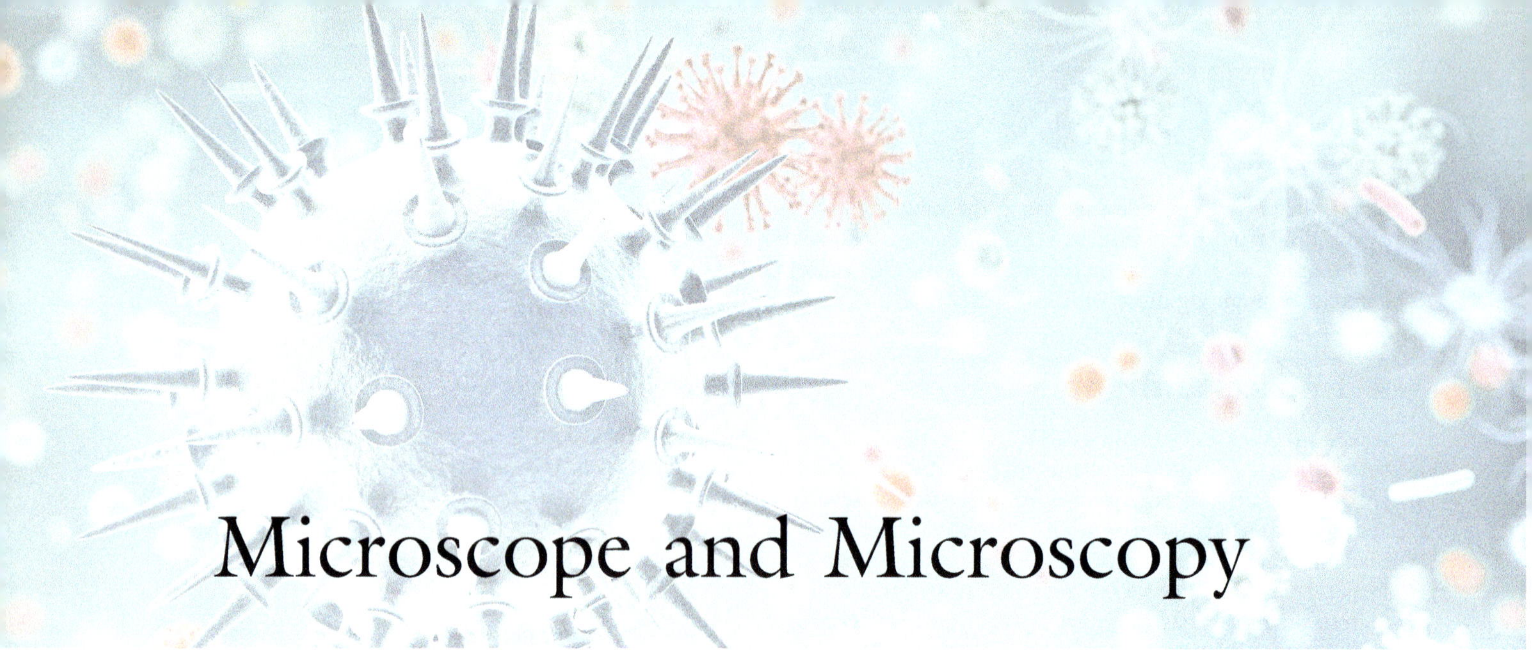

Microscope and Microscopy

Introduction

The microscope is a powerful tool for investigating the complexity of biological life. This includes looking at the identity and structure of microorganisms, which is essential in the diagnosis of many infectious diseases. Microorganisms are not visible to the human eye, owing to their small size. The light microscope focuses visible light on a clinical specimen and allows the microbe to be magnified through a series of lenses.

Staining a specimen that may contain microorganisms is an additional aid to identification. Certain microbes absorb certain stains, whereas others do not. This provides a way of identifying them. Modern microscopic technologies allow for quick and accurate identification of microorganisms involved in human disease. However, microscopic identification is only one part of the investigation required to diagnose an infectious disease. The patient's medical history and biochemical tests on clinical specimens are equally important.

WORDS TO KNOW

ELECTRON A fundamental particle of matter carrying a single unit of negative electrical charge.

LENS An almost clear, biconvex structure in the eye that, along with the cornea, helps focus light onto the retina. It can become infected with inflammation, for instance, when contact lenses are improperly used.

MICROORGANISM With only a single currently known exception (i.e., *Epulopiscium fishelsonia*, a bacterium that is billions of times larger than the bacteria in the human intestine and is large enough to view without a microscope), microorganisms are minute organisms that require microscopic magnification to view. To be seen, they must be magnified by an optical or electron microscope. The most common types of microorganisms are viruses, bacteria, blue-green bacteria, some algae, some fungi, yeasts, and protozoans.

STAINING The use of chemicals to identify target components of microorganisms.

WAVELENGTH A distance of one cycle of a wave, such as the distance between the peaks on adjoining waves that have the same phase.

History and Scientific Foundations

The magnifying power of lenses (curved pieces of glass that can bend light) was first mentioned in the writings of the Roman philosophers Seneca and Pliny the Elder during the 1st century CE. However, they were not put to practical use until the development of spectacles toward the end of the 13th century. Dutch spectacle makers Zacharias Janssen and his son Hans began to experiment with the magnifying properties of combinations of lenses in the late 16th century. News of their work spread to Galileo Galilei (1564–1642), who produced a primitive microscope in 1609. But it was Dutch biologist Antoni van Leeuwenhoek (1632–1723) who first realized the potential of the microscope for the study of the world of microorganisms.

Looking at specimens from many different sources, van Leeuwenhoek described the appearance of what he called animalcules, namely yeast, bacteria, and protozoa. During his life he wrote more than 100 papers on his discoveries for both the Royal Society of England and the French Academy. English scientist Robert Hooke (1635–1703) later confirmed van Leeuwenhoek's work and improved on the design of his light microscope. Toward the end of the 19th century, there were some major advances in microscope manufacture. American science pioneer Charles A. Spencer (1813–1881) founded an industry based on instruments with fine optical systems, similar to the basic light microscopes of the 21st century.

Magnifications of 1,250 are achievable with ordinary white light and up to 5,000 if blue light is used. The microscope is a compound optical system. A condensing lens focuses a bright beam of light on the clinical specimen, which is placed on a platform called a stage and covered with a thin sheet of glass called a cover slip. The objective lens, near the specimen, forms an intermediate magnified image, which is magnified again by the eyepiece, which is close to the eye.

The magnification of a light microscope is limited by the wavelength of the light used to illuminate the specimen. Light microscopes cannot distinguish objects that are smaller than half the wavelength of the light. Because white light has an average wavelength of around 0.55 micrometers, any two lines that are closer together than half of this (0.275 micrometers) will show up as a single line. An object that is smaller than this in diameter will show up as a blur or not at all. Smaller objects, such as viruses, can only be seen with the aid of the electron microscope, in which the beam of illuminating light is replaced by a beam of electrons. Electron microscopes were invented in the late 1940s and are much more expensive than light microscopes. High-powered electron microscopes have allowed the study of viruses and the so-called biological ultrastructure, which comprises the fine details of cells and tissues and their activities in health and disease. Superresolution microscopy can extend resolution to the scale of nanometers.

Applications and Research

The chemical and dyestuffs industry that began in Germany in the 19th century provided microscopists with a range of stains that made the identification of specific microorganisms much easier. Many of these are still used in modern microbiology laboratories. For instance, Gram's stain distinguishes between bacteria on the basis of the thickness and composition of their cell wall. Gram-positive bacteria, such as *Corynebacterium, Listeria*, and *Bacillus* species, which have a more complex cell wall, absorb the stain, trapping it between the cell wall layers. Gram-negative bacteria, such as *Salmonella* and *Shigella* species, do not retain the stain because their walls lack one of the layers.

Ziehl-Neelsen stain is useful for identifying the mycobacteria that cause tuberculosis (TB), and silver methenamine stains chitin, a carbohydrate found in the walls of fungi and *Pneumocystis jirovecii* (formerly known as *Pneumocystis carinii*), the microorganism that causes an otherwise rare form of pneumonia among human immunodefi-

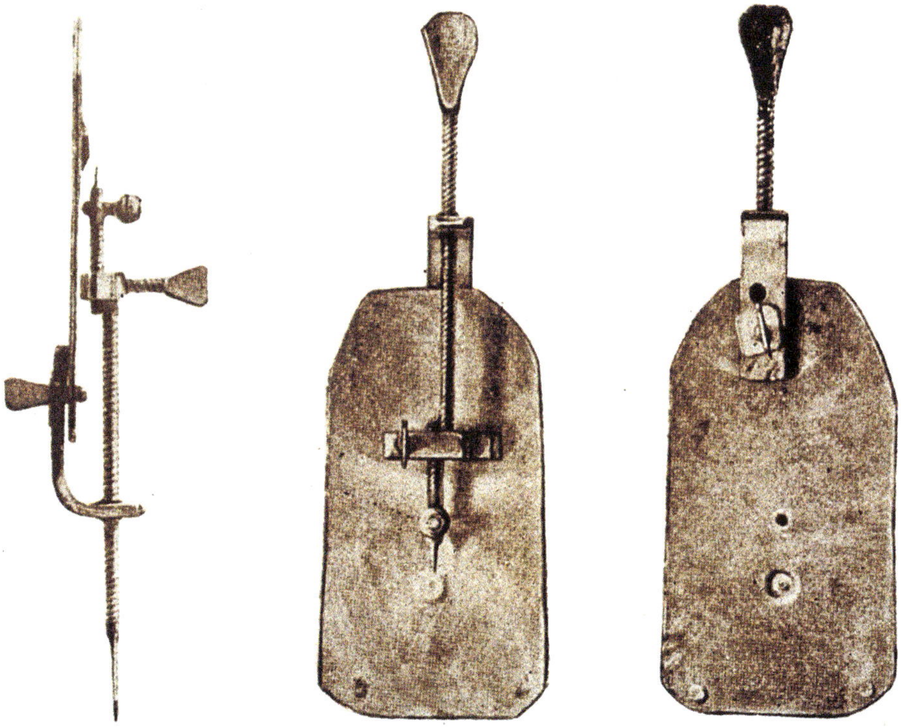

The first microscope invented by Antoni van Leeuwenhoek. Widely credited as the father of modern microscopy, Leeuwenhoek crafted hundreds of microscopes and lenses in his lifetime. *© Wellcome Images/Science Source*

ELECTRON MICROSCOPES

There are two types of electron microscopes, the transmission electron microscope (TEM) and the scanning electron microscope (SEM). The TEM transmits electrons through an extremely thin sample. The electrons scatter as they collide with the atoms in the sample and form an image on a photographic film below the sample. This process is similar to a medical X-ray, where X-rays (very short-wavelength light) are transmitted through the body and form an image on photographic film behind the body. By contrast, the SEM reflects a narrow beam of electrons off the surface of a sample and detects the reflected electrons. To image a certain area of the sample, the electron beam is scanned in a back-and-forth motion parallel to the sample surface, similar to the process of mowing a square section of lawn. The chief differences between the two microscopes are that the TEM gives a two-dimensional picture of the interior of the sample whereas the SEM gives a three-dimensional picture of the surface of the sample. Images produced by SEM are familiar to the public, as in television commercials showing pollen grains or dust mites.

ciency virus/acquired immunodeficiency syndrome (HIV/AIDS) patients. Giemsa stain is found useful in identifying malaria and other parasites, such as *Leishmania*.

Immunofluorescence is a modern microscopy technique that uses antibodies labeled with a fluorescent marker to bind to specific parts of a microbial pathogen. When the specimen is examined under ultraviolet light, the antibody will glow with a green fluorescence if the pathogen is present.

Microscopy aids diagnosis by examining the clinical specimens that are likely to be infected with the causative organism. Therefore, sputum is examined for TB, blood for malaria, stool samples for parasites, and urine to detect bacteria causing urinary tract infections. Viruses are detected, although not routinely, with an electron microscope. There are many other laboratory methods for the detection of microorganisms that complement microscopy.

The optics of a light microscope are adjustable depending on the type of result desired. In light field microscopy, the specimen is visualized by light passing from the condenser through the specimen, whereas dark field microscopy uses oblique illumination that gives higher resolution of detail, if this is needed. Phase contrast microscopy involves modification to the condenser and objective (lens) to give an optical interference pattern in the viewed image. This is valuable for transparent specimens because it makes details appear darker against a light background.

Superresolution microscopy includes a variety of techniques that increase the resolution power of a light microscope. In some cases the light that illuminates the specimen is patterned, and the patterned light is moved relative to the observed object. The resolution is increased by measuring the fringes in the pattern that result from the interference of the illumination pattern and the sample and by then subjecting the results to Fourier transform analysis. Other techniques include photon-tunneling microscopy and improved fluorescence microscopy. In 2014 the Nobel Prize in Chemistry was awarded to Eric Betzig (1960–), Stefan W. Hell (1962–), and William E. Moerner (1953–) for the development of superresolved fluorescence microscopy.

Impacts and Issues

A microscope must be operated by a skilled scientist if findings are to be of clinical value. Some microorganisms are easy to identify under a microscope, especially if the specimen is given the correct preparation, including staining. However, it is not always possible to distinguish between a pathogen and a harmless organism present within the same specimen.

Sometimes inadequate preparation gives faulty results, and therefore an important diagnosis may be missed. Because the microscope is relatively insensitive as a diagnostic tool, as many organisms must be present for a positive result, infections caused by relatively few bacteria may be missed.

It also takes time and experience to come to a correct conclusion based on microscope findings. If lab technicians are handling a large number of specimens, such as from a cervical cancer screening program, they may miss positive findings. Cancer cells have different features under the microscope compared to healthy cells. Sometimes these differences may be missed, leading to a false negative. The microscope is just one of many diagnostic tools at the disposal of the pathology laboratory for the diagnosis of infectious and other diseases.

See Also *Microorganisms; Rapid Diagnostic Tests for Infectious Diseases*

BIBLIOGRAPHY

Books

Gillespie, Stephen, and Kathleen Bamford. *Medical Microbiology and Infection at a Glance.* Malden, MA: Blackwell Science, 2000.

Websites

"Basic Concepts in Microscopy." Zeiss. http://zeiss-campus.magnet.fsu.edu/articles/basics/index.html (accessed January 29, 2018).

"Introduction to Superresolution Microscopy." Zeiss. http://zeiss-campus.magnet.fsu.edu/articles/superresolution/introduction.html (accessed January 29, 2018).

Susan Aldridge
Anna Marie E. Roos

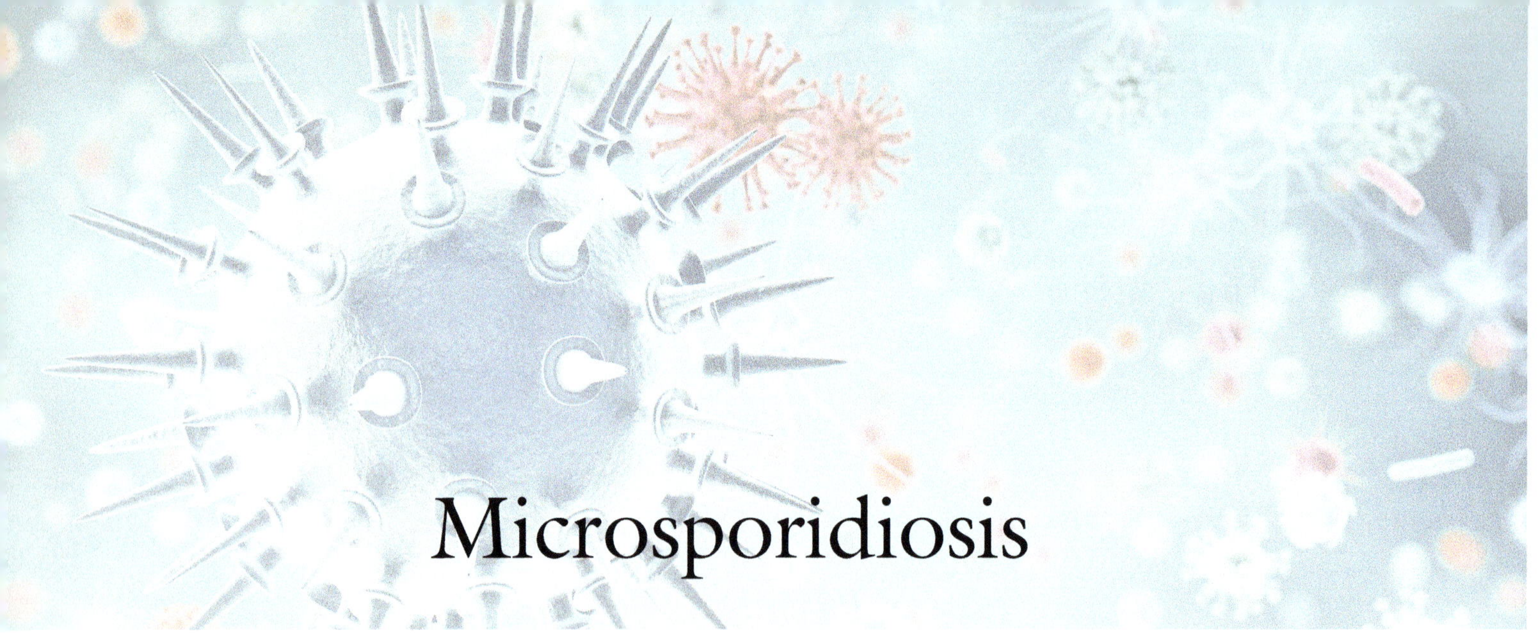

Microsporidiosis

Introduction

Microsporidia are fungi found worldwide that can infect a range of invertebrate and vertebrate hosts, causing microsporidiosis (also known as microsporidiasis). These microorganisms are primarily opportunistic pathogens (those affecting a host with a weak immune system) that cause a variety of conditions, including infections of the intestines, lungs, eyes, muscles, and kidneys. With improved detection methods and the emergence of acquired immunodeficiency syndrome (AIDS), more clinical microsporidiosis cases have been reported in the late 20th and early 21st centuries.

WORDS TO KNOW

HOST An organism that serves as the habitat for a parasite or possibly for a symbiont. A host may provide nutrition to the parasite or symbiont, or it may simply provide a place in which to live.

IMMUNOSUPPRESSION A reduction of the ability of the immune system to recognize and respond to the presence of foreign material.

OPPORTUNISTIC INFECTION An infection that occurs in people whose immune systems are diminished or are not functioning normally. Such infections are opportunistic insofar as the infectious agents take advantage of their hosts' compromised immune systems and invade to cause disease.

PATHOGEN A disease-causing agent, such as a bacterium, a virus, a fungus, or another microorganism.

History, Characteristics, and Transmission

Microsporidiosis is caused by infection from small, spore-forming parasites known as microsporidia. The microbe was first identified in silkworms by Swiss botanist Karl Wilhelm von Nägeli (1817–1891) in 1857. Since then researchers have discovered that microsporidia can infect every animal group, both vertebrate and invertebrate. More than 150 genera and 1,300 species of microsporidia have been identified thus far. The first human case was diagnosed in 1959, when a young boy in Japan began suffering from mysterious headaches, fever, vomiting, and convulsions.

Initially considered a protozoa, microsporidium was later reclassified as a fungus. It has been isolated from sources such as surface water and wild and domestic animals and is known to cause waterborne and foodborne infections in humans. Approximately 15 species of microsporidia are known to cause diseases in humans. The most common is *Enterocytozoon bieneusi*, which is the cause of about 90 percent of human infections, followed by the *Encephalitozoon* species, particularly *E. intestinalis*. Other *Encephalitozoon* species causing human infection are *E. cuniculi* and *E. hellem*.

Microsporidia have two distinct developmental phases. During the intracellular (inside the cell) proliferative phase, asexual replication takes place, which results in a massive increase in the number of spores inside the host cell. During the extracellular and infectious sporogonic phase, spores that are relatively resistant to the environment germinate, and new organisms emerge. When the spores come into contact with the host cell, they pierce the cell through a hollow tube, injecting the infective spores directly into the host. This again restarts the intracellular proliferative phase. Mature spores develop and accumulate inside the host cell, eventually rupturing the host cell to release the spores.

The mode of transmission of microsporidium is not clear, but it is thought to be through ingestion or inhalation of microsporidial spores in the environment and in rare cases through direct contact with an infected person or animal. Consumption or contact with contaminated food or water is another significant risk factor.

The diseases caused by microsporidium vary and are dependent on the species of microsporidium and the status of the host's immune system. In the case of *E. bieneusi* infection, when spores of microsporidium are ingested by hosts with a weak immune system, the microbe penetrates intestinal cells and results in persistent diarrhea, abdominal pain, and weight loss. On rare occasions *E. bieneusi* also causes infection of the lungs, muscles, and brain, including infection of the bile ducts, causing a condition called cholangitis.

In healthy individuals such as travelers, infection may lead to non-chronic diarrhea. Sexual transmission of infection is reported based on observation of microsporidia in the urethra (tube from urinary bladder) and prostate (a gland surrounding the urinary bladder in males) of AIDS patients. Individuals who have undergone kidney transplants have also been shown to be at higher risk of *E. bieneusi* infection.

Scope and Distribution

Microsporidia are found throughout the world, and cases or microsporidiosis have been reported in both developed and developing areas in Africa, the Americas, Asia, Australia, and Europe. Although the worst effects of the disease are concentrated among patients with human immunodeficiency virus (HIV) or AIDS and other people with weakened immune function, immunocompetent (healthy immune system) individuals are also susceptible to infection, though often without symptoms.

The role of microsporidia as a cause of disease in humans and animals has been understood only since the late 20th century based on the discovery of new species of microsporidia and improved diagnostic applications. Most of the cases of microsporidiosis were reported after 1985, when HIV was identified as the cause of AIDS, leading to the isolation of *E. bieneusi* in HIV patients suffering from chronic diarrhea. Since then several new strains of microsporidia have been found to cause opportunistic infection in humans.

The introduction of antiretroviral drugs as a treatment for HIV has helped to significantly decrease the risk of microsporidiosis in patients with HIV. However, the high cost of antiretroviral therapy leaves many HIV patients in developing countries without access to the treatment, and thus rates of microsporidiosis remain high in these areas. A 2018 study, for example, found the prevalence of microsporidiosis among HIV patients to be around 25 percent in low-income countries compared to 8 percent in middle-

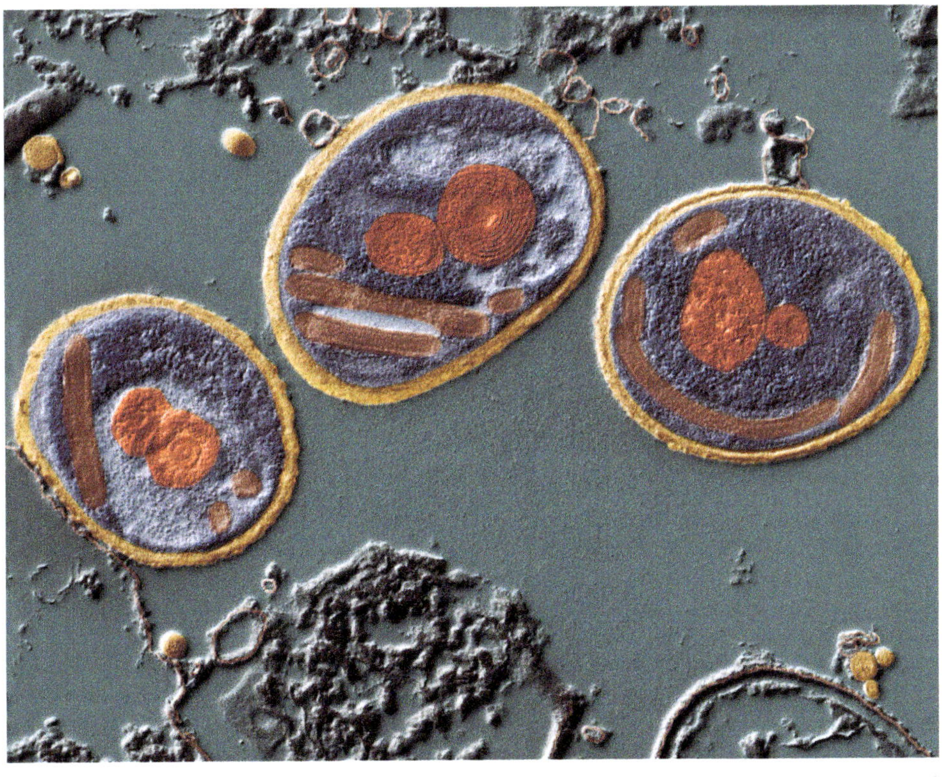

Microsporidia, single-celled parasites that cause the gastrointestinal infection microsporidiosis, viewed under a transmission electron microscope. Microsporidiosis can be life threatening in individuals with a compromised immune system. © *Eye of Science/Science Source*

CONDITIONS CAUSED BY MICROSPORIDIA

Due to multiple genera and species identified as disease-causing pathogens among microsporidia, clinicians often find it difficult to link the symptoms to the pathogen. Some of the conditions caused by microsporidial species are outlined below:

- A fatal case of (inflammation of muscles) due to *B. algerae* infection was diagnosed in a South African woman with diabetes in 2014.
- Six cases of microsporidial keratoconjunctivitis (inflammation of cornea and conjuctiva of the eyes) were reported in healthy individuals who were using topical steroids, which might have initiated the infection.
- A case of microsporidial keratoconjunctivitis was reported in a veterinarian in India after vaccinating a flock of sheep.
- A case of reactive arthritis was reported after microsporidial infection in an otherwise normal man was been reported in 2016.
- In 2014 three cases of neurologic syndrome caused by donor-derived microsporidiosis was reported in the United States after the three patients received a kidney, liver, and heart from a single donor.
- A case of intestinal microsporidiosis was reported in 2017 in an intestinal bowel syndrome patient receiving immunosuppressive medications in Iran.

income and 14 percent in high-income countries. In developed countries an increase in microsporidiosis has been reported among organ transplant recipients with weakened immune function, as well as in healthy individuals, where it commonly manifests as an eye infection. Incidences of *E. bieneusi* infection have also increased among travelers, resulting in diarrhea.

Treatment and Prevention

The antiparasitic medication albendazole is most frequently used and is effective against all species of microsporidia. The antibiotic fumagillin is also recommended to treat microsporidial infection and is particularly effective against *E. bieneusi* when administered systemically at a dose of 20 milligrams three times per day. However, patients should be monitored, as fumagillin can cause blood disorders such as neutropenia (low number of neutrophils) and thrombocytopenia (low number of platelets) in some patients.

There is no vaccine against microsporidiosis. Prevention methods, such as drinking boiled or filtered water and practicing good personal hygiene, are recommended, particularly among those most at risk of developing life-threatening complications from the disease. Experts also recommend practicing proper food safety, as well as avoiding animals that are suspected of carrying the disease.

Histochemical methods (applying stains to cells for easier analysis under microscopy) are routinely used for detecting spores of microsporidia in urine, stool, aspirates, and tissue biopsies. Gram stain is routinely used to stain microsporidia, as the spores stain dark violet and are readily visible under a microscope. Various new staining methods are also available.

Impacts and Issues

Microsporidial spores are found more or less everywhere in the environment and infect a variety of animals, including fish and insects. Before the AIDS pandemic, microsporidial spores were routinely recognized in laboratory animals but rarely in humans. There has been a significant increase in interest in microsporidia as a subject of research among the scientific community in the early 21st century as new species causing opportunistic infections in hosts with a weakened immune system have been discovered. However, the miniscule size of the spores (averaging between 1 and 30 microns) makes them difficult to identify and study with even the most advanced laboratory equipment.

Because an unknown number of microsporidium species are present in nearly every environment and can infect a wide range of hosts, there remains a great deal to be learned about the distribution, transmission pathways, and prevalence of the disease. The World Health Organization classifies microsporidium as an HIV-related opportunistic pathogen, and most research tends to focus on its effects among immunocompromised groups. Yet the US Environmental Protection Agency considers microsporidia an emerging waterborne pathogen constituting a general public health threat, underscoring the need for further study of the parasites and their related risks to the broader population.

BIBLIOGRAPHY

Books

Lindsay, David S., and Louis M. Weiss. *Opportunistic Infections: Toxoplasma, Sarcocystis, and Microsporidia.* New York: Springer, 2011.

Weiss, Louis M., and James J. Becnel, eds. *Microsporidia: Pathogens of Opportunity.* Ames, IA: Wiley Blackwell, 2014.

Periodicals

Didier E. S., and L. M. Weiss. "Microsporidiosis: Current Status." *Current Opinion in Infectious Diseases* 19, no. 5 (2006): 485.

Didier, E. S., et al. "Epidemiology of Microsporidiosis: Sources and Modes of Transmission." *Veterinary Parasitology* 126, no. 1–2 (December 2004):145 –166.

Mathis, Alexander, Rainer Weber, and Peter Deplazes. "Zoonotic Potential of the Microsporidia." *Clinical Microbiological Reviews* 18, no. 3 (July 2005): 423–445.

Santín, M., and R. Fayer. "*Enterocytozoon bieneusi* Genotype Nomenclature Based on the Internal Transcribed Spacer Sequence: A Consensus." *Journal of Eukaryotic Microbiology* 56 (2009): 34.

Websites

Cheng, Lily, and Scott Smith. "Parasites and Pestilence: Infectious Public Health Challenges." Stanford University, 2006. https://web.stanford.edu/class/humbio103/ParaSites2006/Microsporidiosis/microsporidia1.html (accessed February 5, 2018).

"Drugs Used in HIV-Related Infections." World Health Organization, 1999. http://apps.who.int/medicinedocs/en/d/Js2215e/7.3.html#Js2215e.7.3 (accessed February 5, 2018).

"Microsporidiosis." Centers for Disease Control and Prevention, 2017. https://www.cdc.gov/dpdx/microsporidiosis/index.html (accessed February 5, 2018).

Kausalya Santhanam

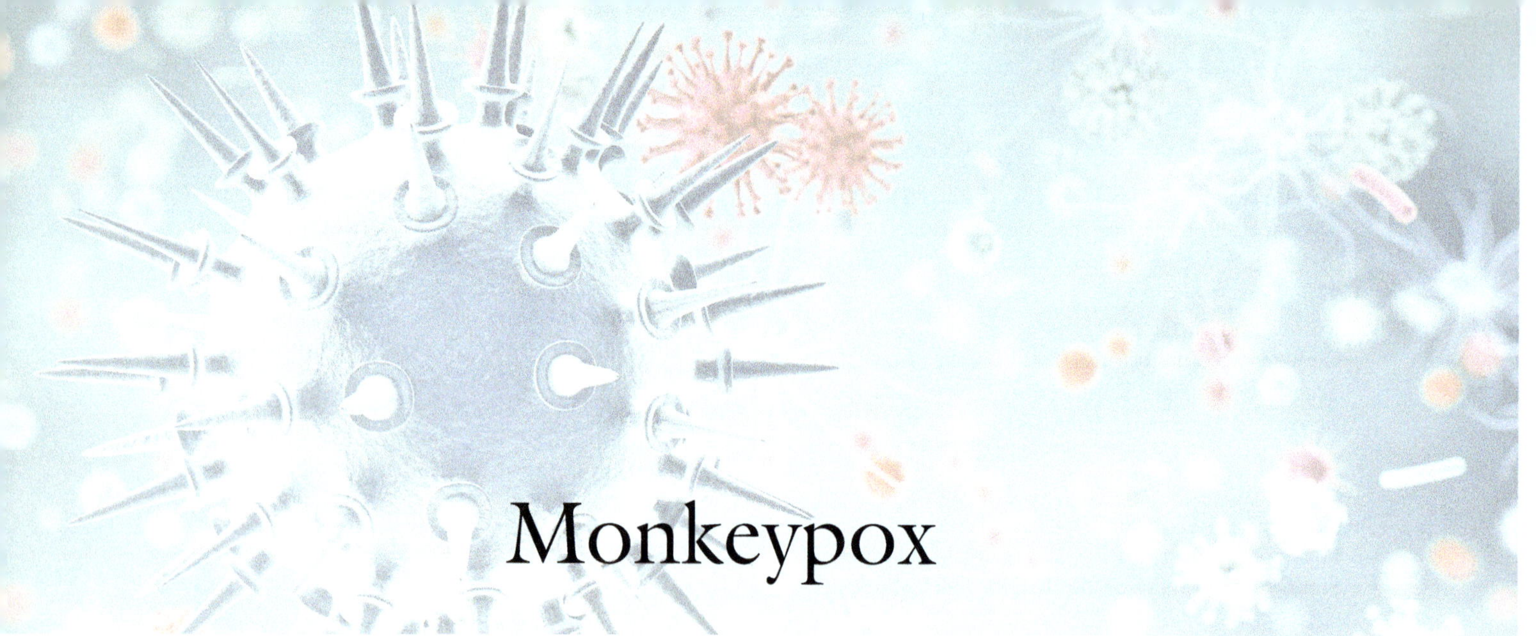

Monkeypox

Introduction

Monkeypox is an infectious viral disease that is similar to but milder than smallpox. This disease has a very low prevalence, with almost all cases occurring in West Africa and central Africa adjacent to tropical rain forests. This disease causes smallpox-like symptoms, including fever, headache, muscle aches, backache, exhaustion, and discomfort, in addition to a papular rash over the body. One symptom common in monkeypox but not in smallpox is swelling of the lymph nodes.

Monkeypox is a zoonotic disease, a disease humans can contract from infected animals. It is usually contracted via an animal bite or by coming into contact with the bodily fluids of infected animals. There is no treatment for monkeypox, but fatality rates are low, with most patients recovering in two to four weeks. Monkeypox can be prevented by controlling the transmission of the disease from animals to humans. This involves reporting diseased animals and taking appropriate action to prevent transfer of the virus to humans.

Disease History, Characteristics, and Transmission

Monkeypox is a rare disease caused by the monkeypox virus. This virus belongs to the *Orthopoxvirus* genus of viruses, which also includes smallpox and cowpox. Monkeypox was first discovered in 1958. It was first identified in laboratory monkeys and later in rodents. The first human case of monkeypox was reported in 1970.

Monkeypox is found in animals. It is hypothesized that rodents are the primary carriers of the disease. All mammals are thought to be susceptible to this virus. Humans become infected with monkeypox when they come into direct contact with an infected animal's bodily fluids, either through an animal bite or by touching lesions on an animal. This virus can also be transmitted by airborne droplets from the respiratory tract. Therefore, face-to-face contact between an infected animal and a human can spread the virus. Contact with contaminated items, such as bedsheets, can also spread the disease.

Monkeypox presents as a milder version of smallpox, with similar, although less severe, symptoms. Approximately 6 to 16 days after infection with the monkeypox virus, a person will develop an illness characterized by fever, headache, muscle aches, backache, exhaustion, and discomfort. Unlike smallpox, monkeypox also causes the lymph nodes to swell. A few days after these initial symptoms, a papular rash (raised bumps on the skin) begins to form. This rash usually develops first on the face and then spreads across the body. The bumps develop, crust over, and finally fall off. The infection usually lasts two to four weeks.

WORDS TO KNOW

CHAIN OF TRANSMISSION The route by which an infection is spread from its source to susceptible host. An example of a chain of transmission is the spread of malaria from an infected animal to humans via mosquitoes.

FOMITE An object or a surface to which an infectious microorganism such as bacteria or viruses can adhere and be transmitted. Papers, clothing, dishes, and other objects can all act as fomites. Transmission is often by touch.

ENDEMIC Present in a particular area or among a particular group of people.

PAPULAR A small, solid bump on the skin; papular means pertaining to or resembling a papule.

ZOONOTIC A disease that can be transmitted between animals and humans. Examples of zoonotic diseases are anthrax, plague, and Q fever.

Between 1 percent and 10 percent of the people in Africa who contract monkeypox will die of the disease. Young children are the most likely to die from the disease. No monkeypox fatalities have been reported outside of Africa.

Scope and Distribution

Monkeypox was first found in Africa. Most cases of monkeypox occur in central Africa and West Africa, particularly in the Democratic Republic of the Congo, where it is endemic. The countries where it occurs are characterized by tropical rain forests. There is a low prevalence of the disease.

In 2003 the first cases of monkeypox occurred in the United States. Of at least 79 reported cases, 29 were confirmed as true cases of monkeypox. It is argued that the virus was transmitted to humans by tame prairie dogs that were earlier in contact with infected Gambian rats from Africa. The tame prairie dogs probably contracted the virus from the Gambian rats.

Although the virus is similar to smallpox, which devastated populations prior to its eradication, monkeypox is not as transmissible as smallpox. The World Health Organization (WHO) reported that as of 2016 there was no proof that "person-to-person transmission alone can sustain monkeypox infections in the human population."

In general, young people are more susceptible to contracting monkeypox. The people most at risk of developing monkeypox are those exposed to infected animals or infected patients. This includes investigators of current monkeypox outbreaks, veterinarians, health care workers, laboratory workers, and friends or family of monkeypox patients.

Treatment and Prevention

There is no safe, specific treatment for monkeypox. However, a good health care system, including adequate supportive care for symptoms, as well as good nutrition, aids recovery. The illness normally lasts two to four weeks, and a person is no longer infectious when the rash lesions have crusted. No monkeypox fatalities have been reported outside of Africa. However, within rural African regions, where health care is generally poor, monkeypox fatalities may reach 10 percent of reported cases.

There is no vaccination against monkeypox, although the smallpox vaccine has been found to be 85 percent effective against monkeypox. The smallpox vaccine has not been commercially available since the global eradication of smallpox in 1980.

In the United States, the Centers for Disease Control and Prevention (CDC) does not recommend widespread smallpox vaccination to prevent monkeypox. Use of the vaccine is recommended only for high-risk individuals, such as those caring for monkeypox patients or people who have been in contact with infected animals and are at risk of becoming infected. Vaccination after exposure to the virus has been found to help prevent or reduce the severity of

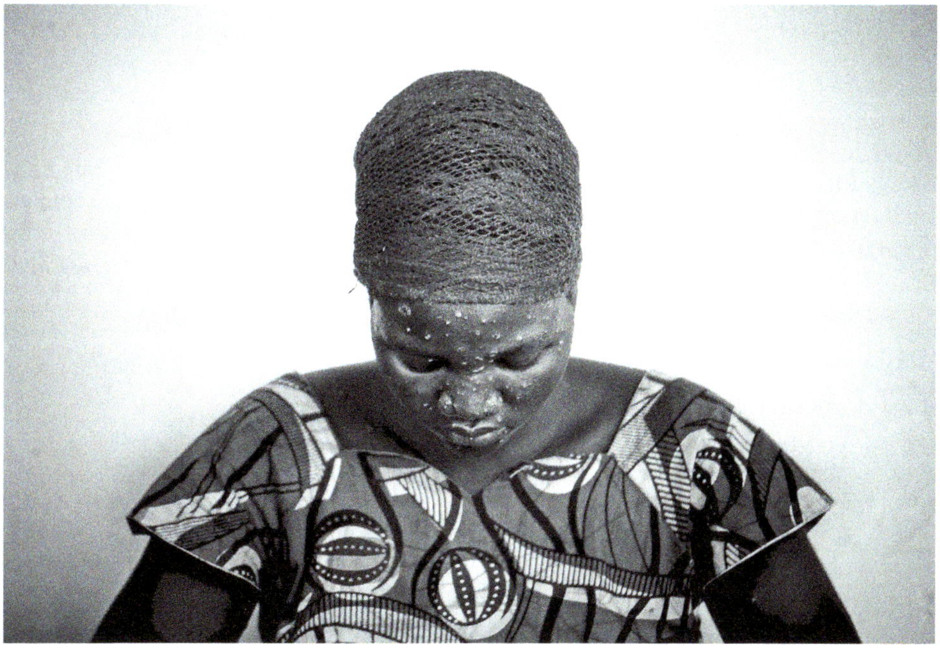

A young woman infected with monkey pox in the Democratic Republic of the Congo. © *Jeff Hutchens/ Getty Images*

REAL-WORLD RISKS

The US Centers for Disease Control and Prevention (CDC) states, "Past data from Africa suggests that the smallpox vaccine is at least 85 percent effective in preventing monkeypox." Nevertheless, the CDC notes that for most people, monkeypox disease carries less risk than would result from taking the smallpox vaccine. This is in part because, although most people only have minor reactions such as fever, fatigue, swollen glands, redness, and itching, the smallpox vaccine carries risk, including the risk of death resulting from complications related to the vaccine. The CDC estimates that between one and two people out of every 1 million die after being vaccinated for smallpox.

When weighing the risk of vaccination, it should be noted that monkeypox is a serious disease that kills between 1 and 10 percent of those infected in central Africa, where access to health care is limited and many people live in remote areas. Although most people experience mild symptoms such as headache, fever, muscle aches, backache, fatigue, rash, and swollen lymph nodes, the disease can result in death, particularly for medically underserved populations.

infection. However, vaccination should be avoided in patients with weakened immune systems or patients with life-threatening allergies to the smallpox vaccine and its ingredients because the smallpox vaccine could be more harmful than the monkeypox virus in these cases. In the United States, a combination of the vaccine, antiviral medications, and vaccinia immune globulin (VIG) medications may be used to treat the disease.

To prevent the spread of this disease, infected animals (if they are known) should be separated from human populations as soon as possible. Because contact with fomites (contaminated surfaces such as clothing) and bedding can also result in transmission of the disease, these items must be washed with hot water and detergent to remove the virus.

■ Impacts and Issues

Monkeypox is not a widespread disease. While low mortality outbreaks occur in Africa, few outbreaks have been reported outside of African countries. Prior to 2003 monkeypox had not appeared in the United States and was not considered a threat. Since 2003 there has been one outbreak of monkeypox in the United States, and, although the disease was contained, it is now considered a possible threat for US citizens.

The outbreak in the United States included at least 29 confirmed cases of monkeypox. However, no deaths occurred due to this disease. The effect of this disease on victims in the United States was noticeably milder than its effect on African populations. A better national health care network is thought to have resulted in a more efficient and thus more effective containment of the disease. This health care network includes better nutrition, access to good supportive care, and availability of a vaccine.

Future outbreaks in the United States and in other countries outside of Africa are still possible. However, not only are the chances of transmission throughout a population low, but it is unlikely that a chain of transmission would be sustained within a human community.

There has been some debate within the United States over the potential for monkeypox to be used by terrorists as a biological weapon. However, the efficient containment of this disease during the 2003 outbreak, coupled with the low likelihood that this disease would spread rapidly through the population, significantly reduces its risk as a bioweapon.

In 2016 and 2017, there were monkeypox outbreaks in the Central African Republic and in Nigeria, respectively. Outbreaks of monkeypox occur on occasion in central Africa and West Africa and do not pose a global health threat.

See Also *Bioterrorism; Smallpox; Smallpox Eradication and Storage; Viral Disease; Zoonoses*

BIBLIOGRAPHY

Books

Bennett, John E., Raphael Dolin, and Martin J. Blaser. *Mandell, Douglas, and Bennett's Principles and Practice of Infectious Diseases.* 8th ed. Philadelphia: Elsevier/Saunders, 2015.

Periodicals

Brown, Katy, and Peter A. Leggat. "Human Monkeypox: Current State of Knowledge and Implications for the Future." *Tropical Medicine and Infectious Disease* 1, no. 8 (2016). This article can also be found online at http://www.mdpi.com/2414-6366/1/1/8/htm (accessed January 24, 2018).

Nolen, Leisha Diane, et al. "Introduction of Monkeypox into a Community and Household: Risk Factors and Zoonotic Reservoirs in the Democratic Republic of the Congo." *American Journal of Tropical Medicine and Hygiene* 93, 2 (August 2015): 410–415. This article can also be found online at http://www.ajtmh.org/content/journals/10.4269/ajtmh.15-0168 (accessed January 24, 2018).

Quiner, Claire A., et al. "Presumptive Risk Factors for Monkeypox in Rural Communities in the Democratic Republic of the Congo." *PLOS ONE* 12, no. 2 (February 13, 2017). This article can also be found online at http://journals.plos.org/plosone/article?id=10.1371/journal.pone.0168664 (accessed January 24, 2018).

Sun, Lena H. "Chasing a Killer." *Washington Post* (November 3, 2017). This article can also be found online at https://www.washingtonpost.com/graphics/2017/national/health-science/monkeypox/?utm_term=.fb1ed3443a41 (accessed January 24, 2018).

Websites

"Monkeypox." Centers for Disease Control and Prevention, May 11, 2015. https://www.cdc.gov/poxvirus/monkeypox/ (accessed January 24, 2018).

"Monkeypox." World Health Organization, November 2016. http://www.who.int/mediacentre/factsheets/fs161/en/ (accessed January 24, 2018).

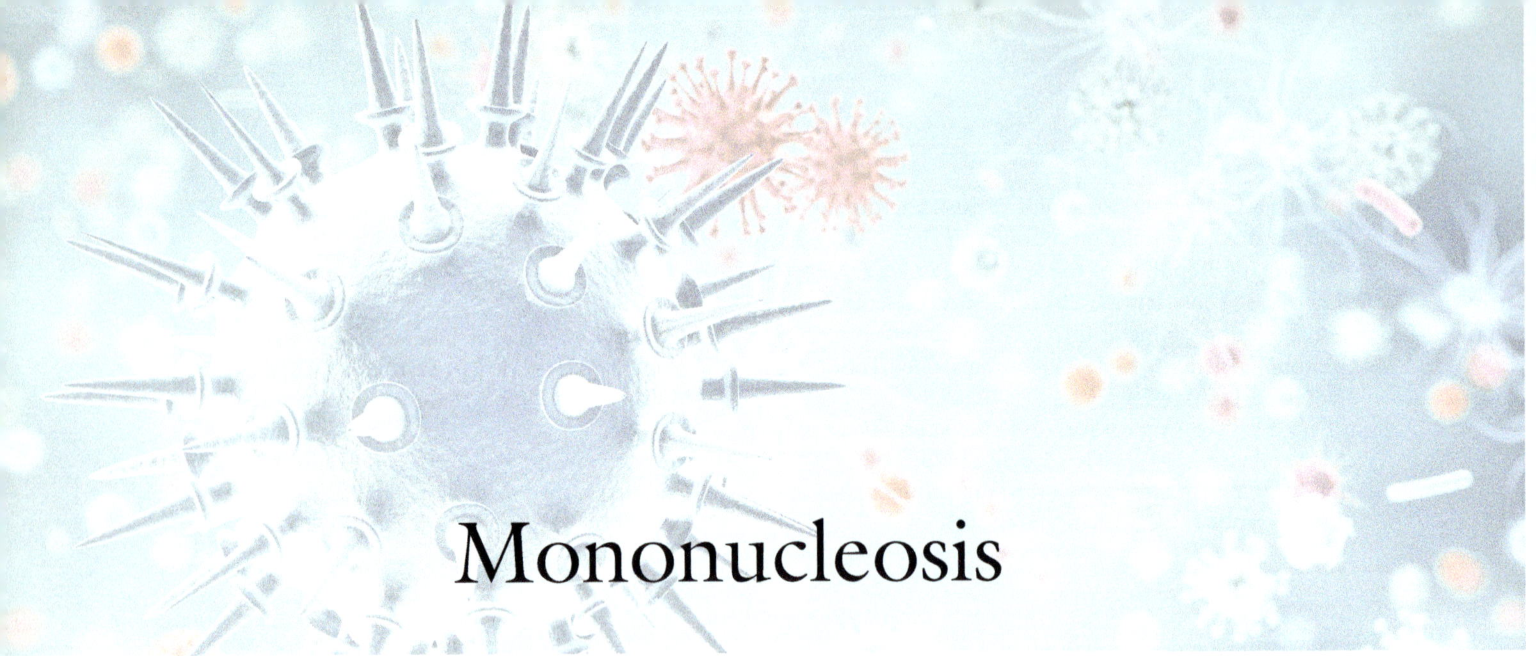

Mononucleosis

Introduction

Mononucleosis is a self-limiting viral disease most commonly, though not only, caused by the Epstein-Barr virus (EBV). EBV is considered to be one of the most common viruses contracted by humans, and most people become infected with the virus at some point during their lives. When infection with EBV occurs during adolescence or young adulthood, the infection develops into mononucleosis more than 25 percent of the time, according to the US Centers for Disease Control and Prevention (CDC). The disease occurs worldwide.

EBV infection during early childhood is usually asymptomatic. When an adolescent or a young adult develops mononucleosis, the symptoms include fever, sore throat, swollen glands, swollen lymph nodes, and general fatigue. In severe cases patients may display symptoms for months, but usually symptoms resolve within four weeks of initial infection. There is no vaccine to prevent mononucleosis, and treatment of symptoms relies largely on rest and rehydration.

No areas have been identified as having an increased risk of infection, and most cases occur sporadically with no

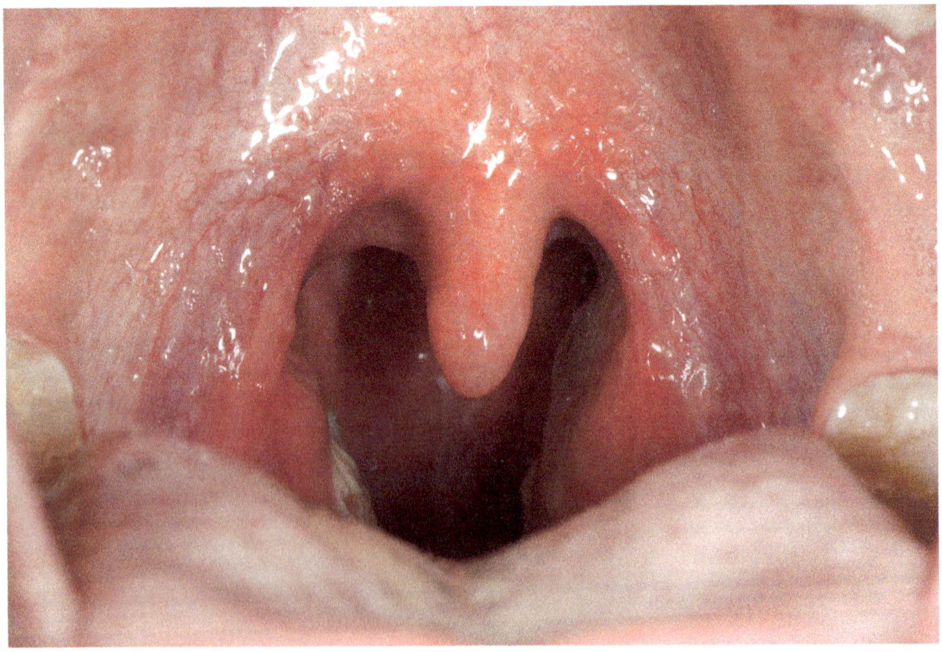

Swollen tonsils resulting from mononucleosis, an infection caused by the Epstein-Barr virus or cytomegalovirus. Also known as glandular fever or the kissing disease, mononucleosis is spread through contact with the saliva or mucus of an infected person. *© Dr P. Marazzi/Science Source*

reports of outbreaks. The long incubation period of infection coupled with the universal presence of the viral agent makes epidemiological control impractical.

WORDS TO KNOW

ANTIBODIES Proteins found in the blood that help fight against foreign substances called antigens. Antigens, which are usually proteins or polysaccharides, stimulate the immune system to produce antibodies, or Y-shaped immunoglobulins. The antibodies inactivate the antigen and help remove it from the body. While antigens can be the source of infections from pathogenic bacteria and viruses, organic molecules detrimental to the body from internal or environmental sources also act as antigens. Genetic engineering and the use of various mutational mechanisms allow the construction of a vast array of antibodies (each with a unique genetic sequence).

CHRONIC FATIGUE SYNDROME A condition that causes extreme tiredness. People with CFS have debilitating fatigue that lasts for six months or longer. They also have many other symptoms. Some of these symptoms are pain in the joints and muscles, headache, and sore throat. CFS appears to result from a combination of factors.

EPSTEIN-BARR VIRUS (EBV) This virus is part of the family of human herpes viruses. Infectious mononucleosis (IM) is the most common disease manifestation of this virus, which, once established in the host, can never be completely eradicated. Very little can be done to treat EBV; most methods can only alleviate resultant symptoms.

MONONUCLEAR LEUKOCYTE A type of white blood cell active in the immune system.

MONONUCLEOSIS (MONO) SPOT TEST A blood test used to check for infection with the Epstein-Barr virus, which causes mononucleosis.

■ Disease History, Characteristics, and Transmission

Mononucleosis is also known as Pfeiffer's disease, Filatov's disease, kissing disease, glandular fever, or simply mono. The disease was first termed glandular fever by a group of German physicians in the 1880s due to the obvious swelling of the lymph nodes and glands. In 1920 scientists discovered that the infection was associated with white blood cells called mononuclear leukocytes, and thus it was also called infectious mononucleosis. The causative agent was not identified as EBV until 1968, when Michael Epstein (1921–) and Yvonne Barr (1932–2016) discovered the virus.

EBV is a member of the family of human herpes viruses. It is one of the most common human viruses and is responsible for 90 percent of mononucleosis cases. Cytomegalovirus is another member of this family of viruses and may cause mononucleosis in a small number of cases. EBV causes mononucleosis by infecting lymphocytes, or white blood cells, which subsequently reduces host immunity for the period of infection. EBV has also been implicated in more severe diseases, such as post-transplant lymphoproliferative disease, Hodgkin's disease, nasopharyngeal carcinoma, and Burkitt's lymphoma.

Mononucleosis has an incubation period of four to seven weeks, during which symptoms may not be present. Most children are exposed to EBV at a young age, which generally results in a mild, asymptomatic infection. If initial infection occurs during adolescence or young adulthood, symptoms may present as a persistent cold or flu and may include fever, enlarged lymph nodes on the neck, sore throat, muscle aches, fatigue, and white patches on the tonsils. Enlargement of the spleen occurs in 25 to 75 percent of cases and poses the threat of further complications due to the possibility of rupture. Other symptoms may include abdominal pain, headache, jaundice, depression, weakness, skin rash, and swollen liver. The broad spectrum of possible symptoms means that almost all cases of mononucleosis are unique to each patient.

Generally the infection is self-limiting within two to four weeks, but in some cases the course of disease is considered chronic, and patients may suffer from symptoms for months or even years. Hospitalization is seldom required unless complications, such as ruptured spleen or liver problems, arise. There have been no indicating factors to suggest why some people develop more serious symptoms than others; however, it is postulated that external stressors in a patient's life could potentially play a key role. The EBV infection does not necessarily affect only people with compromised immunity. Quite often those who contract mononucleosis appear fit and healthy.

Mononucleosis is considered relatively contagious and is transmitted through contact with saliva or mucus, which can occur by kissing or by the sharing of drinks and utensils. In some instances transmission has been linked to blood and may occur through transfusion. Infected people may be contagious while symptomatic, but even asymptomatic people can carry and spread the virus for life and, as such, remain a primary reservoir for transmission.

■ Scope and Distribution

EBV is found worldwide. Mononucleosis most frequently occurs in young adults between ages 15 and 17, but it potentially affects people of all ages. One to 3 percent of college students are affected annually.

Generally, most people will contract EBV at some stage of their life, and, in the United States, 95 percent of 35- to

40-year-olds have previously been infected. In most cases previous infection will have occurred without recognition or diagnosis. This is due to the fact that during early childhood infection is mild, usually producing no symptoms or only mild symptoms similar to the common cold.

The statistics are much the same for developing nations, where 90 percent of children contract asymptomatic EBV when under five years old. These individuals are then not susceptible to mononucleosis caused by EBV. It is interesting to note that mononucleosis is a disease that more commonly affects people in developed countries than those in developing countries. Variations in social etiquette and acceptable social behaviors may account for such differences because mononucleosis is a disease that requires direct contact with saliva for transmission, such as through intimate kissing. Another theory accounting for this difference is that in developing countries individuals are likely to be exposed to EBV while young and so would develop a mild form of the infection. In developed countries individuals may be protected from the virus until adolescence. Without the immunity conferred by prior infection, mononucleosis would develop.

There does not appear to be a strong link between the health status of a person and the likelihood of developing mononucleosis, but potentially people who have a compromised immune system may be at higher risk of developing mononucleosis when infected with EBV.

The global scope of EBV almost certainly ensures the continued transmission of the disease. Most cases of mononucleosis occur sporadically, and outbreaks are rare. Typically, people presenting with symptoms of the disease have no recollection of possible exposure to the virus, and it is uncommon that infection would be transmitted to a group from a single source. In any large adult group, over 90 percent of the people will probably have been exposed to EBV previously, and in such situations an outbreak is unlikely.

There are no known ethnic, racial, or sexual factors that predispose a person to develop mononucleosis. However, it is interesting to note that in developed countries infection more often occurs in people belonging to higher socioeconomic classes. This may be attributed to differences in lifestyle and increased opportunities for the social interactions associated with this disease. In addition, the fact that these individuals receive a higher level of protection from childhood infections may also play a role. The only gender-related factor associated with mononucleosis is that 90 percent of cases of ruptured spleens occur in males.

Treatment and Prevention

Diagnosis of mononucleosis may be confirmed through serological testing to determine the presence of abnormal white blood cells. The mono spot test is a specific test designed to detect the presence of antibodies that have developed as a result of the viral infection. These are known as heterophile antibodies and usually develop about one week after onset of the disease. They peak during the first month of illness but may persist in the blood for several months and up to one year. Some people infected with mononucleosis may never develop these antibodies, so the test may return a false-negative result. Generally, the testing is accurate, with false-positive results occurring in only a small number of patients.

There is no vaccine or preventive medicine available for mononucleosis, largely due to the fact that it results from a viral infection. However, the severity of other infections related to EBV, in addition to a further understanding of the virus, has prompted scientists to investigate avenues for creating a potential vaccine. It is likely that the vaccine would be targeted toward minimizing the clinical manifestations of primary infection with EBV rather than toward malignancies associated with the disease.

The fact that EBV infection in early childhood seldom results in development of mononucleosis, while primary infection occurring after adolescence develops into the disease in 35 to 50 percent of cases, suggests that a vaccine generating a minimized immune response may potentially limit the clinical symptoms of mononucleosis. The limiting factor in this area of research is that such a vaccine requires the use of an attenuated (weakened) virus, which has been deemed unsafe for administration to healthy adolescents. For this reason it is unlikely that the vaccine would meet strict licensing laws.

In most cases mononucleosis resolves within four weeks after symptoms first arise, when treatments are targeted at the symptoms of the infection. Rest is one of the key elements to recuperation, and maintenance of fluid intake is essential. Patients are also advised to avoid heavy activity for at least one month following initial infection to reduce the risk of spleen rupture. Nonsteroidal anti-inflammatory (NSAID) medication may be used to treat pain and reduce fever and swelling, and dietary supplements may help boost the immune system. Antibiotics may be useful in treating throat infections that often accompany mononucleosis but will not be effective against EBV. It is not recommended that patients use aspirin due to the possibility of developing Reye's syndrome, a potentially fatal disease.

The typically benign and self-limiting course of mononucleosis, in addition to the ubiquitous nature of the virus, makes prevention virtually impossible. With over 90 percent of the Western adult population returning positive tests for previous infection, person-to-person infection remains highly likely in societies worldwide.

Prevention of the disease may not be beneficial. As noted, childhood infection with EBV typically results in few or no symptoms. In contrast, infection during adolescence tends to result in a more serious disease. This suggests that intentional early primary exposure could potentially be used as a method of preventing the later onset of mononucleosis.

Impacts and Issues

The statistics show that inevitably, at some stage of their life, almost the entire world population will be exposed to, contract, and harbor EBV. However, the majority of people who encounter infection during early childhood will not develop mononucleosis. It is the omnipresence of EBV that prevents the eradication of the infection.

The impact of mononucleosis may be seen on a personal level. Severe cases may keep patients in bed and away from their normal activities for weeks or even months. This is a particular problem for students because they may miss classes during this time. In addition, being removed from social groups for extended periods may generate emotional issues among adolescents. This is especially significant considering that the disease commonly occurs at an important time in social development.

In addition, social pressures can occur when adults contract mononucleosis. Adults may lose income due to an inability to work, which may put economic pressure on families and strain family relationships. Such concerns may lead individuals to shorten their recovery period and return to their regular activities earlier than recommended. In these cases symptoms of fatigue may persist for longer than usual, resulting in lower productivity.

In some chronic cases of the disease, patients suffer symptoms for more than six months and sometimes for years. In many chronic cases, it is considered that the mononucleosis contributed to the development of chronic fatigue syndrome (CFS). Although the exact causes of CFS have not been identified, approximately 10 percent of mononucleosis patients will go on to suffer from it, so CFS is considered a possible side effect of mononucleosis. People with CFS are unable to work, study, or socialize for long periods of time and sometimes permanently.

Cases of mononucleosis are generally much more severe in people with compromised immune systems, and the complications that develop from such infections may prove fatal. Immunocompromised individuals include those who have undergone organ or marrow transplants, individuals receiving chemotherapy, and those with autoimmune diseases. The development of an immune disorder later in life may also result in a severe relapse of mononucleosis infection among people who previously only carried the virus in a latent form. While fatalities resulting from mononucleosis were previously a rare occurrence, the growing numbers of people suffering from immune disorders make this a potentially significant threat in the future.

Bone marrow has been identified as one site of latent EBV persistence within the body. It has also been observed that an EBV-positive individual who receives a bone marrow transplant from an EBV-negative donor is found to be EBV-negative following transplantation. This means that this recipient is again susceptible to infection and most likely, if the transplant occurs during adulthood, will develop mononucleosis. This raises a new concern: the loss of immunity to certain diseases following transplantation. This could become a more serious problem as organ transplantation becomes more common.

PRIMARY SOURCE

Mono: Tough for Teens and Twenty-Somethings

SOURCE: *Willis, Judith Levine. "Mono: Tough for Teens and Twenty-Somethings."* FDA Consumer *32, no. 3 (May/June 1998): 32–35.*

INTRODUCTION: *A diagnosis of mononucleosis can mean a period of convalescence for about two months, and that is usually a difficult order for otherwise healthy teenagers or young adults, who are the prime ages for infection with the viruses that cause mono. In the following article from the* FDA Consumer, *author Judith Levine Willis discusses mono and its implications for physical and social limitations for young people. At the time the article was published in 1998, Willis was on the public affairs staff of the Food and Drug Administration (FDA). She has since authored, as Judith Levine, books about gender, health, and consumer issues.*

Missed parties. Postponed exams. Sitting out a season of team sports. And loneliness. These are a few of the ways that scourge of high school and college students known as "mono" can affect your life.

The disease whose medical name is infectious mononucleosis is most common in people 10 to 35 years old, with its peak incidence in those 15 to 17 years old. Only 50 people out of 100,000 in the general population get mono, but it strikes as many as 2 out of 1,000 teens and twenty-somethings, especially those in high school, college, and the military. While mono is not usually considered a serious illness, it may have serious complications. Without a doubt your lifestyle will change for a few months.

You've probably heard people call mono the "kissing disease." But if your social life is in a slump, you may wonder, "How did I get this 'kissing disease' when I haven't kissed anyone romantically recently?"

Here's how. Mono is usually transmitted through saliva and mucus—which is where the "kissing disease" nickname comes from. But the kissing or close contact that transmits the disease doesn't happen right before you get sick. The virus that causes mono has a long incubation period: 30 to 50 days from the time you're exposed to it to the time you get sick. In addition, the virus can be transmitted in other ways, such as sipping from the same straw or glass as an infected person—or even being close when the person coughs or sneezes. Also, some people can have the virus in their systems without ever having symptoms and you can still catch it from them.

Two viruses can cause mono: Epstein-Barr virus (EBV) and cytomegalovirus (CMV). Both viruses are in the herpes family, whose other members include viruses responsible for cold sores and chickenpox.

EBV causes 85 percent of mono cases. About half of all children are infected with EBV before they're 5, but at that young age, it usually doesn't cause any symptoms. If you don't become infected with EBV until you're a teen or older, you're more likely to develop mono symptoms. After you're infected, the virus stays with you for life, but usually doesn't cause any additional symptoms. Still, every now and then you may produce viral particles in your saliva that can transmit the virus to other people, even though you feel perfectly fine. By age 40, 85 to 90 percent of Americans have EBV antibodies, indicating they have the virus in their systems and are immune to further EBV infection.

CMV is also a very common virus. About 85 percent of the US population is infected with it by the time they reach adulthood. As with EBV, CMV is frequently symptomless, and mono most often results when infection occurs in the teens and 20s. Sore throat is less common in people who have CMV mono than in those infected with EBV.

As another one of its nicknames—glandular fever—implies, perhaps the most distinguishing mono symptom is enlarged glands or lymph nodes, especially in the neck, but also in the armpit and groin.

Another common mono symptom is fever. A temperature as high as 39.5 degrees Celsius (103 degrees Fahrenheit) is not uncommon. Other symptoms include a tired achy feeling, appetite loss, white patches on the back of the throat, and tonsillitis.

"My tonsils got so swollen they were touching each other in back," says Heidi Palombo of Annandale, VA, who had mono when she was a senior in college. She recalls her throat being "so hot and swollen that the only thing that felt good was ice water."

Cold drinks and frozen desserts are both ways to relieve sore throat symptoms. Doctors also recommend gargling with saltwater (about half a teaspoon salt to 8 ounces of warm water) and sucking on throat lozenges available over the counter in pharmacies and other stores. If throat or tonsils are infected, a throat culture should be taken so the doctor can prescribe an appropriate antibiotic. Ampicillin is usually not recommended because it sometimes causes a rash that can be confused with the pink, measleslike rash that one out of five mono patients develops.

For fever and achiness, you can take acetaminophen (marketed as Tylenol, Datril, and others) or ibuprofen (marketed as Advil, Motrin, Nuprin, and others). If you're under 20, don't take aspirin unless your doctor approves it. In children and teens, aspirin taken for viral illnesses has been associated with the potentially fatal disease Reye syndrome. Sometimes a person with mono may have trouble breathing because of swelling in the throat, and doctors have to use other medications and treatment. A person who has mono—or those caring for the person—should contact a doctor immediately if the person starts having breathing problems.

Some people with mono become overly sensitive to light and about half develop enlargement of the spleen, usually two to three weeks after they first become sick. Mild enlargement of the liver may also occur.

Whether or not the spleen is enlarged, people who have mono should not lift heavy objects or exercise vigorously—including participating in contact sports—for two months after they get sick, because these activities increase the risk of rupturing the spleen, which can be life threatening. If you have mono and get a severe sharp, sudden pain on the left side of your upper abdomen, go to an emergency room or call 911 immediately.

Because its symptoms can be very similar to those of other illnesses, doctors often recommend tests to find out exactly what the problem is.

"I was misdiagnosed at first and told I was bit by a spider," writes John L. Gipson, of Kansas City, MO, in a note he posted to a website. "That's what I thought because I had killed a spider in my room. I figured I'd been bitten by a spider in my sleep. A few days after, I had no energy, a fever, and those pea-sized bumps on the back of my neck." Gipson returned to his doctor, who did blood tests and diagnosed mononucleosis.

Other diagnostic problems can result because enlarged lymphocytes, a type of white cell, are common with mono, but can also be a symptom of leukemia. Blood tests can distinguish between the type of white cell seen in leukemia and that with mono.

If your throat is sore, having a throat culture is usually a good idea for several reasons. First, the symptoms of mono and strep infection (including that caused by Strep A, a particularly serious form of strep) are very similar. Second, strep throat or other throat infections can develop anytime during or shortly after in the disease. In any case, it's important that throat infections be diagnosed as soon as possible and treated with antibiotics that can kill the organism responsible for the infection.

The test most commonly used to tell whether you have mono or some other ailment is the mononucleosis spot test. This blood test detects the antibodies (proteins) that the body makes to fight EBV or CMV. Because it takes a while for antibodies to develop after infection, your doctor may need to order or repeat the test one to two weeks after you develop symptoms. At that time the test is about 85 percent accurate.

Other tests your doctor might order include a complete blood count (CBC) to see if your blood platelet count is lower than normal and if lymphocytes are abnormal, and a chemistry panel to see if liver enzymes are abnormal.

Bed rest is the most important treatment for uncomplicated mono. It's also important to drink plenty of fluids. Mono is not usually a reason to quarantine students. Many people are already immune to the viruses that cause it. But if you have mono you'll want to stay in bed and out of classes for several days, until the fever goes down and other symptoms abate. Even when you've started to get better, you can expect to have to curtail your activities for several weeks, and it can take two to three months or more until you feel like your old self again.

The author of this article had mono herself when she was 16. Though she didn't mind getting out of all that homework (or at least putting it off), having to delay finals only added to her anxiety about college applications that many high school juniors experience. And then there was that guy who never called again.

When you add the time spent recuperating to the fact that most people are not exactly anxious to get close to a person with mono, you can understand why some students find themselves combating loneliness on top of their other troubles.

Getting through mono may be both challenging and depressing—and can seem to take forever. But if you rest when your body tells you to, you can lessen the chances of complications and get back your life.

SEE ALSO *Blood Supply and Infectious Disease; Cancer and Infectious Disease; Childhood-Associated Infectious Diseases, Immunization Impacts; Demographics and Infectious Disease; Viral Disease*

BIBLIOGRAPHY

Books

Bennett, John E., Raphael Dolin, and Martin J. Blaser. *Mandell, Douglas, and Bennett's Principles and Practice of Infectious Diseases.* Philadelphia: Elsevier/Saunders, 2015.

Oxford, John, Paul Kellam, and Leslie Harold Collier. *Human Virology.* New York: Oxford University Press, 2016.

Tselis, Alexandros Constantine, and Hal B. Jenson. *Epstein-Barr Virus.* New York: Taylor & Francis, 2006.

Umar, Constantine S. *New Developments in Epstein-Barr Virus Research.* New York: Nova Science, 2006.

Periodicals

Downham, Christina, et al. "Season of Infectious Mononucleosis as a Risk Factor for Multiple Sclerosis: A UK Primary Care Case-Control Study." *Multiple Sclerosis and Related Disorders* 17 (2017): 103–106.

Jason, Leonard A., et al. "A Prospective Study of Infectious Mononucleosis in College Students." *International Journal of Psychiatry* 2, no. 1 (2017): 1–8. This article can also be found online at https://www.ncbi.nlm.nih.gov/pmc/articles/PMC5510613/ (accessed January 24, 2018).

Sayre, Carolyn. "Students Still Getting Mono After All These Years." *New York Times* (January 21, 2009). This article can also be found online at http://www.nytimes.com/ref/health/healthguide/esn-mono-ess.html (accessed January 24, 2018).

Websites

"Epstein-Barr Virus and Infectious Mononucleosis." Centers for Disease Control and Prevention, September 14, 2016. https://www.cdc.gov/epstein-barr/index.html (accessed January 24, 2018).

"Mononucleosis." Mayo Clinic. https://www.mayoclinic.org/diseases-conditions/mononucleosis/symptoms-causes/syc-20350328 (accessed January 24, 2018).

Mosquito-Borne Diseases

Introduction

Mosquitoes have harmed more humans than any other group of insects. The scientific names conveyed on mosquitoes reflect the torment that they can cause: *Psorophora horrida*, *Culex perfidiosus*, *Mansonia perturbans*, *Aedes vexans*, and *Aedes tormentor*. However, the annoyance caused by mosquitoes pales in comparison to the widespread suffering and millions of deaths that these insects cause. These flies from the order Diptera transmit some of the most devastating diseases.

There are more than 2,500 different species of mosquitoes throughout the world. The vast majority are harmless to humans, feeding only on nectar or other plant juices. Only females of some species consume blood. These mosquitoes transmit such diseases as malaria, yellow fever, dengue, filariasis, Zika, and encephalitis, including St. Louis encephalitis (SLE), Western equine encephalitis (WEE), La Crosse encephalitis (LAC), Japanese encephalitis (JE), Eastern equine encephalitis (EEE), and West Nile virus (WNV), to humans and to animals.

Disease History, Characteristics, and Transmission

A vector-borne disease results from an infection transmitted to humans and other animals by blood-feeding arthropods, such as mosquitoes. Female mosquitoes take a blood meal by bending back a troughlike protec-

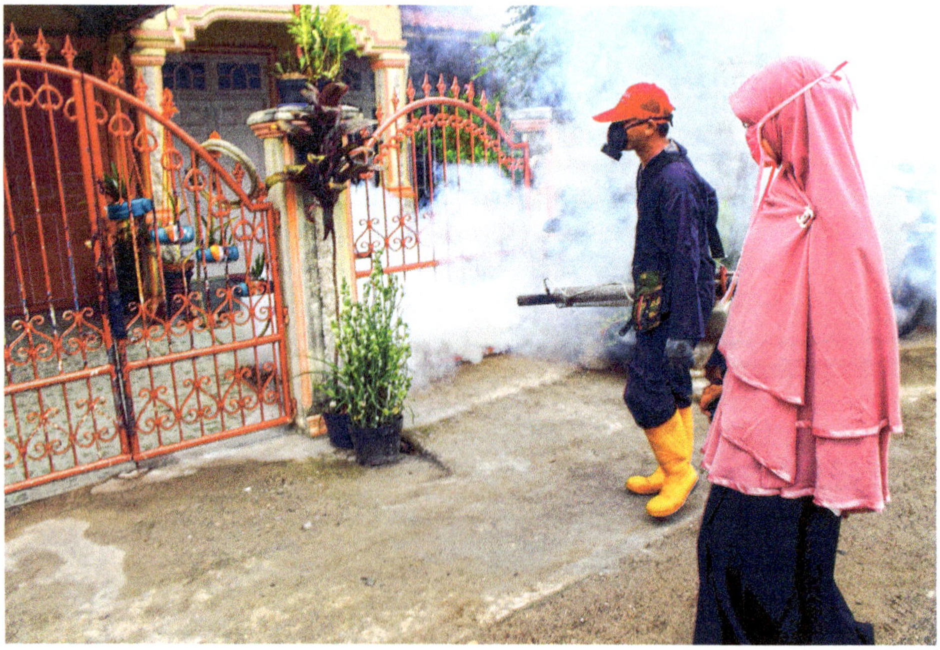

A health worker in Indonesia fumigates a neighborhood. Fumigation is used to kill mosquitoes that spread dengue fever. © *Fachrul Reza/NurPhoto/Getty Images*

tive scabbard to permit other mouthparts to penetrate the skin. The piercing "needle" is a long tube composed of six long, separate, stilettolike stylets wet with saliva that adhere to each other. The tube is traversed by two channels, a wide one through which the blood is sucked into the digestive system and a narrow one through which saliva containing an anticoagulant can be injected into the vertebrate host. Pathogens are transmitted from the mosquito to the host at this point.

In 1878 English parasitologist Patrick Manson (1844–1922) discovered the link between bloodsucking insects and disease. European and American infectious disease experts subsequently focused on the most common mosquito-borne diseases in these regions: malaria and yellow fever. The rapid worldwide movement of goods and people has also helped mosquitoes to cross the globe. By the end of the 20th century, scientists battled mosquito-borne diseases that were worldwide plagues.

West Nile fever, caused by a mosquito-borne virus related to yellow fever, made its first appearance in the Western Hemisphere, in New York City in 1999. First isolated and identified in Uganda in 1937, West Nile came to the United States via an infected mosquito, a sick person, or an infected bird. A human source is improbable because human blood generally contains too little virus to contaminate a mosquito. It may have come to New York in mosquitoes that stowed away on an airplane. However, the most likely scenario is that it arrived in illegally imported birds that had not been quarantined before entering the country. It has subsequently spread by migrating birds and is now present in all 48 contiguous states in the United States.

WORDS TO KNOW

BED NET A type of netting that provides protection from diseases caused by insects such as flies and mosquitoes. It is often used when sleeping to allow air to flow through its mesh structure while preventing insects from biting.

GENETIC ENGINEERING The altering of the genetic material of living cells to make them capable of producing new substances or performing new functions. When the genetic material within the living cells (i.e., genes) is working properly, the human body can develop and function smoothly. However, should a single gene (even a tiny segment of a gene) go awry, the effect can be dramatic: deformities, disease, and even death are possible.

INSECTICIDE A chemical substance used to kill insects.

MOSQUITO COILS Spirals of inflammable paste that, when burned, steadily release insect repellent into the air. They are often used in Asia, where many coils release octachlorodipropyl ether, which can cause lung cancer.

MOSQUITO NETTING Fine meshes or nets hung around occupied spaces, especially beds, to keep out disease-carrying mosquitoes. Mosquito netting is a cost-effective way of preventing malaria.

PESTICIDE A substance used to reduce the abundance of pests or any living thing that causes injury or disease to crops.

Scope and Distribution

Malaria occurs in tropical areas of Central and South America, Africa, Asia, and the East Indies. Until the mid-20th century, it was far more widespread. Malaria was established in virtually all subtropical and tropical areas as well as some temperate areas. Malaria receded because breeding sites for mosquitoes were drained for agricultural and industrial purposes. Meanwhile, people moved into better housing that was less open to mosquitoes. While the disease has been all but obliterated from most of the developed world, it continues to kill elsewhere. More than 1 million people, mostly in Africa, die annually from malaria, with a child succumbing every 30 seconds.

Several different species of the *Aedes* and *Haemogogus* (South America only) mosquitoes transmit the yellow fever virus. The disease is endemic in 47 African countries and 13 Latin American nations. While control programs successfully eradicated mosquito habitats in the past, particularly in South America, these programs have lapsed. As a result, mosquito populations have jumped, and there is an accompanying rise in the risk of yellow fever epidemics.

Dengue and Zika are spread by the *Aedes* mosquito. Dengue hemorrhagic fever (DHF) is a potentially lethal complication. DHF is a leading cause of hospitalization among children, with more than 500,000 requiring such care annually. Dengue, once confined to nine countries, is now endemic to more than 100 countries.

Zika, first identified in 1947, is named after the Zika Forest in Uganda. The first outbreaks occurred in 1952, with the disease subsequently reported throughout the Americas, tropical Africa, Southeast Asia, and the Pacific Islands. The symptoms of Zika are similar to those of other diseases, and the disease can be mild, so it is possible that some cases were not reported. On February 1, 2016, the World Health Organization (WHO) declared Zika to be a public health emergency because of a cluster of cases of severe neurological damage and microcephaly. Zika can be passed by a pregnant woman to her fetus, causing birth defects. It can also be transmitted through sexual intercourse and, possibly, blood transfusions.

SCIENTIFIC, POLITICAL, AND ETHICAL ISSUES

Developed during the 1940s, the pesticide dichlorodiphenyltrichloroethane (DDT) was used to fight malaria and other insect-borne diseases and was considered by many to be a miracle pesticide. During three decades of use, approximately 675,000 tons of DDT were applied in the United States.

Although DDT greatly reduced the burden of mosquito-borne disease in the 1960s, DDT use remains controversial. DDT is an environmentally persistent chlorinated hydrocarbon that accumulates in the food chain and has significant environmental consequences that offset its benefits in the control of disease. Since 1972 the pesticide has been banned in many developed nations, including the United States, because of its potential to damage ecosystems and wildlife. It is, however, still used for disease control in some countries.

Proponents of DDT use assert that its environmental impact has been overstated and that prohibitions on DDT use and manufacturing may have contributed to worldwide deaths from mosquito-borne diseases over the past several decades. It is again recommended for limited use in targeted areas because of its effectiveness in removing this severe public health hazard. Others assert that safer insecticides than DDT should be used in all locations.

American biologist and author Rachel Louise Carson (1907–1964) was a seminal figure in the environmental movement during the 1950s and early 1960s. Carson's book *Silent Spring* was an indictment of overzealous pesticide use and its effects on the environment. It was published in 1962 and quickly became a controversial and enduring contribution to the environmental literature. Carson argued against indiscriminate pesticide use without consideration of its ecological consequences. Largely as a result of *Silent Spring*, DDT was banned by the United States in 1972.

Treatment and Prevention

The best method of preventing mosquito-borne diseases is to kill mosquitoes. To eradicate mosquitoes, public health experts advise emptying containers of standing water that attract egg-laying females. Some governments kill mosquitoes through insecticide-spraying programs or swamp-draining efforts. Exposure to mosquito-borne diseases can be minimized by limiting outdoor movement. Screens are effective at keeping mosquitoes from entering homes.

Infection with the parasite that causes malaria is treated with chloroquine, unless the parasite is resistant to this medication, in which case quinine sulfate and antibiotic combinations are used. As many other mosquito-borne diseases are viral in nature, treatment is mostly supportive or, in some cases, involves antiviral medications. Vaccines are available to protect against Japanese encephalitis, dengue, and yellow fever.

Impacts and Issues

In some regions mosquitoes have shown the ability to become resistant to pesticides. *Anopheles* mosquitoes are no longer killed by applications of DDT in certain areas. Pesticide can also be prohibitively expensive. In 2007 Uganda announced it could not spray DDT to fight malaria because it had failed to raise the $400 million necessary to purchase the pesticide. An estimated 320 Ugandans die of malaria daily.

Several international organizations and charities have been instrumental in the fight against mosquito-borne diseases. The Bill & Melinda Gates Foundation supports mosquito-borne disease research and prevention efforts worldwide, including the development of effective and affordable drugs, improvement of existing preventative measures, and vaccine development. RAPIDS (Reaching HIV-Affected People with Integrated Development and Support), a consortium of several organizations, targets its efforts against mosquito-borne diseases in Zambian communities affected by human immunodeficiency virus (HIV) and acquired immunodeficiency syndrome (AIDS). RAPIDS distributes protective netting and provides in-home follow-up care, ensuring that mosquito netting is properly used.

Promotion of specific sanitation measures is underway in areas where mosquito-borne diseases pose public health threats. Biological control methods, such as wasps that kill mosquitoes, are also being investigated. Researchers are also developing and investigating the use of genetically engineered mosquitoes to fight malaria. The modified mosquitoes are resistant to malaria and breed at a faster rate than unmodified, nonresistant mosquitoes. Researchers hope that such mosquitoes can be introduced into malaria-prone regions and overtake wild disease-carrying mosquito populations. However, little is known about the impact genetically engineered mosquitoes could have on the transmission or development of other diseases.

Outdoor time-released insecticide misting systems are increasing in popularity, particularly in the United States, as a means of controlling mosquitoes. These systems use various synergized formulations of natural pyrethrins or synthetic pyrethroids that are dispensed into the environment at intervals determined by the user. Some systems also use minimum-risk pesticides to control or repel mosquitoes. The American Mosquito Control Association (AMCA) opposes this method of dispensing pesticides as inconsistent with the integrated mosquito management practices approved by the Environmental Protection Agency (EPA) as part of the Pesticide Environmental Stewardship Program. The AMCA specifically fears unnecessary insecticide use, indiscriminate killing of beneficial insects, pesticide exposure to humans, and promotion of insecticide resistance.

The regular use of insecticide-impregnated curtains and bed nets can reduce the rate of such diseases, particularly among children. The success of using bed nets for sustained mosquito control depends on regular treatment of the nets with pyrethroid insecticide once or twice a year. Dip-it-yourself kits have been distributed for this purpose in some countries, and researchers are developing better, longer-lasting insecticide-impregnated fabrics for netting, drapery, and clothing.

Travelers visiting areas known for major outbreaks of mosquito-borne diseases are advised to use mosquito-repellent insecticide. The use of mosquito coils and protective clothing and bedding is also often recommended, along with available vaccinations.

See Also *Dengue and Dengue Hemorrhagic Fever; Eastern Equine Encephalitis; Encephalitis; Filariasis; Japanese Encephalitis; Malaria; St. Louis Encephalitis; Vector-Borne Disease; West Nile Virus; Yellow Fever; Zika Virus*

BIBLIOGRAPHY

Books

Diniz, Debora. *Zika: From the Brazilian Backlands to Global Threat.* London: Zed, 2017.

Speilman, Andrew, and Michael D'Antonio. *Mosquito: A Natural History of Our Most Persistent and Deadly Foe.* New York: Hyperion, 2001.

Periodicals

Arnold, Carrie. "In the Eye of the Tiger: Global Spread of Asian Tiger Mosquito Could Fuel Outbreaks of Tropical Disease in Temperate Regions." *Science News* 183, no. 13 (June 29, 2013): 26–29.

Websites

Division of Vector-Borne Diseases. Centers for Disease Control, National Center for Emerging and Zoonotic Infectious Diseases, April 2, 2016. https://www.cdc.gov/ncezid/dvbd/index.html (accessed February 25, 2018).

Caryn E. Neumann

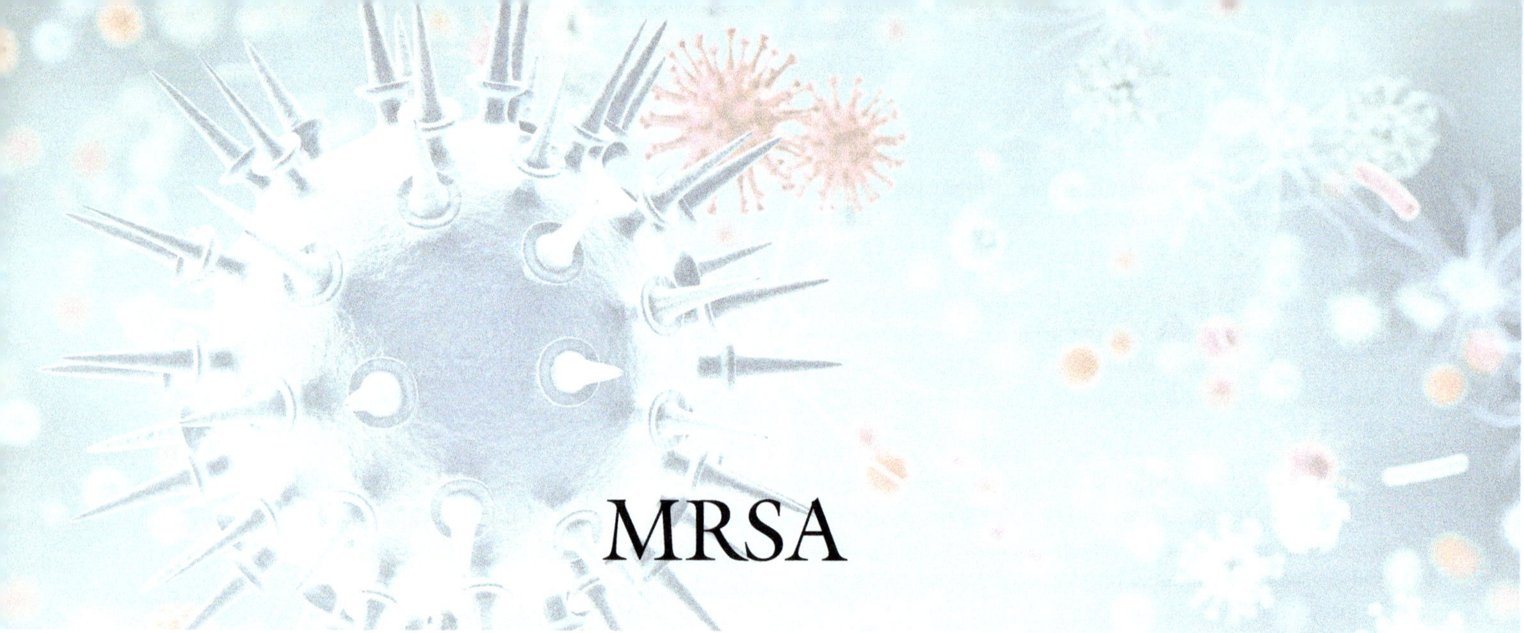

MRSA

Introduction

MRSA is an abbreviation for methicillin-resistant *Staphylococcus aureus*, which is a particular type (strain) of *S. aureus*. The bacterium is important because of its antibiotic resistance and because it can cause a number of severe diseases. One such disease is necrotizing fasciitis, more popularly known as flesh-eating disease. MRSA is also known as oxacillin-resistant *S. aureus* (oxacillin is another antibiotic) and multiple-resistant *S. aureus*.

Until the beginning of the 21st century, MRSA was almost exclusively found in hospitals because the tremendous use of antibiotics in hospitals provided a powerful selection pressure. In other words, only the most resilient bacteria could survive. By 2017 MRSA had become the leading cause of health care–associated infections in the United States and a major problem worldwide. The infection has also become established outside of hospitals. This form of the bacterium is designated as community associated–MRSA (CA-MRSA). In particular, the USA300 type of MRSA has become a significant source of infections that require hospitalization.

WORDS TO KNOW

COLONIZATION The process of occupation and increase in the number of microorganisms at a specific site.

GENE The fundamental physical and functional unit of heredity. Whether in a microorganism or in a human cell, a gene is an individual element of an organism's genome and determines a trait or characteristic by regulating biochemical structure or metabolic process.

PATHOGEN A disease-causing agent, such as a bacteria, virus, fungus, or other microorganism.

RESISTANCE Immunity developed within a species (especially bacteria) to an antibiotic or other drug via evolution. For example, bacteria may acquire genetic mutations that render them invulnerable to the action of antibiotics.

SELECTION PRESSURE The influence of various factors on the evolution of an organism. An example is the overuse of antibiotics, which provides a selection pressure for the development of antibiotic resistance in bacteria.

Disease History, Characteristics, and Transmission

MRSA is resistant to methicillin, a synthetic penicillin antibiotic. It is also resistant to all of the penicillin class of antibiotics. This wide range of resistance makes the bacterium hard to treat because commonly used antibiotics will not kill it.

MRSA has been evident almost as long as methicillin has been in use. Methicillin was introduced in 1959 to treat strains of *S. aureus* that had developed resistance to penicillin. By chemically altering the structure of penicillin, scientists were able to produce methicillin, and the penicillin-resistant *S. aureus* were killed by the newly synthesized antibiotic. But this beneficial effect did not last long. By 1961 MRSA was making a comeback despite the use of methicillin in the United Kingdom. Soon, reports of MRSA came from countries in Europe and North America, as well as Japan and Australia. By 2005 thousands of hospital deaths in the United Kingdom were caused by MRSA, and the organism accounted for almost 50 percent of all hospital-acquired infections. Despite the drop in MRSA infections in US hospitals between 2005 and 2011 because of dedicated efforts to control the infection, the US Centers for Disease Control and Prevention (CDC) reported more than 80,000 MRSA hospital infections and nearly 11,300 deaths in 2011.

Methicillin resistance is caused by the presence of a gene that codes for a protein that binds to the antibiotic and prevents the antibiotic from entering the bacteria. The *S. aureus* that is susceptible to methicillin does not have this gene. The transfer of this gene from one bacterium to another has spread methicillin resistance through populations of *Staphylococcus* around the globe.

The spread of MRSA has been aided by the fact that *S. aureus* is normally found in the environment. The bacterium is present in soil and in the human body. Studies of the bacteria present in certain areas of the body have revealed that approximately 30 percent of healthy adults harbor *S. aureus*, including MRSA, on the surface of their skin or in other places, such as their noses. In these environments the bacterium is harmless. But if MRSA gets into a wound or if a person's immune system is not functioning efficiently, illness can result.

MRSA is sometimes capable of causing necrotizing fasciitis, an extremely invasive disease that progresses rapidly. Sometimes amputation of the infected limb is the only way to save the patient's life. MRSA can also carry genes that code for the production of potent toxins. If these toxins get into the bloodstream, the resulting effects can be devastating to the body.

Scope and Distribution

Because *S. aureus* is found around the world, it is not surprising that MRSA is also ubiquitous. MRSA previously was usually found in hospitals and athletic facilities because both are places where abrasions, cuts, and scrapes occur. By 2017 CA-MRSA had become a significant health threat.

It is estimated that more than 50 million people around the globe carry MRSA in their bodies. In the United States about 32 percent of people are colonized with *S. aureus* in their noses. Colonization refers to bacteria (or other pathogens) that establish a presence on a tissue. Fewer than 1 percent of otherwise healthy individuals colonized with MRSA will develop a MRSA-related disease.

Having another infection can increase the likelihood of developing a MRSA infection. For example, individuals

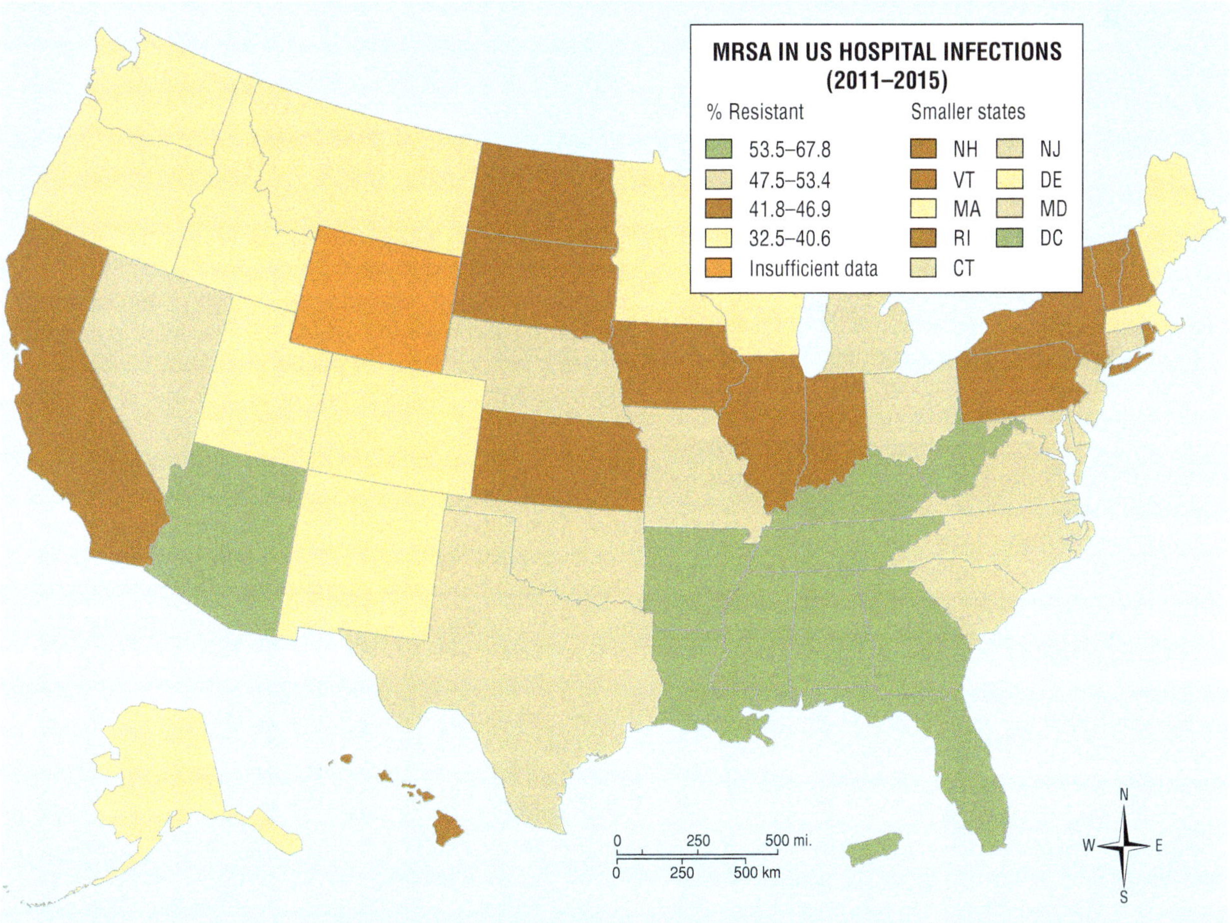

SOURCE: Adapted from "Methicillin-Resistant *Staphylococcus aureas.*" US Centers for Disease Control and Prevention. 2015. Available from: https://gis.cdc.gov/grasp/PSA/MapView.html

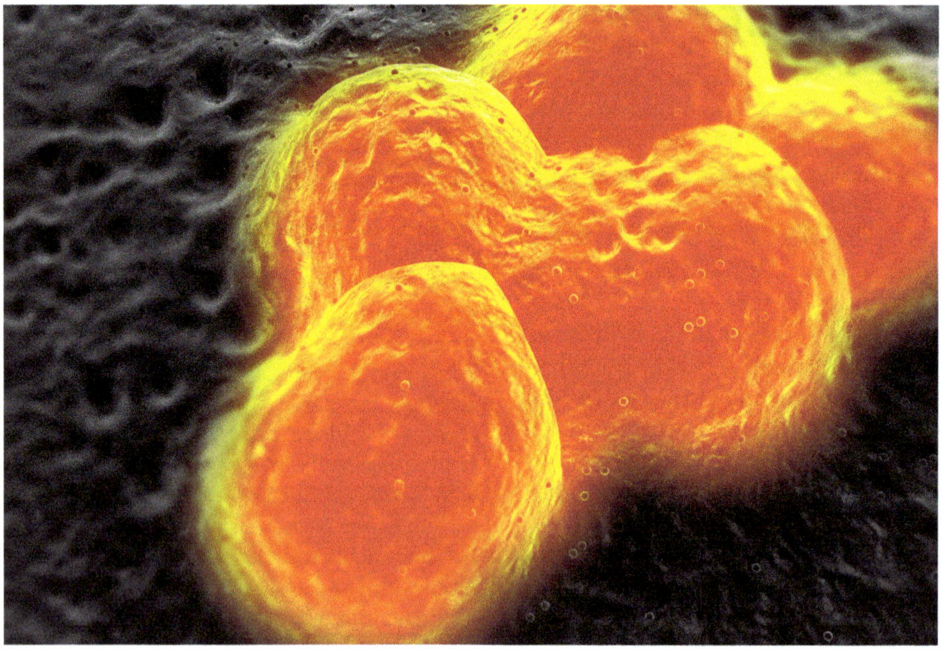

Methicillin-resistant *Staphylococcus aureus*, or MRSA. This bacterium's resistance to commonly used antibiotics makes treating MRSA a challenge. © Science Picture Co/Science Source

with cystic fibrosis often have recurring lung infections that require treatment with a number of different antibiotics. This situation increases the risk that MRSA will be able to gain a foothold in these patients.

Treatment and Prevention

Treating MRSA is challenging. Only a few antibiotics remain effective against the bacterium. One of these is vancomycin. It has the disadvantage of not being absorbed easily into the body. It cannot be given by mouth because there will be little active compound left by the time the antibiotic circulates through the bloodstream to the site of the infection. Rather, vancomycin must be given intravenously (via a needle inserted into a vein). This usually means that a person being treated must be hospitalized.

The search continues for new antibiotics that will be effective against MRSA. In 2017 the most common treatment for people at home involved an oral combination of two antibiotics (trimethoprim and sulfamethoxazole), clindamycin, minocycline, or doxycycline. Patients in hospitals are usually treated intravenously because it is important to rapidly achieve a level of antibiotic in the bloodstream that is effective in killing the bacteria.

Another potential treatment option is called phage therapy. Phage is short for bacteriophage, which is a virus that specifically infects and forms new phage particles inside of a bacterium. The phage-bacterium association is specific. A certain type of phage infects a certain type of bacterium. In doing so the phage ultimately destroys the bacterial cell. Scientists are experimenting with a phage that targets MRSA. If this technique proves successful, it would be a powerful treatment because resistance to a phage does not typically develop. As of 2017 phage therapy remains in the research stage.

Contact precautions, including handwashing, are critical in preventing MRSA infection. In a hospital, washing hands before and after caring for a patient is the most important method of preventing the spread of MRSA from patient to patient. Many hospitals have alcohol-based hand cleansers in each room, sometimes at the patient's bedside. Washing with an alcohol-based wash takes only a few seconds and, thus, is an easy method for busy health care providers. Moreover, MRSA is usually sensitive to alcohol.

Compliance with handwashing precautions is surprisingly low. Surveys in the United States and Europe have confirmed that health care providers only wash their hands about half as much as is optimum for reducing the spread of infection. The CDC has estimated that properly performed handwashing could save the 30,000 lives that are lost each year due to hospital-acquired infections, including MRSA infections.

Outside of hospitals, people can avoid MRSA infection by washing their hands regularly, covering all open wounds with bandages, and avoiding sharing personal care items such as razors and towels. In settings such as gyms and health clubs, it is important to make sure that shared equipment is sanitized with disinfectants before and after use. The chances of contracting MRSA from such equipment can be further reduced by using clothing or a towel as a barrier between skin and workout equipment. Washing towels and athletic clothing in hot water and bleach following a workout can also help prevent MRSA infection.

Impacts and Issues

Studies have indicated that a hospitalized patient who acquires MRSA is about five times more likely to die than a patient in the same hospital that does not carry the bacterium.

Variants of MRSA that are resistant even to vancomycin have appeared. These new forms of the bacterium, which are called vancomycin intermediate-resistant *Staphylococcus aureus*, are especially troublesome because they can be treated with few compounds. With time, further resistance could develop. If newer and more powerful (and likely more expensive) antibacterial agents are not discovered and tested, there could be no means of combating the infections.

MRSA infections that affect the surface of the skin can often respond to antibacterial cream that is rubbed on the skin. Some infections that produce pus-filled lesions can be treated by puncturing the lesions and draining the pus. Some infections that are growing on the surface of a foreign object, such as an artificial heart valve, can be treated by removing the surface. In the heart valve example, this would be major surgery involving the heart.

A lot of effort has gone into trying to devise a vaccine for MRSA. Six trials have failed at the phase 3 stage, which is the stage near the end of development when the treatment is tried on a large number of people with the goal of definitely establishing that the treatment works or does not work. As of 2017 there were several vaccines at the early stages of development. Whether one or more of these is ultimately successful may take years to determine.

CA-MRSA is of great concern. The organism tends to more aggressively invade tissues and produces a more severe infection than that produced by hospital-acquired MRSA for reasons that are not yet clear. In addition, it has been discovered that MRSA can grow and divide inside another microscopic organism called *Acanthamoeba*. *Acanthamoeba* can become airborne and drift for a considerable distance on air currents. This may mean that MRSA has acquired the ability to spread great distances, which would make treatment even more difficult.

SEE ALSO *Antibiotic Resistance; Contact Precautions; Resistant Organisms*

BIBLIOGRAPHY

Books

Kon, Kateryna, and Mahendra Rai. *Antibiotic Resistance: Mechanisms and New Antimicrobial Approaches.* Amsterdam: Elsevier, 2016.

Rosen, William. *Miracle Cure: The Creation of Antibiotics and the Birth of Modern Medicine.* New York: Viking, 2017.

Periodicals

Carrel, Margaret, Eli N. Perencevich, and Michael Z. David. "USA300 Methicillin-Resistant *Staphylococcus aureus*, United States, 2000–2013." *Emerging Infectious Diseases* 21, no. 11 (November 2015): 1973–1980.

Kavanagh, Kevin T., Said Abusalem, and Lindsey E. Calderon. "The Incidence of MRSA Infections in the United States: Is a More Comprehensive Tracking System Needed?" *Antimicrobial Resistance & Infection Control* 6, no. 34 (April 2017). This article can also be found online at https://aricjournal.biomedcentral.com/articles/10.1186/s13756-017-0193-0 (accessed December 7, 2017).

Websites

"Antimicrobial Resistance." World Health Organization, November 2017. http://www.who.int/mediacentre/factsheets/fs194/en (accessed November 20, 2017).

"Methicillin-Resistant *Staphylococcus aureus* (MRSA)." Centers for Disease Control and Prevention, May 16, 2016. https://www.cdc.gov/mrsa/index.html (accessed November 20, 2017).

"Patient Education: Methicillin-resistant *Staphyloccocus aureus* (MRSA) (Beyond the Basics)." UpToDate, August 15, 2017. https://www.uptodate.com/contents/methicillin-resistant-staphylococcus-aureus-mrsa-beyond-the-basics (accessed November 20, 2017).

Brian Hoyle

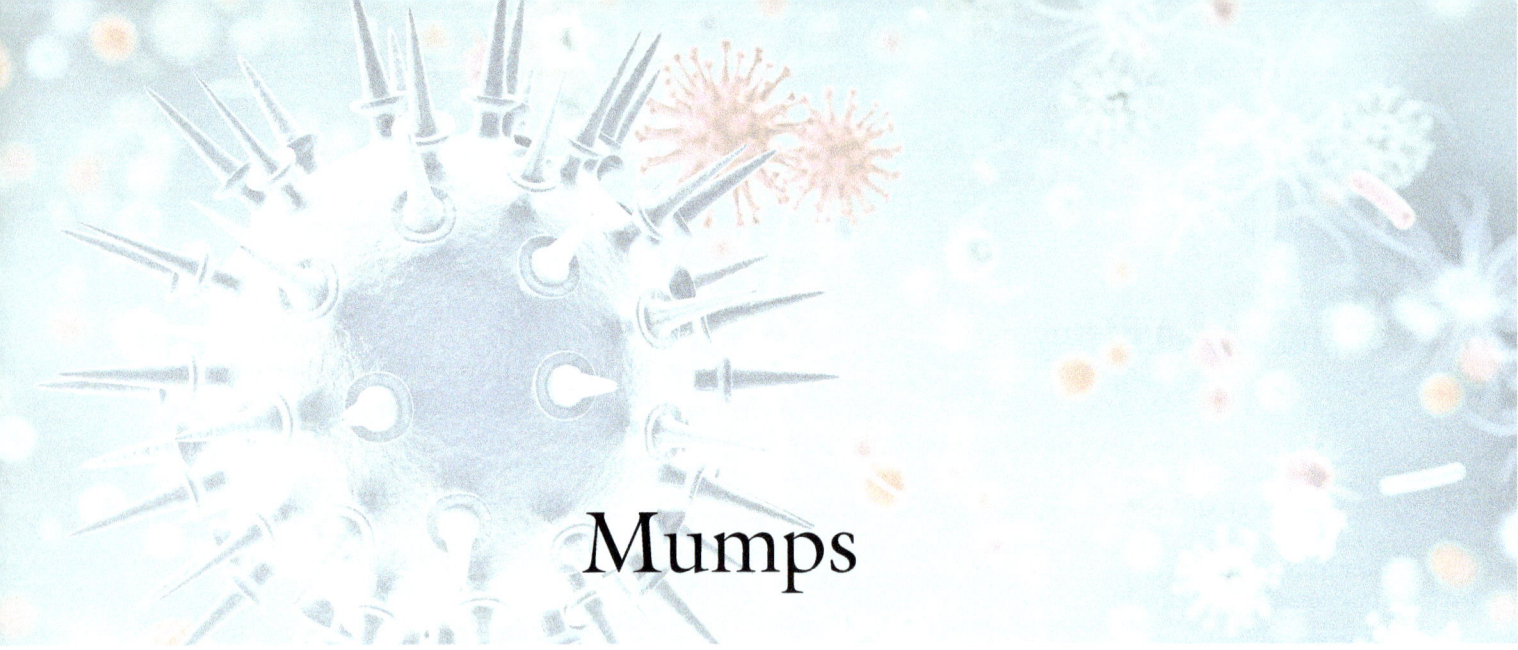

Mumps

Introduction

Mumps is an acute viral illness whose main symptom is parotitis, an inflammation of the salivary glands in the neck. It was first described by the great Greek physician Hippocrates (460 BCE–370 BCE) in the 5th century BCE. Before an effective vaccination program was introduced in 1968, mumps was one of the most significant childhood diseases in the world.

Mumps is as infectious as influenza and rubella (German measles) but somewhat less so than measles and chickenpox. Many of those infected with the virus have no symptoms at all. Mumps usually clears up within a week or so, and those infected then have lifelong immunity. However, the virus can spread through the lymph glands to cause a number of complications, including permanent deafness, so protecting children from mumps through vaccination is important. The introduction of vaccination for mumps has cut the rate of infections in the United States by 99 percent. However, local epidemics still sometimes occur and have happened with increased frequency in the United States during the early 21st century.

Disease History, Characteristics, and Transmission

Mumps, also known as infectious parotitis, is caused by a paramyxovirus, which consists of single-stranded ribonucleic acid (RNA) surrounded by a protein envelope.

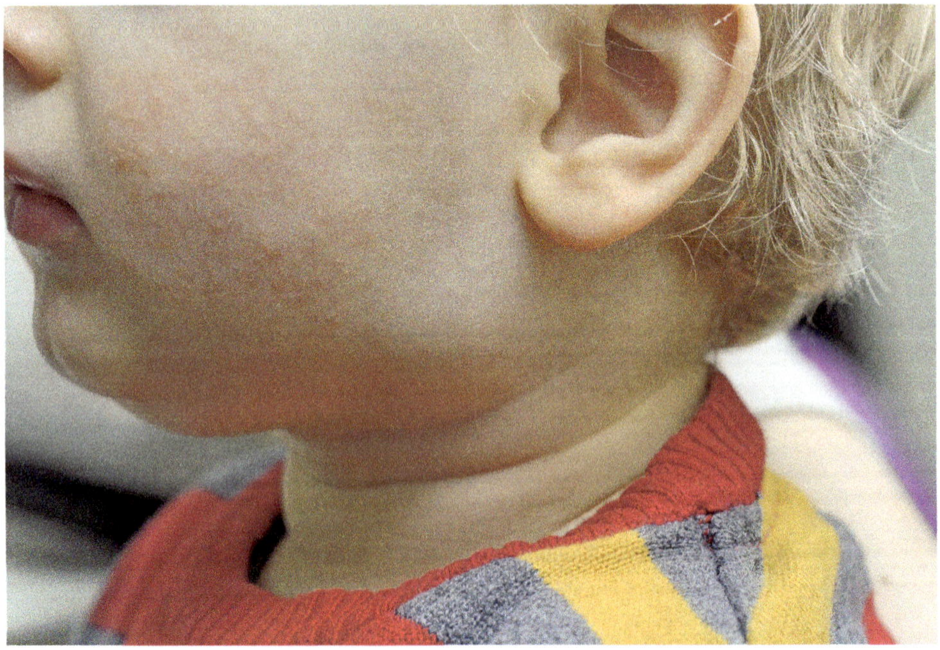

A child exhibiting parotitis, a swelling of the salivary glands beneath the ear. Parotitis is the most common symptom of mumps. *© SPL/Science Source*

WORDS TO KNOW

MALAISE A general or nonspecific feeling of unease or discomfort, often the first sign of disease infection.

OOPHORITIS Inflammation of the ovary, which happens in certain sexually transmitted infections.

ORCHITIS Inflammation of one or both testicles, with swelling and pain as typical symptoms. May be caused by various sexually transmitted infections or escape of sperm cells into the tissues of the testicle.

PANCREATITIS Inflammation of the pancreas, an organ that is important in digestion. Pancreatitis can be acute (beginning suddenly, usually with the patient recovering fully) or chronic (progressing slowly with continued, permanent injury to the pancreas).

PARAMYXOVIRUS A type of virus that contains ribonucleic acid as the genetic material and has proteins on its surface that clump red blood cells and assist in the release of newly made viruses from the infected cells. Measles virus and mumps virus are two types of paramyxoviruses.

PAROTITIS Inflammation of the parotid gland. There are two parotid glands, one on each side of the jaw, at the back. Their function is to secrete saliva into the mouth.

REPORTABLE DISEASE By law, occurrences of some diseases must be reported to government authorities when observed by health care professionals. Such diseases are called reportable diseases or notifiable diseases. Cholera and yellow fever are examples of reportable diseases.

RIBONUCLEIC ACID (RNA) Any of a group of nucleic acids that carry out several important tasks in the synthesis of proteins. Unlike DNA (deoxyribonucleic acid), it has only a single strand. Nucleic acids are complex molecules that contain a cell's genetic information and the instructions for carrying out cellular processes. In eukaryotic cells, the two nucleic acids, ribonucleic acid (RNA) and deoxyribonucleic acid (DNA), work together to direct protein synthesis. Although it is DNA that contains the instructions for directing the synthesis of specific structural and enzymatic proteins, several types of RNA actually carry out the processes required to produce these proteins. These include messenger RNA (mRNA), ribosomal RNA (rRNA), and transfer RNA (tRNA). Further processing of the various RNAs is carried out by another type of RNA called small nuclear RNA (snRNA). The structure of RNA is similar to that of DNA, however, instead of the base thymine, RNA contains the base uracil in its place.

The incubation period of the virus is 12 to 25 days, during which time it infects the upper respiratory tract and may pass to the glandular tissue of the ovaries, testes, or pancreas through the lymphatic system.

The most common symptom of mumps is parotitis, an inflammation of the salivary glands. The patient will experience pain, tenderness, and swelling in the jaw area, which may be accompanied by an earache. Approximately half of mumps infections are accompanied by parotitis. However, bacterial infection by *Staphylococcus* species can also cause parotitis, and that may be confused with mumps on diagnosis. Headache is another common symptom of mumps, and malaise, fever, and loss of appetite may also occur, especially in the early stages. Parotitis peaks about two days after its onset, and the infection begins to clear within a week, with the vast majority of patients making a full recovery. One attack of mumps confers lifelong immunity; therefore, the illness does not recur.

However, mumps does sometimes cause complications and, indeed, is responsible for one death a year, on average, in the United States. When the virus spreads to the glands, it can cause orchitis (inflammation of the testicles), oophoritis (inflammation of the ovaries), pancreatitis, arthritis, and encephalitis. Central nervous system involvement in the form of asymptomatic meningitis is common, and symptomatic meningitis with headache and stiff neck occurs in up to 15 percent of patients, although this usually resolves itself within several days. Around 1 in 10,000 to 20,000 cases of mumps will lead to permanent deafness, with sudden onset. In 80 percent of these cases, the deafness is confined to one ear.

The mumps virus is spread by airborne transmission and through the droplets created by coughs and sneezes. Those infected will spread the virus about a week before they develop symptoms—if any occur—and will remain infectious for up to 10 days after the symptoms begin. People without symptoms may still be infectious.

Scope and Distribution

The mumps virus affects both children and adults around the world, with the peak of infection occurring in late winter and early spring, although cases occur throughout the year as well. However, mass vaccination, when and where used, has had a dramatic impact

SCIENTIFIC, POLITICAL, AND ETHICAL ISSUES

With regard to a potential connection between the measles, mumps, and rubella (MMR) vaccine and autism, the Centers for Disease Control and Prevention (CDC) stated in 2015, "Because signs of autism may appear around the same time children receive the MMR vaccine, some parents may worry that the vaccine causes autism. Vaccine safety experts, including experts at the CDC and the American Academy of Pediatrics (AAP), agree that MMR vaccine is not responsible for recent increases in the number of children with autism."

The question of whether the MMR vaccine could raise the risk of autism in children has been addressed by numerous studies since a paper published in the *Lancet* in 1998 (and retracted in 2010) claimed to find a link in children who had chronic intestinal disorders. Though the paper was widely debunked, the theory was revived in 2014 when a former CDC scientist who had worked on a 2004 study published in *Pediatrics* claimed to have suppressed data that showed a 340 percent increase in autism risk among African American boys who received the MMR vaccine as normally scheduled. The CDC subsequently released the data from the study, which showed the link was most likely due to the fact that the slightly higher vaccination rates among children with autism could be attributed to more stringent vaccination requirements in preschool programs for children with developmental disorders. A number of subsequent studies, including those published in *Vaccine* (2014) and the *Journal of the American Medical Association* (2015), found no evidence of increased autism risk associated with the MMR vaccine.

Although the theoretical link between the MMR vaccine and autism has been roundly rejected by scientists, public health officials worry about the effects of such rumors on global vaccination rates. In its response to the 2014 controversy, the CDC noted, "Our 2014 measles count is the highest number since measles was declared eliminated in 2000. We do not want to lose any opportunity to protect all of our children when we have the means to do so." Although the sharp rise in mumps cases in 2016 and 2017 occurred in areas where vaccination rates remained high, the most severe complications of mumps infections were concentrated among individuals who had not received the MMR vaccine.

on the number of cases of mumps. In World War I (1939–1945) only gonorrhea and influenza caused more hospitalizations among the military than mumps.

When it comes to the complications of mumps, adults appear to be more susceptible than children. Men ages 15 to 29 are the most susceptible to orchitis, which affects 20 to 50 percent of those developing mumps. In 30 percent of these cases, both testicles are affected, which raises the threat of infertility. However, although shrinkage of the testicles does occur in some cases of orchitis, infertility rarely results, with around 13 percent of cases experiencing impaired fertility or complete infertility. Around 5 percent of young women with mumps will develop oophoritis, which may cause severe pelvic pain, but this complication is not linked to infertility. Pregnant women who develop mumps run an increased risk of spontaneous abortion. Mumps has been a reportable disease in the United States for several years.

Treatment and Prevention

Treatment of mumps infection includes hydration and painkillers such as ibuprofen or naproxen. If headache is severe, a lumbar puncture (insertion of a needle into the spinal canal, otherwise known as a spinal tap) may bring relief. In the case of orchitis, cold compresses may also reduce pain. Children and adults with mumps should be excluded from school or work during the infectious period.

Mumps can be prevented by immunization with a live mumps vaccine. This is part of the measles, mumps, and rubella (MMR) vaccine, which is given as childhood immunization—once at 12 to 15 months and again between four and six years of age. In October 2017, amid a resurgence of mumps cases in the United States, the CDC's Advisory Committee on Immunization Practices also recommended that anyone at high risk of contracting mumps because of an outbreak in their area should receive a third dose of the vaccine. Although the mumps vaccine is generally safe, it should not be given to pregnant women, those with a fever, or patients with weakened immunity. There have been occasional side effects of the mumps vaccine on the central nervous system, some of which have led to deafness.

As with all airborne diseases, good personal hygiene helps prevent transmission. Therefore, people should always cover their nose and mouth when they cough or sneeze and should wash their hands regularly.

Impacts and Issues

Mumps was once a major childhood disease with occasional serious complications, such as deafness and infertility. Vaccination has changed that. Mumps became a reportable disease in the United States in 1968, when vaccination was introduced. Before that, there were an estimated 212,000 cases per year. However, between

1983 and 1985, there were only around 3,000 cases reported annually, demonstrating the value of mass vaccination.

In 1986 and 1987, there was a relative resurgence of mumps, with around 13,000 cases being reported in the United States. Most occurred in people ages 10 to 19 who were born before vaccination was introduced. Because mumps can affect adults too, this was not unexpected. There were several outbreaks among highly vaccinated school populations, which suggested that a single dose might not be sufficient to protect children.

After 1989 there was a marked decline in the number of reported cases of mumps, from 5,712 cases to a total of 258 cases in 2004. But childhood infections like mumps can still come back unexpectedly. In 2006 there were outbreaks in several states, mostly among young adults, which led to a total of more than 6,000 reported cases. Most of these cases had received either one or two shots of MMR but possibly had not developed a full immune response. The number of reported cases declined after 2006, although not to the sustained level seen from 2000 through 2005. The potential for mumps outbreak received increased public attention in 2014, when 24 players and 2 referees in the National Hockey League were sidelined with the disease, though the total number of infections across the United States remained relatively low at 1,223. However, the number spiked again in 2016 and was only slightly lower in 2017, according to preliminary estimates. Other developed countries have noted similar outbreaks, with data reported by Australia's Department of Health showing a worrisome 804 cases in 2016.

The increase in the number of US mumps cases, which reached over 6,000 cases in 2016 and roughly 5,500 cases in 2017, has led to a recommendation that a third vaccination should be administered. The CDC reports that one dose of MMR is 78 percent effective at preventing an infection, with a range of 49 percent to 92 percent effective, depending on the study. Two doses of the vaccine are 88 percent effective, with a range of 66 percent to 95 percent. Many of the mumps outbreaks have been seen on college campuses, and the CDC has suggested that the spread of mumps may be associated with dormitory life, including sharing cups and utensils that may have traces of saliva.

In contrast to outbreaks of measles and whooping cough, where outbreaks are typically traced to failure to vaccinate, mumps outbreaks are seen in areas where the population has been vaccinated. European outbreaks have been similar, with the European Centre for Disease Control and Prevention noting that two-fifths of the 13,519 reported European cases in 2015 were previously vaccinated. According to the CDC, the outbreaks of mumps are probably due to a combination of factors, such as the known limits of effectiveness of the vaccine, declaiming immunity after vaccination, and the intensity of exposure to the virus in close-contact settings.

Introduction of mumps vaccine has been associated with a shift in the age at which people get the disease. Previously, 90 percent of cases occurred among children age 15 or younger. But since 1990 those ages 15 or older have accounted for 30 to 40 percent of cases each year, with males and females being affected equally. These trends may reflect the effect of vaccine coverage in the population and also the tendency of mumps to affect both children and young adults. Mumps is a disease that should not be taken lightly. Any lapse in vaccination coverage could lead to more outbreaks, with the attendant—albeit rare—complications.

See Also *Childhood-Associated Infectious Diseases, Immunization Impacts; Measles (Rubeola); Rubella*

BIBLIOGRAPHY

Books

Kaplan, Justin L., et al. *The Merck Manual of Medical Information.* New York: Pocket Books, 2008.

Petersen, Eskild, Lin H. Chen, and Patricia Schlagenhauf-Lawlor. *Infectious Diseases: A Geographic Guide.* Chichester, UK: Wiley Blackwell, 2017.

Remington, Jack S., and Christopher B. Wilson. *Infectious Diseases of the Fetus and Newborn Infant.* Philadelphia: Elsevier Saunders, 2016.

Periodicals

Anjali, Jain, et al. "Autism Occurrence by MMR Vaccine Status Among US Children with Older Siblings with and without Autism." *Journal of the American Medical Association* 313, no. 15 (April 21, 2015): 1534–1540.

Bowerman, Mary. "Mumps Outbreaks Reported across USA." *USA Today* (March 10, 2017). This article can also be found online at https://www.usatoday.com/story/news/nation-now/2017/03/10/mumps-outbreaks-reported-across-country/99002254/ (accessed February 6, 2018).

Chang, Daniel. "Florida Has Reported More Mumps Cases in 2017 Than the Last Five Years Combined." *Miami Herald* (December 19, 2017). This article can also be found online at http://www.miamiherald.com/news/health-care/article190625819.html (accessed February 6, 2018).

Klass, Perri. "Mumps Makes a Comeback, Even among the Vaccinated." *New York Times* (November 6, 2017). This article can also be found online at https://www.nytimes.com/2017/11/06/well/family/mumps-makes-a-comeback-even-among-the-vaccinated.html (accessed January 24, 2018).

Sun, Lena H. "Rise in Mumps Outbreaks Prompts U.S. Officials to Weigh Third Vaccine Dose." *Washington Post* (February 23, 2017). This article can also be found online at https://www.washingtonpost.com/news/to-your-health/wp/2017/02/23/rise-in-mumps-outbreaks-prompts-u-s-officials-to-weigh-third-vaccine-dose (accessed January 26, 2018).

Taylor, L. E., A. L. Swerdfeger, and G. D. Eslick. "Vaccines Are Not Associated with Autism: An Evidence-Based Meta-Analysis of Case-Control and Cohort Studies." *Vaccine* 32, no. 29 (June 17, 2014): 3623–3629.

Tutty, Jacinda. "Country Faces Largest Mumps Outbreak in 20 Years." *Sunshine Coast Daily* (March 16, 2017). This article can also be found online at https://www.sunshinecoastdaily.com.au/news/country-faces-largest-mumps-outbreak-in-20-years/3155104/ (accessed February 6, 2018).

Websites

"Measles, Mumps, and Rubella (MMR) Vaccine Safety Studies." Centers for Disease Control and Prevention, August 28, 2015. https://www.cdc.gov/vaccinesafety/vaccines/mmr/mmr-studies.html (accessed February 6, 2018).

"Mumps." Centers for Disease Control and Prevention, November 20, 2017. https://www.cdc.gov/mumps/index.html (accessed January 24, 2018).

"Mumps—Annual Epidemiological Report for 2015." European Centre for Disease Control and Prevention, November 28, 2017. https://ecdc.europa.eu/en/publications-data/mumps-annual-epidemiological-report-2015 (accessed February 6, 2018).

"Mumps—Number of Reported Cases (Vaccine-Preventable Communicable Diseases)." World Health Organization. http://apps.who.int/gho/data/node.imr.WHS3_53?lang=en (accessed January 21, 2018)

Susan Aldridge
Sam Uretsky

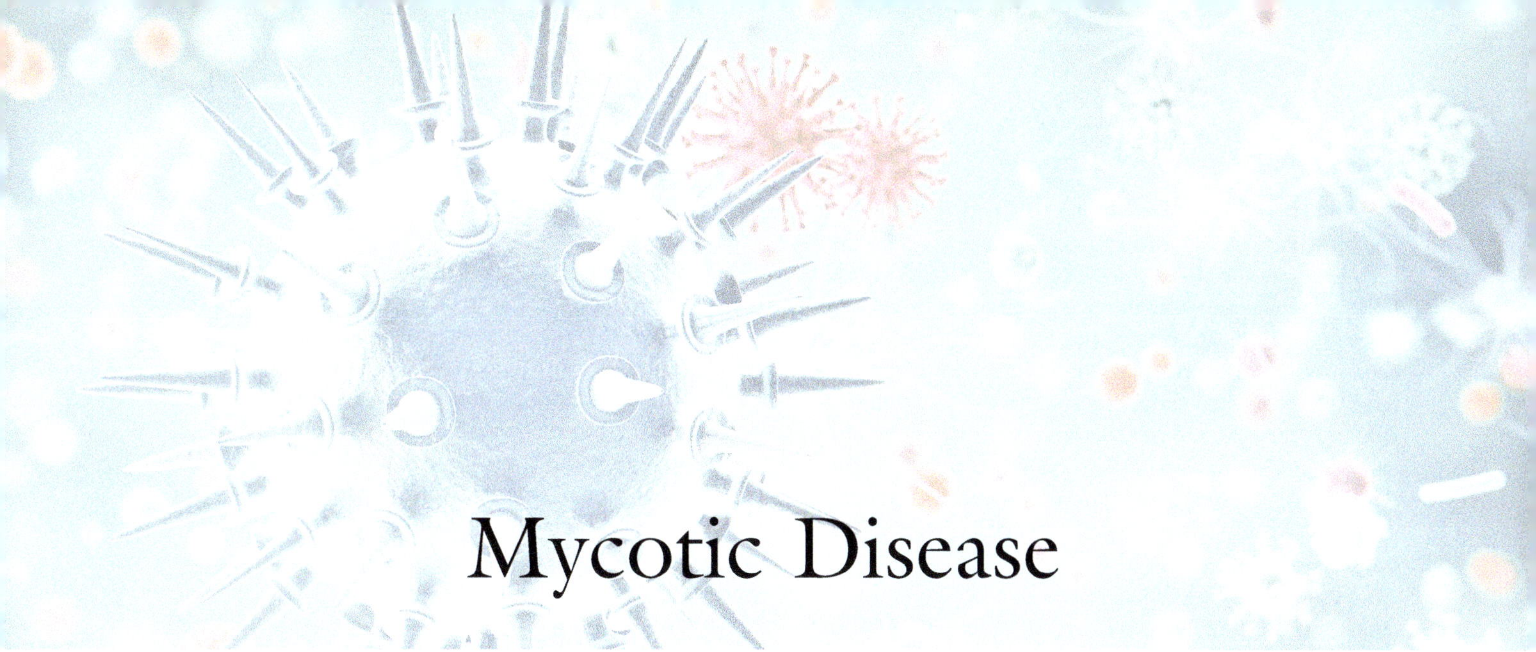

Mycotic Disease

Introduction

Mycotic diseases are caused by fungi, which are present in a number of forms in the environment. Many fungi are found in soil and are transmitted to humans via cuts in the skin or by inhalation of the spores or cells of the fungi. Fungi can also inhabit moist environments, such as damp clothing, shoes, and showers. Transmission occurs when a person's skin comes in contact with the fungi. Other fungi may already be present in the human body at a certain population level and cause infection only when the fungal population grows. An example of this is thrush, a common fungal infection of the mouth.

Symptoms of a fungal disease can range from skin irritation to organ damage, such as lung disease. Fungi are characterized by the area of the body that they affect. Some fungi affect the outer layer of the skin (the epidermis), while others affect the cutaneous and subcutaneous layers of the skin. Furthermore, some fungi develop first in the lungs before spreading to other regions, while other fungi are opportunistic and develop wherever they can. Fungal infections are generally treated with antifungal drugs taken internally or applied externally. However, many of these drugs are toxic and cause unpleasant or harmful side effects. In addition, some fungi are beginning to develop resistance to treatment, making it difficult to eradicate an infection. Mycotic infections are also likely to rise as a result of climate change, which is expanding the geographic zone in which fungi can survive and flourish. As of 2017 an estimated 1.5 million people per year died of mycotic disease, and many observers expect that number to rise.

Disease History, Characteristics, and Transmission

Different types of fungi affect different regions of the body, and mycotic diseases are characterized according to the region being affected. Superficial infections involve the outer layers of the skin and hair. Cutaneous infections involve the epidermis, hair, and nails. Subcutaneous infections involve the dermis, subcutaneous tissues, and muscle. There are also systemic infections that are caused by either primary fungi or opportunistic fungi. Primary fungi originate in the lungs before spreading infection to other organ systems. Opportunistic fungi can originate anywhere in the body. Opportunistic fungal infections tend to occur most commonly in people with a suppressed or weakened immune system, when their health is already compromised.

WORDS TO KNOW

COLONIZATION The process of occupation and increase in number of microorganisms at a specific site.

CUTANEOUS Pertaining to the skin.

IMMUNOCOMPROMISED A reduction of the ability of the immune system to recognize and respond to the presence of foreign material.

OPPORTUNISTIC INFECTION An infection that occurs in people whose immune systems are diminished or are not functioning normally. Such infections are opportunistic insofar as the infectious agents take advantage of their hosts' compromised immune systems and invade to cause disease.

SPORE A dormant form assumed by some bacteria, such as anthrax, that enables the bacterium to survive high temperatures, dryness, and lack of nourishment for long periods of time. Under proper conditions, the spore may revert to the actively multiplying form of the bacteria.

Fungal infections cause a range of symptoms depending on the body region they infect. Cutaneous infections such as tinea, which is a disease of the skin, tend to result in itchy, peeling skin, sometimes with pus or inflamed areas. These symptoms are usually not life threatening but can cause discomfort and irritation. Subcutaneous infections tend to occur when fungi enter under the skin and form lesions as they grow. Systemic fungi originate in the lungs and eventually spread to other organs, potentially causing tissue damage, ulcers, and pulmonary symptoms. Opportunistic fungi can potentially cause disease in any region of the body.

Humans develop fungal infections when they come in contact with a fungus. Some fungi are present in the soil. Therefore, when soil is disturbed (for example, during an earthquake or while gardening), fungal spores can become airborne and be inhaled. The fungi can then cause infection. Other fungi thrive in moist, dark conditions. Therefore, moist clothing, shoes, or rooms such as bathrooms can harbor fungi. When humans come in contact with these fungi, infection can occur. One example is athlete's foot, a type of tinea. Often the fungi responsible for this disease will develop in shoes or in showers and can be spread from these sources. One common fungi from the genus *Candida* can cause thrush, a common infection that results in an itchy rash. This infection can occur in the genital area, mouth, or bloodstream. The fungus is already present in humans in small amounts, and infection occurs when the fungus grows out of control, often in response to a hormonal imbalance.

Scope and Distribution

There are a range of mycotic diseases worldwide. A common fungal infection is tinea, which refers to cutaneous infection of various parts of the body. This infection is common on the feet, where it is known as athlete's foot, and in the genital region, where it is known as jock itch. Both of these infections can be present in men and women, and spread of this disease is facilitated by shared locker rooms or showers where people tend to walk around barefoot.

Some infections occur more commonly in certain people or in people with certain conditions. Genital thrush, which is caused by the fungus *Candida*, is common in women and is also more common during pregnancy, in women with diabetes mellitus, and in women using broad-spectrum antibiotics or corticosteroid medications.

Immunocompromised people appear to be at a significantly greater risk of developing fungal infections. Even fungi that normally do not cause infections in healthy people have been found to cause illness in people with compromised immune systems, such as are caused by conditions including cancer, diabetes, and acquired immunodeficiency syndrome (AIDS). Some fungal infections can also cause more severe symptoms when they develop in these people. For example, human immunodeficiency virus (HIV)–infected people may develop severe pulmonary disease leading to death following infection by the fungus *Coccidioides immitis.* Other factors, such as stress, can also increase the likelihood of a fungal infection.

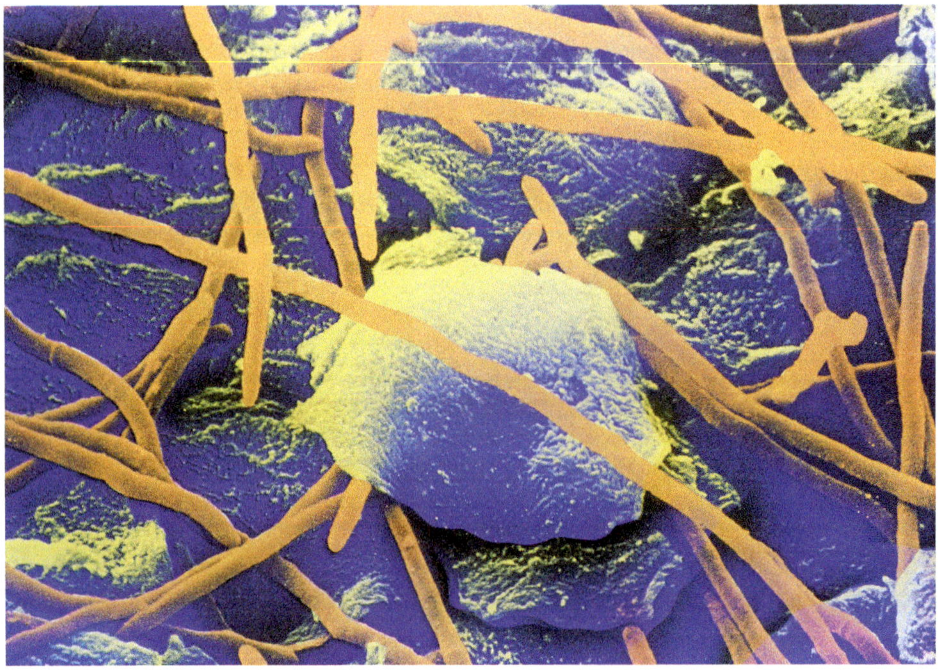

The fungus *Trichophyton interdigitale*, which causes the common mycotic disease athlete's foot, resulting in itchy, peeling skin between the toes. © Biophoto Associates/Science Source

Fungal infections occur worldwide, although specific infections may be found only in some locations. Cryptococcosis, a fungal infection that causes potentially fatal meningitis, can be found in soils throughout the world. Coccidioidomycosis, by contrast, is endemic to areas in the United States, Mexico, and South America. The potential to pick up a fungal infection depends on whether it is present within the country and whether living or working conditions promote the growth and transmission of the fungus. For example, sporotrichosis occurs in hay and is transferred via cuts in the skin. Therefore, farmers and other individuals who handle hay on a regular basis are more susceptible to this fungal infection.

Treatment and Prevention

Fungal infections are generally treated using antifungal drugs. These drugs can be taken orally, inserted in the genital tract, or applied externally. Some common antifungal treatments contain azole derivatives and actively prevent the fungus from producing ergosterol. Ergosterol is a steroid alcohol used by fungal cells to produce a cell membrane, and lack of ergosterol results in cell death and death of the fungus. However, many treatments for fungal infections are extremely toxic and can cause serious side effects if used incorrectly.

Because no vaccines are available for mycotic diseases, avoidance or removal of fungi is the best method of prevention. Maintaining high sanitary standards can help people avoid coming into contact with potentially dangerous fungi. For example, wearing bath shoes in communal showers, avoiding wearing moist clothes, and drying damp shoes can all help prevent contracting the fungus responsible for athlete's foot. Thorough cleaning of contaminated items, such as clothing and bedclothes, using hot water and detergent, may remove the fungi from these items and prevent infection.

For fungi that can be transmitted via airborne spores or cells, avoiding areas in which soil has been disturbed will help minimize contact with fungal spores. For example, in an area where soil fungi are a potential problem, wearing a face mask following an earthquake may help prevent infection. Wearing gloves can also provide protection against soil fungi that are transmitted via cuts in the skin. This is one way to avoid sporotrichosis, which is caused by fungi present in bales of hay or other plant materials that are often harvested and used by humans.

Impacts and Issues

The US Centers for Disease Control and Prevention's (CDC) Mycotic Diseases Branch notes that fungal infections "pose an important threat to public health." According to the CDC, there are three primary kinds of mycotic infections of concern: opportunistic infections, hospital-associated infections, and community-acquired infections.

Opportunistic infections occur in patients with compromised immune systems, either as a result of existing illness or treatments for existing illnesses. Immunocompromised people, including cancer patients, HIV-infected individuals, and people with diseases such as diabetes, are at a high risk of developing opportunistic fungal infections, such as aspergillosis, candidiasis, and cryptococcosis. Furthermore, new forms of old fungal infections, such as coccidioidomycosis, are occurring in these patients. In addition, previously harmless fungi, which normally grow in rotting food, soil, or plants, can cause potentially fatal or debilitating infections in immunocompromised individuals. Opportunistic mycotic infections are on the rise in the early 21st century in large part because the population of immunocompromised individuals is increasing.

Hospital-associated mycotic infections are also of growing concern, according to the CDC, as "advancements and changes in health care practices can provide opportunities for new and drug-resistant fungi to emerge in hospital settings." Such advancements include the use of more effective antifungal treatments for fungal infections, which has led some fungi to develop resistance to antifungal drugs. For example, in some people *Candida* fungi, which cause thrush, have developed resistance to the anti-

FUNGI

Fungi play an essential role in breaking down organic matter and thereby allowing nutrients to be recycled in nature. As such, they are important decomposers, and without them living communities would become buried in their own waste. Some fungi, the saprobes, get their nutrients from nonliving organic matter, such as dead plants and animal waste, clothing, paper, leather, and other materials. Other fungi, the parasites, obtain nutrients from the tissues of living organisms. Both types of fungi obtain nutrients by secreting enzymes from their cells that break down large organic molecules into smaller components. The fungi cells can then absorb the nutrients.

Although the term *fungus* invokes unpleasant images and can be a source of disease, fungi are also a source of antibiotics, vitamins, and industrial chemicals. Yeast, a form of fungi, is used to ferment bread and alcoholic beverages.

In addition to causing human diseases, fungi have also contributed to food spoilage, wheat and corn diseases, and, perhaps most well known, the Irish potato famine of 1843–1847 (caused by the fungus *Phytophthora infestans*), which contributed to the deaths of 250,000 people in Ireland.

fungal treatments used to eradicate this infection. Therefore, fewer treatment options are available as the fungi become resistant to the certain drugs. In 2009 a particularly deadly strain of the *Candida* fungi known as *Candida auris* emerged in Japan and, as of 2016, had spread around the world, including to Kuwait, India, South America, England, and the United States. By mid-2017 nearly 100 cases of *Candida auris* infection had been documented in the United States, a majority of them in New York, and four deaths in the United States had been attributed to the fungi. In response, the CDC sent out multiple alerts to health care facilities about the dangers of this mycotic infection.

Community-acquired mycotic infections are those that result from fungi growing in the environment. While researchers have been able to pinpoint areas where such fungi are endemic, climate change will likely alter where and how such fungi grow. With few exceptions, fungi cannot survive in conditions of extreme heat or cold. But global warming is leading to an expansion of the globe's temperate zone —and that has led to an expanded range in which fungi can survive. Scientists have already detected an expansion of the range of fungal diseases in crops and animals. In addition, as temperatures rise, fungi will likely become increasingly well adapted to surviving within the human body, where temperatures will be increasingly similar to those of the external environment.

The rise in the number of mycotic infections has led to increased research into the control and prevention of fungal diseases. Mycotic disease research involves determining the cause of outbreaks, risk of outbreaks, outbreak trends, and methods of control.

SEE ALSO *Antibiotic Resistance; Aspergillosis; Blastomycosis; Candidiasis; Coccidioidomycosis;* Cryptococcus neoformans *Infection; Histoplasmosis; Opportunistic Infection; Ringworm; Sporotrichosis*

BIBLIOGRAPHY

Books

Dismukes, William E., Peter G. Pappas, and Jack D. Sobel. *Clinical Mycology.* New York: Oxford University Press, 2003.

Howard, Dexter H. *Pathogenic Fungi in Humans and Animals.* New York: Marcel Dekker, 2003.

Periodicals

Badiee, Parisa, and Zahira Hashemizadeh. "Opportunistic Invasive Fungal Infections: Diagnosis & Clinical Management." *Indian Journal of Medical Research* 139, no. 2 (2014): 195–204. This article can also be found online at https://www.ncbi.nlm.nih.gov/pmc/articles/PMC4001330/ (accessed January 25, 2018).

Lesho, Emil, et al. "Mitigating *Candida auris* at a Busy Community Hospital: A Quasi-Experimental Near Real-Time Approach." *Open Forum Infectious Diseases* 4, suppl. 1 (2017): S72. This article can also be found online at https://doi.org/10.1093/ofid/ofx163.001 (accessed January 25, 2018).

McKenna, Maryn. "Fatal Fungus Linked to 4 New Deaths—What You Need to Know." *National Geographic* (November 7, 2016). This article can also be found online at https://news.nationalgeographic.com/2016/11/deadly-fungus-drug-resistance-candida-auris-health-science/ (accessed January 25, 2018).

McNeil, Michael M., et al. "Trends in Mortality Due to Invasive Mycotic Diseases in the United States, 1980–1997." *Clinical Infectious Diseases* 33, no. 5 (2001): 641–647. This article can also be found online at https://doi.org/10.1086/322606 (accessed January 25, 2018).

Websites

Branswell, Helen. "A 'Perfect Storm' Superbug: How an Invasive Fungus Got Health Officials' Attention." STAT, July 31, 2017. https://www.statnews.com/2017/07/31/superbug-fungus-candida-auris/ (accessed January 25, 2018).

"Fungal Diseases." Centers for Disease Control and Prevention, September 6, 2017. https://www.cdc.gov/fungal/index.html (accessed January 25, 2018).

Konkel, Lindsey. "Fungal Diseases Are on the Rise. Is Environmental Change to Blame?" Ensia, April 26, 2017. https://ensia.com/features/19036/ (accessed January 25, 2018).

"Mycotic Diseases Branch." Centers for Disease Control and Prevention, Division of Foodborne, Waterborne, and Environmental Diseases, January 27, 2017. https://www.cdc.gov/ncezid/dfwed/mycotics/index.html (accessed January 25, 2018).

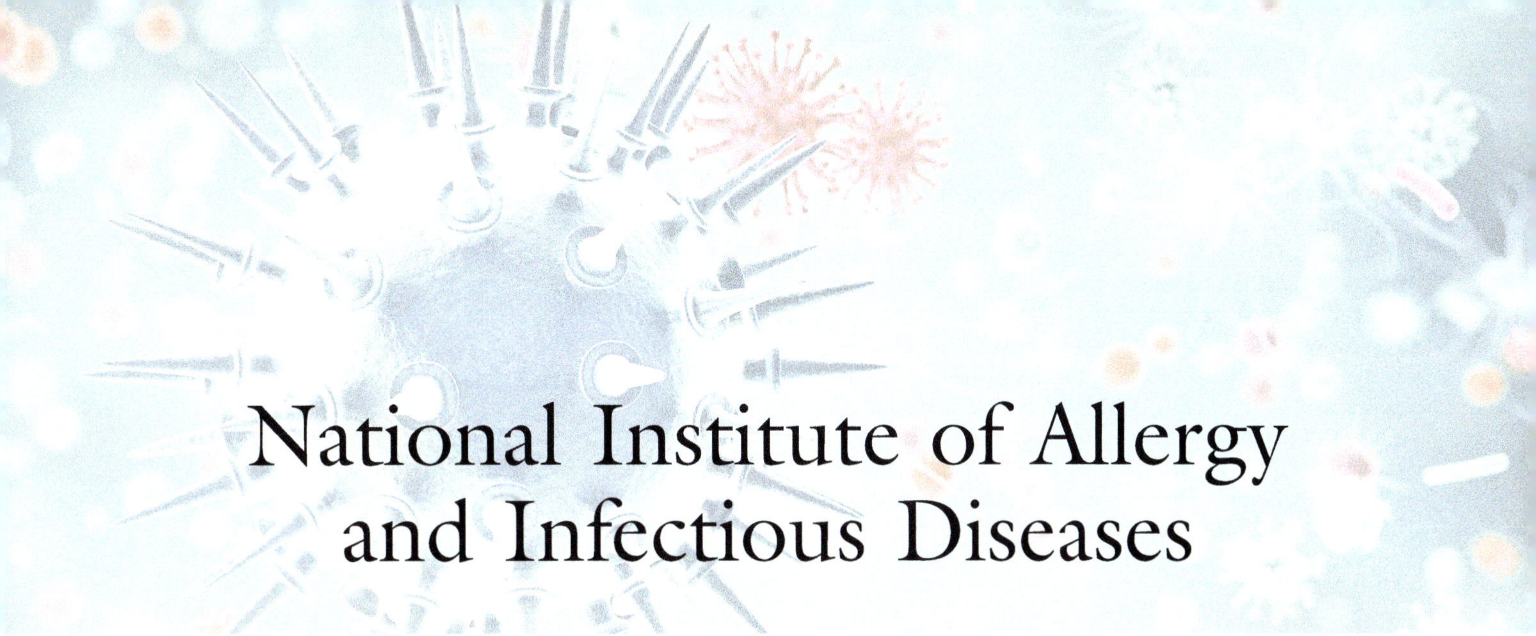

National Institute of Allergy and Infectious Diseases

Introduction

The National Institute of Allergy and Infectious Diseases (NIAID), one of 27 institutes and centers that compose the US National Institutes of Health (NIH), conducts and supports research into the causes of allergic, immunologic, and infectious diseases to develop better ways to prevent, diagnose, and treat such illnesses. The NIH, in turn, is an arm of the US Department of Health and Human Services (HHS) of the US federal government. NIAID both funds its own researchers and grants billions of dollars annually to researchers in universities and industry to pay for research. Scientists wishing to receive grants must apply to NIAID, and grants are competitive.

Some of NIAID's many areas of investigation are human immunodeficiency virus (HIV) and acquired immunodeficiency syndrome (AIDS), allergic diseases, defense of the public against possible terrorism using bacteria or viruses, radiation exposure, emerging infectious diseases, genetics and transplantation, immune-mediated diseases such as asthma and organ rejection, vaccine development, sexually transmitted infections (STIs), and malaria. The institute has been credited with leading highly successful efforts to combat disease in many of these areas—most notably, perhaps, in its work to create treatments for HIV/AIDS. As of 2017 NIAID research and funding was devoted to an array of issues, with the priorities of furthering research into HIV/AIDS, combating Ebola and Marburg viruses, and understanding ways to fight the growing threat from resistant organisms (bacteria, viruses, and other microbes that have developed means of preventing or reducing the effectiveness of antimicrobial drug therapies).

History of Organization

Though NIAID was not officially established until the mid-20th century, the institute's origins can be traced back some six decades through the complex history of federally funded research into infectious diseases in the United States in the late 19th and early 20th centuries. In 1891 the US Congress provided funding for researcher Joseph J. Kinyoun (1860–1919) to move his Laboratory of Hygiene, where he had been studying cholera and other bacterial infections among immigrants to the United States since 1888, from Staten Island, New York, to Washington, D.C. In its new home, the laboratory was renamed the Hygienic Laboratory and Kinyoun was given a broad mandate to study "infectious and contagious diseases and matters pertaining to

WORDS TO KNOW

EMERGING INFECTIOUS DISEASE A new infectious disease such as severe acute respiratory syndrome (SARS) or West Nile virus, as well as a previously known disease such as malaria, tuberculosis, or bacterial pneumonia that is appearing in a new form that is resistant to drug treatments.

GENOME All of the genetic information for a cell or organism. The complete sequence of genes within a cell or virus.

PANDEMIC An epidemic that occurs in more than one country or population simultaneously. *Pandemic* means "all the people."

STRAIN A subclass or a specific genetic variation of an organism.

T CELL VACCINE A vaccine that relies on eliciting cellular immunity, rather than humoral antibody-based immunity, against infection. T cell vaccines are being developed against the human immunodeficiency virus (HIV) and hepatitis C.

the public health." In 1930 the laboratory was renamed the National Institute of Health. In 1948 the National Institute of Health grew to include medical research institutes, leading to another name change and becoming the National Institutes of Health.

Among the new institutes placed under the NIH umbrella was the National Microbiological Institute, which combined four existing laboratories and divisions: the Rocky Mountain Laboratory, the Biologics Control Laboratory, NIH's Division of Infectious Diseases, and NIH's Division of Tropical Diseases. In 1951 the National Microbiological Institute began distributing cash grants to support research by scientists, and in 1955 it was renamed NIAID.

In the following decades, the types of research supported by NIAID multiplied, and its organizational structure was repeatedly reorganized to deal with this widening range of concerns. For example, in 1986 the organization established an Acquired Immunodeficiency Syndrome Program to coordinate the institute's support of research into AIDS, then a recently discovered disease.

A number of research laboratories have been established by NIAID over the years, including the Laboratory of Immunoregulation in 1980, the Laboratory of Molecular Microbiology in 1981, the Laboratory of Immunopathology in 1985, and the Laboratory of Allergic Diseases in 1994. In 2002, as part of the national response to the terrorist attacks of 2001, an Office of Biodefense Research Affairs was established within the Division of Microbiology and Infectious Diseases.

As of March 2018, NIAID was organized into seven divisions: Division of AIDS; Division of Allergy, Immunology, and Transplantation; Division of Microbiology and Infectious Diseases; Division of Extramural Activities; Division of Clinical Research; Division of Intramural Research; and Vaccine Research Center.

Several of these divisions are devoted specifically to supporting medical research:

- The Division of AIDS was founded in 1986. Its mission is to increase basic scientific knowledge of the disease to end the AIDS epidemic. (As of 2017 approximately 37 million people were living with AIDS worldwide, including 1.2 million in the United States.)
- The Division of Allergy, Immunology, and Transplantation supports research to unravel the mechanisms underlying disease of the immune system, with the goal of more effective treatment and prevention.
- The Division of Intramural Research oversees research by the NIAID's laboratories.
- The Division of Microbiology and Infectious Diseases supports research to control and prevent diseases caused by infectious agents other than HIV (the cause of AIDS). For example, this division funds projects to sequence the genomes of infectious agents. NIAID-funded researchers have sequenced the genomes of the bacterium that causes Lyme disease (*Borrelia burgdorferi*) and a number of others.

Impacts and Issues

Due to the scope of NIAID's efforts, basic scientific knowledge of many diseases has been greatly increased. Further, a number of vaccines have been developed using NIAID funds.

In 2005 NIAID made its first cash research grants under Project Bioshield, the federal program to defend the public against possible bioterrorism. Its attempt to fund private-sector development of a vaccine for anthrax, one of the candidate organisms for use as a terror weapon, has not proved successful as of 2018, as the vaccine was not successfully developed by its original target date.

Other vaccine challenges for the NIAID include the pursuit of a vaccine to protect against HIV/AIDS. The current NIAID-sponsored candidates for an HIV vaccine are not formulated to prevent infection as do most vaccines but instead could delay the onset of AIDS by keeping the levels of HIV in the blood in check. Called T cell vaccines, these types of vaccines could also reduce the ability of an infected individual to transmit the HIV virus to others. Several T cell vaccines have undergone expanded clinical trials, and, although they have potential benefits in the battle against HIV/AIDS, the NIAID continues to pursue a traditional-type vaccine that would prevent the establishment of HIV infection altogether. In May 2016 the NIAID reported that developing an HIV vaccine has remained a challenge. Progress has been made, however. Results from a landmark clinical trial in Thailand, reported in 2009, gave researchers their first indication of HIV vaccine efficacy, including a 31 percent reduction in HIV infection among those vaccinated. The NIAID has used these promising results to continue its efforts to create an HIV vaccine, and as of 2016 several investigational vaccines were at various stages of development.

While the institute has helped lead to breakthroughs that have radically improved treatment of people with HIV/AIDS, NIAID continues to promote research into these conditions. In January 2018 alone, for example, the institute launched an international research study designed to understand whether antiretroviral treatment regimens for HIV are safe and effective for pregnant women and their fetuses, announced results of a study that connected the presence of a certain protein with increased risk of HIV infection, and released findings that showed the benefits of brief pauses in HIV antiretroviral treatments.

In 2014 the institute released a report designed to help chart future directions in combating the spread, and threat, of resistant organisms. The report, "NIAID's Antibacterial Research Program: Current Status and Future Directions," provided an updated vision first outlined in the institute's 2008 "Research Agenda of the National Institute of Allergy and Infectious Diseases for Antimicrobial Resistance" and called for "improved surveillance and infection control, more judicious use of antibiotics, new prevention measures, and new therapeutic strategies to combat resistant bacteria remain essential to mitigate this global threat."

Influenza, in both its seasonal and potential pandemic forms, is also a major focus of NIAID research and resources. In February 2018 NIAID announced a new strategic plan for developing a so-called universal flu vaccine that would improve on existing flu vaccines, which protect only against a single influenza strain, by preventing patients from contracting multiple strains of influenza. According to an article by NIAID scientists published in the *Journal of Infectious Diseases*, "NIAID will use this plan as a foundation for future investments in influenza research and will support and coordinate a consortium of multidisciplinary scientists focused on accelerating progress towards this goal."

As of 2018 NIAID was also prioritizing research into fevers caused by Ebola and Marburg, related viral diseases that are highly contagious and have extremely high rates of mortality. The institute is funding various initiatives designed to improve understanding of how these fevers are transmitted, to create tools for diagnosing infection, to treat those who contract Ebola and Marburg, and to create vaccines that will prevent infection.

PRIMARY SOURCE

At Rocky Mountain Labs, "Virus Ecology" Helps Scientists Understand Threats Such as Zika

SOURCE: *Nixon, Lance. "At Rocky Mountain Labs, 'Virus Ecology' Helps Scientists Understand Threats Such as Zika."* Missoulian *(August 29, 2016). This article can also be found online at http://missoulian.com/lifestyles/health-med-fit/at-rocky-mountain-labs-virus-ecology-helps-scientists-understand-threats/article_8f13f9c8-1d99-53fe-a51d-c90d63bfa13d.html (accessed February 28, 2018).*

INTRODUCTION: *This article from the* Missoulian, *a newspaper located in Missoula, Montana, near NIAID's Rocky Mountain Laboratory, describes researchers' efforts to understand the connection between ecology and the spread of infectious diseases.*

He's not the only person in western Montana who cares about ecology.

But Marshall Bloom, associate director for scientific management at Rocky Mountain Laboratories in Hamilton, may be different from most in that a growing preoccupation for him and for many of his scientific colleagues in Hamilton is a far more specialized discipline: "virus ecology."

At Rocky Mountain Laboratories – a laboratory of the National Institute of Allergy and Infectious Diseases, which in turn is one of 27 institutes that make up the National Institutes of Health – it's all part of the job. Scientists say finding out how a virus behaves on its home turf can help understand how viral disease outbreaks occur and how to better respond. It's one of the ways scientists study current health threats such as the Zika virus, and before that, Ebola virus and West Nile virus.

"Like with Ebola virus, you have outbreaks every once in a while, so where is that virus when it's not in an outbreak? Where does it exist in nature? What is the reservoir species? How does it spill over?" Bloom says.

Just as with ecologists studying, say, reptiles or amphibians or birds or mammals, scientists who study diseases are taking into consideration factors such as climate change. Mosquito-borne Zika virus is the current case in point.

"It's been around since the late 1940s, but only when it got into Brazil did it become such a big problem and people are trying to figure out what the causes of its sudden emergence as a problematic disease are there," Bloom said. "Many people feel that climate change is a cause for emergence of some of these infectious diseases."

As the climate changes, the boundary between tropical and temperate zones gets a little "blurred," Bloom explained, meaning the mosquitoes that transmit some diseases such as Zika are no longer confined to smaller areas in tropical regions.

Scientists who study infectious disease also share other concerns of conventional ecologists. For example, the destruction of habitat and incursion of settlements into previously remote areas puts humans in contact with animals and insects which might be carrying infectious diseases.

In addition, factors such as global trade and global travel, and cultural practices, even sexual practices, affect how diseases spread.

Unfortunately for public health, Bloom sees no shortage of work for the scientists of Rocky Mountain Laboratories. Infectious disease may, in fact, be a greater concern than in the past.

"It's going to be an ongoing problem. The key is having a robust basic research program to understand the basic molecular biology of the infectious agents, and also a robust research program to understand how the bodies of animals or people react to those infectious diseases so that we can quickly come to a realization, 'This virus is able to evade this part of the human response against it, how can we help the human response against it do a better job?'"

Fortunately, that's what the scientists of Rocky Mountain Laboratories have been doing since the lab got its start from work more than a century ago.

"You can trace the antecedents of Rocky Mountain Lab back to over a hundred years ago to the hunt for the etiology of Rocky Mountain spotted fever right around 1900. That became a big issue. It was what we would now call an 'emerging infectious disease' and Dr. Howard T. Ricketts was sent out here to try to figure out what was going on. In a few short years he figured out that it was an infectious disease and it could be transmitted by the bite of a tick."

The bacterium that causes Rocky Mountain spotted fever, Rickettsia rickettsii, is named for Rickets.

In 1910 Ricketts died of typhus while studying an outbreak in Mexico City, so although his work directly led to the creation of Rocky Mountain Labs, he never saw that happen. The state of Montana and the federal government continued the work in various ways and in 1928, the first building of The Rocky Mountain Labs was completed.

In the years since then there's been "virtually an encyclopedia" of important infectious disease work done in Hamilton, Bloom says, with work continuing on Rocky Mountain spotted fever, but also on Q fever, tularemia, Salmonella, staph infections, Chlamydia, relapsing fever, bubonic plague and others.

"In World War II, all of the yellow fever vaccine which was used in Allied troops was made here on this site – millions of doses over the course of the war," Bloom said.

Lyme disease – named after Lyme, Connecticut – was understood to be carried by ticks, but researchers in the East turned to the lab in Hamilton for help understanding it better.

"The people on the East Coast weren't able to identify an infectious agent so they sent some of the infected ticks to Rocky Mountain Labs to be studied by Dr. Willy Burgdorfer, who was an expert in the infections of ticks. He was able to identify by microscopy some bacteria that looked kind of like little corkscrews. He saw those and he realized those looked like what are called borrelia, and immediately drew the tentative conclusion that they were probably the causative agent of Lyme disease."

Subsequent work with other scientists at Rocky Mountain Labs proved him right. Borrelia burgdorferi, as the bacterial species is known, is named in his honor.

In 2001 the federal government decided to construct one of the few Biosafety Level 4 laboratories in the United States in Hamilton at Rocky Mountain Laboratories, taking the Hamilton lab's work to a new level. Bloom can demonstrate the level of security it involves by donning a "positive pressure suit" in the training lab of the facility. Rigorous training and specialized equipment such as this are necessary for scientists who work with some infectious diseases.

But are emerging diseases become more of a problem?

"In my own personal opinion, the answer to that question would be yes. I think there's more infectious diseases emerging because of the reasons we listed," Bloom said.

In addition, Bloom said, the ability to identify new infectious agents is improving, meaning scientists may be able to identify some diseases even before they become serious threats to the public.

"Using the new next-generation sequencing methods are going to enable us to identify infectious agents which have not been previously described or a new variant of some existing infectious disease."

That could give scientists a head start in understanding infectious diseases as they emerge.

"Ecology and that kind of disease modeling is prediction is going to become an important part of the armamentarium against emerging infectious diseases," Bloom said.

SEE ALSO *CDC (Centers for Disease Control and Prevention); Epidemiology; Public Health and Infectious Disease*

BIBLIOGRAPHY

Books

Brower, Jennifer, and Peter Chalk. *The Global Threat of New and Reemerging Infectious Diseases: Reconciling U.S. National Security and Public Health Policy.* Santa Monica, CA: RAND, 2003.

Periodicals

Erbelding, Emily J., et al. "A Universal Influenza Vaccine: The Strategic Plan for the National Institute of Allergy and Infectious Diseases." *Journal of Infectious Diseases* (February 28, 2018). This article can also be found online at https://academic.oup.com/jid/advance-article/doi/10.1093/infdis/jiy103/4904047 (accessed February 28, 2018).

Kaiser, Jocelyn. "Quick Save for Infectious-Disease Grants at NIAID." *Science* 303 (2004): 941.

Nixon, Lance. "At Rocky Mountain Labs, 'Virus Ecology' Helps Scientists Understand Threats Such as Zika." *Missoulian* (August 29, 2016). This article can also be found online at http://missoulian.com/lifestyles/health-med-fit/at-rocky-mountain-labs-virus-ecology-helps-scientists-understand-threats/article_8f13f9c8-1d99-53fe-a51d-c90d63bfa13d.html (accessed February 28, 2018).

Websites

"Infographic: Progress Toward an HIV Vaccine." National Institute of Allergy and Infectious Diseases, May 18, 2016. https://www.niaid.nih.gov/news-events/progress-toward-hiv-vaccine (accessed March 14, 2018).

National Institute of Allergy and Infectious Diseases, 2018. https://www.niaid.nih.gov/ (accessed February 27, 2018).

"NIAID's Antibacterial Research Program: Current Status and Future Directions." National Institute of Allergy and Infectious Diseases, 2014. https://www.niaid.nih.gov/sites/default/files/arstrategicplan2014.pdf (accessed February 28, 2018).

Necrotizing Fasciitis

Introduction

Necrotizing fasciitis is a rare, and often fatal, infection that is commonly described as "flesh-eating bacteria," a "flesh-eating disease," or a "flesh-eating infection." But bacteria that causes necrotizing fasciitis is not actually flesh-eating. Rather, the bacteria releases toxins that cause the body's own immune system to dissolve certain tissues. To necrotize tissue is to kill it, and the word *fasciitis* signifies inflammation of the fascia, which are the thin sheaths of fibrous connective tissue that cover the muscles and other organs. In necrotizing fasciitis, bacteria infect the deeper layers of the skin and the fascia in the tissue underneath the skin. This can kill an infected person quickly.

While antibiotics can help slow an infection, surgery is typically required to stop the spread of necrotizing fasciitis before it proves fatal. A variety of bacteria can cause necrotizing fasciitis. The most common of these is group A *Streptococcus*, but *Staphylococcus aureus*, *Clostridium*, *Klebsiella*, *Escherichia coli*, and *Aeromonas hydrophila* are among the other bacteria that can cause this disease. A fearsome disease due to the nature of the symptoms as well as its high fatality rate, cases of necrotizing fasciitis are often reported in the media. While the disease's relative prominence has led to concerns that it will become widespread and evidence suggests incidence of infection are on the rise, necrotizing fasciitis remains rare as of early 2018.

Disease History, Characteristics, and Transmission

Joseph Jones (1833–1896), a surgeon serving in the Confederate army during the American Civil War (1861–1865), is credited with providing the first description of what was then known as hospital gangrene and is now known as necrotizing fasciitis in 1871. Some two decades later, Jean Alfred Fournier (1832–1914), a French doctor of venereology, described cases of necrotizing fasciitis affecting the penis and scrotum of young male patients. This form of necrotizing fasciitis, which affects the perineal, perianal, or genital areas and is

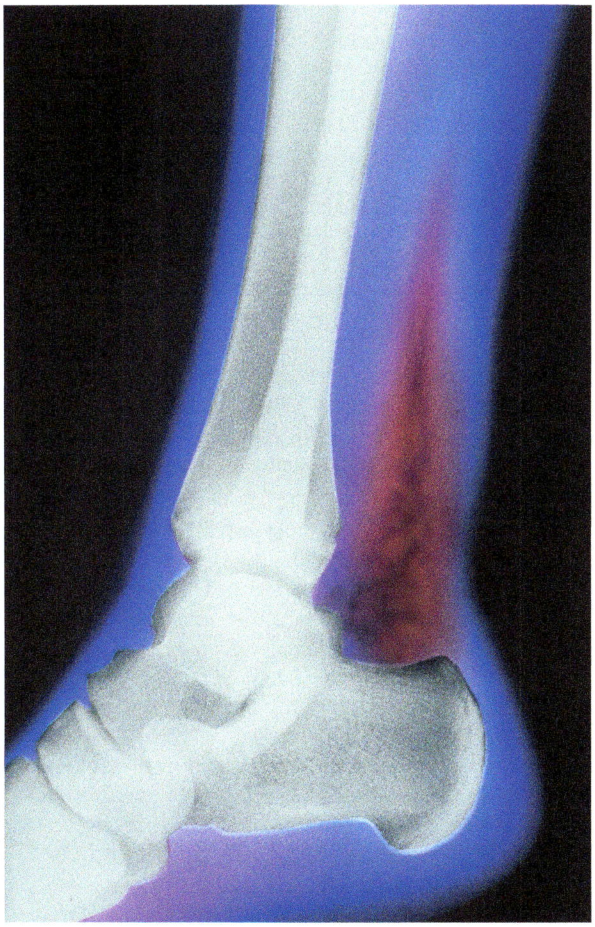

An X-ray shows a deep cut on the heel of a patient suffering from necrotizing fasciitis, a rare but often fatal infection that causes the body's own immune system to dissolve certain tissues. © Chris Bjornberg/Science Source

WORDS TO KNOW

CLINICAL TRIALS According to the National Institutes of Health, a clinical trial is "a research study to answer specific questions about vaccines or new therapies or new ways of using known treatments." These studies allow researchers to determine whether new drugs or treatments are safe and effective. When conducted carefully, clinical trials can provide fast and safe answers to these questions.

FASCIA A type of connective tissue made up of a network of fibers. It is best thought of as being the packing material of the body. Fascia surrounds muscles, bones, and joints and lies between the layers of skin. It functions to hold these structures together, protecting them and defining the shape of the body. When surrounding a muscle, fascia helps prevent a contracting muscle from catching or causing excessive friction on neighboring muscles.

GANGRENE The destruction of body tissue by a bacteria called *Clostridium perfringens* or a combination of *Streptococci* and *Staphylococci* bacteria. *C. perfringens* is found widespread in soil and the intestinal tracts of humans and animals. It becomes dangerous only when its spores germinate, producing toxins and destructive enzymes, and germination occurs only in an anaerobic environment (one almost totally devoid of oxygen). While gangrene can develop in any part of the body, it is most common in fingers, toes, hands, feet, arms, and legs, the parts of the body most susceptible to restricted blood flow. Even a slight injury in such an area is at high risk of causing gangrene. Early treatment with antibiotics, such as penicillin, and surgery to remove the dead tissue will often reduce the need for amputation. If left untreated, gangrene results in amputation or death.

HEMOLYSIS The destruction of blood cells, an abnormal rate of which may lead to lowered levels of these cells. For example, hemolytic anemia is caused by destruction of red blood cells at a rate faster than which they can be produced.

M PROTEIN An antibody found in unusually large amounts in the blood or urine of patients with multiple myeloma, a form of cancer that arises in the white blood cells that produce antibodies.

MUTATION A change in an organism's deoxyribonucleic acid (DNA) that occurs over time and may render it less sensitive to drugs that are used against it.

NECROTIC TISSUE Dead tissue in an otherwise living body. Tissue death is called necrosis.

STREPTOCOCCUS A genus of bacteria that includes species such as *Streptococci pyogenes*, a species of bacteria that causes strep throat.

caused by multiple bacterium (polymicrobial), is known as Fournier gangrene. The term *necrotizing fasciitis* was not coined until 1952, when it appeared in an article in *American Surgery*.

The understanding of the relationship between necrotizing fasciitis and its bacterial causes can be traced to the work of the German-Austrian surgeon Theodor Billroth (1829–1894), who first described the *Streptococci* bacterium in 1874. Billroth discovered *Streptococcus pyogenes* growing in infected wounds. The *Streptococci* are Gram-positive bacteria that tend to clump in pairs or chains and are classed into two basic types based on their ability to cause partial or complete hemolysis (breakdown of blood cells): Group A and Group B. Group A *Streptococci* causes a wide range of infections that can be mild or severe, including common illnesses such as strep throat and rare diseases like necrotizing fasciitis.

While Group A *Streptococci* is the primary cause of necrotizing fasciitis, other bacteria also play a role in causing infections, including *Clostridium perfringens* and *C. septicum*. Necrotizing fasciitis is classified as one of two main types: type 1, which is polymicrobial, meaning multiple aerobic and anaerobic bacteria are involved in the infection, and type 2, which is monomicrobial, meaning only one organism causes the infection. Monomicrobial infections are less common than polymicrobial infections. Polymicrobial infections tend to infect the torso or the perineum, while monomicrobial infections tend to infect the limbs. In addition, polymicrobial infections typically occur in immunocompromised people, whereas monomicrobial infections occur most often in patients who are otherwise healthy.

Infections typically begin when bacteria penetrate the skin at the site of a major injury or even an invisible breakage. The bacteria initially infect deep tissue and fascia, spreading rapidly. Infections in limbs and the torso move especially quickly, due to a lack of cartilage and other fibrous material that can effectively slow or stop infection in parts of the body such as the feet and hands that feature higher concentrations of such material. As infections persist, bacteria can spread to the lymphatic system, the brain, and muscle.

The first signs of necrotizing fasciitis are often difficult to identify as being characteristic of this kind of infection, with patients typically exhibiting symptoms such as fever, confusion, weakness, tiredness, increased heart rate, and altered mental states. In most cases patients also develop a skin lesion or sore spot at the wound site that is red, hot, and painful to the touch. Such skin inflammation aids in the diagnosis of necrotizing fasciitis. In addition, unlike similar infections, there is typically a significant amount of deeply felt pain associated with the relatively minor and superficial skin inflammation that occurs as a result of necrotizing fasciitis.

Over a period of about 24 to 48 hours, as the infection spreads, a patient will develop increasingly severe pain, swelling, and discoloration. The lesion often becomes purple, violet, blue, or patchy. Fluids may swell or discharge a grayish-brown substance. In about 5 to 25 percent of cases, patients develop blisters. In about 18 percent of cases, patients also develop crepitus, which is the sound and feeling of bone and cartilage grating due to the deterioration of fascia, tissue, and possibly muscle. In three to four days, gangrene may appear, with the entire limb in some cases appearing necrotic. In subacute cases a patient's life can be saved—though doing so typically requires the removal of infected tissue through amputation or other surgical means. In hyperacute cases the disease can cause death through shock, organ failure, and respiratory arrest.

Most often people contract necrotizing fasciitis when they receive a wound or some less obvious puncture of the skin. The break may be a large wound or a pinprick; in half of all cases, the break through which the pathogen entered cannot be identified. Whether the bacteria that enters the skin through such a wound or puncture develops into a case of necrotizing fasciitis is apparently random. In addition, a person with necrotizing fasciitis can, in rare cases, spread the infection to other people by direct contact or via airborne saliva droplets released by sneezing or coughing.

Scope and Distribution

Necrotizing fasciitis is primarily found in Europe and North America, though cases have also been reported in Africa, Asia, and Australia. According to the Centers for Disease Control and Prevention (CDC), there were approximately 600 to 1,200 reported cases annually in the United States between 2010 and 2017. However, the CDC considers this number "likely an underestimate." Researchers have had difficulty identifying the factors that increase the likelihood of contracting a necrotizing fasciitis infection, but evidence suggests that people with chronic conditions such as cancer, diabetes, and kidney disease are at heightened risk due to the fact that their immune system is weakened, reducing the body's ability to fight bacterial infection.

Treatment and Prevention

The successful treatment of necrotizing fasciitis requires that a patient immediately seek medical assistance. In the 1990s, when public concern over this disease was at its height, physician Vincent Fischetti of Rockefeller University in New York advised the public that, "if you see a rapidly progressing reddening area that is hot and quite sore to the touch and if you are running a fever, I would go to the doctor very quickly."

When a patient pursues treatment, the first step is typically surgery that aims to remove infected tissue, both for the purpose of understanding the extent of the infection and to help stop further spread of the infection. As Rukshini Puvanendran, Jason Chan Meng Huey, and Shanker Pasupathy observe in their 2009 article in *Canadian Family Physician*, "Patients are often incredulous at the preoperative briefing when told they need an extensive operation for their skin infection; it is important to educate them about the gravity of their condition and the risk of increased mortality if surgical debridement [removal of unhealthy tissue] is not performed." As the authors note, "Without surgical intervention, mortality approaches 100%."

In addition to surgery, necrotizing fasciitis is treated with antibiotics, including penicillin, erythromycin, and clindamycin. While antibiotics and surgery can help slow or stop infection, they are not always successful. Even with treatment, the death rate from necrotizing fasciitis is 16.4 percent for community-acquired infections and 36.3 percent for infections that occur after undergoing invasive medical procedures, according to Puvanendran, Huey, and Pasupathy.

There is no known means of preventing necrotizing fasciitis.

Impacts and Issues

Public consciousness of invasive group A streptococcal disease, including necrotizing fasciitis, has been out of proportion to the number of deaths it causes compared to many other diseases and behaviors. Undoubtedly, one reason for this is the dramatic nature of the disease. A bacterial infection that "eats flesh" and has a significant fatality rate even with the best medical care is certainly attention-getting. In addition, there have been a number of well-publicized deaths from the disease, including leading British economist David Walton (1963–2006), who died within 24 hours of diagnosis.

PRIMARY SOURCE

8-Year-Old Dies from Rare Flesh-Eating Bacteria: Doctors "Kept Cutting and Hoping," Mother Says

SOURCE: *Hahn, James Duaine. "8-Year-Old Dies from Rare Flesh-Eating Bacteria: Doctors 'Kept Cutting and Hoping,' Mother Says."* People

(January 25, 2018). This article can also be found online at http://people.com/human-interest/flesh-eating-bacteria-kills-boy/ (accessed February 13, 2018).

INTRODUCTION: *This article from* People *tells the story of a child who contracted a fatal case of necrotizing fasciitis in 2018 after falling off his bike.*

When Sara Hebard's 8-year-old son suffered a minor injury after falling off his bicycle, she never expected her boy would be fighting for his life just days later.

Just as he's done so many weekends before, Liam Flanagan spent January 13 playing on his bicycle in the driveway of his family's home in Pilot Rock, Oregon. But as he was careening down the hill that Saturday, Liam crashed into the dirt, and his bike's handlebar cut through his jeans, causing a deep laceration on his thigh.

He was quickly taken by family to a nearby emergency room, where doctors gave the second-grader seven stitches to close his wound and sent him on his way. Though the cut was painful, doctors felt it was minor enough not to give Liam antibiotics, Hebard says, and they fully expected for him to recover. Still, Hebard said her son kept complaining about a continuous ache around the area of his gash in the days that followed.

"He said it hurt, but it was his very first accident and he never had stitches before," Hebard, 37, tells PEOPLE of Liam, who she says always had a smile that made others smile. "I don't think he was complaining any more than other kids would when they had their first stitches."

Hebard and Liam's step-father, Scott Hinkle, gave Liam Tylenol to soothe his discomfort over the next three days, but the pain grew increasingly unbearable for the young boy. That's when the couple examined Liam's thigh and groin-area and saw they had become gravely discolored.

"My husband instantly freaked," Hebard recalls. "He immediately said Liam had gangrene and he needed to go to the emergency room—and straight to the emergency room we went."

The couple rushed Liam to the hospital where he underwent emergency surgery to remove the infected tissue.

The next morning, Liam was airlifted from the small town hospital to Doernbecher Children's Hospital in Portland, where doctors performed multiple surgeries, amputating more and more of the boy's body to stay ahead of the infection that was making its way through his tissue.

"Each time they did a surgery, they kept telling us that they thought they got it," Hebard says. "He was on three of the highest doses of antibiotics that you could get. They were pouring everything at them that they could, but they just kept cutting and hoping. Cutting and hoping."

Doctors discovered Liam had contracted a rare flesh-eating bacteria known as necrotizing fasciitis, which they believe entered Liam's body through his wound from the soil he landed on.

Necrotizing fasciitis quickly kills the body's soft tissue found around muscles, nerves, fat, and blood vessels and it can turn lethal in a short period of time, according to the Centers for Disease Control. Since 2010, about 600 to 1,200 Americans are diagnosed with necrotizing fasciitis each year, though the CDC notes this may be an underestimate.

The infection can be successfully treated with antibiotics and surgery to remove infected tissue if it's caught early, which is important to a patient's survival. According to an NCBI study, the infection has about a 27 percent mortality rate.

Liam's doctors worked hard to control the infected area that stretched from ankle to armpit.

"The pain was so bad that he was screaming," Hebard says. "It's horrific. It is a horrific torture, that's what it is. The last things I got to hear from my son was him screaming because it hurt so bad."

Doctors soon placed Liam under sedation and life support, and on January 21, they transferred him to Randall Children's Hospital to be examined by another medical team. About a half-hour later, doctors informed Hebard that they had "done everything that they could do," and Liam passed away later that day. Before the accident, Liam —who Hebard says was a "ray of sunshine" who was loved by so many—was a completely healthy boy.

Today, Hebard is warning other families to watch for the symptoms of necrotizing fasciitis, such as chills, fever, fatigue and vomiting. A key sign, she says, is if a cut or a swollen area on the body is more painful than what is expected.

The family set up a GoFundMe account to help with expenses, and it has raised $16,000 so far.

"Even though this is my worst nightmare, I want to believe his death had a reason, it had a purpose. Maybe it's to save other's lives, because no one deserves to go through what we went through," Hebard says through tears. "Hold your babies tight and listen to them. Just pay attention, and don't just pass things off as if things will be okay."

SEE ALSO *Impetigo; Puerperal Fever; Scarlet Fever; Streptococcal Infections, Group A; Streptococcal Infections, Group B*

BIBLIOGRAPHY

Periodicals

Bulger, Eileen M., et al. "A Novel Drug for Treatment of Necrotizing Soft-Tissue Infections: A Randomized Clinical Trial." *JAMA Surgery* 149, no. 6 (2014): 528–536. This article can also be found online at https://jamanetwork.com/journals/jamasurgery/fullarticle/1859986 (accessed February 12, 2018).

Factor, Stephanie H., et al. "Invasive Group A Streptococcal Disease: Risk Factors for Adults." *Emerging Infectious Diseases* 9, no. 8 (2003): 970–977. The article can also be found online at https://www.ncbi.nlm.nih.gov/pmc/articles/PMC3020599/ (accessed February 12, 2018).

Factor, Stephanie H., et al. "Risk Factors for Pediatric Invasive Group A Streptococcal Disease." *Emerging Infectious Diseases* 11, no. 7 (2005): 1062–1066. This article can also be found online at https://wwwnc.cdc.gov/eid/article/11/7/pdfs/04-0900.pdf (accessed February 21, 2018).

Hahn, James Duaine. "8-Year-Old Dies from Rare Flesh-Eating Bacteria: Doctors 'Kept Cutting and Hoping,' Mother Says." *People* (January 25, 2018). This article can also be found online at http://people.com/human-interest/flesh-eating-bacteria-kills-boy/ (accessed February 13, 2018).

Kolata, Gina. "A Dangerous Form of Strep Stirs Concern in Resurgence." *New York Times* (June 8, 1994). This article can also be found online at http://www.nytimes.com/1994/06/08/us/a-dangerous-form-of-strep-stirs-concern-in-resurgence.html?pagewanted=all (accessed February 12, 2018).

MacMillan, Amanda. "A New Mom Became a Quadruple Amputee from Flesh-Eating Bacteria. Here's What You Need to Know." *Time* (October 16, 2017). This article can also be found online at http://time.com/4984752/flesh-eating-bacteria-necrotizing-fasciitis/ (accessed February 12, 2018).

Musher, Daniel M., et al. "Trends in Bacteremic Infection Due to *Streptococcus pyogenes* (Group A Streptococcus), 1986–1995." *Emerging Infectious Diseases* 2 (1996): 54–56. This article can also be found online at https://wwwnc.cdc.gov/eid/article/2/1/96-0107_article (accessed February 12, 2018).

Puvanendran, Rukshini, Jason Chan Meng Huey, and Shanker Pasupathy. "Necrotizing Fasciitis." *Canadian Family Physician* 55, no. 10 (2009): 981–987. This article can also be found online at https://www.ncbi.nlm.nih.gov/pmc/articles/PMC2762295/ (accessed February 12, 2018).

Stevens, Dennis L. "Streptococcal Toxic-Shock Syndrome: Spectrum of Disease, Pathogenesis, and New Concepts in Treatment." *Emerging Infectious Diseases* 1 (1995): 69–76. This article can also be found online at https://www.ncbi.nlm.nih.gov/pmc/articles/PMC2626872/pdf/8903167.pdf (accessed February 12, 2018).

Websites

National Necrotizing Fasciitis Foundation, January 28, 2007. http://www.nnff.org/ (accessed February 14, 2007).

"Necrotizing Fasciitis." Centers for Disease Control and Prevention, October 26, 2017. https://www.cdc.gov/features/necrotizingfasciitis/index.html (accessed February 12, 2018).

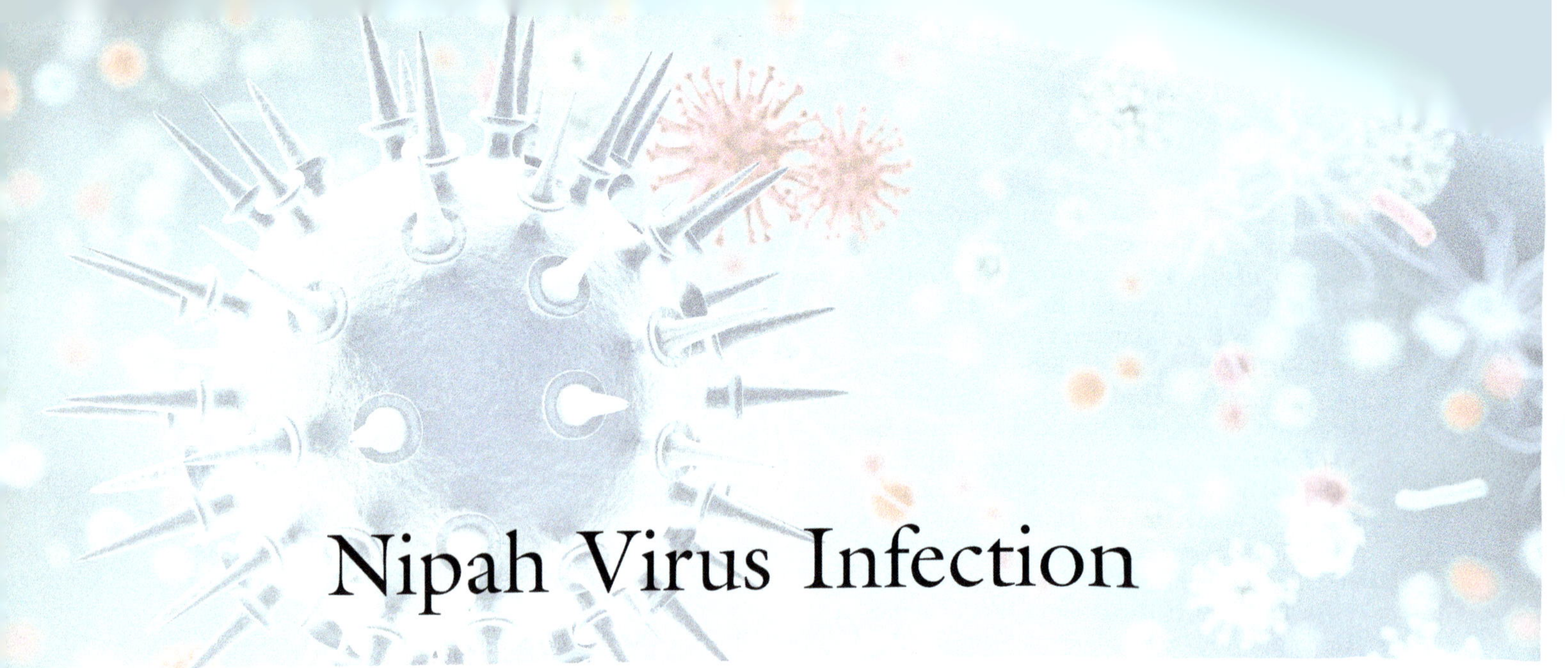

Nipah Virus Infection

Introduction

Nipah virus (NiV) is best known as the causative agent of a large outbreak of disease among pigs in Malaysia and Singapore in 1998 and 1999. It is a member of the Paramyxoviridae family of viruses and is naturally harbored in fruit bats of the *Pteropus* genus in Malaysia.

The virus may be transmitted from bats to pigs in contact with bat urine or feces and subsequently spread to humans through contact with the pig's body fluids on pig farms and in slaughterhouses. The virus can also be transmitted from bat to human via raw date palm sap and from human to human. In humans, NiV infection presents as encephalitis and respiratory disease and carries a significant mortality rate. Treatment is limited to reducing symptoms, but appropriate preventive measures may be implemented to limit spread. For example, in areas where NiV is endemic, it is strongly recommended that people refrain from drinking the raw sap of date palms.

NiV is considered an emerging infectious disease and is argued to pose a significant potential threat to human health. The impact of this viral infection is evident both economically and socially.

Disease History, Characteristics, and Transmission

NiV was first isolated in 1999 during an outbreak of encephalitis and respiratory illness among a group of men in Malaysia. The outbreak resulted in 265 cases of encephalitis, 105 of which were fatal. The virus was named after the location in which it was first detected, Sungai Nipah New Village in Malaysia. Affecting pigs and humans, NiV is a member of the *Henipavirus* genus of the Paramyxoviridae family. The virus's natural reservoir is argued to be *Pteropus* fruit bats.

Transmission from bats to pigs is thought to occur when pigs are exposed to the urine and feces of the bats.

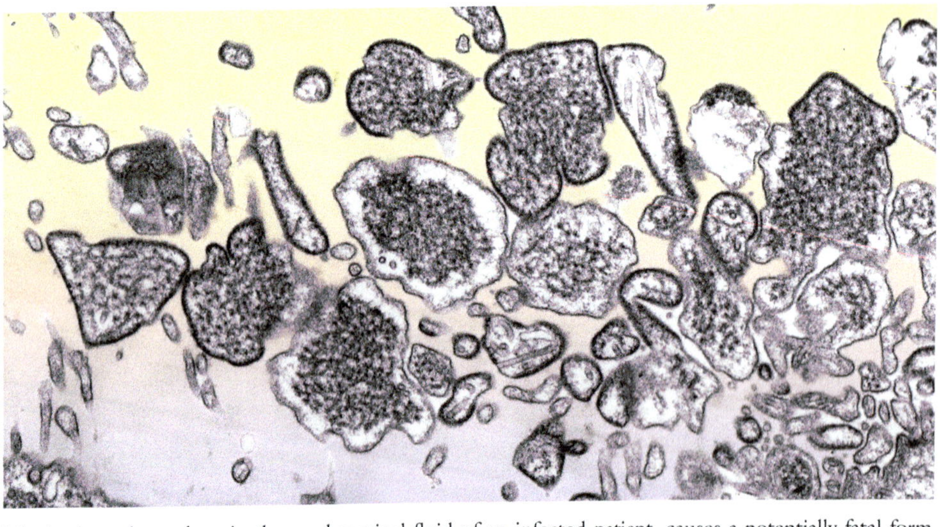

Nipah virus, shown here in the cerebrospinal fluid of an infected patient, causes a potentially fatal form of encephalitis in humans. *© BSIP/UIG/Getty Images*

Humans may contract the disease following exposure to contaminated tissue and body fluids of infected pigs. Person-to-person transmission is possible. Humans can also contract the disease by ingesting raw sap of date palms that has come in contact with the fecal material of infected bats.

In humans, infections are primarily encephalitic after an incubation period of 4 to 18 days. Symptoms initially include fever and headache followed by drowsiness and disorientation, nausea, weakness, and, in some cases, respiratory illness. These signs and symptoms may progress to coma within 24 to 48 hours.

About 40 percent of NiV cases during the Malaysian outbreaks resulted in death, compared to about 75 percent of cases during outbreaks in India and Bangladesh from 2001 to 2013.

WORDS TO KNOW

EMERGING DISEASE A new infectious disease such as severe acute respiratory syndrome (SARS) and West Nile virus, as well as a previously known disease such as malaria, tuberculosis, or bacterial pneumonias that is appearing in a new form that is resistant to drug treatments.

ENDEMIC Present in a particular area or among a particular group of people.

HOST An organism that serves as the habitat for a parasite or possibly for a symbiont. A host may provide nutrition to the parasite or symbiont, or it may simply provide a place in which to live.

PATHOGEN A disease-causing agent, such as a bacterium, a virus, a fungus, or another microorganism.

RESERVOIR The animal or organism in which a virus or parasite normally resides.

STRAIN A subclass or a specific genetic variation of an organism.

ZOONOTIC A disease that can be transmitted between animals and humans. Examples of zoonotic diseases are anthrax, plague, and Q fever.

■ Scope and Distribution

It has been observed that the *Pteropus* genus of fruit bats are susceptible to NiV infection but do not develop illness. Populations of these bats are distributed across a wide area, including the northern, eastern, and southeastern regions of Australia, Indonesia, Malaysia, the Philippines, and other Pacific Islands.

This disease has a wide host range, which accounts for the emergence of NiV as a zoonotic pathogen. Those people most at risk of contracting the disease are those working in close association with infected pigs in areas where the virus is endemic.

NiV was first implicated in encephalitis in the outbreak of neurological and respiratory disease that occurred on Malaysian pig farms in 1998 and 1999. Cases also occurred in Singapore in 1999 and were attributed to pigs that had been imported from the infected Malaysian pig farms. Between 2001 and 2013, NiV outbreaks occurred each year in Bangladesh, with a mortality rate exceeding 70 percent. A handful of outbreaks occurred in India during that time as well. These outbreaks were located in areas where *Pteropus* fruit bats live, suggesting that the spread of the virus is limited to areas where these fruit bats are found.

■ Treatment and Prevention

During the initial outbreaks of NiV infection, the antiviral drug ribavirin was used, which was deemed helpful in reducing the duration of fevers and overall severity of the disease. However, the precise clinical usefulness of the drug remains uncertain. The usual treatment for infected persons is intensive supportive care. Researchers have made progress in identifying the way in which the virus enters cells and replicates, and this knowledge could potentially lead to an effective treatment for the virus.

NiV may be prevented by avoiding contact with animals known to harbor the infection and by using appropriate personal protective equipment when handling infected tissue. Transmission of the virus from bats to pigs may be avoided by minimizing the overlap of the habitats of these animals, thus reducing the likelihood that pigs will come in contact with bat urine, feces, or partially eaten fruits. Bat-to-human transmission can be reduced by avoiding the ingestion of raw date palm sap.

■ Impacts and Issues

NiV is classified as an emerging infectious disease by the US Centers for Disease Control and Prevention. It is considered a cause for public concern due to the significant mortality rates observed following infection. Later outbreaks of the disease in Bangladesh among humans were characterized by a high rate of respiratory disease, which increases the chances of person-to-person transmission. It is assumed the virus did not emerge suddenly but has been slowly adapting to humans as a host; therefore, it is considered to pose an even greater threat. Continuous outbreaks in Bangladesh emphasize the dangers of foodborne illness and the need for increased surveillance of this disease.

NiV infection among pigs also carries a significant economic impact. The 1998 to 1999 outbreak caused 1.1 million pigs to be slaughtered. This loss of potential income exacts an economic toll on both individual farmers and the community as a whole.

PRIMARY SOURCE

Nipah: Fearsome Virus that Caught the Medical and Scientific World Off-Guard

SOURCE: *Boseley, Sarah. "Nipah: Fearsome Virus That Caught the Medical and Scientific World Off-Guard."* Guardian *(January 18, 2017). This article can also be found online at https://www.theguardian.com/world/2017/jan/18/nipah-fearsome-virus-that-caught-the-medical-and-scientific-world-off-guard (accessed January 22, 2018).*

INTRODUCTION: *In the following article from the* Guardian, *author Sarah Boseley recounts the first human outbreak of the Nipah virus that occurred in Malaysia and Singapore in 1998 and 1999 and describes how the disease travels from fruit bats in Southeast Asia to humans. Boseley also shows the connection between the destruction of the rainforest and the first outbreak of the Nipah virus.*

In 1998, with no explanation or signal of danger, a fearsome disease took off in Malaysia. Pigs died in large numbers and then men slaughtering infected animals also fell ill. They passed it to their families at home. Nearly half of those who got sick died.

It was not Ebola – it was a virus that became known as Nipah, after the Malaysian town of Kampung Sungai Nipah where it was first identified. But there are resemblances to Ebola in the way the disease suddenly emerged from the animal world and then spread between humans, causing a threat to life that caught the medical and scientific world off-guard.

The story of the outbreak of Nipah in Malaysia was told – and embellished – in the 2011 film *Contagion*, starring amongst others, Kate Winslet, Gwynneth Paltrow and Matt Damon. There, the disease became a global pandemic, killing 26 million people.

In reality, the death toll from Nipah in Malaysia and Singapore, where it had spread, was 105 out of 265 cases, but could have been much worse had it been more easily transmitted. It also caused the collapse of the $1bn pig industry. The disease seemed to come from nowhere, but as with other such viruses, the emergence and spread was caused by a cocktail of human behaviour and environmental change.

The virus is endemic in fruit bats – also known to carry Ebola virus. The bats were on the move, leaving rainforests where slash-and-burn logging was causing massive haze, shutting out sunlight and preventing the fruit they ate from growing. Drought caused by El Niño made things worse.

Large numbers of bats were later seen in the orchards around the pig farms of northwest Malaysia. The virus from their saliva was in the half-eaten fruit they dropped – which was devoured by the pigs.

The Malaysian outbreak was finally stopped by mass culling of pigs in May 1999. But since then there have been regular Nipah outbreaks in Bangladesh, where transmission occurs directly from fruit bats to humans.

"We know how it happens," said Professor John Clemens, executive director of the International Centre for Diarrhoeal Disease Research, Bangladesh. "The fact that it has established itself as an endemic focus in Bangladesh with regular, albeit infrequent, transmission to man suggests that it could cause broader problems for humanity at large. I would add as well that similar to Ebola virus, people in intimate contact with Nipah patients can acquire the infection, human to human.

"I'm sure you see the parallels there with Ebola, except unlike Ebola, which has its traditional homeland in sub-Saharan Africa, Nipah is here in Asia."

Nipah was at first misdiagnosed in Malaysia as Japanese encephalitis, because of the swelling of the brain that occurs.

"When it is transmitted to man, it can cause an extremely serious encephalitis, sometimes with pneumonia, and when people get sick with this, the case fatality rate is about 50%, with substantial serious neurological impairment of a fraction also who survive," said Clemens.

In Bangladesh, the outbreaks occur because of the traditional drinking of palm wine, a delicacy made from date palm sap. Fruit bats like to hang upside down in the palm trees, with the result that their excretions – urine and saliva can find their way into the sap.

There should be ways to avoid this route of transmission – if not through persuading people to avoid palm wine, then by putting skirts on the trees to keep the bats away, said Clemens.

But that would not end the hidden risk. Changes in people's behaviour or alterations we make to our environment can precipitate a small outbreak – perhaps with a different and unexpected route of transmission – that becomes something far more dangerous. It happened with Ebola, which spread from rural villages into the cities, where large numbers of people lived close together and were easily infected. That is also the danger with other zoonotic diseases, including Nipah, said Clemens.

SEE ALSO *Antiviral Drugs; Emerging Infectious Diseases; Viral Disease; Zoonoses*

BIBLIOGRAPHY

Books

Bennett, John E., Raphael Dolin, and Martin J. Blaser. *Mandell, Douglas, and Bennett's Principles and Practice of Infectious Diseases*. 8th ed. Philadelphia: Elsevier/Saunders, 2015.

Halpin, Kim, and Paul Rota. "A Review of Hendra Virus and Nipah Virus Infections in Man and Other Animals." In *Zoonoses—Infections Affecting Humans and Animals: Focus on Public Health Aspects*, edited by Andreas Sing. Dordrecht, Netherlands: Springer Netherlands, 2015.

Periodicals

Chakraborty, A., et al. "Evolving Epidemiology of Nipah Virus Infection in Bangladesh: Evidence from Outbreaks during 2010–2011." *Epidemiology and Infection* 144, no. 2 (January 2016): 371–380. This article can also be found online at https://www.cambridge.org/core/journals/epidemiology-and-infection/article/evolving-epidemiology-of-nipah-virus-infection-in-bangladesh-evidence-from-outbreaks-during-20102011/B613FF64EDFA3F105C7FAC390F32FB4B (accessed January 19, 2018).

Gurley, Emily S., et al. "Convergence of Humans, Bats, Trees, and Culture in Nipah Virus Transmission, Bangladesh." *Emerging Infectious Diseases* 23, no. 9 (September 2017): 1446–1453. This article can also be found online at https://www.ncbi.nlm.nih.gov/pmc/articles/PMC5572889/ (January 19, 2018).

Kulkarni, D. D., et al. "Nipah Virus Infection: Current Scenario." *Indian Journal of Virology* 24, no. 3 (December 2013): 398–408. This article can also be found online at https://www.ncbi.nlm.nih.gov/pmc/articles/PMC3832692/ (accessed January 22, 2018).

Websites

"Nipah Virus (NiV)." Centers for Disease Control and Prevention, March 20, 2014. https://www.cdc.gov/vhf/nipah/index.html (accessed January 19, 2018).

"Nipah Virus (NiV) Infection." World Health Organization. http://www.who.int/csr/disease/nipah/en/ (accessed January 19, 2018).

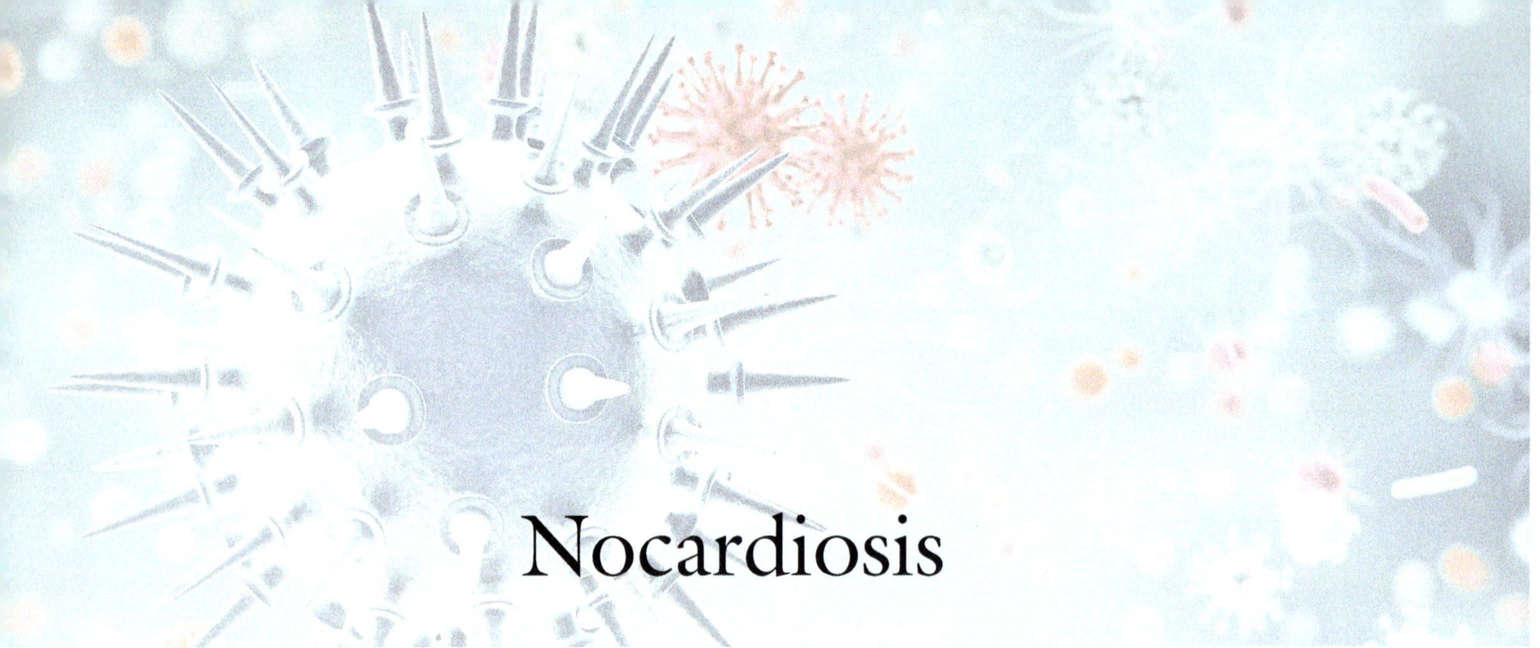

Nocardiosis

■ Introduction

Nocardiosis is a serious infectious disease with a high mortality rate that mostly affects people with weakened immune systems. It is caused by fungus-like bacteria that affect the lungs (pulmonary nocardiosis), skin (nocardiosis), or the entire body (disseminated or systemic nocardiosis), especially the brain and meninges. According to the US Centers for Disease Control and Prevention (CDC), about 80 percent of cases involve lung infections, brain abscesses, or systemic infection. The other 20 percent of cases involve the skin.

The infection itself is caused by bacteria of the genus *Nocardia*. At least 87 species have been identified, with new species still being found. Of the 87 species, about 50 are associated with disease. The bacteria that cause infection most frequently are *N. farcinica, N. nova, N. cyriacigeorgica, and N. pseudobrasiliensis.*

WORDS TO KNOW

CUTANEOUS Pertaining to the skin.

IMMUNOCOMPROMISED A reduction of the ability of the immune system to recognize and respond to the presence of foreign material.

MORTALITY The condition of being susceptible to death. The term *mortality* comes from the Latin word *mors*, which means death. Mortality can also refer to the rate of deaths caused by an illness or injury (e.g., "Rabies has a high mortality rate").

SYSTEMIC Any medical condition that affects the whole body (i.e., the whole system).

■ Disease History, Characteristics, and Transmission

Nocardia are often found in soil and dust particles. They cause occasional disease in humans and animals around the world. Transmission of pulmonary nocardiosis is usually accomplished by inhalation of the organisms when they are within airborne dust particles. Transmission of systemic nocardiosis usually occurs by direct contact with soil through puncture wounds. Abrasions (scrapes) can also be a route for transmission but less frequently than the other two means. Nocardiosis can also be transmitted through medical equipment or during surgery, particularly in immunocompromised organ transplants.

Symptoms of the pulmonary form are usually chills, fever, cough (similar to pneumonia or tuberculosis), thick (often bloody) sputum, night sweats, and chest pain. When the bacteria affect the brain, symptoms usually include severe headaches, lethargy, disorientation, confusion, dizziness, nausea and seizures, problems with walking, and sudden neurological problems. These symptoms are often more severe in patients with compromised immune systems. If a brain abscess (a localized area of infection) ruptures, the infection can often lead to meningitis (infection of the outer covering of the brain, or meninges). When the skin is affected, rashes, lumps, and sores are usually present, along with swollen lymph nodes. They are often located in the skin or directly underneath the skin. Lesions may also form in the kidneys, liver, and bones.

According to the CDC, up to 44 percent of people with nocardiosis that affects the brain or spinal cord die.

■ Scope and Distribution

Nocardiosis is found throughout the world. People of all ages can contract the infection. Nocardiosis is more common in males than in females by a three-to-one ratio. It is especially common in people with impaired immune systems and people who have chronic lung problems, such as emphysema.

According to the CDC, about 500 to 1,000 new cases are reported annually. No accurate statistics are available internationally.

Immunocompromised people are at increased risk from *Nocardia*. Those at higher risk include people with cancer, connective tissue disorders, bone marrow transplants, solid organ transplants, high-dose corticosteroid use, and human immunodeficiency virus (HIV)/acquired immunodeficiency syndrome (AIDS). However, people with no history of serious diseases can also contract nocardiosis.

Treatment and Prevention

The diagnosis is sometimes difficult because *Nocardia* grow more slowly than most bacteria, and so cultures are often not analyzed for a sufficient amount of time in the clinical laboratory. In addition, the infection inside cultures of sputum or discharge is not easily identifiable. It is most often identified from respiratory secretions, abscess aspirates, skin biopsies, and special staining techniques. In addition, they take a complete medical history to help evaluate the patient. Lung biopsies and chest X-rays are also sometimes taken. For brain infections, computer tomography (CT) or magnetic resonance imaging (MRI) scans are usually used.

A treatment usually lasts at least 6 months, but sometimes 12 to 18 months or longer is needed to cure the

REAL-WORLD RISK

People with weakened immune systems are more likely to contract nocardiosis than the general population. Weakened immune systems can occur after organ and bone marrow transplants or can be caused by certain diseases. According to the US Centers for Disease Control and Prevention, the following diseases can weaken the immune system and increase the likelihood of contracting nocardiosis:

1. Alcoholism
2. Cancer
3. Connective tissue disorders
4. Diabetes
5. HIV/AIDS
6. Pulmonary alveolar proteinosis

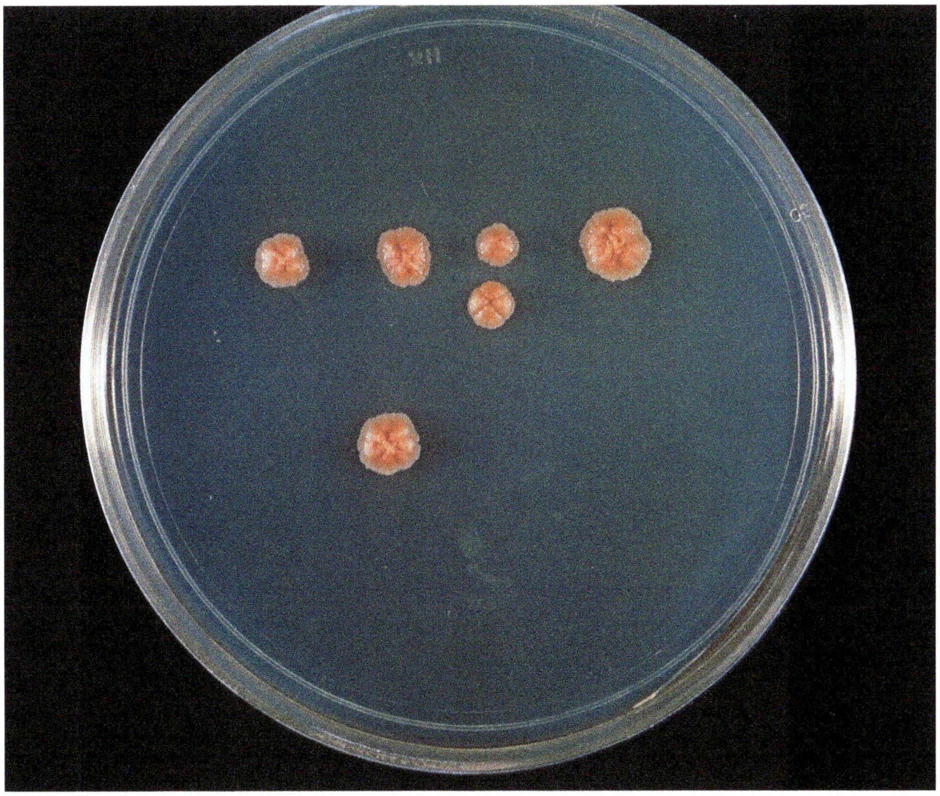

Culture of *Nocardia asteroides*. The bacteria is the cause of nocardiosis. *© Smith Collection/Gado/Getty Images*

infection. Bed rest is recommended during antibiotic drug treatment. Short-term antibiotic treatment does not work. Sometimes co-trimoxazole or sulfonamide drugs (in high doses) are used. Sulfadiazine is often prescribed. The combination of trimethoprim-sulfamethoxazole (TMP-SMX) is generally the drug treatment preferred by the medical community. If patients do not respond to these medicines, ampicillin, erythromycin, or minocycline may be added to them.

According to the CDC Division of Bacterial and Mycotic Diseases, the drug combination of sulfonamide, ceftriaxone, and amikacin has shown promising results, especially when TMP-SMX is difficult to administer. Treatment sometimes also includes surgery to excise dead tissue and drain abscesses. Bed rest is recommended while the patient recovers; however, activity may slowly resume. Sometimes with chronic cases, chronic suppressive therapy is used. This includes prolonged low-dose antibiotic therapy. The prognosis is best for the patient when nocardiosis is diagnosed early and before it reaches the brain.

Diagnosis has been difficult in the past. However, new diagnostic tools, including molecular diagnostic and subtyping methods, are helping to better identify the infection.

■ Impacts and Issues

Nocardia infections, especially in immunocompromised patients, are difficult for physicians because they cause a wide variety of diseases that require extra expertise. The number of cases has been increasing. However, this increase in numbers is generally attributed to improvements in diagnostic techniques and to the overall increase in the number of severely immunocompromised people throughout the world. Recovery may be slow. Treatments are usually able to control the infection. But recurrence of the disease is possible. Sometimes allergies to the antibiotics prescribed to treat the infection occur, and alternatives may need to be provided. The prognosis is generally good when the diagnosis and treatment are prompt and on target. However, the outcome is generally poor after the infection has spread widely in the body and treatment has not been prompt.

SEE ALSO *Antibacterial Drugs; Bacterial Disease; CDC (Centers for Disease Control and Prevention)*

BIBLIOGRAPHY

Books

Bennett, John E., Raphael Dolin, and Martin J. Blaser. *Mandell, Douglas, and Bennett's Principles and Practice of Infectious Diseases.* 8th ed. Philadelphia: Elsevier/Saunders, 2015.

Periodicals

Ambrosioni, J., D. Lew, and J. Garbino. "Nocardiosis: Updated Clinical Review and Experience at a Tertiary Center." *Infection* 38, no. 2 (April 2010): 89–97. This article can also be found online at https://link.springer.com/article/10.1007/s15010-009-9193-9#citeas (accessed January 19, 2018).

Wilson, John W. "Nocardiosis: Updates and Clinical Overview." *Mayo Clinic Proceedings* 87, no. 4 (April 2012): 403–407. This article can also be found online at http://www.sciencedirect.com/science/article/pii/S0025619612002042 (accessed January 19, 2018).

Woodworth, M. H., et al. "Increasing *Nocardia* Incidence Associated with Bronchiectasis at a Tertiary Care Center." *Annals of the American Thoracic Society* 14, no. 3 (March 2017): 347–354. This article can also be found online at https://www.ncbi.nlm.nih.gov/pubmed/28231023 (accessed January 19, 2018).

Websites

Bell, Melissa, Michael M. McNeil, and June M. Brown. "*Nocardia* species (Nocardiosis)." Antimicrobe, 2014. http://www.antimicrobe.org/b117.asp (accessed January 19, 2018).

"Nocardiosis." Centers for Disease Control and Prevention, October 13, 2005. https://www.cdc.gov/nocardiosis/ (accessed January 19, 2018).

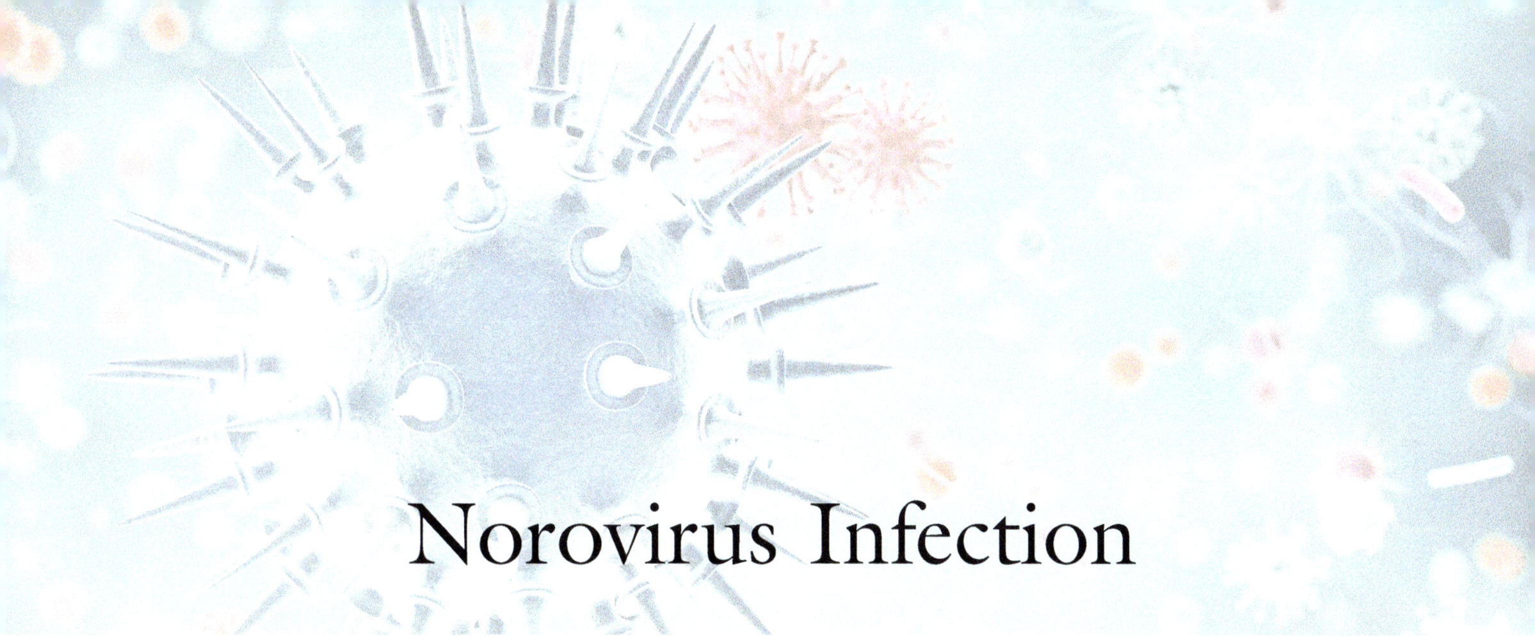

Norovirus Infection

Introduction

A norovirus infection is a type of stomach ailment known as viral gastroenteritis. The infection is also commonly (and incorrectly) known as the stomach flu and is not related to the respiratory symptoms caused by the influenza virus.

The infection is caused by noroviruses, which have also been termed Norwalk-like viruses and caliciviruses.

Disease History, Characteristics, and Transmission

Noroviruses are named after the Norwalk virus, which was the cause of a gastroenteritis outbreak in a school in Norwalk, Ohio, in 1968. Once called Norwalk-like viruses, these viruses have since been officially designated as noroviruses.

An infection caused by a norovirus is usually not life-threatening but can cause a person to feel miserable. Typically, a person develops the symptoms of infection suddenly and becomes ill for several days. Vomiting and diarrhea occur many times during the illness, and the loss of fluids can cause dehydration. Dehydration can be serious in infants, the elderly, and people whose immune systems are not functioning efficiently.

Recovery is usually complete, with no lingering symptoms or infection. However, as different strains (types) of the norovirus exist, repeated gastrointestinal infections throughout a person's life are possible.

Noroviruses are found in the intestinal tract. A norovirus infection can occur when fecal material is transferred to food, liquid, or an object. Most often this occurs when food has been handled improperly or an object such as a doorknob is handled by someone who has not properly washed his or her hands after defecating. The virus is ingested by eating the contaminated food or handling the object and then touching the mouth, known as the fecal-oral route. A person is contagious from the moment he or she displays symptoms to up to two weeks after the symptoms have ended.

There is no evidence that the virus can be transferred by inhaling virus-laden air, even though it has been shown that vomiting can release virus particles into the air.

Scope and Distribution

Norovirus infection is common. As of 2017 the US Centers for Disease Control and Prevention (CDC) estimated that between 19 million and 21 million cases of norovirus infection occur in the United States each year, with over 50 percent of all food-borne disease outbreaks due to noroviruses. Norovirus infections hospitalize 56,000 to 71,000 people annually and kill up to 800 people every year. Most of the food-borne outbreaks are due to the handling of food by someone whose hands are contaminated with virus-laden fecal material.

Globally, an estimated one of every five cases of acute gastroenteritis is due to norovirus. The number of cases each year globally is estimated as 685 million. Of these, 200 million involve children under five years of age. There are an estimated 50,000 child deaths due to norovirus infection annually, mostly in developing countries.

A wide variety of foods can be contaminated, including salad dressing, deli-style meats, bakery items, cake ic-

WORDS TO KNOW

GASTROENTERITIS An inflammation of the stomach and the intestines. Commonly called the stomach flu.

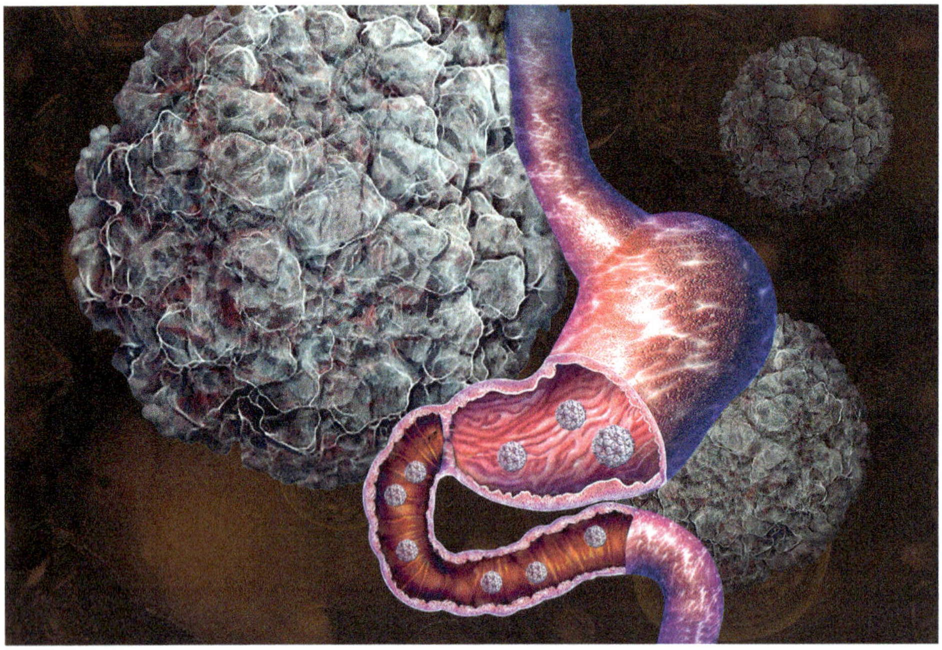

Noroviruses are found in the intestinal tract. Norovirus infection is the primary cause of gastroenteritis, or the stomach flu. *© Carol and Mike Werner/Science Source*

ing, fruits, and vegetables. Seafoods such as oysters can become contaminated and can concentrate the virus when they filter norovirus-laden water. Eating raw oysters can transmit the virus to people. Drinking water contaminated with norovirus can also cause infection.

Norovirus infections can occur anywhere in the world. Because the virus is easily spread and difficult to kill, large-scale outbreaks repeatedly occur.

Treatment and Prevention

Treatment for a norovirus infection consists of keeping a person hydrated and as comfortable as possible while waiting for the infection to subside.

Good personal hygiene is the best prevention strategy. Proper handwashing is crucial in preventing transfer of the virus. Like the viral infections that cause the common cold and influenza, a norovirus infection does not produce immunity because there are many slightly different versions of norovirus. An immune response to one version does not protect against other versions of the virus.

Washing fruits and vegetables before eating them, especially those labeled as organically grown, is wise, as some organic produce is fertilized with manure. Because virus particles require a host cell before they can replicate, norovirus particles that adhere to produce can remain capable of causing an infection for a long time.

Impacts and Issues

The intensity of the symptoms of a norovirus infection is of most concern when the infection occurs in a day care, cruise ship, school, hospital, or similar setting. In an infant or an infirm person, the combination of the infection and the dehydration caused by diarrhea and vomiting can be dangerous.

The consequences of the immune response to a new version of norovirus can be enormous. An example involves the high number of norovirus infections that occurred in the United States and Europe in 2002 with the appearance of a new norovirus variant. The majority of cases occurred in hospitals, cruise ships, and nursing homes. The CDC monitors reports of outbreaks of gastroenteritis aboard cruise ships on a daily basis and works to identify the causative agent.

Another outbreak of norovirus among people in close quarters occurred in the Astrodome in Houston, Texas, during September 2005, when it was used to house evacuees from Hurricane Katrina. Approximately 1,500 evacuees and relief workers received treatment for gastroenteritis at the Astrodome complex between September 2 and 12. The causative agent was later identified as a norovirus. Despite the rapidly changing population of evacuees, the outbreak was contained within one week by isolating persons with symptoms within one area of the complex, distributing hand sanitizer, conducting handwashing awareness campaigns, and installing additional portable sinks in the facility.

Despite knowledge of how norovirus spreads and how it can be prevented, outbreaks remain relatively common. In January 2014 nearly 700 people became ill on a Royal Caribbean cruise ship. The CDC later confirmed that the patients tested positive for norovirus. In May 2017 2,800 cases of norovirus were reported in Yolo County, California, schools.

Many norovirus outbreaks are ultimately traced to restaurants. In 2015 two norovirus outbreaks were tied to Chipotle Mexican Grill restaurants in Simi Valley, California, and Boston. The California outbreak caused more than 200 people to become ill. In Massachusetts more than 120 people, mostly Boston College students, were affected. The restaurant chain later apologized for the Boston outbreak in a series of newspaper advertisements that also addressed a recent outbreak of *E. coli* that had affected Chipotle diners in nine states. Despite the chain's efforts to reassure customers, in July 2017 another norovirus outbreak occurred at a Chipotle restaurant in Sterling, Virginia. This outbreak caused more than 130 people to become ill. The restaurant later reported that the outbreak may have been caused by a sick employee. In August 2017 an outbreak of norovirus was traced to a doughnut shop in Toledo, Ohio. More than 300 customers reported becoming ill after eating at the shop during the first week of August.

Protection against noroviruses in the form of a vaccine is not available, although at least one pharmaceutical company is attempting to develop an inhalable vaccine. Norovirus infection also has consequences for the military. The debilitating and contagious nature of the infection can lessen troops' combat readiness. Recognizing this, US defense agencies have been the main sponsors of the vaccine development effort.

PRIMARY SOURCE

Chipotle Is Subpoenaed in Criminal Inquiry over Norovirus Outbreak

SOURCE: *Abrams, Rachel. "Chipotle Is Subpoenaed in Criminal Inquiry over Norovirus Outbreak."* New York Times *(January 7, 2016): B3. This article can also be found online at https://www.nytimes.com/2016/01/07/business/chipotle-outbreak.html (accessed November 20, 2017).*

INTRODUCTION: *Following an outbreak of norovirus at a California Chipotle Mexican Grill restaurant in 2015, the chain was investigated by the US Attorney's Office for the Central District of California. The following* New York Times *article discusses the investigation and considers the implications of a potential criminal suit based on a single outbreak.*

Chipotle Mexican Grill said on Wednesday that it had been served a federal grand jury subpoena as part of a criminal investigation seeking information about a norovirus outbreak at a California restaurant.

The move could represent a highly unusual step by the federal authorities, which generally have tended to focus on manufacturers or farmers, rather than restaurants, in investigations of food-borne illnesses, food safety experts said. In the past, the authorities have intervened when contaminated food crosses state lines, they said.

But it was unknown whether Chipotle was a target of the inquiry or whether it centered on some part of the food supply chain. Federal officials declined to comment.

The inquiry was yet another setback for Chipotle, which has been struggling to contain the damage to its sales and reputation from a series of food-related illnesses among customers and employees, including outbreaks of *E. coli* in other states in which it closed some restaurants, and, last month, a norovirus outbreak in Boston.

Chipotle said in a filing with the Securities and Exchange Commission that news of additional food-related illnesses and outbreaks in the last several weeks of 2015 had caused a drop in sales in December alone of about 30 percent in stores that had been open more than a year. Its stock has tumbled since news of the outbreaks began.

The company declined to comment beyond the filing.

Bill Marler, a food safety lawyer representing plaintiffs in cases involving the California norovirus outbreak and others involving food contamination, said the federal inquiry was unusual. "It's perplexing, because I've never seen this before," he said of the investigation, which so far seemed focused on only one Chipotle restaurant.

Two hundred and seven people, including 18 Chipotle employees, reported falling ill after eating at one of its restaurants in Simi Valley, Calif., in mid-August, according to Doug Beach, manager of the community services program at the Ventura County Environmental Health Division. He said that workers had closed and cleaned the restaurant, but did not notify his agency until after it reopened.

"I do not know why Chipotle chose not to tell us until everything was done," he said, adding that restaurants typically contact the department as soon as they are aware of food-borne illness cases.

The subpoena was issued by the United States attorney's office for the Central District of California in an inquiry it is conducting with the Food and Drug Administration's Office of Criminal Investigations, Chipotle said in the filing. The subpoena seeks "a broad range of documents," the filing said, although Chipotle did not say whether it was the target of the investigation.

"Whenever there's an investigation of a target, many, many people who do business with that target get a subpoena," said James F. Neale, a partner at the law firm McGuireWoods and co-author of "Food Safety Law." "We're just looking through a very limited keyhole."

Representatives of the Food and Drug Administration and the United States attorney's office declined to comment.

Experts said it was unclear what might have prompted the inquiry. In the past, such investigations have been opened when contaminated food crosses state lines, Mr. Neale and Mr. Marler said, and typically center on food producers.

"It doesn't look to me like this California outbreak goes beyond one restaurant," Mr. Neale said. "We haven't typically seen federal law enforcement activity for localized outbreaks."

Norovirus was also at the center of an episode in which about 120 Boston College students reported getting sick in December after eating at a Chipotle restaurant near the campus.

The company had already been in the spotlight after various restaurants around the country reported outbreaks of *E. coli* bacteria. In early November, Chipotle voluntarily closed 43 restaurants in Washington State and Oregon because of an outbreak. The bacteria are common in the intestines of animals and people, but some strains can cause illness or even death.

Chipotle's reputation—and sales—fell further the week of Dec. 21, after the Centers for Disease Control and Prevention said it was investigating five new cases of *E. coli* reported in November.

All told, more than 500 people were sickened after eating in a Chipotle restaurant in the last half of 2015, according to *Food Safety News.*

Shares of Chipotle fell nearly 5 percent on Wednesday, to close at $426.67. The stock had been trading above $700 a share in the summer.

SEE ALSO *Gastroenteritis (Common Causes); Handwashing; Viral Disease*

BIBLIOGRAPHY

Books

Stone, Carolyn. *Norovirus: How to Stay Safe.* New York: Eternal Spiral, 2014.

Periodicals

Cardemil, Cristina V., Umesh D. Parashar, and Aron J. Hall. "Norovirus Infection in Older Adults: Epidemiology, Risk Factors, and Opportunities for Prevention and Control." *Infectious Diseases Clinics of North America* 31 (December 2017): 839–870.

Lindstrom, Lauren. "More Than 300 People Now Affected by Norovirus Outbreak." *Toledo Blade* (August 11, 2017). This article can also be found online at http://www.toledoblade.com/Medical/2017/08/11/Officials-to-keep-an-eye-on-outbreak-of-novovirus.html (accessed November 20, 2017).

Websites

"Norovirus: U.S. Trends and Outbreaks." Centers for Disease Control and Prevention. https://www.cdc.gov/norovirus/trends-outbreaks.html (accessed November 20, 2017).

"Norovirus Worldwide." Centers for Disease Control and Prevention. https://www.cdc.gov/norovirus/worldwide.html (accessed November 20, 2017).

Brian Hoyle

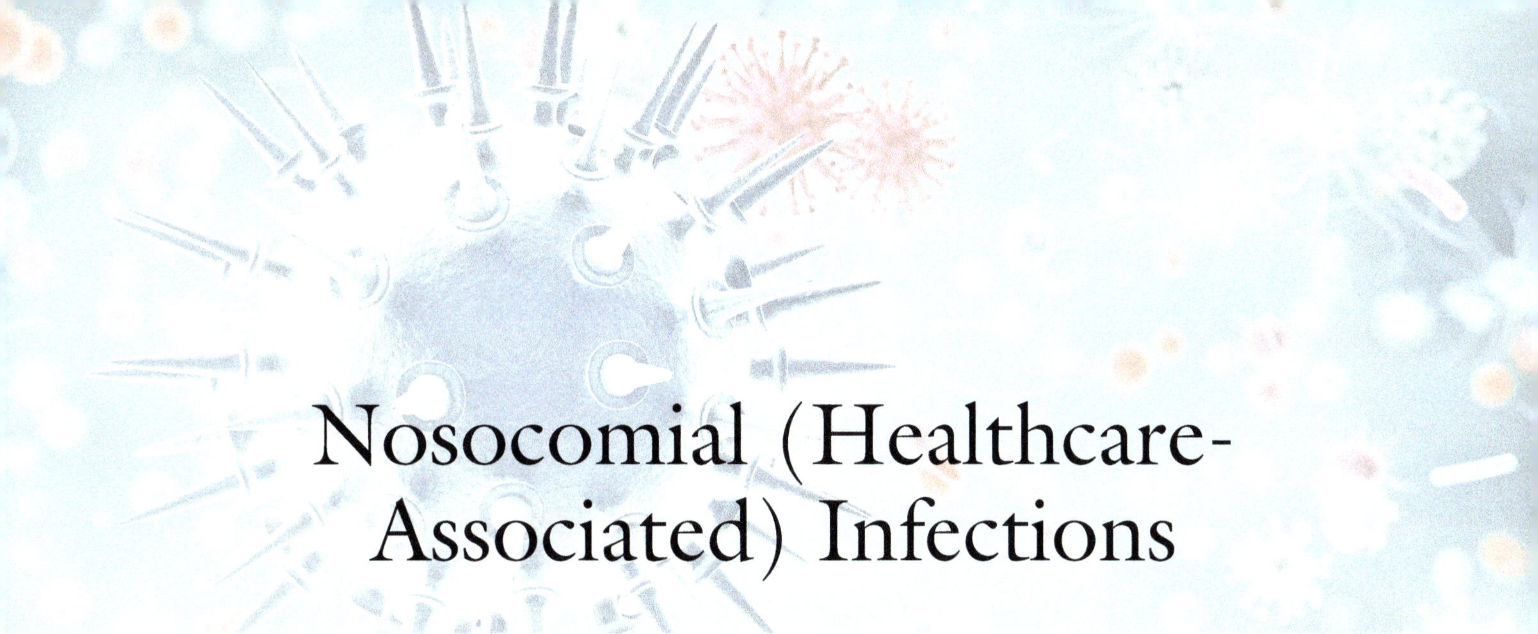

Nosocomial (Healthcare-Associated) Infections

Introduction

Nosocomial infections, also called health care–associated infections (HAIs), are bacterial, viral, or fungal infections contracted in health care settings, usually hospitals. Such infections have occurred for as long as doctors have handled patients. The source of HAIs only began to be widely understood in the mid- to late 19th century. Hundreds of millions of people worldwide acquire HAIs at any given time. These infections claim many tens of thousands of lives every year and occur in both developed and developing nations.

HAIs are found primarily at sites where objects such as catheters, scalpels, needles, breathing tubes, and similar devices are introduced into the body, providing a place for bacteria to grow. Infections caused in this way are an increasing problem, partly due to the ongoing evolution of resistance to many antibiotics by bacteria. Countermeasures include handwashing, glove wearing, increasing blood supply safety, improvement of injection practices, immunization of health care workers and others, and improvement of water supply quality and waste management.

Disease History, Characteristics, and Transmission

The word *nosocomial* comes from the Greek word *nosokomos*, meaning "person who tends the sick." The idea that physicians might themselves be a major cause of disease did not occur until the 1790s, when a few doctors began to notice that puerperal fever, a disease caused by the group A *Streptococcus* bacterium *Streptococcus pyogenes*, was afflicting women after childbirth and seemed to be transmitted to patients by doctors. These observations received little attention from the medical world as a whole, however, until the mid-19th century. At that time puerperal fever was common in hospitals, where *S. pyogenes* was transmitted by physicians' unwashed hands as they went from patient to patient. During childbirth women were often infected with the *S. pyogenes* that contaminated their doctors' hands as they moved between patients or from the autopsy room, which was located near the delivery room. This commonly resulted in death rates in maternity wards of 10 to 25 percent, with occasional epidemics wiping out entire wards.

In 1843 writer and physician Oliver Wendell Holmes (1809–1904) published a seminal essay titled "The Contagiousness of Puerperal Fever." In it he argues forcefully against the widespread medical opinion that puerperal fever is not a contagious disease. "The disease known as Puerperal Fever," he writes, "is so far contagious as to be frequently carried from patient to patient by physicians and

WORDS TO KNOW

PUERPERAL FEVER A bacterial infection present in the blood (septicemia) that follows childbirth. The Latin word *puer*, meaning "boy" or "child," is the root of this term. Puerperal fever was much more common before the advent of modern aseptic practices, but infections still occur. Louis Pasteur showed that puerperal fever is most often caused by *Streptococcus* bacteria, which is now treated with antibiotics.

RESISTANT ORGANISM An organism that has developed the ability to counter something trying to harm it. Within infectious diseases, the organism, such as a bacterium, has developed a resistance to drugs, such as antibiotics.

STANDARD PRECAUTIONS The safety measures taken to prevent the transmission of disease-causing bacteria. These measures include proper handwashing, wearing gloves, goggles, and other protective clothing, proper handling of needles, and sterilization of equipment.

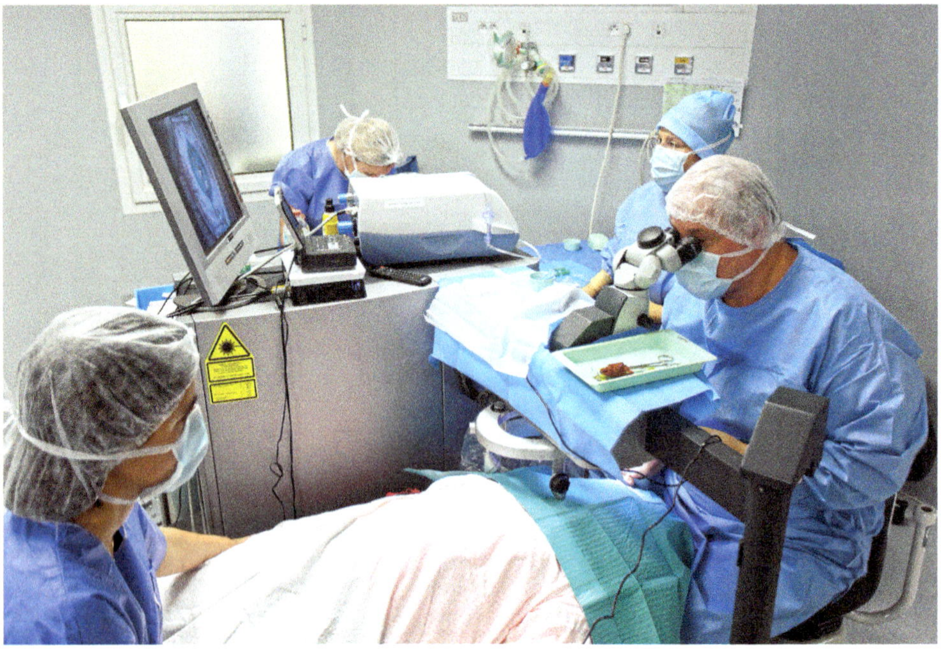

Medical staff wear surgical caps and masks and take other precautions designed to prevent nosocomial infections, which are infections contracted within a health care setting. © Andia/UIG/Getty Images

nurses." He notes that, in case after case, a string of maternal deaths could be traced to a series of visits by a single doctor or midwife. In one instance he documents a string of deaths 40 cases long, all caused by a single doctor.

During the same period, Hungarian German physician Ignaz Semmelweis (1818–1865) documented similar facts in the Vienna General Hospital. The death rate in the section of the hospital in which women in childbirth were attended by doctors was three to five times higher than that of women who were attended by midwives. Semmelweis concluded that doctors were infecting patients by visiting them with unwashed hands after performing autopsies (dissecting corpses). He managed to institute a program of handwashing using a chlorine solution, greatly reducing the death rate. In the 1860s and 1870s, French scientist Louis Pasteur (1822–1895) established that infectious disease was caused by germs, or living organisms too small to be seen by the naked eye. With this discovery he explained the mechanism by which unwashed hands can transmit disease. By the end of the century, medical opinion had shifted toward a nosocomial origin for puerperal fever. However, there were still many doctors who washed their hands after delivering babies but not before.

In the 20th century, nosocomial puerperal fever rapidly became a thing of the past, at least in industrialized countries. However, other forms of nosocomial infection eventually became more common for two reasons. The first is the proliferation of various devices for delivering air or fluid to or from the body, such as hypodermic needles, catheters, intravenous lines, and breathing tubes. The second is the rise, especially in health care settings, of antibiotic-resistant bacteria. Intrusive medical devices and antibacterial drugs have saved many lives that would have otherwise been lost, but not as many as they could have saved without the nosocomial infections that accompanied their use.

Nosocomial infections of the respiratory tract, associated with breathing tubes, are the most common. In particular, ventilator-assisted pneumonia is common in intensive care units. The next most common sources of nosocomial infection, in order of decreasing frequency, are central lines (also called central venous catheters, or tubes inserted into large veins and left in place for days or weeks), urinary drainage catheters, and surgical wounds.

Two factors combine to cause a typical nosocomial infection. The first is decreased immune system function in a patient who is already ill. The second is the introduction of bacteria into the patient, usually by some type of invasive device. The National Nosocomial Infection Surveillance System of the US Centers for Disease Control and Prevention (CDC) has found that about 83 percent of nosocomial pneumonia cases are associated with breathing machines (ventilators), 97 percent of urinary tract infections are associated with catheters, and 87 percent of cases of bacteremia (infection of the bloodstream) are associated with central lines.

The most common cause of nosocomial infection is the *Staphylococcus aureus* bacterium. Some strains of this bacterium have evolved resistance to all penicillin-type antibiotics and others. For example, the USA300 strain of *S. aureus*, first identified in 2000, has evolved resistance to cefalexin, erythromycin, doxycycline, beta lactams, clindamycin, tetracycline, ciprofloxacin, and mupirocin. When a patient is infected with the bacteria, physicians may need to search by trial and error for an antibiotic that will work. During this time an infection may progress and even kill a patient.

Treatment and Prevention

Nosocomial bacterial infections are treated with antibiotics, although antibiotic-resistant strains of bacteria are making this increasingly difficult.

Prevention is accomplished through infection control and standard precautions by health care workers, including handwashing, flushing of catheters and intravenous lines using saline solution or other chemicals, wearing disposable gloves, using disposable needles, and properly sterilizing surgical instruments.

It is also recommended that patients advocate for themselves by expressing their concern about HAIs to their physician and by encouraging the physician to remove catheters as soon as possible.

Scope and Distribution

HAIs are a global problem. However, people are more likely to acquire an HAI in a hospital in a developing country where there are fewer resources. The burden of HAIs, therefore, falls largely on poorer people in poor countries.

Seven out of every 100 patients hospitalized in developed countries will develop at least one HAI, perhaps more, whereas 10 out of every 100 patients in developing countries will. For patients admitted to intensive care, the rate is between around 30 percent in developed countries because such patients are subject to more invasive devices. In developing countries the nosocomial infection rate for intensive care patients is two to three times higher than in developed ones. Infants are more likely to acquire an HAI than older children or adults. Infants are especially at risk for acquiring an HAI in developing countries. The World Health Organization (WHO) states that, "among hospital-born babies in developing countries, health care-associated infections are responsible for 4% to 56% of all causes of death in the neonatal period, and 75% in South-East Asia and Sub-Saharan Africa."

Health care workers may not only transmit nosocomial infections but also acquire them. During the severe acute respiratory syndrome (SARS) epidemic of 2002–2003, health care workers accounted for 20 to 60 percent of cases around the world, depending on location.

Impacts and Issues

In the United States, as of 2011 there were 721,800 HAIs in the United States. Of people who acquired HAIs, some 75,000 died from them. Many of these infections are preventable with proper safety protocols. In many health care settings in industrialized countries, rushed health care workers often comply poorly with rules for hand cleansing. In poorer countries dirty instruments, crowding, lack of safe water sources, and dirty overall conditions also help spread nosocomial infections.

Resistance of bacterial and fungal pathogens to antibiotics and antifungals, respectively, is a concern. In the United States, the CDC notes that *Clostridium difficile* and carbapenem-resistant *Enterobacteriaceae* are particularly troubling antibiotic-resistant bacteria in the health care setting. Spread of resistant fungal pathogens, including species of *Candida*, is an issue in health care settings as well. Because HAIs are so common in hospitals, the rise of drug-resistant bacteria and fungi is worrisome. The best way to combat the problem is for doctors to prescribe antibiotics only to treat infections that require antibiotics and to do so for the appropriate amount of time and at the appropriate dosage. It is also extremely important for people to practice good hygiene so as not to spread drug-resistant bacteria or fungal pathogens to others.

PRIMARY SOURCE

In Soil-Dwelling Bacteria, Scientists Find a New Weapon to Fight Drug-Resistant Superbugs

SOURCE: *Healy, Melissa. "In Soil-Dwelling Bacteria, Scientists Find a New Weapon to Fight Drug-Resistant Superbugs."* Los Angeles Times *(February 13, 2018). This article can also be found online at http://www.latimes.com/science/sciencenow/la-sci-sn-new-antibiotic-soil-20180213-story.html (accessed February 24, 2018).*

INTRODUCTION: *In the following article, the author describes the 2018 discovery of a new antibiotic found in soil that quickly kills drug-resistant bacteria such as methicillin-resistant* Staphylococcus aureus *(MRSA), a serious skin infection. This is hopeful news for health care professionals who treat people with health care –associated infections (HAIs) caused by antibiotic-resistant bacteria.*

It's a new class of antibiotic that promises to live up to its rough Latin translation: killer of bad guys.

In a report published this week in the journal *Nature Microbiology*, researchers describe a never-before-seen antibiotic agent that vanquished several strains of multidrug-resistant bacteria. In rats, the agent—which the researchers dubbed malacidin—attacked and broke down the cell walls of methicillin-resistant *Staphylococcus aureus* and cleared the animals' MRSA skin infections within a day.

Malacidin is short for metagenomic acidic lipopeptide antibiotic-cidins. (Also, "mal" means bad in Latin, and "cide" means to kill.) It is a distant relative of daptomycin, a powerful antibiotic that uses calcium to disrupt bacterial cell walls.

Malacidin appears to work differently than daptomycin, which was introduced in 2003 and has yet to be challenged by resistant bacteria. But scientists have reason to believe it will hold up at least as well. Even after 20 days of continued contact with malacidin—more than enough time for most bacteria to find a way to thwart an antibiotic's effects—samples of MRSA bacteria showed no signs of evolving resistance to the newly discovered agent.

Not bad for a compound that's been hiding in soil for eons.

Indeed, the method used by researchers to find and develop malacidin holds the promise of discovering many more potential medicines that live in soil but whose antibiotic properties elude researchers because they can't be cultured in a lab.

The discovery of a new class of antibiotic medication would be a red-letter event: Researchers haven't brought forth a truly new antimicrobial medication since 1987.

But an even more singular event would be the discovery of a new class of antibiotics that doesn't prompt the development of resistant strains of bacteria.

Ever since the mid-1940s, after penicillin was discovered by microbiologist Alexander Fleming and rushed into development, the introduction of new antibiotics has quickly given rise to disease-causing bacteria capable of eluding their effects.

As a result, many of the workhorses of the world of antibiotics—members of the penicillin, cephalosporin and carbapenem classes—are losing their ability to fight a lengthening list of bacterial diseases.

The result has been called a "slow catastrophe": the Centers for Disease Control and Prevention estimate that each year, at least 23,000 people now die as a direct result of bacterial infections that have become resistant to existing medicines. And many more die from other conditions that were complicated by an antibiotic-resistant infection.

Unless new antibacterial agents are discovered and turned into medicines, mortality rates due to untreatable infections are predicted to rise more than tenfold by 2050.

This is where malacidin becomes most interesting.

More remarkable than what it does is how scientists found it, and that process is described at some length in the new report. The result could be new discoveries, and a new way of sifting the soil for compounds that might make good medicine.

Chemical biologist Sean Brady and his colleagues at Rockefeller University in New York sequenced bacterial DNA extracted from 2,000 soil samples taken from across the United States.

Brady's team was looking specifically for distant relatives of daptomycin, which uses calcium to bust up, break down and generally disrupt the cell walls of target bacteria. They knew that long after the effectiveness of other antibiotics has waned, daptomycin continued to kill its targets, and they surmised that its distinctive use of calcium might be the key to an antibiotic compound's longevity.

They also knew that trying to culture all their soil samples in a lab would take forever, and that most would not replicate themselves under lab conditions anyway. So instead, they used high-speed computer processing to "screen" the soil samples for the distinctive chemical hallmark of calcium dependence.

When they found what they were looking for in a particular sample of desert soil, they captured and cloned the relevant genes, rearranged and inserted them into a host organism, and expanded the resulting sample through fermentation. This process made it possible to test the unique properties of malacidin on MRSA-infected rats.

"They've used a clever approach to mine for antibiotics," said microbiologist Kim Lewis, who directs Northeastern University's Antimicrobial Discovery Center and wasn't involved in the work. By narrowing their search for the DNA signature of calcium dependence, they were able to find a needle in a haystack—and find a promising compound.

"Now we need to say, 'You guys can do even better,'" Lewis said.

To demonstrate that their discovery is more than a one-time event, he said, Brady and his team need to identify and screen for additional DNA signatures that may predict potent antibiotic effects, "and go after them as well."

See Also *Antibiotic Resistance; Blood Supply and Infectious Disease; Infection Control and Asepsis; Streptococcal Infections, Group A*

BIBLIOGRAPHY

Books

Jarvis, William R., ed. *Bennett & Brachman's Hospital Infections.* Philadelphia: Wolters Kluwer Health/ Lippincott Williams & Wilkins, 2014.

Periodicals

Allegranzi, Benedetta, et al. "Burden of Endemic Health-Care-Associated Infection in Developing Countries: Systematic Review and Meta-Analysis." *Lancet* 377, no. 9761 (January 15, 2011): 228–241. This article can also be found online at http://www.thelancet.com/journals/lancet/article/PIIS0140-6736(10)61458-4/fulltext (accessed February 21, 2018).

Piedrahita, Christina T., et al. "Environmental Surfaces in Healthcare Facilities are a Potential Source for Transmission of *Candida auris* and Other *Candida* Species." *Infection Control & Hospital Epidemiology* 38, no. 9 (September 2017): 1107–1109. This article can also be found online at https://www.cambridge.org/core/journals/infection-control-and-hospital-epidemiology/article/environmental-surfaces-in-healthcare-facilities-are-a-potential-source-for-transmission-of-candida-auris-and-other-candida-species/AC2A27472832F4304BD55D24D3B4638F (accessed February 21, 2018).

Sanglard, Dominique. "Emerging Threats in Antifungal-Resistant Fungal Pathogens." *Frontiers in Medicine* (March 15, 2016). This article can also be found online at https://www.frontiersin.org/articles/10.3389/fmed.2016.00011/full (accessed February 21, 2018).

Websites

"Health Care-Associated Infections: Fact Sheet." World Health Organization. http://www.who.int/gpsc/country_work/gpsc_ccisc_fact_sheet_en.pdf?ua=1 (accessed February 21, 2018).

"Healthcare-Associated Infections." Centers for Disease Control and Prevention, July 14, 2017. http://www.cdc.gov/ncidod/dhqp/nnis.html (accessed February 21, 2018).

"Report on the Burden of Endemic Health Care-Associated Infection Worldwide: A Systematic Review of the Literature." World Health Organization, 2011. http://apps.who.int/iris/bitstream/10665/80135/1/9789241501507_eng.pdf?ua=1 (accessed February 21, 2018).

Larry Gilman
Claire Skinner

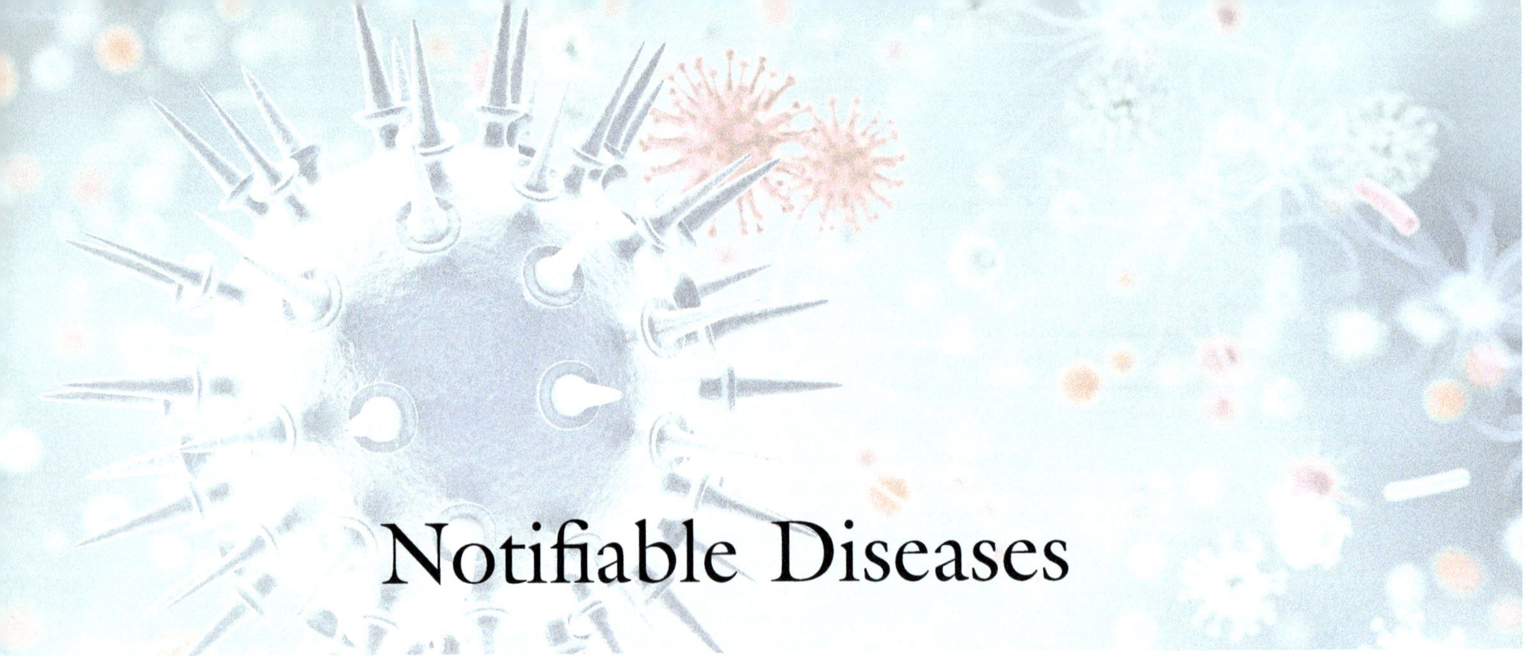

Notifiable Diseases

Introduction

Notifiable diseases are infectious diseases whose occurrence must be reported by physicians and laboratories to a public health agency. This monitoring is necessary to prevent or contain outbreaks of disease and to maintain surveillance of current disease patterns. In the United States, reporting notifiable diseases is mandatory at the state level, and the diseases that must be reported vary slightly by state. Reporting is voluntary at the federal level, although all 50 US states and districts cooperate to report information about cases of notifiable infectious diseases to the US Centers for Disease Control and Prevention (CDC).

Examples of some notifiable diseases in the United States include acquired immunodeficiency syndrome (AIDS), anthrax, cholera, diphtheria, giardiasis, influenza (both bacterial and viral), Lyme disease, malaria, measles, mumps, plague, severe acute respiratory syndrome (SARS), tuberculosis, and yellow fever. The list of notifiable diseases changes as emerging infectious diseases present new public health concerns or as an older disease becomes more prevalent. An example of a newly emerging notifiable disease is SARS, which was added to the list following the outbreak in Asia, Canada, and elsewhere in 2003. An example of a disease that has assumed greater prominence due to its resurgence and development of heightened antibiotic resistance is tuberculosis.

As of 2017 there were 88 notifiable infectious diseases in the United States. Countries including Canada and the United Kingdom have similar lists.

WORDS TO KNOW

NATIONAL ELECTRONIC TELECOMMUNICATIONS SYSTEM FOR SURVEILLANCE (NETSS) A computerized public health surveillance information system that provides the US Centers for Disease Control and Prevention with weekly data regarding cases of nationally notifiable diseases.

NOTIFIABLE DISEASE A disease that the law requires be reported to health officials when diagnosed. Also called a reportable disease.

QUARANTINE The practice of separating from the general population people who have been exposed to an infectious agent but who have not yet developed symptoms. In the United States, this may be done voluntarily or involuntarily under the authority of states or the federal Centers for Disease Control and Prevention.

SURVEILLANCE The systematic analysis, collection, evaluation, interpretation, and dissemination of data. Public health surveillance assists in the identification of health threats and the planning, implementation, and evaluation of responses to those threats.

History and Scientific Foundations

In the United States the history of notifiable diseases dates to 1878, when Congress authorized the predecessor of the modern-day public health service to collect reports of overseas deaths due to the infectious diseases prevalent at the time, such as smallpox, cholera, and yellow fever. The intention was to institute quarantine for people coming into the United States from the affected regions to prevent domestic outbreaks of these diseases.

In 1879 the authority for collection of notifiable disease information was extended to state and local public health officials. By 1928 every US state and territory was contributing information to a national report of 29 designated infectious diseases. The CDC assumed responsibility

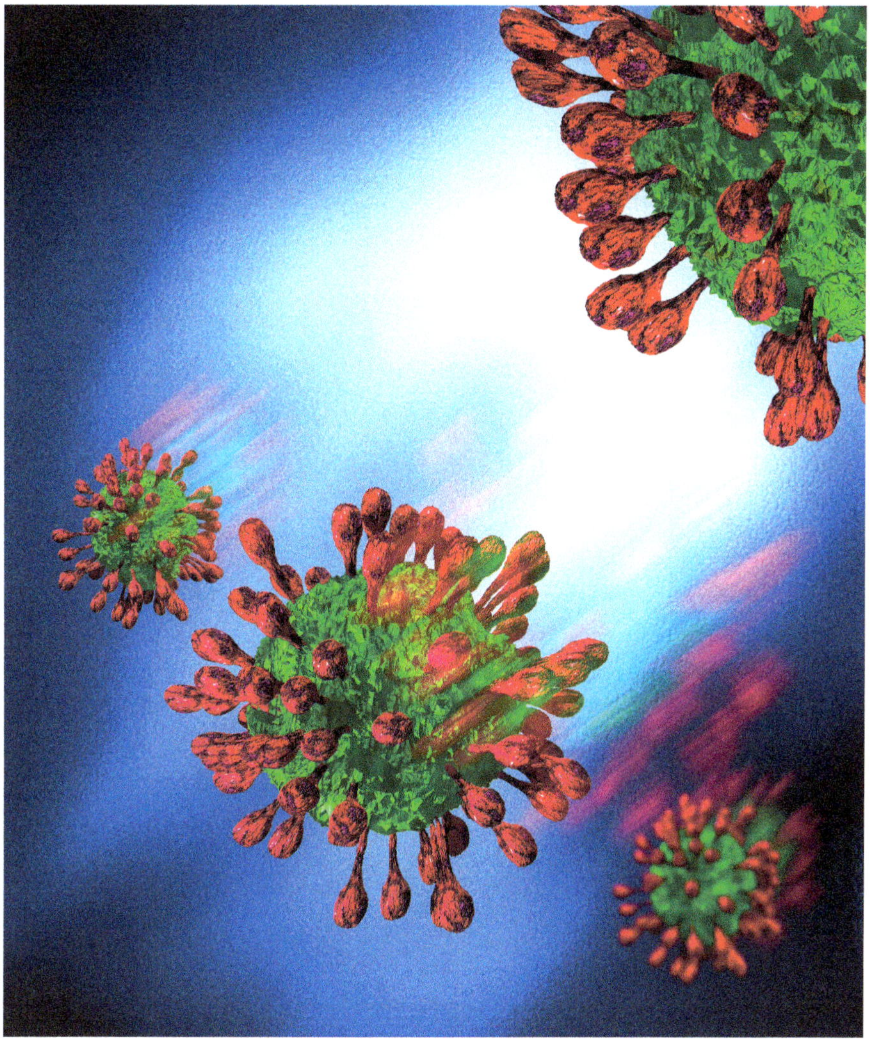

SARS coronavirus particles. SARS was added to the list of notifiable diseases following an outbreak in 2003. © Victor Habbick Visions/Science Source

for the collection and reporting of the information in 1961. Information on some of these diseases is issued weekly in a CDC publication called the *Mortality and Morbidity Weekly Report* and annually in the *Summary of Notifiable Infectious Diseases.*

Applications and Research

A key part of the CDC's National Notifiable Diseases Surveillance System (NNDSS) is a computerized and internet-linked communications network called the National Electronic Telecommunications System for Surveillance (NETSS). The network was established in 1985 as the Epidemiologic Surveillance Project. By 1989 the network was linked to all US states. States and territories convey data to the CDC via NETSS each week. While participation is voluntary, all states, territories, and the District of Columbia were participating in NETSS as of 2017.

The criteria for the reporting of notifiable diseases were published in 1990 by the CDC in collaboration with the US Council of State and Territorial Epidemiologists. The disease-by-disease criteria ensure that the information for a given notifiable disease is sufficient. For example, some diseases require the inclusion of laboratory data, while other diseases, particularly those that can arise due to eating contaminated food, require epidemiological information such as the food eaten at the gathering and the number of cases.

Data gathered on notifiable diseases also typically include information such as the detected date of the illness, geographical information (state, county), and the characteristics of those affected, including age, gender, and race/ethnicity. Information is also gathered on the disease itself, including its type, severity, diagnosis, treatment, and history, as well as the capabilities of the health care facilities and public health response in the affected region. Personal information, including the names and addresses of those who become ill, are recorded with some diseases that re-

REAL-WORLD REPORTING

Below is the Centers for Disease Control and Prevention (CDC) list of nationally notifiable infectious diseases. Beginning in mid-2007 the list was revised to include novel, or unusual, type A influenza. By encouraging states to report a newly observed type A influenza, scientists aimed to recognize a candidate for a pandemic flu virus and respond in its early stages. Physicians, laboratories, and other health providers are mandated to report notifiable diseases to state health authorities. Reporting at the federal level is voluntary. As of 2017 the list included the following diseases:

- Anthrax
- Arboviral diseases, neuroinvasive and non-neuroinvasive
- California serogroup virus diseases
- Chikungunya virus disease
- Eastern equine encephalitis virus disease
- Powassan virus disease
- St. Louis encephalitis virus disease
- West Nile virus disease
- Western equine encephalitis virus disease
- Babesiosis
- Botulism
- Botulism, food-borne
- Botulism, infant
- Botulism, wound
- Botulism, other
- Brucellosis
- Campylobacteriosis
- Chancroid
- *Chlamydia trachomatis* infection
- Cholera
- Coccidioidomycosis
- Congenital syphilis
- Syphilitic stillbirth
- Cryptosporidiosis
- Cyclosporiasis
- Dengue virus infections
- Dengue
- Dengue-like illness
- Severe dengue
- Diphtheria
- Ehrlichiosis and anaplasmosis
- *Anaplasma phagocytophilum* infection
- *Ehrlichia chaffeensis* infection
- *Ehrlichia ewingii* infection
- Undetermined human ehrlichiosis/anaplasmosis
- Giardiasis
- Gonorrhea
- *Haemophilus influenzae*, invasive disease
- Hansen's disease
- Hantavirus infection, non-Hantavirus pulmonary syndrome
- Hantavirus pulmonary syndrome
- Hemolytic uremic syndrome, post-diarrheal
- Hepatitis A, acute
- Hepatitis B, acute
- Hepatitis B, chronic
- Hepatitis B, perinatal virus infection
- Hepatitis C, acute
- Hepatitis C, chronic
- HIV infection (AIDS has been reclassified as HIV Stage III)
- Influenza-associated pediatric mortality
- Invasive pneumococcal disease
- Legionellosis
- Leptospirosis
- Listeriosis
- Lyme disease
- Malaria
- Measles
- Meningococcal disease
- Mumps
- Novel influenza A virus infections
- Pertussis
- Plague
- Poliomyelitis, paralytic
- Poliovirus infection, nonparalytic
- Psittacosis
- Q fever
- Q fever, acute
- Q fever, chronic
- Rabies, animal
- Rabies, human
- Rubella
- Rubella, congenital syndrome
- Salmonellosis
- Severe acute respiratory syndrome–associated coronavirus disease
- Shiga toxin-producing *Escherichia coli*
- Shigellosis
- Smallpox
- Spotted fever rickettsiosis
- Streptococcal toxic shock syndrome
- Syphilis
- Syphilis, primary
- Syphilis, secondary
- Syphilis, early latent
- Syphilis, late latent
- Syphilis, late with clinical manifestations (including late benign syphilis and cardiovascular syphilis)
- Tetanus
- Toxic shock syndrome (other than streptococcal)
- Trichinellosis
- Tuberculosis
- Tularemia
- Typhoid fever
- Vancomycin-intermediate *Staphylococcus aureus* and Vancomycin-resistant *Staphylococcus aureus*
- Varicella
- Varicella deaths
- Vibriosis
- Viral hemorrhagic fever
- Crimean-Congo hemorrhagic fever virus
- Ebola virus
- Lassa virus
- Lujo virus
- Marburg virus
- New World arenavirus—Guanarito virus
- New World arenavirus—Junin virus
- New World arenavirus—Machupo virus
- New World arenavirus—Sabia virus
- Yellow fever
- Zika virus disease and Zika virus infection
- Zika virus disease, congenital
- Zika virus disease, noncongenital
- Zika virus infection, congenital
- Zika virus infection, noncongenital

quire tracing and notifying close contacts who could have been exposed to the disease.

Impacts and Issues

Nationwide networks have been established in the United States, Canada, England, and other countries for the prompt and regular reporting of infectious diseases deemed to have a significant potential to spread and have debilitating or even fatal effects. Such networks have likely saved countless lives, as they have allowed public health officials to detect and respond to infectious illnesses faster and in a more coordinated fashion.

The disease surveillance networks have also become useful in monitoring illnesses that might result from a deliberate release of an infectious agent. By monitoring the pattern of an illness's spread, experts can gauge whether the infection has appeared and progressed naturally (as when cases appear geographically in a bull's-eye pattern, concentrating in one region and then spreading outward) or unnaturally (as when cases suddenly appear in similar numbers in different areas of a region).

The storage of the information in electronic databases is of some concern to those who argue that the databases can be tampered with or that the information can be extracted and used for malicious purposes. As a result, security surrounding the databases is robust. State and federal health authorities must take steps to safeguard as much as possible any personal information collected via the report of a notifiable disease. Typically, names and other personal information are indexed by number or another blind identifier in the relevant databases, allowing access to data on the disease but not specific personal information.

As new diseases emerge, they may be added to the list of notifiable diseases. A recent example is the addition of Zika virus.

The United States also abides by the International Health Regulations (IHR), which were established in 2005 to guide the World Health Organization (WHO) and member states in responding to and reporting international health emergencies. The IHR added novel influenza virus subtypes to the list of diseases that should be immediately reported to WHO.

SEE ALSO *Epidemiology; Public Health and Infectious Disease*

BIBLIOGRAPHY

Books

Bayry, Jagadeesh. *Emerging and Re-emerging Infectious Diseases of Livestock.* New York: Springer, 2017.

Kaslow, Richard A., Lawrence R. Stanberry, and James W. Le Duc, eds. *Viral Infections of Humans: Epidemiology and Control.* New York: Springer, 2014.

Payne, Susan. *Viruses: From Understanding to Investigation.* New York: Academic Press, 2017.

Pulcini, Céline, et al, eds. *Antimicrobial Stewardship.* Vol. 2 of *Developments in Emerging and Existing Infectious Diseases.* London: Elsevier/AP, 2017.

Periodicals

Costerus, Joost M., et al. "Community-Acquired Bacterial Meningitis." *Current Opinion in Infectious Diseases* 30, no. 1 (February 217): 135–141.

Websites

"2017 National Notifiable Infectious Diseases." Centers for Disease Control and Prevention. https://wwwn.cdc.gov/nndss/conditions/notifiable/2017/infectious-diseases/ (accessed November 20, 2017).

"International Health Regulations (IHR)." World Health Organization. http://www.who.int/topics/international_health_regulations/en/ (accessed November 20, 2017).

"NIAID Emerging Infectious Diseases/Pathogens." National Institute of Allergy and Infectious Diseases, October 26, 2016. https://www.niaid.nih.gov/research/emerging-infectious-diseases-pathogens (accessed November 15, 2017).

Brian Hoyle

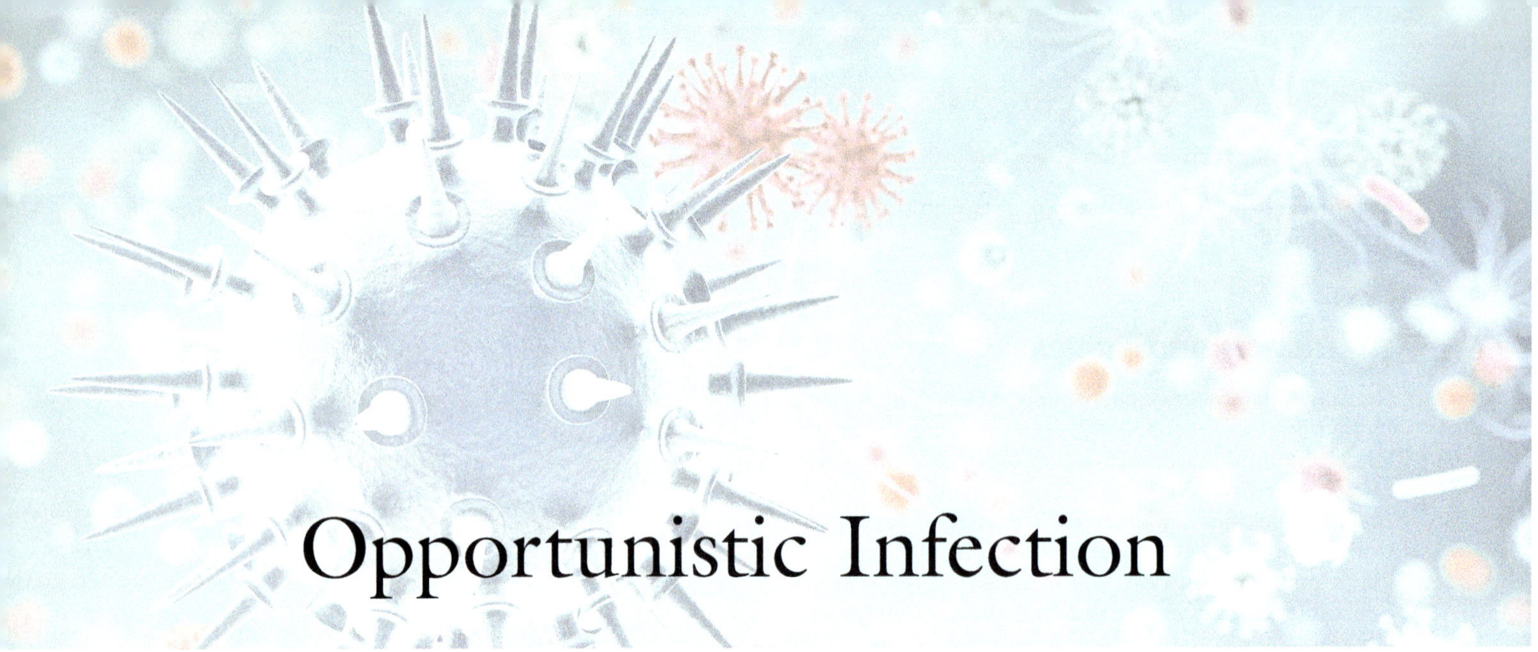

Opportunistic Infection

Introduction

An opportunistic infection is one caused by a bacterium, fungus, protozoan, or virus that would otherwise be kept in check by the immune system. The advent of acquired immunodeficiency syndrome (AIDS) in the late 20th century focused attention on the problem of opportunistic infections. As the name suggests, AIDS results in weakened immunity, giving normally harmless microbes the opportunity to invade the body and cause infection.

Besides AIDS, other medical conditions associated with opportunistic infections include cancer, severe burns, malnutrition, and diabetes. Other patient populations affected by opportunistic infections are those that are critically ill and require intensive care. Medical treatments such as cancer chemotherapy or long-term immunosuppressant drug therapy needed after organ transplantation or critical illness also result in compromised (weakened) immunity. Some common opportunistic pathogens are *Pneumocystis jirovecii*, *Candida albicans*, *Cryptococcus neoformans*, herpes simplex virus, *Toxoplasma gondii*, and cytomegalovirus. Treatment of an opportunistic infection is twofold. The infection is treated with antibiotics or other drug therapy, and the underlying immune problem due to the primary condition is also addressed.

Opportunistic Infections

Fungal Infections
- Aspergillosis
- Candidiasis
- Cryptococcosis
- Pneumocystis jiroveci pneumonia (PJP)

Parasitic Infections
- Cryptosporidiosis
- Giardiasis
- Isosporiasis
- Strongyloidiasis

Bacterial Infections
- Legionnaires' disease
- Mycobacterium avium complex (MAC) infections
- Mycosis
- Tuberculosis

Viral Infections
- Adenovirus
- Cytomegalovirus (CMV)
- Herpes simplex virus (HSV)
- Varicella zoster virus (VZV)

Disease History, Characteristics, and Transmission

Pneumocystis jirovecii (previously known as *Pneumocystis carinii*) is a fungus that infects nearly everyone at some point but is normally harmless. *Pneumocystis jirovecii* causes *Pneumocystis carinii* pneumonia (PCP) in patients with a weak immune system, such as people with human immunodeficiency virus (HIV) The early symptoms of PCP are dry cough, high fever, and difficulty breathing. The reporting of cases of PCP among previously healthy young men in the early 1980s was one of the early warning signs of the emergence of AIDS, as pneumonia due to *Pneumocystis* is normally a rare occurrence. Another microbe that often causes pneumonia in HIV patients is the bacterium *Streptococcus pneumoniae*.

The symptoms of an opportunistic infection depend on the nature of the associated organism. Nearly all microbes, such as bacteria, fungi, viruses, and protozoa, can become pathogenic given the right opportunity. However, certain organisms have a strong association with specific types of impaired immunity.

Tuberculosis infection from *Mycobacterium tuberculosis* may be reactivated among those whose immune systems are impaired because of age or AIDS. Other Mycobacterium species, such as *M. avium*, *M. intracellulare*, and *M. kansasii*, reside in the environment and are generally harmless. However, in people with a defective immune system, infections due to these bacteria may spread throughout the body and can be life-threatening. The fungus *Candida albicans*, which is benign in normal individuals, is often seen in patients suffering from HIV infections and affects the skin, mouth, and vagina, as well as the esophagus and lower respiratory tract. Additionally, the protozoan *Toxoplasma gondii* commonly causes opportunistic infection among AIDS patients, affecting the lungs, retinas, heart, liver, colon, and brain.

The risk of contracting gut infections is also a key concern in critically ill patients and those suffering from HIV infections. Protozoan infections caused by giardia, cryptosporidia, and microsporidia result in persistent diarrhea, leading to weight loss and inflammation of the bladder, bowel, sinuses, and pancreas.

Yet another rare condition associated with HIV infection is progressive multifocal leukoencephalopathy caused by John Cunningham (JC) virus, affecting the brain and spinal cord. Symptoms include loss of muscle control, paralysis, and blindness, often leading to death.

Many cancers are linked to HIV infection, the most prevalent being cervical and anal cancers, Kaposi's sarcoma (KS), and lymphomas (Hodgkin's and non-Hodgkin's). Many of these may be life threatening if not treated in a timely manner. Transmission of an opportunistic infection depends on the organism involved. Many of these organisms are normally present on the skin or in the body in amounts less than necessary to cause infection. This is known as colonization. It is only when the defenses of the immune system are breached that the microorganisms can take hold and cause infection. However, some microbes are transmitted by other modes (through carriers) that readily enter a host whose immunity is compromised or weakened due to an existing condition such as AIDS, severe burns or malnutrition, or other primary disease condition.

WORDS TO KNOW

COLONIZATION The process of occupation and increase in number of microorganisms at a specific site.

HOST An organism that serves as the habitat for a parasite or possibly for a symbiont. A host may provide nutrition to the parasite or symbiont, or it may simply provide a place in which to live.

IMMUNOCOMPROMISED A reduction in the ability of the immune system to recognize and respond to the presence of foreign material.

MORTALITY The condition of being susceptible to death. The term *mortality* comes from the Latin word *mors*, which means "death." Mortality can also refer to the rate of deaths caused by an illness or injury (e.g., "Rabies has a high mortality rate").

PATHOGEN A disease-causing agent, such as a bacterium, a virus, a fungus, or another microorganism.

Scope and Distribution

Many different groups are at serious risk of opportunistic infection. The common factor is an abnormality or defect in the immune system or any related host defense system, such as the skin, which acts as a natural barrier.

Rarely immune deficiency is present from birth. More commonly immune deficiency is acquired, as in AIDS, in which the HIV attacks and destroys the immune system. Certain underlying diseases, including cancer, diabetes, cystic fibrosis, sickle cell anemia, and severe burns, undermine immunity, making a person prone to opportunistic infection. In addition, living conditions in low-income groups across the world may result in infants being undernourished, leading to impaired immunity, which increases the likelihood of opportunistic infections.

Studies indicate that infection due to a microbe is common in critically ill patients. Data suggest that 51 percent of patients in the intensive care unit (ICU) are infected with an opportunistic infection and about 71 percent are treated with antimicrobials.

Various drug treatments impair immunity, such as steroids, immunosuppressants, cancer chemotherapy, and prolonged antibiotic therapy. Medical devices, including catheters and prosthetic heart valves, also attract opportunistic infection. Finally, the very young and very old tend to have weaker immunity, which puts them at higher risk of opportunistic infection.

Treatment and Prevention

Diagnosis of an opportunistic infection can be difficult, as most of the causative agents are normally not harmful. Early diagnosis is important for the management of the disease in patients who already suffer from a primary disease or condition (illness leading to intensive care or AIDS). If the opportunistic infection is caused by a bacterium or fungus, the treatment will generally consist of the appropriate antibiotic or antifungal drug. Cancer in HIV-positive individuals is mostly associated with viruses. For example, cervical and anal cancers caused by human papillomavirus (HPV) and KS is a result of a human herpesvirus-8 (HHV-8) virus infection. Thus, early diagnosis and treatment with specific antiviral drugs are important to control these conditions, as HIV treatment will not improve or resolve these cancers.

Prevention of opportunistic infections depends on the organism involved and the medical condition of the patient. Sometimes antibiotic and antiviral prophylaxis (preventative treatment) may be used. Scrupulous personal hygiene around patients with compromised immunity, such as patients in the ICU and those suffering from HIV, is essential.

Hospital visitors and medical staff should wash their hands thoroughly and regularly before and after touching patients.

Impacts and Issues

Opportunistic infections can be a challenge because they usually involve organisms that are normally not harmful. The incidence of opportunistic infections is likely to increase as the population ages, people with HIV/AIDS live longer, the number of organ transplants increases, and populations of other types of immunocompromised persons grow.

In developing countries malnutrition leaves millions of children with weakened immune systems and, in turn, more vulnerable to infections. Acute infections such as diarrheal diseases, respiratory infections, measles, and malaria account for more than half of childhood mortality in developing countries, and malnutrition is associated with over 50 percent of these deaths. When malnutrition is present, some health authorities broaden the definition of the term *opportunistic infection* to include a synergistic relationship between malnutrition and communicable disease. Malnutrition weakens natural immunity, leading to increased susceptibility to infection and more frequent, severe, and prolonged episodes of infection. The cycle is perpetuated when infection aggravates malnutrition by decreasing intake and increasing the body's metabolic needs. For example, diarrheal diseases in certain communities in Africa are linked to malnutrition and thus may be classified as opportunistic infections.

Data suggest that ICU patients with infection have almost double the mortality rate of those without, and infections in critically ill patients account for 40 percent of total ICU expenditure. Researchers are addressing several key concerns in the management of infections in critically ill patients, including absorption, distribution, metabolism, and excretion of drugs, all of which may be altered due to various disease states.

SEE ALSO *AIDS (Acquired Immunodeficiency Syndrome); Candidiasis;* Pneumocystis carinii *Pneumonia; Toxoplasmosis (Toxoplasma Infection)*

BIBLIOGRAPHY

Books

Galanda, Claudia D. *AIDS-Related Opportunistic Infections.* New York: Nova Biomedical, 2009.

Lindsay, David S., and Louis M. Weiss. *Opportunistic Infections: Toxoplasma, Sarcocystis, and Microsporidia.* New York: Springer, 2011.

Periodicals

Caulfield, Laura E., et al. "Undernutrition as an Underlying Cause of Child Deaths Associated with Diarrhea, Pneumonia, Malaria, and Measles." *American Journal of Clinical Nutrition* 80, no. 1 (July 2004): 193. This article can also be found online at http://ajcn.nutrition.org/content/80/1/193.full (accessed January 30, 2018).

Martin, Steven J., and Raymond J. Yost. "Infectious Diseases in the Critically Ill Patients." *Journal of Pharmacy Practice* 24 (March 2011): 35.

Websites

"5 Opportunistic Infections and Coinfections." HIV i-BASE, January 1, 2016. http://i-base.info/ttfa/5-opportunistic-infections-ois-and-coinfections/ (accessed January 28, 2018).

"Horn of Africa: Emergency-Affected Countries, 2007." World Health Organization, 2007 http://www.who.int/diseasecontrol_emergencies/toolkits/Hoa2.pdf (accessed January 28, 2018).

"Opportunistic Infections." Centers for Disease Control and Prevention, May 30, 2017. https://www.cdc.gov/hiv/basics/livingwithhiv/opportunisticinfections.html (accessed January 28, 2018).

"What Are Opportunistic Infections?" HIV.gov, May 15, 2017. https://www.hiv.gov/hiv-basics/staying-in-hiv-care/other-related-health-issues/opportunistic-infections (accessed January 28, 2018).

Susan Aldridge
Kausalya Santhanam

Outbreaks: Field-Level Response

Introduction

Outbreaks of infectious disease range in size and severity. A prompt response at the local, or field, level can limit the spread of an outbreak and help prevent future episodes. Response is an important component of epidemiology, which involves surveillance and case reporting, so that outbreaks can be identified. Emergency response can include treatment and isolation measures but needs to be coupled with a thorough investigation so that the causes of the outbreak can be recognized and halted.

Health authorities need to put in place advance plans for dealing with outbreaks covering the three components of surveillance, response, and investigation. The World Health Organization (WHO) and the US Centers for Disease Control and Prevention (CDC) have developed structures, guidelines, and networks that allow responses to be mounted to infectious disease outbreaks, including deliberate outbreaks of disease due to a bioterrorist attack.

History and Scientific Foundations

The English physician John Snow (1813–1858) demonstrated one of the earliest recorded responses to a disease outbreak. In 1854 he began to investigate an out-

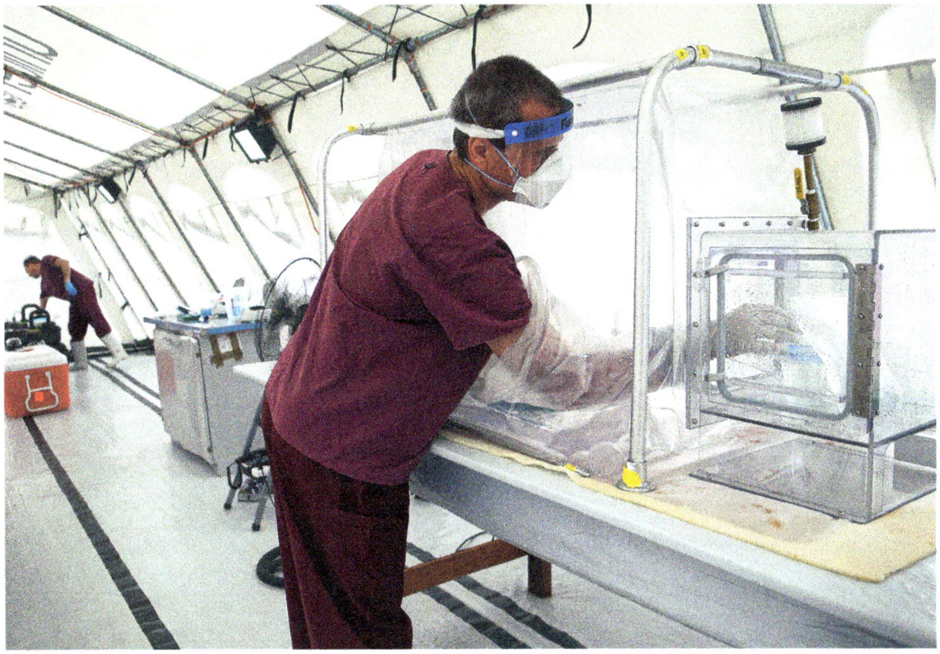

As part of the field-level response to an outbreak of Ebola in Liberia, a virologist handles blood samples in a newly opened mobile laboratory provided by the Centers for Disease Control, the National Institutes of Health, and the Global Outbreak Alert and Response Network. © John Moore/Getty Images

WORDS TO KNOW

EPIDEMIC From the Greek *epidemic*, meaning "prevalent among the people," it is most commonly used to describe an outbreak of an illness or a disease in which the number of individual cases significantly exceeds the usual or expected number of cases in any given population.

EPIDEMIOLOGY The study of the various factors that influence the occurrence, distribution, prevention, and control of disease, injury, and other health-related events in a defined human population. By the application of various analytical techniques, including mathematical analysis of the data, the probable cause of an infectious outbreak can be pinpointed.

GLOBAL OUTBREAK ALERT AND RESPONSE NETWORK (GOARN) A collaboration of resources for the rapid identification, confirmation, and response to outbreaks of international importance.

ISOLATION Within the health community, the precautions taken in the hospital to prevent the spread of an infectious agent from an infected or colonized patient to susceptible people. Isolation practices are designed to minimize the transmission of infection.

NONGOVERNMENTAL ORGANIZATION (NGO) A voluntary organization that is not part of any government and often is organized to address a specific issue or perform a humanitarian function.

PATHOGEN A disease-causing agent, such as a bacterium, a virus, a fungus, or another microorganism.

SURVEILLANCE The systematic analysis, collection, evaluation, interpretation, and dissemination of data. Public health surveillance assists in the identification of health threats and the planning, implementation, and evaluation of responses to those threats.

break of cholera in his local area of London. He constructed a detailed street map showing the location of cases and deduced that the source of the infection was the local water pump.

He either removed the pump handle himself or ordered it to be removed, and shortly afterward the number of cholera cases began to decline. It is not possible to prove that Snow's action, in itself, limited the outbreak, because the outbreak may have been on the decline naturally. But the principle of removing the cause of the infection was correct. It is this same principle that guides effective field response to outbreaks in the 21st century.

A field response to an outbreak occurs at the local level and often involves the facilities of the nearest hospital, particularly its emergency department. In an ideal scenario the hospital would have sufficient capacity to deal with an outbreak in terms of medical supplies, such as vaccines and antibiotics, trained medical staff, and beds to care for seriously ill patients. Some hospitals, especially in developing countries, may not have this capacity on-site and may or may not have the resources to access it.

Adequate and prompt communication between all health care entities, such as the hospital, primary care facilities, emergency services, and relevant public health organization, such as the CDC or a ministry of health, is essential while responding to an outbreak. Media should also be given accurate information from health care entities about the disease, including its prevention and treatment. In most cases local health authorities have detailed plans for responding to an outbreak at the field level, and this is tested in simulation exercises to identify gaps and weaknesses. As infectious agents know no boundaries, states and countries should work together to respond to an outbreak.

■ Applications and Research

Countries, especially developing countries, cannot be expected to deal with outbreaks of infectious disease on their own. In 2000 WHO set up the Global Outbreak Alert and Response Network (GOARN), which is a collaboration of more than 100 technical institutions, nongovernmental organizations, and networks, creating a pooled resource for alert and response operations.

Investigative teams from GOARN arrive at the site of an outbreak within 24 hours. They will offer on-the-spot investigation, confirmation of diagnosis, handling of dangerous pathogens, case detection, patient management, containment, and provision of staff and supplies. All of these elements are needed to safely contain an outbreak, but many may not be available on-site.

Since early 2000 WHO and GOARN have launched international responses to disease outbreaks in countries around the world, including Afghanistan, Bangladesh, India, Pakistan, Sudan, Tanzania, and Uganda. WHO has also strengthened GOARN's outbreak response logistics with specialized transport and communication facilities, which are particularly valuable in areas with weak local infrastructures. Many other nongovernmental organizations (NGOs), such as the humanitarian group Médecins Sans Frontières (MSF; Doctors Without Borders), and national health authorities, such as the CDC, also respond to situations in developing countries

Outbreaks occur across the globe virtually every month. According to a February 2018 report by WHO, for example, international actors worked together to address an outbreak of cholera in Mozambique that began in August 2017 and continued into 2018. As of February 19, 2018, there were 1,799 cases of cholera and one cholera-related death in Mozambique. The cholera outbreak was not unexpected because outbreaks of the waterborne bacterial disease had occurred there for five years. Once it was apparent that another cholera outbreak was underway, the

Mozambique Ministry of Health, WHO, MSF, the international aid agency Red Cross, and the United Nations Children's Fund (UNICEF) worked together to coordinate and manage the public health response, which included rapid assessment of the situation, surveillance of the districts most affected by the disease, and efforts to secure clean drinking water for citizens.

Response to outbreaks in countries with well-developed health infrastructures is usually coordinated by a national body, such as the CDC's Emergency Preparedness and Response Department or the Health Protection Agency in the United Kingdom. Typical incidents might include food poisoning or measles outbreaks, and response would be part of the surveillance, case reporting, and investigation strategy. The response might involve actions such as closing schools, child care centers, or restaurants to eliminate the cause of the infection or limit its spread.

Public information dissemination is an important part of response to an outbreak at field level, including warning people of symptoms and advising them on how to avoid infection. Medical treatments include vaccination, drug administration, and hospitalization, but the specifics depend on the illness involved in the outbreak.

The most testing situation for an outbreak response team is when a new or unusual infection is involved. This was the case with the Zika virus, which erupted in the mid-2010s to the surprise and consternation of the health care authorities who believed that it was a disease of monkeys that rarely infected humans. In March 2015 Brazil reported to WHO 7,000 cases of an unknown disease that was causing mild symptoms and generally could not be explained by another disease. By May 2015 Brazil reported that the Zika virus, which was transmitted by mosquito, was active in the country. Prior to 2015 Zika had never occurred naturally in the Western Hemisphere. In the summer and fall of 2015, it seemed increasingly likely that Zika was causing serious problems, including microcephaly in the fetuses of mothers who were infected with Zika. Meanwhile, the virus was crossing borders. It ultimately reached the United States in 2016. WHO declared Zika a Public Health Emergency of International Concern in February 2016.

The virus, which spread quickly and seemed to cause serious problems, was understudied and, at the beginning of the epidemic, not well understood. It presented a challenge for health care workers and public health officials to effectively react to. Since the outbreak of Zika in Brazil in 2015, international actors, including WHO, have responded by surveilling the extent of the outbreak, helping local communities affected by the disease respond and contain the outbreak, and researching the virus to develop treatments for it. The primary criticism leveled at responders to the Zika virus was that many women in developing countries in Central and South America were not warned forcefully enough that Zika could cause serious birth defects and that infected women should delay pregnancy or abort the fetus.

Current research includes developing vaccines for use before and during outbreaks of disease, developing effective and inexpensive personal protective equipment for responders and community members, and especially developing rapid diagnostic tests to identify particular pathogens and diseases in the field during the initial stages of an outbreak.

Impacts and Issues

When it comes to outbreaks of well-known diseases, such as *Salmonella* food poisoning and meningitis, public health authorities are well practiced in mounting a response. However, there are new threats, from emerging diseases such as H5N1 avian influenza to the possibility of bioterrorist attacks. A major issue is whether the health system has the capacity and preparedness to deal effectively with these. For example, studies have shown that the Ebola virus can spread rapidly and cause mass fatalities only in poor, underresourced health systems. For that reason, to control Ebola outbreaks effectively, international organizations such as WHO and developed countries such as the United States must offer assistance quickly.

This reality was made clear during the 2014–2015 outbreak of the Ebola virus in West Africa. The three countries most affected by the Ebola outbreak (Guinea, Liberia, and Sierra Leone) downplayed the severity of the outbreak during the spring and summer of 2014. This led organizations such as WHO to believe that the outbreak was abating when in fact it was far from over. At the same time, WHO has been criticized for believing the countries' reports, as well as for moving too slowly and cautiously in its response to Ebola's spread. By the time WHO mounted its response effort and by the time the UN Security Council had authorized the UN Mission for Ebola Emergency Response, the outbreak was spiraling out of control.

A major issue that thwarts field-level response to disease outbreaks is misinformation about the disease and local populations' distrust of health care workers. This occurred during the 2014–2015 Ebola outbreak. Many residents of affected communities did not trust health care workers, in part because residents had little experience with health care workers in their daily lives. In some cases community members believed that health care workers were exacerbating the Ebola epidemic. Good communication between community members and outbreak responders is key to a successful response to an infectious disease outbreak.

PRIMARY SOURCE

Ebola Diaries: Hitting the Ground Running

SOURCE: *Hugonnet, Stéphane. "Ebola Diaries: Hitting the Ground Running." World Health Organization, 2015. http://www.who.int/features/2015/ebola-diaries-hugonnet/en/ (accessed February 27, 2018).*

INTRODUCTION: *In the following account, Stéphane Hugonnet, a member of the Global Capacities Alert and Response (GCR) team of the World Health Organization (WHO), recounts his experience coordinating WHO's field level response in Guinea during the first days of the 2014–2015 Ebola virus outbreak. Major challenges were the fact that the Ebola virus crossed international borders and the protests of local community members against health care workers.*

We were following this rumour of a small cluster of unexplained deaths in Guinea. Some thought it could be Lassa fever, but the transmission pattern was very compatible with Ebola. When the lab results came back, we learned that there was Ebola Zaire in West Africa. This was a first.

On March 25, I hit the ground running in Guinea as part of a team made up of logisticians, a medical anthropologist, laboratory technicians, virologists and infection prevention and control specialists. My job was to rapidly assess the situation in the four affected districts, enhance surveillance and support the setting up of a mobile lab.

The day we left Conakry for Guékédou, Conakry confirmed its first case. It immediately became obvious that this outbreak was not like the others. Conakry is more than 1000 kilometres away from Guékédou. Ebola outbreaks are usually quite localized. Person-to-person transmission had quickly spread from a rural area to a large urban city—also unusual. And, the outbreak was becoming multi-national; cases were confirmed in Liberia and were suspected in Sierra Leone.

Managing any outbreak is harder when it crosses borders

Already, when you have a localized outbreak in the middle of nowhere, everything is a problem at the beginning. There is a lack of resources, lack of people to do the job. When an outbreak crosses borders, it's even more difficult to manage, even if those infected are from the same tribe and speak the same language. I was very worried.

We quickly worked to set up a mobile lab in Guékédou to deal with the backlog of samples and new cases to be tested. I believe our maximum capacity was testing 50 samples a day at the beginning, which is funny to think of now. Within two days, we were testing samples from the epicentre. The lab deployment was a success.

Very quickly, we also did social anthropology work, particularly around safe burials. Protests, sometimes violent, had already taken place in Guékédou and Macenta. Public opinion about the outbreak was extremely unstable. There were rumours that international health care workers had brought Ebola with them.

Violent protests made our work difficult

For some, they understood only that their loved ones had been taken to treatment centres and never returned. Infected people refused to be hospitalized; some of them even fled hospital. We recognized the great need for more of a "human touch". Our anthropologist worked with the Ministry of Health and others to persuade them of the importance of showing empathy to families of the infected and of including them in the burial process.

Collaboration with Médecins Sans Frontières was extremely good on surveillance, labs, social mobilization, and anthropological work. At this time, MSF was running treatment centres in Guékédou and Macenta, but centres in Kissidougou and N'Zerekoré were not yet up.

One of my jobs was to convince senior level national staff of the seriousness of this outbreak and get them to stay in Guékédou and take a lead on the response. This was vital.

Through my work I saw that Ebola, in fact, is not so transmissible. A combination of several interventions, even if none is implemented at 100% (isolation, community engagement, social mobilization, preparing healthcare facilities), can be enough to decrease and interrupt transmission. If you can identify the problem and react early, which was the case in the later outbreaks in Mali, Nigeria and Senegal, you can manage.

SEE ALSO *Epidemiology; Public Health and Infectious Disease*

BIBLIOGRAPHY

Books

Dworkin, Mark S., ed. *Cases in Field Epidemiology: A Global Perspective.* Sudbury, MA: Jones & Bartlett Learning, 2011.

Periodicals

Kamradt-Scott, Adam. "WHO's to Blame? The World Health Organization and the 2014 Ebola Outbreak in West Africa." *Third World Quarterly* 37, no. 3 (2016): 401–418. This article can also be found online at https://www.tandfonline.com/doi/abs/10.1080/01436597.2015.1112232 (accessed February 28, 2018).

McNeil, Donald G., Jr. "How the Response to Zika Failed Millions." *New York Times* (January 16, 2017). This article can also be found online at https://www.nytimes.com/2017/01/16/health/zika-virus-response.html (accessed February 28, 2018).

Siedner, Mark J., et al. "Strengthening the Detection of and Early Response to Public Health Emergencies: Lessons from the West African Ebola Epidemic." *PLOS Medicine* 12, no. 3 (March 24, 2015): e1001804. This article can also be found online at http://journals.plos.org/plosmedicine/article?id=10.1371/journal.pmed.1001804 (accessed February 28, 2018).

Websites

"Cholera—Mozambique." World Health Organization, February 19, 2018. http://www.who.int/csr/don/19-february-2018-cholera-mozambique/en/ (accessed February 28, 2018).

"Global Outbreak Alert and Response Network (GOARN)." World Health Organization. http://www.who.int/csr/outbreaknetwork/en (accessed February 27, 2018).

"Guidance for Managing Ethical Issues in Infectious Disease Outbreaks." World Health Organization, 2016. http://apps.who.int/iris/bitstream/10665/250580/1/9789241549837-eng.pdf (accessed February 28, 2018).

"Zika Virus Disease." World Health Organization. http://www.who.int/csr/disease/zika/en/ (accessed February 27, 2018).

Susan Aldridge
Claire Skinner

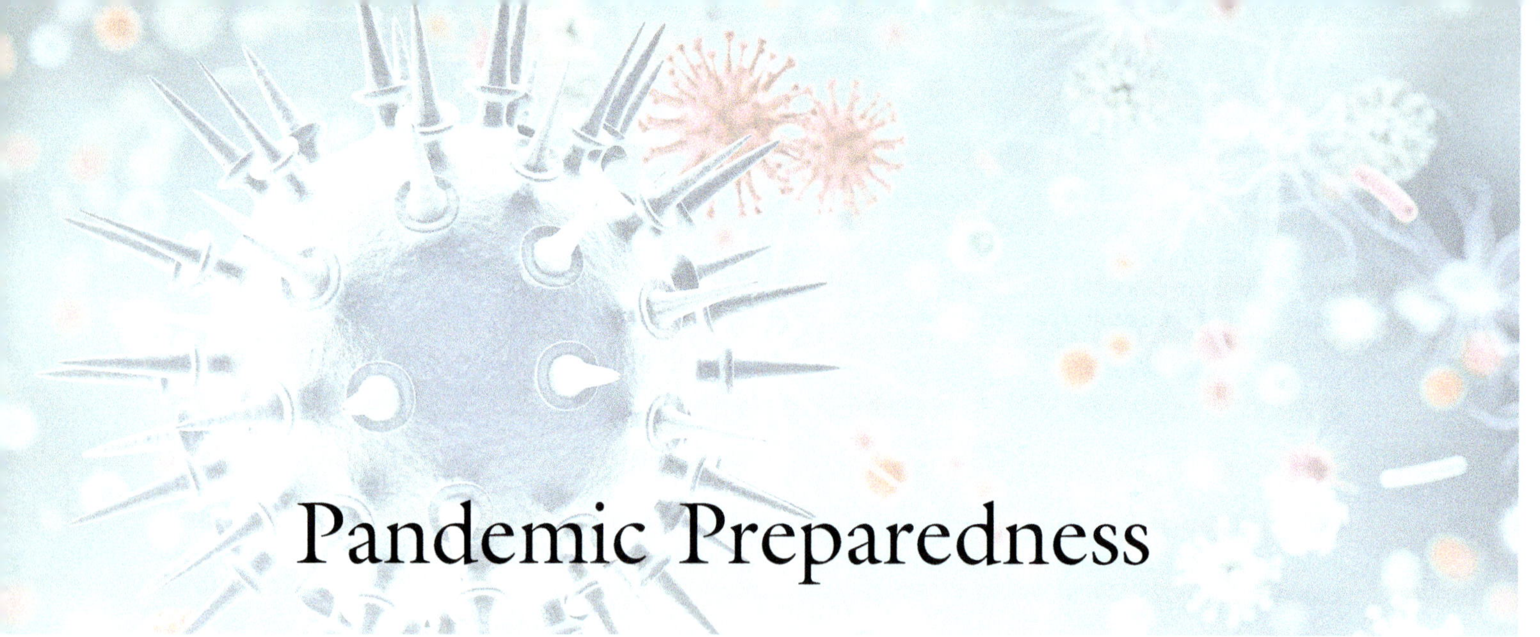

Pandemic Preparedness

Introduction

A pandemic of influenza is one of the greatest infectious disease threats facing the world. A pandemic is a disease epidemic that affects a large proportion of the population over a wide geographic area. Influenza is the virus that is most likely to turn into a pandemic. In the worldwide pandemic influenza attacks of 1918, 1958, and 1968, about 30 percent of the US population developed some degree of illness. It is likely that another pandemic will strike the same percentage of the population.

There is little doubt in the medical community that a pandemic of influenza will strike. However, its timing, severity, and exact microbial strain (type) remain unknown. If a pandemic is severe, the effects of it will be far-ranging. Supplies of life-saving drugs and essential medical supplies may run out. Critical personnel may die. Damage to the infrastructure of nations has both economic and social consequences. Accordingly, a number of governments, mostly in the developed world, along with the World Health Organization (WHO), have created plans to tackle an influenza pandemic.

WORDS TO KNOW

CASE FATALITY RATIO A ratio indicating the number of people who die as a result of a particular disease, usually expressed as a percentage or as the number of deaths per 1,000 cases.

PANDEMIC An epidemic that occurs in more than one country or population simultaneously. *Pandemic* means "all the people."

QUARANTINE The practice of separating from the general population people who have been exposed to an infectious agent but have not yet developed symptoms. In the United States, this can be done voluntarily or involuntarily by the authority of states and the federal Centers for Disease Control and Prevention.

STRAIN A subclass or a specific genetic variation of an organism.

Disease History, Characteristics, and Transmission

Influenza is a respiratory disease that has killed more people than the Black Death (plague). The deceased are usually those with weakened immune systems, typically those who are already ill, the very young, and the very old. However, influenza can affect healthy adults too. The average age of death during the Spanish influenza pandemic of 1918 was 33. During that deadly year, otherwise healthy adults may have produced an intense localized inflammation that overwhelmed their bodies. Transmission of the next pandemic may be from human to human or, in the possible case of avian flu, initially from bird to human.

Scope and Distribution

In the past WHO advised governments to prepare for, respond to, and recover from influenza pandemics. In 2018 WHO updated its checklist for pandemic influenza risk and impact management to focus on preventing and mitigating influenza before it reaches a health emergency. The principles of an emergency risk management for health (ERMH) plan recognize that all sectors of an economy (health care, government, business, and civil society) will need to take a proactive, multidisciplinary approach. Working together, the sectors can

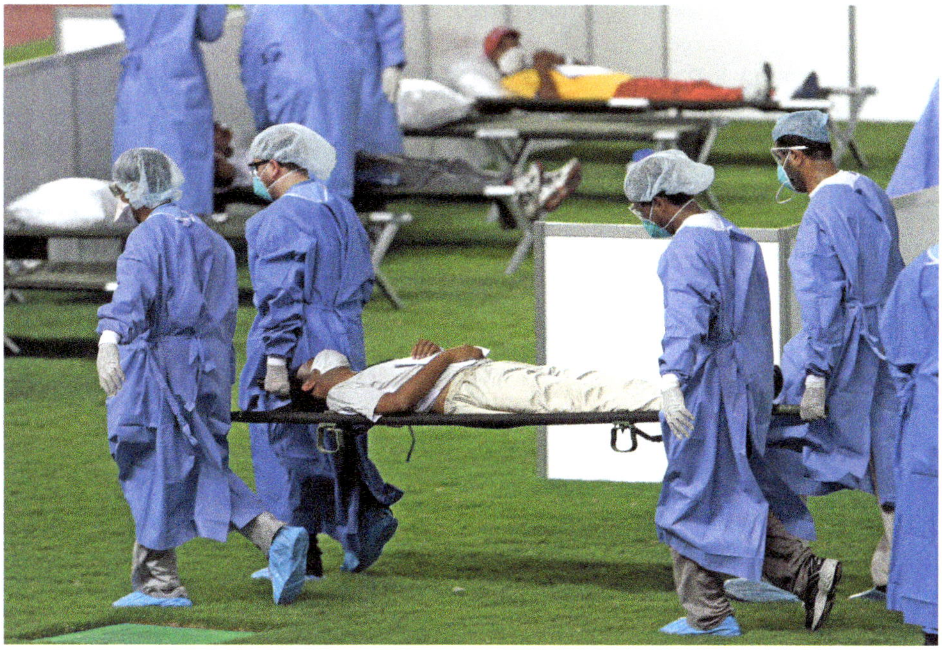

Medical professionals in the United Arab Emirates conduct a bird flu drill. Such drills help health care workers and government agencies prepare for potential pandemics. © AFP/Getty Images

ensure a community strengthens and sustains its capacity to withstand a pandemic. EMRH also considers the ethical principles of health management activities. WHO also advises that a national pandemic response plan needs to involve coordination and communication with neighboring countries and international stakeholders.

Public health experts anticipate a gap between the supply of vaccine and the demand for vaccine during an influenza pandemic. To reduce the impact of an influenza pandemic, WHO recommends a nonpharmaceutical approach, such as infection control, as well as a pharmaceutical approach, such as the use of vaccines and antiviral medications for treatment and prophylaxis. However, the availability of a pandemic vaccine will be delayed for several months after influenza first appears because of the requirements for vaccine formulation and production. The widespread nature of a pandemic means that there will be insufficient production capacity to supply everyone seeking vaccine with medication, at least in the initial months of an outbreak.

For these reasons pandemic planning must include the assumption that a range of individuals will be struck down by disease. The US government estimates that 40 percent or more of workers may be out sick or afraid to go to work for fear of exposure. Community outbreaks may last for six to eight weeks, with multiple waves of disease outbreaks in a calendar year. Further complicating the situation, the highly mobile populations of the 21st century can result in simultaneous disease outbreaks throughout a country or the world.

A pandemic will likely dramatically reduce the number of workers available to provide goods and services. As a result, the critical infrastructure (food, banking, water, energy, telecommunications, transportation, postal and shipping, emergency services, and health care) and key resources (government facilities, dams, nuclear power plants, and commercial facilities) will lack the staff to function without interruption.

Treatment and Prevention

The United States has had a comprehensive plan to prepare for and combat pandemic influenza since 2005. The plan emphasizes the need for all levels of government and the private sector to cooperate in developing a response. In 2006 the US Homeland Security Council distributed the *National Strategy for Pandemic Influenza Implementation Plan*. It requires federal government departments and agencies to develop operational plans addressing the protection of employees, maintenance of essential functions and services, support for federal responses, and communication about pandemic planning and response. State, local, and tribal governments bear responsibility for limiting an outbreak within and beyond a community's borders, establishing plans, educating key spokespersons in risk communication, providing public education on pandemic influenza, and establishing stockpiles of essential goods. The plan also includes a pandemic severity index that uses case fatality ratios (the proportion of deaths among persons with a particular illness) to make specific recommendations for action based on the impact of the pandemic.

In the intervening years, the United States developed a stockpile of vaccines and prepared evidence-based guidance on prevention and treatment. However, the 2009 influenza H1N1 outbreak and the emergency of H7N9 influenza virus in China in 2013 raised concerns that gaps in preparedness remained. The US Department of Health and Human Services updated the pandemic influenza plan in 2017 to emphasize a community response, stress international cooperation, and highlight medical countermeasures beyond vaccines. Communications and public outreach remain critical components of the plan, as does health care system preparedness.

Impacts and Issues

With the majority of critical infrastructure in the United States in the hands of the private sector, developing individual and systemwide business continuity plans are a priority for planning for a possible pandemic. Businesses should assess the regulations and issues that could affect their supply chain, transportation, priority for municipal services, and workplace safety. Companies, such as restaurants, that rely on unavoidable public contact and those with shared workplaces, such as plants, will be especially hard hit by limitations on face-to-face encounters. It is possible that a pandemic response might involve closing places of assembly, isolating those with the disease, quarantining people who have been exposed to the disease, and furloughing nonessential workers. During the 1918 pandemic, the great numbers of sick and deceased overwhelmed the capacity of hospitals and morgues. Another pandemic may also overload the system.

PRIMARY SOURCE

Community Strategy for Pandemic Influenza Mitigation in the United States

SOURCE: *Centers for Disease Control and Prevention.* Interim Pre-pandemic Planning Guidance: Community Strategy for Pandemic Influenza Mitigation in the United States. *Washington, DC: US Department of Health and Human Services, 2007. This report can also be found online at https://www.cdc.gov/flu/pandemic-resources/pdf/community_mitigation-sm.pdf.*

INTRODUCTION: *During a pandemic governmental agencies such as the US Centers for Disease Control and Prevention (CDC) play a key role in tracking the disease, assisting local health agencies, and distributing key personnel and medical supplies. Planning at the community level is also important to maintain vital services during a pandemic while limiting the spread of the disease. In the following excerpt from a guidebook for communities planning for a pandemic, the CDC recommends measures that promote limiting social contact during a pandemic, such as closing schools, and voluntary quarantine for those who are ill with the disease.*

The pandemic mitigation framework that is proposed is based upon an early, targeted, layered application of multiple partially effective nonpharmaceutical measures. It is recommended that the measures be initiated early before explosive growth of the epidemic and, in the case of severe pandemics, that they be maintained consistently during an epidemic wave in a community. The pandemic mitigation interventions described in this document include:

1. Isolation and treatment (as appropriate) with influenza antiviral medications of all persons with confirmed or probable pandemic influenza. Isolation may occur in the home or healthcare setting, depending on the severity of an individual's illness and/or the current capacity of the healthcare infrastructure.
2. Voluntary home quarantine of members of households with confirmed or probable influenza case(s) and consideration of combining this intervention with the prophylactic use of antiviral medications, providing sufficient quantities of effective medications exist and that a feasible means of distributing them is in place.
3. Dismissal of students from school (including public and private schools as well as colleges and universities) and school-based activities and closure of childcare programs, coupled with protecting children and teenagers through social distancing in the community to achieve reductions of out-of-school social contacts and community mixing.
4. Use of social distancing measures to reduce contact between adults in the community and workplace, including, for example, cancellation of large public gatherings and alteration of workplace environments and schedules to decrease social density and preserve a healthy workplace to the greatest extent possible without disrupting essential services. Enable institution of workplace leave policies that align incentives and facilitate adherence with the nonpharmaceutical interventions (NPIs) outlined above.
5. All such community-based strategies should be used in combination with individual infection control measures, such as handwashing and cough etiquette. Implementing these interventions in a timely and coordinated fashion will require advance planning. Communities must be prepared for the cascading second and third-order consequences of the interventions, such as increased

workplace absenteeism related to child-minding responsibilities if schools dismiss students and childcare programs close.

See Also *AIDS: Origin of the Modern Pandemic; Avian Influenza; Influenza; Influenza Pandemic of 1918; Influenza Pandemic of 1957; Isolation and Quarantine*

BIBLIOGRAPHY

Books

Crosby, Alfred W. *America's Forgotten Pandemic: The Influenza of 1918*. 2nd ed. New York: Cambridge University Press, 2003.

Shah, Sonia. *Pandemic: Tracking Contagions, from Cholera to Ebola and Beyond*. New York: Picador, 2017.

Websites

"Pandemic Influenza." US Department of Health and Human Services, January 2, 2018. http://www.pandemicflu.gov/index.html (accessed April 28, 2007).

"Pandemic Preparedness." World Health Organization. http://www.who.int/influenza/preparedness/pandemic/en/ (accessed February 27, 2018).

Caryn E. Neumann

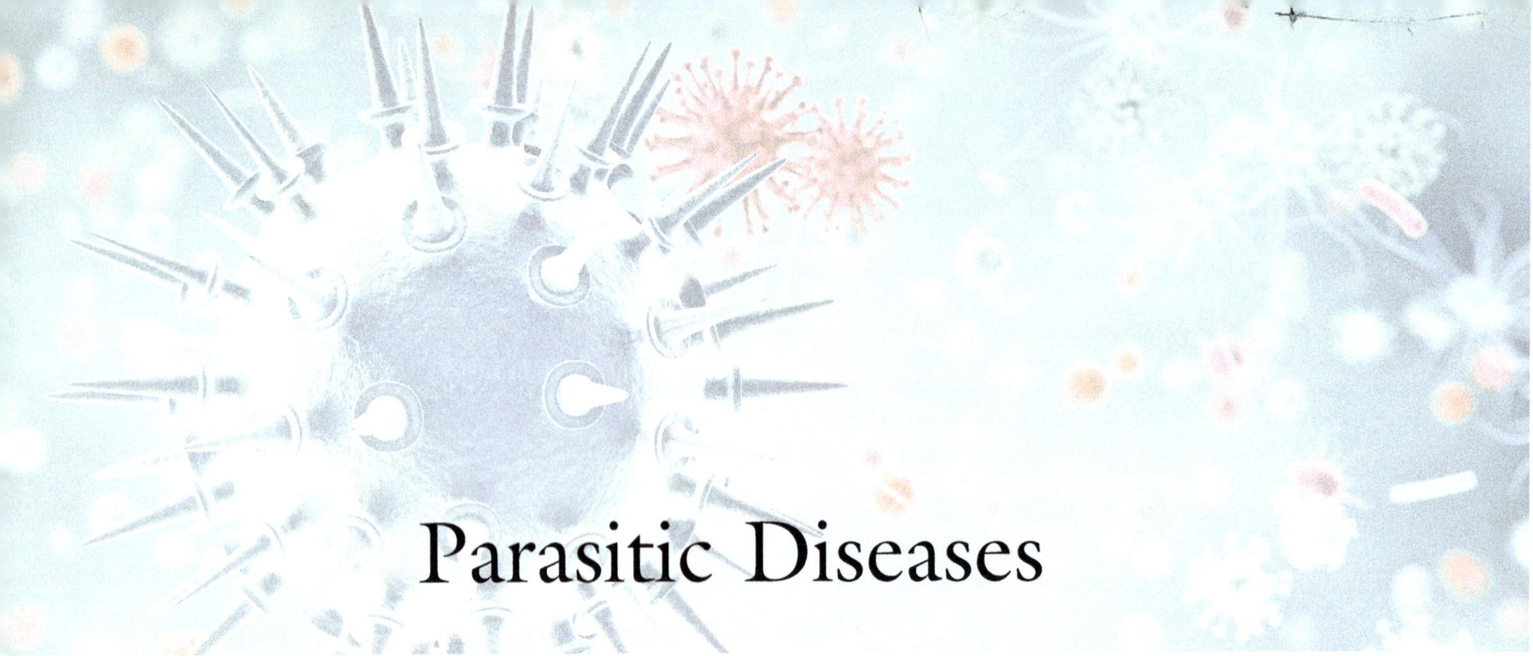

Parasitic Diseases

Introduction

A parasite is an organism that lives on or in a host organism. It is dependent on the host for food and protection. For millions of years, parasites and humans have coexisted. Many parasites do no damage, particularly protozoa in low numbers, but some can cause significant harm. Parasitic infections, such as toxoplasmosis, malaria, and Guinea worm, strike millions of people annually in every region of the world. These infections are often painful, debilitating, or deadly.

There are three main classes of parasites that can cause disease in humans: protozoa, helminths, and ectoparasites. Protozoa are microscopic, one-celled organisms. A serious infection can develop from just a single organism that then multiplies. Helminths are flatworms, thorny-headed worms, and roundworms. Ectoparasites are ticks, fleas, mites, and lice that burrow into the skin. Arthropods, including mosquitos, serve as the vectors of many different pathogens.

Disease History, Characteristics, and Transmission

Transmission of protozoa typically occurs by a fecal-oral route through contaminated food or water or by person-to-person contact. Arthropod vectors, such as ticks, transmit protozoa that thrive in human blood or tissue. Parasitic helminth (worm) infections are spread by ingestion, usually through contaminated meat or water.

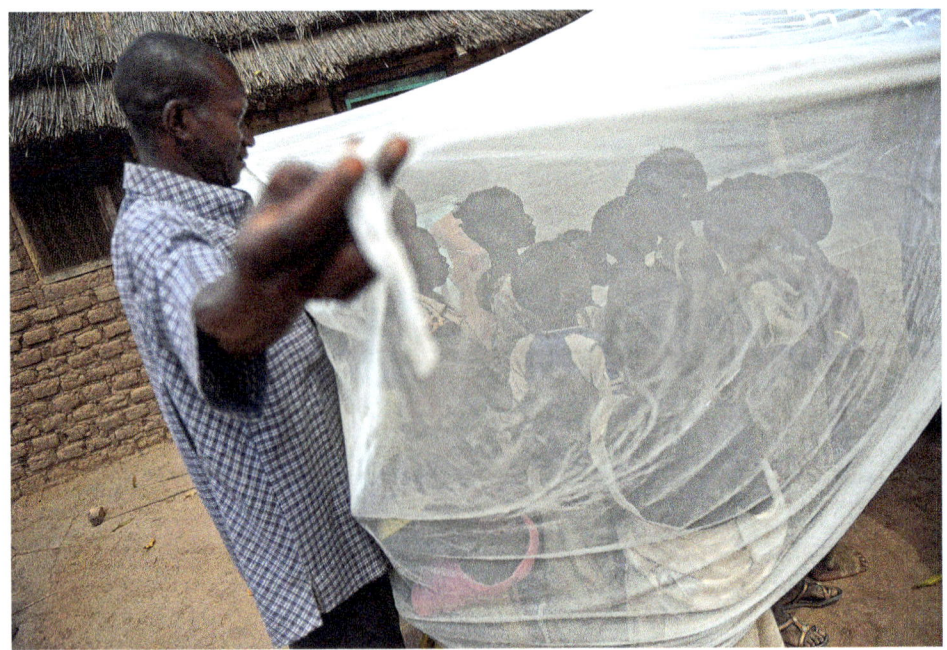

A man demonstrates the use of a long-lasting insecticide-treated net in South Sudan. The nets are used to prevent malaria, a parasitic infection spread by mosquitoes. *© TONY KARUMBA/AFP/Getty Images*

Scope and Distribution

Parasitic diseases occur most often in the tropics and subtropics but can also occur in more moderate climates or anywhere the parasite and its host or vector resides. Worldwide, parasitic diseases, of which malaria is the leader, kill more than 2 million people annually. The World Health Organization (WHO) estimates that 1.5 billion people, or about 25 percent of the global population, are infected with some sort of parasitic helminth. In the United States, trichomoniasis is the most common parasitic infection, with more than 7 million cases diagnosed per year.

The increased movement of people from region to region has also spread parasites. Chagas, an insect-borne parasitic disease, once rarely appeared in the United States. Immigration from Central and Latin America is a contributing factor in an increased incidence of Chagas parasite, *Trypanosoma cruzi*, in the United States. The American Red Cross now screens blood donors for the parasite to prevent transmission.

Another disease, cysticercosis, caused by tapeworm larvae, is also on the rise in the United States, with about 1,000 hospitalizations annually. It is the result of eating uncooked pork that contains larval cysts. It often strikes Hispanics who emigrated from Mexico and Central America, most of whom contracted the disease in their home countries.

Two parasitic infections are linked to common pets. *Toxocara* comes from roundworms found in the intestines of dogs and cats. About 14 percent of Americans have had exposure to *Toxocara*, and at least 70 people, mostly children, die from the infection each year. Toxoplasma is found in cat feces. It is the reason why pregnant women are advised not to clean cat litter boxes. The parasite, which causes birth defects, is also found in undercooked meat and unwashed fruits and vegetables.

WORDS TO KNOW

ARTHROPOD A member of the largest single animal phylum, consisting of organisms with segmented bodies, jointed legs or wings, and exoskeletons.

ECTOPARASITES Parasites that cling to the outside of their host rather than to their host's intestines. Common points of attachment are the gills, fins, or skin of fish.

FECAL-ORAL ROUTE The spread of disease through the transmission of minute particles of fecal material from one organism to the mouth of another. This can occur by drinking contaminated water; eating food exposed to animal or human feces, such as food from plants watered with unclean water; or preparing food without practicing proper hygiene.

HELMINTH A representative of various phyla of wormlike animals.

HOST An organism that serves as the habitat for a parasite or possibly for a symbiont. A host may provide nutrition to the parasite or symbiont, or it may simply provide a place in which to live.

PATHOGEN A disease-causing agent, such as a bacterium, a virus, a fungus, or another microorganism.

PROTOZOA Single-celled, animal-like microscopic organisms that live by taking in food rather than making it by photosynthesis and must live in the presence of water. (Singular: protozoan.) Protozoa are a diverse group of single-celled organisms, with more than 50,000 different types represented. The vast majority are microscopic, many measuring less than 5 one-thousandth of an inch (0.005 millimeters), but some, such as the freshwater Spirostomun, may reach 0.17 inches (3 millimeters) in length, large enough to enable it to be seen with the naked eye.

VECTOR Any agent that carries and transmits parasites and diseases. Also, an organism or a chemical used to transport a gene into a new host cell.

Treatment and Prevention

The first step in treating a parasitic disease is to identify it, but this is complicated by the number of diseases with similar symptoms that exist in the world. If a parasite is detected in a host early enough, strong antiprotozoal drugs such as nifurtimox can bring the parasite to undetectable levels or eliminate it entirely. In other cases, such as the common Latin American and Middle Eastern blight leishmaniasis, medication derived from the chemical element antimony and antifungal drugs have stopped the parasite.

Patients with severe infections must also undergo weekly blood tests and electrocardiograms to make sure that their kidneys, liver, and heart remain healthy throughout treatment. Some parasites, such as the one that causes Chagas, may have multiplied over years and decades. In these cases infected individuals may require treatment with heart-regulating drugs or regulation via an implanted pacemaker.

There are no vaccines for parasitic diseases in humans, though some have been developed to kill helminth diseases in herd animals. Research and development of potential vaccines focus on three distinct ways to stop the spread of

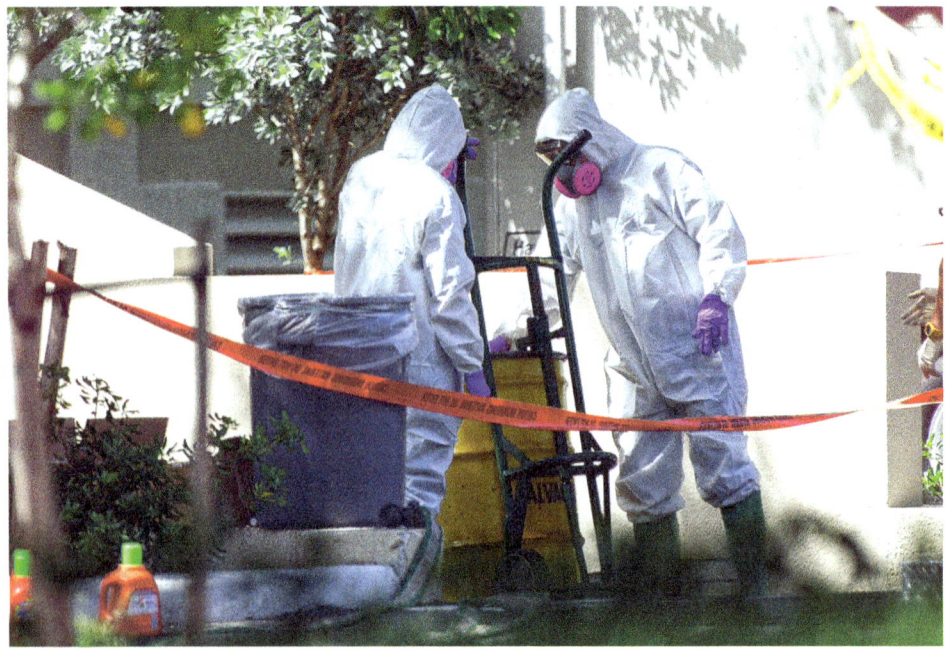

FBI agents wear full body suits to protect themselves from *Bacillus anthracis*, or anthrax, a deadly bacterium. © Eliot J. Schechter/Getty Images

parasitic diseases. Anti-disease vaccines target blood forms and parasite-produced toxins. Transmission-blocking vaccines prevent the development of the parasite within a host. Anti-infection vaccines target parasites in stages where they are most likely to infect.

Impacts and Issues

Many parasitic diseases no longer have geographic borders. Physicians must consider that parasites that are common in distant regions may be seen in immigrants or travelers.

Regular access to potable water for drinking, cooking, and washing can virtually eliminate waterborne parasitic diseases. However, WHO estimates that 1 billion people worldwide live without access to clean water. Improved access to uncontaminated water, personal hygiene and food safety education, and construction of sewer-sanitation systems, even as basic as proper latrines, dramatically reduce incidence of parasite-related illnesses.

Parasitic disease prevention can have environmental consequences. Pesticides are often spread over large areas to reduce parasite-transmitting insect populations. Pesticides are powerful chemicals that can contaminate drinking water and soil. People who work around pesticides must take precautions to avoid exposure.

Use of some pesticides, such as dichlorodiphenyltrichloroethane (DDT), remains controversial, but pesticides are an important part of parasitic disease control that save thousands of lives each year. To minimize environmental damage, researchers are working to develop better pesticides, many directed at killing parasite-transmitting insects or the parasites themselves, while reducing toxicity to humans and animals. Health workers also promote responsible use of pesticides. For example, in the fight against mosquito-borne diseases, health workers advocate the use of insecticide-treated nets to minimize the need for topical insecticides applied directly to the skin.

Research indicates that global climate change may affect the incidence of parasitic infections in humans. Recent studies in Kenya indicate a strong correlation between rising temperatures, more variable rainfall, and a greater incidence of mosquitoes spreading malaria into highland areas previously protected from the parasite. A 2007 report by the Intergovernmental Panel on Climate Change (IPCC) advised that millions of people may be affected by similar shifts in the spread of parasitic diseases. Other studies dispute these findings, asserting that increased migration of people and animals has a more significant impact on parasite distribution.

Malaria remains the top parasitic killer in the world, causing from 1 million to 2 million deaths around the world each year, mostly among children. Primaquine, created in 1946, remains the preferred antimalarial drug. In 2016 the US Centers for Disease Control and Prevention began recommending it as a preventive for people traveling to malaria zones. Avoiding mosquito bites remains the preferred way to halt malaria. Many nations, international agencies, and nongovernment organizations have developed antimalaria campaigns. Among nongovernment charitable entities, the Bill & Melinda Gates Foundation is one of the world's leading sponsors of antimalaria programs and malaria vaccine research.

PRIMARY SOURCE

Climate Change Threatens the World's Parasites (That's Not Good)

SOURCE: *Zimmer, Carl. "Climate Change Threatens the World's Parasites (That's Not Good).* New York Times *(September 13, 2017). This article can also be found online at https://www.nytimes.com/2017/09/13/science/parasites-extinction-climate-change.html (accessed February 26, 2018).*

INTRODUCTION: *Studies show that global climate change is affecting parasite populations. In some cases it is allowing parasites to thrive and move into new habitats. In other cases parasites may be endangered. In this article from the* New York Times, *Carl Zimmer examines why this could have detrimental effects on earth's ecosystems and human health.*

Animals around the world are on the move. So are their parasites.

Recently, scientists carried out the first large-scale study of what climate change may do to the world's much-loathed parasites. The team came to a startling conclusion: as many as one in three parasite species may face extinction in the next century.

As global warming raises the planet's temperature, the researchers found, many species will lose territory in which to survive. Some of their hosts will be lost, too.

"It still absolutely blows me away," said Colin J. Carlson, lead author of the study and a graduate student at the University of California, Berkeley.

He knows many people may react to the news with a round of applause. "Parasites are obviously a hard sell," Mr. Carlson said.

But as much as a tapeworm or a blood fluke may disgust us, parasites are crucial to the world's ecosystems. Their extinction may effect entire food webs, perhaps even harming human health.

Parasites deserve some of the respect that top predators have earned in recent decades. Wolves were once considered vermin, for example—but as they disappeared, ecosystems changed.

Scientists realized that as top predators, wolves kept populations of prey in check, which allowed plants to thrive. When wolves were restored to places like Yellowstone, , as well.

Researchers have begun carefully studying the roles that parasites play. They make up the majority of the biomass in some ecosystems, outweighing predators sharing their environments by a factor of 20 to 1.

For decades, scientists who studied food webs drew lines between species—between wildebeest and the grass they grazed on, for example, and between the wildebeest and the lions that ate them.

In a major oversight, they didn't factor in the extent to which parasites feed on hosts. As it turns out, as much as 80 percent of the lines in a given food web are links to parasites. They are big players in the food supply.

Parasites can control populations of their hosts. Some are killed outright; other hosts, once infected, cannot reproduce, which would divert resources that the parasite craves to eggs or sperm. Some parasites move from host to host by making prey species easier for predators to kill.

So if these horrendous pests are major players in ecosystems that we want to save—what then? "This view requires that parasites be protected alongside their hosts," said Kevin D. Lafferty, an ecologist at the University of California, Santa Barbara, who was not involved in the new study.

A warming climate complicates the picture. Some researchers had already investigated the fate of a few parasite species, but Mr. Carlson and his colleagues wanted to get a global view of the impact of climate change.

They began their work with the National Parasite Collection, founded in 1892 and now maintained by the Smithsonian Institution. One of the world's biggest, it includes 20 million specimens, some preserved in jars of alcohol and some mounted on slides.

By determining the present range of each parasite species, Mr. Carlson and his colleagues were able to estimate the kind of climate in which it can survive and how it might fare in a hotter world.

Building this global geographic database took five years. The researchers often relied on the old tags and cards stored with the specimens to figure out where they lived—often a difficult task.

"Sometimes you'd just get, 'Island, Ocean,'" Mr. Carlson said. "You can imagine the stress that caused."

After he and his colleagues were done sifting through the collection, they ended up with 53,133 parasites they felt confident enough to use in their study. The records come from 457 species of tapeworms, ticks, fleas and other animals.

Parasites typically live in or on their hosts, but that does not protect them from climate change. Rising air temperatures can harm them. Ticks, for instance, risk baking in the heat as they wait in the grass for their next victim. Hookworm larvae require damp soil to survive before slipping into someone's foot.

And parasites need their hosts—if they go extinct, their parasites probably will, too. So Mr. Carlson and his colleagues also evaluated how hosts are expected to fare in response to climate change.

The researchers combined all these factors to estimate the risk that each kind of parasite faced. Some kinds won't lose much in a warming world, the study found. For instance, thorny-headed worms are likely to be protected because their hosts, fish and birds, are common and widespread.

But other types, such as fleas and tapeworms, may not be able to tolerate much change in temperature; many others infect only hosts that are facing extinction, as well.

In all, roughly 30 percent of parasitic species could disappear, Mr. Carlson concluded. The impact of climate change will be as great or greater for these species as for any others studied so far.

Dr. Lafferty said the new results challenged those of much smaller studies, which had come to opposite conclusions. "Our natural tendency is to assume that parasites and the disease they cause will increase as the rest of biodiversity declines," he said.

Mr. Carlson said that climate change would do more than just drive some species extinct. Some parasites would move into new territory.

Deer ticks, for example, spread Lyme disease, and climate change models suggest they have a rosy future as they expand northward. "We're not worried about them going extinct," said Mr. Carlson.

Migrating parasites like these will arrive in ecosystems where other parasitic species are disappearing. With less competition, they may be able to wreak more havoc—and not just on animal hosts. Many human diseases are the result of parasites and pathogens jumping from animal species to our own.

"If parasites are keeping disease down in wildlife, they might also be indirectly keeping them down in humans," Mr. Carlson said. "And we might lose that."

SEE ALSO *Blood Supply and Infectious Disease; Chagas Disease; Climate Change and Infectious Disease; Immigration and Infectious Disease; Malaria; Waterborne Disease*

BIBLIOGRAPHY

Books

McAuliffe, Kathleen. *This Is Your Brain on Parasites: How Tiny Creatures Manipulate Our Behavior and Shape Society.* New York: Eamon Dolan/Mariner, 2017.

Periodicals

Whitty, Christopher J. M., Peter L. Chiodini, and David G. Lalloo. "Investigation and Treatment of Imported Malaria in Non-Endemic Countries." *BMJ* 346, no. 7909 (May 25, 2013): 31–34.

Websites

"Malaria." Centers for Disease Control and Prevention, January 26, 2018. https://www.cdc.gov/malaria/index.html (accessed February 25, 2017)

"Parasites." Centers for Disease Control and Prevention, September 27, 2017. https://www.cdc.gov/parasites/ (accessed February 25, 2018).

Caryn E. Neumann

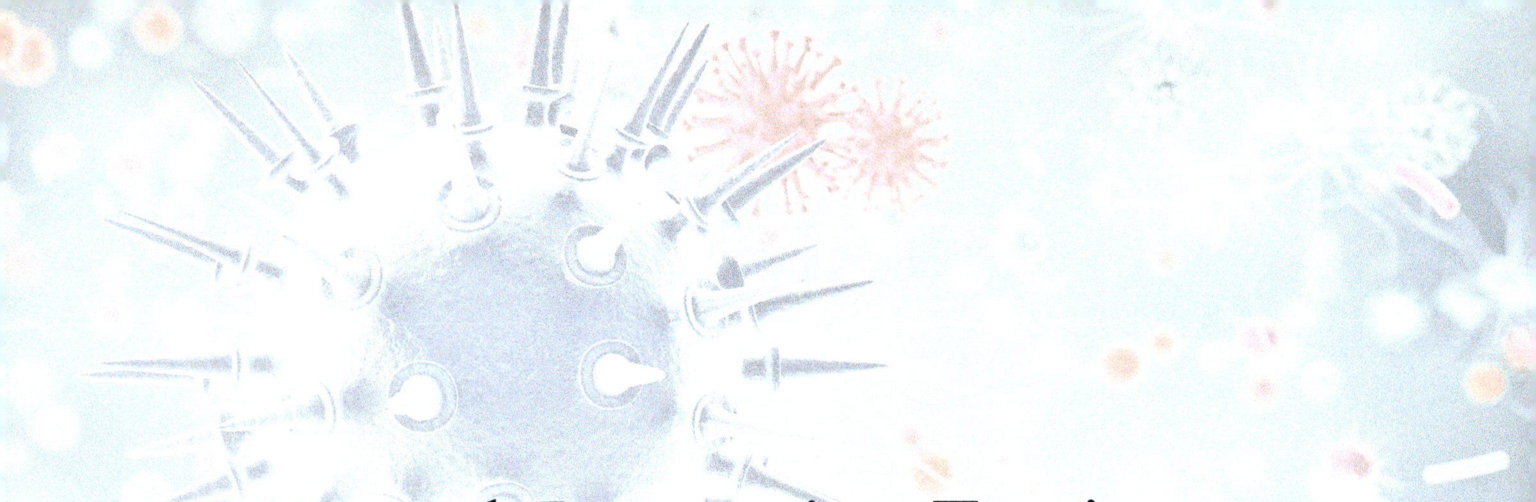

Personal Protective Equipment

■ Introduction

Personal protective equipment is equipment used in a health care setting to prevent direct contact with infectious microorganisms or contact with body fluids that might contain a disease-causing (pathogenic) microorganism.

Gloves, gowns or aprons, masks and respirators, goggles, and face shields are all examples of personal protective equipment. The degree of protection offered by such equipment varies depending on the infectious disease being dealt with. Treating someone who has a common cold may only require the use of medical gloves, for example, while a public health response to the dispersal of *Bacillus anthracis* (the cause of anthrax) requires personnel to wear full body suits, including sealed gloves and respirators that block the inhalation of the tiny bacterial spores.

■ History and Scientific Foundations

The use of personal protective equipment is centuries old. Records from England dating back to the 17th century describe the protective headgear, gowns, and masks worn by physicians treating plague victims. At the time some physicians assumed plague could be transmitted through the air. Although scientists later discovered plague was caused by a bacterium called *Yersinia pestis* that is transmitted by the bite of an infected flea, the use of protective clothing was a wise precaution.

Through the early decades of the 19th century, surgeons did not wear any special clothing when they performed operations. Surgeries were done by physicians who walked in off the street into an open-air operating theater. The realization that dedicated surgical clothing prevented the transmission of infections from patient to patient revolutionized medicine and made postsurgical infections less common. In this sense the clothing was protective to the patient. However, with time the protective value of clothing to health care providers was also recognized.

Then, as in the early 21st century, the premise of personal protective equipment is simple: protective clothing and other gear presents a barrier to the transmission of infectious microorganisms.

WORDS TO KNOW

BIOSAFETY LEVEL FACILITY A specialized biosafety laboratory that deals with dangerous or exotic infectious agents or biohazards that are considered high risks for spreading life-threatening diseases, either because the disease is spread through aerosols or because there is no therapy or vaccine to counter the disease.

MICROORGANISM With only a single currently known exception (i.e., *Epulopiscium fishelsonia*, a bacterium that is billions of times larger than the bacteria in the human intestine and is large enough to view without a microscope), microorganisms are minute organisms that require microscopic magnification to view. To be seen, they must be magnified by an optical or electron microscope. The most common types of microorganisms are viruses, bacteria, blue-green bacteria, some algae, some fungi, yeasts, and protozoans.

PATHOGEN A disease-causing agent, such as a bacterium, a virus, a fungus, or another microorganism.

RESPIRATOR Any device that assists a patient in breathing or takes over breathing entirely for them.

TERRORISM AND BIOLOGICAL WARFARE

Fear of bioterrorism, periodically heightened by news events, sometimes causes the panicked buying of equipment that may be ill designed to meet real threats. For example, military surplus gas masks generally provide only the illusion of protection. In the early days after the 2001 terrorist attacks in New York City and Washington, D.C., there was a reported spike in sales of gas masks and ciprofloxacin (the antibiotic effective against the bacteria that causes anthrax). However, masks offer no real protection against biological agents and should not be bought for that purpose. Stockpiling antibiotics is also unwise. The potency of antibiotics declines with time. Moreover, the inappropriate use of antibiotics can lead to the development of bacterial resistance and a consequential lowering of antibiotic effectiveness.

General preparedness is always prudent. A few days' supply of food and water and the identification of rooms in homes and offices that can be temporarily sealed with duct tape to reduce outside air infiltration is a wise precaution. More specific response plans and protective measures, however, must be based on the specific dangers posed by organisms that produce disease. For example, anthrax (*Bacillus anthracis*), botulism (*Clostridium botulinum* toxin), plague (*Yersinia pestis*), smallpox (*Variola major*), tularemia (*Francisella tularensis*), viral hemorrhagic fevers (e.g., Ebola, Marburg), and arenaviruses (e.g., Lassa) are considered high-risk potential bioterrorism agents. These agents share a common trait of being easily spread from person to person, and all are capable of killing those who are infected. However, the natures of the diseases they cause are very different. A response that is effective against one microorganism may be useless against another.

Applications and Research

The types of personal protective equipment used depend on a number of factors. One factor is the setting. For example, a researcher at a biosafety level 4 (BSL-4) facility, which is designed to deal with dangerously contagious microorganisms, must be completely enclosed in a protective suit that is connected to an air supply. On the other hand, a general practitioner who is examining a person who has a cold may only elect to wear a face mask as a barrier to virus-laden droplets that could be expelled by a cough.

Another factor is the anticipated type of exposure. More extensive face and body coverage is required if there is the potential for splashing or spraying of body fluids. Related to this is the appropriateness of the protective equipment for the task. When confronting a dangerous respiratory infection, a respirator can be more appropriate than a mask because the respirator is designed to exclude small droplets that can pass through the mask fabric. An apron that does not absorb liquids is a safer choice when dealing with a victim of Ebola (where a great deal of bleeding usually occurs) than a surgical gown made of absorbent cotton.

A third factor is the fit of the protective equipment. One size does not fit all. Trying to care for a patient or respond to a medical emergency while wearing protective equipment that is too small or too large is inconvenient and potentially dangerous. Ill-fitting protective gear may restrict movement and, in the case of a respirator that is too large and fits sloppily on the face, may render the equipment useless.

Gloves are the most common personal protective equipment in hospitals and other health care settings. The choice of glove depends on the task. Gloves are available in a variety of materials, may be sterile (free of microorganisms) or non-sterile, and may be intended for single or repeated use. However, gloves are only as effective as the person wearing them. For example, if a health care provider fails to change gloves after leaving one patient and moving on to treat another patient, infections may be spread. Even when treating a single patient, a health care worker should change gloves after examining a body site that is infected and before examining other noninfected sites on the same patient.

The use of approved respirators are required when dealing with certain infections. One example is tuberculosis. The bacterium that is responsible for the respiratory infection (*Mycobacterium tuberculosis*) can be expelled inside small droplets, which can be inhaled by someone close by the patient. Respirators such as the N95, N99, and N100 are designed to exclude droplets that are less than 5 microns (a micron is one-millionth of a meter) in diameter. Avian influenza, a potentially lethal infection caused by the H5N1 virus that has evolved to allow for person-to-person transmission, is another infection that requires a health care provider to use a respirator.

Impacts and Issues

When properly used and worn, personal protective equipment is an efficient means of minimizing the spread of infectious disease from those who are infected to their health care providers, as well as from the health care provider to other patients. For example, before surgeons began to wear surgical garments, operations were a last resort due to the high postsurgical death rate. When surgeons began to wear special clothing that was changed between operations, the rate of postsurgical infection decreased dramatically. In the early 21st century, the Occupational Safety and Health Administration enforces the Bloodborne Pathogens Standard, last updated in 2001, which specifies the personal protective practices and equipment that must be available for health care workers and patients in the United States.

Despite these standards, there are difficulties involved in the use of protective equipment. For example, in an emergency there may not be time to properly clean protective clothing or to maintain the supply of disposable protective equipment, such as gloves or disposable needles. As a result, protective equipment may be reused when it should not be, and the contaminated equipment can continue the spread of infection.

Early outbreaks due to the Ebola virus were a sad example of the lack of proper protective equipment. While personal protection in the field during a viral outbreak continues to be challenging, great strides have been made. Protection for those fighting the Ebola outbreak that began in 2014 was comparatively much improved. Part of the reason for the ferocity of an Ebola outbreak is a lack of understanding of the disease among those most affected by it. More education targeting those who are at risk of acquiring the infection is still needed. In addition, certain cultural beliefs and practices continue to aid the spread of the virus, which can create problems for medical personnel working to contain it. In the epidemic that began in 2014, for instance, residents of villages where people were dying of the infections were advised not to have direct physical contact with their deceased prior to burial, a request that directly conflicted with traditional burial practices.

As shown in the months following the September 11, 2001, terrorist attacks on the United States, the deliberate airborne release of an infectious organism, such as *B. anthracis*, can easily occur. A large-scale release of such a pathogen could affect a wide geographical area, requiring the rapid deployment of many personnel. It is unlikely that their need for protective equipment could be met from a central source, as even facilities dedicated to the study of highly infectious microbes usually have only a limited number of full-body protective suits on hand.

See Also *Bioterrorism; Contact Precautions; Infection Control and Asepsis; Isolation and Quarantine; Standard Precautions*

BIBLIOGRAPHY

Books

Quamenn, David. *Ebola: The Natural and Human History of a Deadly Virus.* New York: Norton, 2014.

Richards, Paul. *Ebola: How a People's Science Helped End an Epidemic.* London: Zed, 2016.

Shah, Sonia. *Pandemic: Tracking Contagions, from Cholera to Ebola and Beyond.* New York: Picador, 2017.

Periodicals

Forrester, Joseph D., et al. "Assessment of Ebola Virus Disease, Health Care Infrastructure, and Preparedness—Four Counties, Southeastern Liberia, August 2014." *Morbidity and Mortality Weekly Report* 63, no. 40 (2014): 891–893.

Rebmann, Terri. "Pandemic Preparedness: Implementation of Infection Prevention Emergency Plans." *Infection Control and Hospital Epidemiology* 31, no. S1 (November 2010): S63–S65.

Websites

"Bloodborne Infectious Diseases: HIV/AIDS, Hepatitis B, Hepatitis C." Centers for Disease Control and Prevention. https://www.cdc.gov/niosh/topics/bbp/genres.html (accessed November 20, 2017).

"Quick Reference Guide to the Bloodborne Pathogens Standard." United States Department of Labor, Occupational Safety and Health Administration. https://www.osha.gov/SLTC/bloodbornepathogens/bloodborne_quickref.html (accessed November 20, 2017).

Brian Hoyle

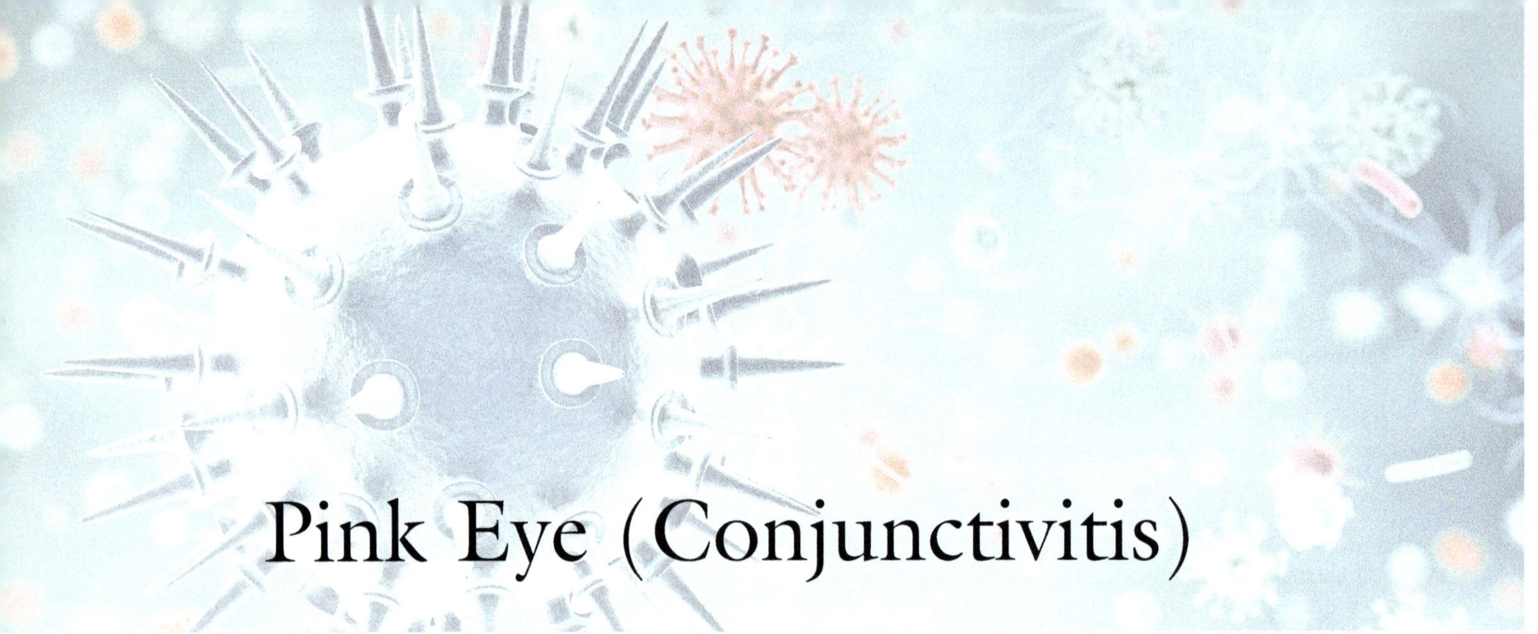

Pink Eye (Conjunctivitis)

Introduction

Pink eye refers to a chemical- or allergy-related inflammation, or a viral or bacterial infection, of the transparent covering of the eyelid and a portion of the eyeball. The transparent covering is called the conjunctiva. The inflammation or infection is known as conjunctivitis.

The designation pink eye indicates the appearance of the inflamed or infected conjunctiva. Due to the increased prominence of blood vessels, the color of the white portion of the eye changes to red or pink.

WORDS TO KNOW

ANTIBIOTIC A drug, such as penicillin, used to fight infections caused by bacteria. Antibiotics act only on bacteria and are not effective against viruses.

EYE DROPS Saline-containing fluid that is added to the eye to cleanse the eye or as the solution used to administer antibiotics or other medication.

HISTAMINE A hormone that is chemically similar to the hormones serotonin, epinephrine, and norepinephrine. A hormone is generally defined as a chemical produced by a certain cell or tissue that causes a specific biological change or activity to occur in another cell or tissue located elsewhere in the body. Specifically, histamine plays a role in localized immune responses and in allergic reactions.

OPPORTUNISTIC INFECTION An infection that occurs in people whose immune systems are diminished or are not functioning normally. Such infections are opportunistic insofar as the infectious agents take advantage of their host's compromised immune systems and invade to cause disease.

OPTIC SOLUTION Any liquid solution of a medication that can be applied directly to the eye.

Disease History, Characteristics, and Transmission

Infection-related conjunctivitis can be caused by the same viruses and bacteria that cause colds, ear infections, sore throats, and sexually transmitted diseases. Bacteria include *Staphylococcus*, *Streptococcus*, *Chlamydia*, and *Haemophilus*, as well as *Neisseria gonorrhoeae*, the bacterium that causes gonorrhea. Viruses include adenoviruses, rhinoviruses, coronaviruses, echoviruses, paramyxoviruses, and coxsackieviruses. Viral conjunctivitis is more common than bacterial conjunctivitis.

Infants can be infected during birth by bacteria in the mother's birth canal. While harmless in the mother, the bacteria can cause an infection in the infant, whose immune system is not yet fully efficient. Such bacteria are known as opportunistic pathogens because they normally cause no harm but can cause disease given the appropriate circumstances. Screening of the mother prior to the birth can detect and treat the infection. Newborn conjunctivitis is treated by the application of an antibiotic ointment to the eyes soon after birth.

The redness of the affected eye(s) is a hallmark of pink eye. Another common symptom is the feeling that something foreign is in the eye. Many people also complain of a gritty or itchy sensation in the infected eye(s). Other symptoms include blurred vision, increased sensitivity to light, increased formation of tears, and a discharge from the infected eye(s) that can become crusty during sleep.

Conjunctivitis can also be caused by an allergic reaction to pollen or some other substance. A part of the allergic response is the production of the antibody immunoglobulin E, which in turn triggers cells in the eyes and airway to release various compounds. One of these compounds, histamine, produces a variety of allergic responses, including allergic conjunctivitis.

While the allergic response cannot be passed from person to person, viral and bacterial conjunctivitis are highly contagious.

Scope and Distribution

Pink eye is global in occurrence and can affect anyone. Pink eye, like most minor contagious infections, spreads easily among groups of children. Viral and bacterial pink eye often affect children who live in group settings or attend school or day care.

Treatment and Prevention

People who develop bacterial or viral pink eye should avoid close contact with others. This is especially important for infants in day care and school-age children.

The cause of pink eye can be determined. If caused by a bacterial infection, pink eye is easily treated using antibiotics. Typically, the antibiotic is applied as an eyedrop solution, although an ointment may be used for infants and younger children. The infection usually clears up within several days, but the antibiotic needs to be used for as long as has been prescribed to ensure all infecting bacteria are killed. If treatment is stopped too early, some bacteria may survive and develop resistance to the antibiotic, making treatment of the recurring infection more difficult.

Allergic pink eye can be treated by use of eye drops containing compounds that reduce symptoms. Rubbing the eye should be avoided, as it can introduce allergens and trigger more symptoms.

Good personal hygiene, especially handwashing and minimizing rubbing of the eyes, reduces the risk of developing pink eye. Frequently washing bathroom and bedroom linens and avoiding sharing pillows and cosmetic applicators further lessen the risk of conjunctivitis.

CONJUNCTIVA AND TEARS

The conjunctiva, a fine mucus membrane, covers the cornea and lines the eyelid. Blinking lubricates the cornea with tears, providing the moisture necessary for the cornea's health. The outside of the cornea is protected by a thin film of tears produced in the lacrimal glands, located in the lateral part of the orbit, below the eyebrow. Tears flow through ducts from this gland to the eyelid and eye and then drain from the inner corner of the eye into the nasal cavity. The aqueous humor, a clear, watery liquid, separates the cornea from the iris and lens. The cornea contains no blood vessels or pigment and obtains its nutrients from the aqueous humor.

Impacts and Issues

While conjunctivitis is usually an inconvenience rather than a health concern, there is a risk that it can lead to

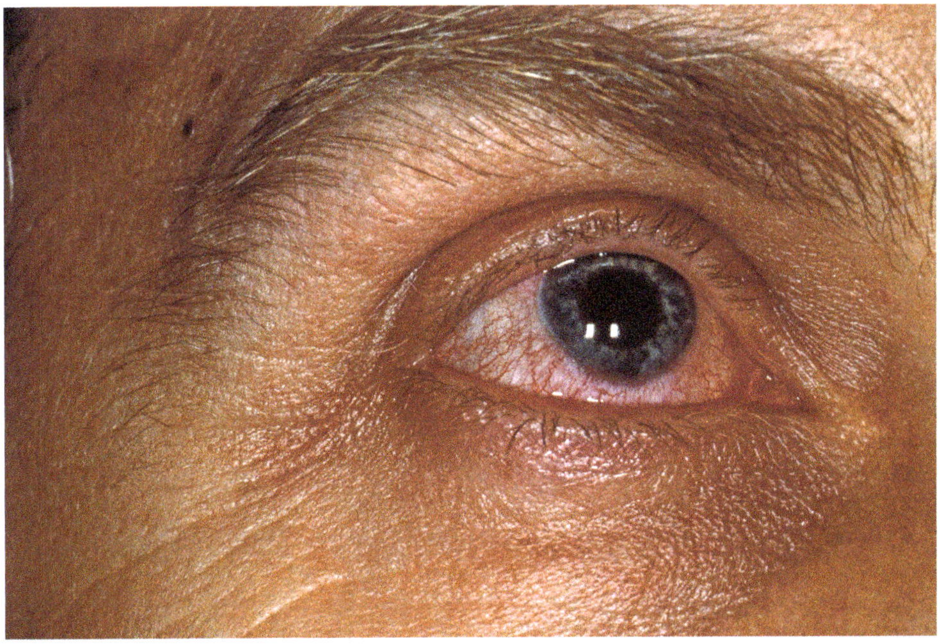

Conjunctivitis, or pink eye, is the inflammation of the transparent covering of the eyelid and a portion of the eyeball. The infection can be caused by viruses, bacteria, or allergies. © *John Watney/Science Source*

problems with the cornea. In addition, the infection in newborns can lead to more serious health issues, including loss of vision. Prompt treatment can eliminate this concern.

UK researchers and public health officials have studied the costs and benefits of changing common medical approaches to the treatment of viral and bacterial conjunctivitis. Because many cases of pink eye can disappear without medical intervention, researchers are developing new protocols for when parents should seek medical attention for children with conjunctivitis and how physicians should treat the disease.

Public health officials have noted that antibiotic eye drops are frequently prescribed, even before clinical diagnosis of bacterial pink eye can be made. Use of antibiotics does not treat viral pink eye and only negligibly reduces recovery time for most cases of bacterial pink eye. Researchers worry that overzealous prescription of antibiotics could lead to bacterial resistance. Health officials note that patient costs associated with treating many mild forms of pink eye, including the cost of eye drops, antibiotics, missed work, missed school, and doctors' visits, may be unnecessarily high.

SEE ALSO *Childhood-Associated Infectious Diseases, Immunization Impacts; Contact Lenses and Fusarium Keratitis*

BIBLIOGRAPHY

Books

Estenson, Joseph. *Conjunctivitis: A Reference Guide.* Washington, DC: Capitol Hill Press, 2015.

Whitcup, Scott M., ed. *Pharmacologic Therapy of Ocular Disease.* New York: Springer Berlin Heidelberg, 2017.

Websites

"Conjunctivitis (Pink Eye)." Centers for Disease Control and Prevention, October 2, 2017. https://www.cdc.gov/conjunctivitis/index.html (accessed November 20, 2017).

"Conjunctivitis (Pinkeye)." WebMD. https://www.webmd.com/eye-health/eye-health-conjunctivitis#1 (accessed November 20, 2017).

Brian Hoyle

Pinworm (*Enterobius vermicularis*) Infection

Introduction

Pinworm infection, or enterobiasis, is a common helminth infection that arises when humans drink water or eat food contaminated by eggs of parasitic pinworms. Enterobiasis is considered the most common roundworm infection in the United States. Although it can affect any human, it is more common in children than in adults.

Pinworms live in the rectum, or lower part of the intestine. The small, thin, white pinworm averages about 0.4 inches (1.0 centimeter) in length, with the adult male ranging from 0.04 to 0.16 inches (0.1 to 0.4 centimeters) and the adult female ranging from 0.32 to 0.50 inches (0.8 to 1.3 centimeters). A pinworm possesses a long, pin-shaped posterior, which gives the worm its common name. Pinworms are nematodes in the family Oxyuridae, genus *Enterobius*. Pinworm infection is most commonly caused by the species *Enterobius vermicularis*, the threadworm. A second species, *E. gregorii*, has been found to cause the infection in Africa, Asia, and Europe.

Disease History, Characteristics, and Transmission

The pinworm is a roundworm, which is the common name of any nonsegmented worm located in freshwater, marine, or terrestrial environments. Roundworms are found almost anywhere around the world, living frequently in the surface layers of the soil.

Pinworms develop to adulthood within the host's intestines, specifically in the lower small intestine and upper colon. Rarely are they found in the abdominal lining, fallopian tubes, liver, uterus, vagina, or bloodstream or in organs other than the intestines.

The male pinworm dies after mating. The female moves from the intestine to the anal area, where she lays 10,000 to 20,000 eggs. Within four to six hours, the eggs mature and, thus, become infectious. The female soon expels a sticky substance that causes itching in the host. Intense itching causes the human to transfer eggs to the fingers, which then transfer the eggs to other objects. The eggs can live outside a host for up to two weeks and in some cases three weeks. The eggs are often accidentally ingested, in which case the larvae hatch and move to the intestine. They mature within 30 to 45 days. Their overall lifespan is about 60 days. The larvae can also hatch outside the host and then move through the anus and into the intestines. In some cases the eggs become airborne and are inhaled by the host.

Symptoms are usually mild. Sometimes there are no symptoms at all. When present, symptoms include itching, intestinal problems, vomiting, nervousness and irritability, restless sleep, and sometimes skin reddening and infection around the anus. The infection usually does not cause permanent damage.

WORDS TO KNOW

HELMINTH A representative of various phyla of wormlike animals.

HOST An organism that serves as the habitat for a parasite or possibly for a symbiont. A host may provide nutrition to the parasite or symbiont, or it may simply provide a place in which to live.

LARVAE Immature forms of an organism (wormlike in insects; fishlike in amphibians) capable of surviving on their own. Larvae do not resemble the parent and must go through metamorphosis, or change, to reach the adult stage.

NEMATODE Also known as a roundworm; a type of helminth characterized by a long, cylindrical body.

Scope and Distribution

Pinworm infection is found worldwide, although it is found more commonly in temperate regions of Western Europe and North America. It is found only occasionally in tropical areas. The infection is frequently found when humans live in crowded environments. It is estimated that between 200 million and 500 million people worldwide are infected annually. The US Centers for Disease Control and Prevention (CDC) estimates that approximately 40 million people are infected each year in the United States. A 2006 study published in *Lancet* estimated that up to 28 percent of the global population could be infected. The most at-risk populations are children and people in institutions, as well as those who care for them. According to the CDC, up to 50 percent of children under age 18 or adults who are institutionalized have pinworm infection. In addition, up to half of all adults who care for children with pinworm infection are infected.

Treatment and Prevention

Diagnosis of pinworm infection is made by an examination of the patient's anal region. A tape test is usually used, which involves placing the sticky side of a transparent adhesive or cellophane tape against the skin around the anus. The procedure should be performed immediately after waking up, before bathing and using the toilet, so that any eggs in the anal area will be picked up. The materials that stick to the tape are then examined under a microscope for the presence of pinworms. The infected person may also see worms crawling on bed sheets or clothing.

Treatment includes various antiparasitic drugs that have been found effective in treating the infection. These drugs include albendazole, mebendazole, piperazine, and pyrantel pamoate. If one person in a household has the infection, all family members are often advised to take the drug treatment.

These medicines kill the worms about 95 percent of the time. However, they do not kill the eggs. To kill the eggs, a second round of medicine is recommended two weeks after the completion of the first round. If this treatment does not eliminate the infection, then additional treatments should be administered. In addition, a thorough search should be made for the source of the infection, including other children, household members, and anyone or anything else that has come in contact with the infected person. Four to six treatments spaced two weeks apart are sometimes recommended for difficult cases.

To avoid becoming reinfected, an array of hygiene practices are advised, including disinfecting eating utensils and bed linens, cleaning the toilet daily, keeping fingers away from the nostrils and mouth, bathing when first waking, changing and washing underwear daily, changing bed clothing frequently and after each treatment, providing plenty of sunlight or artificial light (pinworms are light

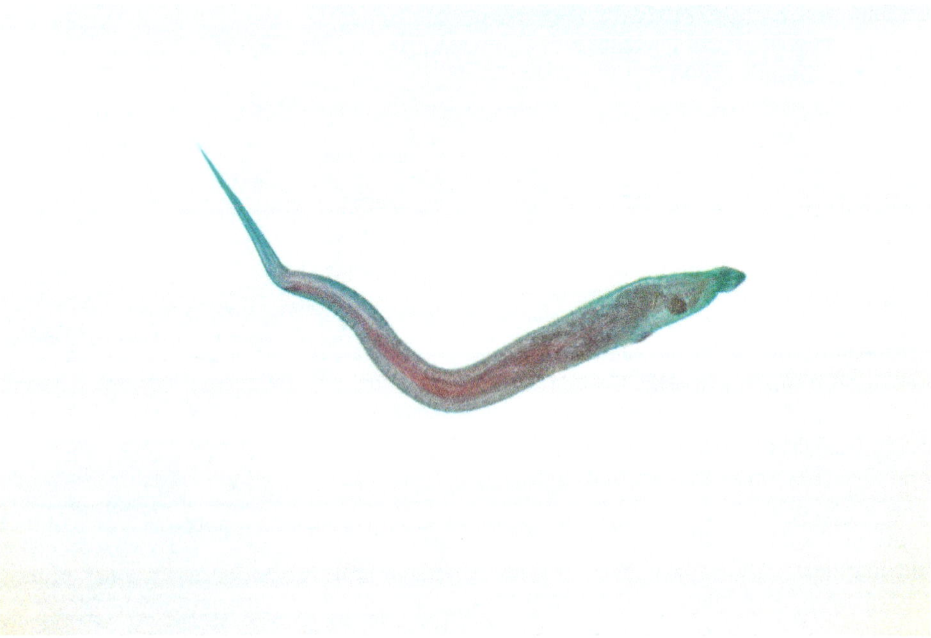

Enterobius vermicularis, also known as the pinworm. Pinworm infection is the most common worm infection in the United States. © E.R. Degginger/Science Source

sensitive), trimming fingernails (scratching of anal area may place pinworms underneath nails), and not scratching bare anal areas.

Impacts and Issues

When treated properly, pinworm infection is fully curable. Even though the prognosis for pinworm infection is very good, complications can set in. Among the most common complications are salpingitis (pelvic inflammatory disease, an infection of the lining of the uterus, fallopian tubes, or ovaries), vaginitis (any infection or inflammation of the vagina), and reinfestation (further reoccurrence of the infection).

Children who are being treated for pinworm infection need not be kept home from school, and it is not appropriate to conclude that a child with pinworms has an unclean environment. Pinworm infections are extremely common among children, with half of all children eventually becoming infected due to the large amount of time spent outdoors playing in dirt and sand. Parents can minimize the chances of their children getting the infection by promoting handwashing and sanitation within and outside the home. Prompt medical care, medication, and preventive hygiene practices will eliminate pinworms from children and adults in a quick and safe manner.

PRIMARY SOURCE

Pinworm Treatments Are an Expensive Drug Mistake You Don't Need to Make

SOURCE: *Skinner, Ginger.* "Pinworm Treatments Are an Expensive Drug Mistake You Don't Need to Make." Consumer Reports *(January 27, 2017). This article is also available online at https://www.consumerreports.org/drugs/pinworm-treatments-expensive-drug-mistake-you-dont-need-to-make/ (accessed January 9, 2018).*

INTRODUCTION: *This 2017* Consumer Reports *article highlights the confusing and contradictory nature of drug pricing using the example of over-the-counter and prescription medications for pinworm.*

When Cheryl Kennedy of Chicago went to fill a pinworm prescription for her 4-year-old daughter, she was astounded to learn that four tablets of the drug Albenza cost almost $700—even with insurance.

"I called the doctor and asked if there was an alternative," Kennedy recalls. "That's when he suggested we try an over-the-counter remedy" called Reese's Pinworm Medicine that costs less than $15.

The OTC drug quickly cleared up her daughter's pinworm, a common and highly contagious infection that affects 40 million Americans each year, most of them schoolchildren. Pinworm attacks the intestines and causes itching and rashes around the anus.

Kennedy's experience isn't unusual. According to medical experts, doctors are routinely prescribing both Albenza (the brand name for albendazole) and another drug called Emverm (the brand name for mebendazole) without realizing how increasingly expensive they are. Both drugs are made by Impax Laboratories.

Albenza, for instance, has shot up from $6 per pill in 2010 to $190 per dose now; that same year mebendazole generic sold for about $16 per pill—and today, Emverm sells for about $430 per dose, according to Symphony Health, which tracks the pharmaceutical market.

Why Do Doctors Prescribe the Pricey Drugs?

"In the case of albendazole, the answer is very simple: Most doctors have no idea that an older, off-patent drug like albendazole could cost $200 per dose," says Jeremy A. Greene, M.D., Ph.D., professor of medicine and the history of medicine at Johns Hopkins University School of Medicine. "That is, until a patient comes back from the pharmacy in shock over the high price."

Because the two drugs are old, "the average prescribing physician is conditioned to think that it must be very cheap," Greene explains. "And they know also that it's a drug that's almost free in other countries. The concept that it could cost $200 per pill is unfathomable."

Consumer Reports' own research suggests that doctors are often in the dark about drug prices. A poll last year of 200 internists showed that the biggest reason doctors have a hard time discussing drug costs with patients is that they don't have access to prices or the patient's insurance coverage. Yet 8 out of 10 doctors said they are concerned about their patient's ability to afford treatments.

"Even when physicians are concerned about prescribing affordable drugs, they have only limited tools available to understand the pricing implication that any given prescription will mean for their patients when they get to the pharmacy," notes Greene of Johns Hopkins.

High Price for a Cheap Cure

How both Albenza and Emverm came to be so expensive—especially when there's a cheap OTC version available—highlights the confusing and contradictory nature of drug pricing in the U.S.

Albendazole was relatively inexpensive until 2010, when the manufacturer stopped making it. Amedra Pharmaceuticals later acquired marketing rights to the drug in 2013 and started raising its price from $6 per pill. Amedra was subsequently acquired by Impax Laboratories in 2015.

Mebendazole, meanwhile, was an inexpensive generic drug for decades, then went off the market in 2011. Amedra also purchased the rights to that drug, so it owned the only two prescription pinworm treatments available. The company was acquired by Impax Laboratories in 2015, and by January 2016 it launched a chewable version called Emverm, pricing it around $400 per pill. The inexpensive version of mebendazole is no longer available.

When Consumer Reports asked why the prices of both prescription drugs are so high, Impax spokesman Mark Donohue had this response:

"Emvern is the only FDA-approved prescription treatment for pinworm, with a 95 percent cure rate in a single tablet," Donohue said. He added that the company offers a savings card on Emvern's website.

Donohue said he couldn't comment on albendazole. (The drug is used "off label," meaning it hasn't been approved by the FDA for pinworm but is legal for doctors to prescribe.)

Consumer advocates—including Consumers Union, the policy and mobilization arm of Consumer Reports—say a lack of federal regulations to curb such price increases means it could happen with other medications.

"The fact that the manufacturers of these once-affordable prescription drugs could get away with engineering such steep price hikes is one more demonstration that our current laws are not giving us a marketplace that works for consumers," says Victoria Burack, health policy analyst at Consumers Union. "We will continue pushing for Congress to fix those broken laws."

SEE ALSO *CDC (Centers for Disease Control and Prevention); Public Health and Infectious Disease; Roundworm (Ascariasis) Infection*

BIBLIOGRAPHY

Books

Cheng, Liang, and David G. Bostwick, eds. *Essentials of Anatomic Pathology*. 3rd ed. New York: Springer, 2010.

Kline, Mark W., et al., eds. *Rudolph's Pediatrics*. 23rd ed. New York: McGraw-Hill Education, 2018.

Periodicals

Bethony J., et al. "Soil-Transmitted Helminth Infections: Ascariasis, Trichuriasis, and Hookworm." *Lancet* 367 (2006): 1521–1532.

Kubiak, K., E. Dzika, and Ł. Paukszto. "Enterobiasis Epidemiology and Molecular Characterization of *Enterobius vermicularis* in Healthy Children in North-Eastern Poland." *Helminthologia* 54, no. 4 (2017): 284–291. This article can also be found online at https://www.degruyter.com/downloadpdf/j/helm.2017.54.issue-4/helm-2017-0042/helm-2017-0042.pdf (accessed January 10, 2018).

Skinner, Ginger. "Pinworm Treatments Are an Expensive Drug Mistake You Don't Need to Make." *Consumer Reports* (January 27, 2017). This article can also be found online at https://www.consumerreports.org/drugs/pinworm-treatments-expensive-drug-mistake-you-dont-need-to-make/ (accessed January 9, 2018).

Van Weyenbeg, S. J. B., and N. K. De Boer. "*Enterobiasis vermicularis*." *Video Journal and Encyclopedia of GI Endoscopy* 1, no. 2 (October 2013): 359–360.

Websites

"Enterobiasis (Also Known as Pinworm Infection)." Centers for Disease Control and Prevention, January 10, 2013. https://www.cdc.gov/parasites/pinworm/index.html (accessed January 9, 2018).

"Pinworm Infection." Mayo Clinic, April 8, 2015. https://www.mayoclinic.org/diseases-conditions/pinworm/symptoms-causes/syc-20376382 (accessed January 9, 2018).

Plague, Early History

Introduction

Plague has shaped the development of all civilizations. In the recorded histories of Chinese civilization, epidemic disease thrice wiped out one-quarter to over one-third of its population. The Black Death transformed the social, political, and economic landscape of medieval Europe.

Most scientists and historians link bubonic plague in antiquity to rats. *Yersinia pestis*, the bacterium that causes bubonic plague, lives inside the guts of a flea. When inside the flea, *Yersinia pestis* can multiply and blocks the flea's throat area, making the flea quite hungry and in search of new hosts, whether rats or humans. When the flea bites, some of the bacteria is spit out into the bite wound, transmitting the disease.

However, pestilence or plague as recorded in the annals of history does not refer to only one disease. "Plague" did not always describe bubonic plague or the Black Death. Measles, smallpox, flu, dysentery, or typhoid all could have produced a sudden rise in mortality and were referred to in antiquity as plague.

Epidemic disease has likely always been part of human history, but the first written account of its devastating ef-

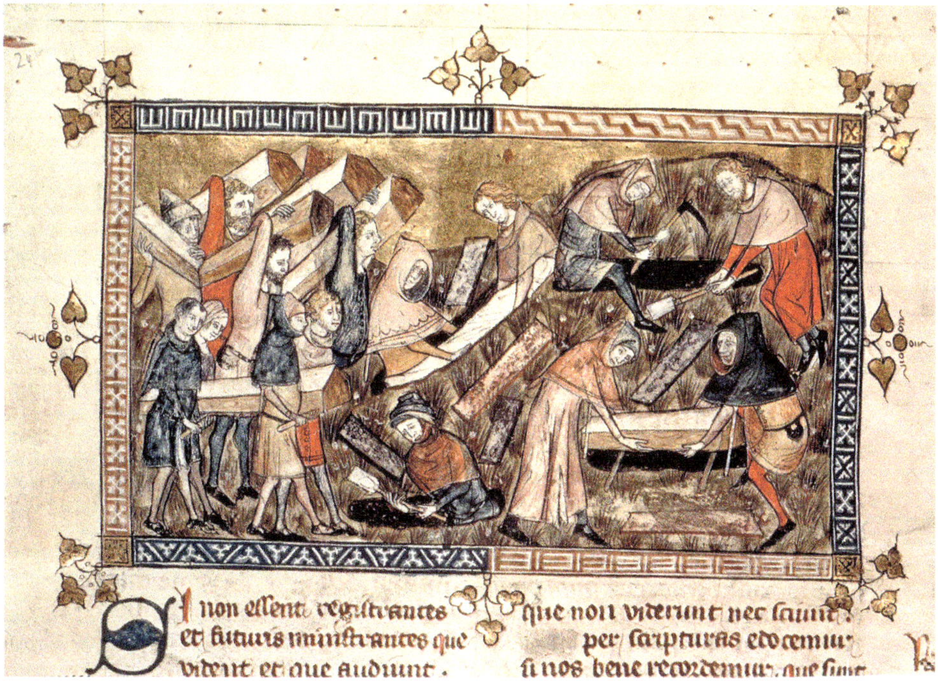

This illustration, from *The Chronicles of Gilles de Muisit* (1272–1352), depicts the burial of the victims of the Plague of Tournai in 1349. The European plague pandemic of 1347–1351 claimed more than 20 million lives, nearly one-third of Europe's total population. Ibliothèque royale. © *Photo 12/UIG/Getty Images*

fects originates in the ancient Middle East. The development of horticulture permitted the development of towns, concentrating populations in relatively small areas and facilitating the spread of some diseases. Many historians assert that infectious disease agents spread and thrived because there was a large supply of nonimmune, disease-susceptible people who diseases could attack. People often shared their living quarters with farm animals. Diseases such as cowpox could affect humans or become genetically modified to create epidemics, such as smallpox.

■ History

Plague in Ancient Egypt, the Middle East, and China

Ancient literature often provides a historical account of ancient epidemics. The Babylonian *Epic of Gilgamesh* from the 7th century BCE claimed that a visit from the god of pestilence was preferable to a flooding disaster, and an Egyptian text from 2000 BCE compared "fear of Pharaoh with fear of the god of disease in the year of pestilence." Biblical texts such as the Book of Exodus also report the plagues in Egypt in the form of skin pustules, and the Plague of the Philistines in I Samuel supposedly killed 70,000 in Israel.

In ancient China references to plague in the Yangtze River Valley were likely endemic malaria or dengue fever, a disease common in low-lying areas borne by mosquitoes. The Chinese also were beset by smallpox, and they invented the first techniques of effective prevention in 590 BCE called pock-sowing. They would grind dried skin scabs from smallpox victims along with musk and apply the mixture to the noses of the healthy. The Chinese also placed matter from the smallpox pustules that arose on the skin into a scratch in the arm of a recipient, in a process called variolation. Exposure to the pathogen usually produced a mild case and gave the recipient immunity, but sometimes a full-blown case would develop. (Effective and safe vaccination for smallpox did not occur until the 18th century.)

However, another Egyptian text, called the Ebers Papyrus, from 1500 BCE, does describe an epidemic disease with symptoms similar to the bubonic plague, a bacterial infection that causes buboes, or swelling of the lymph glands. The Ebers Papyrus mentions an illness that "has produced a bubo, and the pus has petrified, the disease has hit."

Plague in Ancient Greece and Rome

In contrast with Egypt or China, where rivers brought irrigation as well as disease-borne vectors, ancient Greece was relatively free of disease. The Greek agriculture did not alter the environment nearly as much as Chinese rice paddies. As a result, the agricultural revolution in Greece did not bring exposure to new diseases.

Threat of epidemics came from the expansion of cities in Greece, increased population density, and exposure to new pathogens from travelers and trade. Ancient Greece was made up of a number of small independent city-states, and economics was driven by trade; contact with other peoples brought contact with new diseases. In the 5th century BCE, Athens was the most prominent Greek city-state, and it initiated a protracted war with rival city-state Sparta. Expecting to win with its powerful navy, Athens was instead brought to its knees with the appearance of a mysterious epidemic in 430–429 BCE that wiped out one-quarter of the Athenian land forces. The ancient Greek historian Thucydides (460–399 BCE) in his *History of the Peloponnesian War* argues that the epidemic was the main reason for Athens military defeat—a defining event in subsequent Mediterranean political history.

The identity of this epidemic has been a matter of debate, ranging from scarlet fever to smallpox to bubonic plague to the effects of ergot or a mold on the grain supply. Regardless of the source or causative agent of disease, Athenians had little immunity to it. Because the disease entered the Athenian population with sudden ferocity and then disappeared, several scientists and historians theorize that the pathogen came by sea and soon died out after provoking an accelerated immune response in the local population. The Spartans, more geographically isolated on the Peloponnesian peninsula, were untouched, giving them a decisive military advantage.

Ancient Rome was highly prone to plagues. During the reign of emperor Marcus Aurelius (121–180), the Roman Empire was struck by a destructive epidemic that began in 166 CE and occurred with intermittent frequency until 189 CE. The accounts of the Greek physician Galen (c.130–c.200) about the plague, particularly the incidence of skin rash and gastrointestinal bleeding, have led some scholars to conclude it was probably smallpox. The mortality rate was 7 to 10 percent among the local population and 10 to 15 percent in the army, for a total of 5 million deaths over the twenty-three-year period. Unlike in China, treatment in the Western world was relatively ineffectual, though it was common knowledge that smallpox survivors were immune to the disease. As early as 430 BCE, those who had survived the disease were encouraged to nurse others through the illness, and the Romans also advocated this practice.

The Late Roman Empire and the First Pandemic of the Bubonic Plague

The first pandemic of bubonic plague occurred during the reign of Roman emperor Justinian (483–565). The pandemic probably originated in lower Egypt in 542 and spread via trade routes to Alexandria and then to Constantinople, which served as the capital of the eastern part of the Roman Empire (known as Byzantium) at the time. Forty percent of the population in Constantinople perished. The medical writer Procopius of Caesarea (c.500–c.565) clearly identified the disease as bubonic plague, remarking, "The fever made its attack suddenly. Generally on the first or second day, but in a few instances later, buboes appeared, not only in the groin, but also in the armpits and below the ears." The plague then continued to Italy, Spain, Britain, and Denmark and ended up in China in 610 CE, killing an estimated 100 million people, or approximately 50 percent of the human population. As Procopius relates in his *History of the Wars*, doctors had little recourse or understanding of how to treat the disease. They did observe in some patients, however, that their buboes grew to a large size and ruptured. The patient usually recovered but tended to have muscle tremors; doctors therefore would lance the buboes to increase chances of survival.

Land went uncultivated, leading to food shortages; entire villages in rural areas were abandoned; the army shrunk in size; and monastic houses with their close-knit populations were decimated. As the tax base severely declined, civic building projects ceased and public services, including the burial of the dead, virtually disappeared.

Along with these severe cultural effects, the plague in Justinian's reign also greatly affected the history and survival of the Roman Empire. In the West the Roman Empire had been vulnerable to attacks from Germanic tribes such as the Vandals, Goths, and Ostrogoths, and the western part of the empire had been captured in the 5th century CE. Previous to the outbreak of the disease, however, Justinian had made significant inroads in retaking much of Italy from the Ostrogoths and northern Africa from the Vandals. The eastern part of the Roman Empire was prospering, with silk manufacture in Syria adding to its wealth. The population increased in Greece, Asia Minor, and the Balkans. Justinian had also used his increased revenues to engage in a building program in Constantinople, constructing great churches such as Hagia Sophia. As Josiah C. Russell remarked in his article "That Earlier Plague," Justinian's "building program was part of a kind of Golden Age in which literature enjoyed a fine period: Rome still seemed eternal." In 540 the prospect that the empire might be restored without straining its resources seemed entirely probable.

However, the devastation of the plague weakened the eastern Roman Empire at a critical juncture. Justinian's army shrunk from 350,000 men to 150,000 on his death in 565. As the plague tended to be especially fatal to young people over ten years of age and pregnant women, the devastation to the population meant that fresh military recruits were increasingly scarce. The offensive in the West was thus abandoned after 565. The resulting power vacuum, along with the birth of Islam, promoted the rise of the Arabic empires in the 7th century.

The Bubonic Plague in Medieval Europe

After the plague epidemics in the 6th and 7th centuries, the disease reappeared sporadically but did not reemerge with ferocity until the mid-14th century, erupting in the Gobi Desert in the late 1320s. It is not well understood why the bubonic plague reappeared, but the climate of earth had begun to cool at this time, producing a phenomenon known as the Little Ice Age, and this change in environment may have had an effect. It is believed that the cooler temperatures resulted in poor harvests and that there were famines in Western Europe from 1315 to 1317, which weakened the population and made it vulnerable to epidemic disease. Ultimately, one-third of the population of Western Europe perished, and populations did not return to their previous levels until the 16th century. Urban areas such as Florence lost between one-half and three-quarters of their population.

As in the 6th century, the plague followed trade routes in its spread westward, reaching Sicily by 1347 and, later that year, the Italian mainland. It arrived in Germany via Rhine trade routes and then France and England in 1348 when the plague was at its peak. Warfare also spread the Black Death, notably from the plague-infested Genoese colony of Caffa in Crimea, which was besieged by a Mongol army in 1346. According to primary sources, it seems the plague took two forms in the 14th century: a septice-

WORDS TO KNOW

ENDEMIC Present in a particular area or among a particular group of people.

ETIOLOGY The study of the cause or origin of a disease or disorder.

PLAGUE A contagious disease that spreads rapidly through a population and results in a high rate of death.

QUARANTINE The practice of separating people who have been exposed to an infectious agent but have not yet developed symptoms from the general population. This can be done voluntarily or involuntarily by the authority of states and the federal Centers for Disease Control and Prevention.

VACCINATION The inoculation, or use of vaccines, to prevent specific diseases within humans and animals by producing immunity to such diseases. The introduction of weakened or dead viruses or microorganisms into the body to create immunity by the production of specific antibodies.

VARIOLATION The premodern practice of deliberately infecting people with smallpox to make them immune to a more serious form of the disease. It was dangerous but did confer immunity on survivors.

mic plague, which attacks the blood, and pneumonic plague, which infects the lungs and is an especially virulent airborne disease.

Medical treatment ranged from the sophisticated to the folkloric. Some theologians opined that it was the result of vengeance of God and that nothing could be done, but many of the Italian city-states, such as Milan and Venice, took more practical measures and attempted to quarantine sufferers, walling up houses found to have inhabitants with plague. The quarantine, the pest house, and health boards often just crowded the susceptible poor together, causing higher mortality, while the urban wealthy fled the city, segregating themselves in the country away from plague sufferers.

Many correctly thought the disease was thought to be transmitted by air, but in an era with no knowledge of microorganisms, it was thought bad smells, or *miasmas*, caused infections. Incense and aromatic oils were hawked as cures, as were posies of flowers to be held to the face.

Pope Clement VI (1291–1352) consulted the Parisian medical faculty in 1348 to get their opinion, and they theorized that the disaster was due to astrological events, an unfortunate conjunction of Saturn, Jupiter, and Mars that caused hot, moist conditions, which in turn caused the earth to exhale poisonous vapors. Astrology and medicine were intricately intertwined at this time, with the macrocosm of the universe thought to affect the "little world" or microcosm of the body, so their explanation was taken quite seriously. The physicians advised not to eat any food thought to be hot or moist that would add to the effect of the vapors and particularly thought fish were dangerous to include in the diet.

Some expressed their despair at events via religious fanaticism. Groups of flagellants whipped themselves in public to do penance for sins, some believing the end of the world was approaching. Others blamed religious and ethnic minorities such as Jews, Moors, or Roma, accusing them of poisoning town wells and causing the disease. There were pogroms, or mass killings, of Jews and Roma in the 14th and 15th centuries. In Strasbourg in 1349, nearly 200 Jews were burned to death. In response to this persecution, some of the Jewish population moved to Eastern Europe, including Poland and Lithuania.

The massive population loss also had great economic effects. Labor shortages meant that wages rose, and landlords attempted, often forcefully, to hold on to the serfs they had and to enforce more labor duties. It is little surprise that in the 1380s there were several peasant revolts (including the Jacquerie in 1358, the Peasants' Revolt in England in 1381, and the Catalonian Rebellion in 1395) as laborers asserted their rights in a market that should have been favorable to them.

Landlords shifted production on the land from foodstuffs, the demand for which was declining with a smaller population, to pastoral agriculture (sheep and cattle raising). Grazing cattle or sheep required less farm labor. Women also found their labor in demand. The two centuries after the plague have been described as an "early golden age for women" as several female guild masters and business owners appeared. Marriage rates also decreased after the bubonic plague. The disease seemed to disproportionately kill young men, so many women married late or not at all and thus turned to convents or cottage businesses to earn their livings.

These disruptions and changes to the social and economic fabric of medieval society have caused many historians to claim that the plague was the dividing line between the Middle Ages and the Renaissance. It seems that more secular values that became more important in the Renaissance, as opposed to the spiritual values of the medieval era, began to dominate society. For a variety of political reasons, the popes during the plague also did not live in the spiritual home of Rome and the Vatican but rather in southern France in Avignon, to the scandal of many. The Crusades in the 1290s had also been resolute failures, and the Holy Lands were lost.

Accompanied by the disaster of the plague, the loss of faith in the church may have set the stage for Renaissance secularism. The Catholic Church seemed unable to offer the degree of spiritual comfort required in an era of great loss, and many adopted the "live for today" attitude, enjoying life while they could in uncertain times. For instance, the Italian author Giovanni Boccaccio's (1313–1375) *Decameron*, written shortly after the plague, is a literary masterpiece that has as its premise a group of lords and ladies who escaped Florence to the country town of Fiesole during the epidemic. While in exile they told stories to amuse themselves and pass the time, often displaying themes of lust, love, and a decidedly commercial, urban, and secular ethic.

The bubonic plague, though it never reoccurred in as virulent a manner as in 1348, did return several times in the 15th century, and there were local epidemics until the mid-17th century. This may have been due to a variety of factors, including improved health and nutrition as the centuries passed. In her 2015 article in *PLOS ONE*, Sharon DeWitte discussed archaeological analysis of skeletons from three London plague cemeteries. The research has revealed that there were improvements in mortality after the initial occurrence of the Black Death and, "by inference, improved health at least at some ages in the post-Black Death population." The last occurrence of the bubonic plague in Western Europe was in 1665 in London just before the Great Fire burned the medieval wooden houses and seemingly cleansed the capital of fleas and rats responsible for the disease.

■ Current Issues

Another great pandemic of plague spread through China, Southeast Asia, and India beginning in 1855. The advent of the railway and increased migration helped the disease spread rapidly in Asia, India, and parts of Russia. Over the following fifty years, plague (predominantly pneumonic) spread to every inhabited continent. The so-called Third Pandemic killed 12 million people, primarily in Manchuria and Mongolia.

Several scientists have theorized that the Second Pandemic, the Black Death, may not have involved bubonic plague but another form of plague that is not present in the 21st century. Others assert that the Black Death was too virulent to have been bubonic plague, suggesting that a highly contagious hemorrhagic fever—akin to modern Ebola or Marburg—was the epidemic disease of the medieval plague. The theories are controversial, and *Yersinia pestis* remains the predominantly accepted culprit of the Black Death. In 2017 there was an outbreak of plague in Madagascar due to *Yersinia pestis* that caused the death of more than thirty people. Its source was traced to a man who traveled to an area known to have infected rodents and fleas. Outbreaks in Madagascar tend to be seasonal, occurring after the end of rice harvest in late summer, when the rat population drops due to decreased food supply and fleas seek new hosts to bite.

While researchers have been scouring written sources for years for clues about ancient plagues, they had been limited to matching described symptoms to known disease behaviors. Archaeological and forensic research may aid the identification of past epidemics. Eva Panagiotakopulu, an archaeologist from the University of Sheffield, theorizes that Egypt was the very source of the deadly bubonic plague, which has been commonly thought by historians to have its origins from the Near East. Panagiotakopulu found fossilized fleas in ancient Egyptian's habitations, as well as remains of Nile rats that could have carried the disease. She speculates that the Nile River Valley was a natural habitat for flea-carrying rats and that endemic flooding drove large rat populations into urban areas.

PRIMARY SOURCE

Yersinia pestis Orientalis in Remains of Ancient Plague Patients

SOURCE: *Drancourt, M., et al. "Yersinia pestis orientalis* in Remains of Ancient Plague Patients." Emerging Infectious Diseases *(February 2007). This article can also be found online at https://wwwnc.cdc.gov/eid/article/13/2/pdfs/06-0197.pdf (accessed May 28, 2017).*

INTRODUCTION: *In this extract from the journal* Emerging Infectious Diseases, *author Michel Drancourt presents his evidence that* Yersinia pestis *was the cause of at least two historical pandemic plagues using the classic form for reporting in scientific journals. Michel Drancourt is the director of Institut Fédératif de Recherche. His research interests are paleomicrobiology of plague and bartonelloses.*

Abstract

Yersinia pestis DNA was recently detected in human remains from 2 ancient plague pandemics in France and Germany. We have now sequenced *Y. pestis* glpD gene in such remains, showing a 93-bp deletion specific for biotype Orientalis. These data show that only Orientalis type caused the 3 plague pandemics.

Three historical pandemics have been attributed to plague. The causative agent, *Yersinia pestis*, was discovered at the beginning of the ongoing third pandemic. The etiology [origin or cause] of the 5th–7th-century first pandemic and the 14th–18th-century second pandemic, however, remained putative until recently.

THE STUDY

We had historical evidence that 3 mass graves excavated in France were used to bury bubonic plague victims. In Vienne, 12 skeletons, including 5 children, buried within the ruins of a Roman temple have been dated from the 7th–9th centuries both by a 5th-century coin and ^{14}C dating. In Martigues, 205 skeletons buried in 5 trenches were dated from 1720 to 1721 on the basis of coins and detailed parish bills that listed the victims. In Marseille, 216 skeletons buried in a huge pit dated from a May 1722 epidemic relapse. We previously confirmed the diagnosis of plague at this site. Eighteen teeth from 5 skeletons in Vienne, 13 teeth from 5 skeletons in Martigues, and 5 teeth from 3 skeletons in Marseille were processed for the search for *Y. pestis* DNA in the dental pulp. The teeth were processed according to published criteria for authenticating molecular data in paleomicrobiology: 1) there should be no positive control; 2) negative controls, as similar as possible to the ancient specimens, should test negative; 3) a new primer sequence targeting a genome region not previously amplified in the laboratory should be used (suicide PCR); 4) any amplicon should be sequenced; 5) a second amplified and sequenced target should confirm any positive result; and 6) an original sequence that differs from modern homologs should be obtained to exclude contamination.

Accordingly, DNA samples were submitted for suicide-nested PCR conducted by using 1 negative control (18th-century teeth from skeletons of persons without anthropologic and macroscopic evidence of infection) for every 3 specimens. The sequences were compared in the GenBank database (www.ncbi.nlm.nih.gov/GenBank) using the multisequence alignment Clustal within the BISANCE environment.

Conclusions

In this study, contamination of the ancient specimens is unlikely because of the extensive precautions we took, including use of the suicide PCR protocol excluding positive controls. Accordingly, glpD gene had never been investigated in our laboratory before this study, and negative controls remained negative. The specificity of the amplicons was ensured by complete similarity of experimental sequences with that of the *Y. pestis Orientalis* glpD gene. One site (Marseille, 1722) was previously positive for *Y. pestis* after sequencing of 2 different targets (chromosome-borne *rpob* and plasmid-borne *pla* genes) in other specimens collected in other persons' remains.

These results therefore confirm the detection of *Y. pestis*-specific DNA in plague patients' remains from the first and second epidemics. We observed a 93-bp in-frame deletion within the glpD gene sequences obtained from ancient dental pulp specimens. This deletion has been found only in Orientalis biotype isolates in 2 independent studies comprising a total of 77 and 260 *Y. pestis* isolates, respectively, of the 4 biotypes.

After previous demonstration of *Y. pestis* Orientalis biotype multiple spacer type sequences in Justinian and medieval specimens, we now have cumulative evidence using 2 different molecular approaches that *Y. pestis* closely related to the Orientalis biotype was responsible for the 3 historical plague pandemics.

BIBLIOGRAPHY

Books

Boccaccio, Giovanni. *The Decameron*. Translated by Mark Musa. New York: Signet, 1992.

Bollet, Alfred J. *Plagues and Poxes: The Impact of Human History on Epidemic Disease*. New York: Demos Medical, 2004.

Carmichael, Anne G. *Plague and the Poor in Renaissance Florence*. Cambridge, UK: Cambridge University Press, 1986.

McNeill, William Hardy. *Plagues and Peoples*. New York: Doubleday, 1998.

Procopius. *History of the Wars*. Translated by H. B. Dewing. Cambridge, MA: Harvard University Press, 1914.

Varlik, Nükhet. *Plague and Empire in the Early Modern Mediterranean World: The Ottoman Experience, 1347–1600*. New York: Cambridge University Press, 2015.

Wrigley, E. A., and R. S. Scofield. *The Population History of England, 1541–1871: A Reconstruction*. Cambridge, MA: Harvard University Press, 1984.

Periodicals

DeWitte, Sharon. "Mortality Risk and Survival in the Aftermath of the Medieval Black Death." *PLOS ONE* 9, no. 5 (2015): e96513.

Eltagouri, Marwa, and Cleve R. Wootson Jr. "Rats Used to Spread the Black Death. Now, Poverty Plays a Role." *Washington Post* (October 7, 2017). This article can also be found online at https://www.washingtonpost.com/news/to-your-health/wp/2017/10/05/black-death-outbreak-strikes-madagascar-killing-30-and-triggering-panic/?utm_term=.a3517d7c2c49 (accessed November 6, 2017).

Gross, C. P., and K. A. Sepkowitz. "The Myth of the Medical Breakthrough: Smallpox, Vaccination, and Jenner Reconsidered." *International Journal of Infectious Disease* 3 (1998): 54–60.

Littman, R. J., and M. L. Littman. "Galen and the Antonine Plague." *American Journal of Philology* 94, no. 3 (Autumn 1973): 243–255.

Morgan, Thomas E. "Plague or Poetry? Thucydides on the Epidemic at Athens." *Transactions of the American Philological Association* 124 (1994: 197–209.

Russell, Josiah C. "That Earlier Plague." *Demography* 5, no. 1 (1968): 174–184.

Websites

Walker, Cameron. "Bubonic Plague Traced to Ancient Egypt." National Geographic News, March 10, 2004. http://news.nationalgeographic.com/news/2004/03/0310_040310_blackdeath.html (accessed May 17, 2007).

Anna Marie E. Roos

Plague, Modern History

Introduction

Plague is a greatly feared disease that has killed millions of people since medieval times. It is caused by the bacterium *Yersinia pestis*, which is carried by flea-infested rodents. Bubonic plague has a case-fatality ratio of 30 to 60 percent, and the pneumonic plague is always fatal if left untreated. The third pandemic of plague extended into the 20th century and stimulated research into the cause and transmission of the disease.

There have been no major epidemics of plague in the United States for many years, although occasional cases still occur in the Southwest. From 2010 to 2015, the World Health Organization (WHO) reported 3,248 cases globally, including 584 deaths. The three most endemic countries are Madagascar, Peru, and the Democratic Republic of the Congo (DRC), and most outbreaks occur in Africa, Southeast Asia, and Latin America. It may not be possible to eradicate plague, but outbreaks can be prevented by reducing rodent populations. Constant vigilance regarding plague is also necessary because it has some potential as an agent of a bioterrorist attack.

Disease History, Characteristics, and Transmission

Yersinia pestis is a Gram-negative bacillus (rod-shaped) bacterium that was discovered as the cause of plague by Swiss researcher Alexandre-Emile-John Yersin (1863–1943) in 1894. The term *Gram-negative* refers to the way in which the bacterium absorbs the Gram stain used to prepare bacterial cultures for microscopy. The incubation period of *Y. pestis* is between two and eight days, and the microbe produces three types of plague: bubonic, pneumonic, and septicemic.

Bubonic plague accounts for 90 to 95 percent of all cases and is marked by sudden onset of fever, chills, weakness, and headache. Initially, these could be mistaken for flu symptoms. Shortly after, multiplication of the bacteria within the lymph glands of the armpits and groin causes characteristic swellings, called buboes, which are extremely tender, typically between 0.8 inches (2 centimeters) and 4.0 inches (10 centimeters) in diameter, and hot to the touch.

The disease often progresses to bleeding from the gastrointestinal, respiratory, or genitourinary tract, leading to the name "Red Death." Gangrene may occur on the nose or penis, leading to the name "Black Death." This name was also given to some of the plague epidemics in history. These complications are caused by the spread of the bacterium throughout the bloodstream and the effects of associated toxins. Untreated bubonic plague has a death rate of more than 50 percent.

Pneumonic plague may occur as a complication of bubonic plague and also accounts for 5 percent of primary cases. Symptoms include bloody sputum, chest pain, coughing, and breathlessness. The disease is highly infectious. Septicemic plague has similar symptoms to bubonic plague—apart from the buboes—and accounts for around 5 percent of cases, with extensive bloodstream infection being the most significant feature.

Plague is a zoonosis, a disease of animals that can infect humans. Rodents act as the animal reservoir for the disease. When fleas bite an animal infected with *Y. pestis*, they can carry the disease to other rodents. The animals become sick, and, when they start to die, the fleas will seek out human hosts as an alternative source of blood meals. The main flea vector is the Oriental rat flea, *Xenopsylla cheopis.*

Humans generally become infected with plague through the bite of an infected flea or from handling an infected animal and coming into contact with its tissues or body fluids. In the United States, wild rodents are the most common animal reservoirs for plague, with the rock squirrel being implicated in the majority of cases in the Southwest. In the Pacific states, the California ground squirrel is the most important source of plague. Prairie dogs, wood rats, chipmunks, and other burrowing rodents have also been involved in US cases of plague. Other, less frequent sources include wild rabbits, wild carnivores, and

WORDS TO KNOW

BIOWEAPON A weapon that uses bacteria, viruses, or poisonous substances made by bacteria or viruses.

BUBO A swollen lymph gland, usually in the groin or armpit, characteristic of infection with bubonic plague.

EPIDEMIC An outbreak of an illness or disease in which the number of individual cases significantly exceeds the usual or expected number of cases in any given population.

FLEA Any parasitic insect of the order *Siphonaptera*. Fleas can infest many mammals, including humans, and can act as carriers (vectors) of disease.

GANGRENE The destruction of body tissue by a bacteria called *Clostridium perfringens* or a combination of streptococci and staphylococci bacteria. *C. perfringens* is widespread; it is found in soil and the intestinal tracts of humans and animals. It becomes dangerous only when its spores germinate, producing toxins and destructive enzymes, and germination occurs only in an anaerobic environment (one almost totally devoid of oxygen). While gangrene can develop in any part of the body, it is most common in fingers, toes, hands, feet, arms, and legs, the parts of the body most susceptible to restricted blood flow. Even a slight injury in such an area is at high risk of causing gangrene. Early treatment with antibiotics, such as penicillin, and surgery to remove the dead tissue will often reduce the need for amputation. If left untreated, gangrene results in amputation or death.

GRAM-NEGATIVE BACTERIA Bacteria whose cell walls are composed of an inner and outer membrane that are separated from one another by a region called the periplasm. The periplasm also contains a thin but rigid layer called the peptidoglycan.

MULTIDRUG RESISTANCE A phenomenon that occurs when an infective agent loses its sensitivity against two or more of the drugs that are used against it.

NOTIFIABLE DISEASE A disease that the law requires be reported to health officials when diagnosed. Also called a reportable disease.

PANDEMIC An epidemic that occurs in more than one country or population simultaneously. *Pandemic* means "all the people."

RESERVOIR The animal or organism in which a virus or parasite normally resides.

ZOONOSES Diseases of microbiological origin that can be transmitted from animals to people. The causes of the diseases can be bacteria, viruses, parasites, or fungi.

domestic cats and dogs, which pick up infected fleas from wild rodents. In addition, pneumonic plague can be spread from person to person through inhalation of infected secretions.

The *Y. pestis* bacteria quickly enter white blood cells in the bloodstream, where they multiply and produce toxins. They spread throughout the blood and may cause disseminated intravascular coagulation (multiple tiny blood clots), which leads to the complications of plague.

■ Scope and Distribution

Plaque has been responsible for three known pandemics during the course of human history. The first began in the middle of the 6th century and is known as the Justinian plague. It was followed in the middle of the 14th century by the pandemic popularly known as the Black Death. The third, or Modern, pandemic of plague began in the mid-1800s in China and spread throughout the world to cause nearly 30 million cases and more than 12 million deaths between 1896 and 1930.

By the time of the third pandemic, scientists had developed methods for investigating microbial causes of disease that could be applied to this serious public health problem. Yersin discovered *Y. pestis* in 1894, and the transmission of plague via fleas was reported by Paul-Louis Simond (1858–1947) in 1890. This new understanding, together with the later introduction of antibiotics, meant that plague began to exact less of a toll on human life in many countries. Twenty-first-century techniques of analyzing DNA have led to new insights into ancient cases of plague from previous pandemics, using samples from the dental pulp of victims' remains.

Plague continues to cause both sporadic cases and epidemics involving hundreds of people, with the numbers involved depending on geographical location. The disease is found in Africa, Southeast Asia, Latin America, and in the southwestern United States. In Africa there have been severe outbreaks since 1980 in Tanzania, South Africa, the DRC, Zimbabwe, Mozambique, Malawi, Namibia, Kenya, and Uganda.

Smaller outbreaks have occurred in other East African countries. Sporadic cases have been reported from North and West Africa. The disease also occurs regularly in Madagascar, where multidrug resistance has been reported. In Asia countries that are particularly affected by plague include Burma (Myanmar), Vietnam, and Indonesia. In Latin America plague is found in the Andean mountain region and in Brazil. However, there is no plague in Australia or Europe.

In North America most human cases of plague occur in two specific regions. One is in northern New Mexico, northern Arizona, and southern Colorado. The other is in California, southern Oregon, and far western Nevada. The highest rates are in Native Americans, particularly Navajos, as well as among hunters, veterinarians and pet owners handling infected animals, and campers or hikers entering areas with outbreaks of animal plague. The last urban epidemic of plague in the United States occurred in Los Angeles between 1924 and 1925.

In the United States, there is an average of 15 cases of plague each year, of which one in seven proves fatal. In Africa, Asia, and Latin America, there were major outbreaks each year in the 1980s. These cases tend to be associated with domestic rats and were more common among those living in small towns, villages, and agricultural areas than among the population in urban areas.

The major risk factor for epidemic plague is poor living conditions with rodent and flea infestation, coupled with human overcrowding. Lab workers handling plague bacteria are also at high risk.

WHO received reports of outbreaks of pneumonic plague in the DRC in 2005 and 2006. The disease has long been endemic in the Ituri region. In mid-2005 there was an outbreak near the town of Zobia in a forest area that had attracted several thousand people responding to reports of the discovery of diamonds there. The outbreak involved 124 cases of pneumonic plague and 56 deaths. Investigators from WHO found suspect rodents and poor sanitary conditions at the affected site. The situation was made worse by panic, with many people fleeing the outbreak and dying along forest trails, spreading this highly infectious disease. It was no surprise, therefore, when there were further outbreaks in the DRC in the months following.

In October 2006 there were 626 more suspected cases of pneumonic plague, including 42 deaths, in the DRC. However, because this would be an unusually low death rate for pneumonic plague, WHO believed there might have been an overestimation of the number of cases. A team from the humanitarian group Médecins sans Frontières (Doctors Without Borders) worked with WHO and the local health authority in the DRC doing lab tests, case management, and contact tracing to bring the outbreak under control.

In November 2014 WHO was notified about an outbreak of plague in Madagascar. Cases of pneumonic and bubonic plague occurred in nearly half its districts, with the Analamanga Region the most affected. From August 1 through November 22, a total of 2,348 cases were confirmed, with 202 deaths. With the support of WHO, the Ministry of Public Health and Institute Pasteur of Madagascar coordinated the response, training more than 1,800 community health workers. Plague treatment centers were established, and exit screening was instituted at airports. Proximal countries such as Ethiopia, Kenya, Mozambique,

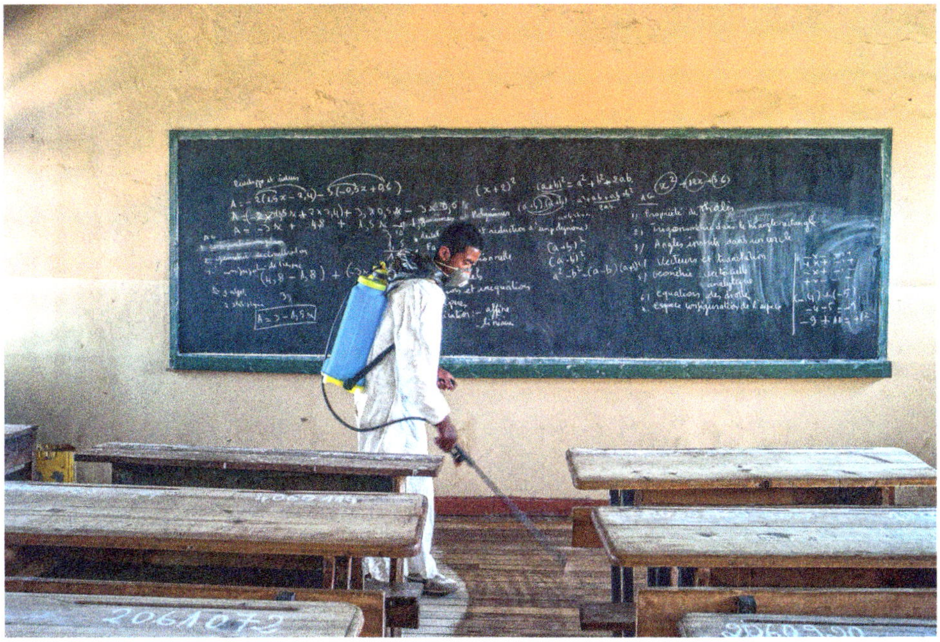

A worker from Madagascar's Department of Emergency and Response to Epidemics and Disasters (SURECA) disinfects a school during a plague outbreak in October 2017. *© Henitsoa Rafalia/Anadolu Agency/Getty Images*

South Africa, Tanzania, Comoros, and the Seychelles were put on health alerts and implemented readiness activities. As a result of these efforts, no travel or trade restrictions were in force against Madagascar as of November 2017, though WHO advised travelers to take precautions to protect their health. Insect repellent, avoiding contact with sick or dead animals, and avoiding contact with ill people are ways travelers can protect themselves.

Plague is notifiable to the Centers for Disease Control and Prevention (CDC). Its location in Fort Collins, Colorado, is a WHO Collaborating Center for Reference and Research on Plague Control, reporting all human plague cases in the United States to WHO. Also, the National Notifiable Disease Surveillance System carries out surveillance on animal plague, reports human cases, and carries out lab testing on fleas, animal tissues, and blood samples.

■ Treatment and Prevention

Antibiotic treatment reduces the mortality rate of plague from more than 50 percent to around 10 percent. Streptomycin and gentamicin are the preferred drugs, but doxycycline, tetracycline, or chloramphenicol can be used as an alternative. Levofloxacin and ciprofloxacin have been approved by the Food and Drug Administration for treatment based on animal studies. Anyone with plague must be isolated and hospitalized. However, with prompt diagnosis and treatment, nearly everyone with plague can expect to recover.

The contacts of plague cases must be traced and treated with antibiotics to help stop the infection from developing. They should also be disinfested of any fleas they may be carrying. Passengers traveling back from plague-endemic areas are generally subject to quarantine regulations in case they are incubating the disease.

Preventive antibiotics can be taken if someone has been exposed to the bites of wild rodent fleas during an outbreak or to the tissues or fluids of a plague-infected animal. The same treatment is appropriate for those who have been exposed to a person or pet with suspected plague, especially if it is pneumonic plague. However, because multidrug resistance has begun to emerge in Madagascar, it has to be assumed that it could also happen elsewhere.

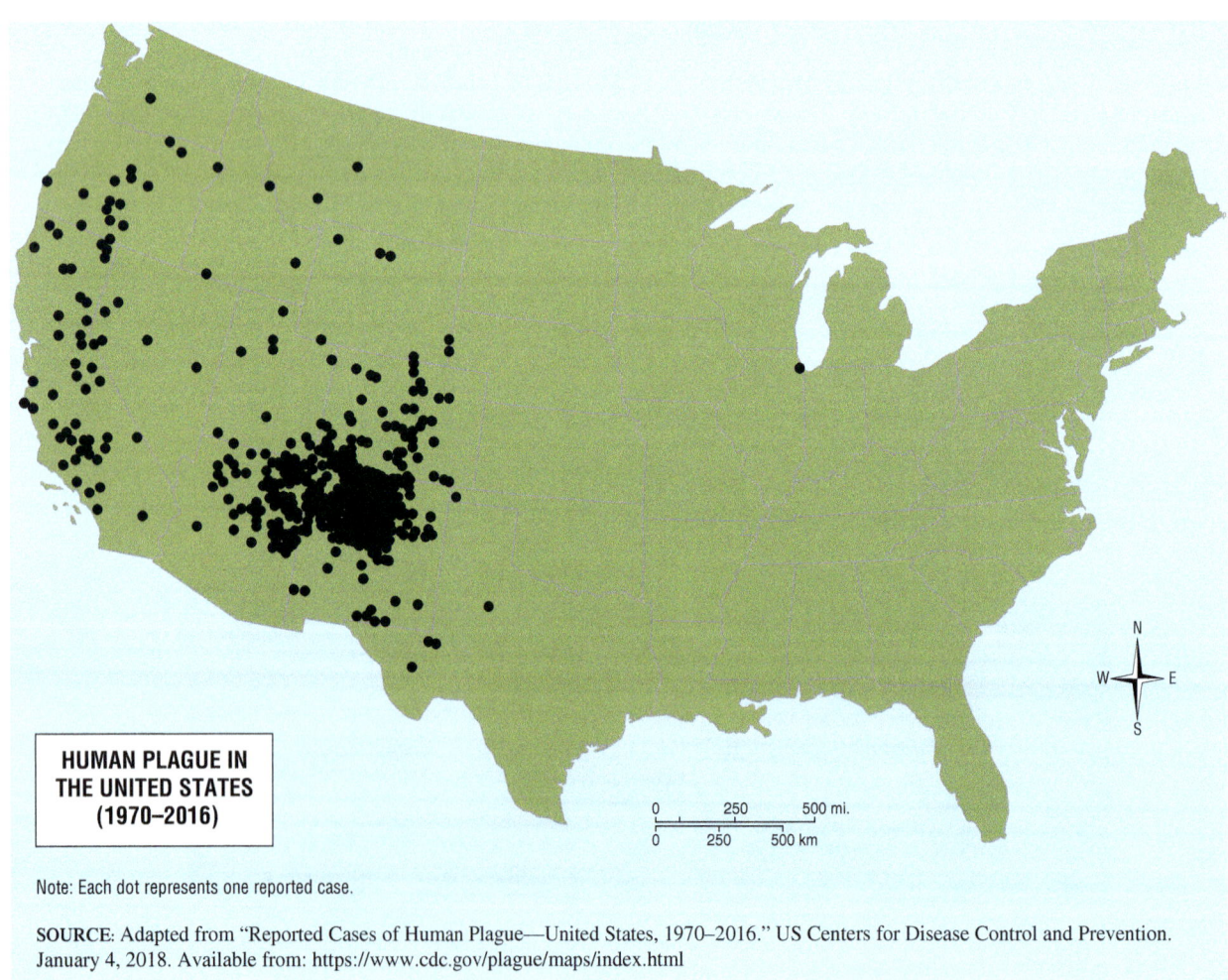

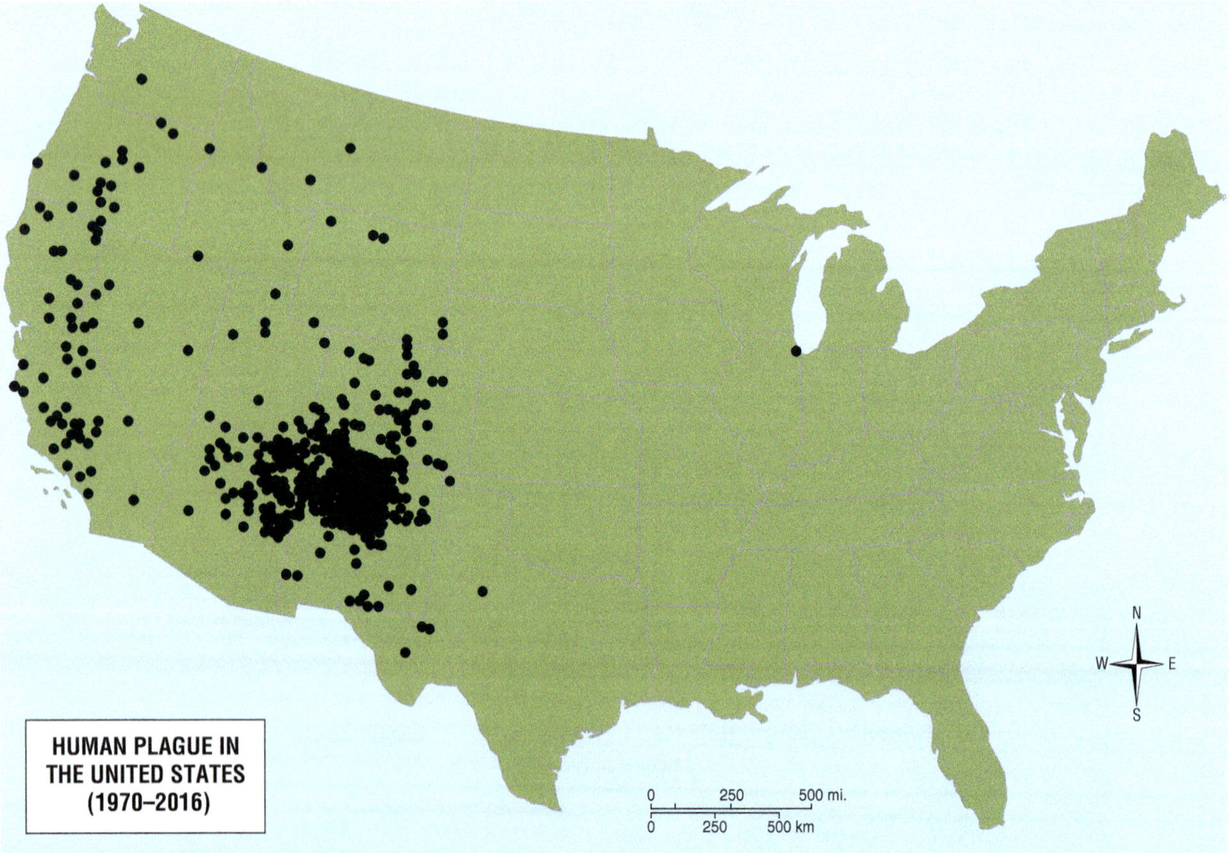

Note: Each dot represents one reported case.

SOURCE: Adapted from "Reported Cases of Human Plague—United States, 1970–2016." US Centers for Disease Control and Prevention. January 4, 2018. Available from: https://www.cdc.gov/plague/maps/index.html

Although vaccines against plague have been used in the past, these are not available in the United States. Research has shown that the vaccine does not help reduce the number of cases or the spread of infection during an outbreak. However, it may have a role to play in protecting those who are repeatedly exposed through lab or health care work.

Prevention of plague among the population depends on controlling fleas and rodents. People living in those regions of the United States where plague infection is active need to take care to avoid exposure. Sick or dead rodents, which may be infected with plague, should be reported to local health authorities and should never be handled.

Keeping homes, workplaces, and recreation areas clear of food and nesting places for rodents is extremely important. Junk, firewood, and rock piles should be removed to make these places rodent-proof. Insect repellents applied to clothing and skin can reduce the risk of exposure to potentially infected fleas. Cats and dogs need to be regularly treated with flea-control agents and should not be allowed to roam freely, in case they come into contact with infected rodents. Investigation of outbreaks and sporadic cases of plague often lead to the identification of a clustered area of animal die-offs that is the exposure source and needs to be disposed of.

Impacts and Issues

Plague has been a public health problem for several centuries, and, unlike polio and smallpox, it is unlikely that it can ever be eradicated. Between outbreaks *Y. pestis* lives on in certain rodent populations without actually wiping them out, thereby constituting a silent, long-term reservoir of infection. The best that can be hoped for is to employ control and precautionary measures in those places where humans and flea-infested rodents are likely to interact.

Although sporadic cases of plague do occur in the southwestern United States, these can be avoided with commonsense precautions regarding contact with potentially infected rodents. Efforts to control plague probably need to be focused where conditions create a risk of disease outbreak or even epidemics. This means managing unsanitary rat-infested environments to make places where people live, work, or play safer.

Control of rat populations in rural and urban areas of many developing countries has not yet been achieved to the extent that it has in most developed countries. Close surveillance of both rodents and humans for plague is the first step in tightening controls. Insecticides can be used to control rodent fleas in danger areas, and efforts can be made to reduce the local population of rodents in human-inhabited areas by removing potential food sources and nesting sites.

In the future, however, plague may become even more unpredictable. Changing climate due to global warming and population movements may create new environments where flea-infested rodents can flourish and put people at risk of plague.

A further threat of the spread of plague comes from its potential use as a bioweapon. The concern centers on pneumonic plague, which is highly infectious and can spread rapidly from person to person. An aerosol-based biological weapon could introduce *Y. pestis* into the population without warning, causing a severe epidemic within just a few days. Containment would depend on rapid detection of cases and treatment of these people, and their contacts, with antibiotics within 24 hours. Public health authorities in the United States hold large stocks of the appropriate antibiotics, and the CDC says these could be made available to any location where they are needed within 12 hours.

There is no plague vaccine available in the United States. Research into such a vaccine by academics and the US Army is ongoing.

The threat of bioterrorism has refocused attention on plague as a problem that has been largely absent from developed countries, including the United States, for many years except in sporadic form. In many African countries and in parts of Southeast Asia, plague is still an endemic public health issue that leads to hundreds of deaths each year. The US bioterrorism effort can learn from what is known of the natural history of plague in other countries and use molecular technologies to better understand the disease. A bioterrorist attack with *Y. pestis* may never happen, but the knowledge gained in preparing for a potential attack may help better diagnosis, treatment, and prevention efforts in those places where the disease occurs naturally.

SEE ALSO *Bioterrorism; CDC (Centers for Disease Control and Prevention); Médicins Sans Frontièrs (Doctors Without Borders); Plague, Early History; World Health Organization*

BIBLIOGRAPHY

Books

Török, Estée, Ed Moran, and Fiona J. Cooke. *Oxford Handbook of Infectious Diseases and Microbiology.* Oxford, UK: Oxford University Press, 2017.

Periodicals

Butler, T. "Plague History: Yersin's Discovery of the Causative Bacterium in 1894 Enabled, in the Subsequent Century, Scientific Progress in Understanding the Disease and the Development of Treatments and Vaccines." *Clinical Microbiology and Infection* 20, no. 3 (March 2014): 202–209.

Drancourt, M., and D. Raoult. "Molecular Insights into the History of Plague." *Microbes and Infection* 4, no. 1 (January 2002): 105–109.

Websites

"Plague." Centers for Disease Control and Prevention. https://www.cdc.gov/plague/index.html (accessed January 29, 2018).

"Plague: Fact Sheet." World Health Organization, October 2017. http://www.who.int/mediacentre/factsheets/fs267/en (accessed January 29, 2018).

"Plague Outbreak Highlighted Ongoing Problem in Africa." Center for Infectious Disease Research and Policy, May 27, 2005. http://www.cidrap.umn.edu/cidrap/content/bt/plague/news/may2705plag.html (accessed January 29, 2018).

Susan Aldridge
Anna Marie E. Roos

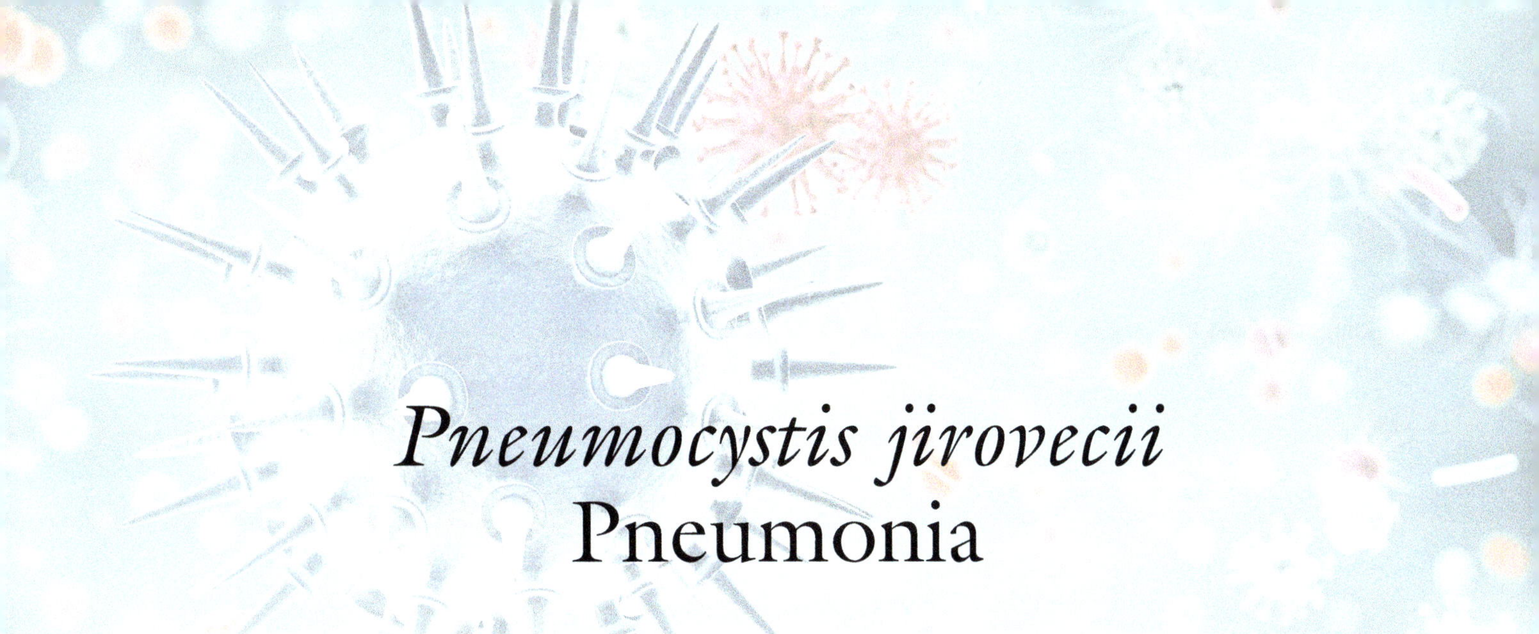

Pneumocystis jirovecii Pneumonia

Introduction

Pneumocystis jirovecii pneumonia is a potentially fatal infection that affects patients with compromised immune systems. *Pneumocystis jirovecii* pneumonia was previously known as *Pneumocystis carinii* pneumonia. The acronym PCP is still used to refer to the infection despite the name change. PCP is the most common opportunistic infection among people with human immunodeficiency virus (HIV) and remains a leading cause of mortality in this patient group within the United States. However, rates of infection have declined since the development of antiretroviral therapy for HIV patients. In patients who do not have HIV, PCP presents with more subtle symptoms.

P. jirovecii is a fungus that is found in the respiratory tract of humans and other mammals. Its distribution is widespread, and evidence suggests that approximately 80 percent of children between the ages of two and four are exposed to it. However, *P. jirovecii* only causes disease among those with impaired immunity. Its appearance among previously healthy homosexual men in the early 1980s was an early warning sign of the emergence of HIV and acquired immunodeficiency syndrome (AIDS). Although infections in older HIV patients have declined, rates of PCP remain high in HIV-infected children. Other at-risk groups include those who have cancer and those receiving immunosuppressive drugs following an organ transplant. PCP is treatable with antibiotics, and survival rates have improved as antiretroviral therapy has become increasingly available. Physicians have also begun to treat PCP preemptively (prophylaxis) by administering preventive drugs to at-risk patients to prevent PCP infection from taking hold.

Pneumocystis jirovecii Pneumonia Symptoms

Dry cough
Dyspnea (difficult breathing)
Hypoxia (lack of oxygen reaching tissue)
Chest pain
Fever
Fatigue (tiredness)

In people infected with human immunodeficiency virus (HIV) or suffering from acquired immunodeficiency syndrome (AIDS), *Pneumocystis jirovecii* pneumonia symptoms tend to develop gradually. In those who have weakened immune systems due to other causes, such as cancer or organ transplantation, symptoms usually develop more suddenly.

SOURCE: US Centers for Disease Control and Prevention

Disease History, Characteristics, and Transmission

PCP was first noted during World War II (1939–1945) among malnourished and premature infants in Central and Eastern Europe. Infections were also observed in malnourished children in Iranian orphanages in the 1950s. In the 1960s PCP infections were described primarily in adults and children with both acquired and congenital immune-system deficiencies. As organ transplants became increasingly common in the second half of the 20th century, organ recipients were also identified as at risk for PCP due to drug regimens that deliberately weaken the immune system to reduce the likelihood that donor organs will be rejected.

Prior to the 1980s, PCP was rare in the United States, with fewer than 100 cases a year, mainly among patients undergoing chemotherapy or in those who had received a solid organ transplant. However, in 1981 the US Centers for Disease Control and Prevention (CDC) reported an unusual finding: five cases of PCP in homosexual men who had no known immunodeficiency. As researchers examined these patients, they discovered a novel underlying cause: a condition that became known as acquired immunodeficiency syndrome (AIDS). PCP acted, therefore, as the first warning of the AIDS epidemic. HIV, the causative agent

WORDS TO KNOW

AIRBORNE TRANSMISSION The ability of a disease-causing (pathogenic) microorganism to be spread through the air by droplets expelled during sneezing or coughing.

CD4+ T CELLS A type of T cell found in the immune system that are characterized by the presence of a CD4 antigen protein on their surface. These are the cells most often destroyed as a result of HIV infection.

MORTALITY The condition of being susceptible to death. The term *mortality* comes from the Latin word *mors*, which means death. Mortality can also refer to the rate of deaths caused by an illness or injury (e.g., "Rabies has a high mortality rate").

OPPORTUNISTIC INFECTION An infection that occurs in people whose immune systems are diminished or are not functioning normally. Such infections are opportunistic insofar as the infectious agents take advantage of their hosts' compromised immune systems and invade to cause disease.

PROPHYLAXIS Pre-exposure treatment (e.g., immunizations) to prevent the onset or recurrence of a disease.

PROTOZOA Single-celled, animal-like microscopic organisms that live by taking in food rather than making it by photosynthesis and must live in the presence of water. (Singular: protozoan.) Protozoa are a diverse group of single-celled organisms, with more than 50,000 different types represented. The vast majority are microscopic, many measuring less than 5 one-thousandth of an inch (0.005 millimeters), but some, such as the freshwater Spirostomum, may reach 0.17 inches (3 millimeters) in length, large enough to enable it to be seen with the naked eye.

of AIDS, attacks and destroys the immune system, leaving those infected susceptible to PCP, an opportunistic infection.

The increase of AIDS cases in the 1980s led to more research into the characteristics, causes, and treatment of PCP. In the early 20th century, *P. jirovecii* was thought to be protozoan and was classified as such. In 1988, however, more detailed biochemical studies established that the organism was structured like a fungus.

P. jirovecii is spread by airborne transmission. Most people have been infected by *P. jirovecii* in early childhood. It is harmless in a healthy person, but if immunity is weakened for any reason, it can invade the lungs, causing pneumonia. Although physicians long believed that PCP occurred as a result of a latent infection being reactivated as a patient's immune system deteriorated, research conducted in the 1990s and bolstered by research in the 21st century indicates that PCP actually occurs as a result of a new infection.

According to David Crockett and Nicole Shonka in *Infections in the Immunosuppressed Patient* (2016), "The clinical presentation [of PCP] is different in HIV-infected patients and patients not infected with HIV, notably those with cancer." The authors noted that HIV-infected patients with PCP have "insidious" symptoms "with subtle findings of progressive dyspnea [difficult breathing], and dry cough," whereas in cancer patients and others with immunosuppression, the onset of symptoms usually occurs "more abrupt in the manner of a few days with dyspnea, hypoxia [deficiency in oxygen reaching tissue], dry cough, and low-grade fevers." Although treatment is often effective, PCP proves fatal in approximately 10 to 20 percent of mild to moderate cases and in 65 percent of severe cases. Overall, survival rates for PCP have improved greatly over the past decade as antiretroviral therapy has become increasingly available for patients with HIV.

The organism that actually causes PCP was renamed *P. jirovecii* after Otto Jirovec (1907–1972), the researcher who first isolated it in human subjects. The proposal to change the organism's name was first made in 1976 but did not begin to catch on until 1999, when a second proposal to change the name was made.

Scope and Distribution

Between the early 1980s and the mid-1990s, rates of PCP soared due to the HIV/AIDS epidemic. By the late 1980s approximately three-quarters of people with AIDS had also developed PCP. As the AIDS epidemic reached its peak in the late 1990s, with nearly a million new HIV infections reported each year and high rates of fatality, researchers discovered a promising new treatment known as highly active antiretroviral therapy (HAART). HAART can dramatically suppress HIV replication in patients, allowing their immune systems to function properly and preventing opportunistic infections such as PCP.

Since HAART was first developed in 1996, it has gradually become more widely available. In the process, it has enabled people with HIV/AIDS to live longer lives and has significantly reduced rates of PCP in HIV-positive people, even as the number of people living with HIV and AIDS reached a peak of 36.7 million in 2016. A lack of reporting, however, makes it impossible to determine the exact rate of PCP infection in HIV-positive people as of 2017.

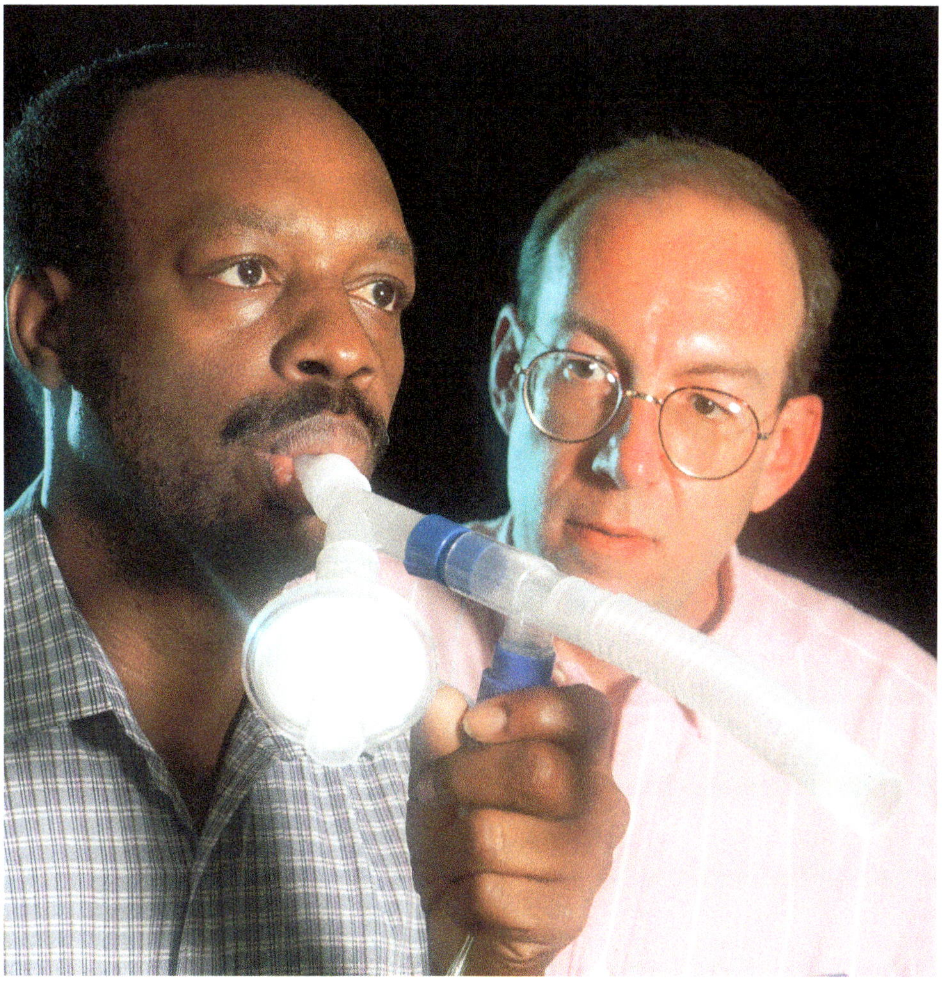

A man being treated for AIDS inhales aerosol pentamidine. The drug is given to prevent *Pneumocystis carinii* pneumonia. © *Roger Ressmeyer/Corbis/VCG/Getty Images*

Despite an overall decline in rates of PCP in people with HIV/AIDS, evidence suggests PCP infection in children with HIV in the developing world are on the rise. According to a 2013 report from the National Institutes of Health, "autopsies done in Africa revealed PCP in 16% of children who died with HIV/AIDS during 1992 and 1993, in 29% of those who died during 1997 and 2000, and in 44% of those who died during 2000 and 2001." Evidence suggests up to four-fifths of HIV-positive children in Africa who present with pneumonia have PCP.

Among immunocompromised people who do not have HIV/AIDS, rates of PCP have also fallen. However, a lack of data makes it difficult to determine the exact rates.

Treatment and Prevention

Although it is a fungus, *P. jirovecii* does not actually respond to antifungal drugs. However, there are a number of antibiotics that can be used to treat it. These include trimethoprim and sulfamethoxazole, which are typically used together. Steroids may be added as an adjunctive therapy to reduce dangerous inflammation in the respiratory tract. If infection persists, doctors may have to intubate (introduce a tube into the trachea) a patient to aid in respiration. When this occurs, the chances of mortality rise to as much as 60 percent.

Although there is no PCP vaccine, preventive drug therapies have been shown to reduce the risk of infection and mortality in high-risk groups, such as cancer patients and transplant recipients. Such prophylactic drug regimens typically include corticosteroids and antibiotics.

Impacts and Issues

PCP is an ongoing threat to people with HIV/AIDS, especially in children. Evidence suggests it mainly affects those whose CD4+ T cell count is less than 200 per microliter. CD4+ T cells are a type of white blood cell that is targeted by the HIV virus. CD4+ T cell counts are an essential monitor of the condition of someone with HIV, and a drop in the count indicates a vulnerability to PCP that should be addressed. Although treatment, both to prevent and cure the infection, is available, epidemiologists and physicians continue to seek ways to reduce PCP and other opportunistic infections in immunocompromised populations.

SEE ALSO *AIDS (Acquired Immunodeficiency Syndrome); CDC (Centers for Disease Control); HIV; Opportunistic Infection; Pneumonia*

BIBLIOGRAPHY

Books

Crockett, David, and Nicole Shonka. "Case 1.15: Cough and Dyspnea in a Sarcoma Patient: Appetite for Infection." In *Infections in the Immunosuppressed Patient*, edited by Pranatharthi H. Chandrasekar. New York: Oxford University Press, 2016.

Periodicals

Castro, Jose G., and Maya Morrison-Bryant. "Management of *Pneumocystis jirovecii* Pneumonia in HIV Infected Patients: Current Options, Challenges and Future Directions." *HIV/AIDS—Research and Palliative Care* 2 (2010): 123–134. This article can also be found online at https://www.ncbi.nlm.nih.gov/pmc/articles/PMC3218692/ (accessed February 14, 2018).

Kelly, Michelle N., and Judd E. Shellito. "Current Understanding of *Pneumocystis* Immunology." *Future Microbiology* 5, no. 1 (2010): 43–65. This article can also be found online at https://www.ncbi.nlm.nih.gov/pmc/articles/PMC3702169/ (accessed February 15, 2018).

Morris, Alison, et al. "Epidemiology and Clinical Significance of *Pneumocystis* Colonization." *Journal of Infectious Diseases* 197, no. 1 (2008): 10–17. This article can also be found online at https://academic.oup.com/jid/article/197/1/10/795412 (accessed February 15, 2018).

Robert-Gangneux, Florence, et al. "Diagnosis of *Pneumocystis jirovecii* Pneumonia in Immunocompromised Patients by Real-Time PCR: A 4-Year Prospective Study." *Journal of Clinical Microbiology* 52, no. 9 (2014): 3370–3376. This article can also be found online at https://www.ncbi.nlm.nih.gov/pmc/articles/PMC4313164/ (accessed February 14, 2018).

Websites

Bennett, Nicholas John. "*Pneumocystis jiroveci* Pneumonia (PJP) Overview of *Pneumocystis jiroveci* Pneumonia." Medscape, August 8, 2017. https://emedicine.medscape.com/article/225976-overview (accessed February 14, 2018).

"*Pneumocystis jirovecii* Pneumonia." AIDS Info, National Institutes of Health, November 6, 2013. https://aidsinfo.nih.gov/guidelines/html/5/pediatric-opportunistic-infection/415/pneumocystis-jirovecii-pneumonia (accessed March 13, 2018).

"*Pneumocystis* pneumonia." Centers for Disease Control and Prevention, April 26, 2017. https://www.cdc.gov/fungal/diseases/pneumocystis-pneumonia/index.html (accessed February 14, 2018).

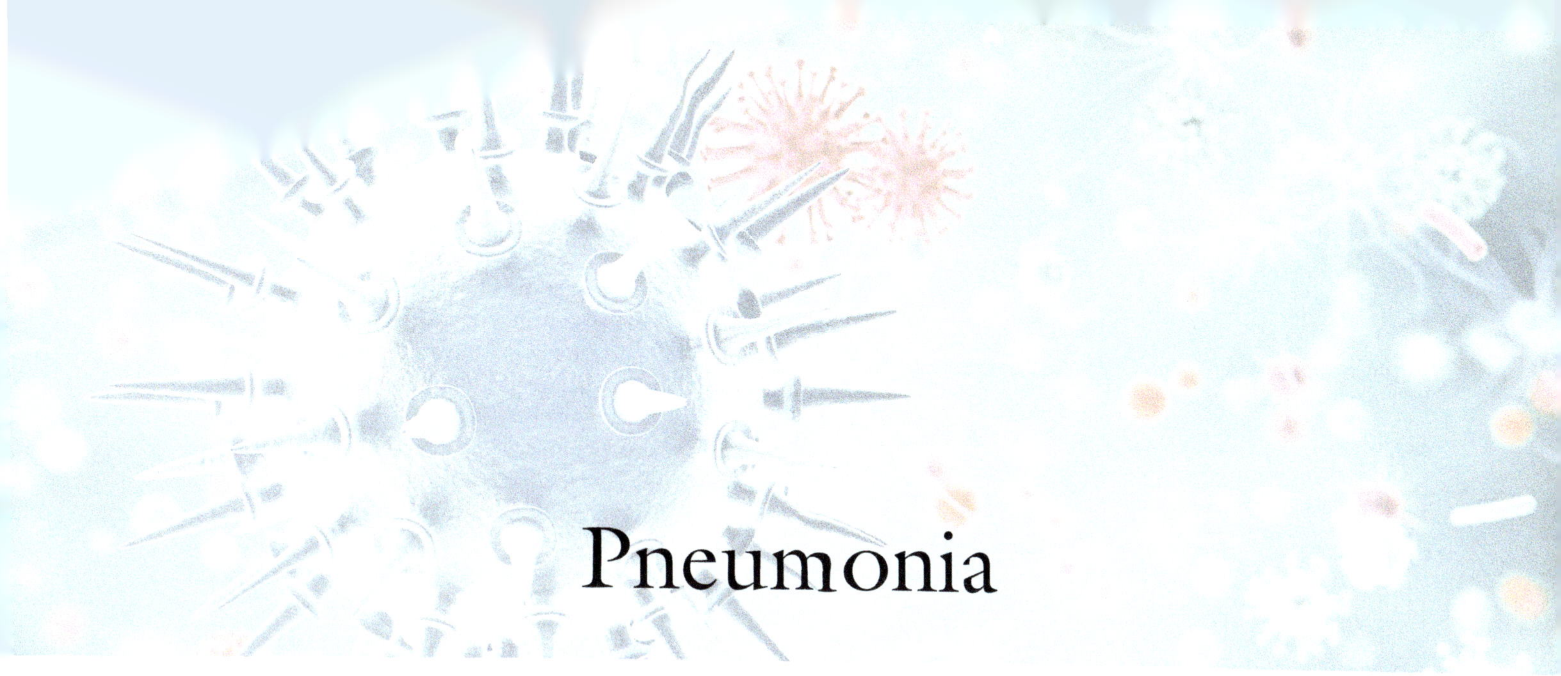

Pneumonia

Introduction

Pneumonia is an inflammatory response of the lungs to the entry of an infective organism or other foreign material. It is the leading cause of death among children worldwide and the eighth-leading cause of death among adults in the United States. It is also the leading cause of death from infection.

A complex disease with many different causes and risk factors, pneumonia can affect people of any age, anywhere, although the very young and very old are most vulnerable to an attack. Pneumonia is classified in two ways, according to its cause and according to its setting.

The cause of pneumonia can be viral, bacterial, mycobacterial, fungal, or even noninfective irritants. The setting may be either within the community or in the hospital. These distinctions are important because they influence the choice of treatment. Before the advent of antibiotics, pneumonia was a greatly feared disease because it could kill so easily. By the 21st century, with effective treatment, most people could expect to make a full recovery from pneumonia.

Disease History, Characteristics, and Transmission

Pneumonia is unlike many other infectious diseases in that it cannot be attributed to infection by one, or just a few, specific microbes. The respiratory tract, consisting of the nose, pharynx (back of the throat), trachea (windpipe), and lungs, has various mechanisms to protect itself from microbes and foreign bodies such as particulate pollution, food, liquid, or gas. The nose and trachea are lined with mucous membranes, which bear tiny beating hairs called cilia. The thick mucous traps any microbes or foreign particles as they enter through the nose and mouth, and the cilia propel them back to the nose and mouth, where they are expelled by nose blowing or are swallowed. This mechanism protects the bronchi, which are the tiny tubes fanning out to connect the trachea with the alveoli, the tiny air sacs making up the lung tissue.

The cough reflex is another of the lungs' defenses against infection, expelling foreign material before it enters the lungs. Added to this is the immune system, which triggers cells or antibodies to destroy any threatening microbes or other material. Therefore, microorganisms may colonize the upper part of the respiratory tract without causing disease, or they may cause an infection such as a cold or influenza. With the usual defenses in place, they do not invade the lungs.

If these defenses break down for any reason, such as because of the use of a mechanical ventilator in the intensive care unit (ICU) or because of weakened immunity, infection may spread to the lungs. The alveoli mediate gas exchange between the lungs and the blood, letting oxygen in and carbon dioxide out. They deal with anything that threatens this function, such as invading microbes or particulate matter, with a strong inflammatory response, which is the underlying mechanism of pneumonia. One of the main features of this inflammation is the production of a thick secretion by the lung tissue.

More than 100 different organisms can cause pneumonia, and the most significant of these depends on patient characteristics and the setting, whether in the community or in the hospital. Some of the most important viral causes of pneumonia include adenovirus, respiratory syncytial virus, influenza virus, parainfluenza virus, and cytomegalovirus. Among the bacteria that cause pneumonia are *Streptococcus pneumoniae, Chlamydia pneumoniae, Haemophilus influenzae, Klebsiella pneumoniae*, and *Pseudomonas aeruginosa*. Mycoplasma, which are organisms that have some of the characteristics of both bacteria and viruses, can also cause pneumonia.

Among patients with acquired immunodeficiency syndrome (AIDS), *Pneumocystis carinii* is a major cause of pneumonia as an opportunistic infection. Before the advent of AIDS, *P. carinii* pneumonia was rare. Its sudden appearance alerted researchers to the emergence of a new disease.

WORDS TO KNOW

ANTIBIOTIC RESISTANCE The ability of bacteria to resist the actions of antibiotic drugs.

ASPIRATION The drawing-out of fluid from a part of the body, which can cause pneumonia when stomach contents are transferred to the lungs through vomiting.

CILIA Specialized arrangements of microtubules that have two general functions. They propel certain unicellular organisms, such as paramecium, through the water. In multicellular organisms, if cilia extend from stationary cells that are part of a tissue layer, they move fluid over the surface of the tissue.

NOSOCOMIAL INFECTION An infection that is acquired in a hospital. More precisely, the US Centers for Disease Control and Prevention (CDC) in Atlanta, Georgia, defines a nosocomial infection as a localized infection or an infection that is widely spread throughout the body that results from an adverse reaction to an infectious microorganism or toxin that was not present at the time of admission to the hospital.

OPPORTUNISTIC INFECTION An infection that occurs in people whose immune systems are diminished or not functioning normally. Such infections are opportunistic insofar as the infectious agents take advantage of their hosts' compromised immune systems and invade to cause disease.

P. carinii is a fungus-like organism. Other fungi that cause pneumonia include *Histoplasma capsulatum* and *Cryptococcus neoformans.*

Pneumonia may follow an attack of influenza or even a cold, but it can also arise on its own. Anyone who suddenly starts to feel worse after the flu or a cold must get medical advice immediately. The symptoms of pneumonia vary from mild to very severe, and they may have either a gradual or a sudden onset. The nature of the symptoms also varies depending on the infecting microbe and patient characteristics. A cough, which may be either dry or productive with green or rust-colored phlegm (a discharge from the lungs), is probably the most common symptom of pneumonia. Sometimes the patient will even cough up blood. Fever, chills, and breathlessness may also occur, and there may be chest pain. However, older people may have few symptoms other than mental confusion.

Bacterial pneumonia tends to come on suddenly with fever, shaking chills, sweating, and chest pain. The cough usually produces thick greenish or yellow phlegm. The symptoms are usually more dramatic among those previously in good health.

In viral pneumonia, which is more common in the winter months, there is a dry cough, headache, fever, muscle pain, and fatigue. Breathlessness tends to develop as the disease goes on and the cough starts to produce white phlegm. Viral pneumonia is a threat in particular to people with heart or lung disease. If it does not clear up, a secondary bacterial pneumonia may take hold.

Mycoplasma pneumonia is sometimes called walking pneumonia because the symptoms are gradual and mild. Indeed, patients are not always aware they are ill. This form of pneumonia often strikes schoolchildren and young adults. It may account for up to one-third of all childhood cases.

The examining doctor will look for signs of pneumonia, such as an increase in respiration and pulse rate. Pneumonia also is associated with characteristic chest sounds that indicate the presence of fluid within the alveoli. These include bubbling, crackling sounds called rales and rumblings called ronchi, which can be heard when the doctor puts a stethoscope to the chest. Chest X-rays, and possibly computed tomography (CT) scanning, are an important part of the diagnosis of pneumonia because they reveal characteristic opacities or shadows on the affected lung. (Pneumonia may affect one or both lungs.)

The complications of pneumonia include blood poisoning, pleural effusion, and lung abscess. The alveoli are in close contact with the bloodstream, so the infection may enter the bloodstream, causing what is commonly known as blood poisoning or septicemia. When bacteria enter the bloodstream, they can reach the other organs of the body in a short time, possibly resulting in multiorgan failure and death. In pleural effusion, fluid leaks from the lungs into the space between the pleura, which are the membranes covering the lungs and the inner surface of the chest wall. This fluid could become infected, a condition known as empyema, and may have to be drained or removed surgically. Finally, an abscess, which is a cavity containing pus-infected material, may form within the lungs due to pneumonia. Although treatable with antibiotics, a lung abscess occasionally must be removed surgically.

The complications of pneumonia are more common among the elderly, the frail, and those with weakened immunity, such as HIV/AIDS patients. The prognosis of pneumonia depends on the setting and the patient. As of 2015 approximately 85 percent of all pneumonia-related deaths in the United States (44,236 out of 51,811 deaths, according to the US Centers for Disease Control and Prevention [CDC]) occurred in those over age 65. Mortality rates ranged from 0.01 per 100,000 in children and adolescents aged 5 to 14 to 378.1 per 100,000 in adults aged 85 or older. The overall death rate for community-acquired pneumonia (CAP) was less than 3 percent but exceeded 50 percent in those requiring treatment in the ICU. Overall mortality for hospital-acquired, or nosocomial, pneumonia (HAP) was around 30 percent but exceeded 70 percent among those hospitalized in the ICU. For both CAP and

HAP, the risk of death is significantly higher among patients requiring mechanical ventilation.

Pneumonia is the leading infectious cause of death in children worldwide. According to the World Health Organization (WHO), in 2015 pneumonia killed 920,136 children under the age of five, accounting for 16 percent of all deaths among this age group. Childhood pneumonia is most common in developing regions, particularly South Asia and sub-Saharan Africa. WHO notes that childhood pneumonia is relatively easy to treat and prevent. Treatment requires common pharmaceuticals, whereas prevention depends on good hygiene and nutrition.

Pneumonia is not transmitted from one person to another. Instead, it involves aspiration of microbes into the lungs from a previously colonized airway, implying that the normal defense mechanisms of the respiratory tract have broken down. It can also develop through aspiration of stomach contents, gas, or particulate pollution, all of which may inflame lung tissue.

■ Scope and Distribution

Although pneumonia is most often seen in less developed countries, it is also a major public health burden in the United States. The US National Vital Statistics report for 2014 listed influenza and infectious pneumonia as the eighth-most common cause of death among adults. It accounted for 55,227 deaths, with another 18,792 deaths ascribed to pneumonitis due to solids and liquids. Although the death rates for the two most common causes, heart disease and cancer, declined in 2014, there were significant increases in chronic lower respiratory disease, diabetes, influenza, pneumonia, and hypertension.

Respiratory problems were also the eighth-most common cause of death among newborns. The six most common causes are due to congenital problems or complications of the birth process.

Pneumonia can strike at any age, but infants and children under age four and adults over 65 are most at risk. The elderly account for almost 90 percent of all deaths from pneumonia and influenza. In adults strong risk factors for pneumonia include existing illnesses such as congestive heart failure, kidney disease, diabetes, chronic obstructive pulmonary disease (COPD), removal of the spleen, malnutrition, alcoholism, institutionalization, and dementia. Children and young adults with cystic fibrosis are especially at risk of pneumonia. For infants, low birth weight and low maternal age have been found to be risk factors for pneumonia.

Community-acquired pneumonia (CAP) refers to pneumonia contracted outside a hospital setting, such as the home, the community, a nursing home, a day care setting, a school, or another place where people congregate. The cause of CAP is often viral, but bacteria are also significant causes of CAP. Different species of bacteria are involved in causing CAP in different age groups. *Streptococcus* and pneumococcus are the most common causes of

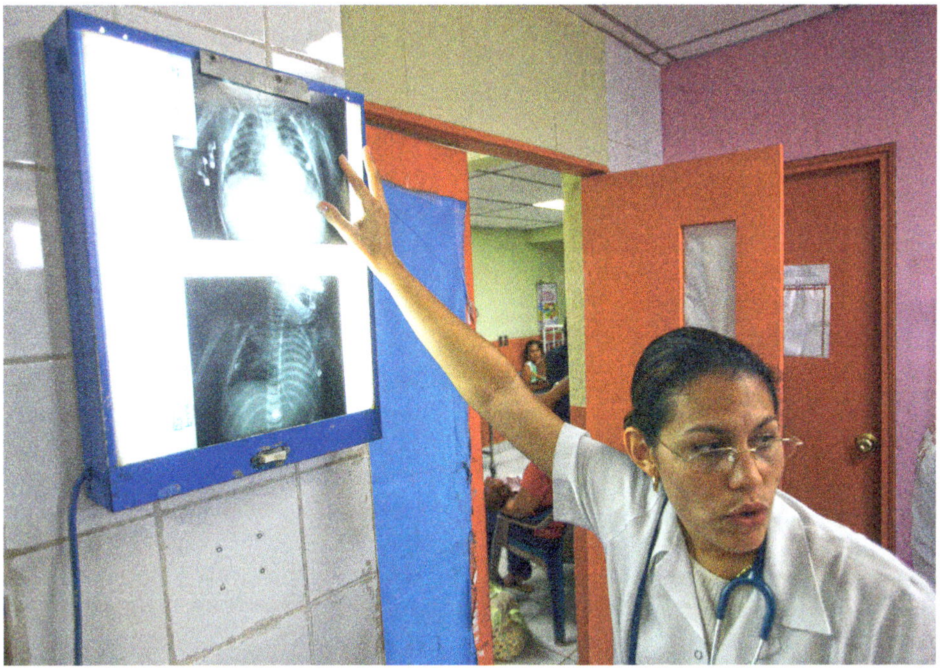

A doctor points out pneumonia on a child's X-ray in Managua, Nicaragua. The country has been working to reduce child mortality from the disease through education and vaccination programs. © *Adrian Brooks/Imagewise/Getty Images*

pneumonia, accounting for up to 35 percent of all cases. *Streptococcus* and *Staphylococcus* species of bacteria are found to be especially important in cases of pneumonia in newborns, whereas *S. pneumoniae* and *H. influenzae* infections are common in older children. *S. pneumoniae* infection is also found often in elderly people with pneumonia.

Hospital-acquired pneumonia (HAP) is one of the most significant nosocomial infections. It refers to pneumonia that develops 48 hours after hospital admission. HAP occurs at a rate of 5 to 10 per 1,000 hospital admissions in the United States. Most cases occur in the ICU or in postsurgical recovery. The risk of HAP is 6 to 20 times greater among those on mechanical ventilation. This is because ventilation involves inserting a tube into the trachea, which disrupts the natural defenses of the respiratory tract. The microbiology of HAP has been found to differ from that of CAP. Most often involved are *Klebsiella pneumoniae*, *Pseudomonas aeruginosa*, and *Serratia* and *Enterobacter* species, all of which are Gram-negative bacilli. The term *Gram-negative* or *Gram-positive* refers to the way a bacterial species reacts with a common stain used in microscopic studies.

Treatment and Prevention

Some cases of pneumonia need to be treated in the hospital. Prompt assessment by a physician is needed because the condition can progress rapidly. Increased respiratory rate, decreased blood pressure, increased temperature, and confusion are all potential indicators for hospital admission. Microbiological tests are often needed to confirm the infective organism. However, the physician often needs to start empiric antibiotic treatment before the microbiology results are available.

There is no effective treatment for viral pneumonia, which usually clears up on its own. In particular, antibiotics will not work against viruses. For those recovering from pneumonia at home, bed rest is important, along with plenty of fluids to help loosen mucus in the lungs. These patients should avoid anyone with weakened immunity, which may mean not visiting the hospital.

Many different antibiotics can be used to treat pneumonia. The American Thoracic Society (ATS) has established guidelines to help physicians choose an antibiotic for pneumonia based on the patient and the setting. For outpatients, amoxicillin, azithromycin, and levofloxacin are often used. Levofloxacin is one of a relatively new group of antibiotics known as the fluoroquinolones, which were initially thought to be useful against drug-resistant bacteria. Unfortunately, many pathogens have developed resistance to the fluoroquinolones. The Clinical Practice Guidelines by the Pediatric Infectious Diseases Society and the Infectious Diseases Society of America recommend that levofloxacin be reserved for treatment of patients who have failed a course of more traditional antibiotics.

Inpatients not in intensive care may be given the antibiotic cefotaxime, whereas intensive care patients may be treated with a combination of drugs, such as cefotaxime with a fluoroquinolone. Sometimes treatment is given by injection to reach the infection as quickly as possible. Patients with cystic fibrosis often need antibiotics in high doses and in combination.

Although the ATS guidelines remain unchanged, the widely respected Merck Manual Professional Edition has suggestions for presumptive therapy, which may be started before the pathogen has been identified and cultured. These recommendations largely follow the ATS guidelines. For children, amoxicillin would be an appropriate start. If there is evidence of an atypical pathogen, an antibiotic from the macrolide group, such as azithromycin or clarithromycin, might be preferred. If methicillin-resistant *Staphylococcus aureus* is suspected, other antibiotics, such as vancomycin or clindamycin, should be added.

For adult patients, the use of a macrolide drug is recommended. The older drugs in this class, most notably erythromycin, may cause severe gastrointestinal irritation. Therefore, the newer variants azithromycin and clarithromycin are preferred.

A meta-analysis of studies, published in 2017 on Medscape, listed additional antibiotics and anti-infectives with their appropriate use. The following is not a complete list but covers the drugs most widely used for presumptive therapy of pneumonia:

- Azithromycin: a member of the macrolide class, considered the drug of choice for initial treatment.
- Aztreonam: a monobactam, or drug with a limited spectrum, that may be useful for patients with allergies to penicillins and cephalosporins.
- Cefepime: a cephalosporin that may be administered intramuscularly.
- Cefotaxime: a cephalosporin that may be useful against resistant pathogens.
- Cefuroxime: a cephalosporin that may be useful against resistant pathogens.
- Ciproflozacin: a fluoroquinolone. Some resistance to this class of drugs has been reported, and treatment should be continued for at least two days after all symptoms have resolved.
- Doxycyline: a derivative of tetracycline that may be useful in patients with allergies to penicillins and cephalosporins who cannot tolerate macrolides.
- Levofloxacin: a fluoroquinolone that has become popular for initial use, but some pathogens have shown resistance. Other drugs in this chemical class may be equally effective.

A number of other anti-infective drugs may be useful based on culture and sensitivity reports and the patient's condition, including severity of infection, age, and other medical conditions.

With appropriate initial therapy, 90 percent of pneumonia patients improve, showing improved breathing, relief of pain and cough, and lowering of the white blood cell count. If the patient fails to improve, it may be necessary to obtain a specialist's consultation

Immunization against *H. influenzae* and pneumococcus is valuable in the prevention of CAP in people over 65 and in those otherwise at risk, such as patients with cystic fibrosis. The latter protects against 23 different types of pneumococcus. HAP is preventable through good hospital hygiene, especially relating to mechanical ventilation. Elevation of the bed has been found useful in protecting the lower respiratory tract from infection. Prevention of pneumonia is important because the complications of the condition can be serious. With the growth of drug-resistant strains of bacteria that cause pneumonia, effective treatment can no longer be relied upon.

Pneumococcal vaccines are recommended as part of standard vaccinations in children under age 5 and adults aged 65 or older. These vaccines are also recommended for individuals who have impaired immune systems, such as patients who have AIDS, cancer, or renal disease; those who are taking drugs that affect the immune system; and those who have inactive spleens, cerebrospinal fluid leaks, or cochlear implants.

There are two types of pneumonia vaccines, pneumococcal vaccine 13-valent and pneumococcal vaccine polyvalent. Pneumococcal conjugate (13-valent) (PCV13) has the brand name Prevnar 13®. This vaccine protects against 13 strains of *Streptococcus* pneumonia. Pneumococcal polysaccharide (23-valent) (PPSV23) has the brand name Pneumovax® 23 and protects against 23 strains of *Streptococcus* pneumonia, although most of them are covered by the 13-valent vaccine. The 13-valent vaccine is approved for children above the age of six weeks as part of a routine immunization schedule. The 23-valent vaccine is approved for administration to children over the age of two who are at high risk for exposure to pneumococcal infection. The vaccine should also be given to adults between ages 19 and 50 who have diabetes, chronic heart disease, or chronic lung disease. Recommendations call for patients over the age of 65 to have one dose of the 23-valent vaccine.

Household air quality has also been shown to affect the incidence and severity of pneumonia, particularly among children. According to WHO, more than half of pneumonia deaths among children age five or younger can be attributed to indoor air pollution related to the use of solid fuels (such as wood) for cooking or heating. This is a major concern in developing countries, where a lack of reliable electricity necessitates the use of solid fuels. A number of international organizations have undertaken efforts to encourage the use of clean-burning fuels and more efficient cooking technologies to areas most affected by pollution-related pneumonia.

Impacts and Issues

William Oster, the great 19th-century Canadian physician, called pneumonia "the old man's friend" because it often releases an elderly, frail, terminal patient from a catalog of severe medical complaints. However, not all patients with pneumonia fall in this category. HAP is the second-most common nosocomial infection in the United States and the most serious in terms of morbidity and mortality, with 300,000 new cases a year, accounting for approximately $3 billion in health care costs.

The causes of HAP need addressing when they are preventable, as in the case of insufficient handwashing and the use of equipment that could be contaminated. However, the risk of HAP is inextricably linked to the nature of modern medicine, especially when it comes to intensive care. Mechanical ventilation may save the lives of the desperately ill, but it is also the leading cause of HAP because of the way in which it breaches the natural defenses of the respiratory tract against infection. Other invasive procedures linked with a high risk of HAP include nasogastric intubation (a tube leading from the nasal passages to the stomach) for feeding an unconscious patient, and chest, abdominal, head, or neck surgery. Because these can be life-saving treatments, health care workers and researchers are attempting to develop technologies and practices within the intensive care and surgical setting that can minimize the risk of pneumonia.

Another major concern arising from HAP is that the cause is often a multidrug-resistant organism. This means that the patient's upper respiratory tract has been colonized with a resistant organism, and it may be difficult to find an antibiotic within the armory available to the physician that can treat the pneumonia successfully. Antibiotic resistance is also a concern in CAP, as penicillin-resistant *S. pneumoniae* is increasingly common. The fight against antibiotic resistance is twofold. Researchers must develop new classes of antibiotic, which act by mechanisms not previously known. Both existing and new antibiotics must be used sparingly. Overuse or misuse of antibiotics promotes the emergence of resistant strains. On exposure the weaker strains die, leaving the more resistant ones to flourish. This is especially likely to happen when a patient does not finish a prescribed course because symptoms of the infection clear up. This is as true of pneumonia as of any other infection. Patients must be responsible and take their medication exactly as prescribed. Only then are the chances of killing resistant bacteria maximized.

International efforts to reduce global mortality rates from pneumonia have increased in the 21st century. In 2009 WHO declared November 12 World Pneumonia Day and announced the formation of the Global Coalition Against Child Pneumonia, a collection of more than 100 international organizations dedicated to reducing the incidence of childhood pneumonia around the world. In 2013, in conjunction with the United Nations Children's Fund (UNICEF), WHO also implemented a Global Action Plan for the Prevention and Control of Pneumonia and Diarrhoea that aimed to eliminate preventable deaths from pneumonia and diarrhea by 2025. Due in part to these efforts, the number of pneumonia deaths among children under age five fell from approximately 1.7 million in 2000 to 0.9 million in 2015. But experts cautioned that more work was needed to ensure broader vaccine and antibiotic use in health systems around the world.

PRIMARY SOURCE

In Disaster's Wake: Tsunami Lung

SOURCE: *Potera, Carol. "In Disaster's Wake: Tsunami Lung."* Environmental Health Perspectives *113 (2005): 11, 734.*

INTRODUCTION: *In the following journal article, author Carol Potera discusses a type of aspiration (inhalation) pneumonia seen after the 2004 Asian tsunami, which was termed "tsunami lung." Potera is a contributor to* Environmental Health Perspectives, *a journal devoted to the interaction between environmental factors and human and animal health.*

When the Asian tsunami struck on 26 December 2004, health authorities braced for an onslaught of waterborne illnesses including malaria and cholera, which often follow such disasters. But saltwater flooded the freshwater breeding grounds of the mosquitoes that spread malaria, and relief agencies quickly distributed bottled water, thwarting a cholera epidemic. Instead, a type of aspiration pneumonia named "tsunami lung" emerged and afflicted some survivors.

Tsunami lung occurs when people being swept by tsunami waves inhale saltwater contaminated with mud and bacteria. The resulting pneumonia-like infections normally are treated with antibiotics. However, the 2004 tsunami "wiped out the medical infrastructure, and antibiotics were not available to treat infections in the early stages," says David Systrom, a pulmonologist at Massachusetts General Hospital in Boston. Consequently, victims' lung infections festered, entered the bloodstream, and spread to the brain, producing abscesses and neurological problems such as paralysis.

Systrom and colleagues volunteered to work on a medical disaster team with Project HOPE (Health Opportunities for People Everywhere) aboard the hospital ship U.S. Naval Ship *Mercy* off the coast of Banda Aceh, Sumatra. When they arrived three weeks after the tsunami hit, "we saw infections not seen in the United States since before the development of antibiotics," says Systrom. Among them were about 25 cases of tsunami lung. "No one expected the number of tsunami lung cases we saw," says Systrom. "It was not on the radar screen."

The diagnosis of tsunami lung requires a chest radiograph and computed tomography scan of the brain to confirm abscesses. This sophisticated equipment was available on the hospital ship. "Only the most severe cases with central nervous system involvement made it to the ship," says Systrom. The team suspects that hundreds of milder cases went unreported.

In the 23 June 2005 issue of the *New England Journal of Medicine*, the team describes the case of a 17-year-old girl who aspirated water and mud while engulfed by a wave and carried about half a mile. She developed pneumonia two weeks later and was treated at a local clinic with unknown medicines. A week later, the right side of her face drooped, her right arm and leg became paralyzed, and she stopped talking.

A chest radiograph revealed air and pus outside the lining of the lung (a condition known as hydropneumothorax), and a brain scan showed four abscesses. After the doctors treated her with a combination of intravenous antibiotics (imipenem until the stock of that drug ran out, then vancomycin, ceftazidime, and metronidazole), her speech and facial movement recovered first. When she moved her right leg and arm for the first time, she "burst into peals of laughter," according to the report. She was transferred to an International Committee of the Red Cross-Crescent field hospital. "I suspect she'll fully recover," says Sydney Cash, a neurologist at Massachusetts General Hospital and member of the team, who has since received pictures of her walking.

A combination of microbes likely contributes to tsunami lung, but no lab facility was available to culture and identify those found in the Indonesian patients before the Mercy arrived. However, in a letter published in the 4 April 2005 issue of the *Medical Journal of Australia*, Anthony Allworth, director of infectious diseases at Royal Brisbane and Women's Hospital, describes culturing *Burkholderia pseudomallei* from two tsunami lung patients in a land-based hospital and *Nocardia* species from a third.

B. pseudomallei lives in the Asian soil and water. Mark Pasternack, an infectious disease specialist at Massachusetts General Hospital who also served on the Mercy, says, "You do not have to directly aspirate *Burkholderia* to produce pneumonia.... After the tsunami, people had soft tissue injuries from being forced into objects, so they could have gotten *Burkholderia* from wounds or aspiration."

Cash echoes this thought: "Natural disasters produce odd combinations of pathogens and unexpected ways for the body to be damaged that lead to unexpected clinical circumstances. [Medical disaster physicians need to] keep an open mind and expect the unexpected."

Could an infection like tsunami lung emerge in victims of Hurricane Katrina? Probably not, speculates Pasternack. Although the water sweeping the Gulf Coast area may have been contaminated, "it was not forced down peoples' lungs by high-speed waves," he says. Therefore, aspiration pneumonia and its complications are unlikely to appear commonly during the Gulf Coast relief efforts.

See Also Chlamydia pneumoniae; Haemophilus influenzae; *MRSA; Nosocomial (Health Care–Associated) Infections;* Pneumocystis carinii *Pneumonia*

BIBLIOGRAPHY

Books

Suárez, Micaela L., and Steffani M. Ortega, eds. *Pneumonia: Symptoms, Diagnosis and Treatment.* New York: Nova Science, 2011.

Torres, Martí Antoni, and Catia Cillóniz. *Clinical Management of Bacterial Pneumonia.* New York: Springer, 2015.

Wardlaw, Tessa, Emily White Johansson, and Matthew Hodge. *Pneumonia: The Forgotten Killer of Children.* New York: United Nations Children's Fund/World Health Organization, 2006. This report can also be found online at http://apps.who.int/iris/bitstream/10665/43640/1/9280640489_eng.pdf (accessed January 29, 2017).

Periodicals

AlOtair Hadil A., et al. "Severe Pneumonia Requiring ICU Admission: Revisited." *Journal of Taibah University Medical Sciences* 10, no. 3 (September 2015): 293–299. This article can also be found online at https://www.sciencedirect.com/science/article/pii/S1658361215000682 (accessed January 24, 2018).

Mandell, L. A., et al. "Infectious Diseases Society of America/American Thoracic Society Consensus Guidelines on the Management of Community-Acquired Pneumonia in Adults." *Clinical Infectious Diseases* 44, suppl. 2 (2007): S27–S72.

McCollum, Eric D., et al. "Reduction of Childhood Pneumonia Mortality in the Sustainable Development Era." *Lancet Respiratory Medicine* 4, no. 12 (December 2016): 932–933. This article can also be found online at http://www.thelancet.com/journals/lanres/article/PIIS2213-2600(16)30371-X/fulltext (accessed January 24, 2018).

Restrepo, Marcos I., Paola Faverio, and Antonio Anzuetoa. "Long-Term Prognosis in Community-Acquired Pneumonia." *Current Opinion in Infectious Diseases* 26, no. 2 (April 2013): 151–158. This article can also be found online at https://www.ncbi.nlm.nih.gov/pmc/articles/PMC4066634/ (accessed January 24, 2018).

Websites

Brady, Virginia A., Chad R. Marion, and Charles S. Dela Cruz. "Hospital Acquired Pneumonia." Clinical Advisor, 2017. https://www.clinicaladvisor.com/pulmonary-medicine/hospital-acquired-pneumonia/article/625521/ (accessed January 24, 2018).

Gamache, Justina. "Bacterial Pneumonia Medication." Medscape, June 20, 2017. https://emedicine.medscape.com/article/300157-medication (accessed January 24, 2018).

"National Vital Statistics Reports." Centers for Disease Control and Prevention, November 27, 2017. https://www.cdc.gov/nchs/products/nvsr.htm (accessed January 22, 2018).

"Pneumonia." Mayo Clinic, August 11, 2017. https://www.mayoclinic.org/diseases-conditions/pneumonia/symptoms-causes/syc-20354204 (accessed January 22, 2018).

"Pneumonia." World Health Organization, September 2016. http://www.who.int/mediacentre/factsheets/fs331/en/ (accessed January 24, 2018).

Stop Pneumonia. https://stoppneumonia.org/ (accessed January 24, 2018).

Susan Aldridge
Sam Uretsky

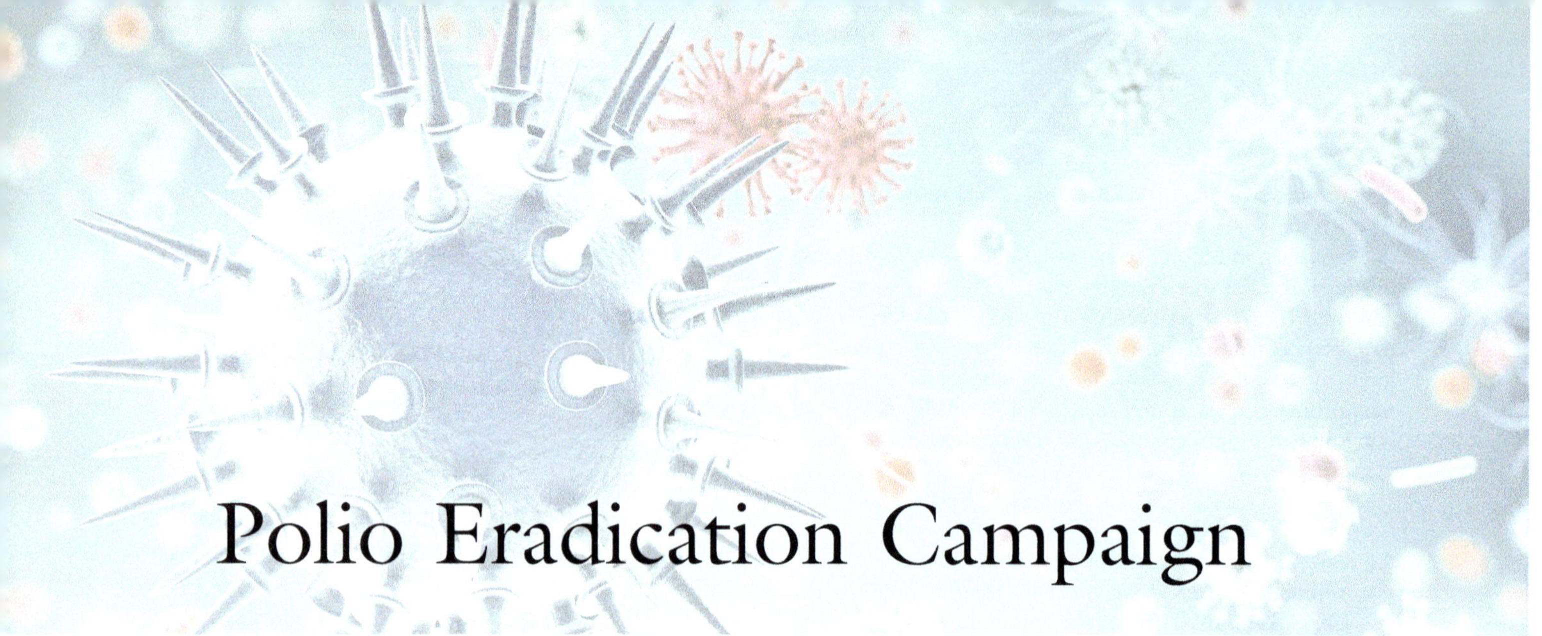

Polio Eradication Campaign

■ Introduction

Polio, short for poliomyelitis, is a viral disease that primarily affects children under the age of five. It is highly infectious and can cause rapid and irreversible paralysis of the limbs and the muscles used in breathing. In the 20th century, polio began to reach epidemic proportions in the United States and more so around the world. The introduction of an effective vaccine in the 1950s began to reduce childhood deaths and disability from polio.

Inspired by the initial success of the polio vaccine, the World Health Organization (WHO) and its partners launched the Global Polio Eradication Initiative in 1988. According to WHO, the campaign has led to a sharp drop in polio cases around the world—from around 350,000 cases in 1988 to only 22 reported cases in 2017. That year polio was endemic in only two countries, and the campaign was entering its final phases.

WORDS TO KNOW

ENDEMIC Present in a particular area or among a particular group of people.

ERADICATION The process of destroying or eliminating a microorganism or disease.

LIVE ATTENUATED VACCINE A vaccine created by reducing the virulence of a pathogen but still keeping it viable (or "live"). Attenuation takes an infectious agent and alters it so that it becomes harmless or less virulent. These vaccines contrast to those produced by "killing" the virus (inactivated vaccine).

MONOVALENT VACCINE A vaccine that is active against just one strain of a virus, such as the one that is in common use against the poliovirus.

WILD VIRUS A genetic description referring to the original form of a virus, first observed in nature. It may remain the most common form in existence but mutated forms develop over time and sometimes become the new wild-type virus.

■ History and Scientific Foundations

By the 1900s localized polio attacks were reported in the United States and Europe. The first polio epidemic, which affected 132 people, was reported in 1894 in the United States. Another epidemic several years later, in 1916, claimed around 6,000 lives and paralyzed 27,000 people. When vaccination began in the mid-1950s, there were approximately 20,000 cases reported per year. Five years later the number had dropped to around 3,000. In 1979 there were only 10 cases of polio in the United States. Similarly dramatic reductions in polio cases were seen around the world.

WHO declared the global eradication of smallpox in 1980. Encouraged by this success, the organization turned its attention to another major infectious disease in 1988 when it announced the Global Polio Eradication Initiative (GPEI). This is a major public-private partnership initially involving WHO, Rotary International, the US Centers for Disease Control and Prevention (CDC), and the United Nations Children's Fund (UNICEF). The prime objective of the campaign is to interrupt the transmission of the wild poliovirus by mass vaccination and thereby achieve global eradication of the disease. In doing so, WHO and its partners hope for the added and long-lasting benefit of strengthening health systems everywhere and promoting routine immunization against other infectious diseases.

GPEI focuses on vaccinating every child, no matter how remotely located or poorly served by his or her country's health system. Since its launch the number of polio cases has fallen by over 99 percent—from more than 1,000 affected cases per day in 1988 to just 22 reported cases for all of 2017. In 1988 the number of countries where polio was endemic totaled 125. In 1994 the WHO region of the Americas, comprising 36 countries, was certified polio-free. Then, in 2000, the WHO Western Pacific Region, consisting of 37 countries and areas, including China, followed. In June 2002 the WHO European region, consisting of 51 countries, was also declared polio-free. Although these were important milestones, there was a resurgence in polio transmission in 21 polio-free countries between 2002 and 2005. Quick and effective strategies by GPEI resulted in successful intervention. As of early 2018, polio was endemic in only two countries in the world—Pakistan and Afghanistan. India was removed from the list of countries with active endemic polio virus transmission in February 2012 by WHO, one year after its last case was reported, and Nigeria was removed from the list in 2015.

The polio eradication campaign has globally witnessed about 20 billion doses of vaccine administered by more than 20 million volunteers. The program encompasses localized efforts and health initiatives, which includes hundreds of national and subnational immunization days across hundreds of countries. For example, China launched its first national immunization day, vaccinating 80 million children in 1994. The next year a similar initiative immunized 87 million in India.

The task that WHO and its partners set out to achieve is not yet complete. According to WHO, pockets of transmission remain a threat. Even if a single child remains infected, all children are at risk of contracting the disease.

Applications and Research

There are three strains of wild poliovirus. These strains cannot survive and replicate without a host (human body). The polio eradication strategy has focused on immunizing infants with four doses of oral polio vaccine (OPV) during the first year of life. Supplementary doses of OPV are also given to all children under the age of five in areas where the wild poliovirus remains in circulation. Once wild poliovirus transmission is limited to a specific area within a country, a targeted "mop up" campaign is initiated. Surveillance for the presence of polio infection is a vital part of the campaign. For example, all cases of acute flaccid (floppy) paralysis, which could be a sign of polio, need to be reported and tested.

In September 2015 WHO declared that wild polio virus type 2 had been eradicated, with no new cases reported since 1999. Likewise, as of 2018, no cases of type 3 had been reported since 2012, giving researchers hope that a similar eradication was on the horizon. However, vaccine-derived polio virus infection (infection caused by a mutated strain of the weakened virus used in vaccines) remains a cause for concern in areas with low rates of immunization. In 2017 there were 91 reported cases of vaccine-derived polio worldwide, 70 of which occurred in Syria, where immunization rates fell from around 95 percent to 60 percent after the outbreak of civil war in 2011.

To prevent the spread of vaccine-derived polio, many governments have introduced inactivated polio vaccines (IPVs), which contain only inactive (dead) strains of the virus. In places where wild poliovirus has been eliminated,

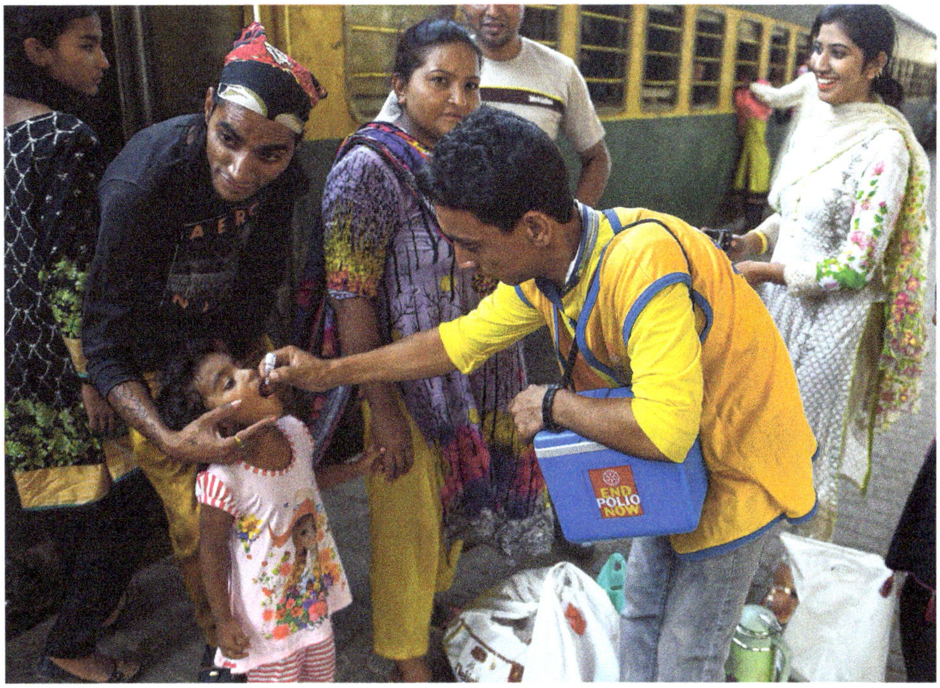

A health care worker administers polio vaccine to a child in Karachi, Pakistan, in October 2017. The nation is one of only two in the world where the disease remains endemic. *© RIZWAN TABASSUM/AFP/Getty Images*

GPEI—REAL-WORLD DETERRENTS

Even though most governments and political organizations around the world support the work of the Global Polio Eradication Initiative (GPEI), there has been significant opposition grounded in religious and political conflicts in some countries. In 2003, for example, five states in northern Nigeria, the source of 80 percent of all polio cases in Africa at the time, banned polio vaccinations over fears that the vaccine was being used by Western countries in an effort to sterilize Muslims. In 2012 nine vaccination workers were murdered by Taliban militants in Pakistan, which led to the suspension of a three-day vaccination program sponsored by WHO. In 2013 and 2014, there were reports of polio workers being killed in northwestern Pakistan and the major city of Karachi. In Afghanistan, vaccination teams were prevented from entering the southern region of the country in 2014 over fears that the teams contained spies following reports that the United States had used a fake vaccination program in the region as a front for its hunt for terrorist leader Osama bin Laden (1957–2011).

In each of these three countries, emergency vaccination programs were eventually introduced, but only after the number of infections began to increase, in some cases spreading to neighboring countries. As of 2018 Nigeria, Afghanistan, and Pakistan remain the only countries where polio has not been eradicated.

IPV is often given in place of OPV (the United States, for example, has used only IPV since 2000). In other places, where wild poliovirus remains a concern alongside vaccine-derived polio, both OPV and IPV may be given in combination. Once all three types of wild poliovirus have been eradicated from the world, it will become important to transition all immunization programs from OPV to IPV to prevent against the continued spread of vaccine-derived polio.

Since 2006 more than 97 percent of all vaccine-derived cases of polio have been type 2. With the wild type 2 virus declared eradicated in 2015, WHO recommended that the live type 2 virus be eliminated from the OPV beginning in April 2016. At the same time, WHO recommended that countries introduce the inactivated type 2 vaccine to reduce the risk of further vaccine-derived infections. A stockpile of type 2–specific live monovalent vaccines was also created for use in response to an unexpected outbreak of wild type 2 poliovirus.

■ Impacts and Issues

To be certified as polio-free, a region must not have any cases of the disease for at least a year and show that it has a high standard of surveillance for three years. It must also be able to show it can deal effectively with imported cases of polio. As of 2018 the Americas (certified in 1994), Western Pacific (2000), Europe (2002), and Southeast Asia (2014) regions had been certified polio free, while the Africa and Eastern Mediterranean regions required further work before the goal of polio eradication could be achieved.

Ensuring every child is vaccinated can be challenging. The involvement and commitment of the local community is essential. In Afghanistan, Nigeria, and Pakistan, anti-vaccination disinformation campaigns and direct violence against vaccination teams perpetrated by extremist groups such as the Taliban and Boko Haram have disrupted immunization efforts, leading to polio resurgences in all three countries between 2014 and 2016. Moreover, awareness of the benefits of vaccination may wane in communities where polio is in decline. Therefore, continual efforts to engage local people in the campaign are needed. UNICEF supports and engages about 2,000 social mobilizers who work directly with local community members to discuss and monitor intervention programs.

There are a number of other challenges to achieving global eradication of polio. About 1 percent of the infected cases are asymptomatic or with mild symptoms, allowing the disease to be spread before these cases are identified. Medical teams also struggle to maintain the potency (strength) of the live attenuated OPV in hot and remote areas. The OPV needs to be maintained at 36°F to 46°F (2°C to 8°C) for the vaccination to work properly in the receiving population. Perhaps the largest hurdle, however, is a lack of accountability by public officials stemming from political or religious objections to vaccination in areas where risk of the disease remains high.

The work of GPEI is ongoing, and it needs substantial financial support as well as political willingness. Concerns remain regarding transmission of the vaccine-derived form of the disease or from asymptomatic carriers in recently polio-free areas. Monitoring and prevention of the virus continues to be a critical factor in making the program a worldwide success.

SEE ALSO *Polio (Poliomyelitis)*

BIBLIOGRAPHY

Books

Sass, Edmund J. "The History of Polio." In *Polio's Legacy: An Oral History*, edited by Sass. Lanham, MD: University Press of America, 1996.

Periodicals

Jegede, Ayodele Samuel. "What Led to the Nigerian Boycott of the Polio Vaccination Campaign?" *PLOS Medicine* 4, no. 3 (2007). This article can also be found online at http://journals.plos.org/plosmedicine/article?id=10.1371/journal.pmed.0040073 (accessed February 2, 2018).

Kluger, Jeffrey. "Is 2018 the Year for Polio's Extinction?" *Time* (December 18, 2017). This article can also be found online at http://time.com/5068516/is-2018-the-year-for-polios-extinction/ (accessed February 2, 2018).

Lahariya, Chandrakant. Global Eradication of Polio: The Case for "Finishing the Job." *Bulletin of the World Health Organization* 85 (2007): 421. This article can also be found online at http://www.who.int/bulletin/volumes/85/6/06–037457/en/ (accessed February 6, 2018).

McNeil, Donald G., Jr. "For Polio Vaccines, a Worldwide Switch to a New Version." *New York Times* (April 11, 2016). This article can also be found online at https://www.nytimes.com/2016/04/12/health/for-polio-vaccines-a-worldwide-switch-to-new-version.html (accessed February 2, 2018).

Walsh, Declan, and Donald G. McNeil Jr. "Female Vaccination Workers, Essential in Pakistan, Become Prey." *New York Times* (December 20, 2012). This article can also be found online at http://www.nytimes.com/2012/12/21/world/asia/un-halts-vaccine-work-in-pakistan-after-more-killings.html-?pagewanted=all (accessed February 2, 2018).

Websites

Graham-Harrison, Emma. "Afghan Taliban Bans Polio Vaccination Teams from Southern Helmand." *Guardian* (July 8, 2014). This article can also be found online at https://www.theguardian.com/world/2014/jul/08/afghan-taliban-bans-polio-vaccination-teams-southern-helmand-province (accessed February 2, 2018).

"Gunmen Kill Police Officer Protecting Polio Workers in Pakistan." *Guardian* (January 29, 2013). This article can also be found online at https://www.theguardian.com/world/2013/jan/29/pakistan-polio-vaccines-gunmen-shooting (accessed February 2, 2018).

Mastny, Lisa. "Eradicating Polio: A Model for International Cooperation." Worldwatch Institute, January 25, 1999. https://web.archive.org/web/20060608165205/http://www.worldwatch.org/node/1644 (accessed February 2, 2018).

"Pakistan Polio Workers Shot Dead in Karachi." BBC News, January 21, 2014. http://www.bbc.com/news/world-asia-25823154 (accessed February 2, 2018).

"Poliomyelitis." World Health Organization, April 2017. http://www.who.int/mediacentre/factsheets/fs114/en/ (accessed February 1, 2018).

"Pulse Polio Programme." National Health Portal, April 6, 2015. https://www.nhp.gov.in/pulse-polio-programme_pg (accessed February 2, 2018).

"10 Facts on Polio Eradication." World Health Organization, April 2017. http://www.who.int/features/factfiles/polio/en/ (accessed February 2, 2018).

UNICEF's Engagement in the Global Polio Eradication Initiative. UNICEF, 2012. https://www.unicef.org/partners/files/Partnership_profile_2012_Polio_revised.pdf (accessed February 2, 2018).

Wild Poliovirus List. Global Polio Eradication Initiative, 2018. http://polioeradication.org/polio-today/polio-now/wild-poliovirus-list/ (accessed February 1, 2018).

Susan Aldridge
Kausalya Santhanam

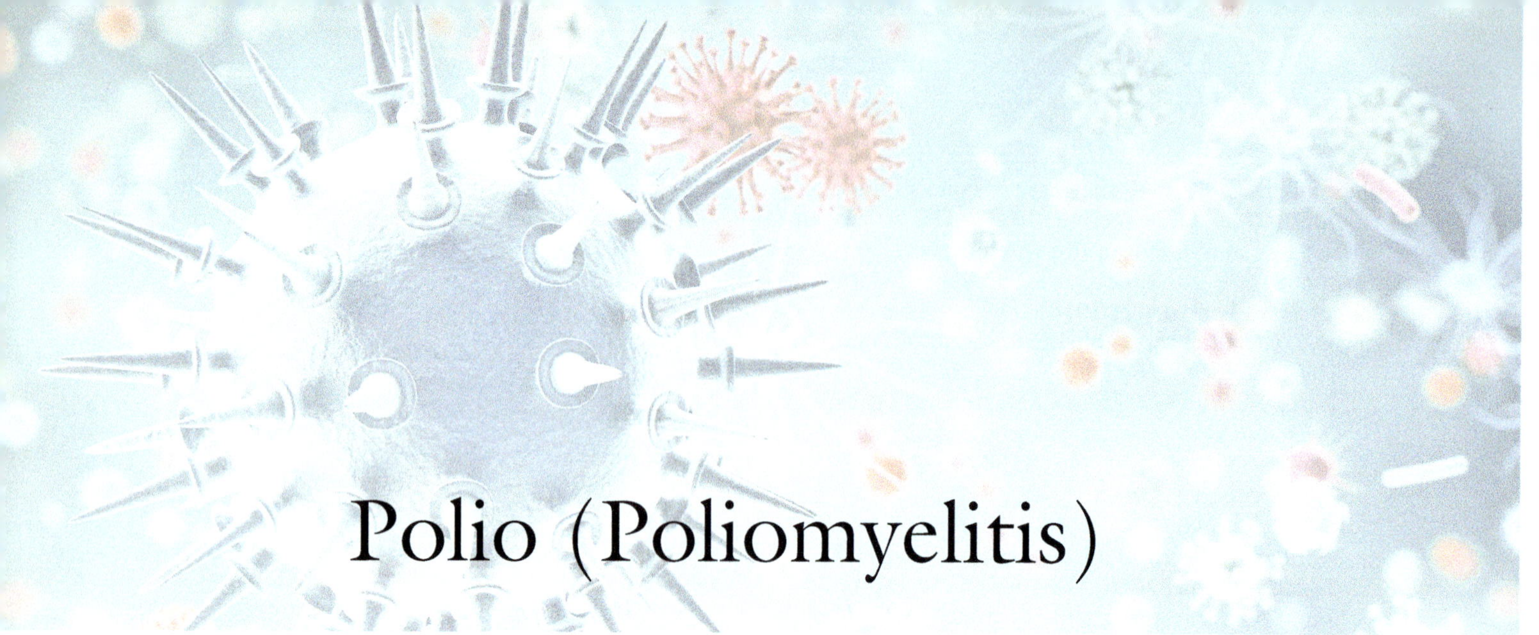

Polio (Poliomyelitis)

Introduction

Polio, short for poliomyelitis, is a highly infectious viral disease that can cause rapid paralysis of the limbs and the muscles used in breathing. Also known as infantile paralysis, polio mainly affects children under the age of five, although it can also affect adults. It was first described at the end of the 18th century.

There have been many epidemics of polio both in the United States and in other countries around the world. However, once an effective vaccine was introduced in 1955, the number of polio cases began to fall dramatically. In 1988 the World Health Organization (WHO), along with other nongovernmental organizations, launched the Global Polio Eradication Initiative (GPEI). This relies on ensuring that all children are vaccinated against polio. The initiative has led to a dramatic drop in the number of cases of polio around the world, from around 350,000 in 1988 to 22 reported cases in 2017.

Disease History, Characteristics, and Transmission

The word *poliomyelitis* comes from *polio*, the Greek word for "gray," and *myelon*, the Greek word for "marrow" (indicating the spinal cord). It is the effect of the poliovirus on the spinal cord that causes the paralysis associated with this disease. There are three types of poliovirus—1, 2, and 3—all of which cause similar infections. Polioviruses belong to the enterovirus group and are part of the picornavirus family of ribonucleic acid (RNA viruses)—that is, their genetic material is composed of RNA rather than deoxyribonucleic acid (DNA). Poliomyelitis virus was first identified by Austrian physicians Karl Landsteiner (1868–1943) and Erwin Popper (1879–1955) in 1908. John F. Enders (1897–1985), Thomas Weller (1915–2008), and Frederick Robbins (1916–2003) of Harvard School for Public Health were the first to grow poliovirus in tissue culture in 1948, and they were awarded the Nobel Prize for this work in 1954.

Polio occurs mainly in the summer and fall in temperate climates but has no seasonal pattern in tropical climates. The incubation time of poliovirus is 7 to 14 days, during which time it multiplies in the cells lining the intestines and in the respiratory tract. In most people the infection causes no symptoms at all. In approximately 25 percent of cases, minor symptoms include headache, fever, fatigue, and vomiting, as well as stiffness of the neck and pain in the limbs. Approximately 1 to 2 percent of polio infections result in nonparalytic aseptic meningitis, which causes stiffness of the neck, back, or legs. This condition tends to clear up within a week or so, and complete recovery is typical. In 1 percent of cases, however, poliovirus spreads from the intestines through the blood to the nervous system, where it can destroy nerve cells in the spinal cord and the base of the brain.

Polio infection in the nervous system leads to paralytic polio, which is the most feared type of the disease. The severity of paralytic polio depends on how many neurons are affected, but onset of paralysis can be rapid. Commonly, a child might go to bed with minor symptoms and wake up unable to walk.

There are three forms of paralytic polio. Spinal polio causes a flaccid (floppy) paralysis of one or more of the limbs, without any loss of feeling. Complete recovery is quite possible, however, and tends to happen within the first six months. Any weakness or paralysis remaining after a year is likely to be permanent, and the child is left with some degree of disability. Spinal polio accounted for 79 percent of all cases of paralytic polio between 1969 and 1979.

Another, less common, form of paralytic polio is called bulbar polio, in which the poliovirus affects the cranial nerves in the upper spinal cord. This leads to paralysis of the pharynx (back of the throat), vocal cords, and respiratory (breathing) muscles. Bulbar polio is the most dangerous form of the disease, killing 75 percent of those affected. Pure bulbar polio accounted for only 2 percent of cases between 1969 and 1979. The rest were bulbospinal polio, which is a combination of the two forms.

The complications of paralytic polio include urinary tract infection and pneumonia, which are common in any condition where a patient is immobilized. The overall death rate from paralytic polio is 2 to 5 percent for children and 15 to 25 percent for adults.

Most doctors will never see a case of polio. However, they may see a condition known as post-polio syndrome, which affects 25 to 40 percent of those who had paralytic polio in childhood. The syndrome is characterized by fatigue, new muscle pain, and exacerbation of any existing weakness. It is more common in those left with residual disability caused by the original infection. It is not clear what causes post-polio syndrome, but it may result from nerve damage occurring during the original recovery process. Post-polio syndrome is not a reactivation of polio infection, and those affected are not infectious to others.

Poliovirus is transmitted from person to person by the fecal-oral route (through consumption of contaminated food and water). It enters the body through the mouth and multiplies in the throat and the gastrointestinal tract, the latter being confirmed through laboratory examination of the feces of people with polio. People with no symptoms, or only mild symptoms, can still transmit the infection. The disease is highly infectious. Therefore, in communities where even one child remains unvaccinated, all are at risk of developing the disease.

Rarely, someone may contract paralytic polio through vaccination when the attenuated (weakened) virus used in the vaccine undergoes a genetic mutation in the intestines. Vaccine-associated paralytic polio (VAPP) occurs in around one person for every 2.7 million doses of live vaccine administered, and its reach is usually limited to the vaccinated individual and his or her unvaccinated immediate contacts. In the case of vaccine-derived poliovirus (VDPV), the mutated vaccine virus may become capable of causing a sustained and widespread outbreak. In 2017 there were 91 cases of VDPV compared to just 22 cases of wild poliovirus.

WORDS TO KNOW

ATTENUATED STRAIN A bacterium or virus that has been weakened. Often used as the basis of a vaccine against the specific disease caused by the bacterium or virus.

ENDEMIC Present in a particular area or among a particular group of people.

ERADICATION The process of destroying or eliminating a microorganism or disease.

INACTIVATED VACCINE A vaccine that is made from disease-causing microorganisms that have been killed or made incapable of causing the infection. The immune system can still respond to the presence of the microorganisms.

LIVE VACCINE A vaccine that uses a virus or a bacterium that has been weakened (attenuated) to cause an immune response in the body without causing disease. Live vaccines are preferred to killed vaccines, which use a dead virus or bacteria, because they cause a stronger and longer-lasting immune response.

WILD VIRUS A genetic description referring to the original form of a virus, first observed in nature. It may remain the most common form in existence but mutated forms develop over time and sometimes become the new wild-type virus.

Scope and Distribution

Children younger than age five have always been most at risk for polio, although it can affect people of any age. For instance, American President Franklin D. Roosevelt (1882–1945) contracted the disease in 1921 at the age of 39. Polio was first described in England in 1789 and was only a sporadic disease during the 18th and 19th centuries.

In the early years of the 20th century, Scandinavia, the United Kingdom, and North America were especially affected by polio. According to data released by the Health Section of the League of Nations (the forerunner of the United Nations), of 178,328 cases of polio occurring between 1919 and 1934, 54.3 percent were in the United States and Canada. However, the peak year for polio in the United States was 1952, with more than 57,000 cases, including 21,000 paralytic cases.

In England there were more than 1,000 cases of polio in 1928 and in 1938, but between these years the annual average was around 640. Polio became more of a problem in Britain after World War II (1939–1945), with almost 8,000 cases reported in 1947. There was also a severe outbreak in 1952 that affected 238 per 100,000 of the population in Copenhagen, Denmark. The majority of these cases were bulbar polio, the most dangerous form of the disease.

The introduction of polio vaccine in the 1950s began to bring the disease under control. However, in 1988, when WHO initiated the GPEI, the disease was still endemic in 125 countries around the world. In 1988 there were about 1,000 cases per day; the WHO initiative drastically decreased the number to 5 cases per day in 2006. Polio was endemic in only two countries—Pakistan and

Afghanistan—as of 2017. That year there were only 22 reported cases of polio spread between the two countries.

■ Treatment and Prevention

There is no treatment for polio. The cure has been somewhat focused on relieving the symptoms and preventing complications, which may lead to quicker recovery. Although the paralysis itself cannot be cured, supportive medications may prevent infections in the weakened muscles. Long-term rehabilitation including physiotherapy and occupational therapy are some modern treatment methodologies advocated in many parts of the world.

Prevention is the key mode to disrupt transmission of polio, and WHO's GPEI program has seen enormous success. Jonas Salk (1914–1995) introduced an inactivated polio vaccine (IPV) in 1955, following testing and trials. This had to be given by injection. Then Albert Sabin (1906–1993) developed an attenuated (weakened) live vaccine (oral polio vaccine, OPV) that could be given orally, which was much more convenient. Oral polio vaccine was introduced in the early 1960s and was used widely in the United States and in many developing countries. Beginning in 1988 more advanced versions of OPV were subsequently used in countries where GPEI was rigorously implemented.

However, although OPV has been largely responsible for the elimination of wild poliovirus infections in the United States and globally, vaccine-derived polio virus infection in areas with low population immunity is increasingly becoming a cause for concern. To avoid OPV-induced transmission, IPV administration is suggested, especially in areas where the wild poliovirus has been eradicated. The United States, for example, has used IPV rather than OPV since 2000. However, OPV remains in use in areas where the risk of wild poliovirus outbreaks is high. Because type 2 poliovirus was eradicated in 1999, WHO introduced a new OPV vaccine in April 2016 that contained attenuated strains of just the type 1 and type 3 viruses and suggested that the type 2 IPV be used as a supplement.

Per the new polio vaccination protocol, children born in areas where polio has been eradicated should receive three doses of IPV within the first 18 months of life and a fourth dose at, or before, school entry. Travelers to the few remaining countries affected by polio, and certain laboratory workers, may need to have a booster dose of IPV vaccine to protect them. But a routine vaccination of adults is not necessary in areas where polio is considered to be completely eradicated.

■ Impacts and Issues

WHO reported a widespread global disease emergence between 1975 and 1985 even though polio vaccine was available. By 1985 the success of the polio vaccine gave the Pan American Health Organization the confidence to set the goal of eradicating polio from the Americas by 1990. Meanwhile, WHO had declared the official eradication of smallpox in 1980 and decided to build

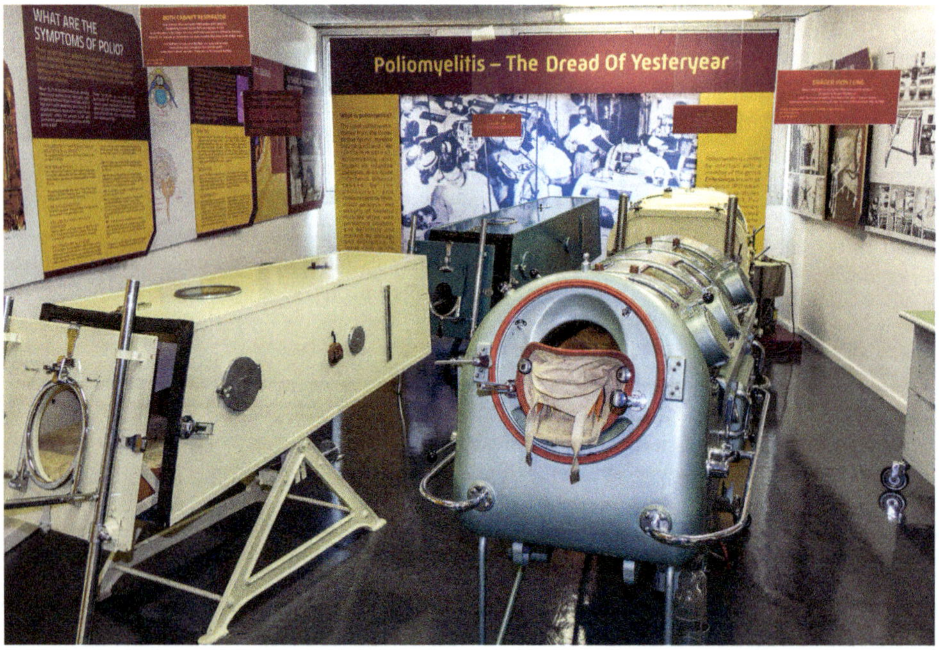

Iron lungs on display at the Adler Museum of Medicine at the University of the Witwatersrand in Johannesburg, South Africa. These mechanical respirators were commonly used to treat polio patients in the 1940s and 1950s. *© Jeff Greenberg/UIG/Getty Images*

SCIENTIFIC, POLITICAL, AND ETHICAL ISSUES

The eldest son of Orthodox Jewish-Polish immigrants, Jonas Salk (1914–1995) earned his medical degree in 1939. After his internship and work on a flu vaccine, Salk devoted his energies to writing scientific papers on a number of topics, including the polio virus. Some of these came to the attention of Daniel Basil O'Connor (1892–1972), the director of the National Foundation for Infantile Paralysis, an organization that had long been involved with the treatment and rehabilitation of polio victims. O'Connor eyed Salk as a possible recruit for the polio vaccine research his organization sponsored. When the two finally met, O'Connor was so taken by Salk that he put almost all of the National Foundation's money behind Salk's vaccine research efforts.

Salk's first challenge was to obtain enough of the virus to develop a vaccine in doses large enough to have an impact. This was particularly difficult because viruses, unlike culture-grown bacteria, need living cells to grow. The breakthrough came when the team of John F. Enders (1897–1985), Thomas Weller (1915–2008), and Frederick Robbins (1916–2003) found that the polio virus could be grown in embryonic tissue, a discovery that earned them a Nobel Prize in 1954. Salk subsequently grew samples of all three varieties of polio virus in cultures of monkey kidney tissue, then killed the virus with formaldehyde. Salk argued that it was essential to use a killed polio virus (rather than a live virus) in the vaccine, as the live-virus vaccine would have a much higher chance of accidentally inducing polio in inoculated children. As such, he exposed the viruses to formaldehyde for nearly 13 days. Though after only three days he could detect no virulence in the sample, Salk wanted to establish a wide safety margin. After an additional 10 days of exposure to the formaldehyde, he reasoned that there was only a one-in-a-trillion chance of there being a live virus particle in a single dose of his vaccine. Salk tested it on monkeys with positive results before proceeding to human clinical trials.

Despite Salk's confidence, many of his colleagues were skeptical, believing that a killed-virus vaccine could not possibly be effective. His dubious standing was further compounded by the fact that he was relatively new to polio vaccine research. Some of his chief competitors in the race to develop the vaccine—most notably Albert Sabin (1906–1993), the chief proponent for a live-virus vaccine—had been working for many years. As the field narrowed, the division between the killed-virus and the live-virus camps widened, and what had once been a polite difference of opinion became a serious ideological conflict. Salk and his chief backer, the National Foundation for Infantile Paralysis, were lonely in their corner. Salk failed to let his position in the scientific wilderness dissuade him, and he continued, undeterred, with his research. To test his vaccine's strength, in early 1952 Salk administered a type I vaccine to children who had already been infected with the polio virus. His results clearly indicated that the vaccine produced large numbers of antibodies. Buoyed by this success, the clinical trial was then extended to include children who had never had polio.

In May 1952 Salk initiated preparations for a massive field trial in which more than 400,000 children would be vaccinated. The largest medical experiment that had ever been carried out in the United States, the test finally got under way in April 1954, sponsored by the National Foundation for Infantile Paralysis. More than 1 million children between the ages of six and nine took part in the trial, each receiving a button that proclaimed them a "Polio Pioneer." At the beginning of 1953, while the trial was still at an early stage, Salk's encouraging results were made public in the *Journal of the American Medical Association*. Predictably, media and public interest were intense. On April 12, 1955, the vaccine was officially pronounced effective, potent, and safe in almost 90 percent of cases. The meeting at which the announcement was made was attended by 500 of the world's top scientists and doctors, 150 journalists, and 16 television and movie crews.

Just two weeks after the announcement of the vaccine's discovery, however, 11 of the children who had received it developed polio; more cases soon followed. Altogether, about 200 children developed paralytic polio, 11 fatally. For a while it appeared that the vaccination campaign would be railroaded. However, it was soon discovered that all of the rogue vaccines had originated from the same laboratory in California. Following a thorough investigation, it was found that the lab used faulty batches of virus culture, which were resistant to the formaldehyde. After furious debate and the adoption of standards that would prevent a recurrence, the inoculation resumed. By the end of 1955, 7 million children had received their shots, and over the course of the next two years, more than 200 million doses of Salk's polio vaccine were administered, without a single instance of vaccine-induced paralysis. By the summer of 1961, there had been a 96 percent reduction in the number of cases of polio in the United States, compared to the five-year period prior to the vaccination campaign.

After the initial inoculation period ended in 1958, Salk's killed-virus vaccine was replaced by a live-virus vaccine developed by Sabin. Use of this new vaccine was advantageous because it could be administered orally rather than intravenously and because it required fewer "booster" inoculations.

The battle between Sabin and Salk persisted well into the 1970s, with Salk writing an op-ed piece for the *New York Times* in 1973 denouncing Sabin's vaccine as unsafe and urging people to use his vaccine once more.

on this success by launching the Global Polio Eradication Initiative in 1988. This was supported by Rotary International, the US Centers for Disease Control and Prevention (CDC), and the United Nations Children's Fund (UNICEF). The Bill & Melinda Gates Foundation has also participated in and contributed hugely to the GPEI.

The GPEI has had considerable success. Since 1988 the number of cases of polio worldwide has fallen by 99 percent. In 1994 the WHO Americas region, consisting of 36 countries, was declared polio-free, followed by the WHO Western Pacific region, consisting of 37 countries, in 2000; the WHO European region (51 countries) in 2002; and the WHO Southeast Asia region (11 countries) in 2014. As of 2017 polio remained endemic in only Pakistan and Afghanistan. In 2016 only 37 cases of polio were reported worldwide, and at the end of 2017 only 22 cases were reported. Despite the enormous success of the GPEI, WHO indicates that failure to eradicate the last few cases in the remaining regions could result in as many as 200,000 new cases in the next 10 years due to transportation of the virus.

Mass vaccination is the key to eradication of polio. The GPEI has seen more than 20 billion doses of the vaccine administered by 20 million volunteers across 125 countries on various national and subnational immunization days. In 2013 the GPEI announced a plan for completely eradicating polio by 2018, though a resurgence of wild poliovirus transmissions in Pakistan and Afghanistan led to an extension of the target date to 2019. The projected total cost of eradicating the disease from 1988 to 2019 was approximately $15 billion, whereas the economic benefit of eradicating the disease was expected to reach $40 or $50 billion by 2035.

However, the total eradication of polio remains a challenge. It can be difficult, even under normal conditions, to access children living in remote areas. Where war and poverty compromise or destroy a country's infrastructure, achieving vaccination goals is even more challenging.

SEE ALSO *CDC (Centers for Disease Control and Prevention); Childhood-Associated Infectious Diseases, Endemicity; Immunization Impacts; Polio Eradication Campaign; Smallpox; World Health Organization (WHO)*

BIBLIOGRAPHY

Books

Closser, Svea. *Chasing Polio in Pakistan: Why the World's Largest Public Health Initiative May Fail.* Nashville: Vanderbilt University Press, 2010.

Renne, Elisha P. *The Politics of Polio in Northern Nigeria.* Bloomington: Indiana University Press, 2010.

Wilson, Daniel J. *Living with Polio: The Epidemic and Its Survivors.* Chicago: University of Chicago Press, 2007.

Periodicals

Hyland, Ryan. "Polio's Last Stand: Frantic Effort to Eradicate Pakistan's 'Badge of Shame.'" *Guardian* (March 15, 2017). This article can also be found online at https://www.theguardian.com/global-development-professionals-network/2017/mar/15/polio-in-pakistan-the-frantic-effort-to-eradicate-the-countrys-badge-of-shame (accessed February 2, 2018).

McNeil, Donald G., Jr. "A Step Closer to the Defeat of Polio." *New York Times* (November 23, 2015). This article can also be found online at https://www.nytimes.com/2015/11/24/health/a-move-closer-to-total-disappearance-of-polio.html (accessed February 2, 2018).

"Polio Vaccines: WHO Position Paper, March 2016." *Vaccine* 35, no. 9 (March 2017): 1197–1199.

Websites

"GPEI: Wild Poliovirus List. Global Polio Eradication Initiative, 2018. http://polioeradication.org/polio-today/polio-now/wild-poliovirus-list/ (accessed February 1, 2018).

"Poliomyelitis." World Health Organization, April 2017. http://www.who.int/mediacentre/factsheets/fs114/en/ (accessed February 1, 2018).

"Poliomyelitis. Immunization, Vaccines and Biologicals." World Health Organization, February 2017. http://www.who.int/immunization/diseases/poliomyelitis/en/ (accessed February 4, 2018).

"Pulse Polio Programme." National Health Portal (NHP), April 6, 2015. https://www.nhp.gov.in/pulse-polio-programme_pg (accessed February 2, 2018).

Resnick, Brian. "The Entire World Has 2 Weeks to Switch Over to a New Oral Polio Vaccine. Here's Why." Vox, April 18, 2016. https://www.vox.com/2016/4/18/11450362/polio-opv-eradication (accessed February 2, 2018).

"10 Facts on Polio Eradication." World Health Organization, April 2017. http://www.who.int/features/factfiles/polio/en/ (accessed February 2, 2018).

"UNICEF's Engagement in the Global Polio Eradication Initiative." UNICEF. https://www.unicef.org/partners/files/Partnership_profile_2012_Polio_revised.pdf (accessed February 2, 2018).

Susan Aldridge
Kausalya Santhana

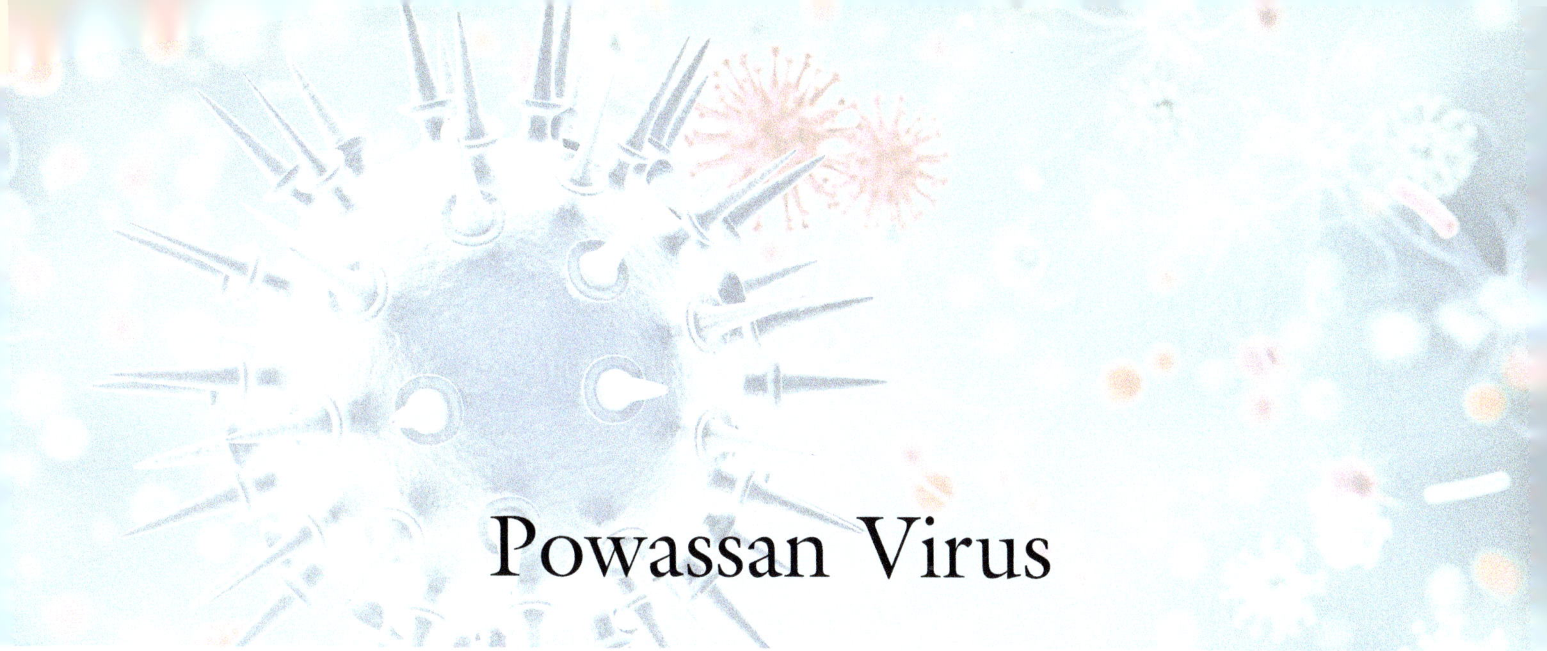

Powassan Virus

Introduction

Powassan virus (POWV) disease is a rare, tick-borne viral infection in humans resulting in severe cases of encephalitis or meningitis, predominantly present in the northeastern United States, Canada, and Russia.

History, Characteristics, and Transmission

The Powassan virus is named after the town of Powassan, Ontario, where it was discovered in 1958. It belongs to the genus *Flavivirus* and family Arbovirus. Of the more than 130 species of known arboviruses, POWV is the only one found in North America and transmitted by tick bite.

Humans contract Powassan virus infection through the bite of ticks carrying the virus. The subsequent infection of the central nervous system affects the brain, causing encephalitis and meningitis. Six species of ticks belonging to genus *Ixodes* (*I. cookei, I. scapularis, I. marxi*, and *I. spinipalpus*) and *Dermacentor* (*D. andersoni* and *D. variabilis*) are known to transmit the virus. The incubation period for POWV infection varies from one week to one month. Infection may be asymptomatic in many people. Symptoms of the disease vary widely, from fever, headache, vomiting, and weakness to confusion, loss of coordination, speech difficulties, seizures, and memory loss.

The POWV life cycle is maintained by blood-sucking ticks and animals such as woodchucks, foxes, raccoons, skunks, and other small mammals. Three main cycles of infection between ticks and animals are identified in North America: *I. cookei* and woodchucks, *I. marxi* and squirrels, and *I. scapularis* and white-footed mice. Depending on the tick species that transmit infection, POWV that infect humans can be categorized under lineage 1 or lineage 2. *I. cookei* and *I. marxi* transmit lineage 1 virus, and *I. scapularis* transmits lineage 2 POWV. The Powassan virus load is not high in human blood. Hence, infected humans do not act as a source of fresh infection to ticks. Consequently, humans are considered "dead-end" hosts of the virus, meaning humans cannot pass the virus on to mosquitoes.

WORDS TO KNOW

ASYMPTOMATIC A state in which an individual does not exhibit or experience symptoms of a disease.

ENCEPHALITIS A type of acute brain inflammation, most often due to infection by a virus.

INCUBATION PERIOD The time between exposure to a disease-causing virus or bacterium and the appearance of symptoms of the infection. Depending on the microorganism, the incubation time can range from a few hours, such as with food poisoning due to *Salmonella*, to a decade or more, such as with acquired immunodeficiency syndrome (AIDS).

MENINGITIS An inflammation of the meninges, the three layers of protective membranes that line the spinal cord and the brain. Meningitis can occur when there is an infection near the brain or spinal cord, such as a respiratory infection in the sinuses, the mastoids, or the cavities around the ear. Disease organisms can also travel to the meninges through the bloodstream. The first signs may be a severe headache and neck stiffness followed by fever, vomiting, a rash, and, then, convulsions leading to loss of consciousness. Meningitis generally involves two types: nonbacterial meningitis, or aseptic meningitis, and bacterial meningitis, or purulent meningitis.

SEROLOGIC TEST A test of the blood or other body fluid, such as spinal fluid, in which serum or the body fluids collected are used to look for antibodies.

INCIDENCE OF POWASSAN VIRUS INFECTIONS IN THE 21ST CENTURY

Sporadic cases of Powassan virus (POWV) have been a cause for concern in the north and northeastern regions of the United States. Three cases of POWV infection were reported in Wisconsin between 2003 and 2007. In 2014 a man from Massachusetts was diagnosed with POWV and survived after being in a coma for a week. In 2016 an infant in eastern Connecticut was diagnosed with POWV infection after a tick bite.

Living close to a wooded area with potential exposure to infected ticks, particularly around the northeastern or Great Lakes regions of the United States, is a high-risk factor for contracting POWV disease.

Scope and Distribution

POWV infection is mostly restricted to the northeastern United States, including Massachusetts, New York, and New Jersey, and regions of the Great Lakes during the late spring, when ticks are most active. POWV has also been recorded in Pennsylvania, Virginia, Wisconsin, and midwestern parts of the United States. In addition, POWV infection has been reported during warmer periods in the Russian Far East. Approximately 10 to 15 percent of infected cases are fatal if not treated. Half of the survivors have permanent symptoms that affect the brain.

Encephalitis caused by POWV infection is difficult to diagnose. Symptoms of POWV are similar to those of acute disseminated encephalomyelitis, an autoimmune disease marked by inflammation in the brain and spinal cord. The availability of serologic testing for POWV is limited, making the diagnosis challenging.

Treatment and Prevention

As of 2018 there were no medications or vaccines available for the treatment or prevention of POWV. Symptomatic individuals with POWV need supportive hospital care such as respiratory support, intravenous fluids, and medications to reduce swelling in the brain.

Avoiding tick habitats such as dense woods and areas with tall grass is the best preventive measure against POWV. Light-colored clothing that covers all parts of skin and insect repellent should be used when visiting areas where ticks may be present. Thorough checking of the body for ticks after spending time outdoors is also an important preventive measure.

Unlike other tick-borne infections such as Lyme disease, in which infection is not acquired if the tick is removed within 24 hours, POWV can be transmitted within 15 minutes of tick attachment. Patients are not generally brought to the hospital until they have entered the encephalic phase of the disease. However, by this point the virus has been cleared from the blood and cerebrospinal fluid (CSF), making diagnosis more difficult. In such cases

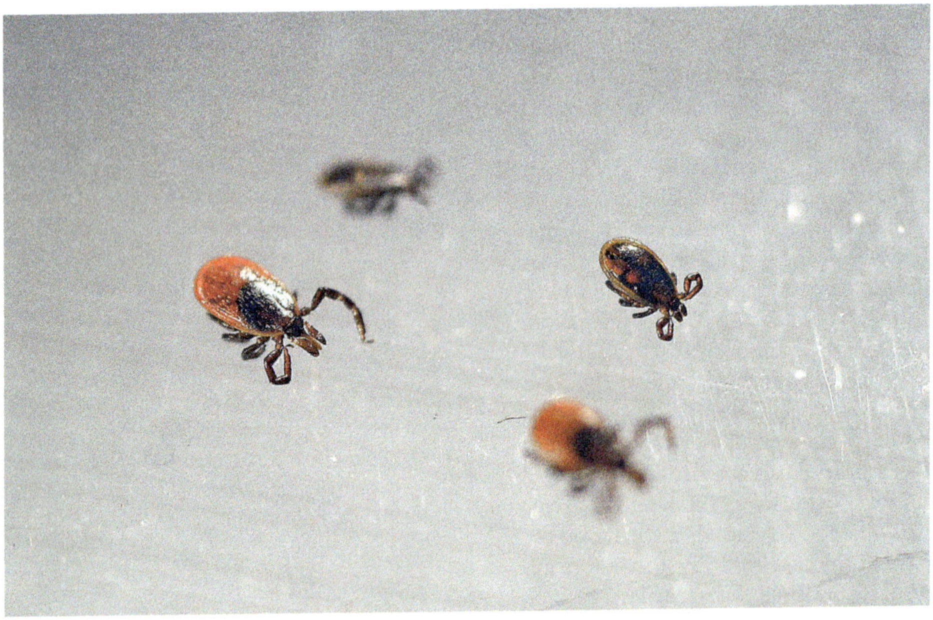

Deer ticks are carriers of Powassan virus, a rare but serious illness most commonly found in the Great Lakes and Northeast regions of the United States. *© Shawn Patrick Ouellette/Portland Press Herald/Getty Images*

the specific diagnosis can be made only through the detection of POWV-specific antibodies in the blood.

Diagnosis of POWV infection is typically done by careful evaluation of clinical symptoms alongside circumstantial evidence such as a history of visiting an endemic area and possible exposure to tick bites. Other diagnostic approaches include isolation of the virus from a patient's blood or CSF, detection of virus-specific antibodies in patient serum or CSF by serologic testing, or demonstration of the ability of patient serum to reduce virus infectivity under experimental settings (plaque neutralization assay).

■ Impacts and Issues

POWV disease cases are rare, but there has been an increase in the reported number of cases in the United States, from 27 cases of human infection between 1958 to 1998 to 88 cases between 2007 to 2016. Because many infected individuals are without symptoms, it is believed that the number affected is underestimated. Although POWV infection is not a serious public health problem, general awareness and prevention of infection are gaining importance, especially due to lack of specific treatment.

See Also *Emerging Infectious Diseases; Encephalitis; Meningitis, Bacterial; Vector-Borne Disease*

BIBLIOGRAPHY

Periodicals

Ebel, G. D. "Update on Powassan Virus: Emergence of a North American Tick-Borne Flavivirus." *Annual Review of Entomology* 55 (2010): 95–110.

Ebel, G. D., and L. D. Kramer. "Short Report: Duration of Tick Attachment Required for Transmission of Powassan Virus by Deer Ticks." *American Journal of Tropical Medicine and Hygiene* 71 (2004): 268–271.

Ebel, G. D., A. Spielman, and S. R. Telford. "Phylogeny of North American Powassan Virus." *Journal of General Virology* 82 (2001): 1657–1665.

Hicar, Mark D., Kathryn Edwards, and Karen Bloch. "Powassan Virus Infection Presenting as Acute Disseminated Encephalomyelitis in Tennessee." *Pediatric Infectious Disease Journal* 30, no. 1 (2011): 86–88.

Johnson, D. K., et al. "Tickborne Powassan Virus Infections among Wisconsin Residents." *Wisconsin Medical Journal* 109, no. 2 (2010): 91–97.

Piantadosi, A., et al. "Emerging Cases of Powassan Virus Encephalitis in New England: Clinical Presentation, Imaging, and Review of the Literature." *Clinical Infectious Diseases* 62 (2016): 707–713.

Tutolo, Jessica W., et al. "Notes from the Field: Powassan Virus Disease in Infant—Connecticut, 2016." *Morbidity and Mortality Weekly Report* 66 (April 2017): 408–409. This article can also be found online at https://www.cdc.gov/mmwr/volumes/66/wr/mm6615a3.htm (accessed February 12, 2018).

Websites

"CDC Report: CDC Arboviral Disease Case Definition." Centers for Disease Control and Prevention. https://wwwn.cdc.gov/nndss/conditions/arboviral-diseases-neuroinvasive-and-non-neuroinvasive/case-definition/2015/ (accessed February 12, 2018).

"Man 'Lucky' to Be Alive after Getting Powassan Virus from Tick Bite." CBS News, June 12, 2017. https://www.cbsnews.com/news/tick-bite-coma-powassan-virus-cape-cod-man/ (accessed February 12, 2018).

"Powassan Virus." Centers for Disease Control and Prevention, November 2, 2017. https://www.cdc.gov/powassan/index.html (accessed February 13, 2018).

Kausalya Santhanam

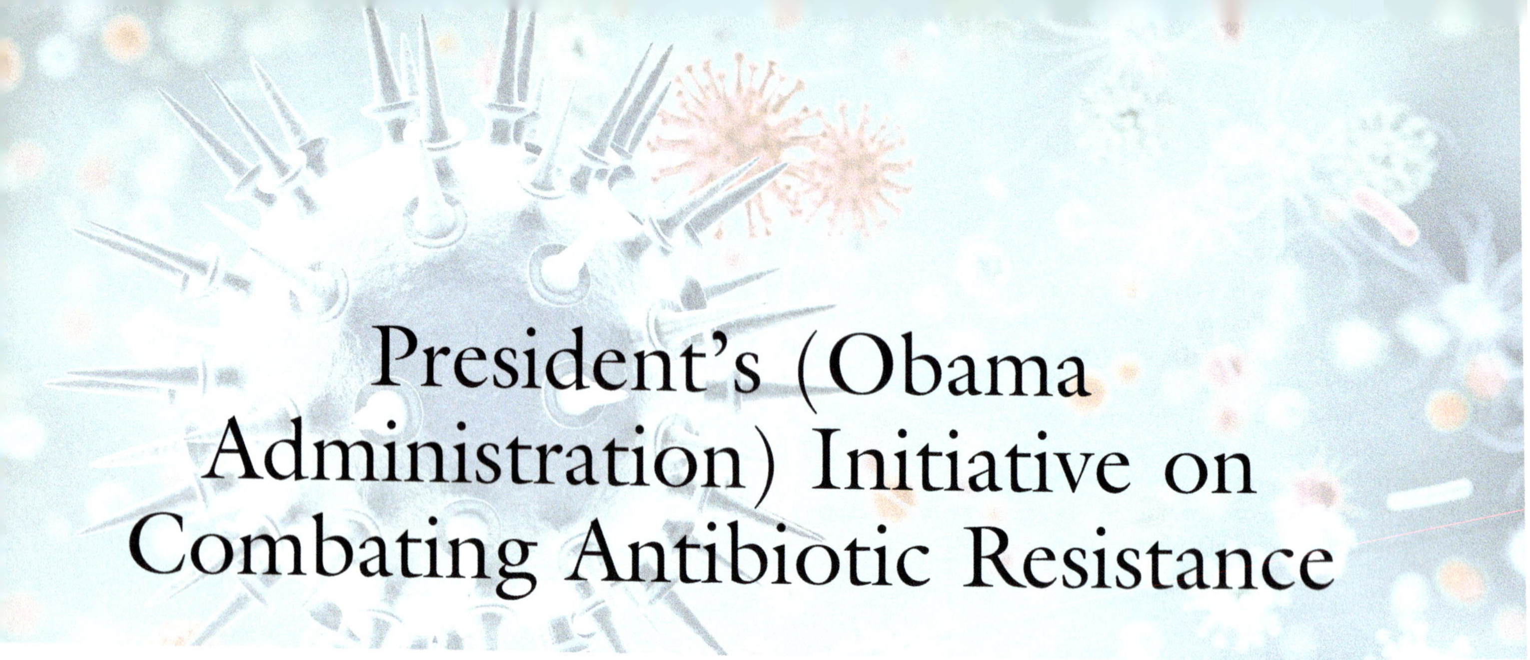

President's (Obama Administration) Initiative on Combating Antibiotic Resistance

■ Introduction

On September 18, 2014, US President Barack Obama (1961–) signed Executive Order 13676: Combating Antibiotic-Resistant Bacteria. This order directed various federal agencies to address the growing prevalence of bacteria that had become resistant to treatment with antibiotic drugs. In 2013 the US Centers for Disease Control and Prevention (CDC) estimated such bacteria to cause at least 2 million illnesses and 23,000 deaths a year within the United States. Among the order's provisions was the creation of a task force charged with devising a five-year road map to implement the objectives of the Obama administration's *National Strategy on Combating Antibiotic-Resistant Bacteria*, a 33-page document released by the White House the same day the executive order was signed.

The task force's plan, unveiled in March 2015 as the *National Action Plan for Combating Antibiotic-Resistant Bacteria*, identified five key goals. These included slowing the emergence of resistant bacteria and preventing the spread of infections; strengthening national surveillance efforts; innovating relevant diagnostic tests; accelerating research and development for new antibiotics, other treatments, and vaccines; and improving international cooperation on the issue. The plan also outlined various activities and policies the US government should pursue over the next five years to meet these goals. The road map was praised as an indication of the government's commitment to addressing the public danger posed by antibiotic-resistant bacteria, though it was criticized in some quarters for not being comprehensive or aggressive enough.

WORDS TO KNOW

ANTIBIOTIC A drug, such as penicillin, used to fight infections caused by bacteria. Antibiotics act only on bacteria and are not effective against viruses.

ANTIBIOTIC RESISTANCE The ability of bacteria to resist the actions of antibiotic drugs.

CENTERS FOR DISEASE CONTROL AND PREVENTION (CDC) One of the primary public health institutions in the world. The CDC is headquartered in Atlanta, Georgia, with facilities at nine other sites in the United States. The centers are the focus of US government efforts to develop and implement prevention and control strategies for diseases, including those of microbiological origin.

MRSA Methicillin-resistant *Staphylococcus aureus* are bacteria resistant to most penicillin-type antibiotics, including methicillin.

■ Historical Context

Although Combating Antibiotic-Resistant Bacteria was the first executive order to address antibiotic resistance, it did not represent the first attempt by the US government to tackle the issue. Throughout much of the 20th century, the surveillance of antibiotic-resistant bacteria was fairly limited. As such, most federal spending related to the subject consisted of tracking and information-gathering activities. The funding of surveillance organizations such as the interagency National Antimicrobial Resistance Monitoring System (NARMS), created in 1996, was instrumental in raising awareness of the increasing prominence of antibiotic-resistant bacteria and the health risks they posed.

As the early 21st century progressed and the spread of resistant bacteria became more severe and better publicized, the problem came to be seen as a major and worsening public health crisis that demanded ongoing and proactive attention. In April 2014 the World Health Organization (WHO) released its first report on antimicrobial resistance (including antibiotics), calling attention to the broad scope of the problem and asserting that "a post-antibiotic era—in which common infections and minor injuries can kill—far from being an apocalyptic fantasy, is instead a very real possibility for the 21st century." The Obama administration's initiative against antibiotic resistance was in part a response to this growing international consensus.

The multipronged approach to combating antibiotic resistance outlined in the 62-page action plan reflected an awareness of the complex nature of the problem. The proliferation of resistant bacteria is believed to have multiple significant contributing factors, some of which are largely inevitable. For example, the use of antibiotics contributes to the problem through evolutionary pressure because nonresistant bacteria are killed by the antibiotics, whereas resistant bacteria survive to pass on their genes. However, the problem is thought to be greatly exacerbated by various factors that are preventable, including the overuse of antibiotics in hospital settings, the prescription of unnecessary antibiotics to medical patients, and the nontherapeutic use of antibiotics in livestock. Furthermore, pharmaceutical companies are often disinclined to research antibiotic development because antibiotics tend to be less lucrative than drugs used over a longer period of time. The Obama initiative's road map therefore addresses different aspects of the crisis with a wide variety of actions, such as implementing economic incentives to antibiotic development, establishing antibiotic stewardship programs in the health care industry, and consulting with veterinarians and animal producers about the agricultural use of antibiotics.

■ Impacts and Issues

Although many commentators hailed the Obama initiative as a crucial indication that the antibiotic resistance crisis was being taken seriously, some were displeased by what they saw as a lack of concrete targets, particularly with regard to the use of antibiotics in livestock. Agricultural applications of antibiotics were among the most controversial aspects of the public conversation about antibiotic resistance, in part because of the heavy economic incentive to continue such applications within US agriculture. Ever since it was discovered that feeding antibiotics to farm animals caused them to grow faster, the nontherapeutic use of such drugs for growth promotion had become a mainstay of American livestock husbandry. In his book *Missing Microbes: How the Overuse of Antibiotics Is Fueling Our Modern Plagues* (2014), Martin J. Blaser asserted that "today, an estimated 70–80 percent of all antibiotics sold in the United States are used for the single purpose of fattening up farm animals."

The extent to which such use was relevant to human infection remained somewhat ambiguous, in part because of a relative lack of research on the subject. Nonetheless, multiple instances of farm workers being infected with the same strains of antibiotic-resistant bacteria as the animals on their farms have been cited as evidence that the medi-

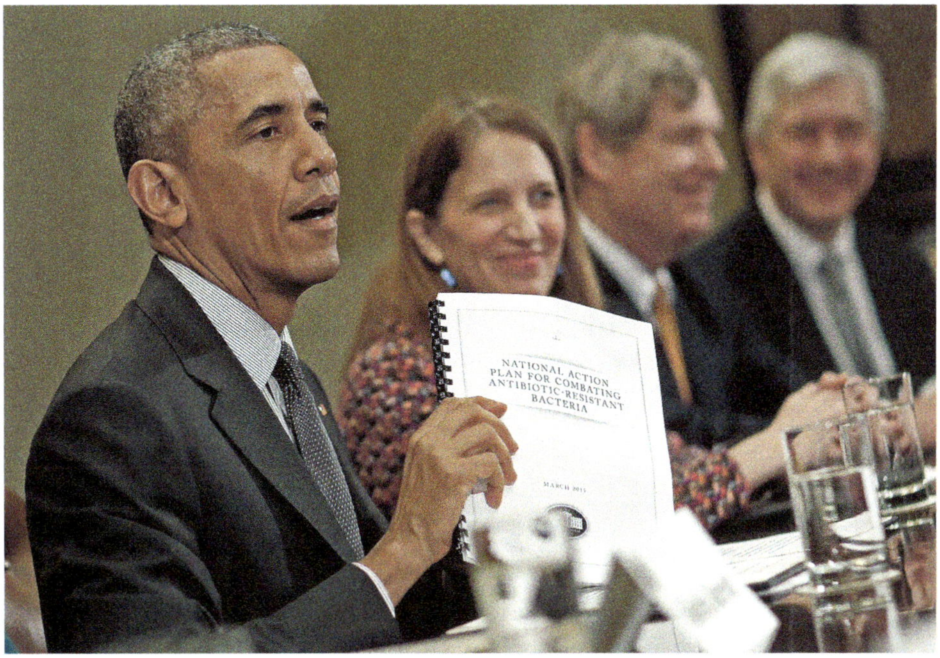

President Barack Obama meets with members of the President's Council of Advisors on Science and Technology after announcing his initiative to combat antibiotic resistance. © Win McNamee/Getty Images cally unnecessary use of antibiotics among animals should be reduced on grounds of public safety. The Obama road map's projected outcome of eliminating "the use of medically important antibiotics for growth promotion in animals" hit a significant milestone in January 2017 when the Food and Drug Administration (FDA) implemented a "judicious use" rule forbidding the agricultural use of antibiotics for the specific purpose of growth promotion. However, many commentators suggested that loopholes in the law continued to allow routine, unnecessary antibiotic use under the guise of "prevention." The efficacy of the new regulations was not immediately clear.

In October 2017 the task force created under Obama released a progress report for the first and second years of its action plan, highlighting the various relevant activities that government institutions had undertaken during that time. The general tenor of the report was optimistic, and it noted that infection rates of two prominent antibiotic-resistant bacteria, *Staphylococcus aureus* (MSRA) and *Clostridium difficile*, had declined in acute care hospitals between 2011 and 2016. It also observed that, "based on preliminary CDC data, the percentage of all U.S. hospitals reporting antibiotic stewardship programs that meet all of CDC's Core Elements rose to 46% in 2015 and 64% in 2016." However, as of early 2018 it remained difficult to evaluate the overall success of the Obama initiative.

PRIMARY SOURCE

Executive Order—Combating Antibiotic-Resistant Bacteria

SOURCE: *"Executive Order—Combating Antibiotic-Resistant Bacteria." Office of the Press Secretary. The White House. September 18, 2014. https://www.cdc.gov/drugresistance/pdf/executive-order_ar.pdf (accessed February 26, 2018).*

INTRODUCTION: *The Initiative on Antibiotic Resistance was created by President Barack Obama's administration to address the dangers posed by bacteria that are resistant to antibiotics. The following excerpt from Obama's executive order introduces the problem of antibiotic-resistant bacteria and provides an overview of plans to combat the problem.*

White House

September 18, 2014

The discovery of antibiotics in the early 20th century fundamentally transformed human and veterinary medicine. Antibiotics save millions of lives each year in the United States and around the world. The rise of antibiotic-resistant bacteria, however, represents a serious threat to public health and the economy. The Centers for Disease Control and Prevention (CDC) in the Department of Health and Human Services (HHS) estimates that annually at least two million illnesses and 23,000 deaths are caused by antibiotic-resistant bacteria in the United States alone.

Detecting, preventing, and controlling antibiotic resistance requires a strategic, coordinated, and sustained effort. It also depends on the engagement of governments, academia, industry, healthcare providers, the general public, and the agricultural community, as well as international partners. Success in this effort will require significant efforts to: minimize the emergence of antibiotic-resistant bacteria; preserve the efficacy of new and existing antibacterial drugs; advance research to develop improved methods for combating antibiotic resistance and conducting antibiotic stewardship; strengthen surveillance efforts in public health and agriculture; develop and promote the use of new, rapid diagnostic technologies; accelerate scientific research and facilitate the development of new antibacterial drugs, vaccines, diagnostics, and other novel therapeutics; maximize the dissemination of the most up-to-date information on the appropriate and proper use of antibiotics to the general public and healthcare providers; work with the pharmaceutical industry to include information on the proper use of over-the-counter and prescription antibiotic medications for humans and animals; and improve international collaboration and capabilities for prevention, surveillance, stewardship, basic research, and drug and diagnostics development.

The Federal Government will work domestically and internationally to detect, prevent, and control illness and death related to antibiotic-resistant infections by implementing measures that reduce the emergence and spread of antibiotic-resistant bacteria and help ensure the continued availability of effective therapeutics for the treatment of bacterial infections.

SEE ALSO *Antibiotic Resistance; CDC (Centers for Disease Control and Prevention); MRSA; World Health Organization (WHO)*

BIBLIOGRAPHY

Books

Blaser, Martin J. *Missing Microbes: How the Overuse of Antibiotics Is Fueling Our Modern Plagues.* New York: Henry Holt, 2014.

Kahn, Laura H. *One Health and the Politics of Antimicrobial Resistance.* Baltimore, MD: Johns Hopkins University Press, 2016.

Periodicals

Davies, Julian, and Dorothy Davies. "Origins and Evolutions of Antibiotic Resistance." *Microbiology and Molecular Biology Reviews* 74, no. 3 (2010): 417–433. This article can also be found online at https://www.ncbi.nlm.nih.gov/pmc/articles/PMC2937522/ (accessed February 25, 2018).

McKenna, Maryn. "After Years of Debate, the FDA Finally Curtails Antibiotic Use in Livestock." *Newsweek* (January 13, 2017). This article can also be found online at http://www.newsweek.com/after-years-debate-fda-curtails-antibiotic-use-livestock-542428 (accessed February 24, 2018).

Potera, Carol. "Obama's Battle Plan for Antibiotic-Resistant Bacteria." *BioScience* 65, no. 7 (2015): 740. This article can also be found online at https://academic.oup.com/bioscience/article/65/7/740/258364 (accessed February 25, 2018).

Websites

"Antimicrobial Resistance: Global Report on Surveillance 2014." World Health Organization. http://www.who.int/drugresistance/documents/surveillancereport/en/ (accessed February 25, 2018).

Executive Order 13676 of September 18, 2014, Combating Antibiotic-Resistant Bacteria. Obama White House. https://obamawhitehouse.archives.gov/the-press-office/2014/09/18/executive-order-combating-antibiotic-resistant-bacteria (accessed February 25, 2018).

"Federal Engagement in Antimicrobial Resistance." Centers for Disease Control and Prevention. https://www.cdc.gov/drugresistance/federal-engagement-in-ar/index.html (accessed February 26, 2018).

National Action Plan for Combating Antibiotic-Resistant Bacteria. Obama White House, March 27, 2015. https://obamawhitehouse.archives.gov/sites/default/files/docs/national_action_plan_for_combating_antibotic-resistant_bacteria.pdf (accessed February 24, 2018).

National Action Plan for Combating Antibiotic-Resistant Bacteria Progress Report for Years 1 and 2. Office of the Assistant Secretary for Planning and Evaluation. https://aspe.hhs.gov/pdf-report/national-action-plan-combating-antibiotic-resistant-bacteria-progress-report-years-1-and-2 (accessed February 24, 2018).

James Overholtzer

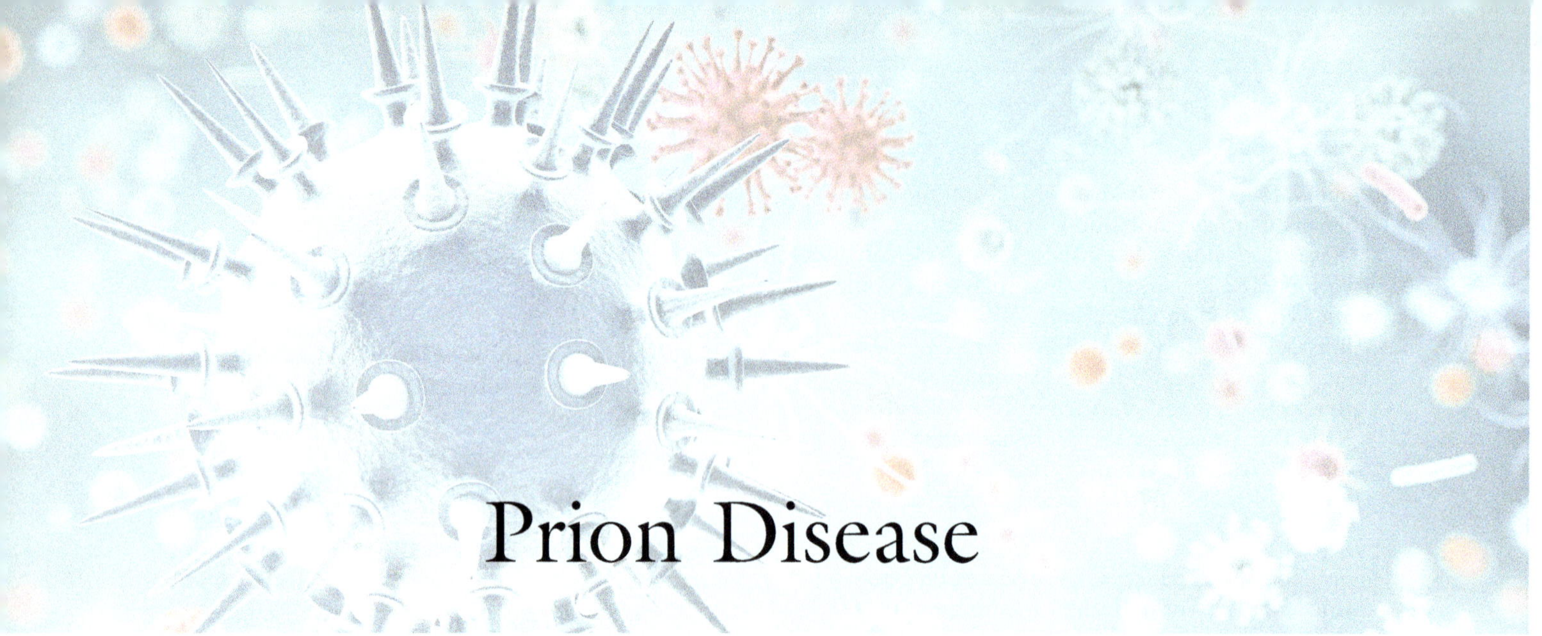

Prion Disease

Introduction

The prion diseases are a group of rare and invariably fatal brain disorders that occur in both animals and humans. They are unusual in that the infective agent is neither a virus nor a bacterium but an abnormal form of the prion protein (PrP) that is normally found in the brain. Prion disease leads to the development of tiny holes within brain tissue, giving it a characteristic spongiform appearance after death. Hence, prion diseases are also known as the transmissible spongiform encephalopathies (TSEs).

The best known of the human prion diseases is Creutzfeldt-Jakob disease (CJD), which affects about one person in 1 million. This rare disease came to public attention in 1996 with the announcement of a new form of CJD in the United Kingdom. Research has suggested that variant CJD is transmitted through exposure to beef contaminated by bovine spongiform encephalopathy (BSE), a prion disease of cattle.

Disease History, Characteristics, and Transmission

There are four forms of CJD, the major form of prion disease. Sporadic CJD accounts for around 85 percent of cases. Familial, or classic, CJD accounts for most of the rest. As of 2017 there had been 228 cases of variant CJD around the world, and three people had contracted

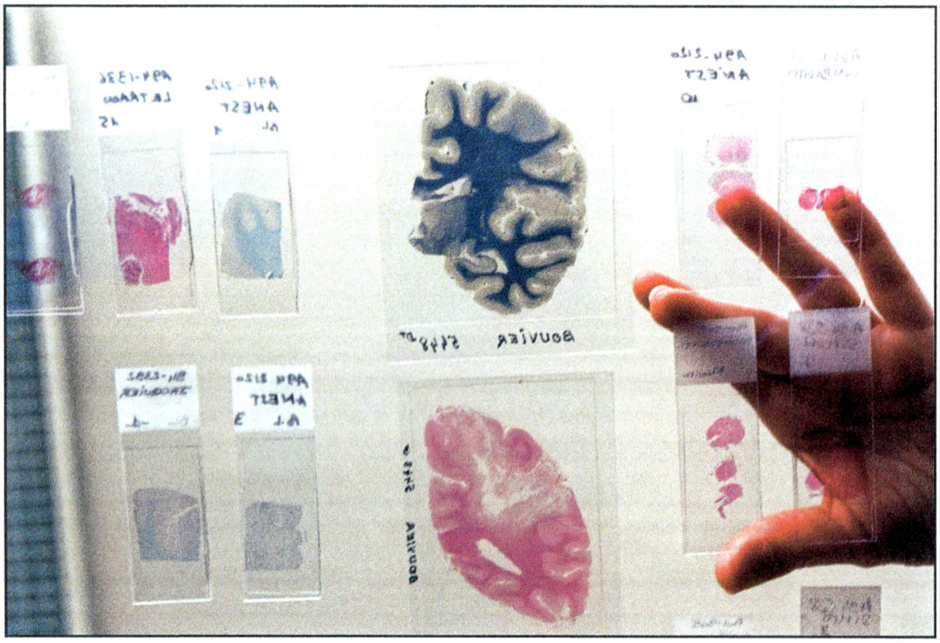

A doctor examines images at the Hôpital de la Pitié-Salpêtrière in Paris. The hospital is a major research center for prion disease. *© Raphael GAILLARDE/Gamma-Rapho/Getty Images*

iatrogenic CJD from prion contamination occurring through medical treatment. The other human prion diseases are Gerstmann-Sträuss-Scheinker (GSS) syndrome and familial fatal insomnia (FFI), which resemble familial CJD, and kuru, an almost extinct disease confined to the Fore people of New Guinea.

Prion diseases are marked by progressive deterioration of brain function that is always fatal. Sporadic CJD affects mainly people over 50 years old and is marked by ataxia, a shakiness and unsteadiness caused by damage to the cerebellum at the base of the brain, which controls movement. Dementia, swallowing difficulties, jerky movements, and blindness rapidly set in, and the patient usually dies within six months.

In familial CJD, GGS, and FFI, the onset of the disease may be at a younger age. The disease's course is measured in years rather than months. In FFI, as the name suggests, a major feature in a progressive and untreatable form of insomnia is caused by damage to the thalamus, the part of the brain regulating sleep-wake cycles.

Variant CJD has a younger age of onset than sporadic CJD and is marked by psychiatric problems and pain and odd sensations in the limbs. The time course of the disease is longer than in sporadic CJD, with ataxia setting in at a later stage. In iatrogenic CJD and kuru, ataxia is the main feature and dementia is unusual.

All prion diseases are transmissible under laboratory conditions, yet only variant CJD, iatrogenic CJD, and kuru are infectious in the way this term is usually understood. The source of abnormal PrP in these disorders is either beef contaminated with BSE or exposure to brain tissue from someone with CJD.

In sporadic CJD and familial CJD, as well as in GGS and FFI, a spontaneous or inherited mutation in the PrP gene leads to the generation of abnormal PrP within the patient's brain without any outside infection. This goes on to interact with normal PrP, causing the characteristic spongiform damage within the brain.

Prion Disease

Human Prion Diseases

Creutzfeldt-Jakob disease (CJD)
Variant Creutzfeldt-Jakob disease (vCJD)
Gerstmann-Straussler-Scheinker (GSS) syndrome
Fatal familial insomnia (FFI)
Kuru

Animal Prion Diseases

Bovine spongiform encephalopathy (BSE)
Chronic wasting disease (CWD)
Scrapie
Transmissible mink encephalopathy (TME)
Feline spongiform encephalopathy (FSE)

SOURCE: US Centers for Disease Control and Prevention, National Center for Infectious Diseases

WORDS TO KNOW

ATAXIA An unsteadiness in walking or standing that is associated with brain diseases such as kuru or Creutzfeldt-Jakob disease.

DEMENTIA A progressive deterioration and eventual loss of mental ability that is severe enough to interfere with normal activities of daily living; lasts more than six months; has not been present since birth; and is not associated with a loss or alteration of consciousness. From the Latin word *dement* meaning "away mind," dementia is a group of symptoms caused by gradual death of brain cells. Dementia is usually caused by degeneration in the cerebral cortex, the part of the brain responsible for thoughts, memories, actions, and personality. Death of brain cells in this region leads to the cognitive impairment that characterizes dementia.

IATROGENIC Any infection, injury, or other disease condition caused by medical treatment.

PRIONS Proteins that are infectious. Indeed, the name *prion* is derived from "proteinaceous infectious particles." The discovery of prions and confirmation of their infectious nature overturned a central dogma that infections were caused only by intact organisms, particularly microorganisms such as bacteria, fungi, parasites, or viruses. Because prions lack genetic material, the prevailing attitude was that a protein could not cause disease.

SPONGIFORM The clinical name for the appearance of brain tissue affected by prion diseases, such as Creutzfeld-Jakob disease or bovine spongiform encephalopathy. The disease process leads to the formation of tiny holes in brain tissue, giving it a spongy appearance.

Scope and Distribution

All prion diseases are rare, occurring with a frequency of about one per 1 million of the population, or fewer, around the world. As of 2017 there were 228 cases of variant CJD in 12 countries to date, 175 of which occurred in the United Kingdom. Kuru has all but disappeared since the Fore people ceased the funeral practices that exposed them to the disease.

Treatment and Prevention

There are no proven cures for any of the prion diseases, although there are a number of drugs being developed for CJD. Drugs can be given to ease the symptoms, such as valproate or clonazepam for jerky movements, and palliative care is employed.

■ Impacts and Issues

American researcher Stanley Prusiner (1942–) was awarded the 1997 Nobel Prize in Physiology or Medicine for his work on prions. But there is still much more to be learned about how prions work. For instance, routes of transmission are not well understood. Prion diseases may be present without symptoms for many years, putting people at risk of infection. Therefore, a better understanding of prions is an important challenge for neurology research.

The emergence of variant CJD in the 1980s in the United Kingdom among mostly young people sparked an epidemiological investigation that garnered worldwide attention. After the disease was linked with contaminated feed consumed by cattle in the United Kingdom, resulting in the cattle contracting BSE, the British beef industry suffered severe losses as more than 150,000 cattle were slaughtered. Many countries banned beef imports, and consumption of beef at home in the United Kingdom dropped dramatically. As other cases of variant CJD were linked to contaminated surgical instruments, stricter controls were put into place for decontamination and disposal of these instruments and tissues that could be infected with prions. In 2000 a British report titled "The BSE Inquiry" concluded that individual cattle were probably infected with BSE in the 1970s and that the disease became epidemic due to an intensive farming practice (the recycling of animal protein, including prions, in ruminant feed). As BSE was transmitted to humans, the new human prion disease known as variant CJD emerged.

See Also *Bovine Spongiform Encephalopathy (Mad Cow Disease); Creutzfeldt-Jakob Disease-nv; Kuru*

BIBLIOGRAPHY

Books

Koata, Gina. *Mercies in Disguise: A Story of Hope, a Family's Genetic Destiny, and the Science That Rescued Them.* New York: St. Martin's, 2017.

Ridley, Rosalind M., and Harry F. Baker. *Fatal Protein: The Story of CJD, BSE, and Other Prion Diseases.* New York: Oxford University Press, 1998.

Periodicals

Carnaud, Claude. "Is There Still Hope after Prions Have Spread within the Brain." *Journal of Infectious Diseases* 204, no. 7 (October 2011): 978–979.

Websites

"The BSE Inquiry." The National Archives. http://webarchive.nationalarchives.gov.uk/20060802142310/http://www.bseinquiry.gov.uk/ (accessed January 29, 2018).

"Creutzfeldt-Jakob Disease, Classic (CJD)." Centers for Disease Control and Prevention, February 6, 2015. https://www.cdc.gov/prions/cjd/index.html (accessed January 29, 2018).

"Creutzfeldt-Jakob Disease Surveillance in the UK." National CJD Research and Surveillance Unit, University of Edinburgh, 2016. https://www.cjd.ed.ac.uk/sites/default/files/report25.pdf (accessed January 29, 2018).

"Variant CJD Cases Worldwide." University of Edinburgh, December 4, 2017. https://www.cjd.ed.ac.uk/sites/default/files/worldfigs.pdf (accessed January 29, 2018).

"Variant Creutzfeldt-Jakob Disease." Centers for Disease Control and Prevention, February 6, 2015. https://www.cdc.gov/prions/vcjd/index.html (accessed January 29, 2018).

Susan Aldridge
Anna Marie E. Roos

ProMED

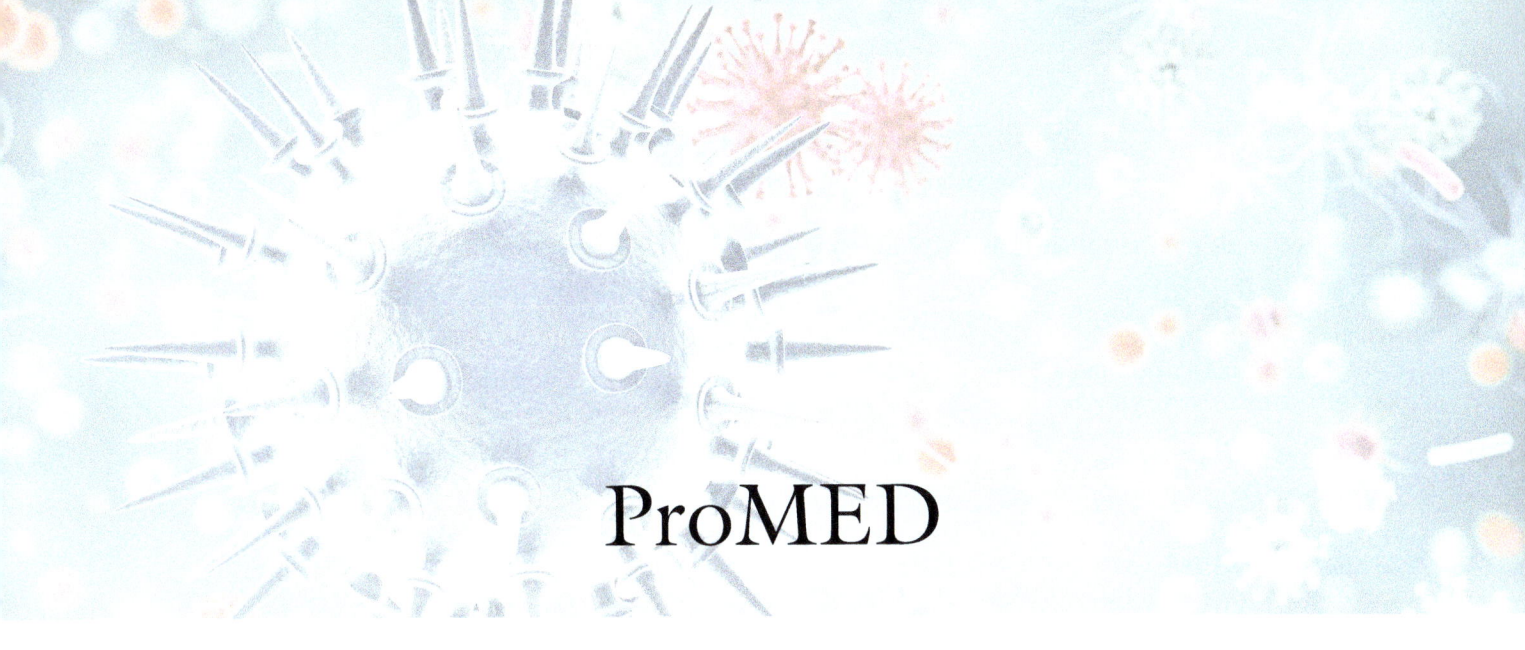

ProMED, or the Program for Monitoring Emerging Diseases, originated at a meeting in 1993 in Geneva, Switzerland, cosponsored by the World Health Organization (WHO). Attendees proposed the idea of a worldwide chain of institutes capable of sending teams to the site of any unusual local disease outbreak. The objective would be to determine whether the outbreak was of natural or unnatural origin.

Since then the concept of emerging diseases, or diseases that were previously unknown, or present only rarely, but have increased in prevalence or geographic scope, has become an important aspect of global disease monitoring. Emerging diseases include Ebola, severe acute respiratory syndrome (SARS), avian influenza, Zika virus infection, and Chikungunya virus infection.

The uniqueness of ProMED is its stable of experts in the fields of clinical and veterinary medicine, microbiology, and plant pathology, all of whom serve on a part-time basis. ProMED is the only free disease reporting system to cover human, livestock, wildlife, and food and feed crop diseases in one place. The latter is important because of the potential impact of animal and vegetable diseases on nutrition and therefore on human health.

In October 1999 ProMED became a program of the International Society for Infectious Diseases (ISID), which guarantees the program's freedom from political constraints

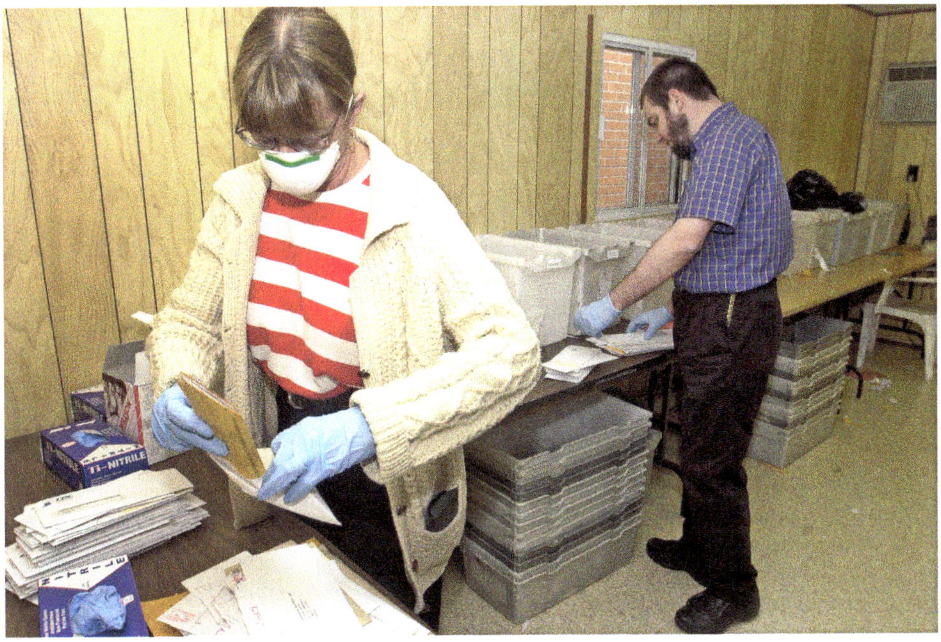

During an anthrax-by-mail scare in 2001, the internet-based infectious-disease reporting system known as the Program for Monitoring Emerging Diseases (or ProMED) served an important role in providing information to government officials in charge of the response to the scare. *© Tannis Toohey/Toronto Star/Getty Images*

that often cause delays in outbreak reporting. In fact, WHO has said it uses ProMED reports of a disease to convince recalcitrant countries to report outbreaks officially.

As of 2017 the subscriber list to ProMED exceeded 70,000. ProMED also had parallel lists in Spanish, Portuguese, Russian, and French, though these are mainly reports of regional interest rather than straight translations of the English reports. Chinese and Japanese translations of many ProMED reports are found on the travel health websites of Hong Kong and Tokyo international airports.

SEE ALSO *Emerging Infectious Diseases; GIDEON; Globalization and Infectious Disease; Reemerging Infectious Diseases; SARS (Severe Acute Respiratory Syndrome); Virus Hunters*

BIBLIOGRAPHY

Books

Dingwall, Robert, Lily M. Hoffman, and Karen Staniland, eds. *Pandemics and Emerging Diseases: The Sociological Agenda*. Chichester, UK: Wiley, 2013.

Shah, Sonia. *Pandemic: Tracking Contagions, from Cholera to Ebola and Beyond*. New York: Sarah Crichton Books/Farrar, Straus and Giroux, 2016.

Periodicals

Hugh-Jones, Martin. "Global Awareness of Disease Outbreaks: The Experience of ProMED-Mail." *Public Health Reports* 116, no. 2 (2001): 27–31.

Madoff, Lawrence C. "ProMED-Mail: An Early Warning System for Emerging Diseases." *Clinical Infectious Diseases* 39, no. 2 (July 2004): 227–232.

Websites

"Disease Outbreak News." World Health Organization. http://www.who.int/csr/don/en (accessed December 11, 2017).

ProMED-Mail. http://www.promedmail.org (accessed December 11, 2017).

Jack Woodall
Brian Hoyle

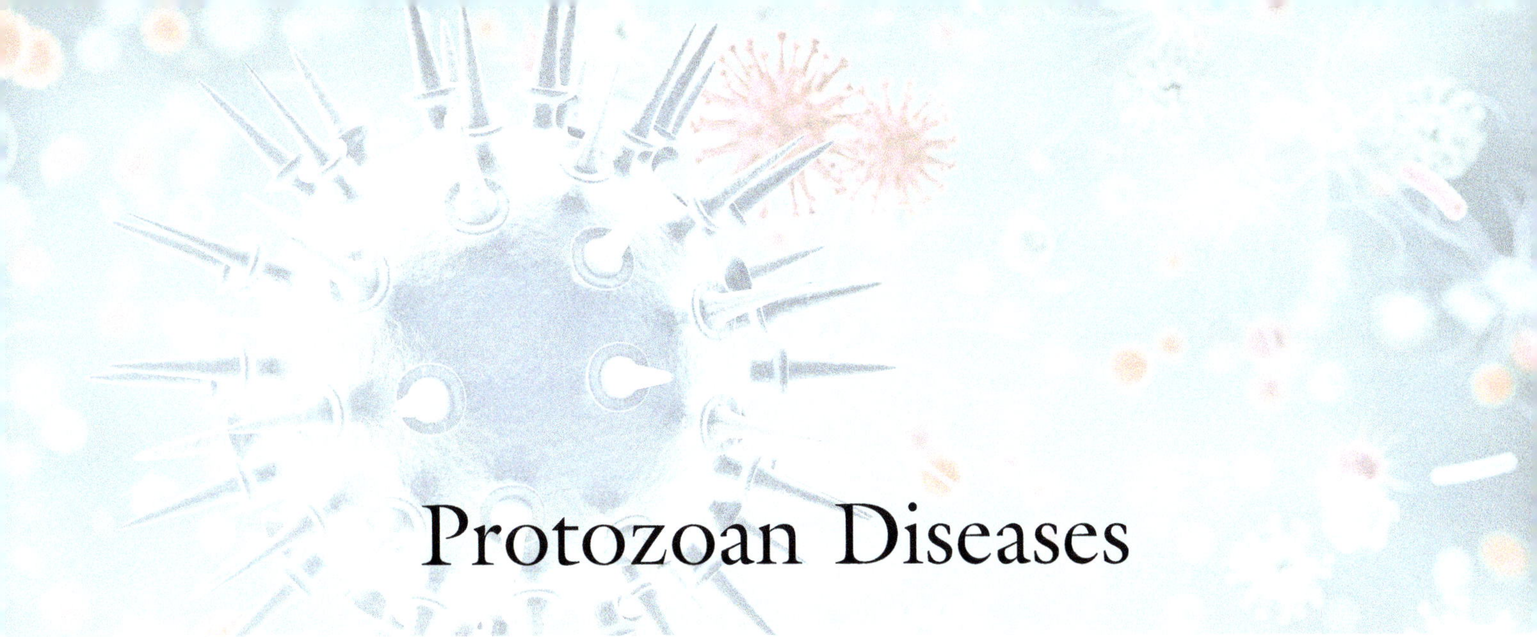

Protozoan Diseases

Introduction

Protozoan diseases are infectious diseases transmitted to humans by parasitic protozoa, single-celled microorganisms that can be seen using a microscope. The method of transmission varies depending on the life cycle of the parasite and can result in both benign and life-threatening conditions. Enteric protozoan parasites, such as *Entoemeba* and *Giardia*, multiply in the human intestine and are transmitted from one person to another through the fecal-oral route. Other protozoan parasites, such as *Leishmania, Trypanosoma*, and *Plasmodium*, are transmitted through infected insect bites and multiply in blood or other tissues. Some protozoan parasites, such as *Toxoplasma*, are also opportunistic pathogens that cause infection only in individuals with weak immune systems, such as individuals with acquired immunodeficiency syndrome (AIDS).

There are four main groups of protozoa that cause infection in humans. They are grouped according to their movement pattern: Sarcodina (e.g., *Entoemeba*), Mastigophora (e.g., *Giardia* and *Leishmania*), Ciliophora (e.g., *Balantidium*), and Sporozoa (e.g., *Plasmodium* and *Cryptosporidium*). Protozoan diseases that inflict a significant medical burden on humans include malaria, African sleeping sickness, Chagas disease, leishmaniasis, giardiasis, amebiasis, toxoplasmosis, balantidiasis, cryptosporidiasis, and trichomoniasis.

History, Characteristics, and Transmission

Proto-zoa means "first animals," and protozoa are one of the earliest known organisms in the animal kingdom. They are classified under the Protozoa kingdom with more than 30,000 species. They are eukaryotic organisms, meaning that they have a nucleus. Protozoa have membrane-bound nuclei and are 10 to 100 microns long (a micron is one-millionth of a meter). Not all protozoan species are pathogenic to humans or animals. Some of the parasites may exist as a cyst during their life cycle.

Numerous protozoans are associated with human disease. Four species of plasmodium, *P. falciparum, P. ovale, P. vivax*, and *P. malariae*, cause malaria in humans. The malarial parasite is introduced into the body by the bite of a female mosquito and enters liver cells. After a few weeks the parasite is released into the blood. The parasite multiplies inside red blood cells and is released to the blood to infect new cells. A small percentage of parasites undergo sexual reproduction (gametocyte stage) and infect mosquitos when they feed on the infected individual's blood, completing the life cycle. Signs and symptoms of malaria include shivering, headache, chills, fatigue, muscle aches, and sweating. Severe cases of malaria include cerebral malaria, severe anemia, respiratory abnormalities, jaundice, and renal failure.

African sleeping sickness, also called trypanosomiasis, is a deadly disease caused *Trypanosoma brucei.* Ninety percent of African sleeping sickness is caused by a variant of *Trypanosoma brucei gambiense.* The other 10 percent is caused by *Trypanosoma brucei rhodesiense.* The infection is transmitted by the bite of the tsetse fly, which is found in Africa. Tsetse flies get infected upon biting infected humans or other animals and multiply over a period of two to three weeks. The trypanosomes reach the salivary gland and infect humans during their next blood meal. They further mature and divide in the blood and lymphatic system of the new host, resulting in clinical symptoms such as malaise, intermittent fever, and rashes. Eventually the parasite reaches the brain, causing severe behavioral and neurologic changes such as progressive confusion, seizures, irritability, personality changes, weight loss, loss of concentration, slurred speech, and difficulty in talking and walking, eventually leading to death if not treated.

Trypanosoma cruzi causes Chagas disease, also known as American trypanosomiasis, which is found mostly in the American subcontinent. The infection is transmitted by blood-sucking triatomine insects also known as kissing

WORDS TO KNOW

CUTANEOUS Pertaining to the skin.

ENTERIC Involving the intestinal tract or relating to the intestines.

FECAL-ORAL ROUTE The spread of disease through the transmission of minute particles of fecal material from one organism to the mouth of another. This can occur by drinking contaminated water; eating food exposed to animal or human feces, such as food from plants watered with unclean water; or preparing food without practicing proper hygiene.

PARASITE An organism that lives in or on a host organism and that gets its nourishment from that host. The parasite usually gains all the benefits of this relationship, whereas the host may suffer from various diseases and discomforts or show no signs of the infection. The life cycle of a typical parasite usually includes several developmental stages and morphological changes as the parasite lives and moves through the environment and one or more hosts. Parasites that remain on a host's body surface to feed are called ectoparasites; those that live inside a host's body are called endoparasites. Parasitism is a highly successful biological adaptation. There are more known parasitic species than nonparasitic ones, and parasites affect just about every form of life, including most all animals, plants, and even bacteria.

RESERVOIR The animal or organism in which a virus or parasite normally resides.

VISCERAL Pertaining to the viscera. The viscera are the large organs contained in the main cavities of the body, especially the thorax and abdomen—for example, the lungs, stomach, intestines, kidneys, or liver.

bugs. The parasite spreads to various parts of the body and multiplies, causing a variety of symptoms, with the heart being the most commonly affected organ in people with chronic Chagas disease.

Leishmaniasis is caused by a blood parasite of the *Leishmania* species. The infection is acquired by the bite of a sand fly. *L. donovani* causes visceral leishmaniasis (also called kala-azar) affecting endothelial cells, bone marrow, liver, lymph glands, and blood vessels of the spleen. Symptoms include weight loss, fever, liver enlargement, spleen enlargement, and abnormal blood counts. *L. tropica* causes cutaneous leishmaniasis affecting the skin. *L. brasiliensis* causes American leishmaniasis, producing multiple sores over large areas of the skin and mucosa.

Toxoplasmosis is caused by *Toxoplasma gondii*, found worldwide in a range of animals and humans. Toxoplasmosis is usually asymptomatic, although it may cause flu-like illness. It can, however, cause serious complications in individuals with weak immune systems, such as patients suffering from AIDS, and may result in stillbirth if a woman is infected early in her pregnancy. Infection is acquired by ingestion of infected meat, unwashed vegetables, or accidental ingestion of feces. Cats are the primary host, contracting infection by eating contaminated raw meat. Infected cats release the cysts through their feces, the primary source of infection for humans.

Babesia causes babesiosis and is transmitted by infected tick bites. It is generally seen around New England, New Jersey, New York, Minnesota, and Wisconsin. Symptoms of babesiosis include fatigue, nausea, body aches, headache, loss of appetite, chills, fever, and sweats.

Amoebiasis, also called amoebic dysentery, is caused by *Entamoeba histolytica*, which infects human intestinal tracts. Infection is acquired by ingestion of contaminated food or water that contains cysts of *Entamoeba*. These cysts release the parasite after reaching the intestine. The parasite may spread to other organs, such as the liver, spleen, lungs, and skin. Amoebiasis is generally without any symptoms. When present, symptoms include diarrhea with mucus and blood and abdominal pain. If left untreated, it may cause abscesses in parts of the body, including the liver and colon.

Giardiasis is caused by a parasite *Giardia intestinalis*, which spreads through the oral route by the intake of food and water contaminated with parasite cysts. In the intestine the parasite attaches itself to the epithelial cells with the help of a sucking disc and resulting in disturbance of intestinal function. Symptoms of giardiasis include greasy stools, diarrhea, nausea, flatulence, and abdominal cramps.

Trichomoniasis is caused by the *Trichomonas* species. *T. hominis, T. lenax*, and *T. vaginalis* are three common species known to infect humans. *T. vaginalis* inhabits the vagina, where it causes vaginitis characterized by inflammation of vaginal mucosa, a burning sensation, and abnormal discharges. Men act as intermediaries. In men infection may cause urethritis (inflammation of the urethra). Infection is usually through sexual contact.

Balantidial dysentery is a disease of the large intestine in humans and is caused by *Balantidium coli.* Pigs are the primary reservoir, and pig handlers are at risk of infection. The parasites exist both as a trophozite and a cyst. Other than diarrhea, symptoms include abdominal pain, nausea, fluid loss, and mild colitis.

■ Scope and Distribution

Amebiasis is found worldwide, with the highest incidences in developing countries with inadequate sanitary infrastructure. Approximately 50 million cases of invasive amoebiasis due to *E. histolytica* are reported worldwide, with 100,000 deaths each year. However, frequency of infection is believed to be far higher, as only

10 to 20 percent of infected individuals develop symptoms. In the United States, the overall prevalence of symptomatic amebiasis is less than 1 percent.

Toxoplasmosis is found worldwide, with the exposure rate as high as 50 to 90 percent in adult individuals and up to 50 percent infection in women of childbearing age. Individuals with weakened immunity, such as HIV/AIDS patients or patients who undergo organ transplant and immunosuppressive medication, are at potential risk for toxoplasmic encephalitis.

Malaria is endemic across Central America, South America, sub-Saharan Africa, the Indian subcontinent, Southeast Asia, and the Middle East. Malaria is responsible for 300 million to 500 million infections annually worldwide with 1 million to 3 million deaths per year. Predominantly children in sub-Saharan Africa are infected with *P. falciparum*. Additionally, 25 million to 30 million people from the United States and Europe travel to endemic areas and acquire malaria, with 10,000 to 30,000 cases every year in this population.

Leishmaniasis is endemic in India, China, Africa, southern Europe, South America, and Russia. The disease is divided into Old World leishmaniasis found in Africa, Asia, the Middle East, the Mediterranean, and India, and New World leishmaniasis found in Central and South America. Old World leishmaniasis produces cutaneous or visceral disease. New World leishmaniasis produces cutaneous and mucocutaneous disease. More than 12 million cases of leishmaniasis are reported worldwide, with 900,000 to 1.3 million new cases each year.

African trypanosomiasis is restricted to tropical Africa, affecting millions of people in 36 countries. An estimated 50,000 to 70,000 cases of African trypanosomiasis are reported, although the exact prevalence rate of the disease is difficult to assess due to the remoteness and lack of active surveillance available to monitor the disease. Chagas disease caused by *T. cruzi* is endemic in Mexico and countries of Central America and South America, with an estimated 6 million to 8 million people infected and 12,000 deaths each year, according to the World Health Organization (WHO) in 2016.

Treatment and Prevention

Amoebiasis is diagnosed by identifying the parasite containing ingested red blood cells in a patient's stool. Metronidazole is the primary drug of choice to treat invasive amebiasis such as amebic liver abscess. Tinidazole has been approved by the US Food and Drug Administration (FDA) for intestinal or extraintestinal amebiasis. Improved sanitation and hygiene that prevents fecal contamination of food and water are the best methods of preventing amebiasis. Efforts should be made to identify and treat disease carriers who otherwise act as a constant source of infection to others.

Toxoplasmosis is diagnosed by the identification of the parasite in blood, body fluids, or tissues. Pyrithramine along with Leucovorin (folinic acid) is used for the treatment of toxoplasmosis. Other drugs used against toxoplasmosis include sulfadiazine and clindamycin. Protecting children's play areas from cat litter and educating pregnant women about the threat posed to the fetus by toxoplasmosis infection may be effective in controlling the disease.

Treatment of malaria is based on the type of infection. Specific treatment options include quinine-based drugs such as quinine sulfate plus doxycycline or clindamycin or pyrimethamine-sulfadoxine. Chloroquine, primaquine, and mefloquine are also used to treat malaria. Malaria is diagnosed through patient history of visiting an endemic area and a blood smear examination for malarial parasites inside the red blood corpuscles.

Leishmaniasis is diagnosed by isolation and visualization of parasites from infected tissues as well as serum-based specific assays. Pentavalent antimony (sodium stibogluconate or meglumine antimonate), liposomal amphotericin B, oral miltefosine, and pentamidine are some of the drugs commonly used to treat leishmaniasis. Treatment for malnutrition, and intervention with the concurrent illness such as AIDS or tuberculosis, is critical to managing leishmaniasis.

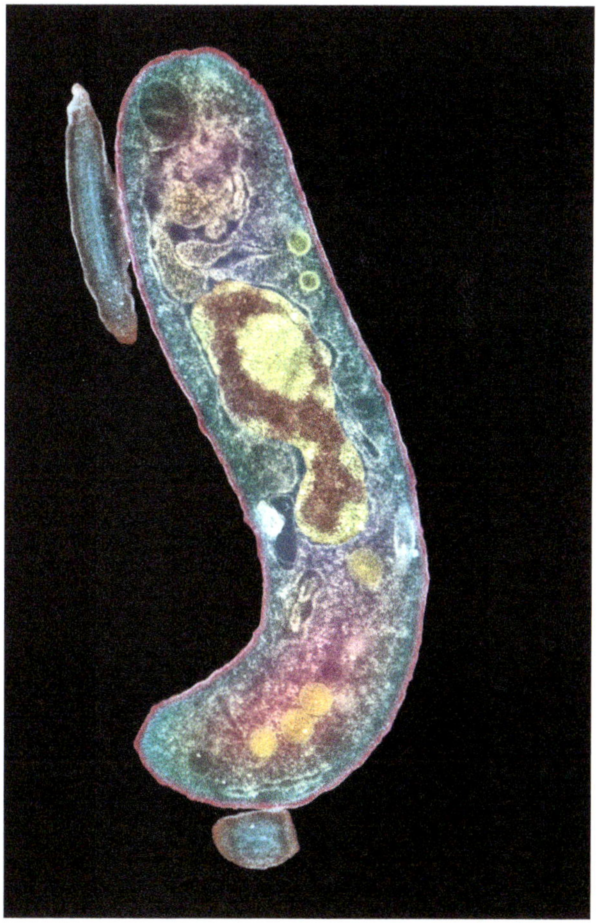

A large number of infectious diseases are caused by microscopic, single-celled organisms known as protozoa, such as the one shown here. © *London School of Hygiene & Tropical Medicine/Science Source*

Trypanosomiasis is diagnosed by histology of blood smear and lymph node or bone marrow aspiration during the early stage of the disease. Benznidazole and Nifurtimox are drugs of choice for the treatment of trypanosomiasis.

Impacts and Issues

There is enormous concern with regard to the prevalence of protozoan diseases across the globe. The Global Burden of Disease Study 2013 indicates malaria is the most prominent parasitic disease, with global deaths of more than 850,000. The study also points out that other protozoan diseases cause fatalities globally: leishmaniasis (62,500 deaths), Chagas disease (10,600 deaths), and African sleeping sickness (6,900 deaths). Among enteric protozoan parasites, 41,900 suffered death due to cryptosporidiosis, whereas 11,300 deaths occurred due to amebiasis.

According to WHO, leishmaniasis is endemic in 98 countries in Africa, Asia, Europe, North America, and South America, with an annual incidence of 0.7 million to 1.3 million cases of cutaneous disease and 0.2 million to 0.4 million cases of visceral disease. However, there has been significant progress in control of visceral leishmaniasis in Southeast Asia.

The Centers for Disease Control and Prevention (CDC) warns that parasitic diseases thought to be prevalent only in developing countries are becoming more common in the United States. For example, in 2014 it was reported that 300,000 US citizens contracted Chagas disease caused by *Typanosoma cruzi* and more than 60 million suffered chronically from toxoplasma infection. Toxoplasmosis is also a significant health concern due to congenital toxoplasmosis. Furthermore, about 3.7 million people in the United States are affected by *Trichomonas*, which is sexually transmitted.

In developed countries infections with enteric protozoa are not particularly researched because of better hygienic conditions. However, due to a shifting environmental landscape such as climate change and changing ecosystems, increases in atmospheric temperature, and flooding, experts believe that even developed countries are at risk of contracting otherwise rare infections. Such infections thus require further research and education.

PRIMARY SOURCE

Climate Change Contribution to the Emergence or Re-emergence of Parasitic Diseases

SOURCE: *Short, Erica E., Cyril Caminade, and Bolaji N. Thomas. "Climate Change Contribution to the Emergence or Re-emergence of Parasitic Diseases."* Infectious Diseases: Research and Treatment *(September 25, 2017).*

INTRODUCTION: *Although most parasitic protozoa can survive only in limited areas of the globe, scientists project that they will spread to new areas as global climate change progresses. In the following excerpt from an article in the journal* Infectious Diseases: Research and Treatment, *the authors offer an overview of the impact of climate change on parasitic disease in general and on ingested protozoa specifically.*

Introduction

Climate change is a naturally occurring event, but human activities have significantly contributed to changes in atmospheric conditions, resulting in an accelerated change in this process, and the current precarious state. Climate change is increasingly threatening as we continue to realize its potential impacts on global health and security. Global climate experts agree that anthropogenic activities have significantly contributed to the increasing concentration of atmospheric greenhouse gases and destruction of ecosystems. Direct consequences of climate change are not difficult to notice through the occurrence of extreme weather events or changes in temperature and precipitation, but indirect consequences are not as easily seen. An increase or change in the endemic range of parasitic diseases as a result of climate change will have very serious repercussions. Now, it is not only our physical footprints prompting the spread of disease through habitat destruction and ecological disruption but possibly our carbon footprints as well. Climate change directly causes increases in temperature and affects weather patterns, which indirectly can change spatial patterns of disease vectors and human populations. Increases in temperature facilitate the development of arthropod vectors that carry many parasitic organisms and the parasites themselves. A warm climate also increases the range of reservoir hosts, vector abundance, biting rates and overall survival, and parasitic transmission rates of vectors such as mosquitoes, ticks, and tsetse flies.

Parasitic diseases are often the burden of tropical and subtropical communities because those climates promote species richness and therefore can support a multitude of potential hosts to sustain parasitic diseases. Complex host interactions are key to survivability and thrivability of parasites, and these complex interactions can be altered by a changing climate to promote infectious diseases. Climate change has the potential to alter or extend the natural ranges of these organisms and make regions of our globe that were previously uninhabitable for parasites habitable. Increases in temperature affect the life cycles of parasites, which can directly affect how prevalent the organism is within the area, considering many parasitic organisms have a temperature-dependent developmental baseline, either within their host or in the environment.

Although less recognized than some other climate change consequences, emergence and reemergence of parasitic diseases are very concerning. These diseases often go deeper than just directly declining human health by promoting a positive feedback loop of poverty and economic stagnation in the communities they are most likely to affect, ultimately declining overall quality of life. This review will explore some of the different parasites whose distributions, severity, or reemergence, in cases that have been previously eradicated, would be affected by climate change as well as some of the risks their associated diseases pose to local and global economies. We will examine vector-borne infections, ingested protozoa, soil-transmitted helminthiasis, and the economic implication of these diseases.

[...]

Parasites in the Environment

Ingested protozoa

Protozoa that are exposed directly to the environment undergo a cyst or oocyst stage as a part of their life cycle, these stages providing varying degrees of resilience for the parasite and allowing its viability outside of a host species. Giardiasis, cryptosporidiosis, amebiasis, and toxoplasmosis can all be transmitted through contaminated drinking water. Climate change may place a strain on agricultural industries as they try to retain crop productivity during droughts or periods of intense precipitation. To compensate for these crop stresses, increased fertilizer use is encouraged. Animal fertilizers, as well as human biosolids used as fertilizers, have the potential to contain parasitic cysts and oocysts. Heavy rainfall events, which may increase in frequency and intensity due to climate change, will more often wash fertilizers into local waterways. Heavy rainfall events can also simply extract cysts and oocysts from soil and grass, and these events have been associated with outbreaks of cryptosporidiosis and giardiasis.

A couple of scenarios can take place once these parasites are in a waterway. First, extreme rainfall events and flooding may render some wastewater treatment plants unable to accommodate the amount of influent sewage. Wastewater treatment plants are typically equipped with overflow systems that allow excess sewage to bypass treatment, other than a primary filter that removes large debris. This sewage then gets returned to the waterway untreated and with parasitic organisms still infective. This issue is augmented for island nations that flood easily during extreme weather events, such as hurricanes, and the groundwater may even be contaminated. In 1987, people living on the Chuuk Islands of the Federated States of Micronesia experienced a sudden increase in amebiasis due to flooding from Typhoon Nina. Second to overflows, parasites may not be killed by common disinfectants used at wastewater and drinking water treatment facilities and remain in the water. For example, chlorine is a common disinfectant that is not capable of killing *Cryptosporidium* spp. in oocyst form. Even a more revered disinfection method, the usage of UV light, is not always effective at killing these oocysts. Water temperature and UV exposure time play a role in parasite mortality, and for maximum effectiveness, these parameters must be carefully determined. In either case discussed, humans ultimately come into contact with these contaminated waters and drink or otherwise ingest parasites because of climatic events.

SEE ALSO *African Sleeping Sickness (Trypanosomiasis); Arthropod-Borne Diseases; Climate Change and Infectious Disease; Malaria; Mosquito-Borne Diseases; Tropical Diseases*

BIBLIOGRAPHY

Books

Castillo, Victor, and Rodney Harris, eds. *Protozoa: Biology, Classification and Role in Disease.* New York: Nova Biomedical, 2013.

Wiser, Mark F. *Protozoa and Human Disease.* New York: Garland Science, 2011.

Periodicals

Avasthi R., S. C. Chaudhary, and S. Khanna. "Visceral Leishmaniasis Simulating Chronic Liver Disease: Successful Treatment with Miltefosine." *Indian Journal of Medical Microbiology* 27, no. 1 (January–March 2009): 85–86.

Fletcher SM, et al. "Enteric Protozoa in the Developed World: A Public Health Perspective." *Clinical Microbiology Reviews* 25, no. 3 (July 2012): 420–449

Franco, Jose R., et al. "Epidemiology of Human African Trypanosomiasis." *Clinical Epidemiology* 6 (2014): 257–275.

Gonzales, Maria Liza M., Leonila F. Dans, and Elizabeth G. Martinez. "Antiamoebic Drugs for Treating Amoebic Colitis." *Cochrane Database of Systematic Reviews* (April 15, 2009). This article can also be found online at http://onlinelibrary.wiley.com/doi/10.1002/14651858.CD006085.pub2/abstract;jsessionid=F46287E3F4291C657AAA1B8E09315CD4.f02t02 (accessed March 15, 2018).

Morillo C. A., et al. "Randomized Trial of Benznidazole for Chronic Chagas' Cardiomyopathy." *New England Journal of Medicine* 373 (October 2015): 1295–1306. This article can be found online at http://www.nejm.org/doi/full/10.1056/NEJMoa1507574.

Rassi, A., Jr., A. Rassi, and J. A. Marin-Neto. "Chagas Disease." *Lancet* 375, no. 9723 (April 17, 2010): 1388–1402.

Rico-Torres C. P., et al. "Molecular Diagnosis and Genotyping of Cases of Perinatal Toxoplasmosis in Mexico." *Pediatric Infectious Disease Journal* 31, no. 4 (December 14, 2011).

Websites

"CDC Warns of Common Parasites Plaguing Millions in U.S." CBS News, May 8, 2014. https://www.cbsnews.com/news/parasites-causing-infections-in-the-us-cdc-says/ (accessed March 2, 2018).

"Chagas Disease (American Trypanosomiasis)." World Health Organization, March 2017. http://www.who.int/mediacentre/factsheets/fs340/en/ (accessed March 1, 2018).

"Leishmaniasis Fact Sheet." World Health Organization, April 2017. http://www.who.int/mediacentre/factsheets/fs375/en/ (accessed March 1, 2018).

"Malaria." Centers for Disease Control and Prevention, January 26, 2018. http://www.cdc.gov/malaria (accessed March 1, 2018).

"One Million Deaths by Parasites." *PLOS* Speaking of Medicine Community Blog, January 16, 2015. http://blogs.plos.org/speakingofmedicine/2015/01/16/one-million-deaths-parasites/ (accessed March 2, 2018).

"Parasites—Babesiosis." Centers for Disease Control and Prevention, May 24, 2016. https://www.cdc.gov/parasites/babesiosis/index.html (accessed March 1, 2018).

"Parasites—Leishmaniasis. Epidemiology & Risk Factors." Centers for Disease Control and Prevention, January 10, 2013. http://www.cdc.gov/parasites/leishmaniasis/epi.html (accessed March 1, 2018).

"Protozoan Parasites." Parasites in Humans. http://www.parasitesinhumans.org/protozoa.html (accessed March 1, 2018).

Kausalya Santhanam

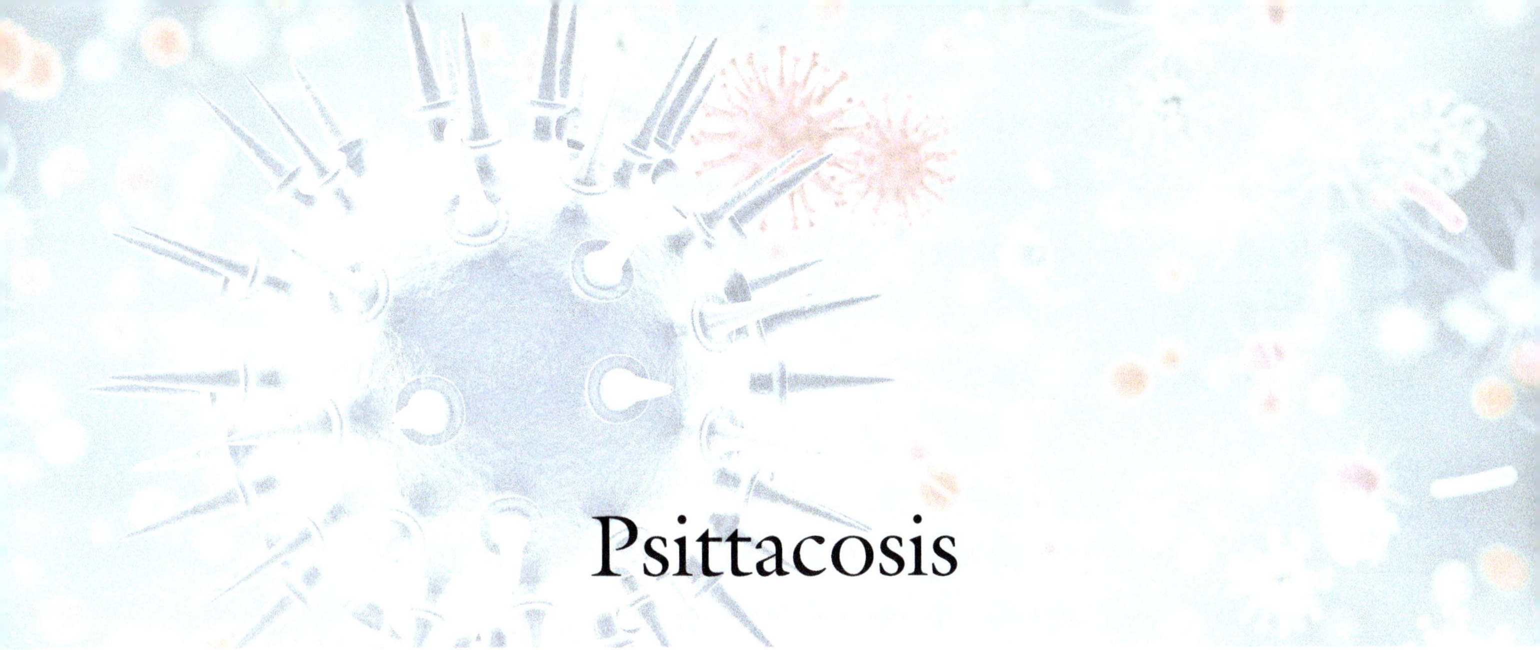

Psittacosis

Introduction

Psittacosis is a bacterial zoonotic (passed from animals to humans) infection caused by the bacterium *Chlamydia psittaci*. This bacterium is present in birds and passed to humans when they inhale airborne infectious particles such as feather dust or bird secretions. Psittacosis causes acute symptoms of fever, headache, body aches, and a dry cough. Respiratory conditions such as pneumonia may also arise. Left untreated, psittacosis has a mortality rate as high as 10 to 20 percent. However, with treatment, the disease is not usually fatal, with approximately a 1 percent mortality rate in the United States. Treatment using tetracycline antibiotics usually leads to a full recovery.

Psittacosis occurs worldwide, but outbreaks are rare. Importation of birds helps to spread the disease. People who come in close contact with birds, including veterinarians, pet store owners, pet owners, and poultry producers, are most at risk of contracting psittacosis. Psittacosis can be prevented by avoiding contact with infected birds or by wearing protective gear such as gloves and masks when handling infected birds.

Disease History, Characteristics, and Transmission

Psittacosis was first identified in 1879 as a bacterial disease that infected birds and was later confirmed to also infect humans and other animals. During 1929 and 1930, a shipment of infected parrots from Argentina caused a worldwide outbreak. There were approximately 1,000 cases, 200 to 300 of which were fatal. The outbreak prompted a ban on bird importation in many major countries, including the United States, but this ban was lifted in 1973.

Psittacosis is a bacterial disease caused by the bacteria *Chlamydia psittaci* and is common in many bird species, both wild and tame. Humans become infected with *C. psittaci* if they inhale dried secretions from infected birds. These secretions may include aerosolized feces, feather dust, and droplets from sneezing or coughing birds.

Psittacosis symptoms include fever, headache, body aches, and a dry cough. Pneumonia may also develop. Severe or untreated cases of psittacosis may result in complications such as a heart valve infection (endocarditis), liver inflammation (hepatitis), and neurologic complications. With treatment, the mortality rate for psittacosis is approximately 1 percent.

Scope and Distribution

The organism that causes psittacosis can be found worldwide. Importation of birds increases the risk of infection spreading from one region to another. The

WORDS TO KNOW

AEROSOL Particles of liquid or solid dispersed as a suspension in gas.

IMMUNOCOMPROMISED Having an immune system with reduced ability to recognize and respond to the presence of foreign material.

MORTALITY The condition of being susceptible to death. The term *mortality* comes from the Latin word *mors*, which means death. Mortality can also refer to the rate of deaths caused by an illness or injury (e.g., "Rabies has a high mortality rate").

ZOONOTIC A disease that can be transmitted between animals and humans. Examples of zoonotic diseases are anthrax, plague, and Q fever.

REAL-WORLD RISKS

Although it is a reportable condition in most states, psittacosis is a rare disease. Within the United States there have been fewer than 10 confirmed cases of psittacosis each year since 2010. However, the Centers for Disease Control and Prevention suggests that some cases of psittacosis may go undiagnosed or misdiagnosed.

bird industry, including poultry farming and the pet trade, provides another route for the infection to spread.

In 2002 an outbreak in the Blue Mountains of Australia involved 59 probable cases. The source of the infection was wild birds. The outbreak prompted the Australian Department of Health to raise public awareness about psittacosis. In 1995 an outbreak occurred involving customs officers in Belgium. The source of the infection was imported parakeets.

Most cases of psittacosis occur in people who have a close association with birds. This includes pet owners, pet store owners, bird fanciers, and poultry producers. In addition, young children, older adults, smokers, alcoholics, and immunocompromised people tend to be more susceptible to infection.

■ Treatment and Prevention

Infection with *Chlamydia psittaci* is effectively treated using antibiotics. The antibiotics most commonly prescribed to treat *C. psittaci* are tetracycline, doxycycline, and erythromycin. Treatment is normally administered for two weeks, after which a full recovery is expected.

The best way to prevent infection with *C. psittaci* is to avoid contact with infected birds and to ensure birds are kept free from infection. Investigating the cause of sickness in ill birds will help determine whether *C. psittaci* is present. Once an infected bird is found, measures can be taken to prevent the disease from spreading to other birds or to humans. Avoidance measures such as wearing face masks and gloves and frequently washing hands can help reduce the chance of inhaling or ingesting contaminated particles. As of 2017 no vaccine was available to prevent contraction of psittacosis.

■ Impacts and Issues

Some cases of psittacosis may go undiagnosed or be misdiagnosed because diagnosis can be difficult. Respiratory symptoms can lead a practitioner to misdiagnose the illness as a case of pneumonia rather than psittacosis. Therefore, the prevalence of psittacosis may be underestimated.

Another issue surrounding psittacosis is the difficulty associated with tracing the disease to its source. First, infected birds may be asymptomatic, making it difficult to

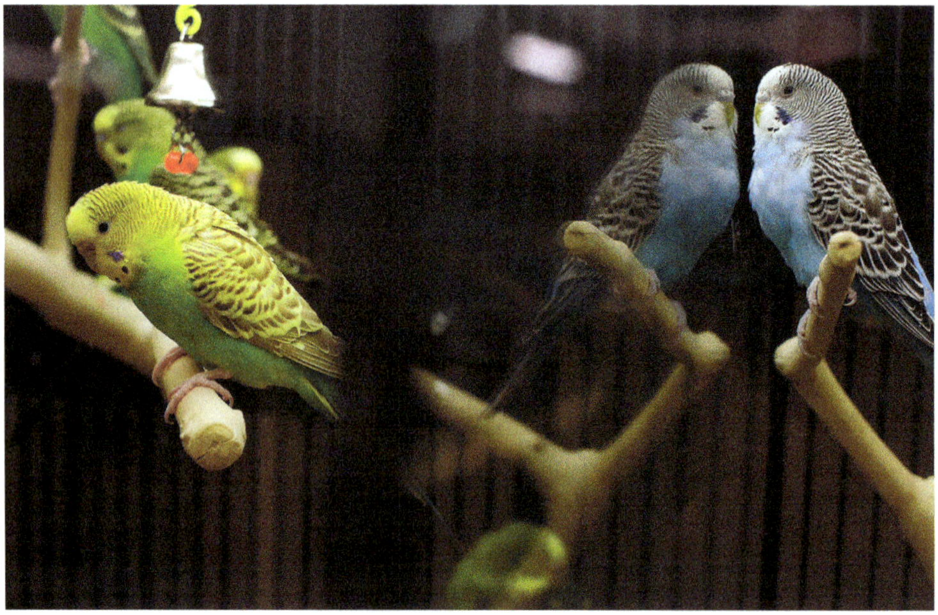

The importation of foreign birds facilitates the spread of psittacosis from one part of the globe to another. Lack of regulation in the pet bird industry makes it difficult to determine the origins of psittacosis outbreaks. *© Victor J. Blue/Bloomberg/Getty Images*

determine whether they are a source of infection. Second, the pet bird industry is not heavily regulated, making it difficult to track the exchange of birds and trace the origin of an outbreak. Wildlife trade, including exotic bird trade, also spreads the disease to new areas. This makes it problematic to effectively control psittacosis and prevent outbreaks.

SEE ALSO *Animal Importation; Bacterial Disease; Pneumonia; Zoonoses*

BIBLIOGRAPHY

Books

Bennett, John E., Raphael Dolin, and Martin J. Blaser. *Mandell, Douglas, and Bennett's Infectious Disease Essentials.* Philadelphia: Elsevier, 2017.

Murray, Patrick R., Ken S. Rosenthal, and Michael A. Pfaller. *Medical Microbiology.* Philadelphia: Elsevier, 2016.

Schmidt, Robert E., Drury R. Reavill, and David N. Phalen. *Pathology of Pet and Aviary Birds, Vol. 2.* New York: Wiley-Blackwell, 2015.

Wilson, Walter R., et al. *Current Diagnosis & Treatment in Infectious Diseases.* New York: McGraw-Hill, 2011.

Periodicals

Hogerwerf, L., et al. "Chlamydia Psittaci (Psittacosis) as a Cause of Community-Acquired Pneumonia: A Systematic Review and Meta-Analysis." *Epidemiology & Infection* 145, no. 15 (2017): 3096–3105.

Kaiser, Pete. "Advances in Avian Immunology—Prospects for Disease Control: A Review." *Avian Pathology* 39, no. 5 (2010): 309–324.

Pal, Mahendra. "Chlamydophila Psittaci as an Emerging Zoonotic Pathogen of Global Significance." *International Journal of Vaccines and Vaccination* 4, no. 3 (2017): 80.

Websites

Lessnau, Klaus-Dieter. "Psittacosis (Parrot Fever)." eMedicine, September 8, 2017. https://emedicine.medscape.com/article/227025-overview (accessed December 8, 2017).

"Psittacosis." Centers for Disease Control and Prevention, June 29, 2017. https://www.cdc.gov/pneumonia/atypical/psittacosis.html (accessed December 8, 2017).

"Psittacosis." Medline Plus, December 5, 2017. https://medlineplus.gov/ency/article/000088.htm (accessed December 8, 2017).

"Psittacosis Fact Sheet." NSW Government Health, July 1, 2012. http://www.health.nsw.gov.au/Infectious/factsheets/Pages/psittacosis.aspx (accessed December 8, 2017).

Laura J. Cataldo

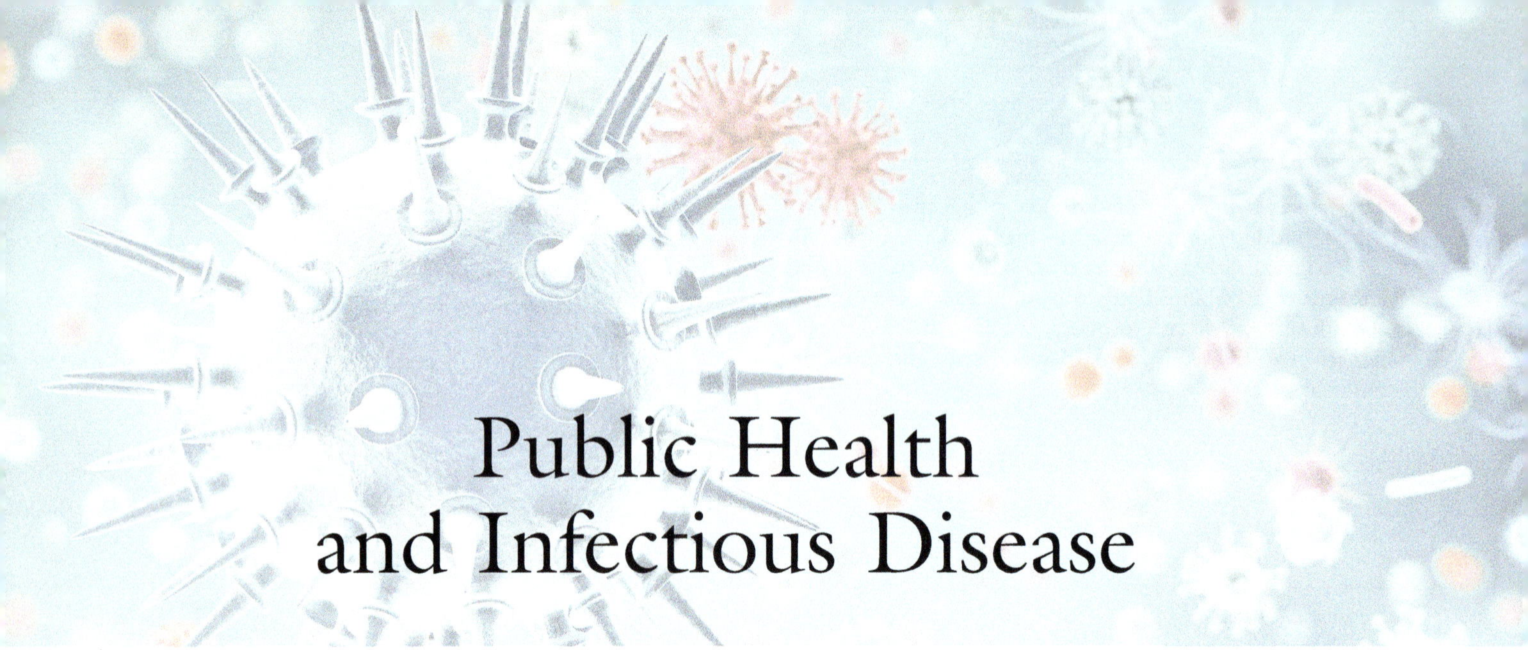

Public Health and Infectious Disease

Introduction

An effective response to an infectious disease outbreak, epidemic, or pandemic requires a coordinated approach from all parts of the public health system. Public health units play an important role in disease control and response, including planning for emergencies, surveillance, education, communication, case identification, case management, infection control, contact tracing, monitoring contacts in quarantine, border surveillance, epidemiological studies, and immunization.

The disease surveillance system must ensure that the first cases of the outbreak are quickly identified. Next, control strategies must be implemented to slow down the transmission of the pathogen while a vaccine or effective treatments are being developed. Surveillance would also detect the final case, indicating an end to the outbreak.

The rise of social media and the ubiquitous presence of the internet in everyday life in many parts of the world may help the public health authorities learn about and respond more quickly to infectious disease outbreaks. The internet can also be used by public health authorities to rapidly disseminate disease prevention and control information to the public.

Reporting and Control of Infectious Disease

When a known "notifiable" disease or an unknown infectious disease is suspected to be a public health threat, clinicians should immediately notify the local health

WORDS TO KNOW

INFECTION CONTROL Policies and procedures used to minimize the risk of spreading infections, especially in hospitals and health care facilities.

MORBIDITY From the Latin *morbus*, "sick," it refers to both the state of being ill and the severity of the illness. A serious disease is said to have high morbidity.

MORTALITY The condition of being susceptible to death. The term *mortality* comes from the Latin word *mors*, which means death. Mortality can also refer to the rate of deaths caused by an illness or injury (e.g., "Rabies has a high mortality rate").

NOTIFIABLE DISEASE A disease that the law requires must be reported to health officials when diagnosed. Also called a reportable disease.

QUARANTINE The practice of separating from the general population people who have been exposed to an infectious agent but have not yet developed symptoms. In the United States, this can be done voluntarily or involuntarily by the authority of states and the federal Centers for Disease Control and Prevention.

PANDEMIC An epidemic that occurs in more than one country or population simultaneously. *Pandemic* means "all the people."

SURVEILLANCE The systematic analysis, collection, evaluation, interpretation, and dissemination of data. Public health surveillance assists in the identification of health threats and the planning, implementation, and evaluation of responses to those threats.

authority. Reporting requirements vary greatly from one region to another because of different conditions and different disease frequencies.

Infectious disease reporting is necessary to provide accurate and timely information for the initiation of investigation and control measures. It also encourages uniformity in morbidity and mortality reporting so that data among different health jurisdictions within a country and among nations will be consistent and comparable.

A reporting system functions at four levels:

- Collection of basic data on incidence, geographic dispersion, and patient outcomes in the local community where the disease occurs
- Assembly of data at district, state, or provincial levels
- Aggregation and analysis of the information at the national level
- For certain designated diseases, the national public health agency reports data and analysis to the World Health Organization (WHO)

Each local health authority determines what diseases should be routinely reported. Physicians are required to report all notifiable illnesses that come to their attention. In addition, the statutes or regulations of many localities require reporting by hospital infectious disease officers, householders, or other people having knowledge of a case of a reportable disease. These may be individual case reports or reports of groups of cases (collective reports). Case findings can be passive or active. A passive case finding is when the physician initiates the report as required. An active case finding is when the public health officer regularly contacts clinicians, clinics, or hospitals to request the desired information.

Although diseases are often made reportable, the information gathered is not put to practical use, with no feedback being given to those who provided case data. This can lead to deterioration in the general level of reporting, even for diseases of critical importance. Better case reporting results when official reporting is restricted to those diseases for which control services are provided or potential control procedures are under evaluation or epidemiologic information is needed for a definite purpose.

Each country has its own reporting protocols and their own classifications of disease. WHO's International Health Regulations state that countries must develop surveillance systems at the local, intermediate, and national levels. The responsibility of the local level is to "detect events involving disease or death above expected levels for the particular time and place" and to report these events to the relevant health care responder. The responsibility at the intermediate level is to confirm the events reported by the local level and coordinate a response. The responsibility of the national level is to assess the events reported by the local and intermediate levels within two days to notify WHO, if appropriate, and then to implement the public health response.

Once an outbreak of infectious disease has been detected, public health agencies must consider a range of disease control measures from the control of patient contacts and the immediate environment of the outbreak to mass vaccination programs or mass prophylaxis using anti-infective medication.

There are risks associated with mass vaccination and prophylaxis as disease control measures. As public health experts consider the implications of serious infectious disease outbreaks, they must balance the potential benefits of control measures such as mass immunization. One consideration that leads to caution in implementing such measures is the occurrence of relatively rare but predictable adverse reactions or events due to vaccination or medication, known as medication-related adverse events (MRAEs). For example, it is generally considered unacceptable to incur predictable mortality by using vaccines that have a rate of adverse reactions, however low, unless there is an actual outbreak of a dangerous disease. In addition, the duration of a mass prophylaxis campaign could have a significant impact on the timing and peak number of serious MRAEs, with brief campaigns overwhelming existing emergency department (ED) capacity to treat real or suspected adverse reactions. Although these results could be refined by further study of adverse reaction rates, the results of modeling underline the necessity for coordinating public health and emergency medicine planning for infectious disease outbreaks to avoid preventable surges in ED use.

Travel restrictions can also be an effective disease control measure. Travel restrictions have often been suggested as an efficient way to reduce the spread of a communicable disease that threatens public health. Swedish researchers conducted a computer simulation of the effect of different levels of travel restrictions on the rapidity and geographical spread of an outbreak of a disease similar to SARS. They tested scenarios of travel restrictions in which travel over distances greater than 30 miles (50 kilometers) and 12 miles (20 kilometers) would be banned, taking into account different compliance levels. They found that a ban on journeys over 30 miles (50 kilometers) would drastically reduce the speed and geographical spread of outbreaks, even when compliance is less than 100 percent. Their study supported the use of travel restrictions as an effective way to mitigate the effect of a future disease outbreak, at least when the infectivity of a disease is moderate, as in the case of severe acute respiratory syndrome (SARS). It is not known how effective travel restrictions are for airborne and animal-borne infections with greater transmissibility such as a potential mutant H5N1 virus.

In addition, medication stockpiles are a potential control measure. Much of the discussion and research regarding infectious disease control measures has happened in the context of concern about a potential new worldwide influ-

STAGES OF A FLU PANDEMIC

According to the US Centers for Disease Control and Prevention (CDC), there are six major stages of an influenza pandemic. The six stages are referred to as the Pandemic Intervals Framework (PIF). The PIF allows for public health agencies and health care workers to plan for a pandemic and address it once it arrives. How long each stage lasts depends on the influenza virus at play, as well as the public health response. The six components of an influenza pandemic are as follows:

1. Investigation of cases of novel influenza A virus infection in humans
2. Recognition of increased potential for ongoing transmission of a novel influenza A virus
3. Initiation of a pandemic wave
4. Acceleration of a pandemic wave
5. Deceleration of a pandemic wave
6. Preparation for future pandemic waves

enza pandemic, such as happens about three times each century. The worst of these pandemics on record was the 1918 pandemic, which killed at least 20 million people. There were 860 human cases of H5N1, including 454 deaths, between 2003 and early 2018. International health officials lacked the resources to monitor avian flu in a population of hundreds of millions in the parts of Asia likely to become the epicenter of such a new pandemic, including some countries with rudimentary or no public health systems.

Most researchers agree that pandemic influenza will recur. The world's surveillance systems and countermeasures are likely inadequate, and current control measures may not significantly slow a pandemic once it has begun.

■ Issues and Impacts

Public Health Response to SARS

In 2003 the world experienced the sudden onset of an epidemic of the virulent disease SARS. The response to this outbreak was the first opportunity for new global public health surveillance and control agencies to act in anticipation of a potential avian influenza outbreak. The infectious agent was a highly pathogenic virus known as a coronavirus. Like the anticipated pattern for avian flu, the outbreaks spread from Asia to the rest of the world. Thus, the SARS epidemic was a trial run of emerging international public health protocols to identify and respond to infectious disease threats.

The largest outbreak of SARS began in March 2003 in Beijing, China. This outbreak was resolved within six weeks of its peak in late April. Chinese public health agencies recorded case data from SARS cases observed in Beijing and their close contacts between March 5 and May 29, 2003, onto standardized surveillance forms, which were subsequently reviewed by epidemiologists. The epidemiological investigation focused on (1) the response of public health agencies to the SARS outbreak in terms of the timeline for implementing major control measures; (2) the number of reported cases and quarantined close contacts; (3) the calculated attack rates, with changes in infection control measures, management, and triage of suspected cases; and (4) the time lag between illness onset and hospitalization with information dissemination.

The investigation found that health care worker training in use of personal protective equipment and the isolation of patients with SARS, along with the establishment of fever clinics and designated hospital SARS wards, predated the steepest decline in cases. During the outbreak 30,178 exposed persons were quarantined in China. Attack rates among quarantined individuals were calculated by type of relationship to known victims and the age of the contact. Among 2,195 quarantined close contacts in five districts, the attack rate was 6.3 percent, with a range of 15 percent among spouses to less than 0.5 percent among work and school contacts. The attack rate among quarantined household members was found to increase with age from 5 percent in children younger than 10 years to 27 percent in adults aged 60 to 69 years.

Among nearly 14 million people screened for fever at airports, train stations, and roadside checkpoints, only 12 were found to have probable SARS. After initial reticence the national and municipal governments adopted a policy of full disclosure, holding 13 press conferences about the SARS outbreak. Following the installation of strict screening and control procedures, the time interval between illness onset and hospitalization decreased from a median of five to six days on or before April 20, 2003, the day the outbreak was announced to the public, to two days after April 20. The rapid resolution of the SARS outbreak was due to multiple factors, including improvements in patient isolation and triage in both hospitals and communities of patients with suspected SARS and the propagation of information to health care workers and the public.

On the other side of the globe, the largest SARS outbreak in North America occurred in Toronto, Canada. Again, epidemiologists analyzed the patterns of transmission and the public health effects of control measures, and the findings and disease patterns closely paralleled those in China. Toronto Public Health examined 2,132 potential SARS cases, ascertained that 23,103 contacts of SARS patients required quarantine, and logged 316,615 calls on a hotline dedicated to SARS. According to the investigators, 225 Toronto residents met the case definition of SARS.

Only three travel-related cases were not linked to the index patient, who came to Toronto from Hong Kong.

A resurgence of the outbreak occurred due to unrecognized SARS among hospitalized patients. This was eventually controlled using active surveillance of hospitalized patients. The control measures of Toronto Public Health brought about a reduction in the number of persons exposed to SARS in nonhospital and nonhousehold settings from 20 before the control measures were implemented to zero after implementation. The number of patients exposed while in a hospital ward rose from 25 before the measures were taken to 68 afterward, while the number exposed during a stay in the intensive care unit dropped from 13 to 0. The spread of the outbreak in the community (outside of hospital settings) was significantly reduced after instituting the control measures.

Toronto SARS transmission was mostly limited to hospitals and households where patients had contacts. Epidemiologists determined that, for every case of SARS, public health authorities could expect to quarantine up to 100 patient contacts and investigate eight potential cases. Active in-hospital surveillance for SARS-like illnesses and heightened infection control measures were essential in bringing the outbreak under control.

Although the public health response to SARS was successful within a short time frame, it is far from clear that a similar response to an avian flu outbreak would be as successful, mainly because influenza mortality and infectivity could be much greater, while current treatments could be considerably less effective. For this reason the production of an effective avian flu vaccine is seen as essential for controlling an avian flu outbreak.

Public Health Response to Ebola

In December 2013 public health officials believe a boy in the West African country of Guinea contracted the Ebola virus from a bat. The virus, which causes a deadly fever, quickly spread through Guinea and beyond, into Sierra Leone and Liberia. While the virus itself is highly contagious, a lack of public health infrastructure in the affected countries made it difficult for medical personnel to diagnose infections and implement measures that might prevent the virus's transmission, leading to Ebola's rapid spread in early 2014.

On March 25, 2014, as reports of both suspected and confirmed Ebola infections were on the rise, WHO declared that an epidemic had erupted in West Africa. This declaration helped bring international attention to the outbreak, which in turn helped mobilize resources. The US Centers for Disease Control and Prevention (CDC) and Public Health England were among the numerous national health organizations from outside West Africa that joined with WHO, various nongovernmental organizations, private philanthropists, and the governments of Guinea, Sierra Leone, and Liberia to organize a response to the disease. Among the first steps was establishing incident management systems that sought to organize and coordinate a system for diagnosing, treating, and combatting the virus's further transmission.

In July 2014 Liberia's Ministry of Health collaborated with various other outside organizations to create a national incident management system comprising numerous emergency operations centers scattered throughout the country. Guinea organized its response through a newly established national coordination cell, which WHO, the CDC, and Canada's Public Health Agency helped operate. Meanwhile, the United Kingdom helped Sierra Leona set up Ebola response centers in various locations.

Over the span of about two years, the combination of local and international, public and private resources led to a coordinated and concerted effort to stamp out Ebola in West Africa. While the disease infected some 28,000 people and killed more than 11,000 of them, the public health response was ultimately successful. On June 9, 2016, more than 40 days after the last confirmed patient tested negative for the disease, WHO officially declared the epidemic was over.

In a 2017 CDC report, Barbara J. Marston and her coauthors noted, like many other observers, that the world health community's response to the 2014–2016 Ebola outbreak "facilitated improvements in the public health systems in West Africa." Such improvements included not only the expansion of public health infrastructure in the affected countries, including the development of new laboratories and surveillance tools, but also an improvement in the trust that exists between West African nations and the international public health community. According to Marston and her coauthors, the Ebola epidemic offered evidence of an important lesson: "In settings with limited public health capacity or in which the magnitude of a health threat overwhelms local capacity and requires international support, response efforts provide a unique opportunity for strengthening public health systems and can serve as a further catalyst to accelerate progress toward global health security goals."

■ US Case Example: A State Prepares for a Flu Pandemic

In June 2006 a panel of national, state, and local experts met in Massachusetts to assess the threat of an avian influenza pandemic. In particular they discussed the readiness of state and local officials' response to such a pandemic. The conference leaders suggested that political entities, the public health system, and the medical community need a "seamless network of protection" against this potentially lethal threat. Three major challenges to pandemic planning and preparedness were noted: (1) the scale of the challenge, (2) connectivity of communication, and (3) the danger of complacency.

The current threat posed by avian influenza was described at the conference as requiring monitoring for mutations in the virus and its ability to transmit efficiently among people, particularly because there is no immunity among human populations against H5N1. In addition, the ease and frequency of international travel and transportation of goods mean that an evolving threat anywhere in the world is a threat everywhere.

Attendees noted that the response to the SARS epidemic conveyed some valuable public health lessons. Among these was that travel advisories seemed to help to contain the SARS pandemic. Interventions such as social distancing (for example, canceling large gatherings, quarantining persons infected with influenza, and using cough etiquette and masks) could be helpful in mitigating the effects of an influenza pandemic. The federal government has made it clear that, in the event of a pandemic, it will not be able to respond to every community. Rather, state and local jurisdictions must take responsibility for preparedness planning and response efforts. Basic public health tools, including good communication about risk, individual/family/community preparedness, identification and quarantine of confirmed cases, and social distancing, could be most useful during the initial stages of a pandemic. Schools and businesses could choose to temporarily close and use technology to reduce direct contact between people.

Effective communication during a pandemic is essential. Because it is possible that the supply chain of services, goods, and food will be disrupted during a severe pandemic, it is recommended that individuals and families store at least a two-week supply of water and food, nonprescription drugs, and other health supplies including pain relievers, stomach remedies, cough and cold medicines, fluids with electrolytes, and vitamins. The CDC addresses these concerns and provides a number of preparedness checklists and other tools on its website www.pandemicflu.gov.

In Massachusetts the state's pandemic preparedness plan is "intended to ensure that essential services are maintained, there is minimal discomfort and loss of life, the most vulnerable are cared for and that individuals, families and first responders are protected." The plan addresses hospital and health care facility surge capacity and staffing issues, surveillance and identification of influenza, the health and safety of vulnerable populations, timely and effective communication, and continuity of government and essential services during a crisis.

SEE ALSO *Epidemiology; Food-Borne Disease and Food Safety; Notifiable Diseases; Pandemic Preparedness*

BIBLIOGRAPHY

Books

Heymann, David L., ed. *Control of Communicable Diseases Manual.* 20th ed. Washington, DC: APHA, 2014.

Rosen, George. *A History of Public Health.* Baltimore, MD: Johns Hopkins University Press, 2015.

Periodicals

Lewis, Katharine Kranz. "The Pandemic Threat: Is Massachusetts Prepared?" *Massachusetts Health Policy Forum* (June 2006): 1–8. This article can also be found online at https://masshealthpolicyforum.brandeis.edu/publications/pdfs/29-Jun06/PolicyBrief29.pdf (accessed March 6, 2018).

Marston, Barbara J., et al. "Ebola Response Impact on Public Health Programs, West Africa, 2014–2017." *Emerging Infectious Diseases* 23, no. 13 (December 2017): S25–S32. This article can also be found online at https://wwwnc.cdc.gov/eid/article/23/13/17-0727_article (accessed March 6, 2018).

Sands, Peter, Carmen Mundaca-Shah, and Victor J. Dzau. "The Neglected Dimension of Global Security—A Framework for Countering Infectious-Disease Crises." *New England Journal of Medicine* 374 (2016): 1281–1287. This article can also be found online at http://www.nejm.org/doi/full/10.1056/NEJMsr1600236 (accessed March 6, 2018).

Wójcik, Oktawia P., et al. "Public Health for the People: Participatory Infectious Disease Surveillance in the Digital Age." *Emerging Themes in Epidemiology* 11, no. 7 (June 20, 2014). This article can also be found online at https://ete-online.biomedcentral.com/articles/10.1186/1742-7622-11-7 (accessed March 6, 2018).

Websites

"Cumulative Number of Confirmed Human Cases for Avian Influenza A (H5N1) Reported to WHO, 2003–2018." World Health Organization, 2018. http://www.who.int/influenza/human_animal_interface/2018_01_25_tableH5N1.pdf?ua=1 (accessed March 7, 2018).

"International Health Regulations." World Health Organization, 2005. http://www.who.int/csr/ihr/voluntarycompliancemay06EN%20.pdf (accessed March 6, 2018).

"National Notifiable Diseases Surveillance System (NNDSS)." Centers for Disease Control and Prevention, February 16, 2018. https://wwwn.cdc.gov/nndss/ (accessed March 6, 2018).

"Pandemic Intervals Framework (PIF)." Centers for Disease Control and Prevention, November 30, 2016. https://www.cdc.gov/flu/pandemic-resources/national-strategy/intervals-framework.html (accessed March 7, 2018).

Kenneth T. LaPensee

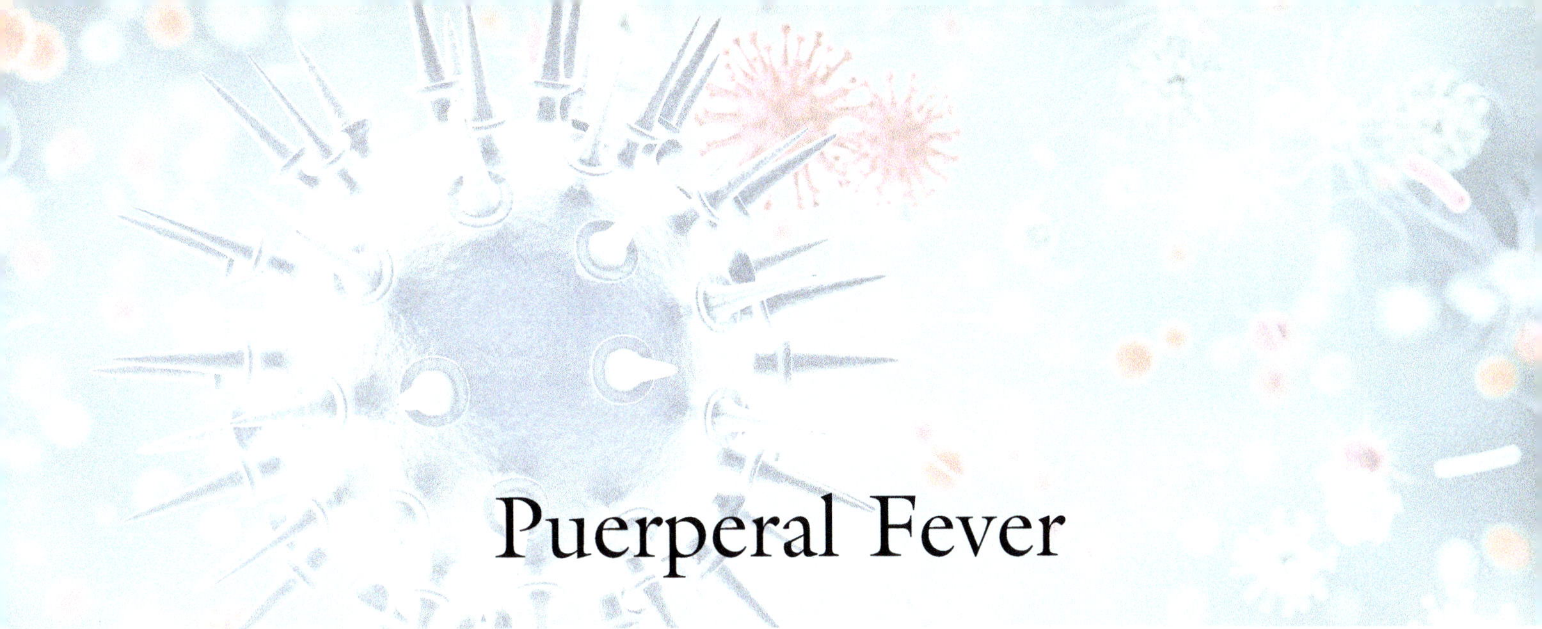

Puerperal Fever

Introduction

Puerperal fever is a highly infectious disease that resulted in significant maternal mortality from the 17th to the 19th centuries and remains a potential threat in developing nations. It is caused most often by infection from Group A streptococcal bacteria during or immediately following childbirth and is transmissible between patients. During historic epidemic periods, infection almost always proved fatal, and mothers exhibited symptoms of fever, abdominal pain, and vaginal hemorrhage.

Puerperal fever was not prevalent in developed nations until the 17th century, when it became common for women to give birth and recover in hospitals. Hospital physicians were responsible for the examination and deliveries of many pregnant women each day. Analysis of these routines eventually indicated that doctors and nurses were responsible for transmitting the disease between patients. American physician and professor Oliver Wendell Holmes (1809–1894) and Hungarian physician Ignaz Semmelweis (1818–1865) were each independently responsible for increasing awareness of this mode of transmission and for implementing preventive measures against further spread of infection. In developed nations puerperal fever poses little significant risk to expecting mothers.

Disease History, Characteristics, and Transmission

Puerperal fever, also referred to as childbed fever or puerperal sepsis, commonly affected mothers during or shortly after childbirth up until the 20th century. The first documented case of puerperal fever occurred in Paris in 1646, but it was not until 1879 that Louis Pasteur (1822–1895) identified the causative agent as bacteria belonging to the *Streptococcus* group.

Following childbirth the placental attachment site in the uterus remains an open wound highly susceptible to infection from bacteria that occur normally on the skin, nose, throat, and vagina. Following infection by *Streptococcus* bacteria, puerperal fever presents with rapid onset of fever, abdominal pain, abnormal vaginal discharge, and bleeding. Infection usually occurs within 10 days of birth and progresses to septicemia (bacterial infection in the blood) or peritonitis (generalized infection of the lining of the abdomen). During historic epidemics puerperal fever carried a fatality rate of up to 100 percent.

The significant prevalence of puerperal fever began only after the establishment of lying-in hospitals, where physicians completed many deliveries and treated many postpartum women each day. Practitioners at that time were attending a number of patients each day without using sterilization procedures between patients. In 1843 Holmes concluded that physicians and nurses were responsible for transmitting the infection through their hands and clothing.

Unaware of this prior conclusion, Semmelweis noticed that one ward of physicians in his hospital in Hungary had a 16 percent fatality rate compared with the midwife wards, which had a 2 percent fatality rate. Semmelweis recognized

WORDS TO KNOW

MORTALITY The condition of being susceptible to death. The term *mortality* comes from the Latin word *mors*, which means death. Mortality can also refer to the rate of deaths caused by an illness or injury (e.g., "Rabies has a high mortality rate").

PUERPERAL An interval of time around childbirth, from the onset of labor through the immediate recovery period after delivery.

SEPTICEMIA Prolonged fever, chills, anorexia, and anemia in conjunction with tissue lesions.

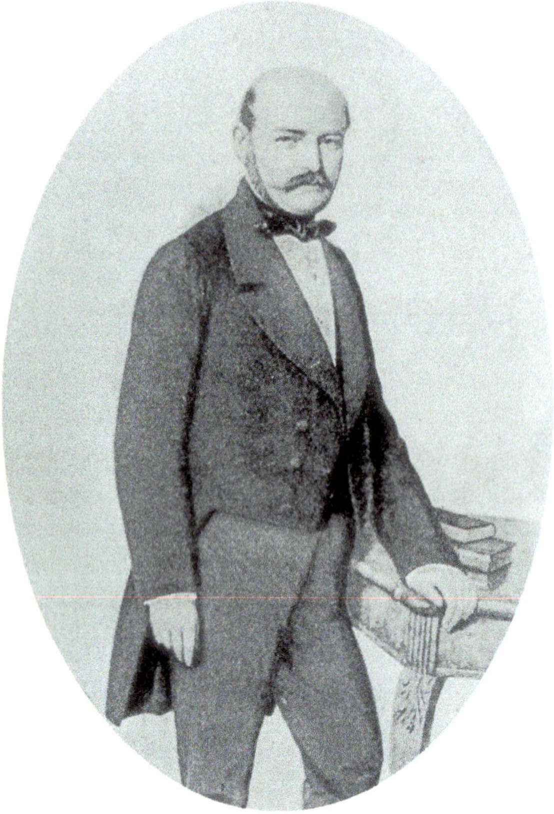

Hungarian doctor Ignaz Philip Semmelweis. Semmelweis is credited with discovering the cause of puerperal fever. © *Universal History Archive/UniversalImagesGroup/Getty Images*

that the physicians had been performing autopsies on puerperal fever patients prior to delivering babies and concluded that the physicians were spreading the infection from patient to patient. Semmelweis then introduced mandatory washing with chlorinated lime at the beginning of shifts and prior to vaginal examination. Mortality was subsequently reduced to less than 3 percent.

Scope and Distribution

Although puerperal fever had a period of significant endemicity during the 18th and 19th centuries, it has been recognized for thousands of years that delivering women may be at risk of a fever that could be fatal. However, the mortality rates of puerperal fever in ancient and medieval times were lower because women generally gave birth at home and were therefore not at risk of exposure to infection carried by attending medical staff.

As of 2010, in developed countries, deaths from puerperal fever were rare, and the mortality rate was about 0.1 to 0.6 per 1,000 births. This significant reduction in fatalities is largely attributed to improvements in sanitation and hygiene during birth, as well as the use of antibiotics to treat bacterial infections. Those at increased risk of developing puerperal fever are women with compromised immune systems, women who are anemic, and women who endure a long labor.

In developing nations childbirth-related fatalities remain a considerable threat to women, with 95 percent of maternal deaths occurring in Africa and Asia. In developing countries around 1 in 16 births is fatal compared to 1 in 2,800 among developed countries. The exact causes of these deaths are often not determined, but puerperal fever is often a significant contributing factor. This substantial risk is due to a lack of health care training and facilities, which increases the risk of patients developing puerperal fever. Substandard health care facilities also reduce the chances that the infection will be effectively treated.

Treatment and Prevention

During periods when puerperal fever was epidemic, the rapid onset of infection, the ease of transmission between patients, and the lack of knowledge regarding causation made both treatment and prevention impossible. Until the causative agent and mode of transmission were understood, puerperal fever remained an almost certain threat among maternity wards.

The discovery by Holmes and Semmelweis that medical birth attendants were responsible for transmitting infection between patients was revolutionary in the fight against puerperal fever. After these realizations practices were estab-

Countries Where Fewer Than Half of All Births Are Attended by Skilled Health Personnel

Country	Percentage of Attended Births	Date
Somalia	9.4	2006
South Sudan	19.4	2010
Chad	20.2	2014
Ethiopia	27.7	2016
Timor-Leste	29.3	2009
Eritrea	34.1	2010
Nigeria	35.2	2013
Niger	39.7	2015
Central African Republic	40.0	2010
Lao People's Democratic Republic	40.1	2011
Bangladesh	42.1	2014
Madagascar	44.3	2012
Togo	44.6	2013
Yemen	44.7	2013
Guinea-Bissau	45.0	2014
Guinea	45.3	2012
Angola	47.3	2006
Haiti	48.6	2013
United Republic of Tanzania	48.9	2010
Mali	49.0	2006

SOURCE: "WHO Database on Skilled Attendant at Delivery." World Health Organization. Available from: http://www.who.int/gho/maternal_health/skilled_care/skilled_birth_attendance/en/

lished to ensure physicians did not spread the infection. These practices included changing clothing between births, washing hands with chlorinated solutions before and after attending to patients, and sterilizing implements used during childbirth. These practices are still followed as a defense against childbirth infections.

Once it was established that puerperal fever was a result of infection by *Streptococcus* bacteria, treatment of the infection also became possible. The use of intravenous antibiotic regimens from the onset of labor through to delivery, especially in prolonged and complicated labors, can effectively treat mothers at risk for puerperal fever.

Impacts and Issues

Although the impacts of puerperal fever have been diminished in the developed world since physicians gained an appreciation of the nature of the disease, it remains a significant threat to expecting mothers in developing nations.

One of the main issues of this disease is that the *Streptococcus* bacteria responsible for causing infection are part of the normal flora of the skin, nose, throat, and vagina. This means that potentially every woman is at risk of developing infection during or following childbirth, even in the absence of an outside reservoir of the contagion. In developed countries problematic births are often predicted prior to the event, and physicians can take a suitable course of action to prevent further complications associated with such infections. Such measures are not available to the majority of women in developing nations.

There is also a lack of health care training in many developing countries, including training of medical personnel who do not entirely understand the mechanisms of disease transmission. This can lead to medical personnel passing the infection from patient to patient, which makes it more likely for women in developing nations to develop puerperal fever. Reduced health care resources also make it more likely that the infection will be fatal.

Further issues exist for the children born from maternally fatal deliveries because they are often instantly subject to disadvantage. During early childhood they are unable to contribute to labor and productivity but remain a strain on essential resources such as food and water. The society may view such a child as a liability rather than as a member of the community, which results in significant social impact.

At the United Nations Millennium Summit in 2000, world leaders established a set of goals to combat certain sources of poverty, illness, illiteracy, hunger, and environmental problems. These goals are commonly referred to as the UN Millennium Development Goals. One of the primary development and health goals was to reduce the maternal mortality rate by 75 percent by 2015. As of 2015 ratings included "Fair Progress" for western Asia, Latin America, and the Caribbean; "Good Progress" for northern and sub-Saharan Africa, Southeastern and southern Asia, and Oceania; and "Target Met or Excellent Progress" in East Asia, Caucasus, and Central Asia. Worldwide, maternal mortality is highest among poor and rural women in developing nations.

While noticeable improvements in the maternal mortality rate have occurred since the inception of the Millennium Development Goals, maternal mortality remains high in the regions where women are most likely to die from childbearing, especially sub-Saharan Africa and southern Asia. Puerperal sepsis continues to be a significant problem. Researchers and health care providers found that women who had a skilled attendant during childbirth, along with access to emergency care if needed, were less likely to die or suffer debilitating complications. Overall, only 56 percent of women in developing regions have a skilled health care attendant during childbirth. In sub-Saharan Africa only 36 percent of women have a skilled attendant assist their birth, compared to 88 percent of women in Latin America.

SEE ALSO *Bacterial Disease; Contact Precautions; Disinfection; Handwashing; Sterilization*

BIBLIOGRAPHY

Books

Bennett, John E., Raphael Dolin, and Martin J. Blaser. *Mandell, Douglas, and Bennett's Infectious Disease Essentials.* Philadelphia: Elsevier, 2017.

Carter, K. Codell, and Barbara R. Carter. *Childbed Fever: A Scientific Biography* of *Ignaz Semmelweis.* New York: Routledge, 2017.

Murray, Patrick R., Ken S. Rosenthal, and Michael A. Pfaller. *Medical Microbiology.* Philadelphia: Elsevier, 2016.

Wilson, Walter R., et al. *Current Diagnosis & Treatment in Infectious Diseases.* New York: McGraw-Hill, 2011.

Periodicals

Benenson, S., et al. "Cluster of Puerperal Fever in an Obstetric Ward: A Reminder of Ignaz Semmelweis." *Infection Control & Hospital Epidemiology* 36, no. 12 (2015): 1488–1490.

Graham, W. J., et al. "Childbed Fever: History Repeats Itself?" *British Journal of Obstetrics and Gynaecology* 122, no. 2 (2015): 156–159.

Khan, K., et al. "WHO Analysis of Causes of Maternal Death: A Systematic Review." *Lancet* 367, no. 9516 (2006):1066–1074.

Van Dillen, J., et al. "Maternal Sepsis: Epidemiology, Etiology and Outcome." *Current Opinion in Infectious Diseases* 23, no. 3 (2010): 249–254.

Websites

"Maternal Deaths Disproportionately High in Developing Countries." World Health Organization, October 20, 2003. http://www.who.int/mediacentre/news/releases/2003/pr77/en/index.html (accessed December 9, 2017).

"Millennium Development Goals Report." United Nations. http://www.un.org/millenniumgoals/reports.shtml (accessed January 7, 2018).

"Modern History Sourcebook: Oliver Wendell Holmes (1809–1894): Contagiousness of Puerperal Fever, 1843." Fordham University, August 1998. http://www.fordham.edu/halsall/mod/1843holmes-fever.html (accessed December 9, 2017).

"Multiple Cause of Death Data." Centers for Disease Control and Prevention, December 20, 2017. https://wonder.cdc.gov/mcd.html (accessed January 7, 2108).

Laura J. Cataldo

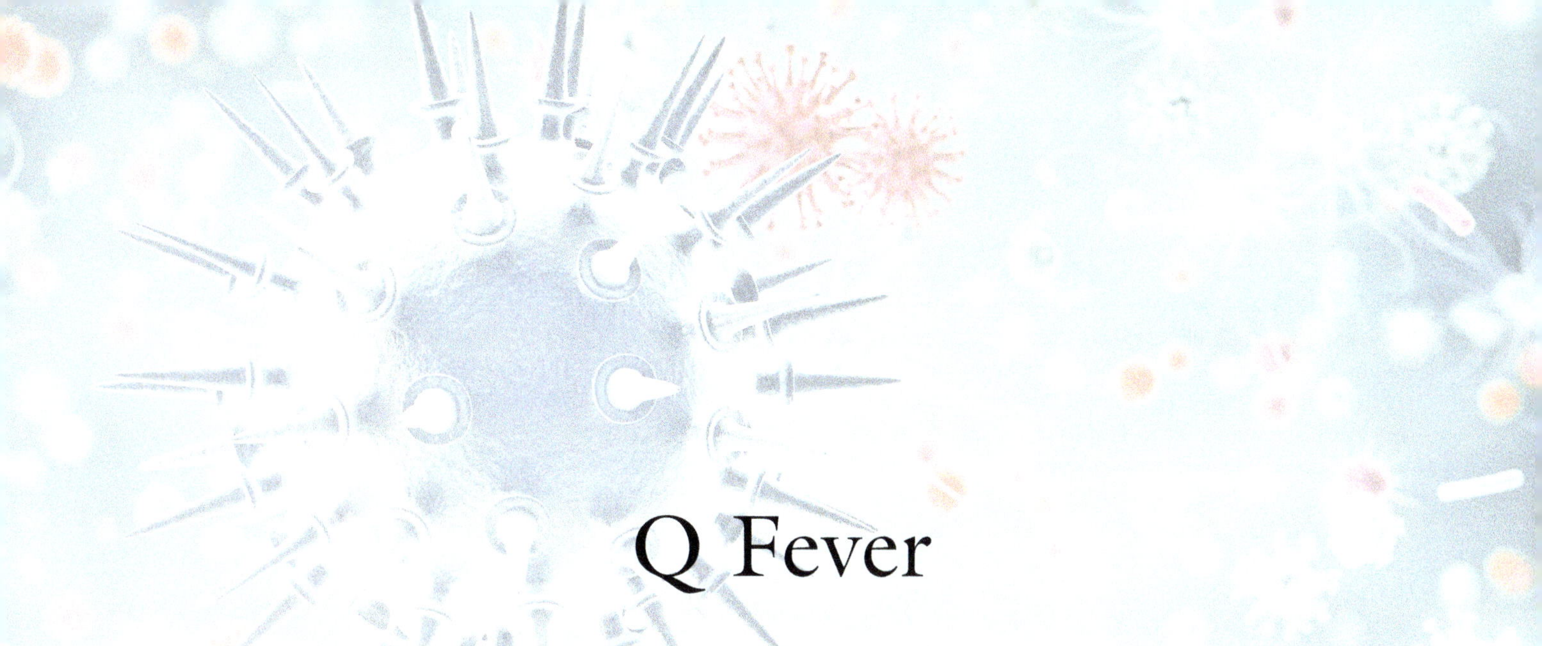

Q Fever

Introduction

Q fever is a disease of humans and some animals that is caused by a bacterium called *Coxiella burnetii*. The infection is a zoonosis, meaning it is passed to humans by contact with infected animals that are not usually harmed by the organism. The animals typically affected are sheep, cattle, and goats. Q fever can occur and clear quickly in the case of an acute infection, or it can persist for a much longer time in the case of a chronic infection.

Disease History, Characteristics, and Transmission

Q fever was first described in Australia in 1935 by physician Edward H. Derrick (1898–1976) in people working in an Australian slaughterhouse. The letter *Q* is short for *query*, alluding to the fact that, at the time, the cause for the illnesses was unknown. In 1937 *C. burnetii* was isolated and identified. The following year the same organism was isolated from ticks in Montana, leading researchers to suspect a tick-mediated animal-human connection. The US researchers also showed that the microbe was a type of bacterium called rickettsia. Rickettsia is important from the standpoint of infectious diseases and is responsible for the potentially serious diseases Rocky Mountain spotted fever and trench fever.

C. burnetii is a Gram-negative organism, meaning it has two membranes surrounding the inner contents of the cell. In addition, the bacterium requires a host cell to grow and divide. This is similar to viruses. However, unlike viruses, which are not considered to be alive, *C. burnetii* is living and can survive but cannot grow and divide when not in a host cell.

The bacteria can survive for a long time in their natural environment. They are not easily killed by heat, dryness, and even chemical compounds that readily kill other bacteria. This increases the likelihood that the bacteria will be spread to those who come into contact with them.

Q fever results from inhalation of the bacteria. Infections have been traced to the inhalation of bacteria dislodged into the air from dry hay or a dusty barnyard. Only a few living organisms need be inhaled to establish an infection. This route of infection is different from other rickettsial diseases, where the bacteria are transferred from animal to human by tick bites.

People who are most at risk of acquiring Q fever are those who are around animals such as goats, sheep, and cattle, which naturally harbor the bacterium. The bacteria may be present in the milk, urine, amniotic fluid, and feces of these animals. The bacteria may also be present in amniotic fluid and the placenta and so can be spread to people who help in the birth of animals. Veterinarians, processing plant workers, and livestock farmers are more susceptible to Q fever than the general population.

WORDS TO KNOW

ACUTE INFECTION An infection of rapid onset and of short duration that either resolves or becomes chronic.

GRAM-NEGATIVE BACTERIA Bacteria whose cell walls are composed of an inner and outer membrane that are separated from one another by a region called the periplasm. The periplasm also contains a thin but rigid layer called the peptidoglycan.

ZOONOSES Diseases of microbiological origin that can be transmitted from animals to people. The causes of the diseases can be bacteria, viruses, parasites, or fungi.

For reasons that are not clear, only about 50 percent of people who inhale the bacteria display symptoms. The symptoms include a sudden and high fever, a flulike sickness, severe headache, nausea with vomiting, abdominal pain, and a general feeling of being unwell. People can lose weight during their illness, which can take some time to regain following their recovery. Only 1 to 2 percent of those with the milder form of Q fever die of the illness.

A serious lung infection (pneumonia) can develop in 30 to 50 percent of people with Q fever. Liver damage including hepatitis can also occur. These symptoms usually ease in several months. However, a more persistent form of Q fever can develop, resulting in debilitating damage to heart valves due to the longer-lasting infection that kills up to 60 percent of those who acquire the chronic infection.

There are two different forms of *C. burnetii* that differ in the types of molecules present on the outer surfaces of their cells. The two forms have been designated phase 1 and phase 2. The phase 1 form is associated with the chronic form of Q fever.

The short-term form of Q fever does not always immediately lead to the longer form. Indeed, the chronic form of Q fever can develop in the absence of the milder form of the disease. The time lag between the short-term and chronic forms of Q fever can be as long as several decades.

Scope and Distribution

The bacterium responsible for Q fever occurs worldwide. Countries with a heavier emphasis on livestock agriculture or that have a greater prevalence of animals that naturally harbor the bacterium, such as Australia and the United States, have a higher occurrence of the disease.

From 2007 to 2010 an outbreak of Q fever occurred in the Netherlands. The outbreak involved about 4,000 people.

Treatment and Prevention

Diagnosis of Q fever most typically involves the detection of antibodies to *C. burnetii* or genetic material from the bacterium. Growing the organism is difficult, so detection of the bacterium itself is not typically accomplished. Following diagnosis, treatment consists of antibiotic therapy. Typically, this is effective, although the therapy will be necessary for years when the infection is chronic. Heart valve damage can require replacement of the defective tissue.

A vaccine for Q fever exists and was widely available as of 2017. Treatment is usually with doxycycline. Long-term

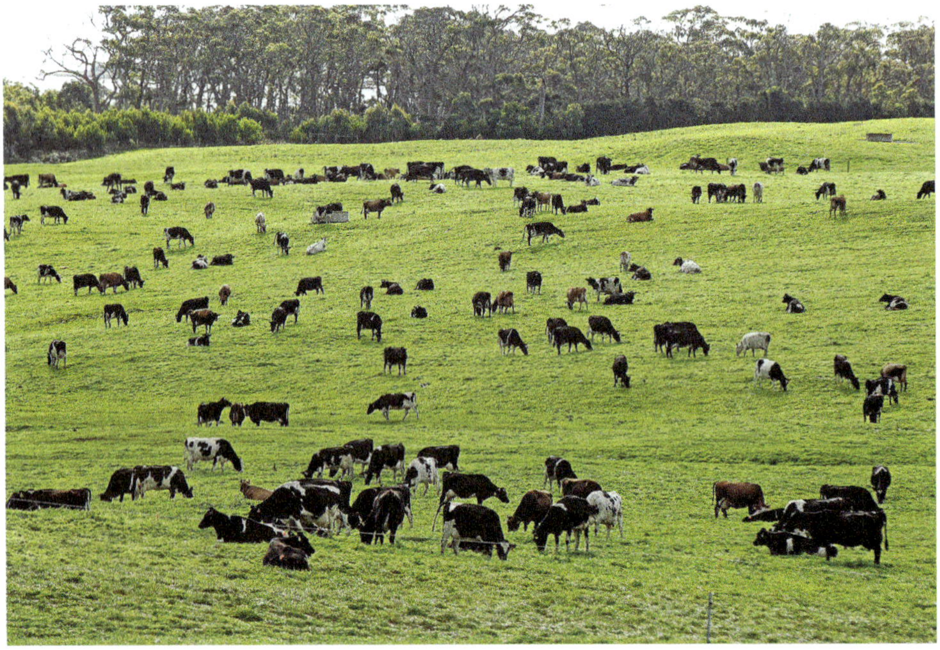

Coxiella burnetti, the bacterium responsible for Q fever, is found in livestock animals such as cows, goats, and sheep. Humans who work with such animals are most at risk of contracting Q fever. © Brendon Thorne/Bloomberg/Getty Images

infections can require additional use of hydroxychloroquine, trimethoprim-sulfamethoxazole, fluoroquinolones, and rifampin.

Prevention of the transmission of the bacterium to humans involves wearing masks when around domestic livestock and the prompt disposal of the placenta and other tissues resulting from the birth process.

Impacts and Issues

Q fever can be a potentially serious disease because it can be spread from animals to people. In the United States cases of the illness have been required to be reported to the US Centers for Disease Control and Prevention (CDC) since 1999. Imported livestock are also monitored for the presence of the bacterium, as transfer to other domestic animals could occur unknowingly in the absence of development of any symptoms in these hosts.

Why only about 50 percent of infected people display symptoms of infection is still unclear, but it is important to learn if vaccines are to be fully protective. Research is underway to try and distinguish factors associated with people, the bacterium, or both that help some people ward off the consequences of infection. Additionally, it is not clear why Q fever does not persist for a long time in some people but becomes a chronic, destructive, and potentially life-threatening condition in others.

PRIMARY SOURCE

The largest Q fever outbreak ever reported

SOURCE: *Speelman, P. "The Largest Q Fever Outbreak Ever Reported."* Netherlands Journal of Medicine *68, no. 12 (December 2010): 380–381. This article can also be found online at https://www.njmonline.nl/getpdf.php?id=990 (accessed November 21, 2017).*

INTRODUCTION: *Since 2007, the Netherlands has experienced the largest Q fever outbreak ever reported in the literature. From 2007 till today approximately 4000 people have been affected and at least 14 of these patients, nearly all of them with severe underlying conditions, have died.*

It all started in May 2007 when medical specialists in a hospital in the southern part of the Netherlands and a general practitioner in the same region reported a substantial number of patients with pneumonia not responding to amoxicillin, whereas patients did well on moxifloxacine. Soon it became clear that these pneumonias were caused by *Coxiella burnetii.* During 2007, 168 patients were reported. Although an association with intense goat farming was already suggested in 2007 and experts warned that the outbreak could recur, a limited number of preventive measures were taken. The experience that earlier reported outbreaks were usually limited in time and did not recur in the following years may have played an important role. In 2008, however, the epidemic recurred and 1000 patients were reported. This prompted more preventive regulations. In June 2008, Q fever finally became a notifiable disease for the veterinary sector as well. A ban on the spread of manure from farms with Q fever was issued and (voluntary) vaccination of non-pregnant goats on dairy goat farms in the region was advised. In 2009 compulsory hygiene measures in farms with more than 50 goats or sheep were instituted and compulsory vaccination of goats and sheep in farms with more than 50 animals was ordered. Later that year testing for *Coxiella burnetii* on bulk milk was started and transport of cattle was prohibited. In December 2009 breeding on infected farms was prohibited. After a lot of political pressure and a critical documentary on national television, it was decided to start culling more than 50,000 pregnant goats on infected farms. In January 2010 compulsory vaccination for all goats and sheep was instituted. In 2010 up to 3 November, 492 patients with Q fever (not confirmed yet) have been reported. Since several measures have been instituted simultaneously it is difficult to speculate which measures have been most effective. It is very likely that the culling of all pregnant goats has had an important impact. It is clear, however, that most interventions were issued too late. Retrospectively, we know that Q fever was already a problem in the veterinary sector in 2005 and 2006 but that this knowledge was not communicated to the human health sector.

SEE ALSO *Animal Importation; Bioterrorism; Opportunistic Infection; Zoonoses*

BIBLIOGRAPHY

Books

Estenson, Joseph. *Q Fever: A Reference Guide.* Washington, DC: Capitol Hill Press, 2015.

Simoes, João Carlos Caetano, Sofia Ferreira Anastácio, and Gabriela Jorge Da Silva. *The Principles and Practice of Q Fever: The One Health Paradigm.* Boston: Nova Science, 2017.

Periodicals

Eldin, Carole, et al. "From Q Fever to *Coxiella burnetii* Infection: A Paradigm Change." *Clinical Microbiology Reviews* 30, no. 1 (January 2017): 115–190.

Websites

"Q Fever." *CDC Health Information for International Travel.* Centers for Disease Control and Prevention, May 31, 2017. https://wwwnc.cdc.gov/travel/yellowbook/2018/infectious-diseases-related-to-travel/q-fever (accessed November 20, 2017).

"Q Fever Fact Sheet." New South Wales Government. http://www.health.nsw.gov.au/Infectious/factsheets/Pages/q-fever.aspx (accessed November 20, 2017).

Brian Hoyle

Rabies

Introduction

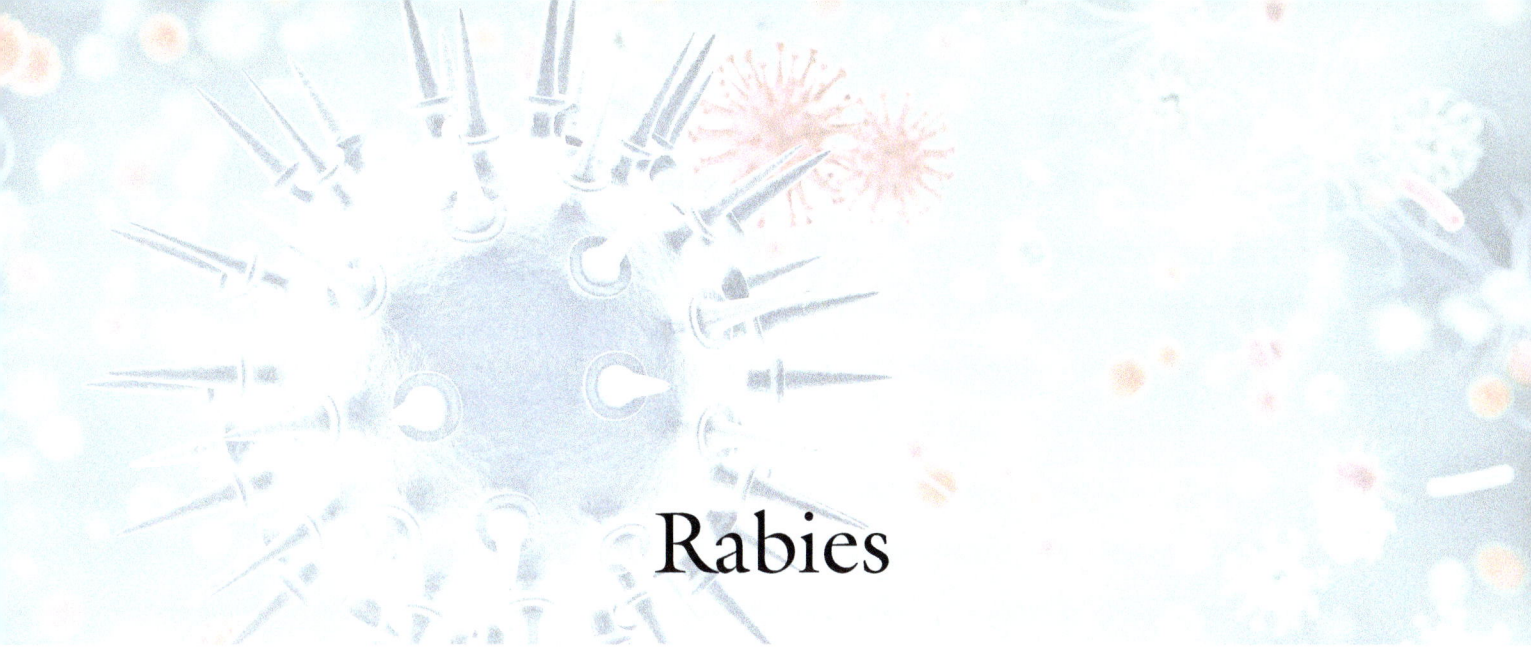

Rabies is an acute viral illness that affects the brain and nervous system of humans and other mammals. Left untreated, it is invariably fatal. From the Latin word *rabies* for "mad," rabies has long been one of the most feared diseases. It was described by the Greek philosopher Aristotle (384 BCE–322 BCE), who realized that humans could contract rabies when bitten by infected dogs, which is still the most common way the disease is transmitted.

In the first few decades of the 21st century, rabies continued to claim the lives of tens of thousands of people around the world each year, mainly in rural parts of Africa and Asia. The World Health Organization (WHO) stated that more than 150 countries and territories, on every continent except Antarctica, reported cases of rabies in any given year, with about 40 percent involving children under 15 years old.

The symptoms of rabies are dramatic and include seizures, hallucinations, foaming at the mouth, and violent throat spasms. Rabies is a zoonosis, a disease of animals that can affect humans. Wild mammals are the reservoir (the animal or organism in which the virus normally resides) of the rabies virus, and they can, in turn, affect domestic animals such as cats and dogs. Humans usually become infected through a bite from a wild or domestic animal with rabies. Fortunately, an effective vaccine against rabies is available, and it can be used either before or after exposure to the virus.

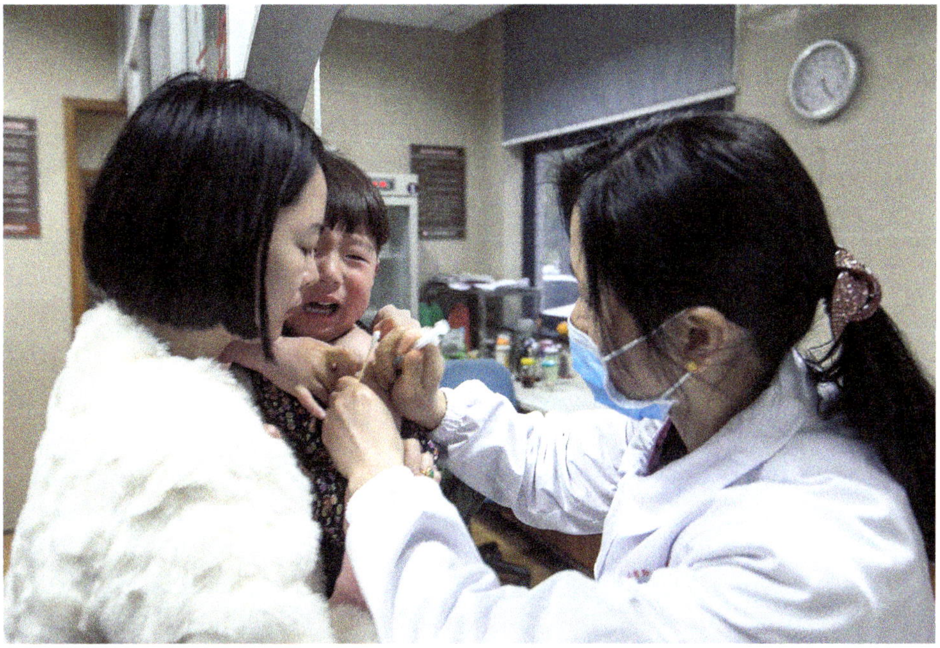

A child receives a rabies vaccine at a hospital in Hangzhou, China, after being scratched by a cat. *© VCG/Getty Images*

Disease History, Characteristics, and Transmission

Rabies is caused by a virus within the genus *Lyssavirus*. The rabies virus (species name *Rabies lyssavirus*) belongs to the rhabdovirus group (family Rhabdoviridae). It is a bullet-shaped enveloped RNA virus; that is, its genetic material is RNA (ribonucleic acid) rather than DNA (deoxyribonucleic acid). The incubation period of the virus is between 10 days and one year, but in most cases the period is from one to three months. Early symptoms are vague and may resemble influenza (flu). They include fatigue and general weakness, fever, headache, tingling at the exposure site(s), and nausea.

Once the rabies virus reaches the brain and nervous system, dramatic neurological symptoms set in. These include hallucinations, agitation, uncontrolled excitement, and violent movements that include muscle spasms, paralysis, seizures, and loss of consciousness. Foaming at the mouth is a classic symptom of rabies and is a combination of increased salivation and difficulty swallowing. The latter produces another classic symptom, hydrophobia (fear of water), where extreme throat spasms may be induced by even the sight of water. Sometimes rabies dominated by agitation is known as furious rabies, while that dominated by paralysis is dumb rabies.

Within days of the onset of these latter, more serious, symptoms, a person with rabies will enter a coma. Death usually results from paralysis of the respiratory muscles. Survival is extremely rare. There have been only a few documented cases, and all survivors had been protected to some extent by vaccination before or after exposure to the rabies virus.

The rabies virus eventually passes through the nervous system to the salivary glands. It is the saliva of an infected animal that transmits the disease to other animals and to humans. Exposure to the rabies virus usually occurs from a bite by an infected animal, although the virus might also sometimes be transmitted through a scratch or lick from the animal. Infections have also occurred through inhaling aerosols (particles of liquid or solid dispersed as a suspension in gas) from the droppings of infected bats.

Wild carnivorous mammals, including bats (both carnivorous and noncarnivorous), skunks, foxes, wolves, jackals, raccoons, and coyotes, act as a reservoir for the rabies virus. The infection may be passed to domestic animals

WORDS TO KNOW

IMMUNE GLOBULIN A type of protein found in blood. The immune globulins (or *immunoglobulins*) are Y-shaped globulins that act as antibodies, attaching themselves to invasive cells or materials in the body so that they can be identified and attacked by the immune system. There are five immune globulins, designated IgM, IgG, IgA, IgD, and IgE.

INCUBATION PERIOD The time between exposure to a disease-causing virus or bacterium and the appearance of symptoms of the infection. Depending on the microorganism, the incubation time can range from a few hours, such as with food poisoning due to *Salmonella*, to a decade or more, such as with acquired immunodeficiency syndrome (AIDS).

NOTIFIABLE DISEASE A disease that the law requires be reported to health officials when diagnosed. Also called a reportable disease.

RESERVOIR The animal or organism in which a virus or parasite normally resides.

SYLVATIC Meaning "pertaining to the woods," the term refers to diseases such as plague that are spread by animals including ground squirrels and other wild rodents.

VACCINATION The inoculation, or use of vaccines, to prevent specific diseases within humans and animals by producing immunity to such diseases. It is the introduction of weakened or dead viruses or microorganisms into the body to create immunity by the production of specific antibodies.

VECTOR Any agent that carries and transmits parasites and diseases. Also, an organism or a chemical used to transport a gene into a new host cell.

VIRUS Essentially nonliving repositories of nucleic acid that require the presence of a living prokaryotic or eukaryotic cell for the replication of the nucleic acid. There are a number of different viruses that challenge the human immune system and that may produce disease in humans. A virus is a small, infectious agent that consists of a core of genetic material—either deoxyribonucleic acid (DNA) or ribonucleic acid (RNA)—surrounded by a shell of protein. Very simple microorganisms, viruses are much smaller than bacteria that enter and multiply within cells. Viruses often exchange or transfer their genetic material (DNA or RNA) to cells and can cause diseases such as chickenpox, hepatitis, measles, and mumps.

ZOONOSES Diseases of microbiological origin that can be transmitted from animals to people. The causes of the diseases can be bacteria, viruses, parasites, and fungi.

such as dogs and cats. Humans can be infected by direct contact with either wild or domestic mammals. The former is sometimes known as sylvatic rabies; the latter, urban rabies. An animal with rabies virus will not be infectious all the time—only when the virus is in its saliva. This can happen late in the incubation period because the virus must pass from the muscle, where infection occurs, through the nervous system to the salivary glands.

Insectivorous (depending on insects as food) and vampire bats can also transmit rabies. Rodents (such as rats, mice, and hamsters) and lagomorphs (such as rabbits and hares) rarely get infected with rabies and have never been shown to transmit it to humans. However, woodchucks and groundhogs have been known to be responsible for a large percentage of rabies among rodents reported to the US Centers for Disease Control and Prevention (CDC). Other herbivorous mammals, including cattle, horses, and deer, can become infected with rabies but very rarely infect humans.

Human-to-human transmission of rabies is rare but not unknown. There have been several cases recorded among recipients of transplanted corneas and some in recipients of solid transplanted organs. In theory, bites could also transmit rabies from one person to another, although no such cases are known. Casual contact, such as touching a person with rabies or coming into contact with noninfectious fluids (such as urine, blood, or feces), does not carry a risk of infection with rabies virus.

Scope and Distribution

Rabies is a global problem that has been recognized for at least 3,000 years. At the turn of the 20th century, there were more than 100 cases of rabies in the United States each year. By the 1990s that number was fewer than 5. The disease is notifiable to the CDC, meaning health care providers are required by law to report any instances of rabies to official health authorities. US states also collect data on rabies cases. According to a survey conducted by WHO in 2004, there were approximately 55,000 deaths from rabies each year worldwide, most of them in rural Africa and Asia. That number was roughly the same as of 2018. Around half of all cases of rabies from dog bites occur among children less than 15 years old.

There is marked geographical variation in the mammal species that pose a threat of rabies. In the United States, sylvatic rabies accounts for most cases, while urban rabies is rare; the reverse is true in developing countries. The bat is the most common reservoir of the disease in Latin America, and the wolf is the most common in Eastern Europe.

Treatment and Prevention

There is no specific treatment for rabies once the symptoms have begun. A rabies vaccine was first developed by French biologist and chemist Louis Pasteur (1822–1895) in the late 1880s. This was a crude preparation made from the dried spinal cord of infected rabbit. Similar vaccines are still used in some countries, although WHO does not recommend them. Rabies vaccines made in cell culture are preferred for safety reasons.

Rabies vaccine can be given either before or after exposure to the virus. A pre-exposure vaccine should be given when a person's occupation brings them into contact with wild animals or with the virus itself (for instance, veterinarians, animal handlers, and certain laboratory workers). Travelers to regions where rabies is common and children living in these countries should also be vaccinated.

Post-exposure prophylaxis (PEP) vaccination is needed if someone has been potentially exposed to rabies virus through an animal bite or other contact. Each year more than 1 million Americans receive an animal bite, and these must always be taken seriously. Although only a few of these bites will pose a risk of rabies infection, each case must be carefully evaluated. An important part of the evaluation process is having an expert examine the animal involved for symptoms and signs of rabies.

The only method approved by the Food and Drug Administration (FDA) for PEP use in humans within the United States is the administration of an inactivated rabies vaccine and immunoglobulin. On its website WHO stated the categories of contact with a suspected rabid animal and whether PEP was recommended. The PEP vaccination prevents the virus from entering the central nervous system of someone potentially bitten by a rabid animal. It consists of the following steps:

- Thorough cleansing of the wound as soon as possible
- Administration of a rabies vaccine that meets WHO requirements
- If indicated, administration of rabies immunoglobulin (RIG; medication consisting of antibodies used to counter the rabies virus)

Two types of RIG may be used: human rabies immunoglobulin (HRIG) and equine rabies immunoglobulin (ERIG). (Immunoglobulin is also called gamma globulin and immune globulin.) ERIG is available in many countries and is considered less expensive than HRIG, which is expensive and available in only limited amounts. WHO suggests that a skin test be performed before the administration of ERIG. When ERIG is administered, the recommended dose is 20 international units per kilogram (IU/kg) of body weight for HRIG or 40 IU/kg of body weight for ERIG. Most of this amount should be positioned around the wound(s) with the remainder administered into the gluteal region (buttocks) of the body. A complete course of vaccination should be followed immediately, according to WHO.

Vaccination of domestic animals against rabies plays an important role in keeping the disease at bay. Some Euro-

LOUIS PASTEUR AND THE RABIES VACCINE

By 1880 French scientist Louis Pasteur (1822–1895) had shown that vaccination against anthrax worked in animals. He used a weakened, or attenuated, form of a culture of the anthrax bacterium as the vaccine and found it protected animals against the disease, compared to control animals that had not been vaccinated. In 1880 Pasteur decided to turn his attention to rabies, a feared disease with a high mortality rate. Pasteur showed that a vaccine made from an attenuated form of the rabies virus could protect dogs that had been bitten by rabid animals. He hesitated, however, before trying his vaccine on humans.

Pasteur's first human patient was a young boy, Joseph Meister, who was brought to him from Alsace on July 6, 1885. Joseph had been bitten 14 times by a rabid dog on his hands, legs, and thighs. Clearly his life was in danger, and Pasteur administered the first dose of vaccine the next day. He used the dried-out spinal cord from a rabid rabbit as the source of the vaccine. The drying process allowed the virus to lose much of its virulent character and helped to allay safety fears. The boy was given increasingly strong doses of vaccine over the next 12 days and was soon able to return to Alsace in good health, having developed no symptoms of rabies or any ill effects from the vaccination.

The development of an effective rabies vaccine was the final, and most dramatic, success of Pasteur's long and distinguished career in medicine, chemistry, and microbiology. Pasteur's work on rabies led to the establishment of the world-famous Pasteur Institute in Paris. The institute was funded through public contributions and was initially devoted to rabies vaccination. Since its launch in 1888, it has been home to many distinguished scientists, including several Nobel Prize winners.

pean countries, such as France, Switzerland, and Belgium, have eliminated rabies in their wildlife through vaccination campaigns, and this is being tried in places where the disease is more common such as India and South Africa.

Impacts and Issues

In 2004 WHO was informed of a case of rabies in a dog owned by a resident of Bordeaux, France. Many people had handled this dog over a five-week period when the animal was potentially infectious. WHO personnel put out a call for these individuals to come forward for assessment and possible PEP vaccination. The dog had been imported illegally from Morocco and had not been vaccinated against rabies.

This incident shows the importance of taking animal import and quarantine regulations seriously. By flouting these regulations on entry to France, the dog's owner put many people's lives at risk. Responsible owners get their pets vaccinated against rabies. In addition, when it comes to wildlife, it is best to admire from afar and never to handle or touch such animals.

Wisconsin teenager Jeanna Giese became the first person known to have survived symptomatic rabies without vaccination. In September 2004 Giese contracted rabies after being bitten on the finger by a bat. One month after the bite, she was admitted to the hospital. Rabies was considered always fatal in unvaccinated patients, but physicians and Giese's family chose an experimental treatment. Physicians put Giese into a drug-induced coma for a week, at the same time giving her several strong antiviral drugs (amantadine and ribavirin).

Giese's immune system fought the infection. She returned to school the following academic year after several months of recovery and intense physical therapy. Physicians and medical researchers continue to debate whether Giese survived because of the experimental treatment or whether other factors, such as a stronger-than-average immune system or a weaker-than-average strain of rabies, played a larger role.

Following the Geise case, there was an increased focus on bats as potential vectors of the disease. Though bats are beneficial in controlling mosquito and insect populations, researchers estimate that 1 percent of bats in the United States carry rabies. Bats rarely bite humans and cause only minor injury at the location of the bite. It is possible for bites on sleeping victims to go undetected. In August 2006 more than 1,000 young girls were advised to obtain rabies vaccinations after attending a Girl Scout camp where bats were present in sleeping quarters. Not all families opted for vaccination, but none of the girls developed rabies.

Cases of rabies are increasing, even in developed urban environments. In 2006 the Chinese government passed a law that forbid dogs in many public places and limited dog ownership to one animal per household. Rabies is endemic in China and is one of the nation's leading causes of death from infectious disease. However, officials cited the popularization of pet ownership and the failure of many pet owners to vaccinate dogs as primary causes for the resurgence of rabies, especially in the nation's cities.

WHO; the Organisation Mondiale de la Santé Animale (World Organisation for Animal Health); the Food and Agriculture Organization (FAO), a part of the United Nations (UN); and the Global Alliance for Rabies Control

(GARC) established a joint agenda in 2015 called United Against Rabies. The agenda, using the slogan "Zero by 30," hopes to eliminate human deaths from rabies by 2030.

In 2016 WHO established the Strategic Advisory Group of Experts on Immunization (SAGE). The group's purpose is to review and advise the UN on rabies vaccines and immunoglobulins. As of February 2018, SAGE was evaluating vaccine delivery times and methods, vaccination schedules, and aspects of new biological products for rabies control and prevention.

From 1983 to 2018, WHO reduced the incidence of rabies in the Americas by more than 95 percent in humans and 98 percent in dogs. Effective policies and vaccination campaigns made this possible. In 2010 WHO implemented a campaign to eliminate rabies in Southeast Asia by 2020. From 2010 to 2013, the incidence of rabies deaths in humans in Bangladesh was reduced by 50 percent, primarily through free vaccines, comprehensive dog vaccinations, and effective management of dog bites.

Several other countries, including the Philippines, South Africa, and Tanzania, have reduced their reported cases of rabies though WHO-sponsored programs, some with assistance from the Bill & Melinda Gates Foundation. WHO has found that succeeding with small programs often leads to successes in other programs in adjacent countries or territories.

In 2015 researchers developed a new vaccine that was effective in protecting mice from rabies, even after they had shown physical symptoms of the disease. To develop the vaccine, researchers inserted a protein from the rabies virus into the parainfluenza virus 5 (PIV5; an upper respiratory virus that is safe for humans). After these trials with mice are completed, testing on humans will be performed. Biao He, an author of a study published in the *Journal of Virology* and professor at the College of Veterinary Medicine at the University of Georgia, stated, "This is the most effective treatment we have seen reported in the scientific literature. If we can improve these results and translate them to humans, we may have found one of the first useful treatments for advanced rabies infection."

Before 2016 the inactivated rabies vaccine was the only rabies vaccine available in the United States. However, that year live-attenuated viruses were introduced as possible ways to immunize for rabies. These potentially new vaccines consist of genetically modified viruses used as immunization agents. Other possibilities for new vaccines introduced in or around this time include monoclonal antibody-based vaccines, nucleic acid–based vaccines, and small interfering RNAs (siRNAs), which interfere with virus replication.

In 2017 the Animal and Plant Health Inspection Service (APHIS), an agency of the United States Department of Agriculture, expanded its field trials to evaluate the effectiveness and safety of the ONRAB rabies vaccine for use in wildlife. One million oral rabies vaccination (ORV) baits were distributed in several US states. APHIS personnel hope to determine whether the ONRAB vaccine is better at controlling rabies in wildlife (specifically, raccoons and skunks) when compared to the currently approved vaccine, RABORAL. Another field trial concentrates on testing the new vaccine in urban and suburban settings.

SEE ALSO *Animal Importation; CDC (Centers for Disease Control and Prevention); Contact Precautions; Handwashing; World Health Organization (WHO); Zoonoses*

BIBLIOGRAPHY

Books

Jackson, Alan C., ed. *Rabies: Scientific Basis of the Disease and its Management.* Amsterdam: Elsevier Academic, 2013.

Kumar, P. Dileep. *Rabies.* Westport, CT: Greenwood, 2009.

Papadakis, Maxine A., and Stephen J. McPhee, eds. *Current Diagnosis and Treatment in Infectious Diseases.* New York: McGraw-Hill, 2017.

Rupprecht, Charles, and Thirumeni Nagarajan, eds. *Current Laboratory Techniques in Rabies Diagnosis, Research and Prevention.* Amsterdam: Elsevier Academic, 2015.

Walls, Ron M., Robert S. Hockberger, and Marianne Gausche-Hill, eds. *Rosen's Emergency Medicine: Concepts and Clinical Practice.* 9th ed. Philadelphia: Elsevier, 2018.

Periodicals

Huang, Ying, et al. "Parainfluenza Virus 5 Expressing the G protein of Rabies Virus Protected Mice after Rabies Virus Infection." *Journal of Virology* (December 31, 2014). This article can also be found online at http://jvi.asm.org/content/early/2014/12/26/JVI.03656-14.full.pdf+html (accessed February 26, 2018).

Lite, Jordan. "Medical Mystery: Only One Person Has Survived Rabies without Vaccine—But How?" *Scientific American* (October 8, 2008). This article can also be found online at https://www.scientificamerican.com/article/jeanna-giese-rabies-survivor/ (accessed February 19, 2018).

Zhu, Shimao, and Caiping Guo. "Rabies Control and Treatment: From Prophylaxis to Strategies with Curative Potential." *Viruses* 8, no. 11 (November 2016): 279. This article can also be found online at https://www.ncbi.nlm.nih.gov/pmc/articles/PMC5127009/ (accessed February 26, 2018).

Websites

"Administration of Rabies Immunoglobulin." World Health Organization. http://www.who.int/rabies/human/adminimmuno/en/ (accessed February 19, 2018).

Hataway, James. "Beating the Clock: UGA Researchers Develop New Treatment for Rabies." UGAToday, January 26, 2015. https://news.uga.edu/beating-the-clock-researchers-develop-new-rabies-treatment-0115/ (accessed February 19, 2018).

Hays, Brooks. "Scientists Develop Potential Late-Stage Rabies Treatment." UPI, January 29, 2015. https://www.upi.com/Science_News/2015/01/29/Scientists-develop-potential-late-stage-rabies-treatment/9691422485373/ (accessed February 20, 2018).

"Rabies." Centers for Diseases Control and Prevention, National Center for Infectious Diseases, September 28, 2017. https://www.cdc.gov/rabies/ (accessed February 19, 2018).

"Rabies." World Health Organization, September 2017. http://www.who.int/mediacentre/factsheets/fs099/en (accessed February 19, 2018).

"USDA Begins 2017 Field Trials to Evaluate New Oral Rabies Vaccine in Raccoons, Other Wildlife." United States Department of Agriculture, August 7, 2017. https://www.aphis.usda.gov/aphis/newsroom/news/sa_by_date/sa-2017/new-rabies-vaccine (accessed February 19, 2018).

"USDA Expands Field Trials of New Oral Rabies Vaccine for Use in Raccoons and Other Wildlife in 5 States." United States Department of Agriculture, August 31, 2016. https://www.aphis.usda.gov/aphis/newsroom/news/sa_by_date/sa_2012/sa_08/ct_rabies_vaccine_expanded (accessed February 20, 2018).

Susan Aldridge
William Arthur Atkins

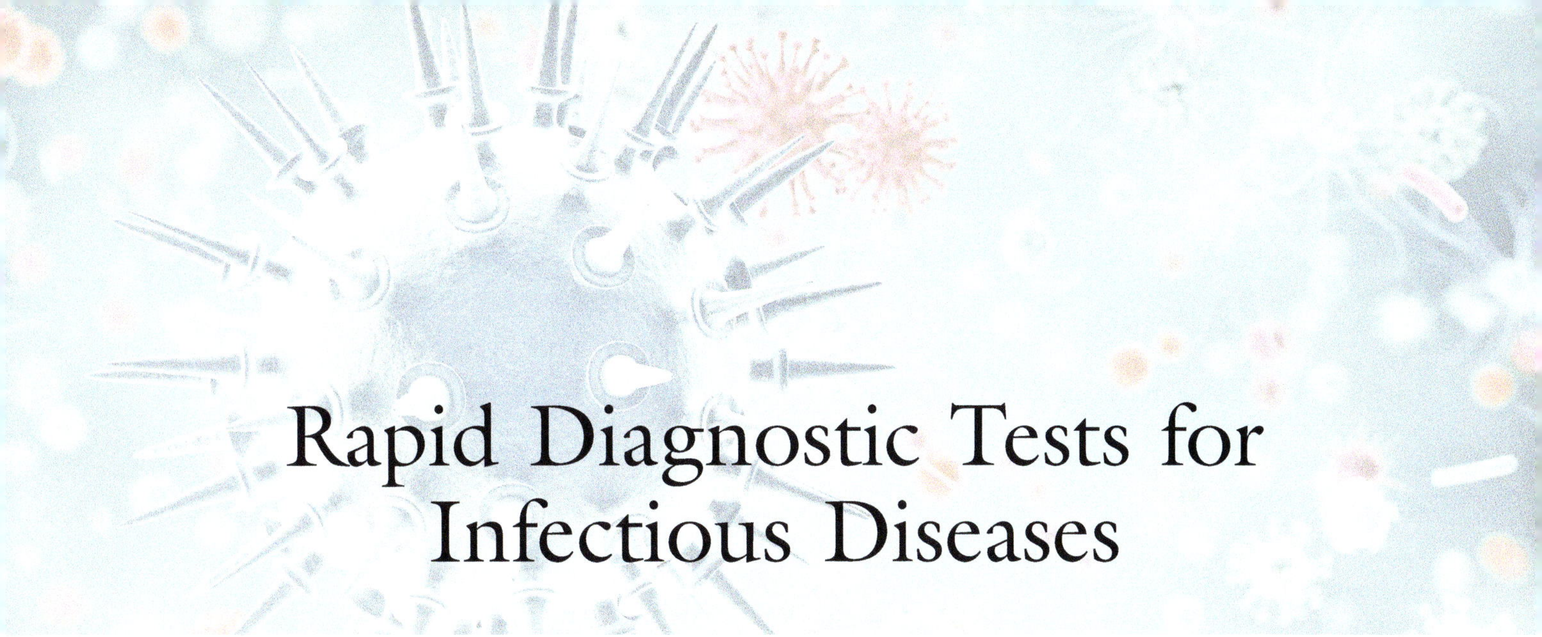

Rapid Diagnostic Tests for Infectious Diseases

Introduction

Before the era of molecular biology, determination of the cause of an infectious disease (the process of diagnosis) involved the observation of the symptoms of the disease; the culturing (growing and identifying) of the responsible bacteria, virus, or protozoa (which still is not always possible or may require a long time); and the results of a variety of biochemical tests. Diagnosis typically took days or weeks.

Since the 1970s the ability to detect target regions of bacterial and viral deoxyribonucleic acid (DNA) or ribonucleic acid (RNA) has made it possible to demonstrate the presence of microorganisms in blood, urine, and tissue samples from an infected person and to identify the microorganism even to the species level. Some of these molecular-based tests can be done in minutes.

Other rapid diagnostic tests are based on the presence of an antibody that is produced by the human immune system in response to the presence of a certain bacterial or

WORDS TO KNOW

ANTIBODIES Proteins found in the blood that help fight against foreign substances called antigens. Antigens, which are usually proteins or polysaccharides, stimulate the immune system to produce antibodies, or Y-shaped immunoglobulins. The antibodies inactivate the antigen and help remove it from the body. While antigens can be the source of infections from pathogenic bacteria and viruses, organic molecules detrimental to the body from internal or environmental sources also act as antigens. Genetic engineering and the use of various mutational mechanisms allow the construction of a vast array of antibodies (each with a unique genetic sequence).

ANTIBODY-ANTIGEN BINDING Antibodies are produced by the immune system in response to antigens (material perceived as foreign). The antibody response to a particular antigen is highly specific and often involves a physical association between the two molecules. Biochemical and molecular forces govern this association.

ANTIGEN A substance, usually a protein or polysaccharide, that stimulates the immune system to produce antibodies. While antigens can be the source of infections from pathogenic bacteria and viruses, organic molecules detrimental to the body from internal or environmental sources also act as antigens.

CULTURE A single species of microorganism that is isolated and grown under controlled conditions. German bacteriologist Robert Koch first developed culturing techniques in the late 1870s. Following Koch's initial discovery, medical scientists quickly sought to identify other pathogens. In the 21st century bacteria cultures are used as basic tools in microbiology and medicine.

IMMUNO-BASED TEST A medical technology that tests for the presence of a disease by looking for a reaction between disease organisms that may be present in a tissue or fluid sample and antibodies contained in the test kit.

PCR (POLYMERASE CHAIN REACTION) A widely used technique in molecular biology involving the amplification of specific sequences of genomic DNA.

viral component, usually a protein, that is generically termed an antigen. These immunotests are based on the detection of the binding of the sample antigen to the antibody.

As of 2017 rapid detection based on DNA sequencing was available and was starting to become adopted more widely for clinical use. In this approach DNA recovered from blood is analyzed to determine all DNA sequences present, and the sequences are compared to databases to identify sequence matches with bacterial pathogens.

Detecting the presence of specific arrangements of nucleic acid that are present in the genetic material of the infecting organism is another testing method. This nucleic acid testing can be combined with the use of molecules that fluoresce when exposed to light of a particular wavelength. If the specific disease-causing organism is present, it is detected by the development of fluorescence that has resulted from the binding of the probe to the specific stretch of nucleic acid. The molecular-based approaches do not require growth of the bacteria.

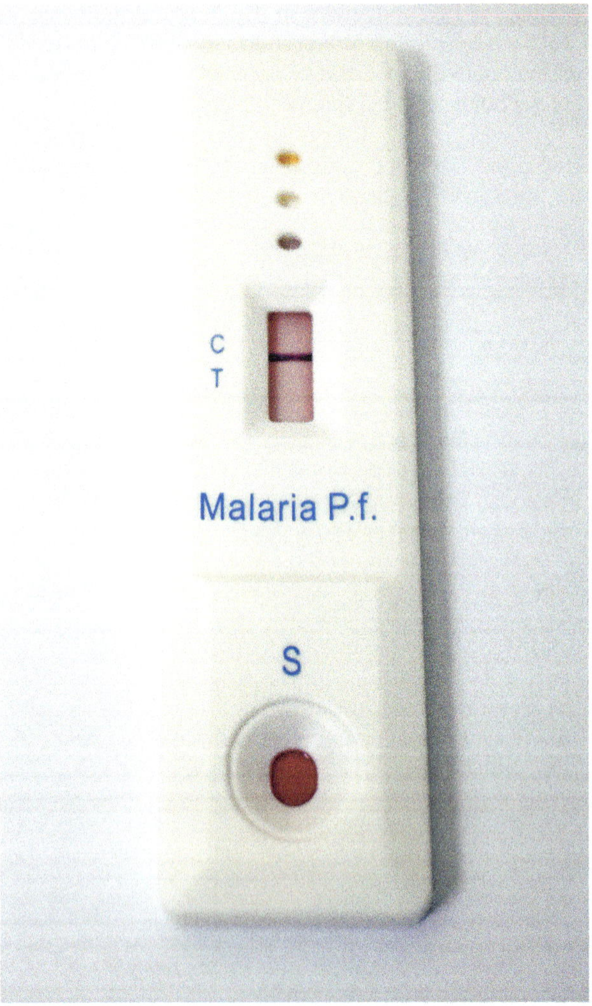

An immunochromatographic test (ICT) for malaria. Rapid tests allow medical professionals to make a diagnosis without access to electricity or specialized equipment. *© Universal Images Group/Getty Images*

History and Scientific Foundations

Rapid molecular tests rely on the detection of target regions of the microbial genetic material. Once the genetic sequence (the arrangement of the building blocks [nucleotides] of the DNA or RNA) of a variety of important microbial pathogens has been determined, target regions that are unique to a given organism or a gene that codes for the presence of an important disease-causing contributor, such as a toxin, can be identified. The detection of these target regions can prove the presence of the microbe even in the absence of the actual isolation of the organism. Furthermore, comparison of the genetic sequence with sequences that have been saved in databases can identify the genus and sometimes even the species of the infecting microorganism.

The target genetic region may only be present in low quantities. A technique called polymerase chain reaction (PCR) was developed in the 1980s and earned its discoverer, Kary Mullis (1994–), the 1993 Nobel Prize in Chemistry. PCR enables the amplification of bits of DNA. Because each PCR cycle doubles the amount of the genetic material, and because cycles can be done quickly (sometimes in minutes), literally billions of copies of the target DNA can be made in a few hours.

Immuno-based tests rely on the binding of a sample antigen to its corresponding antibody that is bound to a support such as a paper strip. Antigen-antibody binding is a specific reaction. Other antigens in a sample will not bind to the bound antibody unless they are almost identical both in the arrangement of amino acids that make up the protein and in the three-dimensional shape adopted by the protein molecules in solution. Commercially available immunostrips also contain controls that verify that the observed antigen-antibody binding, which is detected by the development of a color, is not a mistake.

Applications and Research

Rapid diagnostic tests have become popular in the diagnosis of infectious diseases. Antigen-antibody binding tests have been available for decades for the examination of fluid specimens that include whole blood, the serum and plasma components of blood, saliva, urine, and even fluid recovered from tissues.

The various tests can detect as little as one nanogram (0.000000001 g) of an antigen in the sample. The huge

TERRORISM AND BIOLOGICAL WARFARE

The Advanced Diagnostics Program is funded by the Defense Advanced Research Projects Agency (DARPA) of the US government. Its objective is to develop tools and medicines to detect and treat biological and chemical weapons in the field at concentrations low enough to prevent illness. Challenges to this task include minimizing the labor, equipment, and time for identifying biological agents. One area of interest includes development of field tools that can identify many different agents. To accomplish this goal, several groups funded under the Advanced Diagnostics Program have developed field-based biosensors that can detect a variety of analytes, including fragments of DNA, various hormones and proteins, bacteria, salts, and antibodies. These biosensors are portable, run on external power sources, and require little time to complete analyses.

A second focus of the Advanced Diagnostics Program is the identification of known and unknown or bioengineered pathogens and the development of early responses to infections. A final goal is to develop the ability to continuously monitor the body for evidence of infection. Researchers are addressing this goal in two ways. The first involves engineering monitoring mechanisms that are internal to the body. In particular, groups funded under the initiative are developing bioengineered white blood cells to detect infection from within the body. Often genetic responses to infection occur within minutes of infection, so analysis of blood cells provides a quick indication of the presence of a biological threat. The second method involves the development of a wearable, noninvasive diagnostic device that detects a broad spectrum of biological and chemical agents.

variety of viruses and bacteria that can be detected include hepatitis B, human immunodeficiency virus (HIV), malaria (based on detection of an antigen of the malaria-causing microbe *Plasmodium falciparum*), syphilis (based on detection of a *Treponema pallidum* antigen), *Streptococcus* (a common cause of the infection strep throat), urinary tract infections (based on the enhanced production of several enzymes during an infection), carbapenemase-producing *Enterobacteriaceae*, methicillin-resistant *Staphylococcus aureus* (MRSA), and influenza.

The rapid detection of influenza is noteworthy because influenza viruses are characterized by their changing outer surface, and thus their antigenic composition, from year to year. The rapid test targets a viral component that has proven to be more stable over time.

Research continues to refine the molecular and immuno-based rapid diagnostic tests, both in terms of their accuracy and the spectrum of microbial diseases that can be detected. Projects underway as of 2017 included DNA-based rapid detection of pathogens that are transmitted to humans from insects like mosquitoes and other types of arthropods. Examples include dengue and chikungunya viruses and *Borrelia burgdorferi* (the cause of Lyme disease).

■ Impacts and Issues

Being able to rapidly diagnose infectious diseases can help initiate treatment faster, which can be key in combating a swiftly spreading infection. Furthermore, for diseases such as influenza that are caused by a virus, a rapid diagnosis curtails the misuse of antibiotics, which are useless against viral infections but which can stimulate the development of antibiotic resistance in resident bacteria. Such antibiotic misuse has been a key factor in the development of bacterial antibiotic resistance, which is increasingly making diseases such as tuberculosis more difficult and expensive to treat.

Molecular techniques require specialized (and expensive) equipment and trained personnel. This can be a limitation for smaller clinics in developed countries and can be completely impractical for rural clinics in developing and underdeveloped countries. Immuno-based tests are less expensive, the test strips are easier to transport and store because refrigeration is usually not required, and the results are clear and do not require interpretation.

The use of immuno-based strip tests has brought rapid diagnostic testing to rural clinics in developing and developed regions. Staff at these clinics can be easily trained to carry out and interpret the test results. The tests are also useful to field staff of agencies including the World Health Organization and the US Centers for Disease Control and Prevention, which respond to illness outbreaks. The rapid detection of a disease and its geographical scope can be vital in combating an outbreak.

As of 2017 researchers were refining molecular techniques that enable the rapid detection of the presence of antibiotic resistance in important clinical bacteria, including carbapenem-resistant *Enterobacteriaceae* and extended-spectrum beta-lactamase-producing *Enterobacteriaceae.*

See Also *Food-Borne Disease and Food Safety; Water-Borne Disease*

BIBLIOGRAPHY

Books

Henderson, Cary G. *Enterococci and Bacterial Diseases: Risk Factors, Molecular Biology, and Antibiotic Resistance.* New York: Nova Science, 2017.

Kudva, Indira T., et al. *Virulence Mechanisms of Bacterial Pathogens.* Washington, DC: American Society for Microbiology, 2016.

Mirete, Salvador, and Marcos López Pérez, eds. *Antibiotic Resistance Genes in Natural Environments and Long-Term Effects.* New York: Nova Biomedical, 2017.

Periodicals

Kelley, Shana O. "New Technologies for Rapid Bacterial Identification and Antibiotic Resistance." *SLAS Technology* 22 (April 2017): 113–121.

Nordmann, Patrice, Aurélie Jayol, and Laurent Poirel. "Rapid Detection of Polymyxin Resistance in *Enterobacteriaceae.*" *Emerging Infectious Diseases* 22 (June 2016): 1038–1043.

Nordmann, Patrice, Laurent Poirel, and Laurent Dortet. "Rapid Detection of Carbapenemase-Producing *Enterobacteriaceae.*" *Emerging Infectious Diseases* 18 (September 2012): 1503–1507.

Websites

"Rapid Detection of Methicillin-Resistant *Staphylococcus aureus.*" UpToDate. https://www.uptodate.com/contents/rapid-detection-of-methicillin-resistant-staphylococcus-aureus (accessed November 21, 2017).

Brian Hoyle

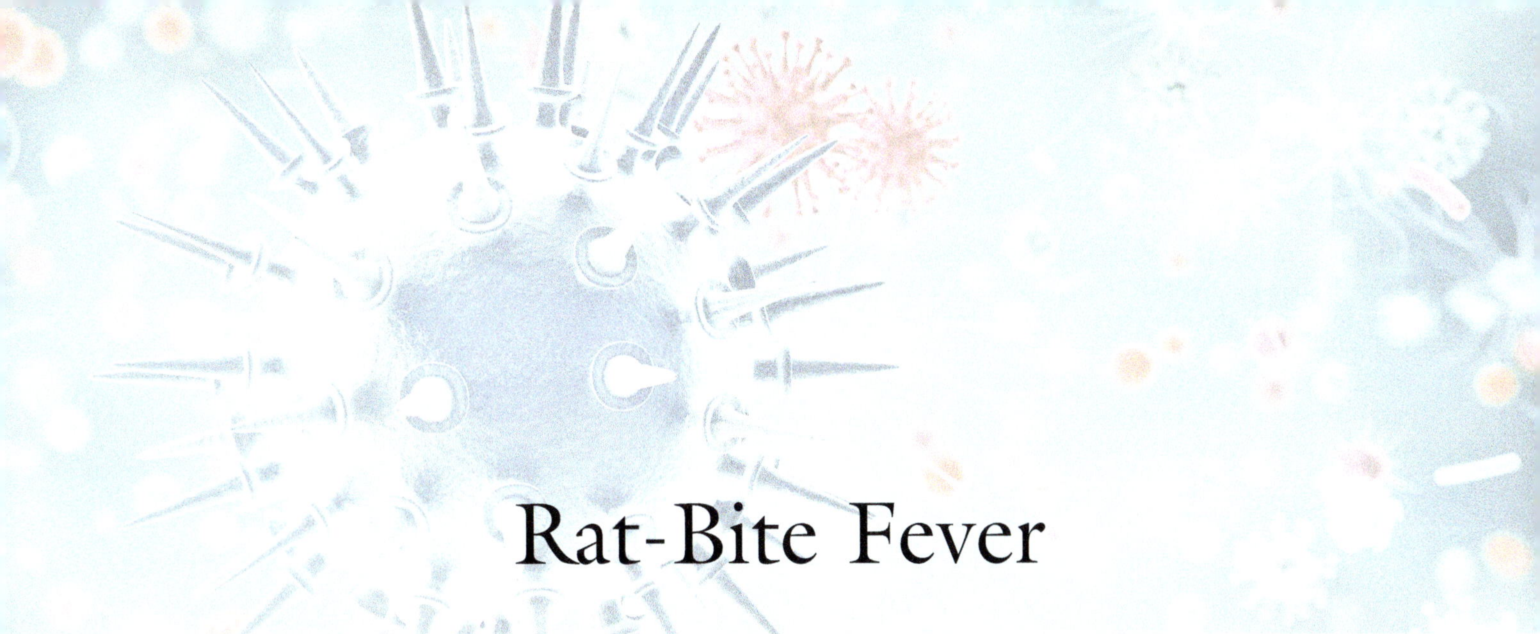

Rat-Bite Fever

Introduction

Rat-bite fever (RBF) is an acute infectious disease in humans caused by the scratch or bite of rodents, mostly rats, infected with one of two types of bacteria, *Streptobacillus moniliformis* or *Spirillum minus.* It is not transmitted from person to person. Scratches and bites are not necessarily the only way to contract the infection. Both bacteria may be passed from rodents to humans through urine or mucous secretions from the eyes or nose of infected rats.

RBF occurs most often among biomedical laboratory technicians, pet store employees who handle rodents, and people who have rodents as pets. It also occurs among people who live in rat-infested conditions. Children are more likely to be infected, both from their time spent inside and outdoors. Other animals that can carry the infectious bacteria are cats, dogs, gerbils, mice, squirrels, and weasels. The disease is also known as Haverhill fever and epidemic arthritic erythema (redness).

Disease History, Characteristics, and Transmission

Symptoms from the bacteria *Streptobacillus moniliformis* begin 2 to 22 days (usually within 10 days) after an initial bite or scratch. The infection can also be acquired by drinking contaminated milk or water, sometimes referred to as Haverhill fever.

Symptoms are similar to those of severe influenza (flu), with moderate fever (101–104°F [38.3–40.0°C]), chills, nausea, vomiting, headache, joint and back pain, gastrointestinal problems, and a reddish-pink rash made of tiny bumps located generally on the palms of the hands and the soles of the feet. The rash usually erupts about three days after initial contact with the bacteria.

Infections from the bacterium *Spirillum minus* are more common than infections with the other bacterium that causes RBF. *Spirillum minus* infections are called spirillary RBF or, sometimes, sodoku. Symptoms do not begin until 4 to 28 days (usually less than 10 days) after exposure and after the wound made by the bite or scratch has already healed. After the wound appears to initially heal, it suddenly becomes swollen and chronically inflamed.

Symptoms of spirillary RBF include fever, chills, and headache. The fever lasts longer than with *Streptobacillus moniliformis* and may also reoccur over a period of months. The gastrointestinal symptoms are less severe than with Haverhill fever. The rash is a light, rosy color; causes itching; and covers most or all of the body. Joint and muscle pain does not usually occur or, if it does, is much less severe than with Haverhill fever.

WORDS TO KNOW

ABSCESS A pus-filled sore, usually caused by a bacterial infection. It results from the body's defensive reaction to foreign material. Abscesses are often found in the soft tissue under the skin in areas such as the armpit or the groin. However, they may develop in any organ, and they are commonly found in the breast and gums. If they are located in deep organs such as the lung, liver, or brain, abscesses are far more serious and call for more specific treatment.

ERYTHEMA Skin redness due to excess blood in the capillaries (small blood vessels) in the skin.

SEPTIC Infected with bacteria, particularly in the bloodstream.

Scope and Distribution

The infection caused by the bacterium *Str. moniliformis* has been found in the past to occur in North America. With this bacterium the infection is commonly called streptobacillary RBF. RBF is rare in the United States. The disease is not a nationally notifiable disease, meaning there is no requirement to report diagnosed cases. Consequently, accurate statistics on the incidence of the disease are not available.

The infection caused by *Sp. minus* is usually found in Asia and Africa.

Treatment and Prevention

Str. moniliformis is identified by a culture of blood or fluid taken from one of the affected joints of the infected human. The culture is then analyzed in a laboratory.

Antibiotics including procaine penicillin G or penicillin V by mouth (orally) are the most common treatments for streptobacillary RBF. If the patient is allergic to penicillin, erythromycin may be provided orally. Treatment is usually successful, although the infection is sometimes eliminated by the human body given sufficient time. If left untreated and the body is unable to eliminate the disease, streptobacillary RBF can develop into serious complications such as septic arthritis, abscesses of any tissue or organ of the body, endocarditis (inflammation of the heart's lining), meningitis (inflammation of the lining surrounding the brain and spine), and pneumonia (inflammation of the lungs). Death is a rare outcome of untreated RBF, occurring in roughly 10 percent of untreated cases.

The disease caused by the bacterium *Sp. minus* is identified by examining blood or tissue removed from the wound of the infected human. Spirillary RBF is usually treated with procaine penicillin G or penicillin V by mouth. If the patient is allergic to penicillin, tetracycline can be given orally. If it is not treated, the fever usually subsides but returns in cycles of two to four days for up to one year. In most circumstances the illness, even without treatment, will resolve itself within four to eight weeks.

To prevent both forms of RBF, the US Centers for Disease Control and Prevention (CDC) recommends humans avoid contact with animals capable of passing on the bacterial organisms. If contact cannot be avoided with rodents, recommendations include wearing gloves, regularly washing hands, and avoiding hand-to-mouth contact while handling rodents and cleaning their cages. Avoiding unpasteurized milk or water from unsafe sources can help prevent streptobacillary RBF.

Impacts and Issues

Rodent infestations contribute greatly to the decline of already poor communities. Rodents cause extensive losses of food and destruction of property when they are present in large numbers. They can cause damage and loss of revenue to grocery stores, warehouses, cargo carriers, and homes. Rodents can also cause loss of property due to fires from the gnawing of electrical wiring.

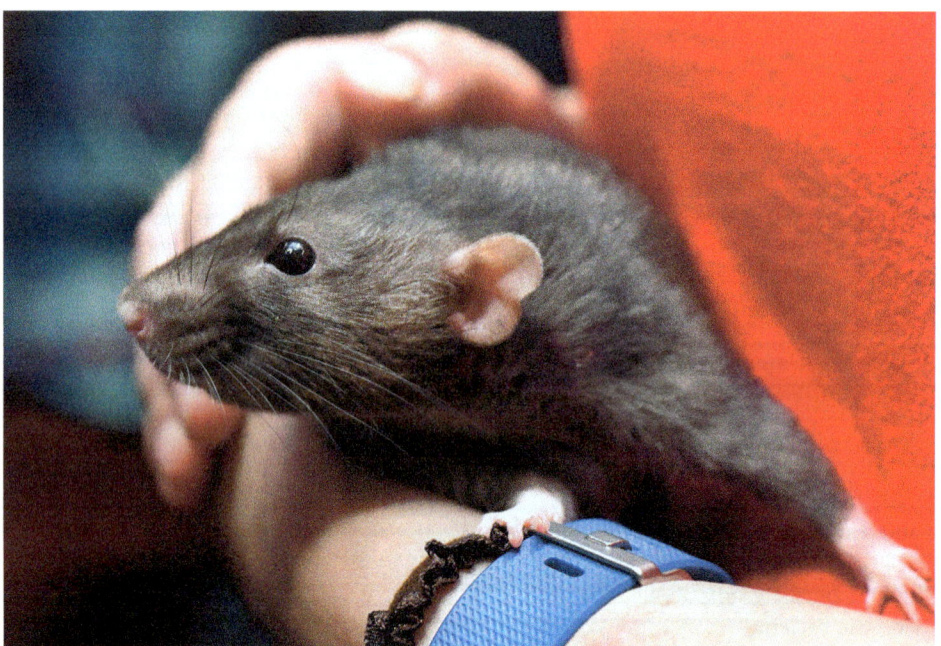

Rats are the primary carriers of rat-bite fever, which causes a moderate fever (101–104°F [38.3–40.0°C]), chills, nausea, vomiting, and other flu-like symptoms. © JOSH EDELSON/AFP/Getty Images

Sometimes rodents are controlled improperly with poisons, which exaggerates the problems already present. Health and safety problems can occur, especially among children, domesticated animals and pets, and the environment due to improper poison use.

Along with RBF, large populations of rats within communities can increase the chance of contracting diseases such as hantavirus, leptospirosis (also called Weil's disease, canicola fever, and seven-day fever), plague, salmonella, and typhoid. These diseases can be potentially deadly, especially among the young and elderly.

PRIMARY SOURCE

Notes from the Field: Fatal Rat-Bite Fever in a Child—San Diego County, California, 2013

SOURCE: *Adam, Jessica K., et al. "Notes from the Field: Fatal Rat-Bite Fever in a Child—San Diego County, California, 2013."* Morbidity and Mortality Weekly Report *63, no. 50 (December 19, 2014): 1210–1211. This article can also be found online at https://www.cdc.gov/mmwr/preview/mmwrhtml/mm6350a8.htm (accessed January 19, 2018).*

INTRODUCTION: *Rats are a popular pet, especially for children. Although the risks of contracting rat-bite fever from a pet rat are low, it is important for all pet owners to understand the risks. In 2013 a 10-year-old boy from San Diego, California, died after contracting the disease from a rat recently purchased from a pet store. The following article from the US Centers for Disease Control and Prevention discusses the child's death and its implications.*

In August 2013, the County of San Diego Health and Human Services Agency was notified of a fatal case of rat-bite fever (RBF) in a previously healthy male, aged 10 years, who owned pet rats. Two days before his death, the patient experienced rigors, fevers, vomiting, headaches, and leg pains. His physician noted a fever of 102.6°F (39.2°C), documented a normal examination, diagnosed viral gastroenteritis, and prescribed antinausea medication. During the next 24 hours, the patient experienced vomiting and persistent fever. He was confused and weak before collapsing at home. Paramedics reported the patient was unresponsive and had dilated pupils; resuscitation was initiated in the field and was continued for >1 hour after arrival at the emergency department but was unsuccessful. A complete blood count performed during resuscitation revealed anemia (hemoglobin 10.0 g/dL [normal = 13.5–18.0 g/dL], thrombocytopenia (platelets 40,000/μL [normal = 140,000–440,000/μL]), leukocytosis (white blood cells 17,900 cells/μL [normal = 4,000–10,500/μL]) with 16% band neutrophils; the patient also had evidence of disseminated intravascular coagulation. No rash or skin breakdown was noted. Lung, liver, and epiglottis tissue collected postmortem was positive for *Streptobacillus moniliformis* DNA by polymerase chain reaction.

During the 10 days before his death, the patient had obtained his second pet rat; *S. moniliformis* was detected by polymerase chain reaction in oropharyngeal tissue from this rat. Oropharyngeal swabs of the first pet rat were negative for *S. moniliformis* by polymerase chain reaction. The autopsy report noted that patient had been scratched by his pet rats.

RBF is a systemic illness of humans caused principally by *S. moniliformis*, a gram-negative bacterium that is commensal among rats. The organism can be transmitted to humans through rodent bites or scratches; approximately one in 10 bites might cause infection. Infection can also occur after handling infected rodents without a bite or scratch, or through ingestion of food or water contaminated with the bacteria. Symptoms include fever, rash, vomiting, and muscle or joint pain. RBF is treatable with antibiotics; approximately 13% of untreated RBF illnesses are fatal.

Nearly all domestic and wild rats carry *S. moniliformis.* An estimated 0.1% of U.S. households owned one or more pet rats during 2011 (Sharon Granskog, American Veterinary Medical Association, personal communication, April 25, 2014).

RBF is not a reportable condition in California or nationally. To estimate RBF incidence in San Diego County, hospitals in San Diego County that discharged any patients during 2000–2012 with *International Classification of Diseases, Ninth Revision* codes 026.0–026.1 (for streptobacillary fever and spirillary fever) were identified based on data from the California Office of Statewide Health Planning and Development. Medical records were requested, and 16 cases were identified. One additional RBF case was reported to the County of San Diego Health and Human Services Agency during 2013 as an occurrence of unusual disease.

Among the 17 cases, the median patient age was 10 years (range = 4–67 years); 59% of patients were female, and 65% were healthy before infection. Most infections (94%) were pet-associated; one patient had an occupational exposure (rat breeder). Sixteen of 17 patients reported exposure to rats. Of these, 44% reported only having handled a rat, 38% reported being bitten, and 13% reported a scratch. All patients had blood drawn for cultures; only 29% tested positive for *S. moniliformis;* the remainder were treated presumptively for RBF on the basis of exposure and clinical presentation. All patients survived except the patient described in this report.

RBF is a rare but potentially fatal illness that should be considered in persons with rash, fever, and joint pain and when a history of rodent exposure is reported. Clinicians suspecting *S. moniliformis* infection should promptly alert laboratory staff because microbiologic diagnosis is difficult, requiring specific media and incubation conditions. Clinicians should also consider requesting diagnosis assistance from their state public health laboratories. Because rapid laboratory confirmation might not be possible, empiric treatment for RBF in the setting of appropriate exposure history might be considered.

Pet rat owners should wear gloves and wash their hands thoroughly after handling rats or cleaning rat cages, avoid rat secretions, and promptly seek medical care if they have RBF symptoms after contact with rats.

SEE ALSO *Bacterial Disease; Vector-Borne Disease; Zoonoses*

BIBLIOGRAPHY

Books

Conover, Michael R., and Rosanna M. Vail. *Human Diseases from Wildlife*. Boca Raton, FL: CRC, 2015.

Periodicals

Elliott, Sean P. "Rat Bite Fever and *Streptobacillus moniliformis*." *Clinical Microbiology Reviews* 20, no. 1 (January 2007): 13–22. This article can also be found online at http://cmr.asm.org/content/20/1/13.full (accessed January 19, 2018).

Elsenberg, Tobias, et al. "Approved and Novel Strategies in Diagnostics of Rat Bite Fever and Other *Streptobacillus* Infections in Humans and Animals." *Virulence* 7, no. 6 (August 2016): 630–648.

Websites

"Rat-Bite Fever." Centers for Disease Control and Prevention, April 24, 2015. https://www.cdc.gov/rat-bite-fever/index.html (accessed January 19, 2018).

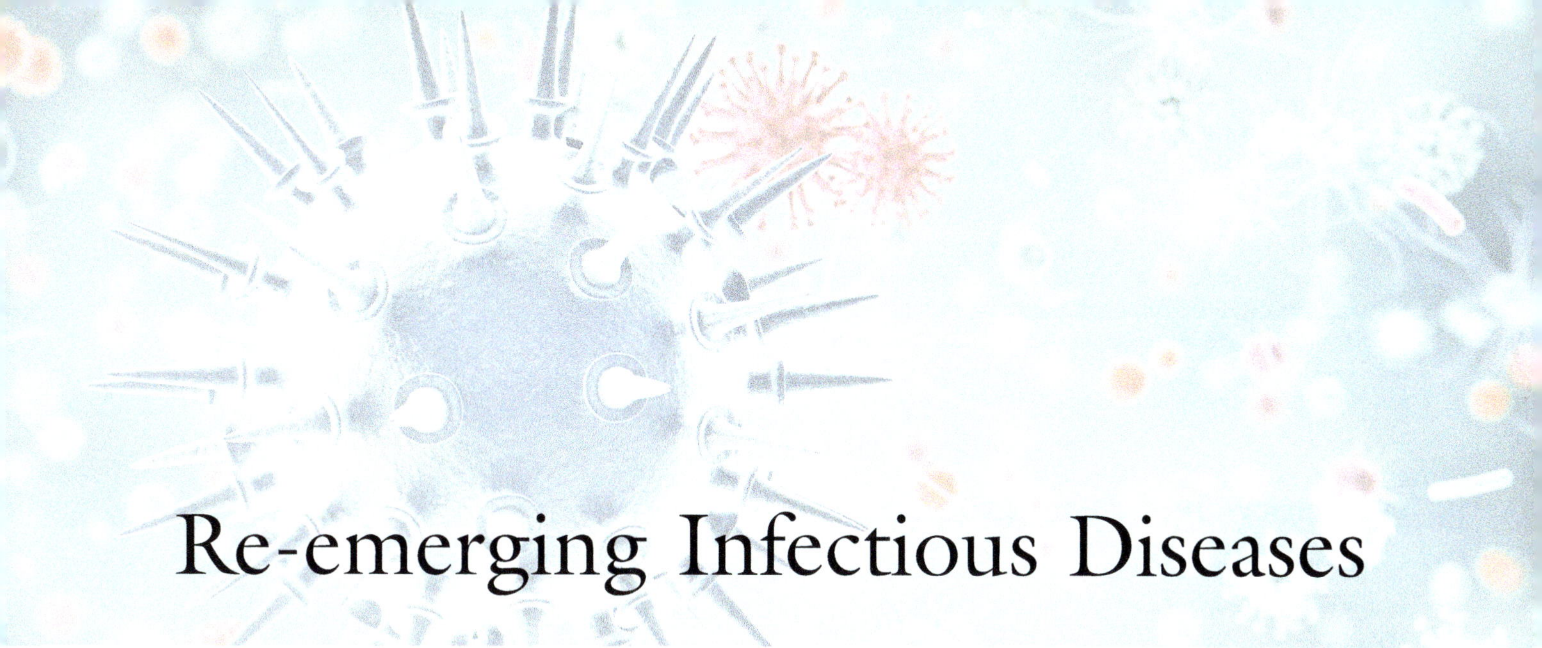

Re-emerging Infectious Diseases

Introduction

In the middle of the 20th century, the development of highly effective antibiotics and the implementation of successful disease prevention and global vaccination programs led to the control or eradication of serious diseases such as polio and smallpox. At the time it was widely assumed that infectious disease would ultimately become a minor problem. However, as of 2018, re-emerging infectious diseases presented a growing public health threat worldwide.

According to a 2012 survey by the World Health Organization (WHO), three infectious diseases ranked among the top 10 causes of death globally: lower respiratory infections, with 3.1 million deaths; human immunodeficiency virus (HIV) and acquired immunodeficiency syndrome (AIDS), with 1.5 million deaths; and diarrheal diseases, with 1.5 million deaths. The rankings varied by national income levels. For example, in low-income countries, malaria and tuberculosis, both of which are reemerging diseases, were among the 10 leading causes of death. Re-emerging infections have gained renewed virulence due to other emerging or chronic diseases that impair the immune system (for example, HIV/AIDS, diabetes, cancer) or the spread of antibiotic, antiviral, and antifungal medication resistance.

WORDS TO KNOW

ADAPTIVE IMMUNITY Another term for acquired immunity, referring to the resistance to infection that develops through life and is targeted to a specific pathogen. There are two types of adaptive immunity, known as active and passive. Active immunity is either humoral, involving production of antibody molecules against a bacterium or virus, or cell-mediated, in which T cells are mobilized against infected cells. Infection and immunization can both induce acquired immunity. Passive immunity is induced by injection of the serum of a person who is already immune to a particular infection.

EMERGING INFECTIOUS DISEASE A new infectious disease such as severe acute respiratory syndrome (SARS) or West Nile virus, as well as a previously known disease such as malaria, tuberculosis, or bacterial pneumonia that is appearing in a new form that is resistant to drug treatments.

ENDEMIC Present in a particular area or among a particular group of people.

ERADICATION The process of destroying or eliminating a microorganism or disease.

GLOBALIZATION The integration of national and local systems into a global economy through increased trade, manufacturing, communications, and migration.

IMMUNOGENICITY The capacity of a host to produce an immune response to protect itself against infectious disease.

INNATE IMMUNITY Resistance against disease that an individual is born with, as distinct from acquired immunity that develops with exposure to infectious agents.

PATHOGEN A disease-causing agent, such as a bacterium, a virus, a fungus, or another microorganism.

VIRULENCE The ability of a disease organism to cause disease. A more virulent organism is more infective and liable to produce more serious disease.

In addition, there is the threat of reemergent infectious disease that is intentionally spread in connection with bioterrorism, as occurred in the United States in the anthrax attacks of 2001. Although only a small number of people were infected and killed in these attacks, the potential for widespread targeted assaults makes the use of bioterrorism agents especially disturbing to consider.

History and Scientific Foundations

In the United States, the National Institute of Allergy and Infectious Diseases (NIAID) and the US Centers for Disease Control and Prevention (CDC) have expanded research funding, information sharing, and clinical support to fight emerging and reemerging infectious disease. Focusing on reemerging diseases, the CDC journals *Emerging Infectious Disease* and *Morbidity and Mortality Weekly Report (MMWR)* feature frequent reports of reemergent infections such as coccidioidomycosis, the incidence of which began to dramatically increase as a consequence of the HIV/AIDS pandemic.

Since 1994 epidemiologists have confronted the reemergence of West Nile fever, human monkeypox, dengue, tuberculosis, and malaria, at times in populations for which these diseases had not previously been a problem. Furthermore, certain infections such as *Staphylococcus aureus* and *Mycobacterium tuberculosis* have developed increasing resistance to drug agents that were previously effective treatments.

Malaria

The ancient plague of malaria has experienced a resurgence due to rising rates of resistance to chloroquine and other drugs used to treat it. According to WHO, malaria affected more than 212 million people in 2015 and resulted in the deaths of more than 429,000 people worldwide, the majority occurring among children in sub-Saharan Africa.

Epidemiologists have discovered a connection between resurgent malaria and the HIV/AIDS epidemic. According to a 2006 study sponsored by the Millennium Fund, HIV has major effects on the incidence of malaria. HIV-induced immunodeficiency may decrease the immune response against malarial infection and increase the risk of parasitemia (parasites in the blood). Illness with malaria has been inversely correlated to CD4+ T cell counts, which are adversely affected by AIDS. These findings were confirmed in other studies and countries, including Malawi, Kenya, and Rwanda.

HIV infection in regions where malaria transmission is endemic increases the risk of clinical malaria in adults and malarial fever in children. In regions where malaria transmission is not yet endemic, high HIV prevalence results in much higher rates of malaria morbidity and mortality. Infection with HIV also affects the treatment and prophylaxis of malaria. Antimalarial therapy is most effective in individuals with some previous immunity to malaria, so immunosuppression due to HIV infection can decrease antimalarial treatment response. Malaria is not, however, classified as an opportunistic infection. Rather, HIV infec-

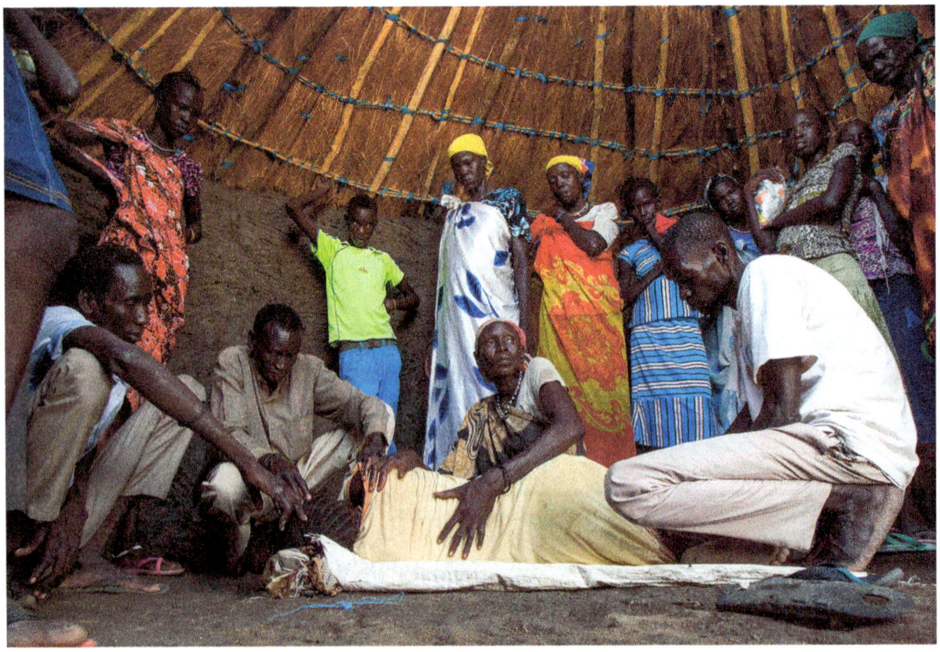

A woman suffers from malaria in South Sudan. Increased rates of malaria in undeveloped parts of the world have been linked to the emergence of HIV/AIDS. © ALBERT GONZALEZ FARRAN/AFP/Getty Images

CLIMATE CHANGE AND MALARIA, A REEMERGING DISEASE

Researchers have shown that climate change will affect the mosquito that harbors *Plasmodia*, the malaria parasite. A 2014 study published in the *Proceedings of the National Academy of Sciences* used numerous mathematical models to show that warming temperatures caused by climate change will enlarge the range of the *Anopheles* mosquito and lengthen the amount of time each year that the disease is transmitted.

According to the modeling, the transmission season will likely be lengthened in Central America, eastern and southern Africa (including Madagascar), eastern Australia, and southern Brazil, along with the border between India and Nepal. Meanwhile, the modeling also suggests that the length of the transmission season will be shortened in other places. Such modeling is helpful because it allows public health authorities, health care workers, and governments to plan for the future. However, predictions made from modeling are far from certain. They are simply educated guesses about the future, made with the information at hand.

Another study published in 2014 in the journal *Science* showed that warm temperatures caused by climate change will push the *Anopheles* mosquitoes to higher elevations (where it has previously been too cold for the mosquito to survive) in countries in Africa and South America that are home to the disease.

tion appears to make people more vulnerable and less resilient to exogenous (external) malaria infection.

Malaria poses formidable scientific and technical hurdles to vaccine development, including issues regarding the appropriateness and accessibility of animal models. Furthermore, the clinical trials themselves are difficult to design because the ultimate measure of efficacy is the interruption of malaria transmission. In spite of these challenges, pharmaceutical companies are engaged in clinical development of a variety of vaccine candidates that show promise. As of 2015 the only approved vaccine was RTS,S. This vaccine required four injections and had a relatively low efficacy rate (26 to 50 percent). Because of this low efficacy, WHO did not recommend its use in babies between 6 and 12 weeks of age.

Tuberculosis

Tuberculosis (TB) is one of the top 10 causes of death worldwide. In 2016 10.4 million people contracted TB, and 1.7 million died from the illness. More than 95 percent of these TB deaths occurred in low- and middle-income nations. In the United States, the CDC reported 9,272 new TB cases (a rate of 2.9 cases per 100,000 people) in 2016, a record low for new case counts in the country. Tuberculosis rates are extremely high among the HIV-infected population.

As of 2018 only one vaccine, Bacillus Calmette-Guérin (BCG), was available for tuberculosis. BCG, which was developed in 1921, offers some protection from TB, but its effectiveness diminishes over time. Human studies of the most advanced new vaccine candidate, a poxvirus-vectored vaccine called modified vaccinia Ankara (MVA) that was developed by the Oxford-Emergent Tuberculosis Consortium, began in South Africa in 2009. Initial results published in 2013 showed little evidence of increased protection in vaccinated infants.

Effective pharmaceutical treatment exists for TB, but the regimen is lengthy, and it is difficult for patients to maintain adherence, which gives rise to multidrug-resistant TB strains. Resistance to rifampicin, an antibiotic used as the first-line drug of choice, is growing. This in turn has added impetus to programs to develop novel vaccines, some of which are now in the preclinical investigation stage. Although TB incidence is falling at about 2 percent per year globally, this number still falls short of WHO's goal of a reduction of 4 to 5 percent to meet the targets of its End TB Strategy.

More than a billion people have dormant tuberculosis infections, however, the disease becomes symptomatic when immune systems are weakened by HIV. TB risk doubles shortly after infection with HIV, and it increases further over time. In the "Growing Burden of Tuberculosis: Global Trends and Interactions with the HIV Epidemic" (2003), Elizabeth L. Corbett and her coauthors estimated that, in 2000, 9 percent of the 8.3 million new adult TB cases worldwide were directly attributable to HIV. Furthermore, a 2018 fact sheet from WHO ranked TB as the leading cause of death among the HIV-positive population, noting that it caused 40 percent of HIV deaths in 2016. HIV infection makes treating active TB much more difficult, leading to an increase in TB rates in areas with a high prevalence of HIV, particularly sub-Saharan Africa. The spread of HIV in sub-Saharan Africa is primarily responsible for driving the number of active TB cases upward by 6 percent each year.

In 2005 a virulent strain of tuberculosis killed all but 1 of 53 infected patients at the Church of Scotland Hospital in South Africa's rural KwaZulu-Natal Province. The strain of TB, named XDR for "extensively drug-resistant," cannot be treated effectively with most tuberculosis drugs and may be incurable. Because XDR TB is resistant to the most effective TB drugs, alternative treatment options are less safe, less effective, and costlier. XDR TB is particularly dangerous for people infected with HIV or for those who have other conditions that impair the immune system.

Since the detection of XDR, additional cases have been found at other South African hospitals. Some epidemiologists and TB experts believe that XDR TB has probably moved beyond the borders of South Africa into Lesotho, Swaziland, Mozambique, and perhaps to Zimbabwe. At least two in three South African TB sufferers are HIV-positive. If XDR TB becomes established in the HIV-positive population, it could devastate tens of millions of HIV-infected people throughout sub-Saharan Africa.

HIV-negative people have a low probability of contracting tuberculosis, even if they are already infected with the TB bacillus. However, because tuberculosis is spread through the air, people in close contact with an active TB victim have some risk of contracting the disease. TB patients who fail to adhere to their physician's prescribed dosing regimens are more likely to develop XDR TB because spotty medication dosing may kill off the more susceptible bacteria while allowing the XDR bacteria to multiply.

It seems likely that all of the 52 people who died in the initial outbreak of XDR TB in the South African hamlet of Tugela Ferry in 2005 and early 2006 had AIDS. Most of the patients died within a few weeks of infection with drug-resistant tuberculosis. According to epidemiologists, this is an unprecedented TB mortality rate.

In 2016 WHO estimated that there were 490,000 new cases of multidrug-resistant TB globally. Many cases of XDR TB go undetected because a number of countries lack the resources to screen for it.

West Nile Virus

West Nile virus (WNV) has been endemic in Africa, West Asia, Europe, and the Middle East for centuries but has only reemerged in the United States since 1999. The first WNV infections occurred in the New York metropolitan area and have continued to spread throughout the United States during the summer season, infecting increasingly larger populations. The inexorable spread of the virus has prompted vaccine and drug therapy development, with some candidates showing prevention or treatment effectiveness in animals. As of 2018 the most immediately promising approach to slowing the spread of WNV was the control of insect vectors. New methods of controlling mosquitoes and countering mosquito resistance to insecticides were under development for use in areas where WNV threatened to become endemic.

Potential Bioterrorism Agents

The use of anthrax in terroristic attacks can be seen as a deliberate effort to promote the reemergence of infectious agents that have otherwise been either eradicated, as in the case of smallpox, or largely controlled, as in the case of anthrax itself. Bioterrorism could also promote the emergence of a pathogen such as the Ebola virus in a setting (the United States, for example) that is radically different and distant from the rural African regions in which such infections have typically occurred. Because a wide variety of pathogens could potentially be used as bioweapons, defensive strategies must rely on research at a broad and basic level, investigating how human immune systems react to them and how infections can be detected, prevented, and treated.

■ Applications and Research

As of 2018, a wide variety of scientific and industrial biodefense research infrastructure projects were under way in the United States. These included the development of regional Centers of Excellence for Biodefense and Emerging Infectious Disease Research, in addition to the building of secure facilities, including two National Biocontainment Laboratories and nine Regional Biocontainment Laboratories.

Research projects included gene sequencing of pathogens considered to be the most potent threats, the screening of chemical compounds that could provide potential treatments, and development of animals to test promising drugs. In addition, immunologists are investigating ways to boost human innate immunity. Innate immunity is the immune system's first line of defense and is represented by monocytes and neutrophils (white blood cells), which react to any and all foreign substances and organisms in the body. This innate immune system is distinct from adaptive immunity, the second line of defense represented by T cells and B cells (lymphocytes), which are influenced by the innate immune system to recognize specific pathogens and foreign organisms and destroy them in a focused attack. Vaccine development is also being fostered under the nation's biodefense program.

Clearly, vaccine development is central to the control of reemerging infections, particularly development of an effective vaccine for HIV, which is key to preventing the spread of tuberculosis and a number of other infections that otherwise would not have been able to regain virulence after decades of effective treatment and prevention. The HIV epidemic, the rapid growth of international travel and commerce, and the danger of the deliberate spread of pathogens into vulnerable new populations due to bioterrorism will continue to foster the reemergence of dangerous pathogens. This threat will pose an ongoing and permanent challenge to public health agencies that must be dealt with by intensified basic biological and clinical research. The best strategy for dealing with the threat of emerging and reemerging infections alike is the funding, implementation, and staffing of an excellent global public health infrastructure, which will require international cooperation on an unprecedented scale.

■ Impacts and Issues

A 2016 report of the CDC's National Center for Emerging and Zoonotic Infectious Diseases described efforts to counter more recent outbreaks of reemerging diseases. These efforts included responding to the Zika outbreak; addressing the threat of carbapenem-resistant *Enterobacteriaceae* infections, dubbed a "nightmare" bacteria by the CDC; and countering resistant bacterial infections including gonorrhea, Salmonella, *Streptococcus pneumoniae*, and *Clostridium difficile*. The agency also listed efforts to control *Candida auris* fungal infections and viral diseases, including Lhasa fever, Rift Valley fever, and Ebola.

Researchers have shown that climate change will likely increase the reemergence of infectious diseases. Although climate change will cause numerous changes to the earth's climate, two changes in particular—namely, increased rainfall and higher temperatures—may allow disease vectors, such as certain species of mosquito, to be more productive in areas where they are already endemic or to increase their range into more temperate areas. In some cases the relationship between climate change and an infectious disease pathogen is not completely understood, beyond the fact that climate change is affecting it in some way. This is the case with cholera, a reemerging bacterial infection that is spread through contaminated water and food.

The human population is becoming increasingly urban. The United Nations (UN) stated that in 2016 more than half of the world's population (54.5 percent) lived in urban areas. This percentage is slated to increase to 60 percent by 2030. Increasing urbanization supports the spread of infectious diseases, including reemerging ones. High-density housing, overcrowding within homes, and poor sanitation systems in poor urban areas that lack resources can also encourage disease transmission.

See Also *Emerging Infectious Diseases; Lyme Disease; Malaria; Pandemic Preparedness; Tuberculosis; War and Infectious Disease; West Nile*

BIBLIOGRAPHY

Books

Heymann, David L., and Vernon J. M. Lee. "Emerging and Re-emerging Infections." In *Oxford Textbook of Global Public Health*, edited by Roger Detels, Martin Gulliford, Quarraisha Abdool Karim, and Chorh Chuan Tan. 6th ed. Oxford, UK: Oxford University Press, 2015.

Rezza, Giovanni, and Giuseppe Ippolito, eds. *Emerging and Re-emerging Viral Infections: Advances in Microbiology, Infectious Diseases and Public Health, Volume 6.* Cham, Switzerland: Springer, 2017.

Periodicals

Caminade, Cyril, et al. "Impact of Climate Change on Global Malaria Distribution." *Proceedings of the National Academy of Sciences* 111, no. 9 (March 2014): 3286–3291. This article can also be found online at http://www.pnas.org/content/111/9/3286 (accessed March 12, 2018).

Corbett, Elizabeth, et al. "The Growing Burden of Tuberculosis: Global Trends and Interactions with the HIV Epidemic." *Archives of Internal Medicine* 163, no. 9 (May 12, 2003): 1009–1021. This article can also be found online at https://www.ncbi.nlm.nih.gov/pubmed/12742798 (accessed March 9, 2018).

Hecht, Robert, et al. "Putting It Together: AIDS and the Millennium Development Goals." *PLOS Medicine* 3, no. 11 (2006): e455. This article can also be found online at http://journals.plos.org/plosmedicine/article?id=10.1371/journal.pmed.0030455 (accessed March 9, 2018).

Kashangura, Rufaro, et al. "Effects of MVA85A Vaccine on Tuberculosis Challenge in Animals: Systematic Review." *International Journal of Epidemiology* 44, no. 6 (December 2015): 1970–1981. This article can also be found online at https://academic.oup.com/ije/article/44/6/1970/2572503 (accessed March 16, 2018).

Kirkland, Theo N., and Joshua Fierer. "Coccidioidomycosis: A Reemerging Infectious Disease." *Emerging Infectious Diseases* 2, no. 3 (July 1996). This article can also be found online at https://wwwnc.cdc.gov/eid/article/2/3/96-0305_article (accessed March 9, 2018).

Short, Erica E., Cyril Caminade, and Bolaji N. Thomas. "Climate Change Contribution to the Emergence or Re-emergence of Parasitic Diseases." *Infectious Diseases: Research and Treatment* 10 (2017): 1–7. This article can also be found online at http://journals.sagepub.com/doi/pdf/10.1177/1178633617732296 (accessed March 12, 2018).

Tong, Michael Xiaoliang, et al. "Infectious Diseases, Urbanization and Climate Change: Challenges in Future China." *International Journal of Environmental Research and Public Health* 12, no. 9 (September 2015): 11025–11036. This article can also be found online at https://www.ncbi.nlm.nih.gov/pmc/articles/PMC4586659/ (accessed March 12, 2018).

Websites

"Drug-Resistant TB: XDR-TB FAQ." World Health Organization. http://www.who.int/tb/areas-of-work/drug-resistant-tb/xdr-tb-faq/en/ (accessed March 7, 2018).

"Malaria Vaccine Development." World Health Organization, May 27, 2016. http://www.who.int/malaria/areas/vaccine/en/ (accessed March 7, 2018).

"National Center for Emerging and Zoonotic Infectious Diseases (NCEZID)." Centers for Disease Control and Prevention, March 8, 2018. https://www.cdc.gov/ncezid/index.html (accessed March 7, 2018).

"Tuberculosis." World Health Organization, January 2018. http://www.who.int/mediacentre/factsheets/fs104/en/ (accessed March 7, 2018).

"Tuberculosis Data and Statistics." Centers for Disease Control and Prevention, February 1, 2018. https://www.cdc.gov/tb/statistics/default.htm (accessed March 7, 2018).

"Warmer Temperatures Push Malaria to Higher Elevations." EurekaAlert!, March 6, 2014. https://www.eurekalert.org/pub_releases/2014-03/uom-wtp030414.php (accessed March 12, 2018).

Kenneth T. LaPensee

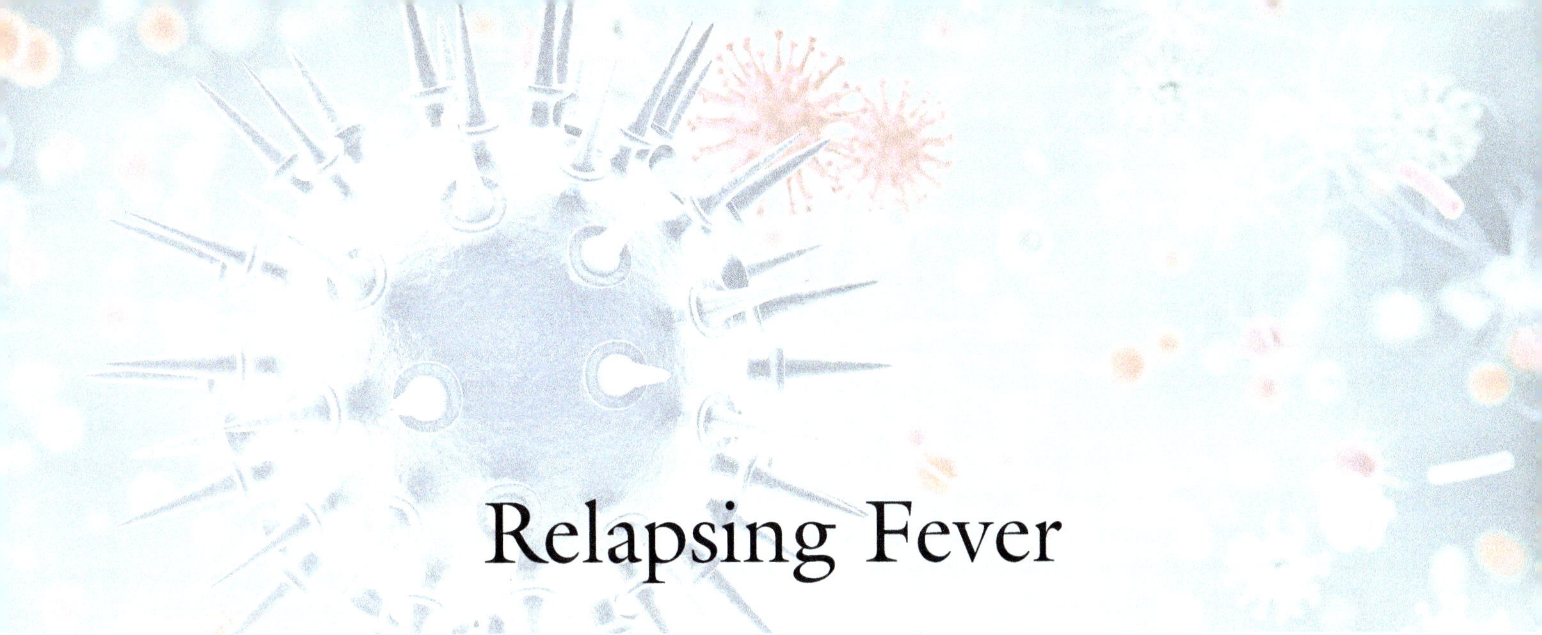

Relapsing Fever

Introduction

Relapsing fever is an acute infectious disease caused by various bacteria within the genus *Borrelia*. The disease is commonly recognized by repetitious bouts of fever. Relapsing fever is a zoonotic disease that is transmitted to humans primarily from parasitic insects called body lice, which enter the body, or from the bites of soft-bodied ticks, which occur on the outside of the body.

Louse-borne relapsing fever (LBRF) is transmitted to humans from lice (specifically, *Pediculus humanus*) that are infected with the bacterium *Borrelia recurrentis*. The lice enter the human body through mucous membranes and then invade the bloodstream. They eventually multiply inside the abdomen of the host.

Tick-borne relapsing fever (TBRF) is transmitted to humans from bites of ticks infected with *Borrelia* bacteria species such as *Borrelia hermsii* and *B. parkeri*. The ticks spread from hosts such as rodents and other animals. *B. hermsii* and *B. recurrentis* cause similar symptoms, but *B. hermsii* causes more relapses and is responsible for more deaths. *B. recurrentis* infection, however, results in longer periods with fever and without fever and with more extended incubation periods.

For both forms of the disease, the first symptoms occur 5 to 15 days after the bite of an infected vector. Symptoms initially include a high and sudden fever followed by chills, shakes, neck stiffness, sweating, low body temperature, low blood pressure, nausea, vomiting, rash, headache, and muscle or joint pain.

When these symptoms become serious, many patients develop central nervous system (CNS) problems such as near-unconsciousness, seizure, facial droop, weakness, and coma. Heart and liver tissues that are invaded by the bacteria often result in hepatitis (inflammation of the liver), meningitis (inflammation of the meninges), or myocarditis (inflammation of the heart muscle). Bleeding and pneumonia are other problems associated with the disease.

Disease History, Characteristics, and Transmission

LBRF was first reported in the United States in 1844. That year there was an outbreak in Philadelphia among recent immigrants from Liverpool, England. The first case of TBRF was reported in the United States in 1905. The patient, who was diagnosed in New York, had recently traveled to Texas. Cases were reported in Colorado in 1915, and in 1939 it was recognized as endemic in the state. During the 1920s and 1930s, cases were recognized in other western states, including California, Montana, Texas, Washington, Arizona, Nevada, Idaho, Kansas, New Mexico, and Utah.

WORDS TO KNOW

HOST An organism that serves as the habitat for a parasite or possibly for a symbiont. A host may provide nutrition to the parasite or symbiont, or it may simply provide a place in which to live.

INCUBATION PERIOD The time between exposure to a disease-causing virus or bacteria and the appearance of symptoms of the infection. Depending on the microorganism, the incubation time can range from a few hours, such as with food poisoning due to *Salmonella*, to a decade or more, such as with acquired immunodeficiency syndrome (AIDS).

VECTOR Any agent that carries and transmits parasites and diseases. Also, an organism or a chemical used to transport a gene into a new host cell.

ZOONOTIC A disease that can be transmitted between animals and humans. Examples of zoonotic diseases are anthrax, plague, and Q fever.

In LBRF the first round of symptoms lasts from three to six days and is followed by other milder rounds of symptoms, with each episode lasting up to three days. Fever may be absent for up to two weeks before another round occurs. Generally, the patient has symptoms when the organism is within the host's blood, then the symptoms disappear when the organism leaves the blood.

The effects of LBRF become critical to the patient when the following occur: severe jaundice (yellowing of the skin and mucous membranes due to impaired liver function), changes in mental status, bleeding, and prolonged QT interval (the measure between the beginning of the Q wave and the end of the T wave on an electrocardiogram). According to the European Centre for Disease Prevention and Control (ECDC), LBRF has a mortality rate of between 2 and 5 percent with treatment and between 10 and 40 percent without treatment.

Scope and Distribution

LBRF occurs primarily in Ethiopia and Sudan in northern Africa. It is also found in Europe and India. The disease is often the cause of epidemics within areas of poor living conditions and regions where famine and war are prevalent. During World War I (1914–1918) and World War II (1939–1945), millions of people died from LBRF. In 2015 LBRF cases began to appear in refugee populations in Europe. Between July and October 2015, 27 cases were reported in Italy, Germany, and the Netherlands. The refugees were believed to have contracted the disease during their voyage from northeastern Africa. LBRF is occasionally seen in the United States in patients who have traveled outside of the country. The last US outbreak of the disease occurred in New York in 1871.

TBRF is found in Africa, Asia, Saudi Arabia, South America, Spain, and certain areas in the western regions of the United States and Canada. In the United States it usually occurs west of the Mississippi River, predominantely in the mountains of the West and the high-elevation deserts and plains of the Southwest. Between 1990 and 2011, 504 cases of TBRF were reported in 12 US states.

Treatment and Prevention

According to the CDC, treatment of TBRF usually involves a one-week course of antibiotics. When treated properly, most people recover, and death only rarely occurs. Tetracycline is often the antibiotic of choice and is generally taken orally every six hours for ten days. Many people with relapsing fever have negative reactions to tetracycline, including anxiety, fever, sweating, rapid heart rate, and low blood pressure. Erythromycin is generally the second choice for those patients. Chloramphenicol, doxycycline, and penicillin are also used to treat the disease.

The duration for antibiotic treatment of LBRF, according to the CDC's Division of Vector-Borne Infectious

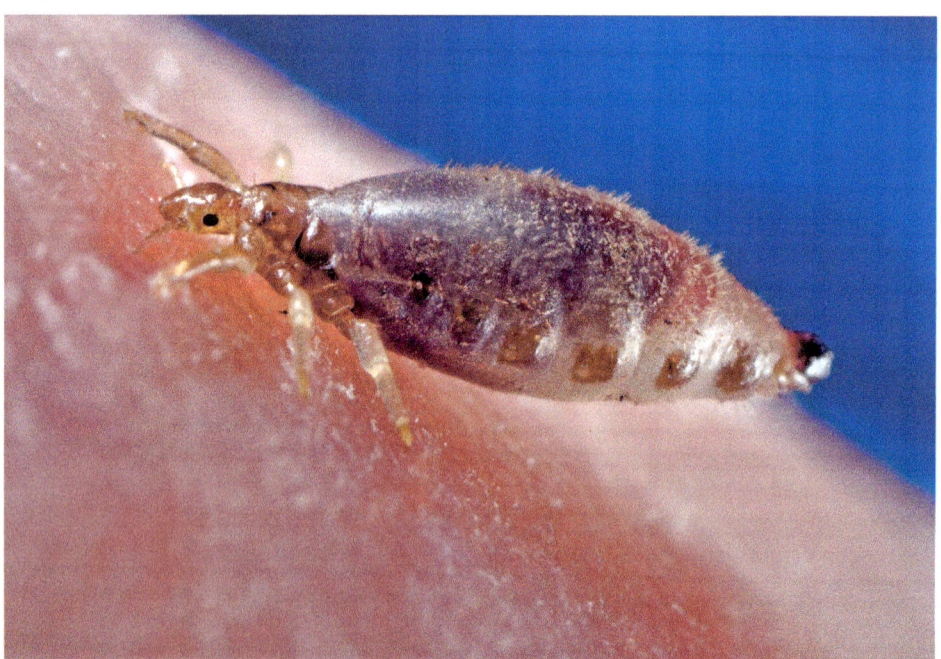

Lice are the primary transmitters of relapsing fever, an acute infectious disease that is commonly recognized by repetitious bouts of fever. The louse-borne relapsing fever (LBRF) is transmitted when lice enter the human body through mucous membranes and then invade the bloodstream. *© BSIP/UIG/ Getty Images*

Diseases, is a single dose of antibiotics, usually tetracycline or doxycycline. Erythromycin may also be used. Both forms of relapsing fever can be prevented by wearing protective clothing and using insect repellent. Comprehensive lice and tick control should be used in areas hardest hit with the infections.

Impacts and Issues

Relapsing fever was once a global concern. However, with antibiotic treatment, it is now restricted mostly to areas of the developing world. Circumstances such as increased worldwide travel by humans, wide-ranging movement of animals, and even the trend toward washing clothes in cold or warm water rather than hot water are causing a reemergence of relapsing fever. According to the CDC, since the 1980s there has been an increase in the number of *Borrelia* species associated with relapsing fever.

Most cases of TBRF have occurred in mountainous areas of the western United States, primarily among vacationers to forests or cabins in elevations above 8,000 feet (2,438 meters). Campers and other persons rarely realize that they are bitten by the soft ticks that carry TBRF, as the ticks feed for a few minutes and then fall off. When experiencing a fever after vacationing in the mountains, therefore, it is advisable to seek medical treatment. TBRF remains on the list of diseases requiring reporting to health officials in many western states to track the prevalence of the disease and the ticks that cause it.

All of these situations demonstrate that the potential for relapsing fever, as with other reemerging infectious diseases, is unpredictable. The potential for it to emerge in areas not recognized before is high. People who are very young, old, pregnant, or in weakened physical condition are at increased risk of the effects and complications of relapsing fever.

PRIMARY SOURCE

"Letter: Louseborne Relapsing Fever in Young Migrants, Sicily, Italy, July–September 2015."

SOURCE: *Ciero, Alessandra, et al. "Letter: Louseborne Relapsing Fever in Young Migrants, Sicily, Italy, July–September 2015."* Emerging Infectious Diseases *22, no. 1 (January 2016): 152–153. This article can also be found online at https://wwwnc.cdc.gov/eid/article/22/1/15-1580_article (accessed December 18, 2015).*

INTRODUCTION: *In the following letter to the editor of the scientific journal* Emerging Infectious Diseases, *a group of scholars reflect on the increase in louse-borne relapsing fever among migrants entering Italy in 2015.*

To the Editor: During the early 20th century, at the end of World War I, and during World War II, louse-borne relapsing fever (LBRF) caused by *Borrelia recurrentis* was a major public health problem, especially in eastern Europe and northern Africa. Currently, poor living conditions, famine, war, and refugee camps are major risk factors for epidemics of LBRF in resource-poor countries, such as those in the Horn of Africa.

Increased migration from resource-poor countries and war/violence create new routes for spread of vectorborne diseases. Recently, several cases of LBRF have been reported among asylum seekers from Eritrea in the Netherlands, Switzerland, and Germany. All of these asylum seekers had been in refugee camps in Libya or Italy. We report 3 cases of LBRF in migrants from Somalia to refugee camps in Sicily, Italy.

Patient 1 was a 13-old-boy from Somalia who arrived in Palermo, Italy, on July 11, 2015, after traveling though Libya. He was admitted to G. Di Cristina Hospital in Palermo 5 days after arrival because of high fever, headache, and general malaise, which developed 2 days after arrival. The patient had skin lesions on his fingers and legs and a conjunctival infection. He had thrombocytopenia (79,000 platelets/μL [reference range 150 platelets/μL−400 platelets/μL]), creatine phosphokinase level 967 mg/L [reference range 0.001 mg/L–0.10 mg/L], aspartate aminotransferase level 30 U/L (reference value 37 U/L), and alanine aminotransferase level 21 U/L (reference value 41 U/L). He was given ceftriaxone (2 g/d) and intravenous hydration. His conditions worsened ≈10 hours after treatment: high fever (temperature 40°C), chills, and profuse sweating (Jarish-Herxheimer reaction). The patient recovered after 15 days of treatment with ceftriaxone. A Giemsa-stained blood smear was negative for *Plasmodium* spp. but showed large numbers of spirochetes. Serologic screening results for *B. burgdorferi* were negative.

Patient 2 was a 17-old-boy from Somalia who arrived in Lampedusa, Italy, on August 27, 2015, after traveling through Libya. Fever and artromyalgia developed 6 days after his arrival, and he was admitted to Hospital Paolo Giaccone in Palermo. Blood analyses showed increased levels of aminotransferases, thrombocytopenia (69,000 platelets/μL), and mild anemia (hemoglobin level 94 g/L [reference range 130 g/L–160 g/L]). A blood smear was negative for *Plasmodium* spp. but positive for spirochetes. Serologic screening results were negative for malaria, leptospirosis, infection with *Rickettsia conorii*, and dengue. An ELISA result was positive for *B. burgdorferi*, and a Western blot result was positive for *Borrelia* spp. proteins p10, p41, and OspC. The patient recovered after treatment with doxycycline (100 mg/d) and ceftriaxone (2 g/d) for 10 days.

Patient 3 was a 17-year-old boy from Somalia who arrived in Trapani, Italy, on September 4, 2015. He reported that he stayed for 5 months in Libya before arriving in Italy. Fever, artromyalgia, severe dehydration, renal failure, and mental confusion developed 3 days after his arrival, and he was admitted to Hospital Paolo Giaccone. He had severe thrombocytopenia (4,000 platelets/μL); mild anemia (hemoglobin level 88 g/L); increased levels of aminotransferases (aspartate aminotransferase 282 U/L, alanine aminotransferase 489 U/L), lactate dehydrogenase (1,041 U/L [reference range 105 U/L−333 U/L]), d-dimer (6,311 ng/mL [reference range 10 ng/mL–250 ng/mL]), C-reactive protein (237.8 mg/dL [reference range 0 mg/dL–10 mg/dL]), and creatinine (2.6 mg/dL [reference range 0.6 mg/dL–1.2 mg/dL]); and azotemia (blood urea nitrogen level 150 mg/dL [reference range 7 mg/dL–20 mg/dL]). A blood smear was negative for *Plasmodium* spp., but a Giemsa-stained thick blood smear was positive for spirochetes. Serologic screening results were negative for malaria, leptospirosis, infection with *B. burgdorferi*, and dengue. The patient recovered after treatment with doxycycline (100 mg/d) and ceftriaxone (2 g/d) for 10 days.

DNA was extracted from blood specimens from the 3 patients and used for molecular identification and characterization of the etiologic agent of LBRF. We used a species-specific real-time PCR for *B. recurrentis* and *B. duttonii*, which targeted an internal region of the *recN* gene. Multispacer sequence typing of the 16S rRNA gene was used for bacterial identification and genotyping. All blood samples were positive for *B. recurrentis* by real-time PCR. Multispacer sequences showed 100% identity with sequences of *B. recurrentis* reference strain A1 (GenBank accession no. CP000993) for isolates from all patients.

We report 3 patients in Italy with LBRF who migrated from Somalia. These patients arrived in Italy after traveling in several countries in Africa and crossing the Mediterranean Sea. The patients did not associate with each other during travel, and the place where they were infected is unknown. However, because they came from a disease-endemic country, they probably had been infested with body lice and were infected with *B. recurrentis* in Somalia or other neighboring countries.

Because the 3 cases we observed might indicate that more migrants and refugees are infected, LBRF should be considered an emerging disease among migrants and refugees. Diagnostic suspicion of LBRF should lead to early diagnosis among refugees from the Horn of Africa and in persons in migrant camps. Furthermore, improved public health measures and hygiene must be implemented for persons in refugee or migrant camps.

See Also *African Sleeping Sickness (Trypanosomiasis); Bacterial Disease; Emerging Infectious Diseases; Travel and Infectious Disease*

BIBLIOGRAPHY

Books

Bennett, John E., Raphael Dolin, and Martin J. Blaser, eds. *Principles and Practice of Infectious Diseases.* 8th ed. Philadelphia: Elsevier Saunders, 2015.

Salman, Mowafak Dauod, Jordi Tarrés-Call, and Agustín Estrada-Peña, eds. *Ticks and Tick-Borne Diseases: Geographical Distribution and Control Strategies in the Euro-Asia Region.* Boston: CAB International, 2013.

Schwartz, Eli, ed. *Tropical Diseases in Travelers.* Hoboken, NJ: Wiley-Blackwell, 2009.

Periodicals

Dworkin, Mark S., et al. "Tick-Borne Relapsing Fever." *Infectious Disease Clinics of North America* 22, no. 3 (September 2008): 449–468.

Kuchinsky, Sarah Catherine, et al. "Assessing the Infection Rates and Pathogenesis of *Borrelia burgdorferi* in Wild Rodents and Ticks in Western Maryland." *Journal of Immunology* 198, no. 1 (May 1, 2017): S7–S13.

Websites

"Facts about Louse-Borne Relapsing Fever." European Centre for Disease Prevention and Control. https://ecdc.europa.eu/en/louse-borne-relapsing-fever/facts (accessed November 16, 2017).

"Tick-Borne Relapsing Fever (TBRF)." Centers for Disease Control and Prevention, October 15, 2015. https://www.cdc.gov/relapsing-fever/index.html (accessed November 15, 2017).

Resistant Organisms

Introduction

Resistant organisms are microbes (bacteria, fungi, viruses, or parasites) that have evolved immunity to one or more of the drugs used to kill them (drugs known as antimicrobials). While some organisms are resistant to only one kind of drug, multidrug-resistant (MDR) organisms are resistant to more than one kind of drug, making them even more difficult to treat. Resistance threatens human health because it reduces or eliminates the efficacy of drugs used to treat infections. If organisms evolve resistance to drugs more quickly than new drugs can be discovered, doctors' choices for treating infections by those organisms dwindle. This has happened for many real-world bacteria, viruses, fungi, and parasites.

Resistance to a drug is more likely to evolve when the drug is widely used. Antibiotic resistance, in particular, has arisen in part because of chronic overuse of antibiotics in medical and agricultural settings. Antibiotics are often prescribed for viral, not bacterial, infections (antibiotics have no effect on viruses), and millions of pounds of antibiotics are given to livestock each year. As of 2017 an estimated 700,000 people died each year as a result of antibiotic resistance, a number that is expected to increase dramatically over the next several decades because of a decline in research, the development of new antibiotics, and growing microbial resistance to existing antibiotic medications. Most experts agree that, in the 21st century, antimicrobial resistance and MDRs, in particular, represent a major public-health crisis.

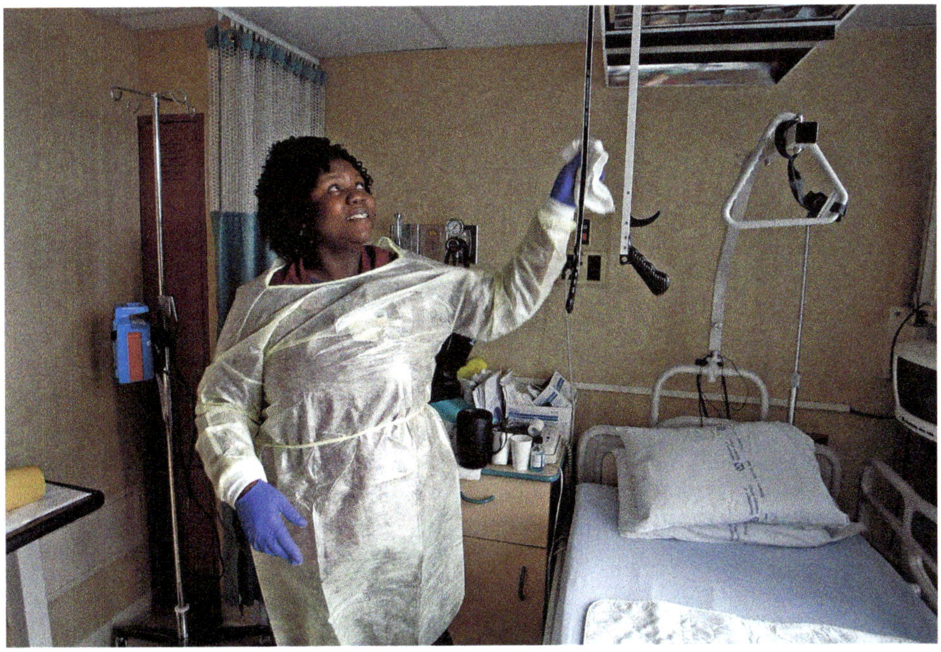

Many hospitals have implemented strict policies designed to stop *Staphylococcus aureus* (or staph) infections, as this bacteria is resistant to nearly all antibiotics. *© Joe Raedle/Getty Images*

WORDS TO KNOW

ANTIBACTERIAL A substance that reduces or kill germs (bacteria and other microorganisms but not including viruses). Also often a term used to describe a drug used to treat bacterial infections.

ANTIBIOTIC A drug, such as penicillin, used to fight infections caused by bacteria. Antibiotics act only on bacteria and are not effective against viruses.

ANTIFUNGAL Also called antifungal drugs, are medicines that are used to fight fungal infections. They are of two kinds, systemic and topical. Systemic antifungal drugs are medicines taken by mouth or by injection to treat infections caused by a fungus. Topical antifungal drugs are medicines applied to the skin to treat skin infections caused by a fungus.

ANTIMICROBIAL Slows the growth of bacteria or is able to kill bacteria. Antimicrobial materials include antibiotics (which can be used inside the body) and disinfectants (which can only be used outside the body).

BACTERIA Single-celled microorganisms that live in soil, water, plants, and animals that play a key role in the decay of organic matter and the cycling of nutrients. Some bacteria are agents of disease. Microscopic organisms whose activities range from the development of disease to fermentation. Bacteria range in shape from spherical to rod-shaped to spiral. Different types of bacteria cause many sexually transmitted diseases, including syphilis, gonorrhea, and chlamydia. Bacteria also cause diseases ranging from typhoid to dysentery to tetanus. Bacterium is the singular form of bacteria.

COHORTING The practice of grouping people with similar infections or symptoms together to reduce transmission to others.

DRUG RESISTANCE Develops when an infective agent such as a bacterium, fungus, or virus develops a lack of sensitivity to a drug that would normally be able to control or even kill them. This tends to occur with overuse of anti-infectives, which selects out populations of microbes most able to resist them, while killing off those organisms that are most sensitive. The next time the anti-infective agent is used, it will be less effective, leading to the eventual development of resistance.

MICROORGANISM With only a single currently known exception (i.e., *Epulopiscium fishelsonia*, a bacterium that is billions of times larger than the bacteria in the human intestine and is large enough to view without a microscope), microorganisms are minute organisms that require microscopic magnification to view. To be seen, they must be magnified by an optical or electron microscope. The most common types of microorganisms are viruses, bacteria, blue-green bacteria, some algae, some fungi, yeasts, and protozoans.

PATHOGEN A disease-causing agent, such as a bacterium, a virus, a fungus, or another microorganism.

VIRUS Essentially nonliving repositories of nucleic acid that require the presence of a living prokaryotic or eukaryotic cell for the replication of the nucleic acid. There are a number of different viruses that challenge the human immune system and that may produce disease in humans. In common, a virus is a small, infectious agent that consists of a core of genetic material (either deoxyribonucleic acid (DNA) or ribonucleic acid (RNA) surrounded by a shell of protein. Very simple microorganisms, viruses are much smaller than bacteria that enter and multiples within cells. Viruses often exchange or transfer their genetic material (DNA or RNA) to cells and can cause diseases such as chickenpox, hepatitis, measles, and mumps.

■ Disease History, Characteristics, and Transmission

History

Resistant organisms arose in the mid-20th century, as antimicrobials potent enough to force the evolution of resistance were first developed. After penicillin, one of the first widely used antibiotics, was discovered in 1928, it gradually entered into wide use. As it did so, penicillin-resistant *Escherichia coli* bacteria emerged and were first observed in 1940. Penicillin-resistant *Staphylococcus* bacteria were reported as early as 1942, and by the 1950s a penicillin-resistant strain of *Staphylococcus aureus* became a worldwide problem in hospitals. By the 1960s most *Staphylococci* were resistant to penicillin.

Another example of resistance development is the malaria parasite and the antimalarial drug chloroquine. Chloroquine was introduced in the 1940s. Ten years later resistance to chloroquine evolved independently in Asia and South America but remained rare. After another 20 years, resistance appeared in East Africa and spread rapidly thereafter. In the 21st century, chloroquine-resistant malaria is found in several regions across the globe. According to the World Health Organization (WHO), despite a 29 percent reduction in the malaria mortality rate since 2010, there were still approximately 212 million malaria cases and an estimated 429,000 malaria deaths worldwide in 2015. WHO noted that "resistance to antimalarial medicines is a threat to global efforts to control and eliminate malaria."

While these two examples of organisms developing drug resistance are illustrative, they are not unique. All bacteria "will inevitably find ways of resisting the antibiotics developed by humans," according to the US Centers for Disease Control (CDC), and no special circumstances are required for this resistance to emerge beyond the use of drugs designed to kill them. As antibiotics and other antimicrobial drug therapies have become increasingly common, organisms have developed greater resistance to them. According to Hiroshi Nikaido in a 2009 article for *Annual Review of Biochemistry*, "antibiotics are manufactured at an estimated scale of about 100,000 tons annually worldwide, and their use had a profound impact on the life of bacteria on earth. More strains of pathogens have become antibiotic resistant, and some have become resistant to many antibiotics and chemotherapeutic agents."

Characteristics

In any wild population of microorganisms, whether bacteria or viruses, there will be small, random, heritable (genetic) differences between individuals. The protein recipe for a microorganism is not rigid and exact; its many proteins can take on slightly different forms without compromising its ability to survive. When a population of microorganisms is exposed to a drug designed to destroy it, the genetic differences between individuals sometimes allow microorganisms to survive. Thus, the entire next generation of microorganisms will tend to be more resistant to that drug. If this evolutionary process of variation and selection is repeated, resistance can evolve.

There is much variation in the traits such resistant organisms possess that allow them to combat the drugs designed to kill them. Any mutation that interferes with the harmful action of the drug on the organism will confer resistance. The features that make an organism resistant to a drug vary widely because the precise ways in which antimicrobials attack organisms vary widely. For example, some bacteria have become resistant to the antibiotic penicillin by evolving the ability to produce beta-lactamases, which are enzymes (a type of protein) that deactivate the antibiotic. In other cases, microorganisms use several methods of antibiotic resistance: learning how to keep drugs from passing into the cell or accumulating there, altering surface molecules that antimicrobial drugs bind to, or evolving alternatives to series of chemical reactions in the cell (metabolic pathways) that are blocked by antimicrobials.

While such drug-resistant bacteria may initially be rare, the use of antibiotics kills off nonresistant organisms, creating an opportunity for the resilient bacteria to multiply and thrive. As a result, when antibiotics are used, they inherently create the opportunity for resistant organisms to emerge and reproduce. In addition, drug-resistant bacteria can transfer their resistant features to other bacteria via transformation, transduction, and conjugation (three mechanisms by which organisms are able to exchange genetic material).

In general, the more often a drug is used, the more quickly resistance can evolve. However, resistance can also advance when insufficient quantities of a drug are used and some microorganisms survive. The fewer survivors there are, the more resistant they may be. Therefore, dosing to the threshold of elimination can be worse than drastically underdosing. Resistance may still evolve even if drugs are dosed appropriately. This has been the case with antivirals, antifungals, and antiparasitics. However, needless or inadequate use of antimicrobials encourages more rapid evolution of resistance.

Since the late 1980s, pathogens resistant to more than one drug—which are even more difficult to treat than organisms with single-drug resistance—have emerged at an accelerating pace. These MDR organisms are considered among the most prominent threats to global public health in the early 21st century, as it can be extremely difficult to identify treatment for infections with such pathogens. In some cases, organisms are resistant to all existing treatments, making them essentially impossible to treat. Perhaps the most prominent example of such a pan-resistant or pan-drug-resistant (PDR) organism is methicillin-resistant *Staphylococcus aureus* (MRSA), a potentially life-threatening infection.

Resistant organisms develop not only in humans but also in animals, which are often treated with antibiotics when being raised as livestock.

Transmission

Transmission of resistant organisms occurs by the same mechanisms as for their nonresistant relatives but is more likely to occur in certain settings. For example, infection by MRSA happens more commonly in hospital intensive care units and long-term care facilities. MRSA has also been detected on pets, having probably been transmitted to them by humans, and may be transmitted back to humans from these animals. It has not been detected in food animals. However, certain strains of resistant bacteria do move from animals to humans, either via meat that is not treated properly, contaminated water, or fecal matter used as fertilizer to grow crops.

■ Scope and Distribution

Resistant organisms are most common in settings where antimicrobial drugs are most widely used. They are

REAL-WORLD RISKS

Acquired adaptation of bacteria to many antibiotics has become a problem since the early 1990s. For example, many hospitals now must cope with the presence of methicillin-resistant *Staphylococcus aureus* (MRSA), which displays resistance to almost all currently used antibiotics. Dealing with infections caused by MRSA and other resistant organisms requires increased hospital staff hours and increased supplies and can restrict the availability of hospital beds when cohorting or isolation is necessary.

The few antibiotics to which antibiotic-resistant bacteria do respond tend to be expensive, with few options for delivery. For example, the drug meropenem is sometimes prescribed for people with pneumonia, meningitis, or serious skin infections that are caused by organisms that are resistant to common antibiotics. Meropenem can be delivered by intravenous injection or infusion only and is two to three times more expensive than the commonly prescribed antibiotics for these conditions.

Additionally, disease-causing organisms can sometimes adapt so that they are able to grow and multiply on solid surfaces, creating a biofilm. A biofilm environment induces many changes in growing bacteria, some of which involve the expression of previously unexpressed genes and deactivation of actively expressing genes. The structure of the biofilm and these genetic changes often make the bacteria extraordinarily resistant to many antibiotics. Biofilms sometimes occur on hospital surfaces and in implanted devices such as artificial joints and long-term intravenous access catheters.

therefore most often encountered in industrialized countries. In the United States, for example, about one-third of all *S. aureus* infections are now methicillin-resistant. Certain organisms that are found and treated almost exclusively in developing countries, such as the malaria parasite, have evolved resistant varieties in those regions.

Treatment and Prevention

When doctors find that they are trying to treat an infection by a resistant organism, they use trial and error to find a drug to which the organism is not resistant. This process usually involves trying one drug after another, starting with those that are least toxic for the patient and most specific for the target organism and working toward drugs that are less desirable or potentially produce greater side effects. Even when a drug that works is found—and some organisms are now resistant to all the agents used against them—the delay involved in this process is dangerous to the patient.

While there is no way to prevent the emergence of resistant organisms, their spread can be slowed by the cautious and prudent use of antibiotics and other drugs. According to the CDC in 2017, antibiotics are improperly prescribed up to 50 percent of the time, with physicians recommending the wrong dose, the incorrect duration of use, or the wrong drug altogether. In addition, many observers have argued that farmers overuse antibiotics. Using antibiotics and other drugs in proper doses, only when necessary, and in minimal doses would help limit the emergence of resistant organisms and reduce infections with such organisms.

Impacts and Issues

Antimicrobial resistance has become a major public health concern in the 21st century. According to the US National Institute of Allergies and Infectious Diseases (NIAID), tuberculosis, gonorrhea, malaria, and childhood ear infections have all been more difficult to treat than they were just a few decades prior, in the late 20th century, because of antimicrobial resistance. Chloroquine resistance evolved by the malaria parasite has threatened millions of lives: since 1978, chloroquine resistance has been reported in all tropical African countries. The impact on public health has been major, with malaria deaths doubling or tripling in some African countries. In Senegal child deaths from malaria have increased by up to a factor of six with the growth of chloroquine resistance. The increased use of artemisinin-based combination therapies (ACTs) in the early 20th century provided a promising alternative for treating drug-resistant malaria. However, emerging artemisinin resistance has itself become a major concern, according to WHO in 2016.

Concerns about the decreasing efficacy of antibiotics led WHO to release the 2014 report "Antimicrobial Resistance: Global Report on Surveillance," which included alarming warnings about what resistant organisms might mean for global disease-control efforts. According to the report, increasing antimicrobial resistance

> means that standard treatments no longer work; infections are harder or impossible to control; the risk of the spread of infection to others is increased; illness and hospital stays are prolonged, with added economic and social costs; and the risk of death is greater—in some cases, twice that of patients who have infections caused by non-resistant bacteria. The problem is so serious that it threatens the achievements of modern medicine. A post-antibiotic era—in which common infections and minor injuries can kill—is a very real possibility for the 21st century.

In 2017 WHO released a list of 12 families of bacteria that pose the greatest risk to human health because of their drug resistance, which include *Acinetobacter*, *Pseudomonas*, and various *Enterobacteriaceae*.

The CDC has stated that antibiotic resistance is a key microbial threat to health in the United States. In 1995 the CDC launched its National Campaign for Appropriate Antibiotic Use in the Community, which was renamed Get Smart: Know When Antibiotics Work in 2003, and Be Antibiotics Aware in 2017. This campaign seeks to slow the evolution of antibiotic resistance primarily by discouraging the unnecessary use of antibiotics for upper respiratory infections. The CDC estimated in 2017 that, while physicians incorrectly prescribed antibiotics for all conditions 30 percent of the time, that number jumped to 50 percent in the treatment of acute respiratory infections such as ear infections, sinus infections, common colds, and pneumonia (most of which are viral and therefore unaffected by antibiotics). To press for reform, the CDC has developed the Antibiotic Resistance (AR) Solutions Initiative, which "supports national infrastructure to detect, respond, contain, and prevent resistant infections across healthcare settings, food, and communities."

Many observers note that the threat from resistant organisms could be most effectively combated through the development of new drugs against which organisms have not yet developed resistance. However, the pace at which pharmaceutical companies develop new antibiotics has slowed due to the difficulty of profiting from these drugs, which would appeal only to a relatively small market of patients infected with resistant organisms. This has led to public initiatives designed to promote antibiotic development, such as the 2016 US 21st Century Cures Act, which eases the approval process for drugs that combat potentially fatal infections, and CARB-X (Combating Antibiotic Resistant Bacteria Biopharmaceutical Accelerator), which provides funding for the clinical development of antibacterial products.

One of the most contentious aspects of antimicrobial resistance today is the use of antibiotics in agriculture. Millions of pounds of antibiotics are fed to livestock annually in the United States and elsewhere, mostly as growth promoters. Studies over the last several decades have shown that this promotes the evolution of resistant organisms. In 2005 the US Food and Drug Administration (FDA) banned the use of enrofloxacin (an antibacterial) in poultry. The European Union (EU) has banned the use of a range of almost all growth-promoting hormones and antimicrobials in agriculture. Despite such concerns, some doubt the connection between antibiotics used in agriculture and the growth of resistant organisms that can affect humans. As the authors of the 2015 article "Antibiotics in Agriculture and the Risk to Human Health: How Worried Should We Be?" noted, "The use of antibiotics in agriculture is routinely described as a major contributor to the clinical problem of resistant disease in human medicine. While a link is plausible, there are no data conclusively showing the magnitude of the threat emerging from agriculture."

Some experts warn that the nearly universal use of antimicrobial household soaps may contribute to the evolution of resistant organisms. Ordinary soap and water wash bacteria away rather than killing them directly and so do not provide selective pressure for evolution of resistance. Moreover, studies in India have found that antimicrobial soaps do not improve health any more than ordinary soaps.

Phage therapy, the use of certain viruses to infect and kill bacteria, shows some promise as an alternative strategy for treating infections by multiply resistant organisms, and research continues in this area.

SEE ALSO *Antibiotic Resistance; Antimicrobial Soaps; Antiviral Drugs; Nosocomial (Healthcare-Associated) Infections; Vancomycin-resistant Enterococci*

BIBLIOGRAPHY

Books

Salyers, Abigail A., and Dixie D. Whitt. *Revenge of the Microbes: How Bacterial Resistance Is Undermining the Antibiotic Miracle.* Washington, DC: ASM, 2005.

Periodicals

Chang, Quizhi, et al. "Antibiotics in Agriculture and the Risk to Human Health: How Worried Should We Be?" *Evolutionary Applications* 8, no. 3 (2015): 240–247. This article can also be found online at https://www.ncbi.nlm.nih.gov/pmc/articles/PMC4380918/ (accessed February 26, 2018).

Cunha, Burke A. "Effective Antibiotic-Resistance Control Strategies." *Lancet* 357 (2001): 1307–1308.

Lipsitch, Marc, and Matthew H. Samore. "Antimicrobial Use and Antimicrobial Resistance: A Population Perspective." *Emerging Infectious Diseases* 8 (2002): 347–354. This article can also be found online at https://www.ncbi.nlm.nih.gov/pmc/articles/PMC2730242/ (accessed February 26, 2018).

Nikaido, Hiroshi. "Multidrug Resistance in Bacteria." *Annual Review of Biochemistry* 78 (2009): 119–146. This article can also be found online at https://www.ncbi.nlm.nih.gov/pmc/articles/PMC2839888/ (accessed February 26, 2018).

Shea, Katherine M. "Antibiotic Resistance: What Is the Impact of Agricultural Uses of Antibiotics on Children's Health?" *Pediatrics* 112 (2003): 253–258. This article can also be found online at http://pediatrics.aappublications.org/content/112/Supplement_1/253 (accessed February 26, 2018).

Simmons, Bryan P., and Elaine L. Larson. "Multiple Drug Resistant Organisms in Healthcare: The Failure of Contact Precautions." *Journal of Infection Prevention* 16, no. 4: 178–181. This article can also be found online at https://www.ncbi.nlm.nih.gov/pmc/articles/PMC5074191/ (accessed February 26, 2018).

Smith, David L., et al. "Agricultural Antibiotics and Human Health" *PloS Medicine* 2 (2005): 731–735. This article can also be found online at http://journals.plos.org/plosmedicine/article?id=10.1371/journal.pmed.0020232 (accessed February 26, 2018).

Van Duin, David, and David Paterson. "Multidrug Resistant Bacteria in the Community: Trends and Lessons Learned." *Infectious Disease Clinics of North America* 30, no. 2 (2016): 377–390. This article can also be found online at https://www.ncbi.nlm.nih.gov/pmc/articles/PMC5314345/ (accessed February 26, 2018).

Willyard, Cassandra. "The Drug-Resistant Bacteria That Pose the Greatest Health Threats." *Nature* (February 28, 2017). This article can also be found online at https://www.nature.com/news/the-drug-resistant-bacteria-that-pose-the-greatest-health-threats-1.21550 (accessed February 26, 2018).

Websites

"About Antibiotic Resistance." Centers for Disease Control and Prevention, September 19, 2017. https://www.cdc.gov/drugresistance/about.html (accessed February 26, 2018).

"Antibiotic Use in the United States, 2017: Progress and Opportunities." Centers for Disease Control and Prevention, October 6, 2017. https://www.cdc.gov/antibiotic-use/stewardship-report/outpatient.html (accessed March 14, 2018).

"Antimicrobial Resistance." World Health Organization, January 2018. http://www.who.int/mediacentre/factsheets/fs194/en/ (accessed February 26, 2018).

"Antimicrobial Resistance: Global Report on Surveillance: 2014 Summary." World Health Organization, 2014. http://apps.who.int/iris/bitstream/10665/112647/1/WHO_HSE_PED_AIP_2014.2_eng.pdf?ua=1 (accessed February 26, 2018).

"A Public Health Action Plan to Combat Antibiotic Resistance." Centers for Disease Control and Prevention, February 9, 2005. http://www.cdc.gov/drugresistance/actionplan/aractionplan.pdf (accessed February 26, 2007).

"10 Facts on Malaria." World Health Organization, December 2016. http://www.who.int/features/factfiles/malaria/en/ (accessed March 14, 2018).

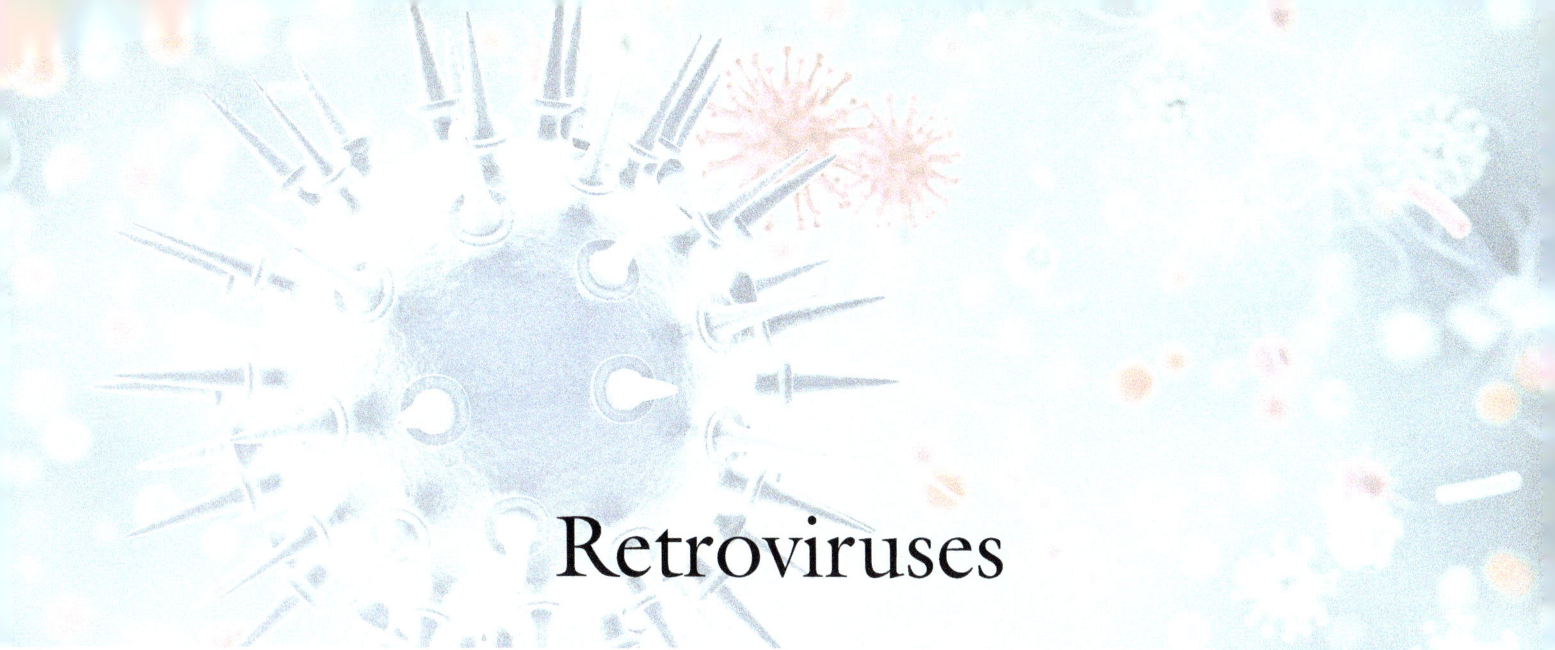

Retroviruses

Introduction

Retroviruses are viruses that contain ribonucleic acid (RNA) as their genetic material. This contrasts with most other microorganisms, which instead contain deoxyribonucleic acid (DNA). Like other viruses, retroviruses create new copies of themselves by infecting a host cell and using the host's genetic replication machinery. To accomplish this, early in the infection process of retroviruses, an enzyme called reverse transcriptase is produced. The enzyme can transform the viral RNA into DNA, which is then inserted into the host DNA. The inserted viral DNA can be replicated along with the host DNA during growth and division of the host cell, and the manufactured viral components assemble to form new copies of the virus.

Retroviruses cause a number of serious infections in humans and other creatures. The most infamous is acquired immunodeficiency syndrome (AIDS), which is considered by most scientists to be caused by several versions of the retrovirus human immunodeficiency virus (HIV). Other retroviruses known as oncogenic viruses can stimulate abnormal cell growth.

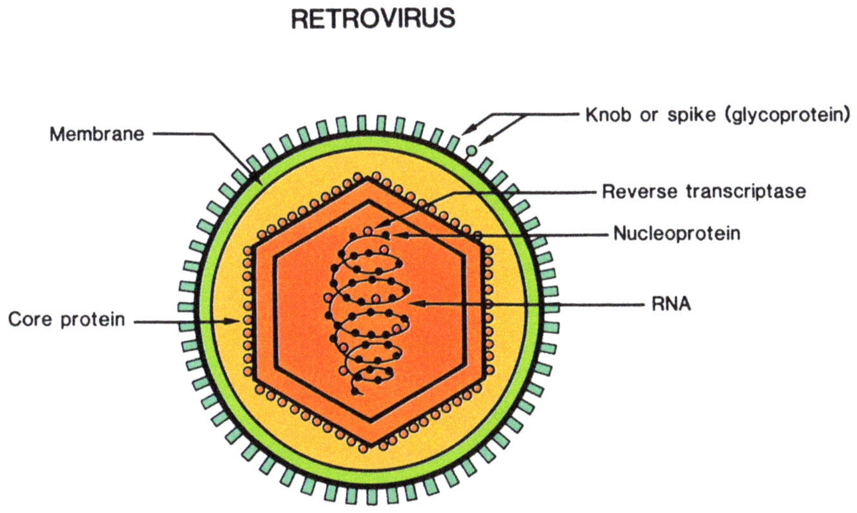

Anatomy of a retrovirus. Unlike other viruses, which contain DNA, retroviruses contain RNA as their genetic material. *© CDC/Science Source*

SCIENTIFIC, POLITICAL, AND ETHICAL ISSUES

In 1980 a US research team headed by Robert Gallo (1937–) reported the discovery of a retrovirus that causes cancer in humans. The virus was designated human T-cell leukemia virus (HTLV). Three years later HIV was reported almost simultaneously in 1983 by two US research teams: Gallo's and a French team. Because the researchers used different designations for the virus, a debate arose over which team was the first to discover HIV. The debate was heated because the discovery was almost immediately recognized as extremely important and likely of Nobel Prize significance. In the end, in the spirit of scientific cooperation, the researchers put aside their debate and agreed to be co-discoverers.

History and Scientific Foundations

The first known retrovirus, the Rous sarcoma virus, was discovered in 1911. It was subsequently shown that the virus caused cancer in some species of chickens. Demonstration of the ability of retroviruses to cause human diseases did not come until almost 70 years later.

In 1980 researchers at the National Cancer Institute discovered the first human retrovirus. They found the virus within leukemic T cells of patients with an aggressive form of T-cell cancer. These patients were from the southern United States, Japan, and the Caribbean. Almost all patients with this form of cancer were found to have antibodies to human T-cell leukemia virus (HTLV).

HTLV and HIV infect and replicate inside of T cells, which are vital to the human immune response. As more T cells are disabled, the immune system becomes progressively less efficient, and microorganisms not normally capable of causing disease are able to do so. These infections are called opportunistic infections. HTLV also causes a lethal cancer called adult T-cell leukemia.

Retroviruses are spherical. An outer structure called a capsule surrounds either one or two strands of RNA. The capsule also contains proteins that can recognize target protein sites on the host cell. The association of the viral and host proteins enables the virus to attach to the host cell, which is necessary before the virus can enter the host. For example, in the case of the HIV retrovirus, the viral proteins bind to T-cell proteins called CD4 receptors.

Once inside the host cell, the retrovirus begins to make more copies. Retroviruses are an exception to the general order of replication, which involves the use of DNA as a template to make a type of RNA called messenger RNA, which in turn provides the information to make proteins. Instead, retroviruses have a preliminary step in which the viral RNA is used to manufacture DNA. From then on the replication process occurs as in other cells.

Retroviruses contain an enzyme called reverse transcriptase, which produces DNA from the viral RNA. The viral-derived DNA can then be integrated into the host's DNA. When the host cell replicates, the viral DNA is read along with the host DNA. The manufactured viral components are then assembled to produce new virus particles. Reverse transcriptase is unique to retroviruses. Drugs that impair this enzyme can interrupt the production of a new retrovirus. As a result, therapies to treat HIV infection usually include a reverse transcriptase inhibitor.

Retroviruses that cause cancer do so when the reverse-transcribed viral DNA is integrated into the DNA of the host. In some cases the viral DNA can insert itself within a gene. This will alter the sequence of the gene, which can in turn alter or completely destroy the genetic information. When disruption occurs in a gene related to regulation of cell division, the result can be the uncontrolled cell growth and division that is the hallmark of cancer.

Applications and Research

Retroviral research has focused on understanding how the viruses infect cells, with the aim of blocking or even preventing the infection. Blocking the attachment of the virus to the host cell by binding an added molecule either to the viral protein involved in binding or to the target site on the host surface can prevent infection. Within the human body, this sequence is not as straightforward as in the laboratory, but progress is being made.

A powerful potential application of retroviruses involves their use as vehicles to insert genes inside of cells. This technique has been explored in gene therapy, where host genes can be disrupted or their activity increased, depending on the aim of the therapy. When the retroviral genetic material enters the host cell and, in turn, enters the host DNA, the target gene is also inserted. This can allow the target gene to be expressed. In another approach, the insertion of the retrovirus can disrupt a host gene. For example, insertion of the viral genetic material can disable a bacterial gene that codes for the manufacture of a destructive toxin. However, the trials of retroviral gene therapy in humans have been plagued with problems.

Impacts and Issues

Retroviruses that cause human diseases sickened and killed millions of people in the 20th century alone. While the best known of these diseases is AIDS, other retroviruses cause paralysis, physical and mental deterioration, at least one type of muscular dystrophy, multiple sclerosis, and arthritis.

WORDS TO KNOW

ANTIBODIES Proteins found in the blood that help fight against foreign substances called antigens. Antigens, which are usually proteins or polysaccharides, stimulate the immune system to produce antibodies, or Y-shaped immunoglobulins. The antibodies inactivate the antigen and help remove it from the body. While antigens can be the source of infections from pathogenic bacteria and viruses, organic molecules detrimental to the body from internal or environmental sources also act as antigens. Genetic engineering and the use of various mutational mechanisms allow the construction of a vast array of antibodies (each with a unique genetic sequence).

DEOXYRIBONUCLEIC ACID (DNA) A double-stranded helical molecule that forms the molecular basis for heredity in most organisms.

GENE THERAPY The treatment of inherited diseases by corrective genetic engineering of the dysfunctional genes. Part of a broader field called genetic medicine, gene therapy involves the screening, diagnosis, prevention, and treatment of hereditary conditions in humans. The results of genetic screening can pinpoint a potential problem to which gene therapy can sometimes offer a solution. Genetic defects are significant in the total field of medicine, with up to 15 out of every 100 newborn infants having a hereditary disorder of greater or lesser severity. More than 2,000 genetically distinct inherited defects have been classified as of 2018, including diabetes, cystic fibrosis, hemophilia, sickle cell anemia, phenylketonuria, Down syndrome, and cancer.

HUMAN IMMUNODEFICIENCY VIRUS (HIV) The virus that causes acquired immunodeficiency syndrome (AIDS).

HUMAN T-CELL LEUKEMIA VIRUS (HTLV) Also known as human T-cell lymphotropic viruses, human T-cell leukemia viruses are divided into two known types: HTLV-1 and HTLV-2. HTLV-1 is often carried by people with no obvious symptoms, though it can cause a number of maladies, such as abnormalities of the T cells and B cells, a chronic infection of the myelin covering of nerves that causes degeneration of the nervous system, sores on the skin, and inflammation of the inside of the eye. HTLV-2 infection usually does not produce any symptoms. However, in some people a cancer of the blood known as hairy cell leukemia can develop.

MESSENGER RIBONUCLEIC ACID (mRNA) A molecule of RNA that carries the genetic information for producing one or more proteins; mRNA is produced by copying one strand of DNA, but in eukaryotes it is able to move from the nucleus to the cytoplasm (where protein synthesis takes place).

ONCOGENIC VIRUS A virus capable of changing the cells it infects so that the cells grow and divide uncontrollably.

OPPORTUNISTIC INFECTION An infection that occurs in people whose immune systems are diminished or are not functioning normally. Such infections are opportunistic insofar as the infectious agents take advantage of their hosts' compromised immune systems and invade to cause disease.

REVERSE TRANSCRIPTASE An enzyme that makes it possible for a retrovirus to produce deoxyribonucleic acid (DNA) from ribonucleic acid (RNA).

RIBONUCLEIC ACID (RNA) Any of a group of nucleic acids that carry out several important tasks in the synthesis of proteins. Unlike deoxyribonucleic acid (DNA), it has only a single strand. Nucleic acids are complex molecules that contain a cell's genetic information and the instructions for carrying out cellular processes. In eukaryotic cells RNA and DNA work together to direct protein synthesis. Although it is DNA that contains the instructions for directing the synthesis of specific structural and enzymatic proteins, several types of RNA carry out the processes required to produce these proteins. These include messenger RNA (mRNA), ribosomal RNA (rRNA), and transfer RNA (tRNA). Further processing of the various RNAs is carried out by another type of RNA called small nuclear RNA (snRNA). The structure of RNA is similar to that of DNA, however, instead of the base thymine, RNA contains the base uracil in its place.

ROUS SARCOMA VIRUS Named after American doctor Francis Peyton Rous (1879–1970), a virus that can cause cancer in some birds, including chickens. It was the first known virus capable of causing cancer.

T CELL An immune-system white blood cell that enables antibody production, suppresses antibody production, or kills other cells. When a vertebrate encounters substances capable of causing it harm, a protective system known as the immune system comes into play. This system is a network of many different organs that work together to recognize foreign substances and destroy them. The immune system can respond to the presence of a disease-causing agent (pathogen) in two ways. Immune cells called the B cells can produce soluble proteins (antibodies) that can accurately target and kill the pathogen. This branch of immunity is called humoral immunity. In cell-mediated immunity, immune cells known as the T cells produce special chemicals that can specifically isolate the pathogen and destroy it.

Multiple sclerosis and arthritis are examples of autoimmune diseases, in which the body's immune system malfunctions and reacts against its own tissues. There is evidence that such autoimmune diseases may be caused by inserted retroviral genetic material. The original insertion that produced the genetic changes behind the immune difficulties may have occurred thousands of years ago, with the inserted DNA being passed from generation to generation ever since. Studies have shown that this ancient retroviral genetic material makes up almost 10 percent of the human genome.

Retroviral diseases are global and affect people in wealthy and poorer nations. The consequences are particularly severe in developing countries because these diseases can disrupt family life due to the need to care for the afflicted person. Retroviral diseases also cause absences from school and the workplace that impair the national economy.

The retroviruses used in gene therapy are altered to cripple their ability to establish an infection in host cells. These disabled retroviruses are able to incorporate their genetic material into the host cell genome but are not able to produce new viruses. These retroviruses have been used in disease therapy in animals. But retroviral gene therapy in humans is still experimental.

In 1999 18-year-old Jesse Gelsinger died of multiple organ failure days after beginning retroviral gene therapy. A severe immune reaction to the retrovirus used is argued to have been responsible for his death. In 2003 the US Food and Drug Administration banned gene therapy trials using retroviruses in blood stem cells. As of 2017 the approach continues to be researched using cultured cells. Clinical applications remain limited.

A gene-editing technique known as Crispr-Cas9 has the potential to selectively recognize and snip out or add genes of interest to genomes. Such technology might someday allow the selective removal of problematic genes rather than disabling the genes using techniques such as the insertion of retroviruses.

A therapy that treats the patient with a drug that stimulates HIV replication has shown promise. In the approach, the drug is given along with conventional antiretroviral drugs. The idea is that the eradication of the formerly dormant virus will deplete the virus. However, because only one patient has been treated as of the end of 2017, it is too early to say whether the approach will be fundamentally important.

SEE ALSO *HIV;* Pneumocystis carinii *Pneumonia; Viral Disease*

BIBLIOGRAPHY

Books

Turksen, Kursad, ed. *Stem Cells: Current Challenges and New Directions.* New York: Humana, 2014.

Periodicals

Coller, Beth-Ann, et al. "Clinical Development of a Recombinant Ebola Vaccine in the Midst of an Unprecedented Epidemic." *Vaccine* 35 (August 16, 2017): 4465–4469.

Henry, Ronnie, and Frederick A. Murphy. "Etymologia: Marburg Virus." *Emerging Infectious Diseases* 23, no. 10 (October 2017): 1689. This article can also be found online at https://wwwnc.cdc.gov/eid/article/23/10/et-2310_article (accessed January 18, 2018).

Websites

"How CRISPR Could Snip Away Some of Humanity's Worst Diseases." *Wired*, May 5, 2017. https://www.wired.com/2017/05/crispr-snip-away-humanitys-worst-diseases (accessed November 21, 2017).

"Rapid Detection of Methicillin-Resistant *Staphylococcus aureus.*" UpToDate, November 20, 2017. https://www.uptodate.com/contents/rapid-detection-of-methicillin-resistant-staphylococcus-aureus (accessed November 21, 2017).

Brian Hoyle

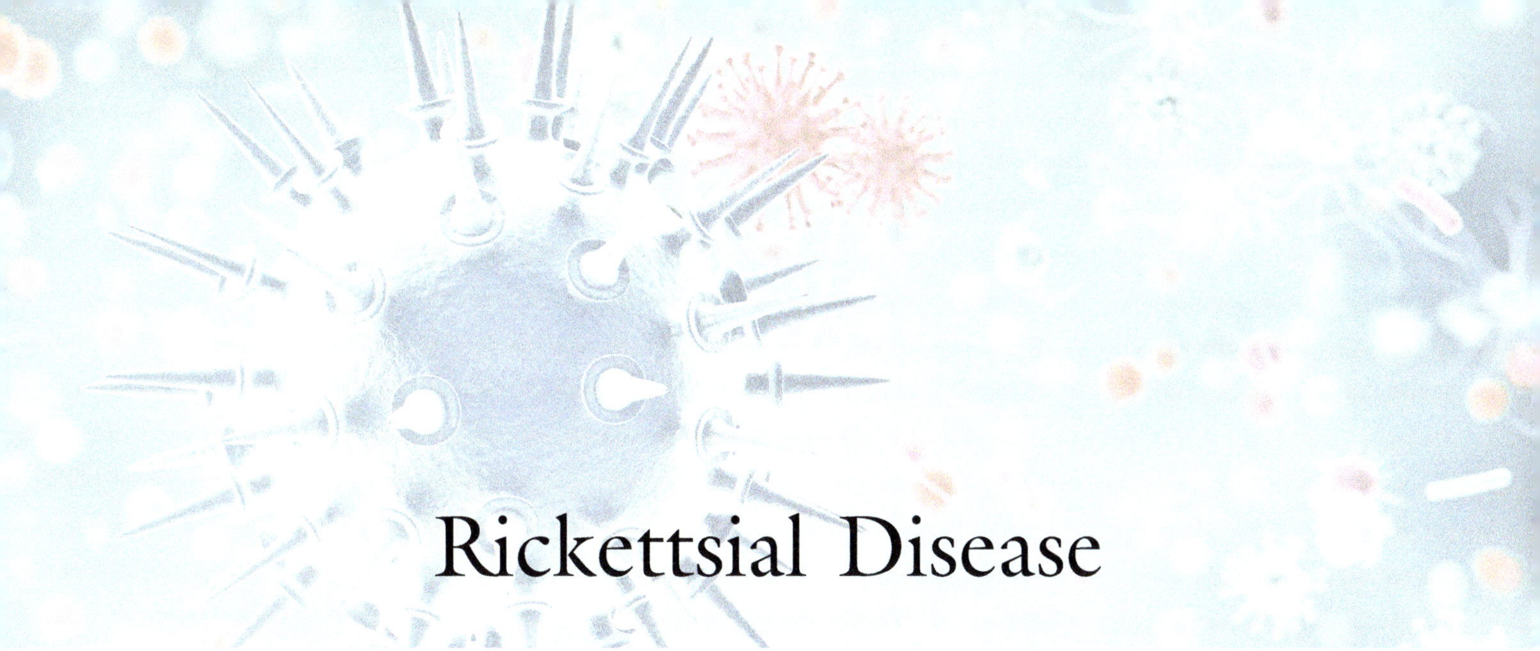

Rickettsial Disease

■ Introduction

Rickettsial diseases result from infection with bacteria from the genus *Rickettsia* or from related genera (such as *Neorickettsia*, *Neoehrlichia*, *Anaplasma*, *Ehrlichia*, and *Orientia*) that are only able to survive within the cells of another organism. These bacteria are typically transmitted from infected mammals to humans via parasitic arthropod vectors, including ticks, fleas, and lice. Once the bacteria are in the host body, they infect the cells lining blood vessels or white blood cells and cause cell death. This results in complications relating to the blood. There are numerous types of rickettsial diseases caused by different species of these bacteria. Common symptoms of rickettsial diseases include fever, headache, depression, and fatigue. In some cases a rash forms on the body, either around the site of infection or elsewhere.

Rickettsial diseases occur worldwide. Some diseases remain limited to certain geographic regions, whereas others are present on almost all continents. The distribution of the arthropod that carries the infectious bacteria determines the distribution of the disease. Rickettsial diseases are generally treated with a course of antibiotics. However, delayed administration of treatment can lead to more serious illness and even death. Although no vaccine is available to prevent contracting rickettsial diseases, prevention is achieved by avoiding contact with arthropods. This involves using repellents or wearing protective clothing.

■ Disease History, Characteristics, and Transmission

Rickettsial diseases are caused by bacteria from the genus *Rickettsia* and from related genera. These bacteria are named after Howard Taylor Ricketts (1871–1910), who conducted pioneering research on two major rickettsial diseases in North America. In 1906 he presented research indicating that ticks were the transmitters of Rocky Mountain spotted fever, a potentially fatal rickettsial disease. Three years later he studied another rickettsial disease, epidemic typhus, in Mexico City. While conducting research that showed the disease was spread via lice, Ricketts contracted typhus himself, which proved fatal soon after. In honor of his work, both the bacteria that cause these diseases and the class of diseases were named after Ricketts. (Rickettsial disease should not be confused with another disease called rickets, which is caused by a deficiency of vitamin D.)

Rickettsial bacteria cause illness in hosts by infecting the cells and causing cell destruction or death. They tend to infect vascular cells (cells lining the blood vessels), thus cell death leads to increased permeability of these vessels.

WORDS TO KNOW

ARTHROPOD A member of the largest single animal phylum, consisting of organisms with segmented bodies, jointed legs or wings, and exoskeletons.

ENDEMIC Present in a particular area or among a particular group of people.

EPIDEMIC From the Greek *epidemic*, meaning "prevalent among the people," is most commonly used to describe an outbreak of an illness or a disease in which the number of individual cases significantly exceeds the usual or expected number of cases in any given population.

INTERMEDIATE HOST An organism infected by a parasite while the parasite is in a developmental, not sexually mature form.

VECTOR Any agent that carries and transmits parasites and diseases. Also, an organism or a chemical used to transport a gene into a new host cell.

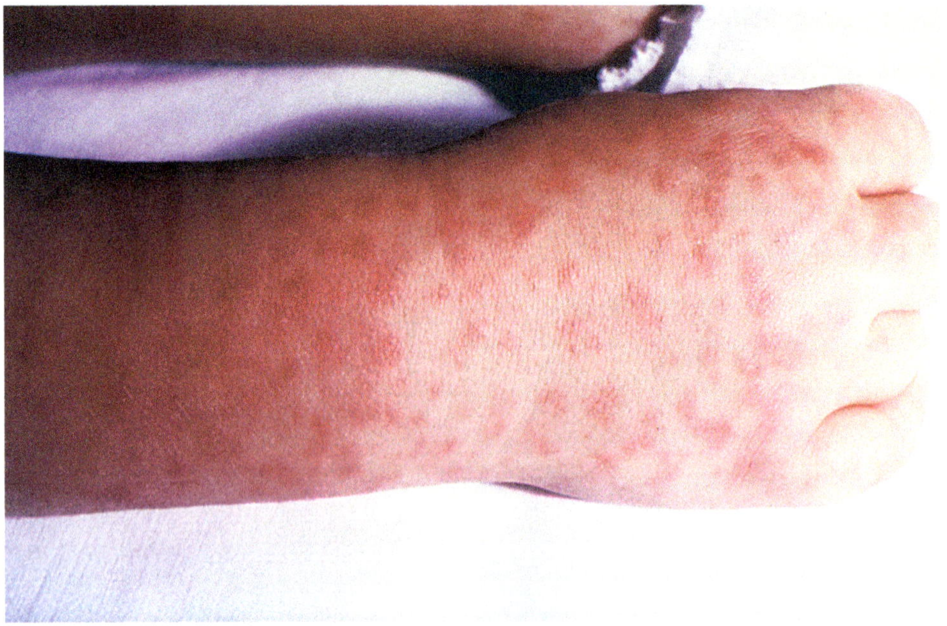

A child displays the spotted rash symptomatic of Rocky Mountain spotted fever, which is the United States' most severe and most common rickettsial disease. © *Smith Collection/Gado/Getty Images*

This causes changes in blood volume, concentration, and pressure, which is debilitating for the host. Two rickettsial diseases, ehrlichiosis and anaplasmosis, infect white blood cells rather than vascular cells.

Rickettsial bacteria are present in arthropods and mammals. Transmission usually occurs when an arthropod feeds on an infected mammal, sometimes becoming the intermediate host, and then feeds on a human. Humans may also become infected if they come in direct contact with the blood or feces of an infected arthropod. One rickettsial disease, Q fever, represents an exception to this rule, as it is transmitted not by arthropods but by airborne droplets containing the bacteria. In addition, ehrlichiosis and anaplasmosis can be transmitted from person to person via organ transplants or blood transfusions, as these diseases infect white blood cells and therefore circulate in the bloodstream.

There are many different types of rickettsial diseases. The main types are grouped into the spotted fever group or the typhus group or with scrub typhus. Most of the diseases share similar symptoms. In general, acute symptoms of fever, headache, depression, and fatigue occur within two weeks of exposure to a bacterium. A rash also often appears a few days after the onset of fever. This rash can appear on various regions of the body, as in Rocky Mountain spotted fever, or may occur specifically as skin lesions that develop at the site of the arthropod bite. In the most severe cases, people with rickettsial diseases can develop gangrene, blood vessel damage, organ damage, and problems with the liver, spleen, or kidneys. These symptoms can prove fatal.

■ Scope and Distribution

Rickettsial diseases occur worldwide. However, not all rickettsial diseases are present in all countries. Endemic and epidemic typhus occur worldwide, whereas North Asian tick typhus, Queensland tick typhus, and scrub

Common Tick-Borne Rickettsial Diseases

Disease	Incubation Period	Early Symptoms	Fatality Rate
Rocky Mountain Spotted Fever	2–14 days	Fever, nausea, vomiting, weight loss, headache, muscle pain	5–10%
Human Monocytic Ehrlichiosis	5–14 days	Fever, headache, exhaustion, muscle pain	2–3%
Anaplasmosis	5–21 days	Fever, headache, exhaustion, nausea, vomiting	Less than 1%
Ehrlichia ewingii Infection	5–14 days	Fever, headache, muscle pain, nausea, vomiting	No documented deaths

SOURCE: Adapted from Huntzinger, Amber. "Guidelines for the Diagnosis and Treatment of Tick-Borne Rickettsial Diseases." *American Family Physician* 76, no. 1 (July 1, 2007): 137–139. Available from: https://www.aafp.org/afp/2007/0701/p137.html

typhus have particular distributions that limit them to certain locations. The distribution of rickettsial diseases is determined by the distribution of their arthropod vectors.

However, cases of specific rickettsial diseases sometimes occur in areas not known to harbor the bacterium. This is a consequence of travel. Due to the long incubation period for these bacteria, travelers infected in one country may not exhibit symptoms until they are in another country.

In the United States, endemic rickettsial diseases include Rocky Mountain spotted fever, rickettsial pox, and cat-flea transmitted infection. The most common tick-borne rickettsial infections in the United States are ehrlichiosis, which is endemic to the country's southeastern and south-central regions, and anaplasmosis, which is found from the West Coast to the mid-Atlantic. Rickettsial diseases tend to be less prevalent in the 21st century than they were when first discovered. This is most likely a result of both improved prevention methods and the introduction of effective treatments. However, despite effective treatments, some rickettsial diseases can still be fatal, including Rocky Mountain spotted fever, which has an approximate mortality rate of 4 percent, or epidemic typhus, which has a mortality rate of approximately 10 percent in young adults and 60 to 70 percent in older patients. In Rocky Mountain spotted fever, a late diagnosis can lead to more serious complications, which contributes to higher mortality rates. In the case of epidemic typhus, increased age can decrease a patient's chance of survival.

Treatment and Prevention

Effective treatment of rickettsial disease usually involves a course of antibiotics. The best results are achieved when treatment is administered within the first week of illness. The longer the illness goes without treatment, the less chance there is of a good recovery. Tetracycline antibiotics effectively destroy rickettsial bacteria, and thus derivatives from this group are most often used for treatment. The preferred tetracycline is doxycycline because it has few negative side effects when used for short periods in low doses. Another form of tetracycline used is chloramphenicol. For patients older than 18 years of age, fluoroquinolones have been shown to be effective against some forms of rickettsial bacteria.

Antibiotic treatment usually takes less than a week. Fever generally disappears one to three days after treatment begins. If the fever does not begin to subside, misdiagnosis is likely. Once a patient no longer has a fever, treatment is stopped. Other treatment, aimed at managing the complications caused by the bacteria, such as hypotension, coagulation, and fluid leakage, is usually given in addition to the antibiotics. This treatment usually lasts about two weeks.

Rickettsial diseases cannot yet be prevented by vaccination. Research is under way to determine a possible vaccination for certain infections. In the absence of a vaccine, the best prevention method is avoidance or elimination of arthropod vectors to decrease the chance of being bitten. Avoidance measures include using repellents when outdoors, avoiding long grass or woodlands, wearing clothing that completely covers the arms and legs, wearing boots, and thoroughly checking the body after walking through arthropod-inhabited areas. Often, quick removal of ticks that have become attached to the body can prevent infection. Elimination of arthropod vectors involves using pesticides in arthropod-inhabited areas.

Impacts and Issues

One of the greatest issues surrounding rickettsial diseases is the impact that late diagnosis has on recovery. The treatments currently used for cases of rickettsial disease usually result in a successful recovery. However, the later treatment is given, the less chance there is of a good recovery. Late diagnosis may occur when patients do not visit their doctor or when medical personnel misdiagnose the disease. Some types of rickettsial disease, such as Rocky Mountain spotted fever, may feature a characteristic red rash. In the absence of this rash, the symptoms of this infection are similar to those of a multitude of other infections. Therefore, Rocky Mountain spotted fever may be misdiagnosed and the wrong treatment administered. Despite effective treatment for this disease, the mortality rate still stands at almost 4 percent, largely due to misdiagnosis and, thus, delayed administration of proper treatment.

SEE ALSO *Arthropod-Borne Disease; Bacterial Disease; Host and Vector; Q Fever; Rocky Mountain Spotted Fever; Typhus; Zoonoses*

BIBLIOGRAPHY

Books

Arguin, Paul, ed. *Health Information for International Travel 2005–2006*. Philadelphia: Elsevier, 2005.

Beers, Mark H., and Robert Berkow. *The Merck Manual of Diagnosis and Therapy*. 18th ed. Whitehouse Station, NJ: Merck Research Laboratories, 2006.

Nicholson, William L., and Christopher D. Paddock. "Rickettsial (Spotted & Typhus Fevers) & Related Infections, including Anaplasmosis & Ehrlichiosis." In *CDC Health Information for International Travel (Yellow Book)*. New York: Oxford University Press, 2018.

Periodicals

Aung, Ar Kar, et al. "Rickettsial Infections in Southeast Asia: Implications for Local Populace and Febrile Returned Travelers." *American Journal of Tropical Medicine and Hygiene* 91, no. 2 (2014): 451–460. This article can also be found online at https://www.ncbi.nlm.nih.gov/pmc/articles/PMC4155544/ (accessed February 15, 2018).

Biggs, Holly M., et al. "Diagnosis and Management of Tickborne Rickettsial Diseases: Rocky Mountain Spotted Fever and Other Spotted Fever Group Rickettsioses, Ehrlichioses, and Anaplasmosis—United States." *Morbidity and Mortality Weekly Report* 65, no. 2 (2016): 1–44. This article can also be found online at https://www.cdc.gov/mmwr/volumes/65/rr/rr6502a1.htm (accessed February 15, 2018).

Websites

Petri, William A. "Overview of Rickettsial Infections." Merck Manual: Consumer Version. https://www.merckmanuals.com/home/infections/rickettsial-and-related-infections/overview-of-rickettsial-infections (accessed February 15, 2018).

Rathore, Mobeen H. "Rickettsial Infection." Medscape, June 14, 2016. https://reference.medscape.com/article/968385-overview (accessed February 15, 2018).

"Rickettsial Infections—including Symptoms, Treatment and Prevention." South Australia Health. http://www.sahealth.sa.gov.au/wps/wcm/connect/public+content/sa+health+internet/health+topics/health+conditions+prevention+and+treatment/infectious+diseases/rickettsial+infections/rickettsial+infections+-+including+symptoms+treatment+and+prevention (accessed February 15, 2018).

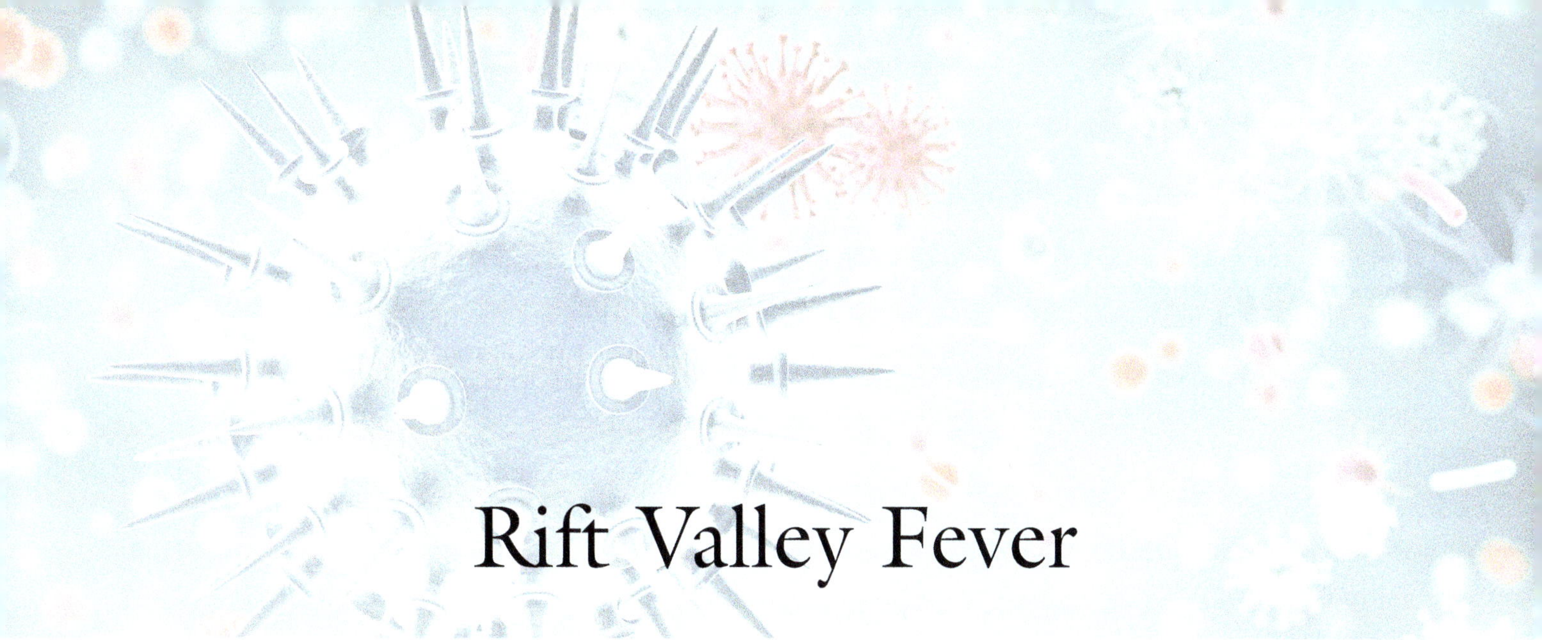

Rift Valley Fever

Introduction

Rift Valley fever (RVF) is a viral disease usually associated with outbreaks among livestock animals, although it also affects humans. It is caused by a virus from the family *Bunyaviridae* and is endemic in areas of Africa but can also spread to surrounding regions.

The virus is passed to animals and humans via mosquitoes. It is naturally occurring in some mosquitoes, and the highest incidence of infection is associated with periods of heavy rain and flooding, when mosquito populations are at peak numbers. Mortality rates among animals are high, but fewer than 1 percent of human cases typically prove fatal. Symptoms generally resolve within a week of illness onset and include fever, headache, and weakness. In some cases complications occur, including inflammation of the eyes, meningoencephalitis (inflammation of the brain), and hemorrhagic fever.

There are currently no preventive treatments available. However, researchers are developing vaccines and treatments for the disease among humans and animals. Increasing evidence of human fatalities has led to Rift Valley fever being termed an emerging virus and one that is considered a significant potential threat to communities.

Disease History, Characteristics, and Transmission

Rift Valley fever is a viral disease primarily affecting domestic livestock (such as cattle, sheep, buffalo, goats, and camels) but can also be passed on to humans. The disease is caused by the RVF virus, which is a member of the genus *Phlebovirus* in the family *Bunyaviridae*. RVF was first reported among livestock in Kenya around 1915. The Rift Valley virus was first isolated in Kenya in 1931.

The Rift Valley fever virus is naturally occurring in some species of mosquitoes, such as the *Aedes*. The virus may lay dormant in the eggs, which are capable of surviving for several years in dry conditions. During periods of heavy rain and flooding, these eggs then hatch and cause a significant increase in the mosquito population. The mosquitoes transfer the virus to the animals on which they feed. The disease can be transmitted to humans via mosquitoes or by exposure to the blood or organs of infected animals.

Incubation of the infection is usually two to six days, after which symptoms commonly present as a flu-like illness including fever, headache, muscle pain, generalized weakness, dizziness, and weight loss. In fewer than 2 percent of cases, the illness progresses and develops into a severe form. In 1 to 10 percent of cases, eye disease occurs and involves ocular swelling and retinal inflammation. This can lead to permanent vision loss, including blindness. In fewer than 1 percent of cases, RVF leads to meningoencephalitis. The most severe complication is hemorrhagic fever, and this occurs in fewer than 1 percent of cases. The hemorrhagic fever complication is responsible for most RVF deaths, with around 50 percent of cases involving hemorrhagic fever proving fatal.

WORDS TO KNOW

ENDEMIC Present in a particular area or among a particular group of people.

EPIDEMIC An outbreak of an illness or a disease in which the number of individual cases significantly exceeds the usual or expected number of cases in any given population.

EPIZOOTIC The abnormally high occurrence of a specific disease in animals in a particular area, similar to a human epidemic.

RVF may also cause miscarriage in women. A 2016 study published in the *Lancet: Global Health* demonstrated that there is an association between RVF and miscarriage in Sudan. The authors of the study wrote, "Our findings have implications for implementation of preventive measures." They continued, "Preventive measures should be introduced to avoid Rift Valley fever virus infection; for example, women at a fertile age could be given information on the effect of Rift Valley fever during pregnancy and how to avoid being infected."

Scope and Distribution

Rift Valley fever was initially limited to the regions of eastern and southern Africa where sheep and cattle are raised. Prior to 2000 RVF was limited to Africa. In late 2000 cases of Rift Valley fever occurred in Saudi Arabia and Yemen. This spread of the virus indicates a potential threat of the virus spreading further into Europe or Asia.

There was one reported case of RVF in China in 2016. The patient, a Chinese man, was infected with RVF in Angola and then returned to China while infected. In 2016 the World Health Organization (WHO) commented on the presence of RVF in China. It stated that, "since there has been no documented human to human transmission of the virus to date, and appropriate vector control measures have been put in place in China, WHO assesses the risk for further disease transmission from a single imported case in China and/or from China to be low."

People at risk of contracting the disease include people in contact with animals, such as animal herders, veterinarians, and slaughterhouse workers. Frequent exposure to mosquito bites in areas where outbreaks occur will also increase risk of contracting the virus. Travelers to areas where the Rift Valley fever virus is endemic are also under threat of infection, particularly during times of viral outbreak.

Epidemics are almost always associated with heavy rainfall periods and localized flooding, which creates breeding

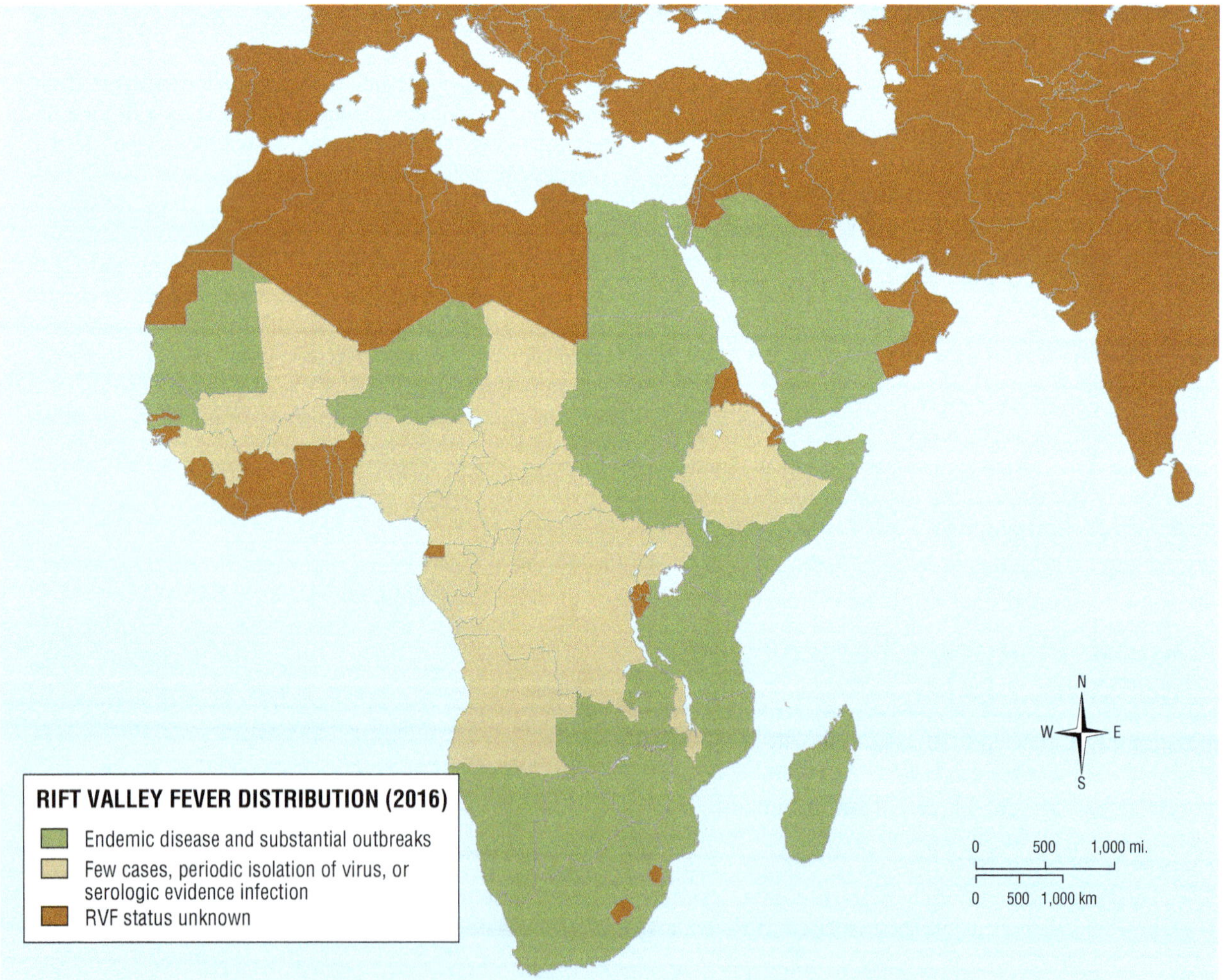

SOURCE: Adapted from "RVF Distribution Map." Centers for Disease Control and Prevention. November 10, 2016. Available from: https://www.cdc.gov/vhf/rvf/outbreaks/distribution-map.html

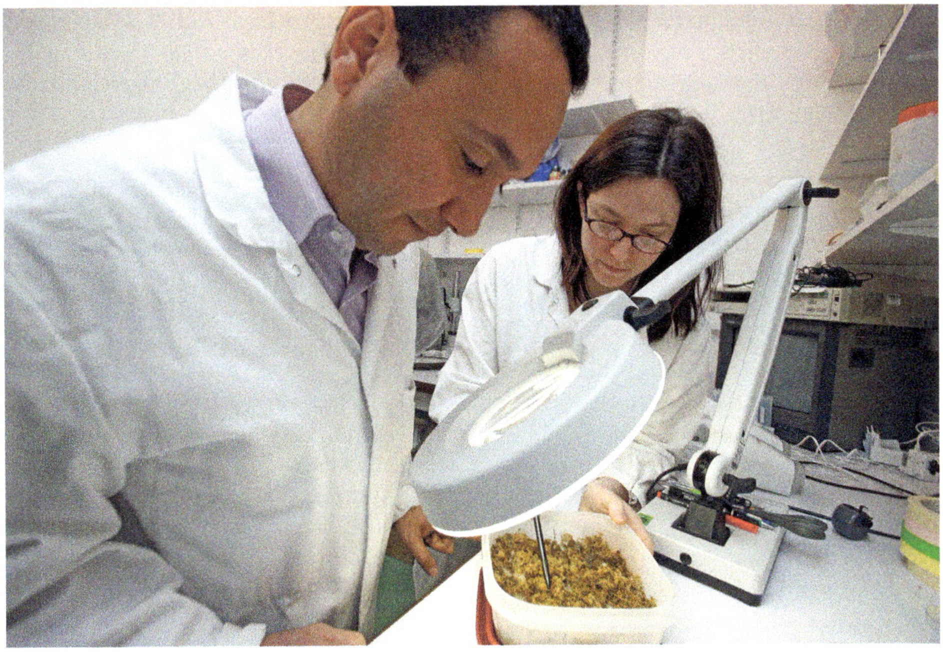

Researchers belonging to a mosquito research team at the Institut Pasteur in Paris examine larvae of *Aedes vexans* bred at the institute. This common mosquito is known to transmit Rift Valley fever. © BSIP/UIG/Getty Images

grounds for the mosquitoes. The first RVF outbreak was reported in Egypt in 1977 and 1978: human infection rates in some parts were as high as 35 percent, and 598 deaths resulted from hemorrhagic fever. An epidemic occurred in 1987 in West Africa due to flooding caused from construction of the Senegal River Project. In 1997 Kenya and Somalia suffered an epidemic that resulted in 300 human fatalities, with much higher rates for livestock. In 2006 to 2007 an epidemic occurred in Kenya, Tanzania, and Somalia following flooding, and from 2007 to 2008 there was an epidemic in Sudan, with 222 people dying.

Between 2006 and 2017 there were nine outbreaks in Africa, ranging in size from a few people infected with RVF to hundreds.

Treatment and Prevention

Diagnosis of Rift Valley fever in humans is performed through laboratory blood analysis identifying antibodies to the virus. In the majority of cases, the causative agent is obvious, due to the epidemic nature of outbreak. There is no treatment available for the infection except for supportive therapy for the symptoms. Researchers are investigating the potential for the use of an antiviral drug in infected humans. However, as of 2017 this is still in its developmental stages.

Many animal vaccines have been developed to protect against RVF infection but are often subject to limitation. One such vaccine was found to deliver immunity to mice for up to three years but led to spontaneous abortion when administered to pregnant ewes. It was found that multiple doses of vaccines may be required to provide immunity. This would prove problematic in areas where successful immunity would be subject to resource availability. A human vaccine had been developed but was not yet commercially available as of 2017.

Preventive measures may be taken by people to avoid contracting the disease. These include reducing possible contact with mosquitoes. This may be achieved by wearing protective clothing such as long pants and long-sleeved shirts in addition to the use of insect repellents and bed nets while sleeping. People in contact with animal blood or tissue can avoid infection by wearing gloves and other protective equipment.

Impacts and Issues

Rift Valley fever poses significant economic impacts on communities due to the fatality rates among livestock and the permanent threat of epidemics in certain areas. In an outbreak of RVF in Kenya in the 1950s, more than 100,000 sheep were killed. This devastated the community, and it took several years to recover. In pregnant livestock, infection by this virus results in abortion of almost all fetuses. This raises the issues of herd sustainability and growth. The mode of transmission of the Rift Valley fever virus makes it virtually impossible for farmers to protect their herds or themselves. With the natural occurrence of the virus in some mosquitoes, a rainy season or flood will almost certainly leave some communities devastated.

The complications associated with infection from RVF among humans can be quite severe, and as such, this disease can also be considered a high risk. Spreading of the disease from Africa to Yemen and Saudi Arabia has raised concern that the disease could spread to new areas, such as Europe. It is considered that stock, mosquitoes, and travelers could all potentially act as carriers of the virus and introduce it into new regions. Various species of mosquitoes act as vectors for the RVF virus, suggesting that the virus could be maintained once in a new region. This may potentially cause animal and human epidemics.

In addition to being spread by mosquitoes, the virus can also be spread by aerosols. This suggests that the virus could be introduced to a new area and spread rapidly within the area. These concerns have led many countries to list Rift Valley fever as a significant biological warfare threat.

Rift Valley fever remains a health threat, especially in Africa. From November 2006 through March 2007, an epidemic of Rift Valley fever in Kenya killed 234 people, according to WHO. There were nearly 700 suspected cases associated with the outbreak. The epidemic hit most acutely in several regions already strained by severe flooding and food shortages. Health officials instituted a quarantine of animals and humans in disease-affected areas, but the disease spread across national borders, infecting 264 and killing 109 in neighboring Tanzania, according to a report from WHO. A 2016 outbreak in Niger caused 33 deaths, the largest number of RVF-associated fatalities since the 2005 to 2007 epidemic in and near Kenya.

SEE ALSO *Airborne Precautions; Antiviral Drugs; Bioterrorism; Emerging Infectious Diseases; Viral Disease*

BIBLIOGRAPHY

Books

Bennett, John E., Raphael Dolin, and Martin J. Blaser. *Mandell, Douglas, and Bennett's Principles and Practice of Infectious Diseases.* Philadelphia: Elsevier/Saunders, 2017.

Guerrant, Richard L., David H. Walker, and Peter F. Weller. *Tropical Infectious Diseases: Principles, Pathogens and Practice.* Philadelphia: Elsevier/Saunders, 2011.

Periodicals

Baudin, Maria, et al. "Association of Rift Valley Fever Virus Infection with Miscarriage in Sudanese Women: A Cross-Sectional Study." *Lancet: Global Health* 4, no. 11 (November 2016): e864–e871. This article can also be found online at https://www.sciencedirect.com/science/article/pii/S2214109X16301760 (accessed January 18, 2018).

Bird, Brian H., and Anita K. McElroy. "Rift Valley Fever: Unanswered Questions." *Antiviral Research* 132 (August 2016): 274–280. This article can also be found online at https://www.sciencedirect.com/science/article/pii/S0166354216302522 (accessed January 18, 2018).

Hartman, Amy. "Rift Valley Fever." *Clinics in Laboratory Medicine* 37, no. 2 (June 2017): 285–301. This article can also be found online at https://www.sciencedirect.com/science/article/pii/S0272271217300069 (accessed January 18, 2018).

Mansfield, Karen, et al. "Rift Valley Fever Virus: A Review of Diagnosis and Vaccination, and Implications for Emergence in Europe." *Vaccine* 33, no. 42 (October 13, 2015): 5520–5531. This article can also be found online at https://www.science-direct.com/science/article/pii/S0264410X15011342 (accessed January 18, 2018).

Websites

"Rift Valley Fever." World Health Organization, July 2017. http://www.who.int/mediacentre/fact-sheets/fs207/en/ (accessed January 18, 2018).

"Rift Valley Fever in China." World Health Organization, August 2, 2016. http://www.who.int/csr/don/02-august-2016-rift-valley-fever-china/en/ (accessed January 18, 2018)/

"Rift Valley Fever (RVS)." Centers for Disease Control and Prevention, October 19, 2016. https://www.cdc.gov/vhf/rvf/ (accessed January 18, 2018).

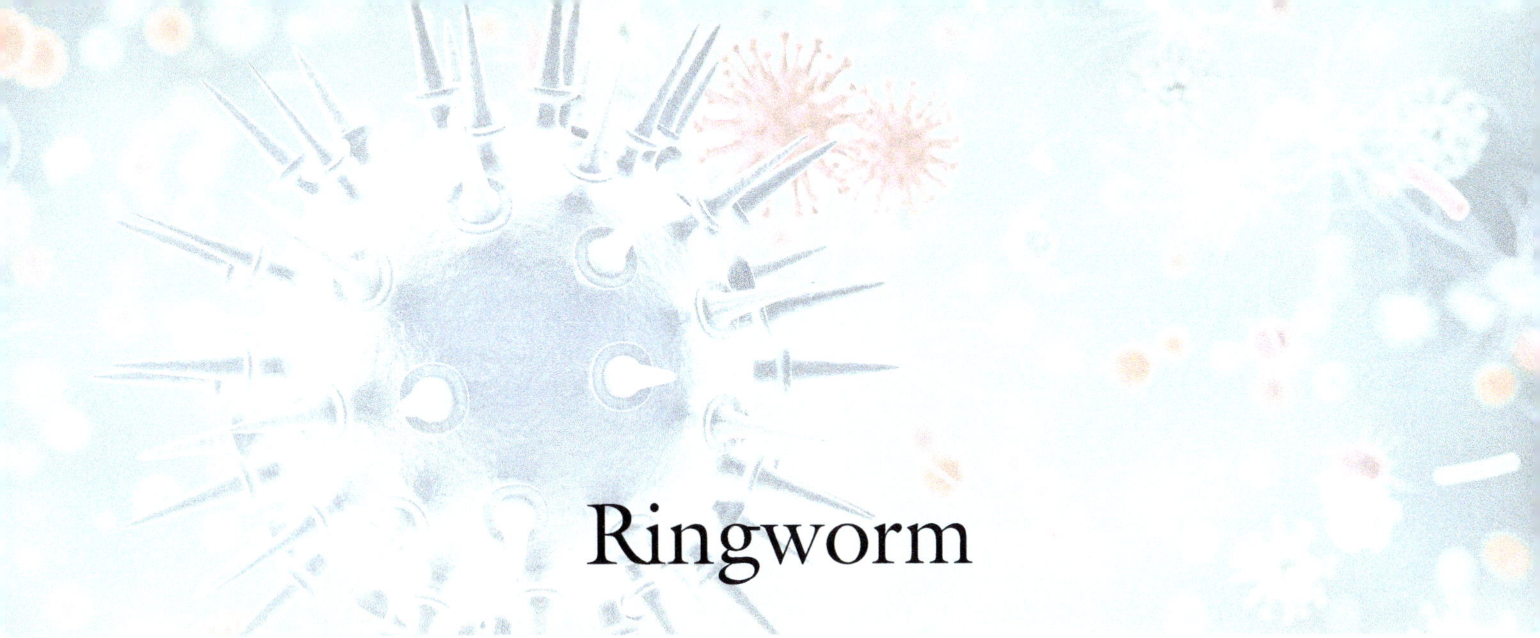

Ringworm

Introduction

Ringworm, also known medically as *Tinea* and dermatophytosis, is a group of contagious, very common cutaneous (skin) infections that can also involve the scalp, hair, or nails. It is caused by dermatophytes, various moldlike fungi that live on dead tissues of the body. Because many different fungi species cause ringworm, an infection with one species will not make a person immune to infection from other species.

Moist areas of the body such as the groin, between the toes, and in the armpits are generally infected most frequently. The infected area often looks inflamed and feels itchy. These symptoms are caused by sensitivity to the fungus or by a secondary bacterial infection. In its most serious forms, ringworm causes an acute infection with blisters on the feet or lesions on the scalp.

Disease History, Characteristics, and Transmission

The most common symptom of ringworm is flat, nearly round lesions. They may be dry and scaly or moist and crusty. Eventually, they turn red and become extended, itchy bumps with edges that blister and secrete fluid. As the infection continues, the color sometimes becomes nearly clear in the center and redder on the outside. This pattern causes the patch to look ringlike in appearance, which gives ringworm its common name.

Ringworm infection is most often spread during human-skin-to-human-skin contact. It becomes contagious to another person even before the infection is evident on the first person. Ringworm is sometimes spread when humans touch infected cats and dogs; when humans care for other domestic animals such as cows and pigs; and when humans touch contaminated clothes, towels, hairbrushes, combs, headgear (such as hats), or other infected objects.

The incubation period is not known for all types of ringworm. However, ringworm of the scalp (*tinea capitis*) usually appears 10 to 14 days after contact, and ringworm of the body (*tinea corporis*) usually appears in 4 to 10 days.

The most contagious form, ringworm of the scalp, is seen primarily in children. Symptoms include growing pimples, itchy scalp, and hair breakage. The scalp may temporarily become bald in patches. In some cases, an allergic reaction to the fungus can result in an abscess known as a kerion. The kerion will resolve when the fungus is treated.

Ringworm can also occur on the arms, legs, and trunk. It causes raised, round patches on the skin. The inner parts heal first, while the outer parts further spread the infection. When ringworm infection reaches other areas of the body, such as the armpit and groin, the shape often changes to resemble butterfly wings, or it may be completely irregular in shape. The condition is called *tinea cruris*, or jock itch, when it affects the groin area.

The fingernails and toenails may also be infected with ringworm. This condition is called *tinea unguium*. When this happens, the nails become yellowish, thickened, and deformed. They may crumble and fall off. When the infection spreads to the feet, ringworm is often called athlete's

WORDS TO KNOW

CUTANEOUS Pertaining to the skin.

DERMATOPHYTE A parasitic fungus that feeds off keratin, a protein that is abundant in skin, nails, and hair and therefore often causes infection of these body parts.

TOPICAL Any medication that is applied directly to a particular part of the body's surface, for example, a topical ointment.

foot (*tinea pedis*). When ringworm affects areas where facial hair grows, it is called *tinea barbae*; when it affects the face, *tinea faciei*; and when it affects hands and palms, *tinea manuum*.

Scope and Distribution

Ringworm can occur almost anywhere in the world. Because the fungi that cause *tinea cruris* and *tinea pedis* thrive in moist and humid areas, these conditions occur most frequently in tropical and subtropical regions.

Treatment and Prevention

Doctors often identify ringworm visually. Because it can resemble other dermatological conditions such as eczema, psoriasis, or seborrheic dermatitis, physicians often take a sample by scraping some material from the infected area. The sample is examined under a microscope to confirm the presence of fungal growth. A fungal culture may be performed if other results are inconclusive. Ringworm of the scalp is diagnosed with an ultraviolet light known as a Wood lamp. The fungus appears to be a bright yellowish-green color under this light, which helps to differentiate *tinea* from other infections. In rare cases, a skin biopsy may be required to examine the cause of lesions that do not respond to treatment.

Ringworm treatment depends on where on the body the infection is located, as well as its severity. Common antifungal creams, lotions, or powders that contain miconazole, econazole, or clotrimazole are often used in either prescription or over-the-counter formulations.

Ringworm on the scalp does not respond to topical treatments. It is therefore commonly treated with a four- to six-week course of oral griseofulvin. Griseofulvin usually eliminates the infection, but side effects, including nausea, dizziness, and diarrhea, can be pronounced. Griseofulvin can also cause complications during pregnancy, including conjoined twins, and so women and men should use birth control during treatment and for six months after being treated. Undecylenic acid is sometimes used as a fungicide. Antibiotics may be necessary to cure bacterial infections.

Although ringworm is unpleasant, it is rarely serious; it usually resolves within four weeks. Antifungal drugs, including fluconazole, itraconazole, ketoconazole, and terbinafine, are sometimes taken by mouth for persistent infections.

The National Institutes of Health (NIH) recommends a variety of measures to prevent contracting or spreading ringworm. These include washing hair regularly; wearing shoes in public areas such as shower stalls, locker rooms, and pools; and avoiding touching pets that have bald spots. The NIH also recommends against sharing personal care items or items of apparel such as towels, hairbrushes, shoes, or hats. Infected children are sometimes isolated from others, especially other children, to prevent further spreading of the infection. Bed linens and pajamas should be washed daily while symptoms are present. A shampoo containing selenium sulfide can help reduce the potential for spreading scalp ringworm by reducing shedding of hair.

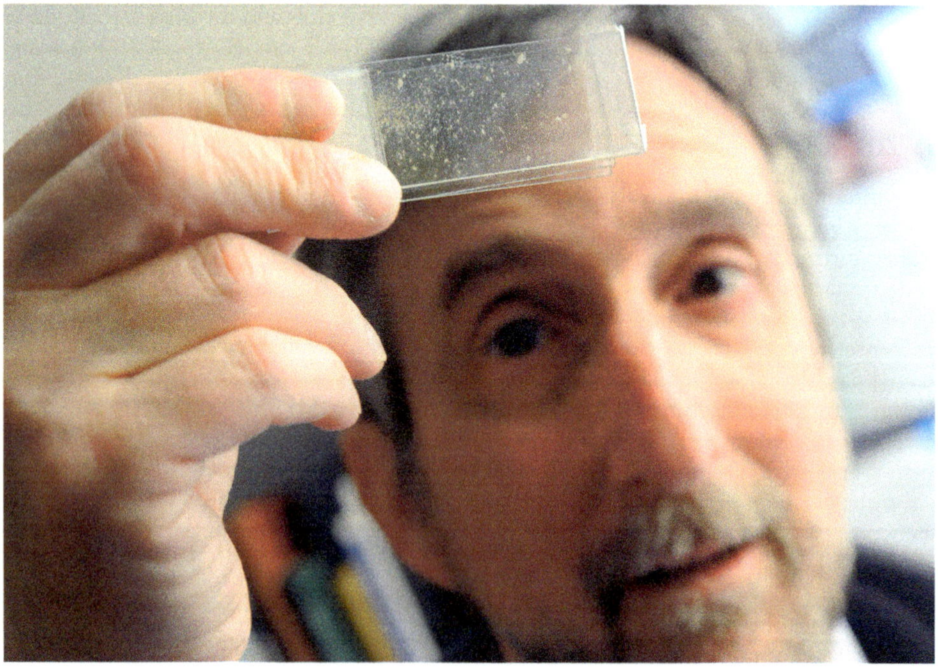

A doctor examines a slide containing hair from a child suffering from ringworm. Ringworm is a fungal infection that affects the skin and scalp. *© Sarah L. Voisin/The Washington Post/Getty Images*

Types of Ringworm

Location	Common Name	Medical Term
Skin	Ringworm	*Tinea corporis*
Soles of feet	Athlete's foot	*Tinea pedis*
Palms of hands	Ringworm	*Tinea manuum*
Groin	Jock itch	*Tinea cruris*
Nails	Nail infection	*Tinea unguium* or *onychomycosis*

Impacts and Issues

Anyone can get ringworm. Children are more susceptible to certain types of ringworm fungi, while other types occur equally in all age groups. Children become more susceptible to ringworm when they are malnourished, live in a warm climate, practice poor hygiene, come into contact with other children or pets with ringworm, or have weak immune systems due to medicines or disease. Complications of ringworm include spreading the infection to other areas than the initial site; bacterial skin infections; skin irritations, such as contact dermatitis; and side effects from drugs used for treatment.

Fungal infections such as ringworm present a concern for patients with weakened immune systems, such as those living with human immunodeficiency virus (HIV)/acquired immunodeficiency syndrome (AIDS). These patients may have difficulty fighting off the infection. Patient education about the risks of such infection is recommended, and patients with any symptoms of ringworm should be immediately evaluated and treated as necessary.

See Also *Mycotic Disease*

BIBLIOGRAPHY

Books

Hospenthal, Duane R., and Michael G. Rinaldi. *Diagnosis and Treatment of Fungal Infections.* Cham, Switzerland: Springer, 2015.

Richardson, Malcolm D., and David W. Warnock. *Fungal Infection: Diagnosis and Management.* New York: Wiley-Blackwell, 2012.

Periodicals

Weinstein, A. "Topical Treatment of Common Superficial Tinea Infections." *American Family Physician* 65, no. 10 (May 15, 2002): 2095–2102.

Websites

"Fungal Diseases: People Living with HIV/AIDS." Centers for Disease Control and Prevention. https://www.cdc.gov/fungal/infections/hiv-aids.html (accessed January 25, 2018).

"Ringworm." American Academy of Dermatology. https://www.aad.org/public/diseases/contagious-skin-diseases/ringworm (accessed January 10, 2017).

"Ringworm." Centers for Disease Control and Prevention. https://www.cdc.gov/fungal/diseases/ringworm/index.html (accessed January 10, 2017).

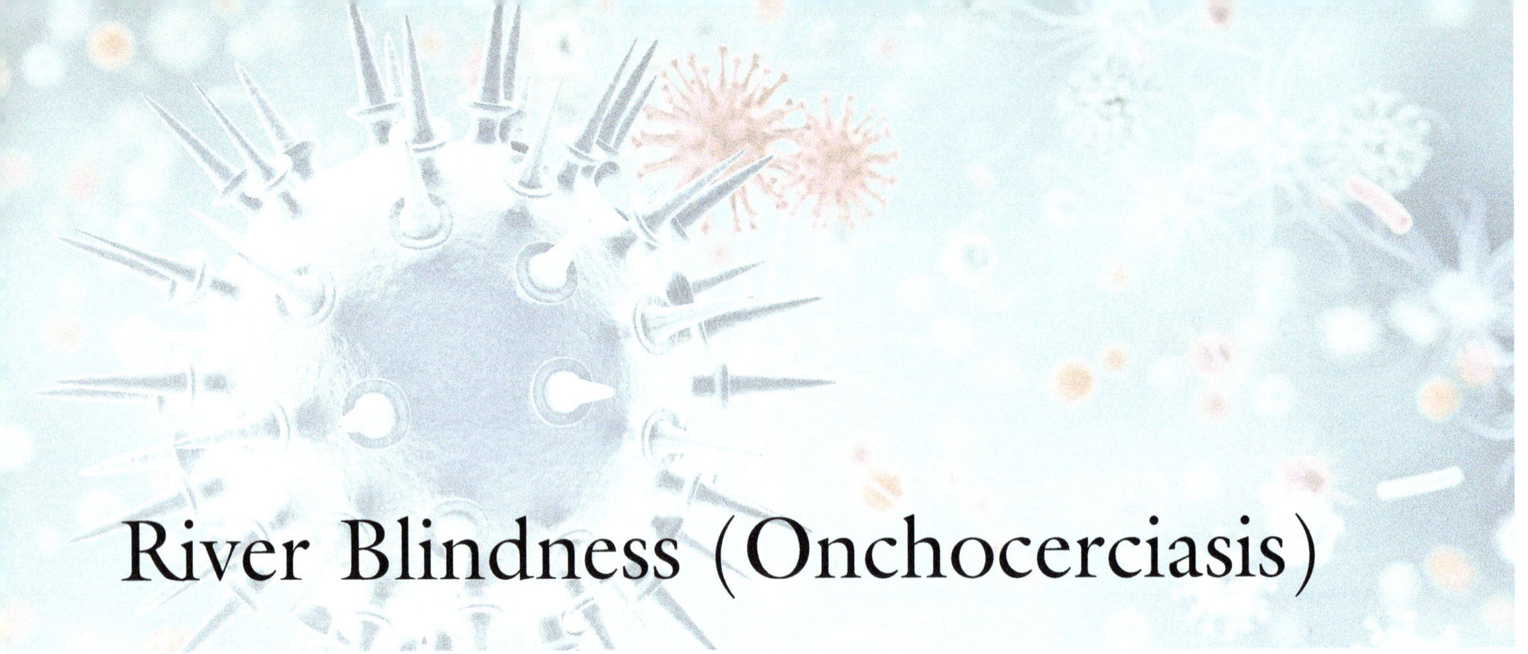

River Blindness (Onchocerciasis)

Introduction

Onchocerciasis (on-kough-sir-KY-A-sis) is caused by a helminth (type of parasitic worm) and occurs mainly in Africa. The worms are spread by the bite of infected black flies, which live mainly near fast-running rivers and streams. Hence, the alternative name for the condition is river blindness.

Once they have invaded the body, the worms reproduce, and millions of microscopic offspring migrate to the eye. When they die the toxic effects cause severe and chronic inflammation of the cornea and related areas of the eye that result in loss of vision. The threat of river blindness led to mass migration of people in West Africa away from areas infested with black flies. This had severe economic consequences as people settled in less productive upland areas.

The antiparasitic drug ivermectin can be used to treat river blindness. Mass treatment programs have decreased the burden of the disease in the 21st century.

WORDS TO KNOW

HELMINTH A representative of various phyla of wormlike animals.

MICROFILIAE Live offspring produced by adult nematodes within the host's body.

VECTOR Any agent that carries and transmits parasites and diseases. Also, an organism or a chemical used to transport a gene into a new host cell.

Disease History, Characteristics, and Transmission

River blindness is caused by a tiny parasitic worm called *Onchocerca volvulus.* The vector of the disease is a black fly belonging to the *Simulium* genus. These flies breed near fast-moving rivers and streams in the savannas and rain forests of several African countries. Therefore, people living in such areas are prone to infection. The incubation period of the parasite varies between 10 and 20 months.

River blindness does not always cause symptoms. But the parasitic worms, known as microfilariae, may accumulate in characteristic nodules under the skin. Dermatitis with severe itching is common, and the skin may become wrinkled and thickened. The resulting disfigurement is sometimes called "leopard" or "lizard" skin. More seriously, the parasites may migrate to the eyes. The microfilariae have been found in all parts of the eye, except the lens. When the microfilariae die, they cause toxic effects such as inflammation and bleeding, which can ultimately lead to blindness.

Transmission of river blindness occurs when someone is bitten by an infected black fly. This introduces the parasitic worms in a larval form under the skin, where they mature. Then the mature female worm releases millions of microfilariae, which migrate toward the eyes. The microfilariae may also move to the surface of the skin, where they may be ingested by other black flies, which may then bite someone else, thereby spreading the infection.

Unlike malaria, which can be transmitted by a single mosquito bite, it usually takes several black fly bites to transmit river blindness. The intensity of infection in an individual depends on the number of microfilariae they are carrying, which, in turn, depends on how many bites they have sustained. Blindness usually occurs in people with intense infection.

Scope and Distribution

River blindness is the second-leading cause of preventable blindness worldwide, after trachoma. According to the World Health Organization (WHO), about 123 million people worldwide are at risk of river blindness. There are nearly 25 million cases of the disease, with about 300,000 cases of blindness and 800,000 cases of visual impairment. The clear majority of these cases occur in Africa, with the remainder occurring in Yemen and in Central and South America.

As of 2017 31 countries in equatorial West, Central, and East Africa are affected by river blindness, especially in areas where there are fast-running rivers and streams frequented by *Simulium* black flies. In Central and South America, the affected regions are some areas in Brazil and Venezuela. In the Middle East, the only affected country is Yemen. The disease was eliminated from Colombia in 2013, Ecuador in 2014, Mexico in 2015, and Guatemala in 2016.

Because infection with river blindness normally requires several bites, the residents of these countries, rather than visitors, are most affected. However, there have been cases among foreign nationals who visit endemic areas for long periods, averaging three months or more.

Treatment and Prevention

The oral antiparasitic drug ivermectin is effective against the microfilariae but is less effective against the adult worms. One dose every six months should clear the infection and relieve dermatitis, as well as prevent blindness. Doxycycline also works against river blindness. A dose of doxycycline must be taken every six weeks.

Ivermectin can cause serious side effects, including death, in people who are infected with both *Onchocerca volvulus* and the parasite *Loa loa*. It is important to screen people for *Loa loa* before administering ivermectin.

There are no vaccines against river blindness, although researchers recommend the development of one. Insecticides can help control black flies in areas where river blindness is a problem. The flies bite during the day, so people at risk should wear long-sleeved shirts and pants and apply insect repellent to avoid being bitten.

A 2018 article published in the *Lancet* reported that the drug moxidectin has similar effects to ivermectin but requires a once-yearly dose as opposed to a twice-yearly one. In addition, it appears that moxidectin is effective for a longer period than ivermectin. The drug may become a useful aid in the fight against river blindness.

Impacts and Issues

Blindness has a profound impact on an individual's earning capacity and quality of life. River blindness has therefore proved a severe obstacle to socioeconomic development in many African countries. According to WHO, in some West African communities in the 1970s, about 50 percent of all men under the age of 40 had been blinded by onchocerciasis. This caused migration away from fertile river valleys infested by black flies to less productive upland country. The resulting economic losses were around $30 million.

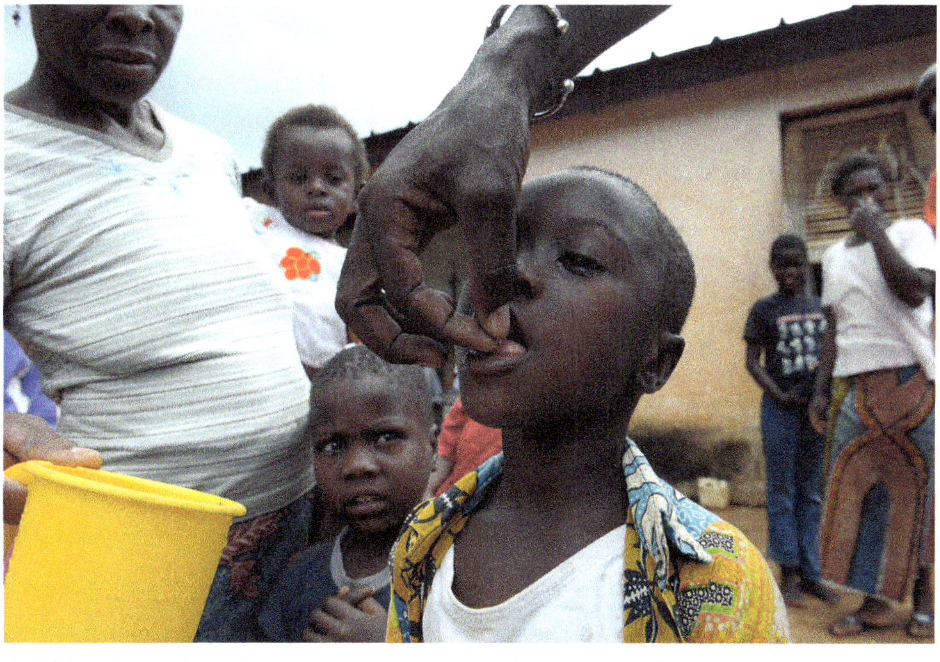

A child is given a dose of ivermectin to prevent river blindness. The disease is spread by black flies.
© ISSOUF SANOGO/AFP/Getty Images

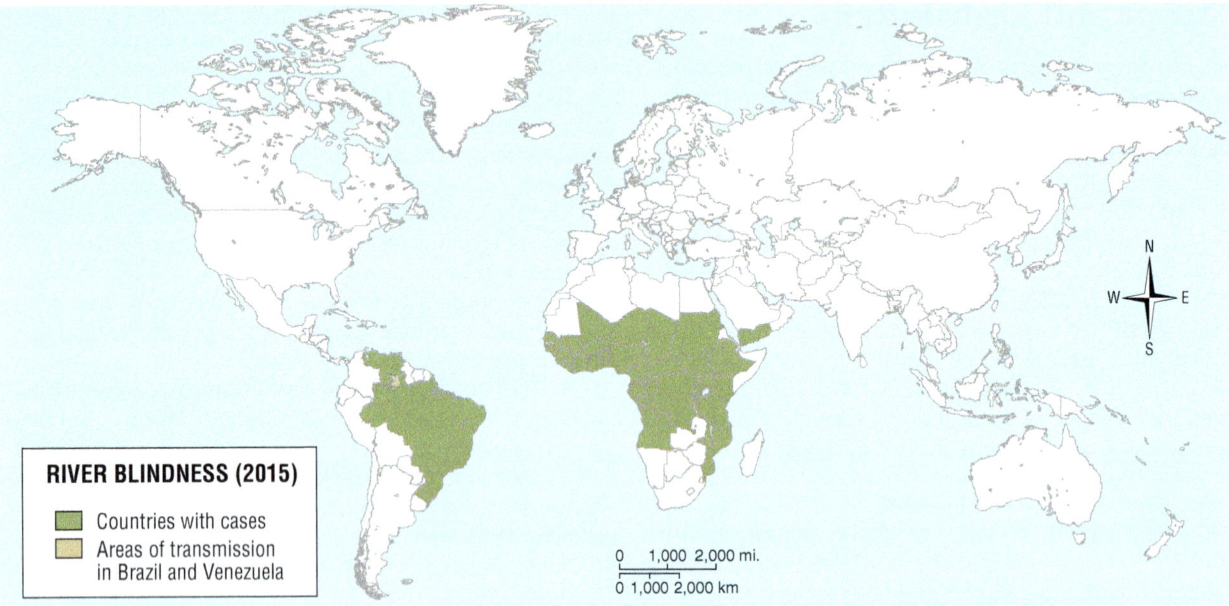

SOURCE: Adapted from "The Range of River Blindness." American Museum of Natural History. 2015. Available from: https://www.amnh.org/var/ezflow_site/storage/images/media/amnh/images/exhibitions/current-exhibitions/countdown-to-zero-superarticle/cz_rv_03_map/1906390-2-eng-US/cz_rv_03_map.png

According to the authors of a 2015 article published in *PLOS Neglected Tropical Diseases*, the elimination and eradication of river blindness would save from $1.5 billion to $1.6 billion between 2013 and 2045. The authors noted that, for this dream to become a reality, "policymakers should keep empowering community volunteers, and pharmaceutical companies would need to continue drug donation."

The world took action to halt the economic and social toll of river blindness in the world's poorest countries. Since the 1970s there have been various coordinated efforts to control the disease. In 1974 the Onchocerciasis Control Program (OCP) began in West Africa. This program was based on vector control by treating the breeding sites of the black fly with larvicides (insecticides that kill fly larvae). OCP expanded over the next several years to cover many river systems in seven countries, and it eventually doubled in size to cover 11 countries. The program ended in 2002, when river blindness had been virtually eliminated as a public health problem in 11 West African countries.

In 1989 a second strategy was added, involving the distribution of drugs to treat river blindness. Then, in 1995, the African Program for Onchocerciasis (APOC) began, with the aim of covering an additional 19 countries, which included the rest of Africa affected by river blindness. In these countries vector spraying was not a viable option because of environmental conditions. Therefore, APOC was based on the distribution of ivermectin, donated by Merck, the company that discovered the drug.

By the end of 2014, APOC was administering around 112.4 million treatments of ivermectin to residents of 22 countries. It was estimated that the program prevented 24.2 million river blindness infections, 9.8 million cases of itching, 500,000 cases of vision problems, and 300,000 cases of blindness. The APOC ended in 2015, and its efforts were absorbed by the Programme for the Elimination of Neglected Diseases in Africa (PENDA). Its goal is to eliminate river blindness, as well as other tropical diseases that are neglected in Africa.

Onchocerciasis is also covered by the WHO initiative VISION 2020: The Right to Sight, which works to eliminate preventable vision problems, including blindness. It is a partnership between WHO and the International Agency for the Prevention of Blindness (IAPB), a coalition of eye care professional groups and nongovernmental organizations involved in eye care. The initiative grew from the positive experience of APOC. Poor communities in developing countries are disproportionately affected by conditions that cause preventable vision problems and blindness. Each condition that causes preventable blindness, from river blindness to trachoma, has a cost-effective solution. The strategy of VISION 2020 is to bring these solutions to as many people as possible.

See Also *Developing Nations and Drug Delivery; Economic Development and Infectious Disease; Parasitic Diseases; Trachoma*

BIBLIOGRAPHY

Books

Despommier, Dickson D. *People, Parasites, and Plowshares: Learning from Our Body's Most Terrifying Invaders.* New York: Columbia University Press, 2013.

Periodicals

Abbasi, Jennifer. "iPhone-Based Device Helps Treat River Blindness." *Journal of the American Medical Association* 319, no. 2 (January 9, 2018): 113. This article can also be found online at https://jamanetwork.com/journals/jama/article-abstract/2668328?redirect=true (accessed February 12, 2018).

Boussinesq, Michel. "A New Powerful Drug to Combat River Blindness." *Lancet* (January 18, 2018). This article can also be found online at https://www.sciencedirect.com/science/article/pii/S0140673618301016 (accessed February 12, 2018).

Kim, Young Eun, Elisa Sicuri, and Fabrizio Tediosi. "Financial and Economic Costs of the Elimination and Eradication of Onchocerciasis (River Blindness) in Africa." *PLOS Neglected Tropical Diseases* (September 11, 2015). This article can also be found online at http://journals.plos.org/plosntds/article?id=10.1371/journal.pntd.0004056 (accessed February 12, 2018).

Websites

"Onchocerciasis." World Health Organization, September 2017. http://www.who.int/mediacentre/factsheets/fs374/en/ (accessed February 12, 2018).

"Onchocerciasis (River Blindness)—Disease Information." World Health Organization. http://www.who.int/blindness/partnerships/onchocerciasis_disease_information/en/ (accessed February 12, 2018).

"Parasites—Onchocerciasis (Also Known as River Blindness)." Centers for Disease Control and Prevention, August 10, 2015. https://www.cdc.gov/parasites/onchocerciasis/index.html (accessed February 12, 2018).

"River Blindness Elimination Program." The Carter Center. https://www.cartercenter.org/health/river_blindness/index.html (accessed February 12, 2018).

Susan Aldridge
Claire Skinner

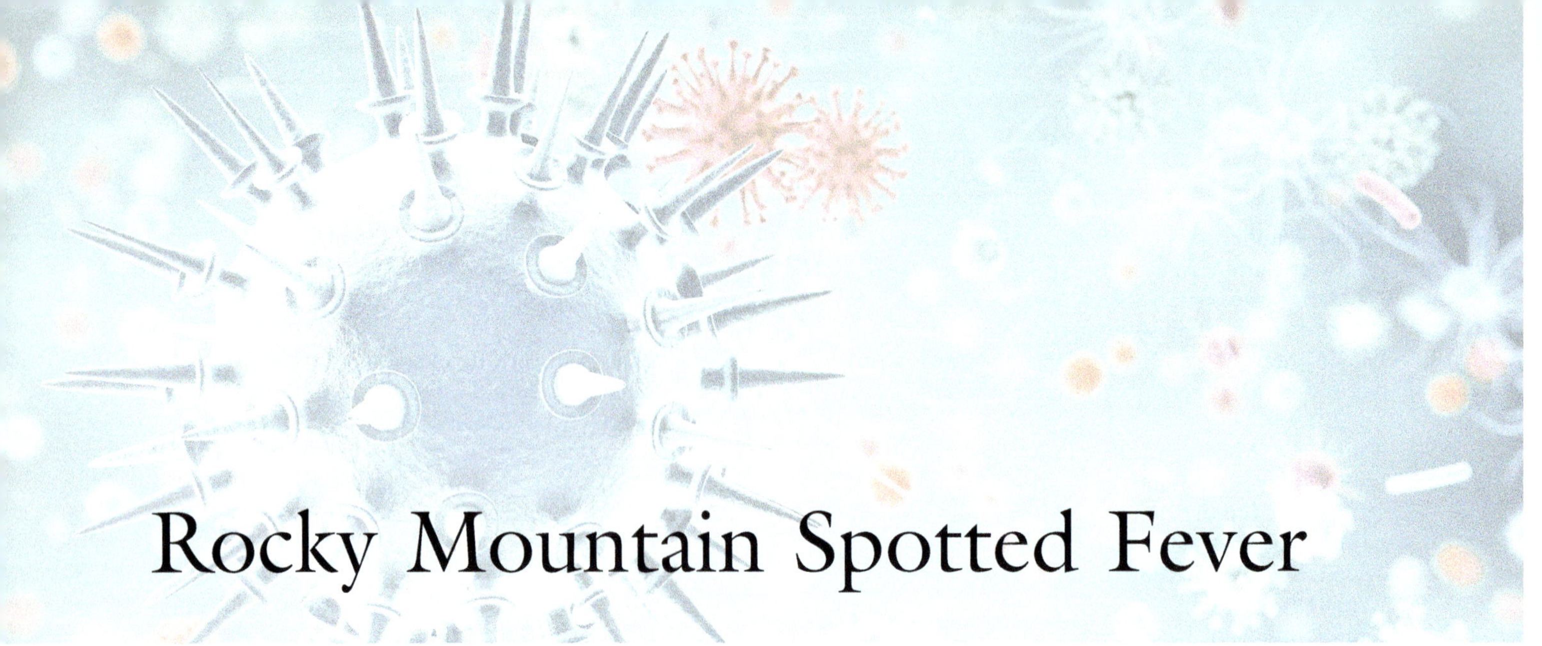

Rocky Mountain Spotted Fever

■ Introduction

Rocky Mountain spotted fever is a bacterial disease caused by *Rickettsia rickettsii*. This bacterium causes holes in blood vessels, which allows blood to leak into tissues and organs, causing damage to these areas. Humans become infected with Rocky Mountain spotted fever following a bite from an infected tick. Infection can also occur after contact with the blood or feces of infected ticks.

This disease usually results in fever, nausea, vomiting, headache, muscle aches, lack of appetite, diarrhea, abdominal pains, and in some cases a characteristic red rash. While recovery is likely for patients who receive early treatment, delayed treatment can result in complications, including death. Treatment involves a course of antibiotics for the duration of the fever. Because there is no vaccine available, the best prevention method is avoidance of ticks. This reduces the chance that a tick bite will lead to transmission of *R. rickettsii*.

WORDS TO KNOW

ACARACIDES Chemicals that kill mites and ticks.

TICK Any blood-sucking parasitic insect of suborder *Ixodides*, superfamily *Ixodoidea*. Ticks can transmit a number of diseases, including Lyme disease and Rocky Mountain spotted fever.

VECTOR Any agent that carries and transmits parasites and diseases. Also, an organism or a chemical used to transport a gene into a new host cell.

■ Disease History, Characteristics, and Transmission

Rocky Mountain spotted fever was first identified as a tick-borne bacterial disease by Howard T. Ricketts (1871–1910) shortly before his death. The disease was initially recognized in 1896 in the Snake River Valley of the US state of Idaho, where it infected hundreds of people and was often fatal. Although it was discovered in the Rocky Mountains, the disease occurs all over the United States, except for Hawaii, Vermont, Maine, and Alaska. Rocky Mountain spotted fever is a potentially fatal disease and prior to 1940 had a mortality rate of 30 percent. This rate decreased to 3 to 5 percent following the introduction of an effective antibiotic treatment.

Rocky Mountain spotted fever is caused by the bacterium *R. rickettsii*. Infection occurs when a tick vector bites an infected animal and then bites a human. Infection can also occur if human skin is contaminated with tick blood or feces. The most common ticks to spread this infection to humans are the American dog tick (*Dermacentor variabilis*) and the Rocky Mountain wood tick (*D. andersoni*). *R. rickettsii* lives and reproduces within cells lining blood vessels. The bacteria cause cell death, which leads to gaps forming in the surface of the blood vessel. Blood leaks through these gaps into surrounding tissue and causes tissue and organ damage.

Various symptoms may arise over the course of a week. Initial symptoms include fever, nausea, vomiting, headache, muscle aches, and lack of appetite. A faint rash may appear within two to five days after fever. Later symptoms include abdominal pain, joint pain, and diarrhea. Around six days after the onset of fever, a red, spotted rash occurs in 35 to 60 percent of patients. Complications can arise in patients suffering severe cases when the respiratory, central nervous, gastrointestinal, and renal systems are affected. Long-term effects of Rocky Mountain spotted fever can include paralysis, amputation of limbs due to gangrene, hearing loss, loss of bowel or bladder control, and development of movement disorders.

Scope and Distribution

Rocky Mountain spotted fever occurs in almost all regions of the United States. It is dominant in the southern Atlantic region, particularly in North Carolina. This fever also occurs in South America, particularly in Argentina, Brazil, Colombia, Costa Rica, and Panama, as well as Mexico. Bacterial strains (types) closely related to *R. rickettsii* also cause spotted fevers worldwide. The type of *Rickettsia* bacterium present in a region determines which type of spotted fever occurs in the area.

The US Centers for Disease Control and Prevention (CDC) recorded 11 cases of Rocky Mountain spotted fever per 1 million people in 2014. This fever predominantly occurs during warm weather when ticks are more active. The summer months in the United States, from April through to September, mark the highest levels of infection throughout the year.

All people can potentially contract Rocky Mountain spotted fever. However, males, Caucasians, and children are infected most often. Increased exposure to ticks increases the likelihood of infection. Therefore, people who live with dogs or people who reside near tick-inhabited areas, such as woodlands, are at risk of infection.

Treatment and Prevention

A course of antibiotics is used to treat Rocky Mountain spotted fever. Doxycycline is recommended by the CDC as an effective drug to eradicate this infection. However, for pregnant women, chloramphenicol should be used as an alternative to doxycycline, as doxycycline is associated with risk of malformation of the teeth and bones in unborn children. Treatment administered immedi-

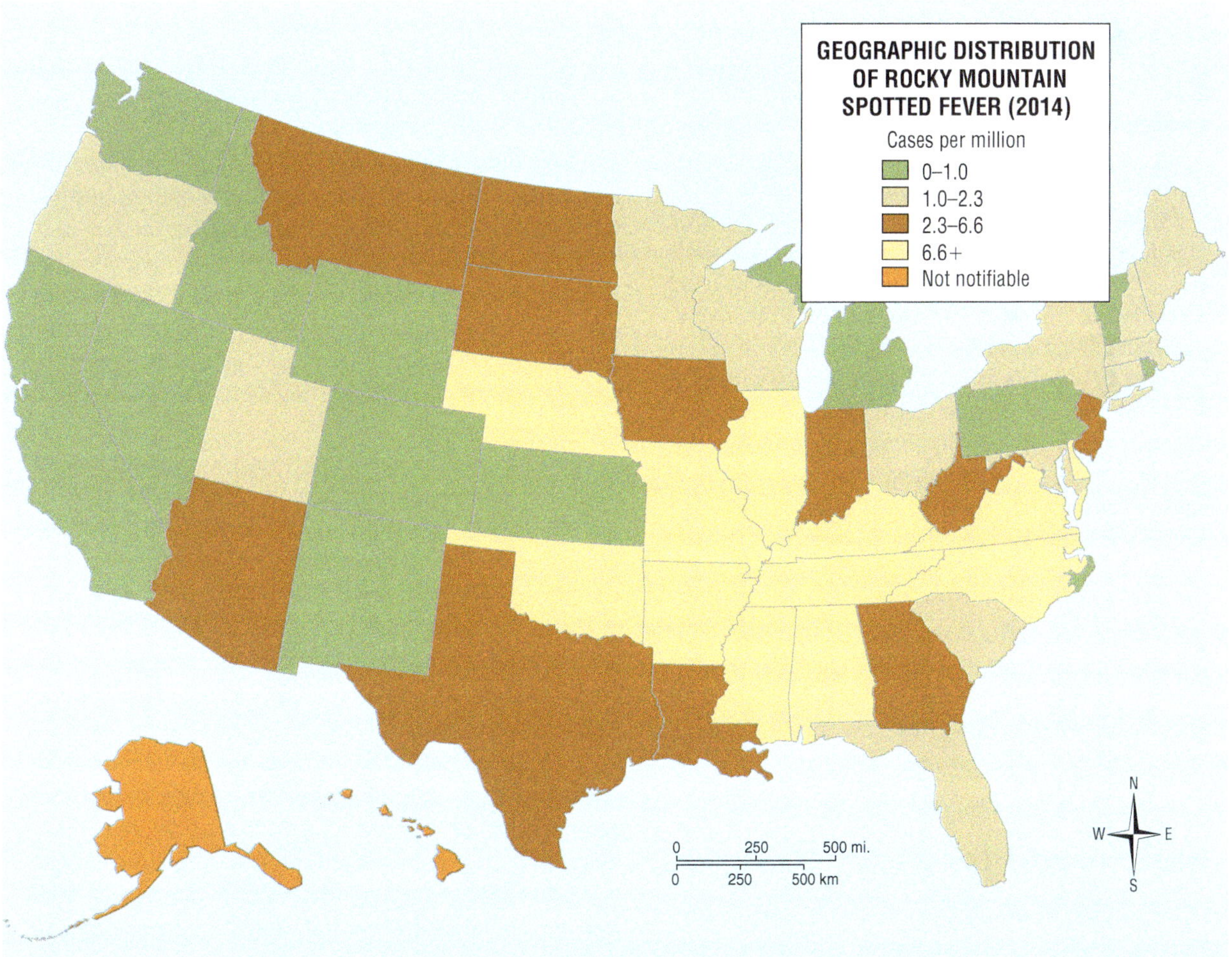

SOURCE: Adapted from "Rocky Mountain Spotted Fever (RMSP): Statistics and Epidemiology." US Centers for Disease Control and Prevention. 2014. Available from: https://www.cdc.gov/rmsf/stats/index.html

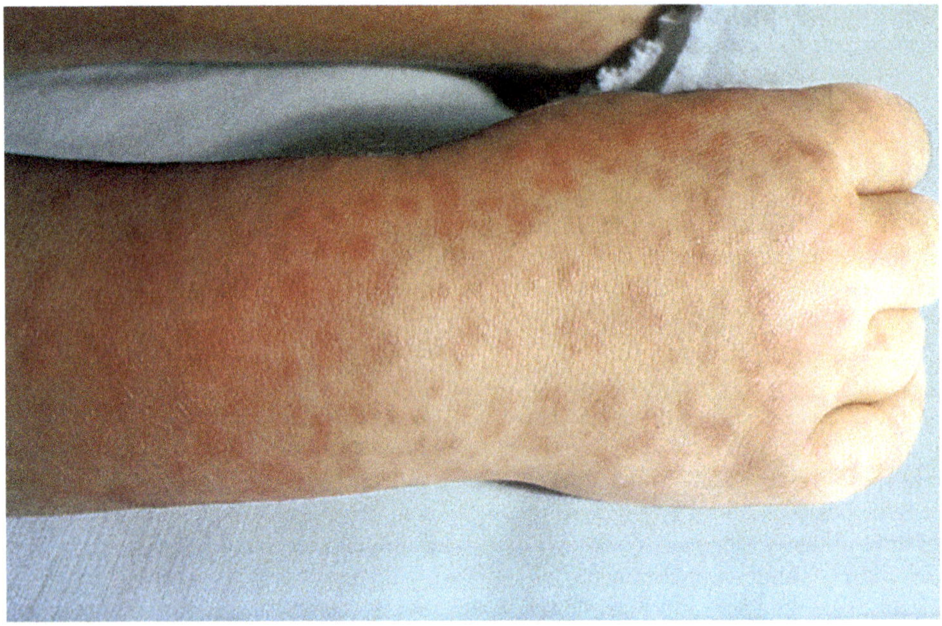

Rocky Mountain spotted fever gets its name from the faint rash associated with the infection. The spotted rash develops in 45 to 60 percent of patients. © CDC/Science Source

ately provides the best results. Fever usually subsides within one to three days following antibiotic treatment given within four to five days of the onset of the disease. However, recovery from fever will take longer in patients who receive treatment later or who suffer from severe illness.

There is no vaccine available for Rocky Mountain spotted fever. Therefore, the best prevention method is to avoid contact with ticks. This can be achieved in several ways. Areas inhabited by ticks, such as long grasslands and woodlands, should be avoided. If these areas cannot be avoided, repellents on clothing or skin can help discourage ticks from biting. In addition, protective clothing, such as long-sleeved shirts, boots, and hats, can be worn to prevent ticks coming in contact with the skin. It is also important to thoroughly check the body for ticks following any activity in tick habitats. This may prevent ticks from biting or, in cases when ticks have already attached to the skin, facilitate early removal and reduce the chances of infection.

Large-scale prevention methods include the use of acaricides (insecticides that kill ticks) in tick-infested areas to reduce the number of ticks. If there are fewer ticks in an area, it is less likely that humans will be bitten.

■ Impacts and Issues

Rocky Mountain spotted fever is a potentially life-threatening disease. Late diagnosis and delayed treatment increase the chances of complications such as kidney failure and even death. Because this disease infects more than 3,000 people a year in the United States and is potentially fatal, the Directors of Health Promotion and Education recommend increased awareness and reminders about prevention.

This disease can be difficult to diagnose during the initial stages due to its wide range of symptoms and the fact that not all cases exhibit the characteristic red rash. This is a problem because late diagnosis increases the chances of severe complications and possible fatalities. To address this problem, treatment is usually given before conclusive evidence confirms the disease. This approach ensures that patients with the disease receive treatment as soon as possible.

Despite prevention methods such as the use of acaricides, the wearing of protective clothing, and the use of repellents, ticks can still come in contact with humans. When people find ticks on their bodies, removal is vital, and the earlier it is done, the less chance there is of infection. However, incorrect removal of ticks can cause complications. If the mouthparts of the tick remain in the body, infection can still occur. Furthermore, handling ticks with bare hands also increases the risk of exposure, as infection can occur when blood or feces come in contact with open skin. The best technique for removing a tick involves grabbing the tick with tweezers as close to the skin as possible and pulling it away from the skin. Coating ticks with petroleum jelly or burning them with a match are not effective techniques for removal, despite the popularity of these methods.

SEE ALSO *Bacterial Disease; Rickettsial Disease; Zoonoses*

BIBLIOGRAPHY

Books

Alotaibi, Mohammed, and Siraj Amanullah. "*Rickettsia rickettsii* (Rocky Mountain Spotted Fever) Attack." In *Ciottone's Disaster Medicine*, edited by Gregory R. Ciottone et al., 724–725. Philadelphia: Elsevier, 2016.

Bennett, John E., Raphael Dolin, and Martin J. Blaser. *Mandell, Douglas, and Bennett's Infectious Disease Essentials.* Philadelphia: Elsevier, 2017.

Bennett, John E., Raphael Dolin, and Martin J. Blaser, eds. *Mandell, Douglas, and Bennett's Principles and Practice of Infectious Diseases.* 8th ed. Philadelphia: Elsevier, 2015.

Murray, Patrick R., Ken S. Rosenthal, and Michael A. Pfaller. *Medical Microbiology.* Philadelphia: Elsevier, 2016.

Wilson, Walter R., and Merle A. Sande. *Current Diagnosis and Treatment in Infectious Diseases.* New York: McGraw-Hill, 2014.

Periodicals

Drexler, Naomi. A., et al. "Fatal Rocky Mountain Spotted Fever along the United States–Mexico Border, 2013–2016." *Emerging Infectious Diseases* 10 (October 23, 2017): 1621–1626.

Kunze, Ursula. "Tick-Borne Encephalitis—Still on the Map." *Ticks and Tick-Borne Diseases* 7, no. 5 (July 2016): 911–914.

Websites

"Rocky Mountain Spotted Fever." Centers for Disease Control and Prevention, June 26, 2017. http://www.cdc.gov/ncidod/dvrd/rmsf/index.htm (accessed December 9, 2017).

"Rocky Mountain Spotted Fever." Illinois Department of Public Health. http://www.idph.state.il.us/public/hb/hbrmsf.htm (accessed December 9, 2017).

Laura J. Cataldo

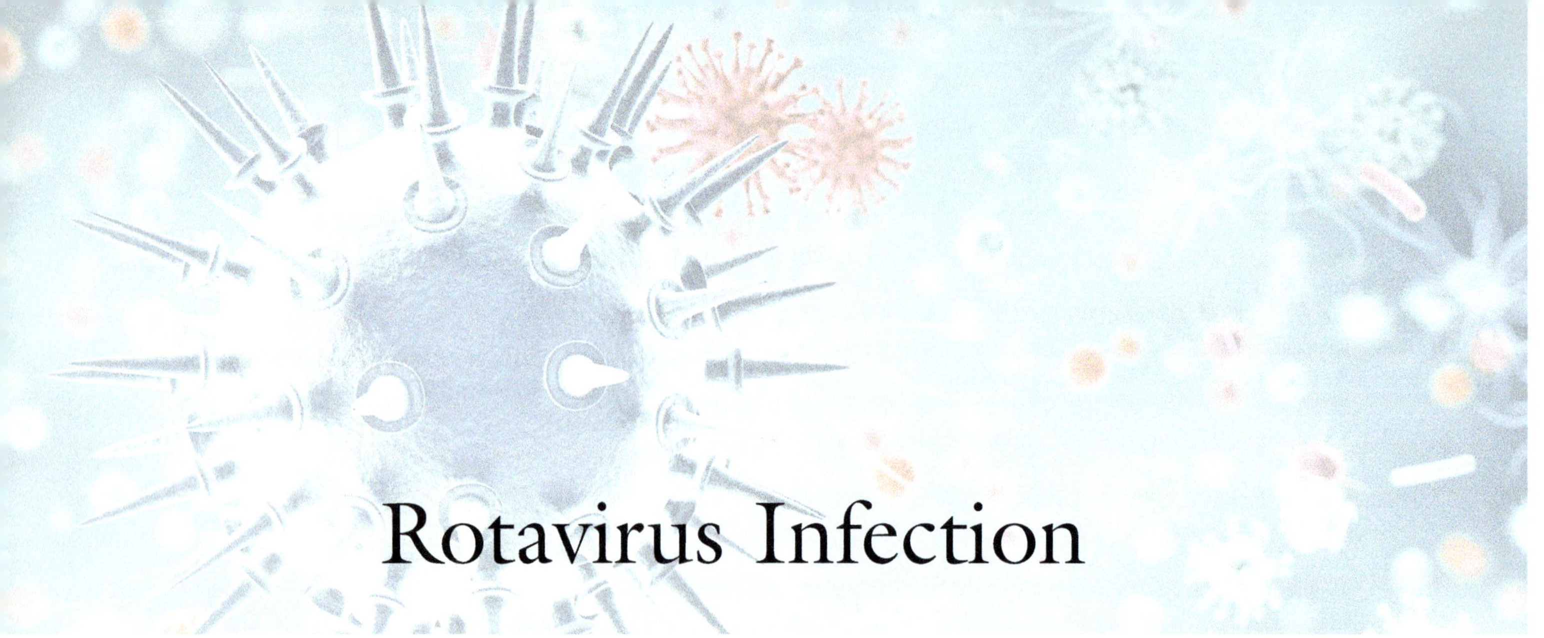

Rotavirus Infection

■ Introduction

Rotavirus is the most common cause of severe diarrhea in children and is one of the primary causes of gastroenteritis among children, accounting for approximately 40 percent of hospitalizations worldwide for children under five years old as of 2017. While rotavirus remains a major cause of sickness, hospitalization, and death in children, the introduction of two rotavirus vaccines in 2006 has helped dramatically reduce the impact of infections globally. According to a 2016 article in *Clinical Infectious Diseases*, the number of rotavirus-caused deaths in children under age five declined by more than 50 percent, from about 528,000 in 2000 to 215,000 in 2013. Other studies have also shown sharp drops in hospitalizations and emergency room visits due to rotavirus.

There are 11 different strains of rotavirus, four of which are known to cause diarrhea in humans. The disease has an incubation period of up to two days. This is followed by symptoms such as fever, stomachache, vomiting, and diarrhea. The disease is usually self-limiting within eight days. However, dehydration is a severe complication and may prove fatal if untreated.

While transmission typically occurs through ingestion of fecally contaminated food or water, the virus is able to live on surfaces for days, so people may also become infected following contact with contaminated surfaces such as toys and benches. Rotavirus is highly contagious, and infection can also come from human-to-human contact, including contact with contaminated hands. However, use of rotavirus vaccine is effective at preventing infection. Through the efforts of governmental and private agencies, as of 2017 rotavirus vaccine had been introduced in more than 80 countries. As access to the vaccine increases, epidemiologists anticipate continued declines in rotavirus-caused diarrhea and gastroenteritis.

WORDS TO KNOW

DEHYDRATION The loss of water and salts essential for normal body function. It occurs when the body loses more fluid than it takes in. Water is very important to the human body because it makes up about 70 percent of the muscles, around 75 percent of the brain, and approximately 92 percent of the blood. A person who weighs about 150 pounds (68 kilograms) will contain about 80 quarts (just over 75 liters) of water. About two cups (0.5 liter) of water are lost each day just from regular breathing. If the body sweats more and breathes heavier than normal, the human body loses even more water. Dehydration occurs when that lost water is not replenished.

FECAL-ORAL ROUTE The transmission of minute particles of fecal material from one organism (human or animal) to the mouth of another organism.

REHYDRATION The restoration of water after dehydration.

STRAIN A subclass or a specific genetic variation of an organism.

■ Disease History, Characteristics, and Transmission

Rotavirus is the causative agent for most cases of gastroenteritis among children globally. It was first shown to cause diarrhea in 1972 and was named the following year based on the wheel-like appearance of the virus. Of the several strains identified, Group A is associated with childhood gastroenteritis, and Groups B and C most often occur in adults. The disease is also called infantile diarrhea and winter diarrhea because outbreaks most commonly occur in infants and during the cooler months of winter.

Symptoms usually appear within 48 hours of infection and include fever, abdominal cramping, vomiting, and watery diarrhea, lasting up to eight days. Conditions may result in severe fluid loss leading to dehydration, which is a common complication associated with gastroenteritis. Signs of dehydration include dry lips, a dry tongue, dry skin, and sunken eyes. While dehydration is readily treatable, it is responsible for the fatalities associated with infections of this kind.

Rotavirus infections are highly contagious and are transmitted via the fecal-oral route. The highest incidence is among infants and children, where good hygiene is difficult to maintain. Following ingestion, the viral particles imbed in the mucosal layers of the small intestine and may be passed in excretions. The virus is stable in the environment, and infection may result from ingestion of contaminated food and water or from contact with contaminated surfaces, such as toys or tables. Prior infection does not produce complete immunity, but subsequent infections are usually less severe than the primary infection.

Scope and Distribution

Rotavirus was responsible for an estimated 130 million cases of diarrhea worldwide annually and more than 500,000 deaths in 2000; however, the introduction of a rotavirus vaccine has brought those numbers down substantially. Despite this, rotavirus remains a leading cause of illness and death in children. According to the World Health Organization, as of 2013 rotavirus caused the death of 215,000 children under the age of five each year. Globally, this represented 3.4 percent of all deaths for children of these ages.

Although the rotavirus vaccine had been approved for use in more than 100 countries as of 2016 and although numerous initiatives worked to provide access to these vaccines around the world, the impact of rotavirus is concentrated in certain countries. In 2013 Nigeria, Pakistan, the Democratic Republic of the Congo, and India accounted for 49 percent of all rotavirus deaths for children under age five. India alone accounted for 22 percent of these deaths. Other countries have almost eliminated fatal rotavirus cases. In the United States, only 163 deaths were attributed to rotavirus in 2013.

Although the vaccine is highly effective, rotavirus infection persists in developing nations where access to the vaccine, clean water, and health care is more difficult to access. Outbreaks occur due to the way in which the virus is transmitted and to the fact that contamination of a major water source often results in infection for everyone using that supply.

The highest rates of infection occur among infants and children. In developed nations rotavirus is most likely to occur before a child's second birthday. Children between the ages of 6 months and 24 months who attend day care are at higher risk for rotavirus infection. This is because these locations commonly harbor diseases transmitted by the fecal-oral route and it is difficult to ensure the maintenance of good hygiene practices, such as handwashing, at this young age.

Adults tend not to develop the disease, and adults in contact with the virus typically only develop a mild infection. Most instances of adult infection occur in elderly people and those with compromised immunity, such as

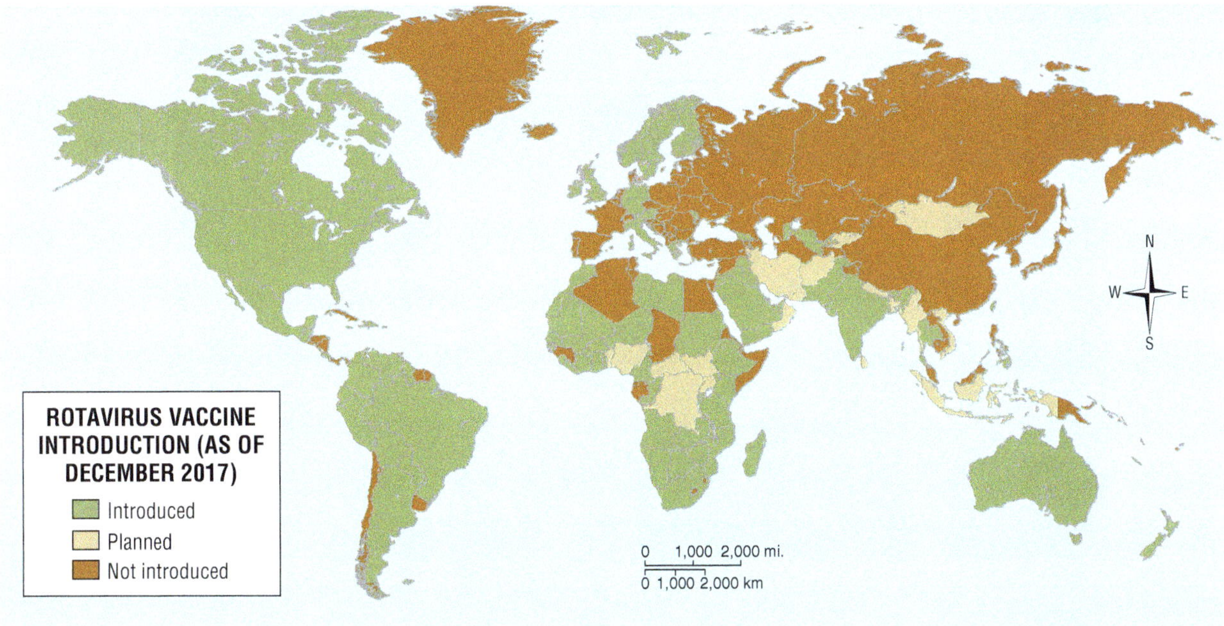

SOURCE: Rotavirus Organization of Technical Allies (ROTA) Council

transplant patients, chemotherapy patients, and people with human immunodeficiency virus (HIV).

Treatment and Prevention

In people with intact immunity, the infection is self-limiting, and symptoms will resolve within a few days of onset. While there is no specific treatment for the infection itself, oral rehydration therapy is essential and acts to restore the fluid lost as a result of severe dehydration. In developed countries electrolyte and fluid replacement solutions are readily available over the counter, although serious cases of dehydration may require hospitalization for intravenous treatment. Substantial rehydration options are much more limited in developing nations and, in cases of contaminated water supply, drinking the contaminated water further contributes to the infection rather than helping to treat the symptoms of the infection.

The environmental stability of rotavirus means that basic hygiene is often not enough to prevent infection. Improvements in food, water, and sanitation do not often reduce disease incidence, although they may be employed to limit the spread of the infection. In day care settings, monitoring children to ensure that they are correctly washing hands after toilet use and during food preparation can reduce the spread of the disease.

A combined vaccine to prevent all four strains of rotavirus known to cause severe gastroenteritis was approved for use in 1998. However, the vaccine was later withdrawn due to potentially fatal side effects involving blocking or twisting of the intestine. In 2006 the US Food and Drug Administration approved a new vaccine for use in the United States. A second vaccine was approved for use in Europe in 2006. The Rotavirus Vaccine Program (RVP) was established in 2003 by PATH with the support of the World Health Organization and the US Centers for Disease Control and Prevention. The goal of RVP was to make the vaccines available in developing countries. RVP was successful enough at expanding access to the rotavirus vaccine that it ended in 2008, having achieved its mission. Since that time the work of helping people access the vaccine has been taken up by a wide variety of organizations, some of them governmental and some of them private. As of January 2018, 45 million children were able to access the vaccine.

Impacts and Issues

While the progress made against rotavirus infections since the 2006 introduction of a rotavirus vaccine has helped drive down hospitalizations and deaths of children under age five, rotavirus remains a problem that disproportionately affects developing countries. In these countries, as of 2018 severe diarrhea was responsible annually for the death of some 500,000 children under age five. Rotavirus was the primary cause of such fatal diarrheal disease. As a result, there are numerous ongo-

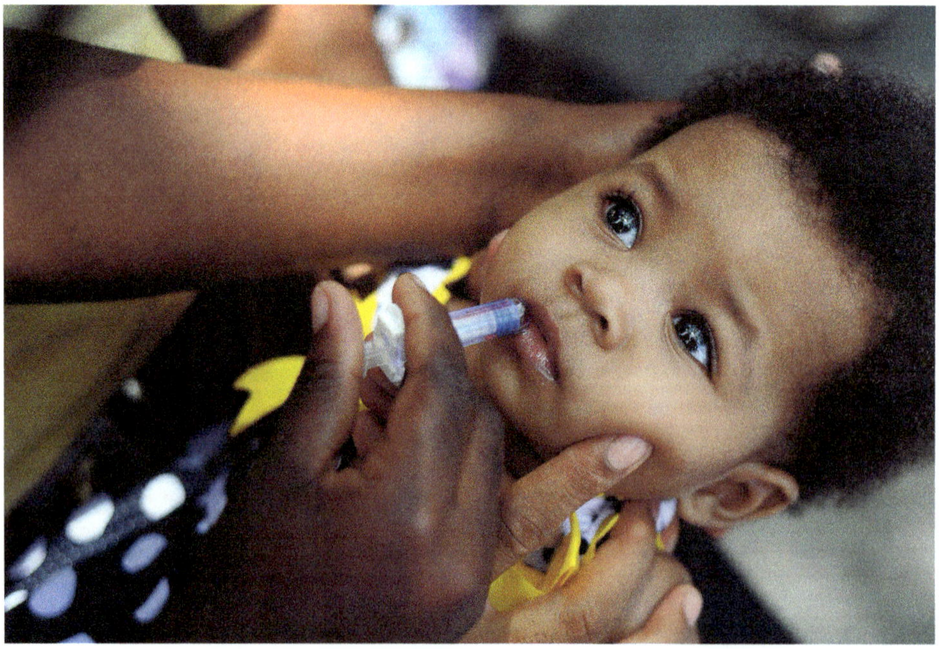

A nurse administers the rotavirus vaccine to a Haitian baby. In 2014 the Ministry of Public Health and Population of Haiti partnered with the Pan American Health Organization and the World Health Organization to make the vaccine freely available to all Haitians. Diarrhea caused by rotavirus is a leading killer of children under the age of five in Haiti. *© HECTOR RETAMAL/AFP/Getty Images*

ing efforts to expand access to the vaccine in countries where rotavirus remains a major public health issue. (PATH, for example, continues to support development of new vaccines to ensure affordability and expansion of coverage.) Such efforts involve both public and private initiatives. In 2009 South Africa became the first country to begin a rotavirus vaccination program. As of 2018 36 African countries had followed suit, adding rotavirus to their public vaccination programs. According to WHO, this has led to a one-third drop in the hospitalizations of children with rotavirus-caused diarrhea. The Indian government began to offer the vaccine to citizens in 2016. The next year the government of Pakistan initiated its own rotavirus-vaccination program. These programs alone will reach 30 million children a year once they are fully implemented. In addition, Nigeria, the Democratic Republic of Congo, Nepal, Bangladesh, and Afghanistan had plans to introduce rotavirus-vaccine programs as of early 2018.

Though the vaccine has become increasingly available, access has been limited by its cost, which is sometimes prohibitive in developing countries. Gavi, an international organization that aims to improve accessibility to various vaccines in poor countries, has helped enable low-income countries to purchase the rotavirus vaccine for only 40 cents per course, according to Mathuram Santosham and Duncan Steele's 2017 article in the *New England Journal of Medicine.*

Another factor that will likely drive down the cost of the rotavirus vaccine is the development of new vaccines, which will increase competition among vaccine manufacturers. As of early 2018, new vaccines were soon expected to receive approval for use in India, with other vaccines in development elsewhere in Asia.

See Also *Childhood-Associated Infectious Diseases, Immunization Impacts; Handwashing; Vaccines and Vaccine Development; Viral Disease; Waterborne Disease*

BIBLIOGRAPHY

Books

Mandell, G. L., J. E. Bennett, and R. Dolin. *Mandell, Douglas, and Bennett's Principles and Practice of Infectious Diseases.* Philadelphia: Saunders, 2015.

Svensson, Lennart, et al. *Viral Gastroenteritis: Molecular Epidemiology and Pathogenesis.* Amsterdam: Elsevier, 2016.

Periodicals

Burnett, Eleanor, et al. "Global Impact of Rotavirus Vaccination on Childhood Hospitalizations and Mortality from Diarrhea." *Journal of Infectious Diseases* 215, no. 11 (2017): 1666–1672. This article can also be found online at https://academic.oup.com/jid/article/215/11/1666/3738521 (accessed January 23, 2018).

Santosham, Mathuram, and Duncan Steele. "Rotavirus Vaccines—A New Hope." *New England Journal of Medicine* 376 (2017): 1170–1172.

Tate, Jacqueline E., et al. "Global, Regional, and National Estimates of Rotavirus Mortality in Children <5 Years of Age, 2000–2013." *Clinical Infectious Diseases* 62 (suppl.2) (2016): S96–S105. This article can also be found online at https://academic.oup.com/cid/article/62/suppl_2/S96/2478843 (accessed January 23, 2018).

Websites

PATH. "Accelerating Access to Rotavirus Vaccine." http://www.path.org/projects/rvp.php (accessed January 23, 2018).

"Rotavirus." Centers for Disease Control and Prevention, August 12, 2016. https://www.cdc.gov/rotavirus/index.html (accessed January 23, 2018).

"Rotavirus." Mayo Clinic. https://www.mayoclinic.org/diseases-conditions/rotavirus/symptoms-causes/syc-20351300 (accessed January 23, 2018).

"Rotavirus." World Health Organization, June 3, 2016. http://www.who.int/immunization/diseases/rotavirus/en/ (accessed January 23, 2018).

Santosham, Mathuram. "5 Reasons the Global Gap in Rotavirus Vaccine Access Is Shrinking. *Impatient Optimists*, January 9, 2018. https://www.impatientoptimists.org/Posts/2018/01/5-reasons-the-global-gap-in-rotavirus-vaccine-access-is-shrinking#.WmexOSOZPGK (accessed January 23, 2018).

"Vaccine Evidence." ROTA Council. http://rotacouncil.org/vaccine-evidence/ (accessed February 15, 2018).

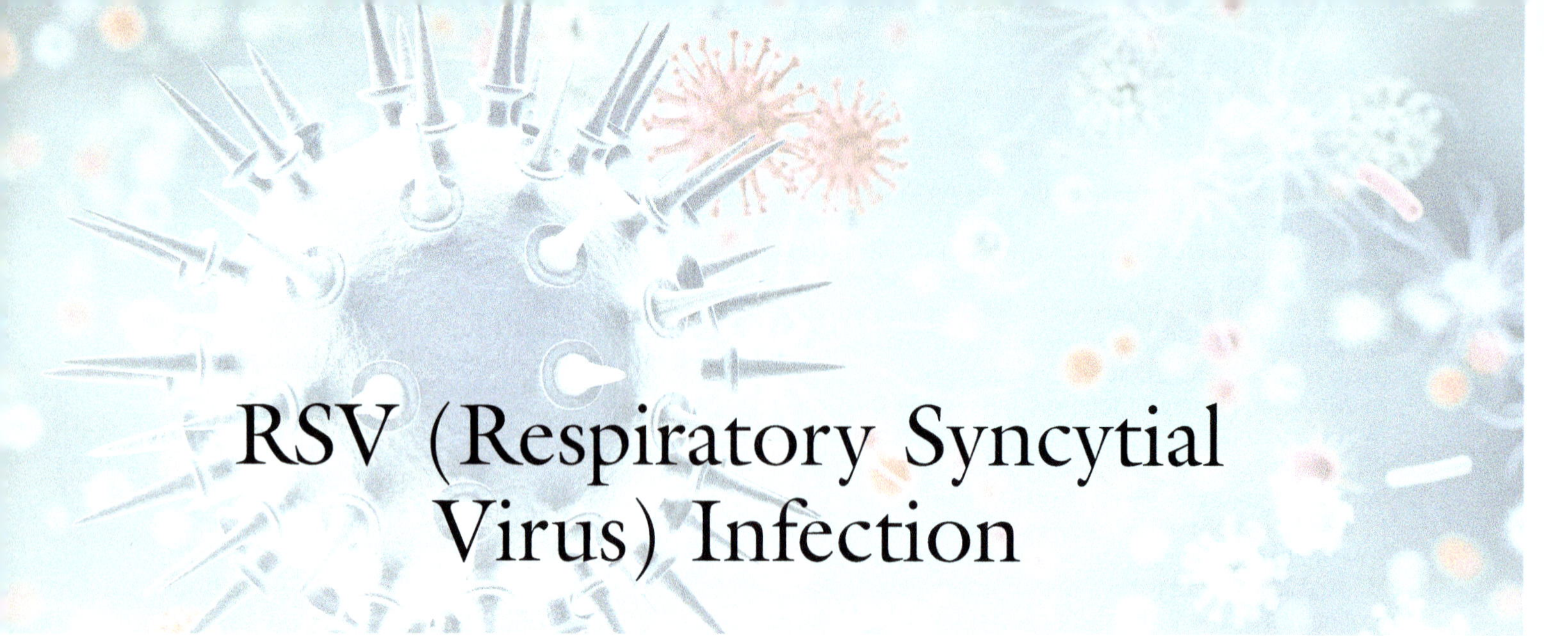

RSV (Respiratory Syncytial Virus) Infection

■ Introduction

Respiratory syncytial virus (RSV) is a ribonucleic acid (RNA)–containing virus that causes a lung infection (pneumonia) that affects the oxygen and carbon dioxide–carrying tubes called the bronchioles. These tubes are tiny and are located deep within the lungs. Because of this, the infection, which is also known as bronchiolitis, can hamper the function of the lungs.

RSV infection can be spread easily from person to person and can occur repeatedly in infants. It is the most common cause of bronchiolitis and pneumonia in newborns and infants under one year of age.

RSV infection can be lethal. As of 2017 the annual number of hospitalizations and deaths due to RSV infection globally (including developed countries) in children under five years was estimated to be 3.2 million and nearly 60,000, respectively.

■ Disease History, Characteristics, and Transmission

The first symptoms of an RSV lung infection are often mistaken for a cold. A child can have a fever and a runny nose. The involvement of the lungs can be evident as a cough and sometimes a wheezing type of breathing.

A lung infection that involves the bronchioles may not occur the first time someone is infected by RSV. However, up to 40 percent of infants experience the more severe lung infection. This can require hospitalization, especially in infants under six months of age.

Most children recover from the infection within a few weeks. However, repeated cold-like infections can then occur throughout life. In addition, the lung infection can be more serious, especially in elderly people or those whose immune systems are less capable of fighting off infections.

WORDS TO KNOW

ANTIBODIES Proteins found in the blood that help fight against foreign substances called antigens. Antigens, which are usually proteins or polysaccharides, stimulate the immune system to produce antibodies, or Y-shaped immunoglobulins. The antibodies inactivate the antigen and help remove it from the body. While antigens can be the source of infections from pathogenic bacteria and viruses, organic molecules detrimental to the body from internal or environmental sources also act as antigens. Genetic engineering and the use of various mutational mechanisms allow the construction of a vast array of antibodies (each with a unique genetic sequence).

ATTENUATED STRAIN A bacterium or virus that has been weakened. Often used as the basis of a vaccine against the specific disease caused by the bacterium or virus.

BRONCHIOLITIS An inflammation (-itis) of the bronchioles, the small air passages in the lungs that enter the alveoli (air sacs).

The virus is spread in the tiny drops of mucus and other fluids that are expelled from the nose during a sneeze and from the lungs when someone coughs. If another person is near, these drops can be inhaled, and the virus may then be able to establish an infection in the new host. Alternatively, the virus-laden droplets can land on inanimate objects such as doorknobs or can be transferred to a hand when the nose is wiped. Touching an object before the hands are washed can also transfer the virus. If the contaminated object is touched within a few hours, the virus can be picked up on the hands, and transfer to the new host can occur.

This route of transmission makes RSV infection especially prevalent in more northern climates during colder months, when people are indoors more often and the chances of person-to-person spread are greater. This sort of pattern is known as a community outbreak. Illness in warmer climates shows less of a seasonal pattern.

Scope and Distribution

RSV infection tends to be more prevalent in climates that have colder seasons because people are in closer indoor contact for part of the year. However, the infection can occur virtually anywhere. Because infants and the elderly are the most susceptible, RSV infection is associated with hospitals, day care centers, and retirement or elder care settings.

Treatment and Prevention

The spread of RSV can be minimized or even prevented by commonsense hygiene. Covering the nose and mouth with a tissue when sneezing or coughing can prevent the spread of virus-laden droplets in the air. Washing the hands with regular hand soap will inactivate any RSV on the skin.

The presence of the virus can be detected by isolation of the virus. In addition, molecular techniques can be used to detect protein components of the virus by the presence of antibodies to these proteins (antibodies are proteins produced by the immune system in response to the presence of a component that is foreign to the host) and by the presence of viral genetic material. These tests are specialized and require trained staff and a laboratory with the

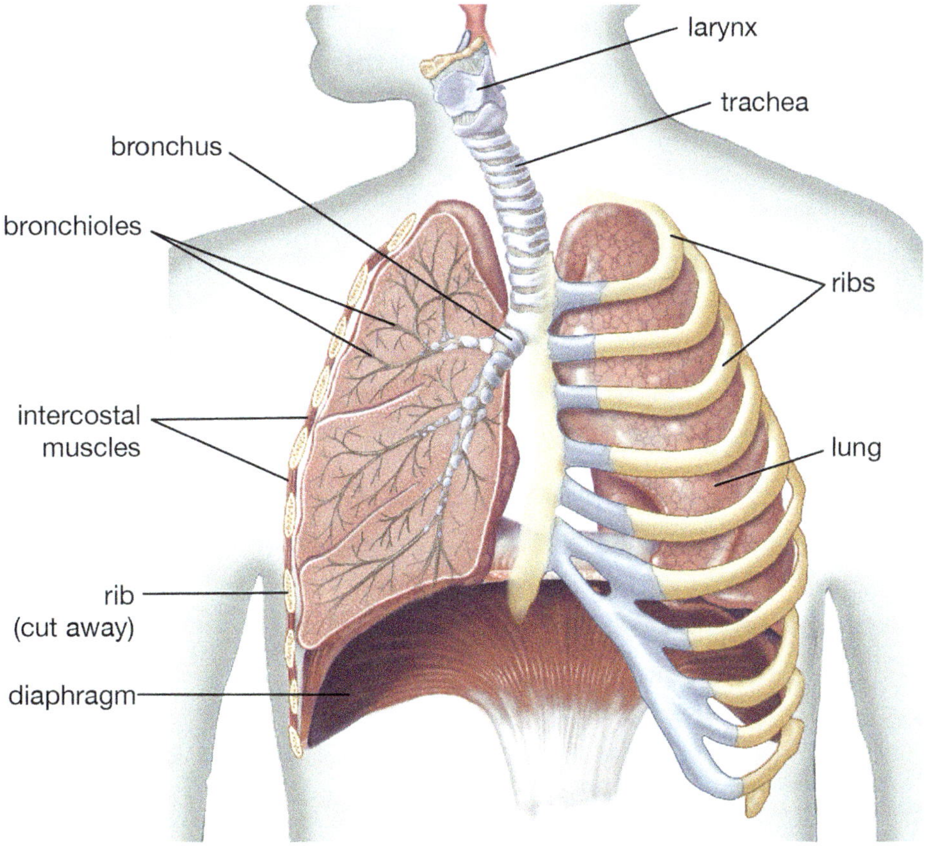

The respiratory syncytial virus (RSV) infects tiny airways in the lungs called bronchioles. Bronchioles, which branch off of larger tubes known as bronchi, carry inhaled air to elastic air sacs, or alveoli. RSV infection is the most common cause of bronchiolitis in newborns and infants under age one year. *© Encyclopaedia Britannica/AFP/Getty Images*

necessary equipment. Tests to monitor the antibody levels are the more common molecular approach.

Diagnosis is usually confirmed only for severe illnesses in hospitalized patients. For most people who have RSV infection, no specific treatment is administered because the illness is limited. In infants and children, treatment typically is aimed at reducing the discomfort caused by fever, and acetaminophen is most commonly used for this purpose.

More severe disease can require the use of supplemental oxygen or even mechanical ventilation (when a tube is inserted down the patient's trachea to deliver oxygen directly to the lungs), as the lungs may not be functioning efficiently. Antiviral drugs such as ribavirin are also administered. The drug is structurally similar to the viral RNA and thus can interfere with the process used by the virus to make new copies of itself.

Another treatment option for more severe RSV infection is the use of immune globulin, a compound produced by the immune system. This strategy is especially useful for people whose own immune systems are malfunctioning and are thus not as capable of producing the compound. Immune globulin is usually given intravenously.

The monoclonal antibody palivizumab can prevent severe RSV illness in infants and children thought to be at high risk of RSV. It cannot cure RSV.

Impacts and Issues

The fact that RSV infection predominantly affects the very young and the elderly makes it a concern for these age groups. In some cases lung function can be affected by RSV infection to the point that hospitalization and mechanical breathing assistance are necessary. In the United States about 80,000 children are hospitalized with RSV infections every year. People with asthma already have respiratory problems, which can be increased by this viral infection. Moreover, there is some evidence indicating that RSV infection could be a cause of the development of asthma, although clinical trials are still needed to make a firm conclusion of this relationship.

Almost half of otherwise healthy babies who are hospitalized with RSV develop asthma later in childhood. Asthma is the number one reason for school absences in children who have a chronic illness, resulting in about 14 million lost school days per year in the United States. In several studies researchers are tracking healthy newborns who develop RSV as they grow to determine genetic and environmental factors that may link RSV with asthma.

RSV infections also highlight the potential for an infectious disease to spread more easily in a crowded indoor environment and the importance of commonsense hygiene. Such hygienic measures as cleaning toys and equipment in day care centers and frequent handwashing can help to significantly minimize the risk of infection.

Efforts are ongoing to develop a vaccine against RSV. Researchers at Vanderbilt University are pursuing one approach that involves using genetic technologies to manipulate genes in the RSV virus. By causing small mutations or deletions in the genes of the virus, an improved attenuated (weakened) form of the RSV virus is produced that could lead to the development of a safe, efficient vaccine. In another approach, the replication of RSV was blocked in the presence of very small particles of gold (nanorods). The method has proven effective for other viruses, including human immunodeficiency virus (HIV), and is thought to trigger the signaling pathways in the infected cell that lead to the clearance of the virus. As of 2018 this approach was still being researched, and a vaccine for RSV was not yet available.

PRIMARY SOURCE

All That Glitters: Gold Nanoparticles Yield Possible Vaccine for Common Childhood Virus

SOURCE: *Akpan, Nsikan. "All That Glitters: Gold Nanoparticles Yield Possible Vaccine for Common Childhood Virus."* Medical Daily *(June 25, 2013). This article can also be found online at http://www.medicaldaily.com/all-glitters-gold-nanoparticles-yield-possible-vaccine-common-childhood-virus-247121 (accessed November 21, 2017).*

INTRODUCTION: *Tiny gold particles coated with sugar molecules could be the perfect vehicle for delivering new vaccines that help humans build immunity against dangerous viruses. Pediatricians at Vanderbilt University used gold nanoparticles to build a possible vaccine for respiratory syncytial virus, one of the most prevalent infections observed in infants. Details of their vaccine candidate were published today in* Nanotechnology.

Respiratory syncytial virus (RSV) is so common in babies, that it is assumed all newborns contract the disease before they are two years old. Most recover without any serious issues, but between 25 to 40 percent require hospitalization for pneumonia or bronchiolitis—inflammation of the lungs' smallest air passages, the bronchioles. In addition, adults who are immunocompromised and those over the age of 65 have an increased risk of severe consequences after RSV infection.

In order to prevent the 1 million worldwide deaths caused by RSV, a vaccine is needed. Gold nanoparticles are an attractive option because their tiny size mimics that of naturally occurring viruses.

"A vaccine for RSV, which is the major cause of viral pneumonia in children, is sorely needed," said lead author Dr. James Crowe.

The theory is that the gold nanoparticles can be coated with certain viral proteins that don't cause disease, but are recognized by cells in the human immune system. This could help people build immunity before contracting the virus.

"This platform could be used to develop experimental vaccines for virtually any virus, and in fact other larger microbes such as bacteria and fungi," remarked Crowe.

Crowe's team coated gold nanoparticles with viral material from respiratory syncytial virus, and then exposed these glittery carriers to human dendritic cells in a petri dish.

Dendritic cells are the immune system's sentinels. When they come across a dangerous germ, they capture it and then present it to more aggressive immune system members—B cells and T cells—that mount a serious attack against the invader.

After being exposed to gold particles, the primed dendritic cells were transferred to a petri dish with T cells. The T cells became active and began multiplying, a sign that they were preparing an immune defense.

The researchers also found that the gold nanoparticles were non-toxic to these human cells.

"The studies we performed showed that the candidate vaccines stimulated human immune cells when they were interacted in the lab," concluded Crowe. "The next steps to testing would be to test whether or not the vaccines work in vivo [in animal models, humans.]"

SEE ALSO *Public Health and Infectious Disease*

BIBLIOGRAPHY

Books

Tripp, Ralph A., and Patricia A. Jorquera. *Human Respiratory Syncytial Virus: Methods and Protocols.* New York: Humana, 2016.

Periodicals

Russell, Clark D., et al. "The Human Immune Response to Respiratory Syncytial Virus Infection." *Clinical Microbiology Reviews* 30, no. 2 (April 2017): 481–502.

Weinberg, Geoffrey A. "Respiratory Syncytial Virus Mortality Among Young Children." *Lancet Global Health* 5 (October 2017): e951–e952.

Websites

"Respiratory Syncytial Virus." Centers for Disease Control and Prevention. January 1, 2005. http://www.cdc.gov/rsv/index.html (accessed November 21, 2017).

"Respiratory Syncytial Virus (RSV)." Mayo Clinic. https://www.mayoclinic.org/diseases-conditions/respiratory-syncytial-virus/symptoms-causes/syc-20353098 (accessed November 21, 2017).

Brian Hoyle

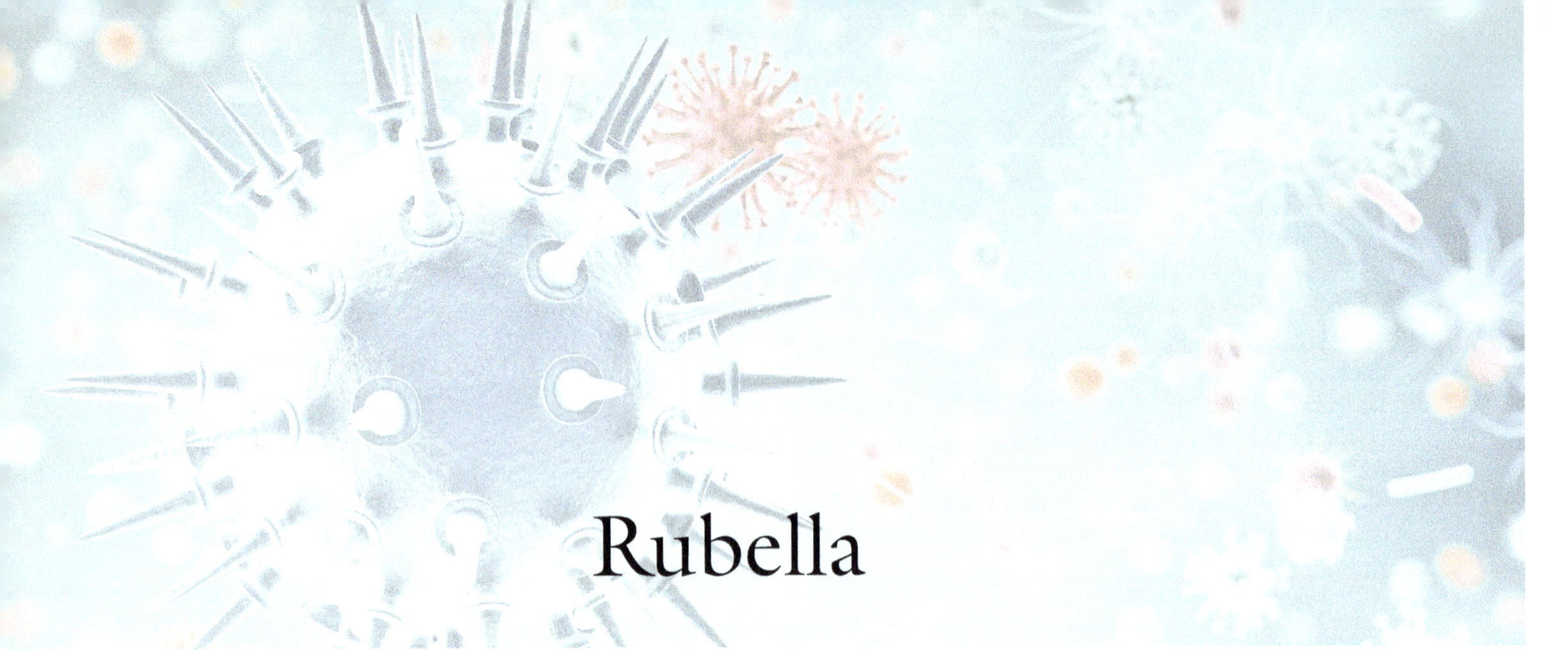

Rubella

Introduction

The word *rubella* comes from the Latin word for "little red" and refers to the characteristic rash that accompanies the disease. It was first described in the early 19th century, when it was thought to be a type of either scarlet fever or measles. German doctors then decided that rubella was a disease in its own right, which is why it is sometimes called German measles.

People of any age can contract rubella, and there were many epidemics in the first half of the 20th century. Rubella only poses a real risk, however, to a developing fetus. Infection during the first three months of pregnancy can cause the child to be born with congenital rubella syndrome (CRS), which may be accompanied by deafness, mental retardation, and blindness. Vaccination has greatly reduced the rate of rubella in the United States and the European Union, and it is especially important that women of childbearing age are protected from the disease.

Disease History, Characteristics, and Transmission

The rubella virus belongs to the togavirus family and is a single-stranded ribonucleic acid (RNA) virus—that is, its genetic material is RNA, not deoxyribonucleic acid (DNA). It only naturally infects humans, although other

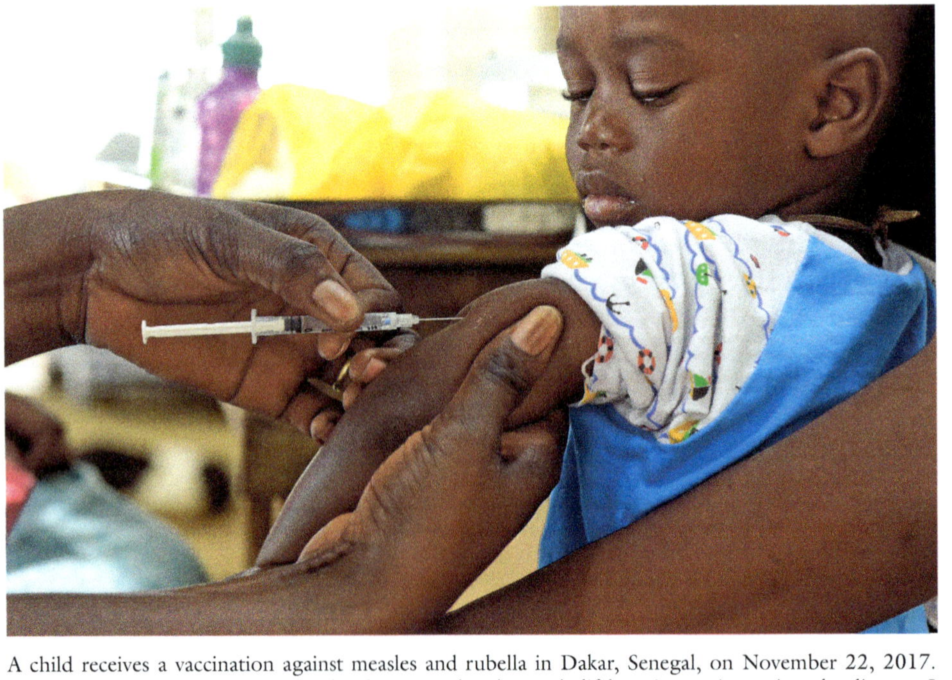

A child receives a vaccination against measles and rubella in Dakar, Senegal, on November 22, 2017. Vaccinations against rubella are widely administered and provide lifelong immunity against the disease. © *SEYLLOU/AFP/Getty Images*

animals can be infected in experimental conditions. The incubation period of rubella virus is around 14 days, and infections are most common in late winter and early spring.

Most people with rubella infection have no, or only mild, symptoms. A rash, which is sometimes the only symptom, appears around 14 to 17 days after exposure to the virus. This rash is fainter than a measles rash and consists of tiny red spots. The rubella rash typically begins on the face and then spreads down the trunk to the rest of the body. Sometimes the rash is preceded by fever and swollen glands; tiny red spots may appear on the soft palate. Generally the rash clears up in three to four days.

Adults are more prone to complications and more severe symptoms of rubella than children. Arthritis in the fingers, wrists, and knees affects 70 percent of adult females with rubella. Encephalitis (inflammation of the brain) is a rare complication, affecting 1 in 6,000 rubella cases, and clinical studies have suggested a mortality rate varying between 0 and 50 percent.

Congenital rubella syndrome occurs among babies born to a mother who was infected with the virus during early pregnancy, particularly in the first 8 to 10 weeks. Rubella can affect all the organs of a developing fetus. Deafness is the most common symptom, but cataracts and other visual defects and neurological abnormalities may also occur. The problems may not appear until the child is two to four years old. Other complications arising from CRS include diabetes, anemia, enlargement of the liver and spleen, and autism. Maternal infections occurring after 20 weeks of pregnancy are far less likely to lead to CRS.

Rubella is transmitted by the respiratory route through coughs and sneezes. It is only moderately contagious. People without symptoms may still be infectious. Those with symptoms are at their most infectious when the rash appears.

WORDS TO KNOW

ENDEMIC Present in a particular area or among a particular group of people.

MEASLES Infectious disease caused by a virus of the paramyxovirus group. It infects only humans, and the infection results in lifelong immunity to the disease. It is one of several exanthematous (rash-producing) diseases of childhood, which include rubella (German measles), chickenpox, and the now-rare scarlet fever. The disease is particularly common in both preschool-age children and young school-age children.

MMR VACCINE A vaccine that is given to protect someone from measles, mumps, and rubella. The vaccine is made up of viruses that cause the three diseases. The viruses are incapable of causing the diseases but still stimulate the immune system.

NOTIFIABLE DISEASE A disease that the law requires must be reported to health officials when diagnosed; also called a reportable disease.

RIBONUCLEIC ACID (RNA) Any of a group of nucleic acids that carry out several important tasks in the synthesis of proteins. Unlike deoxyribonucleic acid (DNA), it has only a single strand. Nucleic acids are complex molecules that contain a cell's genetic information and the instructions for carrying out cellular processes. In eukaryotic cells, the two nucleic acids, RNA and DNA, work together to direct protein synthesis. Although it is DNA that contains the instructions for directing the synthesis of specific structural and enzymatic proteins, several types of RNA actually carry out the processes required to produce these proteins. These include messenger RNA (mRNA), ribosomal RNA (rRNA), and transfer RNA (tRNA). Further processing of the various RNAs is carried out by another type of RNA called small nuclear RNA (snRNA). The structure of RNA is very similar to that of DNA, however, instead of the base thymine, RNA contains the base uracil in its place.

TOGAVIRUS A single-stranded ribonucleic acid (RNA) virus.

Scope and Distribution

Rubella has been known since the 19th century and was long thought to be a trivial disease. Then, in 1941, Australian ophthalmologist Norman Gregg (1892–1966) reported a worrying trend—78 cases of severe cataracts among newborns, all of which could be traced back to rubella infection among the mothers in early pregnancy. Later, other problems such as heart defects, deafness, and mental retardation were noted in such babies. CRS is now diagnosed in about 85 percent of babies who have been exposed to rubella in the womb.

Epidemics of rubella were the norm every 7 to 10 years throughout the first half of the 20th century and were always followed by an increase in the number of cases of CRS. The last major epidemic in the United States was in 1964 when there were 20,000 resulting cases of CRS and many deaths of babies in the womb.

Rubella and CRS became notifiable diseases in the United States in 1966, and a peak of 57,686 cases was noted in 1969, the year in which a vaccine was first introduced. Since then cases have fallen to around 0.5 per 100,000 of the population, although there have been outbreaks in California (1990) and among the Amish people of Pennsylvania (1991). Following these outbreaks, California reported 25 new cases of CRS; Pennsylvania reported 33. The National Congenital Rubella Registry, which is

SCIENTIFIC, POLITICAL, AND ETHICAL ISSUES

In the late 1990s the public began to express concern that the presence of thimerosal, a mercury-containing compound added to vaccines as a preservative, might be causing autism spectrum disorders (ASD). However, a 2004 scientific review by the Institute of Medicine (IOM) concluded, "The evidence favors rejection of a causal relationship between thimerosal-containing vaccines and autism." The US Centers for Disease Control and Prevention (CDC) has also weighed in definitively: "There is no link between vaccines and autism."

To put the question to rest, the CDC has taken part in several studies looking at the issue. In fact, between 2003 and 2015, there were nine CDC-funded or conducted studies that found no link between thimerosal-containing vaccines and ASD, as well as no link between the measles, mumps, and rubella (MMR) vaccine and ASD in children.

For the CDC and other public health groups around the world, emphasizing the safety and importance of vaccines is essential to protecting the population from outbreaks of diseases such as rubella. According to the CDC, "What would happen if we stopped vaccinations? We could soon find ourselves battling epidemics of diseases we thought we had conquered decades ago." Without vaccinating, the CDC further explained, more people will become ill, and some of those people will die.

The MMR vaccination offers a lot of protection against disease, especially rubella. "Because of successful vaccination programs, rubella has been eliminated from the United States since 2004," the CDC states. "However, rubella is still common in other countries. Unvaccinated people can get rubella while abroad and bring the disease to the United States and spread it to others." Two doses of MMR vaccine are 97 percent effective against measles and 88 percent effective against mumps. One dose of MMR vaccine is 93 percent effective against measles, 78 percent effective against mumps, and 97 percent effective against rubella.

managed by the National Immunization Program, carries out the national surveillance of CRS.

In 2004 the Centers for Disease Control and Prevention (CDC) declared that rubella was no longer endemic in the United States. In 2015 the World Health Organization (WHO) certified that endemic transmissions of rubella and CRS had been eliminated throughout the Americas, the first region in the world to successfully eradicate the disease. WHO's Global Measles and Rubella Strategic Plan includes the goal to eliminate measles and rubella from at least five regions by 2020.

Rubella occurs around the world, and it can affect people of any age. However, only about 10 percent of cases occur in people over 40 years old. In the early 21st century, adults between 15 and 39 have accounted for about half of all cases, so rubella is no longer considered a childhood disease.

Treatment and Prevention

There is no treatment for rubella infection. The first live vaccines were introduced in 1969 and were replaced by an improved version in 1979. Rubella vaccine is now given in combination with mumps and measles vaccinations, which is known as the MMR vaccine, or in combination with measles, mumps, and varicella (chickenpox) vaccinations, which is known as MMRV. The MMRV vaccine is only licensed for use in children 12 months through 12 years of age. It is recommended that a child be vaccinated with MMR between the age of 12 and 15 months and that he or she should receive another dose before school entry.

Women of childbearing age should be checked for their immunity to rubella; this is possible through a simple blood test. A test is necessary because other conditions may be mistaken for rubella, making a report of having had the infection in childhood unreliable. The test can be administered as part of regular gynecologic care at a family planning clinic, a sexual health clinic, or a doctor's office.

WHO implemented a program to increase the rate of rubella vaccination worldwide. According to WHO, as of December 2016, 152 countries around the world had introduced a rubella vaccine, though vaccination rates varied widely, from around 13 to 99 percent. The program contributed to a sharp global decline in reported rubella cases, from 670,894 cases across 102 countries in 2000 to 22,361 cases across 165 countries in 2016. Infection rates were highest in regions with the lowest vaccination rates, including Africa and Southeast Asia.

The rubella vaccine is safe, and two doses confer lifelong immunity. Any adverse effects from MMR are likely due to the measles component, not the rubella component. However, there is a small theoretical risk that an unborn child could be affected by rubella vaccine; therefore, it is not recommended for pregnant women or for women who might become pregnant within four weeks of receiving the vaccine. Researchers have also found that, in countries with lower vaccination rates, introduction of the rubella vaccine can raise the average age of rubella infections, making it more likely that a woman will become infected while pregnant and raising the risk of CRS. WHO therefore recommends that the rubella vaccine only be introduced in countries that have vaccination rates of 80 percent or higher.

Impacts and Issues

Despite mass vaccination efforts in the United States, as of 2017 there were still an average of five to six cases of CRS per year. Although the numbers are tiny, each case represents a family tragedy and is costly in terms of health care for the child involved. In fact, costs for rubella and CRS cases vary worldwide, as do the studies of cost effectiveness of the rubella vaccine. Cost effectiveness varies widely depending on the nation where the study was conducted, the type of vaccine used, and the number of doses given. One 2013 US study estimated that a two-dose MMR program would save $231 per rubella case prevented and $683,813 for every CRS case prevented.

Worldwide, rubella continues to cause illness. Outbreaks are common and costly. For example, the state of Maharashtra in India had 94 confirmed outbreaks of measles and rubella in 2013, according to a study in the *Indian Journal of Medical Research.* Indian health workers, much like others around the globe, continued to call for increased vaccine coverage.

See Also *Measles (Rubeola); Mumps; Scarlet Fever*

BIBLIOGRAPHY

Books

Beers, Mark H., ed. *The Merck Manual of Medical Information.* London: Gallery, 2008.

Weston, Debbie, Alison Burgess, and Sue Roberts. *Infection Prevention and Control at a Glance.* Newark, NJ: Wiley, 2016.

Periodicals

Babigumira, Joseph B., Ian Morgan, and Ann Levin. "Health Economics of Rubella: A Systematic Review to Assess the Value of Rubella Vaccination." *BMC Public Health* 13, no. 406 (2013). This article can also be found online at https://bmcpublichealth.biomedcentral.com/articles/10.1186/1471-2458-13-406 (accessed January 16, 2018).

Lessler, Justin, and C. Jessica E. Metcalf. "Balancing Evidence and Uncertainty When Considering Rubella Vaccine Introduction." *PLOS One* 8, no. 7 (July 2013). This article can also be found at http://journals.plos.org/plosone/article?id=10.1371/journal.pone.0067639 (accessed January 16, 2018).

Vaidya, Sunil R., et al. "Measles & Rubella Outbreaks in Maharashtra State, India." *Indian Journal of Medical Research* 143, no. 2 (February 2016): 227–231. This article can also be found online at https://www.ncbi.nlm.nih.gov/pmc/articles/PMC4859132/ (accessed February 12, 2018).

Websites

"Americas Region Is Declared the World's First to Eliminate Rubella." Pan American Health Organization, April 29, 2015. http://www.paho.org/hq/index.php?option=com_content&view=article&id=10798&Itemid=1926 (accessed January 16, 2018).

"Rubella." World Health Organization, January 2018. http://www.who.int/mediacentre/factsheets/fs367/en/ (accessed January 16, 2018).

"Rubella (German Measles, Three-Day Measles)." Centers for Disease Control and Prevention, September 15, 2017. https://www.cdc.gov/rubella/index.html (accessed January 16, 2018).

"Rubella (German Measles) Vaccination." Centers for Disease Control and Prevention, November 16, 2016. https://www.cdc.gov/vaccines/vpd/rubella/index.html (accessed February 12, 2018).

"Vaccine Safety." Centers for Disease Control and Prevention, August 14, 2017. https://www.cdc.gov/vaccinesafety/index.html (accessed February 12, 2018).

Susan Aldridge
Sam Uretsky

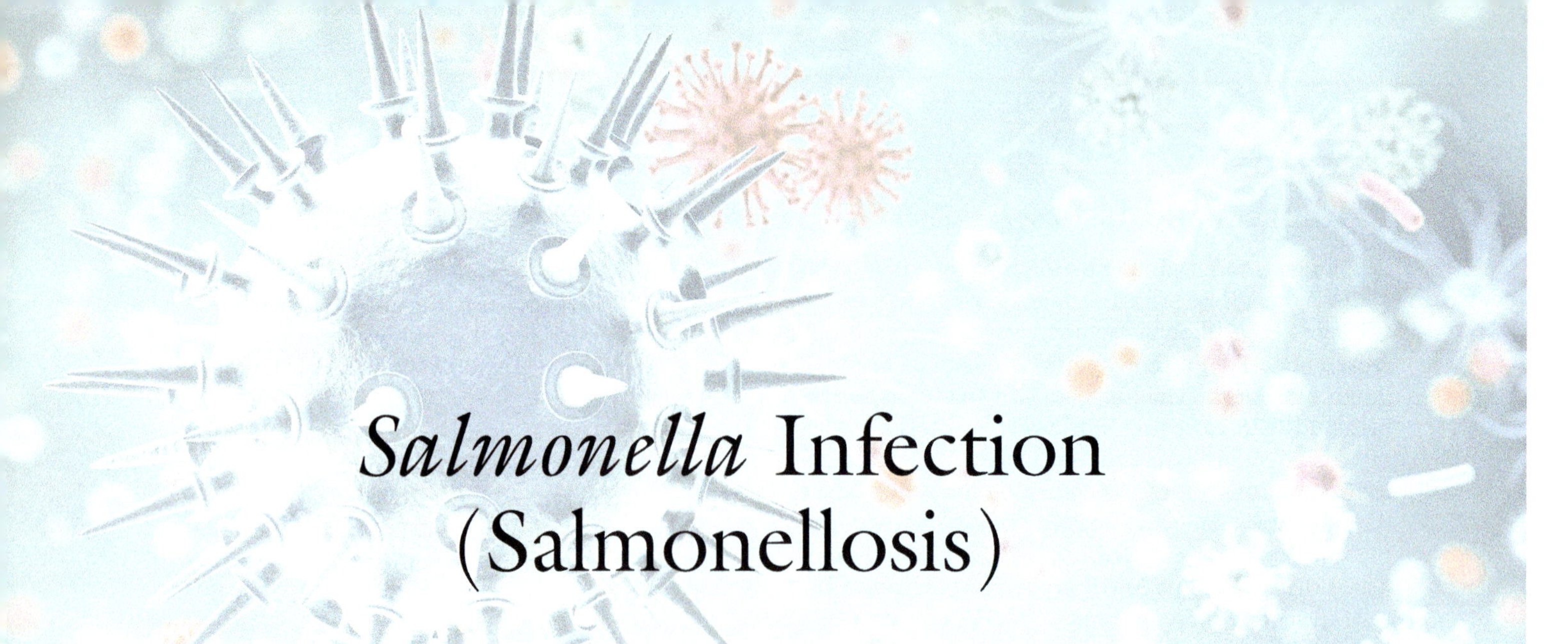

Salmonella Infection (Salmonellosis)

Introduction

Salmonellosis refers to an infection in humans caused by bacteria of the genus *Salmonella*. Contamination of food by the bacteria is a common cause of salmonellosis.

WORDS TO KNOW

CONTAMINATION The unwanted presence of a microorganism or compound in a particular environment. That environment may be a laboratory setting, for example, in a medium being used for the growth of bacteria during an experiment. Another environment is the human body, where contamination by bacteria can produce an infection. Contamination by bacteria and viruses can occur on several levels and their presence can adversely influence the results of laboratory experiments. Outside the laboratory, bacteria and viruses can contaminate drinking water supplies, foodstuffs, and products, causing illness.

ENTEROTOXIN A class of toxin produced by bacteria. Unlike exotoxins, which are released by bacteria, enterotoxins reside with the bacterial cells.

LIPOPOLYSACCHARIDE (LPS) A molecule that is a constituent of the outer membrane of Gram-negative bacteria. LPS is also referred to as an endotoxin. It helps protect the bacterium from host defenses and can contribute to illness in the host.

SEROTYPE Also known as a serovar, a class of microorganism based on the types of antigens (molecules that elicit an immune response) presented on the surface of the microorganism. A single species may have thousands of serotypes with medically distinct behaviors.

TOXIN A poison produced by a living organism.

Salmonellosis may be caused by food infection or food intoxication depending on the antigenic type (serotype) of *Salmonella* involved. Food infection relies on the growth of the bacteria to levels capable of causing symptoms, whereas food intoxication does not require growth of the contaminating strain. Salmonellosis is most often caused by food infection, but it may also be caused by food intoxication if enough toxin-loaded bacteria are ingested.

Salmonellosis is common and widespread. Of particular concern is the emergence of *Salmonella* that are resistant to many commonly used antibiotics.

Disease History, Characteristics, and Transmission

Salmonella is a gram-negative, rod-shaped bacterium named after Daniel Salmon (1850–1914). In 1885 Salmon, along with Theobald Smith (1859–1934), isolated the bacterium from pigs. Since then more than 2,500 serotypes of the bacterium have been found. The term *serotype* refers to the protein composition of the bacterial surface, which produces a distinct immune response by the host. The many different *Salmonella* serotypes indicate that the surface of *salmonella* is highly variable.

Salmonella is commonly found in the gastrointestinal tract of humans and other animals, where it is of no concern. However, if food or water contaminated with *Salmonella*-containing feces is ingested, illness can result. As with other fecal bacteria, food contamination most often occurs when the food is handled by someone who has not properly washed his or her hands after having a bowel movement. Good hygiene is important in minimizing the risk of salmonellosis.

Salmonellosis is caused most often by two strains: *S. typimurium* and *S. enteritidis*. Other serotypes of the bacterium usually cause disease in animals such as cattle and pigs. If these serotypes infect humans, the infection can be severe and even life threatening.

Poultry carcasses can be contaminated with intestinal contents during slaughter of the bird. The bacteria can remain alive long enough for the carcass to be shipped to a grocery store and sold. Although the bacteria are readily killed by heat, if cooking is inadequate, the surviving organisms can cause illness. Eggs can also be contaminated if the shell has a crack or break, which allows the bacteria to enter the egg. Other foods that are often involved in salmonellosis are raw or undercooked meat, processed meat, dairy products, custards and cream-based desserts, and sandwich filling such as tuna or chicken salad.

Symptoms of salmonellosis develop within a few hours of eating contaminated food. The symptoms include abdominal cramping, nausea with vomiting, fever, headache, chills and sweating, a feeling of weakness, and loss of appetite. Some people also develop watery diarrhea or, if cells lining the intestine are damaged, bloody diarrhea. The rapid loss of fluids due to diarrhea can be dangerous to infants and the elderly. Less commonly, the infection may spread to the bloodstream. Some people can develop a painful condition called Reiter's syndrome, which can persist for years and lead to arthritis.

For most people the infection lasts four to seven days. Most people recover without needing medical attention. However, severe diarrhea usually results in hospitalization.

Outbreaks of salmonellosis can occur due to the consumption of contaminated food in a restaurant or at a social gathering. Data from the food-borne outbreak database of the US Centers for Disease Control and Prevention (CDC) indicated that between 2007 and 2016 there were 8,726 outbreaks (in which two or more people experienced salmonellosis) resulting in 159,298 illnesses, 8,726 hospitalizations, and 207 deaths.

Globally, according to the World Health Organization (WHO), one of every four cases of diarrheal illness is due to salmonellosis.

The bacteria that cause salmonellosis possess what are termed virulence factors, or molecules that enable the bacteria to establish an infection. One important virulence factor is called adhesin. This is a molecule that can recognize a target site on the host cell and help the bacterium adhere to the host cell target. An example of a *Salmonella* adhesin are tubes called fimbriae that protrude from the bacterial surface. The end of each fimbriae contains a protein that can bind with a specific host cell surface protein.

Another virulence factor is called lipopolysaccharide (LPS). There are many different structures of LPS. Those that are longer can help shield the bacterial surface from host compounds that can damage or kill the bacteria. Furthermore, a part of LPS called lipid A is a toxin.

Some strains of *Salmonella* also produce enterotoxin. This toxin is located inside the bacteria, so, as the numbers of *Salmonella* increase, the concentration of the enterotoxin in the food increases. Ingesting the food releases the enterotoxin in the intestine, where it ruptures the intestinal cells by forming a hole in their cell membrane.

Scope and Distribution

Salmonellosis is global in occurrence and common. According to data from the CDC, more than 1 million cases of salmonellosis resulting in 19,000 hospitaliza-

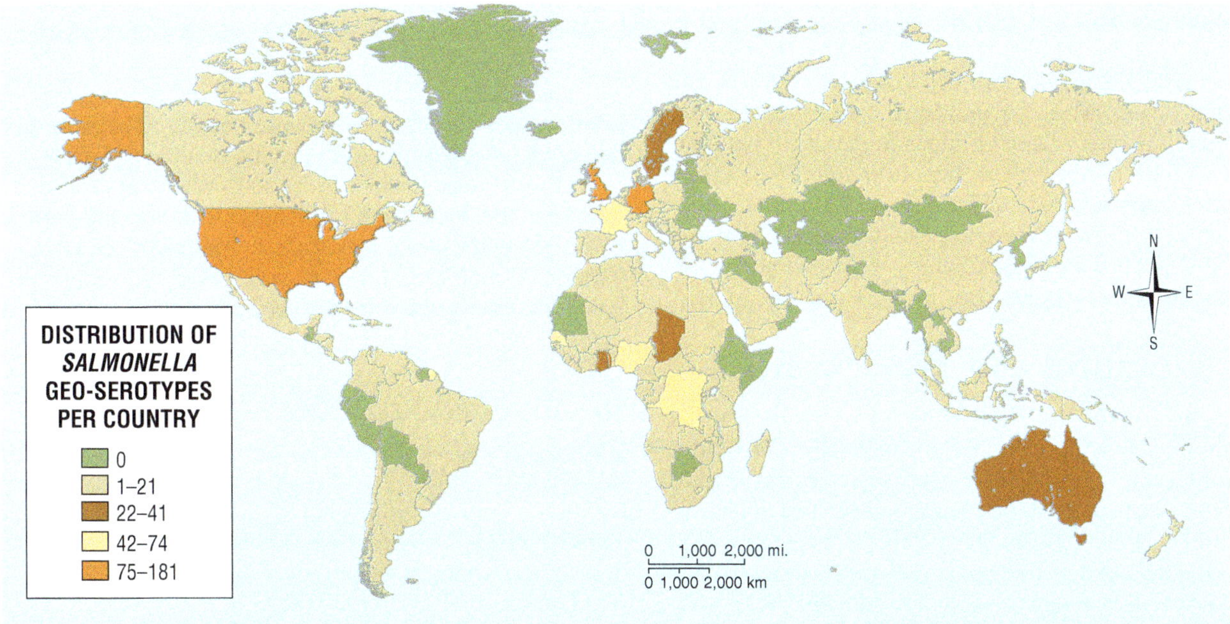

SOURCE: Adapted from "Around the World in 1,475 Salmonella Geo-serotypes." US Centers for Disease Control and Prevention. 2016. Available from: https://wwwnc.cdc.gov/eid/article/22/7/14-1678_article

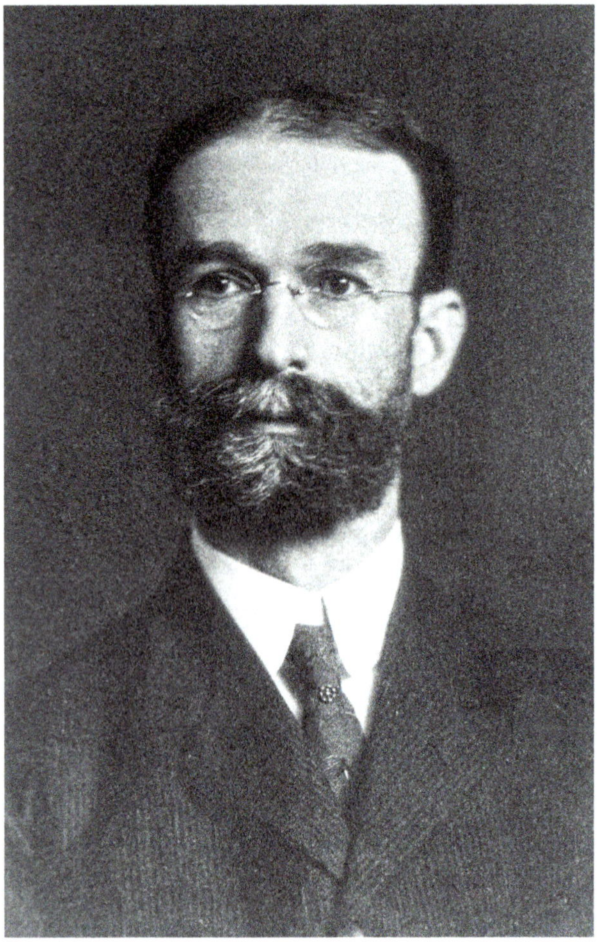

Theobald Smith, American epidemiologist. Smith discovered the genus of bacteria known today as *Salmonella*. The genus was named after Smith's research supervisor, Daniel Elmer Salmon. © NLM/Science Source

tions and 380 deaths are reported each year in the United States. Most are individual cases, which is why the total number of cases is much higher than the number of illnesses reported during outbreaks.

In September 2017 235 people in 26 US states were sickened after eating papayas contaminated with *Salmonella* shipped north from Mexico.

Treatment and Prevention

Diagnosis of salmonellosis relies on recognition of its symptoms and the identification of *Salmonella* from a stool (fecal) sample. Current tests that detect certain *Salmonella* proteins do not require growth of the bacteria and thus can be completed within hours.

Identification of the type of *Salmonella* involved usually helps in determining which antibiotics to use. Salmonellosis usually responds well to antibiotics, though serotypes of *Salmonella* that are resistant to a variety of antibiotics are becoming more common. According to the CDC, in 2013 10 percent of tested *Salmonella* samples were resistant to three or more classes of antibiotics. This was roughly equivalent to the number of multidrug-resistant samples tested in 2012. However, 46 percent of samples of one *Salmonella* serotype were found to be multidrug resistant, which was a rate more than twice as high as the rate for that serotype in 2011. In 2016 the CDC linked resistance to four serotypes: Enteritidis, Newport, Typhimurium, and Heidelberg. These four serotypes were reported to account for 73 percent of all resistant *Salmonella* infections.

Prevention involves good hygiene, including handwashing and the cleaning of cooking utensils and equipment that have been used with foods such as poultry and ground meat before reuse. Foods containing raw eggs should not be eaten. Even if the eggs appeared intact, cracks that are not visible are large enough to allow bacteria to contaminate the egg.

Researchers are exploring the production of a vaccine against salmonellosis. The most promising strategy is to block the adhesion of the bacteria to the intestinal cells. This strategy has proven successful in developing a vaccine that appeared on the market in 2006 for another intestinal bacterium called *Escherichia coli* O157:H7 (*E. coli* O157:H7).

Impacts and Issues

Salmonellosis has major economic impacts. According to the US Department of Agriculture, the costs of treatment for salmonellosis in the United States in 2015 were $3.7 billion. Millions of people each year miss work and school because of the illness. Exact figures for the costs of the disease are difficult to obtain, especially in developing countries, where cases of salmonellosis may not be reported.

The human suffering and economic consequences of salmonellosis are likely to increase with the continuing spread of *Salmonella* serotypes that are resistant to a variety of commonly used antibiotics. In 2001 WHO, in collaboration with the CDC, began the Global Salm-Surv program to determine the global prevalence and antibiotic resistance patterns of multidrug-resistant *Salmonella*. The program name was changed to the Global Foodborne Infections Network in 2009 and was still active in 2017.

SEE ALSO *Food-Borne Disease and Food Safety*

BIBLIOGRAPHY

Books

Barach, Jeffrey T. *FSMA and Food Safety Systems: Understanding and Implementing the Rules.* Hoboken, NJ: Wiley, 2017.

Hackett, Christopher B. *Salmonella: Prevalence, Risk Factors and Treatment Options.* New York: Nova Science, 2015.

Periodicals

DuPont, Herbert L. "The Growing Threat of Foodborne Bacterial Enteropathogens of Animal Origin." *Clinical Infectious Diseases* 45, no. 10 (2007): 1353–1361.

Waters, Andrew E., et al. "Multidrug-Resistant *Staphylococcus aureus* in US Meat and Poultry." *Clinical Infectious Diseases* 52, no. 10 (2011): 1227–1230.

Websites

"Global Foodborne Infections Network (GFN)." World Health Organization. http://www.who.int/gfn/en/ (accessed November 21, 2017).

"Salmonella." Centers for Disease Control and Prevention. https://www.cdc.gov/salmonella/ (accessed November 21, 2017).

Brian Hoyle

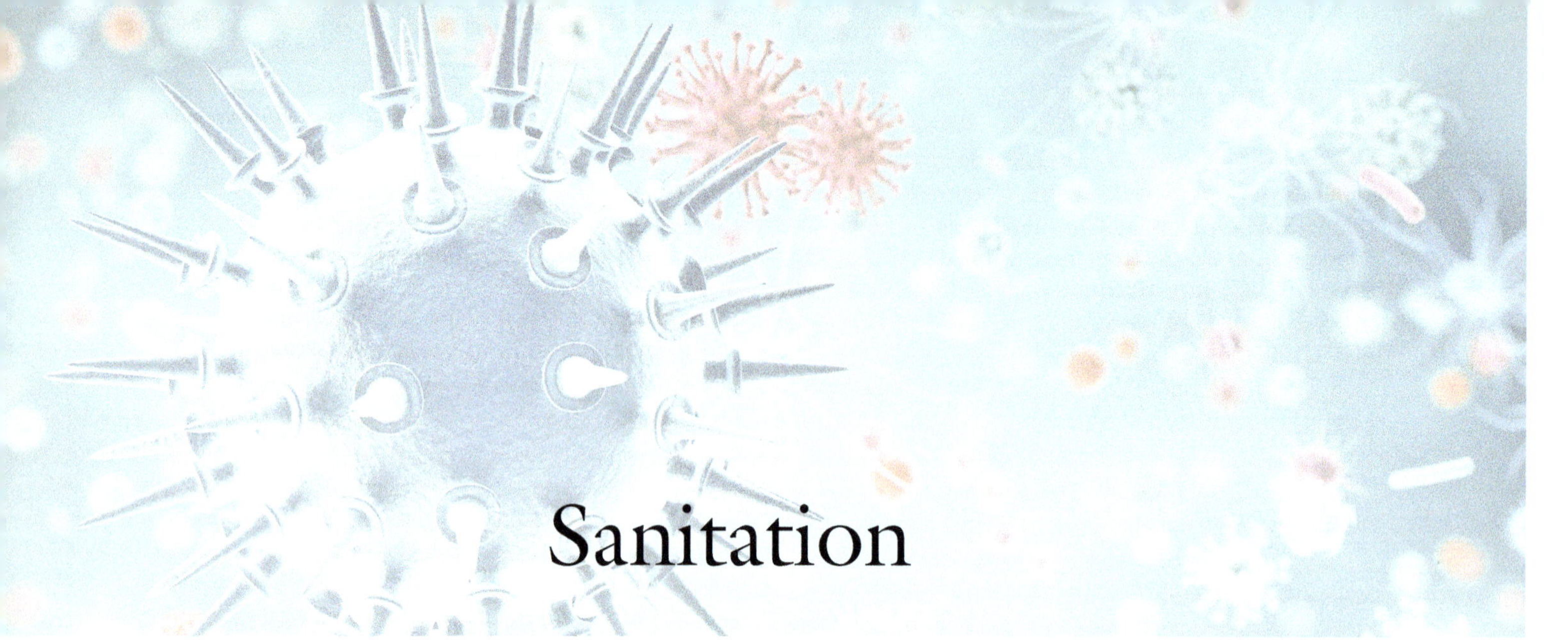

Sanitation

Introduction

Poor sanitation, which involves the contamination of drinking water by fecal matter, permits infectious diseases to spread. In the developed world, water treatment has practically eliminated cholera, typhoid, and dysentery. In the developing world, however, the absence of safe drinking water and latrines is associated with high rates of diarrheal illness. Unimproved sanitation includes public or shared latrines, pit latrines without slabs or open pits, hanging toilets or hanging latrines (a platform for defecation over a body of water), bucket latrines, and an absence of facilities, which forces people to use unsuitable areas for defecation.

People lacking sanitation live primarily in Asia, sub-Saharan Africa, Latin America, and the Caribbean. The World Health Organization (WHO) has identified open defecation as a major worldwide problem, with the combination of population growth and slow sanitation improvements steadily worsening the situation. Diarrhea is suspected to be the cause of the "South Asian enigma," which involves an unusually low rate of child nutrition relative to the region's income level. There is growing evidence that exposure to poor sanitation contributes to stunting, or a low height-to-age ratio. With respect to adults, the elderly are more susceptible and more likely to die from diseases related to sanitation. There is also suspicion that reproductive infections in women may be linked to poor sanitation.

WORDS TO KNOW

FECAL-ORAL ROUTE The transmission of minute particles of fecal material from one organism (human or animal) to the mouth of another organism.

PATHOGEN A disease-causing agent, such as a bacterium, a virus, a fungus, or another microorganism.

SENTINEL An epidemiological method in which a subset of the population is surveyed for the presence of communicable diseases. Also, an animal used to indicate the presence of disease within an area.

TOXIN A poison produced by a living organism.

History and Scientific Foundations

Before the development of microbiology, the specific causes of diseases were unknown. Diseases such as cholera, typhoid, and dysentery were common in the United States, Europe, and other parts of the world. In 1854, during an Asiatic cholera epidemic in London, physician John Snow (1813–1858) linked a contaminated well to deaths. A house privy emptying into a cesspool overflowed to a drain passing close to the well. Feces infected with the bacterium *Vibrio cholerae* contaminated the water and produced a toxin that caused diarrhea, vomiting, and severe fluid and electrolyte loss. Snow's discovery tied poor sanitation directly to disease and death.

In subsequent years links between sanitation and typhoid, typhus, and dysentery were established. Dehydration is the outstanding characteristic of these diseases and the main cause of death. Typhoid is caused by bacterium called *Salmonella typhi*. A different pathogen, *Salmonella paratyphi*, causes paratyphoid fever. *S. typhi* and *S. paratyphi* are passed in the feces and, occasionally, in the urine of infected people. Most cases of typhoid result from contaminated drinking water and poor sanitation. Typhoid causes fever, rash, delirium, and diarrhea.

Dysentery is also known as traveler's diarrhea. The two most common causes of dysentery are *Shigella* bacteria or amebic infection by the *Entamoeba histolytica*. Both forms of dysentery are spread by fecal contamination of food and water. Amebic dysentery is prevalent in regions where human excrement, or "night soil," is used as fertilizer. Cysts (inactive amoebas) are excreted in the feces of an infected person. When these cysts are ingested with contaminated water, they become active amoebas in the intestine, and dysentery results. Dysentery was once known as "the bloody flux" because it produces blood in the feces.

Poor sanitation and hygiene are prime contributors to the spread of schistosomiasis and soil-transmitted helminthiasis (worms). Children are particularly prone to infections because their high level of activity brings them into regular contact with contaminated water and soil.

■ Impacts and Issues

Diarrhea resulting from inadequate sanitation and lack of clean drinking water affects much of the daily life of the world's population, according to WHO. More than 340,000 children under age five die annually from diarrheal diseases connected with poor sanitation, making diarrhea the third-leading cause of death for small children. WHO notes that many health facilities lack access to clean water and modern sanitation. Efforts to stop open defecation have been successful in Ethiopia, but as of 2018 the practice remained common in much of sub-Saharan Africa and southern Asia.

With so few families in developing nations having access to a latrine or to water for hygiene, many people live in an environment that permits disease to spread rapidly. Chronic poor health robs children of the cognitive development necessary for schooling and takes earning power away from adults.

Oral rehydration therapy (ORT) is an inexpensive and effective way of saving lives. The widespread availability of oral hydration salts has contributed to significant reductions in infant deaths from diarrhea in the developing world. However, ORT does not address the root causes of diarrhea.

Improved sanitation reduces deaths from diarrhea by an average of 32 percent. Accordingly, WHO advises the construction of flush/pour-flush facilities to piped sewer systems, septic tanks, or pit latrines; pit latrines with slabs; and composting toilets. Communal facilities for groups of homes are not, as a rule, maintained in a clean and sanitary condition. They are not recommended. WHO further advises that the political environment in developing nations needs to be changed to support improved sanitation. WHO seeks legislation and regulations in support of sanitation; an increase in national capacity in the form of sanitation engineers and stronger institutions; governmental allocation of financial resources; educational programs that link sanitation, hygiene, health, and economic development; and improved information flow from producers to users.

The US Centers for Disease Control (CDC) recommends that travelers avoid raw food in areas where sanitation is inadequate. The only foods safe to consume in these regions are cooked foods or fruit that has been washed in clean water and then peeled by the traveler personally. Ad-

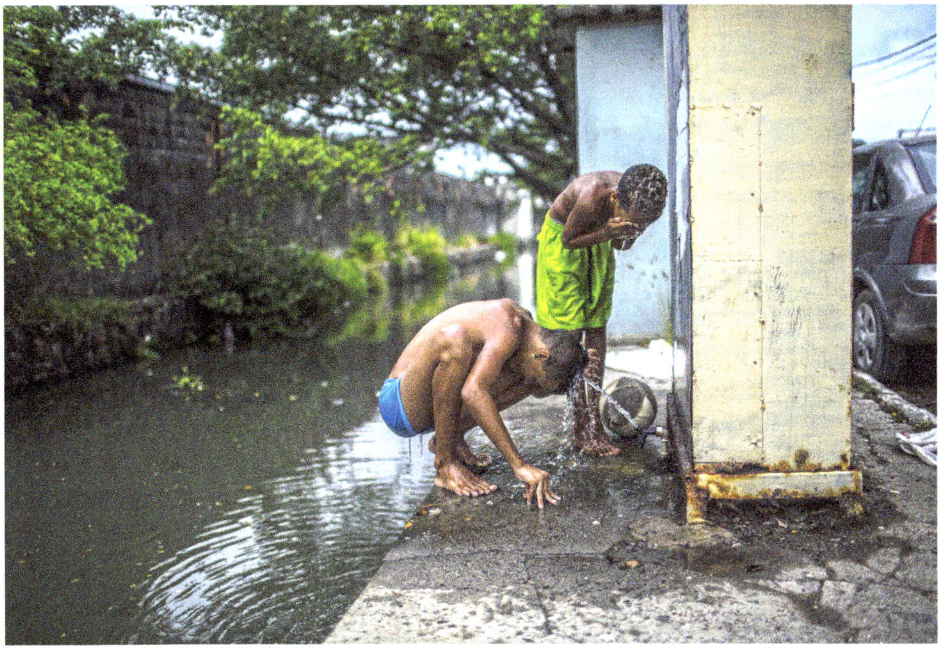

In Recife, Brazil, teenagers rinse off after swimming in an unsanitary canal. Poor sanitation allows infectious diseases to spread as fecal matter contaminates drinking water. *© Dado Galdieri/Bloomberg/Getty Images*

DISEASE IN DEVELOPING NATIONS

According to the World Health Organization (WHO):

- In 2015 2.4 billion people lacked access to improved sanitation. Of them, 946 million defecate in the open.
- Fifty percent of the population in western Asia and 41 percent in North Africa gained access to improved sanitation since 1990. By contrast, less than 17 percent gained access in sub-Saharan Africa.
- Eighty-two percent of the global urban population versus 51 percent of the rural population uses improved sanitation facilities.
- Seven out of 10 people without improved sanitation facilities and 9 out of 10 people still practicing open defecation live in rural areas.

ditionally, accidentally swallowing small amounts of fecally contaminated water can cause illness. Pools that contain chlorinated water are considered safe places to swim if the disinfectant levels and pH are properly maintained. All travelers who have diarrhea are advised to refrain from swimming to avoid contaminating recreational water. Travelers with open cuts or abrasions that might serve as entry points for pathogens are warned to avoid swimming and wading in areas with poor sanitation.

Improvements in sanitation bring immediate and enduring benefits in health and dignity. However, these improvements can be beyond the financial means of some governments, particularly those in third-world nations. In the 1980s Brazil developed a condominial sewer system, which provides less expensive, localized hookups for poor neighborhoods by connecting groups of houses, rather than individual houses, to the larger grid and by using cheaper materials. However, such systems have not been adopted in other developing countries as quickly as is needed. Bolivia built condominial systems only after it received assistance from the Swedish International Development Cooperation Agency and the World Bank's Water and Sanitation Program. These support agencies provided technical skills as well as funds. Other developing nations require the same sort of help.

China has used tightly sealed excreta vats for years to store human excrement for use as fertilizer. The vats produce ammonia and albuminoid nitrogen under anaerobic (without oxygen) conditions, which is reported to kill parasite eggs and reduce transmission of parasitic and infectious diseases. Chinese scientists have developed a biogas tank that is likely the future means of dealing with excrement. The tanks are tightly sealed to permit the fermentation and settling of excreta, livestock manure, crop stalks, weeds, and tree leaves. The tight seal prevents contamination of nearby water sources. About 60 percent of the gas produced in the tanks is methane. The methane from a family unit is used for cooking. This solution is both locally and globally environmentally friendly.

The United Nations (UN) has sponsored a World Toilet Day in November since 2014 to call attention to the need for improved world sanitation. Part of the goal of the UN is to end the stigma surrounding the topic of defecation. UNICEF-India created a children's song called "Take Poo to the Loo" toward this aim, as open defecation is such a serious health threat.

See Also *Cholera; Dysentary; Parasitic Diseases; Typhoid; Waterborne Disease*

BIBLIOGRAPHY

Books

Angelakis, Andreas N., and Joan B. Rose, eds. *Evolution of Sanitation and Wastewater Technologies through the Centuries.* London: IWA, 2014.

Banerjee, Sudeshna Ghosh, and Elvira Morella. *Africa's Water and Sanitation Infrastructure: Access, Affordability, and Alternatives.* Washington, DC: World Bank, 2011.

Websites

"Key Facts from JMP 2015 Report." World Health Organization. http://www.who.int/water_sanitation_health/monitoring/jmp-2015-key-facts/en/ (accessed February 12, 2018).

United Nations–Water. "World Toilet Day." http://www.worldtoiletday.info/ (accessed February 12, 2018).

Caryn E. Neumann

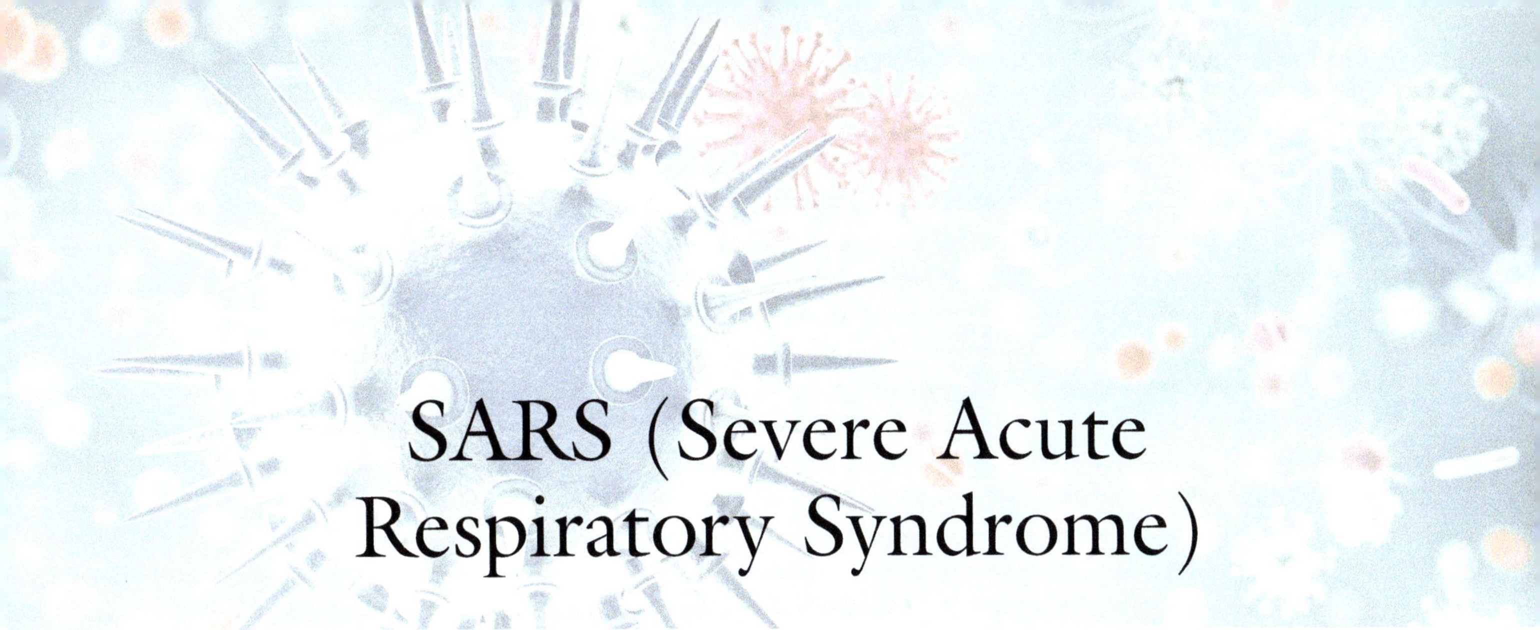

SARS (Severe Acute Respiratory Syndrome)

Introduction

Severe acute respiratory syndrome (SARS) is the first emergent and highly transmissible viral disease to appear among humans during the 21st century. Patients with SARS develop flu-like fever, headache, malaise, dry cough, and other breathing difficulties. Many patients develop pneumonia, and in 5 to 10 percent of cases, the pneumonia and other complications are severe enough to cause death. SARS is caused by a virus that is transmitted usually from person to person—predominantly by the aerosolized droplets of virus-infected material.

Disease History, Characteristics, and Transmission

Many flu-causing viruses have previously originated from Guangdong Province in China because of cultural and exotic cuisine practices that bring animals, animal parts, and humans into close proximity. In such an environment, pathogens can more easily genetically mutate and make the leap from animal hosts to humans. The first cases of SARS showed high rates among Guangdong food handlers and chefs.

Chinese health officials initially remained silent about the SARS outbreak, and no special precautions were taken to limit travel or prevent the spread of the disease. The world health community, therefore, had no chance to institute testing, isolation, and quarantine measures that might have prevented the subsequent global spread of the disease.

Although not discovered until epidemiologists began to probe the subsequent 2003 outbreak, epidemiologists traced the first known case of what was eventually known as SARS to a November 2002 case in Guangdong. By mid-February 2003 Chinese health officials had tracked more than 300 cases, including five deaths in Guangdong from what was at the time described as an acute respiratory syndrome.

On February 21, 2003, Liu Jianlun, a 64-year-old Chinese physician from Zhongshan hospital, traveled to Hong Kong to attend a family wedding despite the fact that he had a fever. Liu was later determined to have been a "super-spreader," or a person capable of infecting unusually high numbers of contacts. Epidemiologists subsequently determined that Liu passed on the SARS virus to other guests at the Metropole Hotel where he stayed, including American businessman Johnny Chen, who was en route to Hanoi; three women from Singapore; two Canadians; and a Hong

WORDS TO KNOW

ASYMPTOMATIC A state in which an individual does not exhibit or experience symptoms of a disease.

DISSEMINATION The spreading of a disease in a population or over a large geographic area or the spreading of disease organisms in the body.

ISOLATION AND QUARANTINE Public health authorities rely on isolation and quarantine as two important tools among the many they use to fight disease outbreaks. Isolation is the practice of keeping a disease victim away from other people, sometimes by treating them in their homes or by the use of elaborate isolation systems in hospitals. Quarantine separates people who have been exposed to a disease but have not yet developed symptoms from the general population. Both isolation and quarantine can be entered voluntarily by patients when public health authorities request it, or it can be compelled by state governments or by the federal Centers for Disease Control and Prevention.

NUCLEOTIDE SEQUENCE A particular ordering of the chain structure of nucleic acid that provides the necessary information for a specific amino acid.

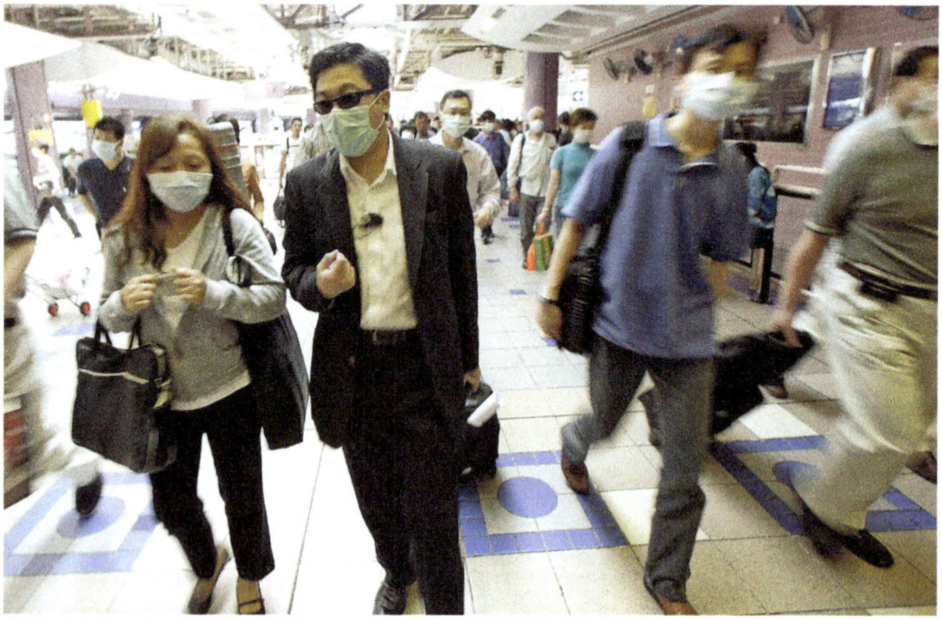

People crossing into mainland China from Hong Kong wear masks to protect against severe acute respiratory syndrome (SARS) during an outbreak in 2003. © PETER PARKS/AFP/Getty Images

Kong resident. Liu's travel to Hong Kong and the subsequent travel of those he infected allowed SARS to spread from China to the infected travelers' destinations.

Chen, the American businessman, grew ill in Hanoi, Vietnam, and was admitted to a local hospital, where he infected 20 health care workers including noted Italian epidemiologist Carlo Urbani, who worked at the Hanoi World Health Organization (WHO) office. Urbani provided medical care for Chen and first formally identified SARS as a unique disease on February 28, 2003. By early March, 22 hospital workers in Hanoi were ill with SARS.

Unaware of the problems in China, Urbani's report drew increased attention among epidemiologists when coupled with news reports in mid-March 2003 that Hong Kong health officials had also discovered an outbreak of an acute respiratory syndrome among health care workers. Unsuspecting hospital workers admitted the Hong Kong man infected by Liu to a general ward at the Prince of Wales Hospital because it was assumed he had a typical severe pneumonia, a fairly routine admission.

The first notice that clinicians were dealing with an usual illness came not from health notices from China of increasing illnesses and deaths due to SARS but from the observation that hospital staff, along with those subsequently determined to have been in close proximity to the infected persons, began to show signs of illness. Eventually 138 people, including 34 nurses, 20 doctors, 16 medical students, and 15 other health care workers, contracted pneumonia.

One of the most intriguing aspects of the early Hong Kong cases was a cluster of more than 250 SARS cases that occurred in a group of high-rise apartment buildings, many of which housed health care workers. The cluster provided evidence of a high rate of secondary transmission. Epidemiologists conducted extensive investigations to rule out the hypothesis that the illnesses were related to some form of local contamination, such as from sewage and bacteria in the ventilation system. Rumors began that the illness was due to cockroaches or rodents, but no scientific evidence supported the hypothesis that the disease pathogen was carried by insects or animals.

Hong Kong authorities then decided that those suffering the flu-like symptoms would be given the option of self-isolation, with family members allowed to remain confined at home or in special camps. Police conducted compliance checks.

One of the Canadians infected in Hong Kong, Kwan Sui-Chu, returned to Toronto, Ontario, and died in a hospital on March 5, 2003. As in Hong Kong, because there were no alerts from China about the SARS outbreak, Canadian officials did not initially suspect that Kwan had been infected with a highly contagious virus until Kwan's son and five health care workers showed similar symptoms. By mid-April 2003 Canada reported more than 130 SARS cases and 15 fatalities.

Increasingly faced with reports that provided evidence of global dissemination, on March 15, 2003, WHO took the unusual step of issuing a travel warning that described SARS as a "worldwide health threat." WHO officials announced that SARS cases, and potential cases, had been tracked from China to Singapore, Thailand, Vietnam, Indonesia, Philippines, and Canada. Although the exact cause of the acute respiratory syndrome had not, at that time, been determined, WHO officials' issuance of the precautionary warning to travelers bound for Southeast Asia about the potential SARS risk served notice to public health officials about the potential dangers of SARS.

Within days of the first WHO warning, SARS cases were reported in the United Kingdom, Spain, Slovenia, Germany, and the United States. WHO officials were initially encouraged that isolation procedures and alerts were working to stem the spread of SARS, as some countries reporting small numbers of cases experienced no further dissemination to hospital staff or others in contact with SARS victims. However, in some countries, including Canada, where SARS cases occurred before WHO alerts, SARS continued to spread beyond the bounds of isolated patients.

WHO officials responded by recommending increased screening and quarantine measures that included mandatory screening of people returning from visits to the most severely affected areas in China, Southeast Asia, and Hong Kong.

On March 29, 2003, Urbani, the scientist who initially identified SARS, died of complications related to SARS contracted while investigating the outbreak. Mounting reports of SARS showed an increasing global dissemination of the virus. By April 9, 2003, the first confirmed reports of SARS cases in Africa reached WHO headquarters, and eight days later a confirmed case was discovered in India. WHO took the controversial additional step of recommending against nonessential travel to Hong Kong and Guangdong. The recommendation, sought by infectious disease specialists, was not controversial within the medical community but caused immediate concern regarding the potentially widespread economic impacts.

In Beijing, China, fear of a widespread outbreak caused a late but intensive effort to isolate SARS victims and halt the spread of the disease. By the end of April 2003, schools in Beijing were closed, as were many public areas. Despite these measures, SARS cases and deaths continued to mount. According to WHO, by the end of the outbreak in July 2003, 8,098 people worldwide had contracted SARS, and 774 had died from complications of the disease. In the United States eight people had laboratory evidence of SARS infection, and all of the patients had recently traveled out of the country to places with SARS outbreaks. The 2003 SARS outbreak then subsided almost as quickly as it arose.

In 2004 Chinese officials reported new cases of possible SARS in Beijing and in Anhui Province, with at least one confirmed death. Almost 100 contacts were placed under medical observation. Chinese authorities reported outbreaks of SARS affecting laboratory workers who were exposed to the virus. In late 2004 four more unlinked, community-acquired cases of SARS were found in Guangdong. Although the source of this outbreak was unconfirmed, it is suspected to have originated in wild animals, most likely those found in food markets.

As of 2017 there had been no further outbreaks.

EFFECTIVE RULES AND REGULATIONS

The 2003 severe acute respiratory syndrome (SARS) outbreak did not spread within the United States. In response to the 2003 SARS outbreak, the US Centers for Disease Control and Prevention (CDC):

- Worked with the World Health Organization (WHO) and other global partners to address the outbreak.
- Activated its Emergency Operations Center. The center was equipped to provide a round-the-clock response to the outbreak.
- Staffed the response effort with more than 800 medical experts and support staff.
- Provided medical officers, epidemiologists, and other specialists to support on-site investigations of possible outbreaks around the globe.
- Assisted in state and local health department investigations of possible cases of SARS.
- Carried out laboratory testing of specimens from patients infected with SARS to investigate the cause of the disease.
- Created a system to disseminate health alerts to travelers who might have been exposed to SARS.

Scope and Distribution

At the end of April 2003, SARS public health officials expressed concern that SARS had the potential to become a global pandemic. Scientists, public health authorities, and clinicians around the world struggled to both treat and investigate the disease.

Global efforts at isolation, quarantine, and observation proved effective, and a pandemic did not occur. In 2017 the Centers for Disease Control and Prevention (CDC) and WHO reported no current cases of SARS anywhere in the world.

Treatment and Prevention

In the 2003 outbreak, scientists scrambled to isolate, identify, and sequence the pathogen responsible for SARS. Modes of transmission characteristic of viral transmission allowed scientists to place early attention on a group of viruses termed coronaviruses, some of which are associated with the common cold. There was a global two-pronged attack on the SARS pathogen, with some efforts directed toward a positive identification and isolation of the virus and other efforts directed toward discovering the genetic molecular structure and sequence of genes contained in the virus. The development of a genomic map of the precise nucleotide sequence of the virus would be key in any subsequent development of a definitive diagnostic test, the identification of effective antiviral agents, and perhaps a vaccine.

The development of a reliable and definitive diagnostic test was considered of paramount importance in keeping SARS from becoming a global pandemic. A definitive diagnostic test would not only allow physicians earlier treatment options but would also allow the earlier identification and isolation of potential carriers of the virus.

Without advanced testing, physicians were initially forced to rely on less sensitive tests that were unable to identify SARS prior to 21 days of infection, in most cases too late to effectively isolate the patient.

In mid-April 2003 Canadian scientists at the British Columbia Cancer Agency in Vancouver announced that they had sequenced the genome of the coronavirus most likely to be the cause of SARS. Within days scientists at the CDC in Atlanta, Georgia, offered a genomic map that confirmed more than 99 percent of the Canadian findings. Both genetic maps were generated from studies of viruses isolated from SARS cases. The particular coronavirus mapped had a genomic sequence of 29,727 nucleotides, which is average for the family of coronavirus that typically contain between 29,000 and 31,000 nucleotides.

Proof that the coronavirus mapped was the specific virus responsible for SARS would eventually come from animal testing. Rhesus monkeys were exposed to the virus via injection and inhalation and then monitored to determine whether SARS-like symptoms developed. If sick, animals exhibited a histological pathology similar to findings in human patients. Other tests, including polymerase chain reaction (PCR) testing, helped positively match the specific coronavirus present in the lung tissue, blood, and feces of infected animals to the exposure virus.

Identification of a specific pathogen can be a complex process, and positive identification requires thousands of tests. All testing is conducted with regard to testing Koch's postulates, the four conditions that must be met for an organism to be determined the cause of a disease. First, the organism must be present in every case of the disease. Second, the organism must be able to be isolated from the host and grown in laboratory conditions. Third, the disease must be reproduced when the isolated organism is introduced into another, healthy host. The fourth postulate stipulates that the same organism must be able to be recovered and purified from the host that was experimentally infected.

SARS has an incubation period range of two to seven days, with an average incubation of about four days. In some cases incubation has taken 10 days and, in a very rare number of cases, as long as 14 days. Much of the inoculation period allows the virus to be both transported and spread by an asymptomatic carrier. With air travel, asymptomatic carriers can travel to anywhere in the world. The initial symptoms are nonspecific and common to the flu. Infected cases then typically spike a high fever 100.4°F (38 .0°C) as they develop a cough, shortness of breath, and difficulty breathing. SARS often fulminates (reaches it maximum progression) in a severe pneumonia that can cause respiratory failure and results in death in about 10 percent of its victims.

No definitive therapy has been demonstrated to have clinical effectiveness against the virus that causes SARS. Antibiotics, antiviral medications, corticosteroids, and supportive therapies such as fluids and ventilation are the mainstays of treatment for SARS.

Isolation and quarantine remain potent tools in the modern public health arsenal. Both procedures seek to control exposure to infected individuals or materials. Isolation procedures are used with patients with a confirmed illness. Quarantine rules and procedures apply to individuals who are not currently ill but are known to have been exposed to the illness, such as those who have been in the company of an infected person or who have come in contact with infected materials.

Isolation and quarantine both act to restrict movement and to slow or stop the spread of disease within a community. Depending on the illness, patients placed in isolation may be cared for in hospitals, specialized health care facilities, or, in less severe cases, at home. Isolation is a standard procedure for tuberculosis patients. In most cases isolation is voluntary, though it may be compelled by federal, state, and some local law.

■ Impacts and Issues

Before the advent of vaccines and effective diagnostic tools, isolation and quarantine were the principal tools to control the spread of infectious disease. The public discussion of SARS-related quarantine in the United States and Europe renewed tensions between the needs for public heath precautions that safeguard society at large and the liberties of the individual.

US state governments have a general authority to set and enforce quarantine conditions. At the federal level, the CDC's Division of Global Migration and Quarantine is empowered to detain, examine, or conditionally release (release with restrictions on movement or with a required treatment protocol) individuals suspected of carrying certain listed communicable diseases.

In 2003 the CDC recommended SARS patients be voluntarily isolated but did not recommend enforced isolation or quarantine. Regardless, CDC and other public health officials, including the US Surgeon General, sought and secured increased powers to deal with SARS. On April 4, 2003, US president George W. Bush (1946–) signed

Presidential Executive Order 13295, which added SARS to a list of quarantinable communicable diseases. The order provided health officials with the broader powers to seek "apprehension, detention, or conditional release of individuals to prevent the introduction, transmission, or spread of suspected communicable diseases."

Other diseases on the US communicable disease list, specified pursuant to section 361(b) of the Public Health Service Act, include "Cholera; Diphtheria; infectious Tuberculosis; Plague; Smallpox; Yellow Fever; and Viral Hemorrhagic Fevers." Another executive order concerning SARS was signed by US president Barack Obama (1961–) on July 31, 2014.

During the 2003 outbreak, passengers arriving in Singapore coming from other countries with SARS were required to undergo questioning by nurses in isolation garb and then required to walk through a thermal scanner calibrated to detect an elevated body temperature. Soldiers immediately escorted those with elevated temperatures into quarantine facilities. Those subsequently allowed to remain in their homes were monitored by video cameras and electronic wristbands.

The 2003 SARS outbreak provided a test of recent reforms in International Health Regulations designed to increase surveillance and reporting of infectious diseases and to enhance cooperation in preventing the international spread of disease. Although not an act of bioterrorism, because the same epidemiologic principles and isolation protocols might be used to both initially determine and initially respond to an act of bioterrorism, intelligence and public health officials closely monitored the political, scientific, and medical responses to the SARS outbreak. In many regards the SARS outbreak provided a real and deadly test of public health responses, readiness, and resources.

See Also *Contact Precautions; Developing Nations and Drug Delivery; Emerging Infectious Diseases; Influenza; Influenza, Tracking Seasonal Influences and Virus Mutation; Influenza Pandemic of 1918; Isolation and Quarantine; Notifiable Diseases; Pandemic Preparedness; Personal Protective Equipment; Standard Precautions; Vaccines and Vaccine Development*

BIBLIOGRAPHY

Books

Delort, Anne-Marie, and Pierre Amato, eds. *Microbiology of Aerosols.* Hoboken, NJ: Wiley, 2017.

Kumar, Sandeep, and Jane C. Benjamin. *Pathogenic Bacteria in Bioaerosol of Hospitals: Important of Airborne Pathogen in Hospital.* New York: Lap Lambert Academic, 2013.

Periodicals

Young, Andrew T. Y., et al. "From SARS to Avian Influenza Preparedness in Hong Kong." *Clinical Infectious Diseases* 64 (May 2017): S98–S104.

Websites

"Severe Acute Respiratory Syndrome (SARS)." Centers for Disease Control and Prevention. http://www.cdc.gov/sars/index.html (accessed December 11, 2017).

"Severe Acute Respiratory Syndrome (SARS)." World Health Organization. http://www.who.int/csr/sars/en (accessed December 11, 2017).

Brenda Wilmoth Lerner
Brian Hoyle

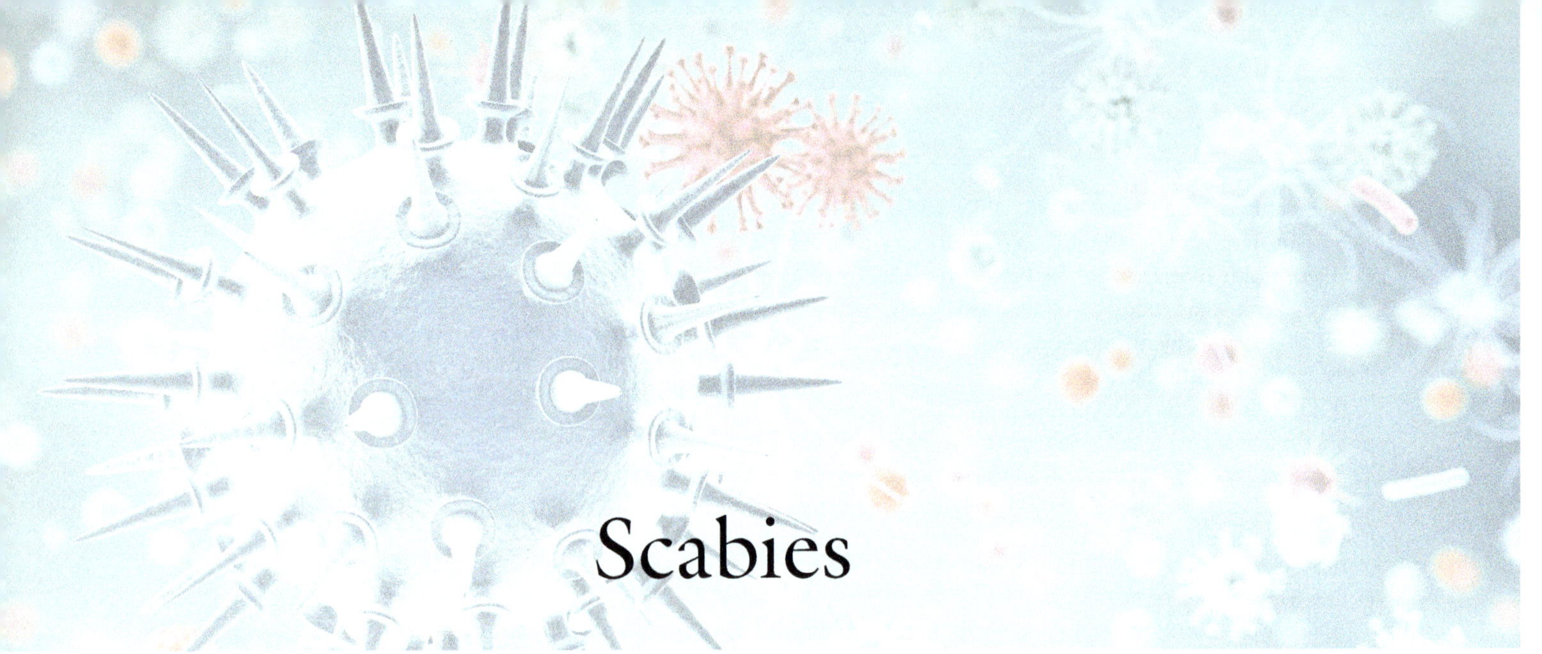

Scabies

Introduction

Scabies is an infestation of the skin by the human itch mite (*Sarcoptes scabiei*). It occurs all around the world and is one of the most common skin problems reported to dermatologists. The word *scabies* comes from the Latin *scabere*, which means "to scratch." There is a variant known as Norwegian scabies, which is very infectious and can lead to epidemics in places such as nursing homes, homeless shelters, and prisons. Scabies is caused by close human contact, including sexual contact, and leads to intense itching because of an immune response to the infestation.

Scabies is an uncomfortable condition that disproportionately affects vulnerable populations including young children, the elderly, and those whose immune systems are compromised. Lack of access to clean water, malnutrition, and overcrowding are strong risk factors for an outbreak of scabies. Treatment is usually by a skin cream or tablets containing a drug that kills the mites. When left untreated, scabies can lead to life-threatening complications, including sepsis and organ failure.

WORDS TO KNOW

ATOPY An inherited tendency toward hypersensitivity toward immunoglobulin E, a key component of the immune system, which plays an important role in asthma, eczema, and hay fever.

MITE A tiny arthropod (insect-like creature) of the order *Acarina*. Mites may inhabit the surface of the body without causing harm or may cause various skin ailments by burrowing under the skin. The droppings of mites living in house dust are a common source of allergic reactions.

PRURITIS The medical term for itchiness.

PUSTULE A reservoir of pus visible just beneath the skin. It is usually sore to the touch and surrounded by inflamed tissue.

Disease History, Characteristics, and Transmission

Mites are tiny organisms (approximately 0.4 millimeters in length) that are barely visible to the human eye. *S. scabiei* mate on human skin, after which the male dies. The fertilized female burrows through the epidermis–the outer layer of the skin—and lays her eggs. Although the mites can only live for a maximum of 72 hours away from a human host, they can live for up to two months on a person. Typically, around 10 to 15 organisms are found in an infestation giving rise to symptoms, although there can be many more in immunocompromised hosts, such as people with HIV/AIDS. Scabies arises from human contact, including sexual intercourse.

The symptoms of scabies come from the human immune response to the feces of the female mite in her burrow. There is severe itching—known clinically as pruritis—which is especially intense at night or after a hot shower or bath. This can occur in any part of the body but is most common between the fingers, in the genitalia, and around the waist or other areas constricted by clothing. Among adults, scabies tends not to cause symptoms on the face, arms, neck, or soles of the feet, but these areas may be affected in children. Pustules—pimples filled with pus, a yellow fluid made up of dead white blood cells, bacteria, and bits of dead tissue—and blisters might occur in areas affected by scabies.

The Norwegian variant of scabies, sometimes also called crusted scabies, often affects the face, scalp, palms of the hands, and soles of the feet. It may be mistaken for eczema or psoriasis, two other subacute to chronic inflammatory skin conditions. Norwegian scabies is very contagious. It can also be especially difficult to treat.

Untreated scabies can lead to complications including recurrent skin infection and can even cause sepsis, streptococcal skin infection by *Streptococcus pyogenes*, and post-streptococcal kidney injury.

Scope and Distribution

Although infection rates are highest in areas with hot, tropical climates, scabies is a worldwide problem. It affects roughly 130 million people at any given time. Populations who live in crowded conditions are most vulnerable to scabies, and it is therefore often seen in institutions such as hospitals, nursing homes, and prisons. Scabies affects people from all races and socioeconomic groups, although the poor, who are most likely to live in the crowded conditions in which it flourishes, are disproportionately affected globally. Malnutrition and lack of access to water and hygiene supplies also increase susceptibility to scabies infection.

Those with reduced immunity, such as patients with HIV/AIDS, are more prone to scabies, and thousands to millions of *S. scabiei* eggs may be found under the skin of these individuals. Those with known atopy—that is, with hereditary, allergy-related symptoms such as asthma or eczema—may be more vulnerable to scabies, because of their sensitivity to the house dust mite, which is related to *S. scabiei.*

Treatment and Prevention

Scabies is diagnosed based on its characteristic rash. Ideally, medical professionals will confirm the diagnosis through identification of the *Sarcoptes scabiei* mite, its eggs, or its fecal matter. Once diagnosed, scabies is treated by a topical medication applied from the neck down to cover the whole body. Popular scabicides include 5 percent permethrin cream, 10–25 percent benzyl benzoate emulsion, 5–10 percent sulphur ointment, or 5 percent malathion. Among young children, treatment of the face might also be needed. The treatment

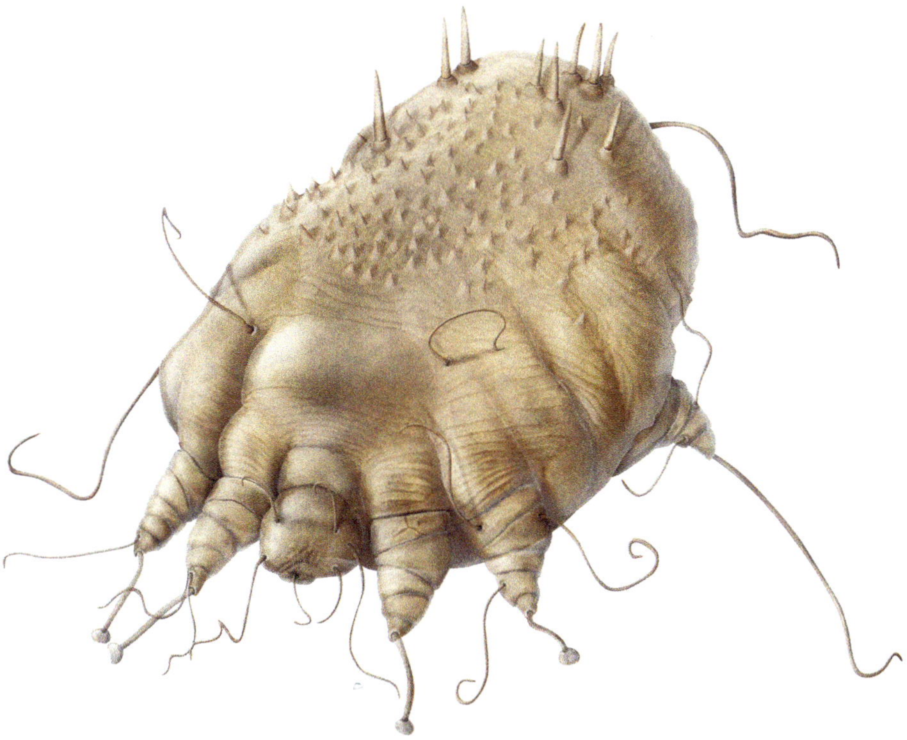

Sarcoptes scabiei, the scabies mite. Scabies infections are the result of the female mite laying her eggs under the epidermis of a human. © QAI Publishing/UIG/Getty Images

PREVENTING SCABIES IN SCHOOL SPORTS

According to the Division of Parasitic Diseases and Malaria at the Centers for Disease Control and Prevention (CDC), scabies is most often caused by prolonged skin-to-skin contact with an infected person. A quick hug or handshake is not generally enough to spread the condition, but contact through sports such as wrestling and football can be. Although it is a less common form of transmission, scabies can be spread by shared clothing, bedding, and towels or by contact with a gym mat or gym equipment that has not been properly cleaned after use by an affected individual. It can thus spread quickly from athlete to athlete.

To prevent the spread of scabies, athletes should avoid sharing towels and clothing. If a team member is diagnosed with scabies, he or she should wait 24 hours after beginning treatment to return to team activities. Individuals should also notify their coaches and teammates so that they can watch for signs of infection. This is especially important in the case of crusted scabies, which spreads quickly and can lead to outbreaks.

is left on for several hours to kill the mites and is then washed away. This cures 90 percent of those infested. Oral ivermectin may also be useful, especially if the all-body topical treatment is hard to administer, as in nursing home residents. Topical anti-itch creams and oral antihistamines can be used to relieve the itching associated with scabies, which sometimes lasts for up to four weeks after the mites have been eradicated due to the continued inflammatory response to feces that have not yet been cleared from the body.

In addition to treating the individuals affected by scabies, it is important to treat the living environment. Clothing, bedding, and other items that might have been in touch with the mites should be dry-cleaned or washed in hot water and dried using high heat. Items that cannot be washed should be placed in sealed plastic bags for several weeks to guarantee that all mites have died. All carpets in an infected person's home should be vacuumed thoroughly. The best treatment outcomes are achieved when all members of a household and all household clothes and linens are treated simultaneously.

Treatment of close contacts is also a good idea to prevent reinfestation.

■ Impacts and Issues

Scabies is an uncomfortable disease that often targets vulnerable populations, including those with compromised immunity, such as people with AIDS or the elderly. Therefore, those at risk need to be aware of the problem of scabies and educated about how best to prevent contracting it. At-risk populations should take action to avoid close and prolonged contact with those who could already be infested.

The International Alliance for the Control of Scabies (IACS) is working to make scabies a global health priority. IACS focuses on making education and prevention a routine part of public health programs. The organization has also been involved in studies of the efficacy of mass drug administration of the oral treatment ivermectin, which is a more promising approach to scabies control than the application of topical scabicides.

Progress on eradicating scabies remains slow. In June 2017 the World Health Organization (WHO) added scabies to its list of neglected tropical diseases. This designation was based on various criteria, including that the disease disproportionately affects the poor, primarily affects those living in tropical and subtropical regions, is immediately treatable, and is neglected by researchers. Both the IACS and WHO have expressed hope that the designation will help focus attention on eradicating scabies.

SEE ALSO *Lice Infestation (Pediculosis)*

BIBLIOGRAPHY

Books

Farrar, Jeremy, et al, eds. *Manson's Tropical Diseases.* 23rd ed. New York: Elsevier, 2013.

Micheli, Lyle J., ed. *Encyclopedia of Sports Medicine.* Vol. 1. Los Angeles: Sage, 2011.

Periodicals

Brody, Jane E. "An Itchy Torment, Often Misdiagnosed." *New York Times* (September 22, 2008): F6. This article is also available online at http://www.nytimes.com/2008/09/23/health/23brod.html (accessed November 13, 2017).

Engelman, Daniel, et al. "Toward the Global Control of Human Scabies: Introducing the International Alliance for the Control of Scabies." *PLOS Neglected Tropical Diseases* 7, no. 8 (August 2013): e2167. This article is also available online at https://www.ncbi.nlm.nih.gov/pmc/articles/PMC3738445/ (accessed November 13, 2017).

Klass, Perri. "When Athletes Share Infections." *New York Times* (October 3, 2017): D4. This article is also available online at https://www.nytimes.com/2017/09/25/well/family/when-athletes-share-infections.html (accessed November 13, 2017).

Websites

International Alliance for the Control of Scabies. http://www.controlscabies.org/ (accessed November 13, 2017).

"Lymphatic Filariasis: Scabies." World Health Organization. http://www.who.int/lymphatic_filariasis/epidemiology/scabies/en/ (accessed November 13, 2017).

"Parasites: Scabies." Centers for Disease Control and Prevention. https://www.cdc.gov/parasites/scabies/index.html (accessed November 17, 2017).

"Scabies." American Academy of Dermatology. https://www.aad.org/public/diseases/contagious-skin-diseases/scabies (accessed November 13, 2017).

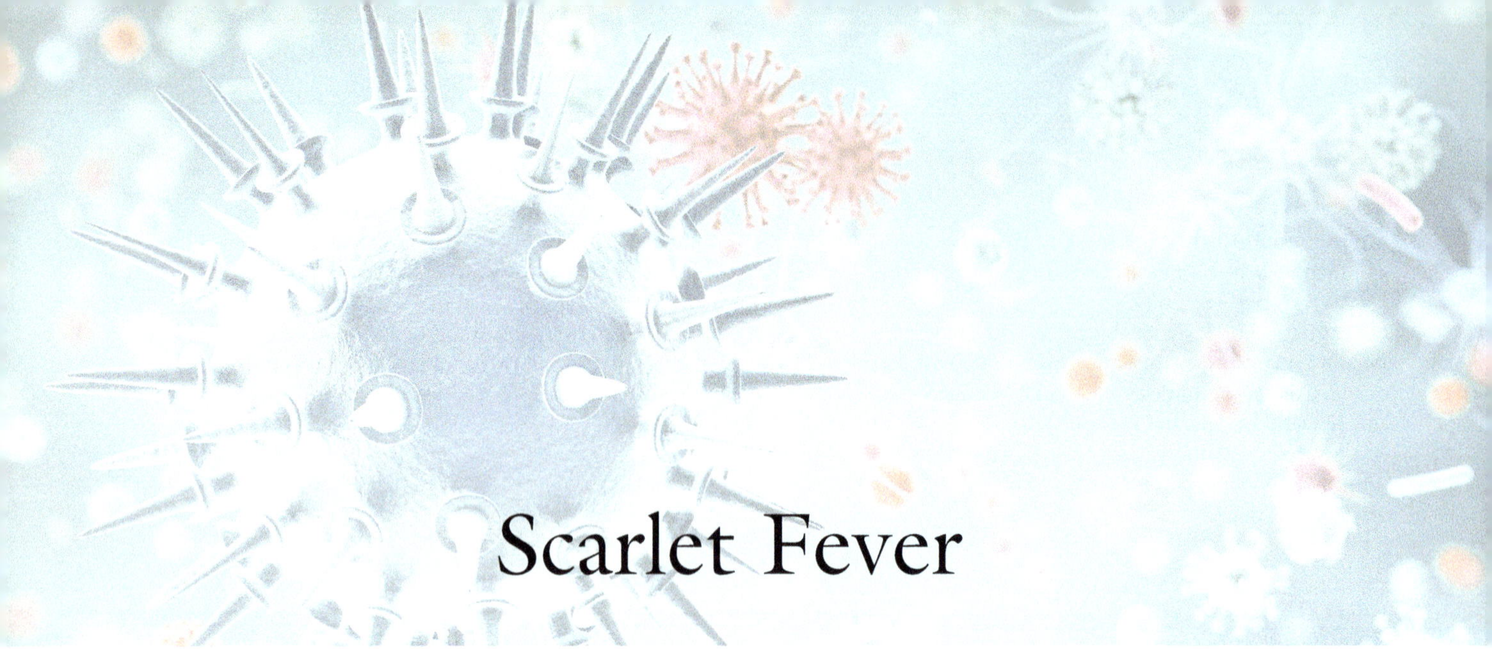

Scarlet Fever

Introduction

In the 19th century scarlet fever was one of the most feared childhood diseases, with a mortality rate of up to 35 percent. The causative agent is the bacterium *Streptococcus pyogenes.* Scarlet fever still exists in the 21st century but tends to be a mild disease in developed countries, although serious complications are still common in developing nations.

The modern, milder form of scarlet fever is sometimes called pharyngitis (throat infection) with rash, or scarlatina. It is not clear why this disease has lost its virulence. Unlike other childhood diseases, vaccination has not played a role in reducing its toll. The microbe may have mutated into a milder pathogen, or improvements in hygiene may have contributed. The advent of antibiotics and drugs to treat seizures and fever has certainly helped deal with the cause and symptoms of scarlet fever.

WORDS TO KNOW

GROUP A STREPTOCOCCUS (GAS) A type (specifically a serotype) of the streptococcus bacteria, based on the antigen contained in the cell wall.

NOTIFIABLE DISEASE A disease that the law requires must be reported to health officials when diagnosed. Also called a reportable disease.

RASH A change in appearance or texture of the skin. A rash is the popular term for a group of spots or red, inflamed skin that is usually a symptom of an underlying condition or disorder. Often temporary, a rash is only rarely a sign of a serious problem.

RESERVOIR The animal or organism in which a virus or parasite normally resides.

TOXIN A poison produced by a living organism.

Disease History, Characteristics, and Transmission

The *S. pyogenes* bacteria causing scarlet fever is known as group A streptococcus (GAS). The "A" refers to a characteristic antigen protein that exists on the surface of the microbe. GAS also causes strep throat (sometimes called bacterial sore throat) and impetigo. It is also responsible for necrotizing fasciitis, which involves the soft tissue under the skin, and toxic shock syndrome, both of which are potentially fatal. Around 40 percent of the population are asymptomatic carriers of GAS, and the bacterium does not have an animal reservoir (an organism that maintains the infective agent). The main symptoms of scarlet fever are a very sore, red throat, possibly with visible white or yellow patches, and the bright red rash that gives the disease its name.

The rash is caused by production of a toxin by the bacteria that spreads into the bloodstream via infected tissue in the throat. It begins as small spots on the neck and upper chest, and then spreads to the rest of the body. When the skin is pressed, it becomes pale, and the rash feels like sandpaper. The cheeks are flushed while the mouth remains pale, as if the patient had a white moustache. The tongue is often coated with a white fur, with tiny projections called papillae poking through. Doctors sometimes call this a "strawberry" tongue due to its appearance. After a few days, it turns into a "raspberry" tongue, becoming red with prominent papillae.

Other symptoms of scarlet fever include headache, vomiting, swollen glands, and poor appetite. As the rash fades, within three to four days of onset, the skin of the face, palms, and tips of the fingers and toes may begin to peel. More serious cases of scarlet fever are rare in the West but more common in the developing world. These cases are divided into two types, known as toxic and septic. In the toxic form, fever can be extreme, accompanied by delirium, convulsions, and rapid pulse, leading to death within 24 hours. In the septic form, the course of the disease is more prolonged, causing death in two to three weeks.

The complications of scarlet fever include upper-airway obstruction, meningitis, pneumonia, mastoiditis, and otitis media (severe ear infection). Later complications, such as kidney disease and rheumatic fever, which weakens the heart in the long term, may also occur.

Scarlet fever is transmitted by coughs and sneezes, as the saliva and nasal fluids are infectious. Touching items contaminated with these fluids therefore carries a risk of infection. Sharing cups and utensils can also transmit infection.

Scope and Distribution

Scarlet fever used to cause pandemics with high mortality in the 19th century in the United States, Western Europe, and Scandinavia. Often, because of a lack of understanding of how the disease was transmitted, all the patient's belongings would be burned for fear of contamination. Long periods of convalescence were common, perhaps because of complications due to rheumatic fever.

Because scarlet fever is now a mild disease in the West, it is no longer notifiable in many countries. The United Kingdom, however, still collects data on scarlet fever cases and noted 2,200 cases occurring in England and Wales in 2004. Ten years previously the number of cases was around 6,000, suggesting the disease was on the decline. However, beginning in 2014 scarlet fever cases rose for three seasons in a row in the United Kingdom, with 2014 seeing the highest number of cases since 1969. A total of 6,157 new cases were reported in 2015. As of 2017 the reasons for the increase remained unclear.

Ninety percent of cases of scarlet fever occur among children between the ages of two years and eight years. In temperate regions the number of cases peaks in the winter months. Complications such as rheumatic fever, ear infections, and pneumonia are relatively common in developing countries.

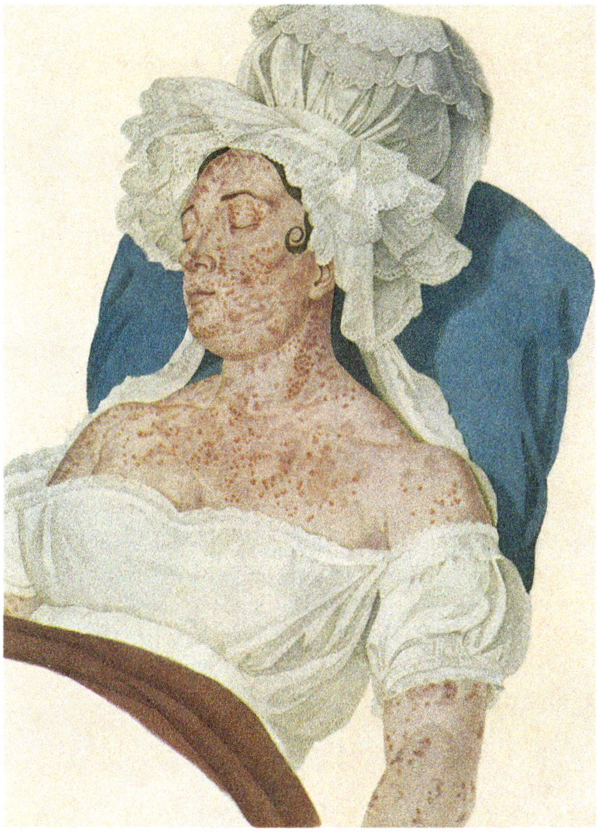

Illustration of woman with scarlet fever in 1883. Deadly epidemics of scarlet fever were common in the 19th century. In the 21st century deaths from the illness are rare in developed countries. The disease remains a threat in developing countries. © New York Public Library/Science Source

Treatment and Prevention

Scarlet fever is treated with antibiotics, with penicillin being the most common drug used. For those allergic to penicillin, erthryomycin or clindamycin are often prescribed instead. Completing the course of treatment is essential to prevent the onset of rheumatic fever or other complications. The majority of patients make an uneventful recovery after treatment.

Paracetamol or ibuprofen are useful for treating the symptoms of scarlet fever. Cold liquids such as milkshakes, ice pops, and warm soup are useful for soothing throat pain. A humidifier placed in the room will help ease dryness of the throat. In general, the patient should be kept well hydrated and get plenty of rest.

Good hygiene, including thorough handwashing, is very important in preventing the transmission of scarlet fever. Therefore, children with the illness, even if the case is mild, should be kept away from school or childcare centers. Utensils belonging to a child who is sick at home should always be kept separate from those used by the rest of the family.

Impacts and Issues

When an infectious disease is notifiable, it allows public health authorities to mount an investigation and stop an outbreak from spreading. In 2006 the UK Health Protection Agency dealt with an outbreak of scarlet fever in the southern county of Wiltshire, where 50 cases were reported during January and February. Six of these cases were in adults aged 18 years or older, while the rest occurred in children aged between eight months and 10 years who were attending childcare centers. Eleven cases had been reported during the same period of 2004 and only four in the same period of 2005, making the outbreak unusual. After the administration of antibiotics to symptomatic children and a hiatus from the childcare centers, no further cases were reported.

The local health protection team sent letters to all doctors in the area, informing them of the outbreaks. All suspected cases were to have throat swabs taken to test for the presence of GAS. This resulted in reports of 30 other cases of scarlet fever. Samples from the throat swabs taken were sent to the Health Protection Agency Centre for Infections for detailed analysis. These actions were taken because previous experience showed that outbreaks of scarlet fever can have serious consequences for young patients if the infection is not treated promptly and adequately.

Another significant upswing of scarlet fever was noted during 2014 in England. According to Public Health England's records, more than 15,000 cases were reported during this time, a dramatic and considerable rise from only 5,000 cases reported the previous year and the highest rate of increase in 50 years. The number of cases continued to rise in subsequent years, with 17,696 cases in 2015 and 19,206 in 2016. Neither medical researchers or public health experts could account for the sudden increase.

PRIMARY SOURCE

Scarlet Fever: A Sudden and Dramatic Outbreak Has Been Recorded in England, and Scientists Can't Explain Why

SOURCE: *Hignett, Katherine. "Scarlet Fever: A Sudden and Dramatic Outbreak Has Been Recorded in England, and Scientists Can't Explain Why."* Newsweek *(November 28, 2017). This article can also be found online at http://www.newsweek.com/unexplained-outbreak-scarlet-fever-england-724257 (accessed December 11, 2017).*

INTRODUCTION: *Although scarlet fever is far less common than it was in the early 1900s, outbreaks continue to occur. The following article from* Newsweek *examines an outbreak of the disease in England and considers the public health implications of the outbreak.*

Public health experts have discovered a dramatic resurgence of scarlet fever in England. A disease in decline since the 19th century, scientists cannot explain the sudden increase.

Rates of scarlet fever have been falling around the world for centuries. Characterized by a red rash like sandpaper, the disease can lead to kidney failure, sepsis and even death. It is caused by bacteria linked to strep throat, and most commonly affects children.

Published in *Lancet Infectious Diseases*, Theresa Lamagni and her team searched through Public Health England's records from 1911 to 2016. They came across a sudden escalation of scarlet fever cases in 2014. More than 15,000 cases were reported that year—three times those in 2013, and the highest rate for 50 years. Rates continued to rise through 2015 and 2016, which saw 17,696 and 19,206 cases respectively.

Following the 1924 development of a scarlet fever test and vaccine by Gladys Henry Dick and George Frederick Dick, the disease declined in the United Kingdom and the United States. The advent of penicillin in the 1940s stifled the disease further, leading to substantially lower rates around the world. Before these interventions, however, the prevalence of the disease had been dropping for at least 200 years. Just like today's increase, the researchers note, no one really knows why this happened.

"Whilst current rates are nowhere near those seen in the early 1900s, the magnitude of the recent upsurge is greater than any documented in the last century," said Lamagni, who works at Public Health England. "Whilst notifications so far for 2017 suggest a slight decrease in numbers, we continue to monitor the situation carefully ... and research continues to further investigate the rise."

International outbreaks of scarlet fever

This is not the first time scarlet fever has reemerged in recent years. Asia has seen epidemics of scarlet fever, with the most recent claiming two lives in Hong Kong in 2011. Academics linked these deaths—the first recorded in Hong Kong for a decade—to an antibiotic-resistant strain of the disease.

Antibiotic resistance is escalating around the world, with multidrug resistant Escherichia coli (E.coli) bacteria recently observed among U.S. children.

Reasons for the sudden English outbreak elude researchers. The researchers speculate that the resurgence could be driven in part by an increase in media coverage of scarlet fever, leading to better reporting. However, concrete evidence for such an explanation is lacking.

Stark impact on public health

The public health implications of the resurgence in England have been "substantial," the authors write. Finding the causes, they say, must be a priority. "We encourage parents to be aware of the symptoms of scarlet fever and to contact their general practitioner if they think their child might have it," Lamagni said.

In a linked comment, also published in *The Lancet*, University of Queensland researchers Mark J. Walker and

Stephan Brouwer urge a global response to local outbreaks of scarlet fever. "Heightened global surveillance for the dissemination of scarlet fever is warranted," they write, citing the unexplained resurgence of the disease.

"The current upsurge is both real and truly falls beyond that previously documented suggesting an exceptional cause and not simply reflecting a natural cycle," they continue. "Further understanding of the drivers behind the rise is essential to guide future prevention strategies."

SEE ALSO *Impetigo; Necrotizing Fasciitis; Strep Throat; Toxic Shock*

BIBLIOGRAPHY

Books

Bennett, John E., Raphael Dolin, and Martin J. Blaser. *Mandell, Douglas, and Bennett's Infectious Disease Essentials*. Philadelphia: Elsevier, 2016.

Bennett, John E., Raphael Dolin, and Martin J. Blaser. *Mandell, Douglas, and Bennett's Principles and Practice of Infectious Diseases*. 8th ed. Philadelphia: Elsevier, 2014.

Murray, Patrick R., Ken S. Rosenthal, and Michael A. Pfaller. *Medical Microbiology*. Philadelphia: Elsevier, 2015.

Wilson, Walter R., and Merle A. Sande. *Current Diagnosis and Treatment in Infectious Diseases*. New York: McGraw-Hill, 2014.

Periodicals

Chalker, V., et al. "Genome Analysis Following a National Increase in Scarlet Fever in England 2014." *BMC Genomics* 18 (2017): 224.

Guy, W., et al. "Increase in Scarlet Fever Notifications in the United Kingdom, 2013/2014." *Eurosurveillance* 19, no. 12 (2014): 1–2.

Ramsey, C. "A Sore Throat, Fever and Rash." *Prescriber* 25, no. 12 (2014): 22.

Silva-Costa, C. "Scarlet Fever Is Caused by a Limited Number of *Streptococcus pyogenes* Lineages and Is Associated with the Exotoxin Genes ssa, speA and speC." *Pediatric Infectious Disease Journal* 33, no. 3 (2014): 306–310.

Websites

"Group A Streptococcal (GAS) Disease." Centers for Disease Control and Prevention, September 16, 2016. https://www.cdc.gov/groupAstrep/index.html> (accessed December 9, 2017).

"Increase in Scarlet Fever across England." Public Health England, March 11, 2016. https://www.gov.uk/government/news/increase-in-scarlet-fever-across-england (accessed December 9, 2017).

Laura J. Cataldo

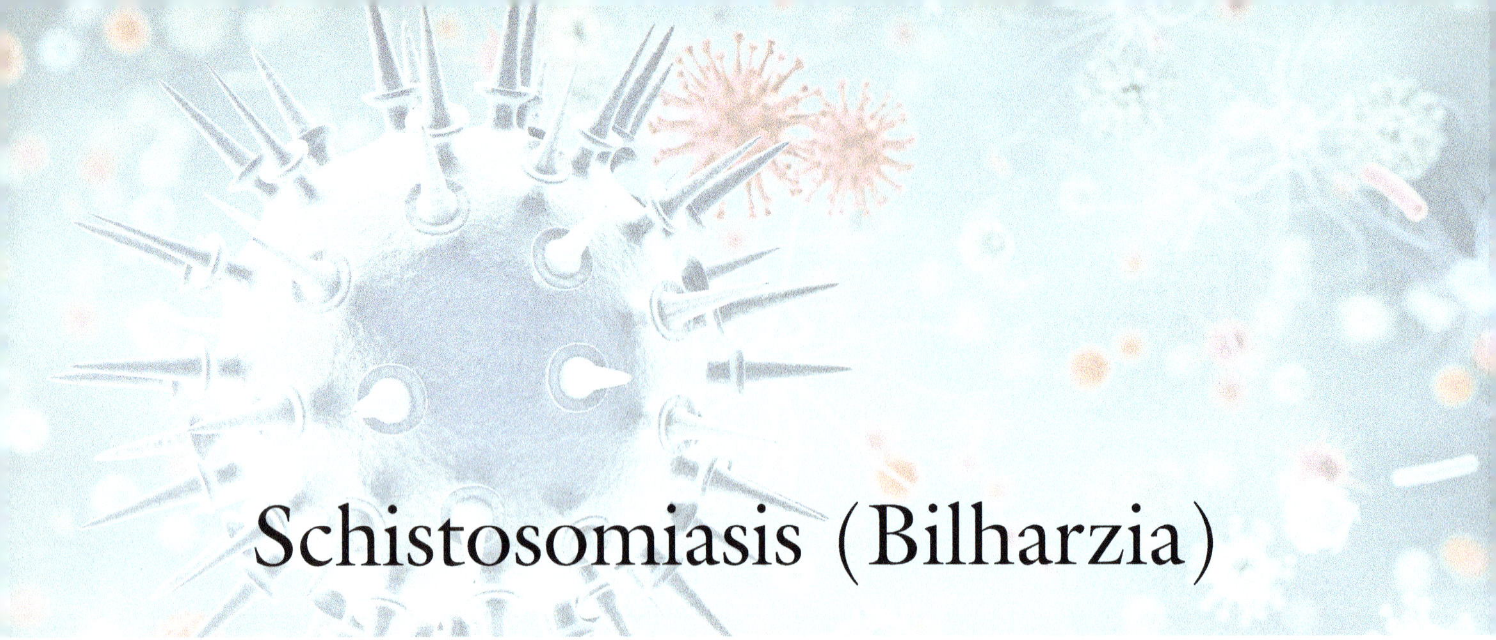

Schistosomiasis (Bilharzia)

Introduction

Schistosomiasis (SHIS-toe-SO-my-uh-sis), or bilharzia (bill-HAR-zi-a), is an infection that usually results in organ damage and is caused by parasitic flatworms (or flukes) of the genus *Schistosoma*. Schistosomiasis is considered the world's second-most devastating parasitic disease, ranked behind only malaria in terms of its negative impact on the global human population. An estimated 200 million people are infected with *Schistosoma* blood flukes, which people typically contract from water containing snails that host the parasites. The disease is known colloquially as snail fever. Cattle and other domesticated animals are also prone to schistosomiasis infection. According to the World Health Organization (WHO), schistosomiasis is endemic in 78 developing countries. Although the disease is mostly restricted to these countries, infections have been recorded in developed countries, usually due to travel, immigration, or the entrance of refugees.

Schistosomiasis can be acute. Acute symptoms commonly include a fever appearing six to eight weeks following infection and disappearing within a few months. Chronic schistosomiasis can cause organ damage as a result of the immune system attacking the parasite eggs retained in the body's organs. Chronic schistosomiasis is more common than acute schistosomiasis and usually does not appear until months or years after infection.

Treatment of schistosomiasis is effective and safe, involving a course of oral medications, typically praziquantel. While such drugs can treat and prevent transmission of schistosomiasis, the cost of such medication is prohibitive for widespread use in many developing nations where infection rates are highest. As a result, epidemiologists have emphasized the need to focus on methods of preventing infection of bodies of water, treating water, improving sanitation and hygiene, and controlling snails that host the parasitic flukes. While attempts to treat infected populations and to control infection had positive results in the early 21st century, observers called for a renewed focus on preventing transmission in 2017.

WORDS TO KNOW

ANTHELMINTIC Medicines that rid the body of parasitic worms.

ENDEMIC Present in a particular area or among a particular group of people.

HOST An organism that serves as the habitat for a parasite or possibly for a symbiont. A host may provide nutrition to the parasite or symbiont, or it may simply provide a place in which to live.

INTERMEDIATE HOST An organism infected by a parasite while the parasite is in a developmental, not sexually mature form.

SCHISTOSOMES Blood flukes.

Disease History, Characteristics, and Transmission

Humans have suffered from schistosomiasis for thousands of years, with cases recorded in the period of the Egyptian pharaohs. However, the parasite causing this disease was not recognized until the 19th century. In 1851 Theodor Bilharz (1825–1862) discovered the schistosome (a parasitic trematode worm), which caused infection in people. Since then a number of species of this parasite have been found to cause schistosomiasis, and their mode of infection and life cycle have been identified.

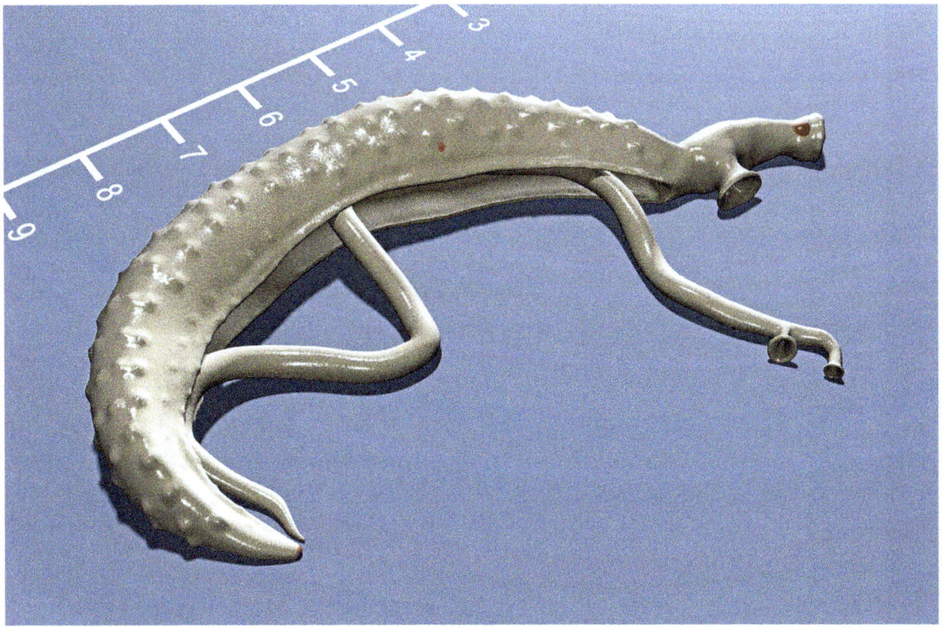

A conceptual image of a parasitic worm from the *Schistosoma* genus. Infection by these parasites, called schistosomiasis, causes organ damage in the regions of the body where the parasites' eggs are laid. Commonly infected areas include the urinary and intestinal systems. In rare cases, the eggs can become lodged in the brain and spinal cord, causing seizures and paralysis. © 3D4Medical/Science Source

In humans schistosomiasis is primarily caused by one of three types of *Schistosoma* parasites: *S. mansoni, S. haematobium*, and *S. japonicum*. There are also more localized species, such as *S. mekongi* in Cambodia and Laos and *S. intercalatum* in Central and West Africa, which can cause human infections. While infection by these parasites usually results in some form of schistosomiasis, some species cause severe dermatitis, notably cercarial dermatitis. Schistosomiasis is also common in cattle and other domesticated animals. There are 19 *Schistosoma* that infect nonhuman animals, some of which can be transmitted to humans.

There are both acute and chronic forms of schistosomiasis in humans. Acute symptoms usually appear six to eight weeks after exposure to the parasite. The most common acute syndrome is Katayama fever, with symptoms including fever, loss of appetite, weight loss, abdominal pain, blood in the urine, weakness, headache, joint and muscle pain, diarrhea, nausea, and cough. An initial symptom, usually occurring within days of exposure, is itchy skin. Acute symptoms usually disappear after a few weeks, although some cases can be fatal.

Chronic symptoms are more common than acute and appear months to years after exposure. Chronic symptoms arise as a result of the body's immune system responding to the parasite's eggs. These eggs become lodged in various areas of the body depending on their species. Organ damage usually occurs as a result of the immune system responding to egg retention. The most commonly infected areas of the body are the urinary and intestinal systems, and damage to the bladder, intestines, spleen, and liver can occur. In rare cases eggs may lodge in the spinal cord or brain, which can lead to seizures and paralysis.

Fresh water becomes contaminated with the eggs of *Schistosoma* parasite when a human who has the disease urinates or defecates in the water. The parasites hatch and are then ingested by freshwater snails, which are intermediate hosts during the parasite's life cycle. Following excretion from the snail, parasites can live in fresh water for 48 hours. During this time they may come into contact with another human host, and they can penetrate human skin within seconds. Once inside a host, the parasite develops into male and female worms that breed and lay eggs within blood vessels. While half of these eggs are excreted in urine or feces, the other half remain in the body and cause schistosomiasis symptoms. Excreted eggs hatch as soon as they enter fresh water, resulting in contamination of the body of water. The cycle begins again if snails are present in the contaminated water.

Scope and Distribution

Schistosoma parasites are endemic to 78 developing countries in Africa, the Caribbean, the Middle East, southern China, and Southeast Asia. Schistosomiasis is a major health risk, particularly within rural areas of central China and Egypt. As of 2017 an estimated 200 million people were infected with *Schistosoma* parasites worldwide. While most of those suffering from the disease were found in countries where the parasite is endemic, some cases were found in other countries as a result of travel, immigration, and entry of refugees into uninfected countries.

Most infected people tend to be rural agricultural workers who come into frequent contact with contaminated fresh water. In addition, a large number of children are infected. In some villages in Lake Volta, Ghana, for example, 90 percent of children were infected in 2007–2008.

■ Treatment and Prevention

Treatment for schistosomiasis is effective and safe, usually involving a one- to two-day course of oral medications. Depending on the type of infection, one of three drugs is usually used. Praziquantel can be used for all forms of infection. Oxamniquine is exclusively used for intestinal infections in Africa and South America. Metrifonate is used to treat urinary infections. Reinfection is possible after treatment, although the risk of serious organ damage is reduced as a result of treatment.

Because schistosomiasis is caused by a freshwater parasite, the most effective prevention methods involve avoiding or treating contaminated water. Because the parasite penetrates the skin within seconds, avoiding contact with potentially contaminated bodies of water, such as lakes, rivers, and dams, will prevent infection. This includes avoiding swimming, bathing, and working in these water bodies. Fresh water that has been filtered or heated to at least 150.0°F (65.5°C) is suitable for bathing. Water held in storage for 48 hours is also suitable for bathing because the parasite cannot survive for this length of time without a host. To ensure drinking water is free of parasites, filtering or boiling for at least one minute removes or kills the parasites.

Vigorous towel drying may also prevent parasite penetration if the body has only been briefly submerged in contaminated water. However, this method is not recommended as a reliable means of prevention. Long-term prevention of parasite infection involves controlling the occurrence of infection. Methods of control include educating people on parasite transmission, supplying clean water to regions where the parasite is endemic, diagnosing and treating infected people, controlling freshwater snails (the parasite's intermediate host), and increasing sanitation in infected regions.

■ Impacts and Issues

Schistosomiasis infection primarily occurs in developing countries for several reasons. The parasites that cause schistosomiasis are endemic to developing countries, and the conditions of life in these regions play an important role in the incidence and spread of the disease. Poverty, lack of awareness of the mode of infection and treatment methods, absent or inadequate public health facilities, and unsanitary conditions all contribute to an increased risk of infection in developing countries. Furthermore, transmission of the disease to different

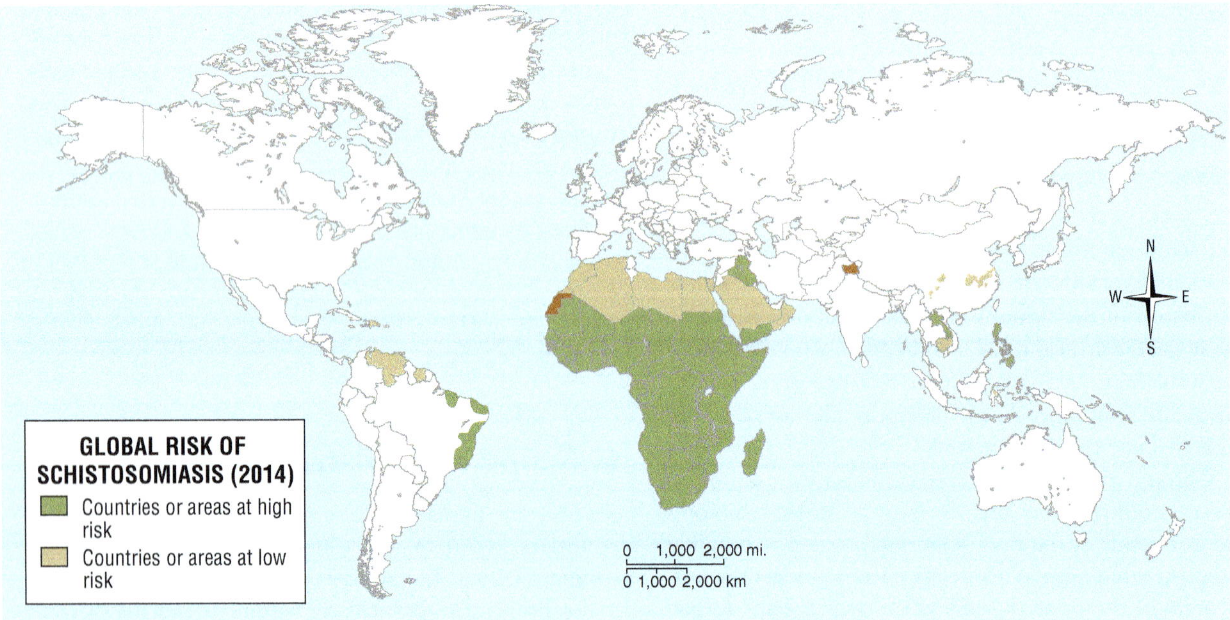

SOURCE: Adapted from "Schistosomiasis, Countries or Areas at Risk, 2014." World Health Organization. 2015. Available from: http://gamapserver.who.int/mapLibrary/Files/Maps/Global_ShistoPrevalence_ITHRiskMap.png

areas is facilitated by the movement of populations and refugees. In both rural central China and Egypt, schistosomiasis poses a major health risk to populations.

Schistosomiasis can result in symptomatic infections and fatalities. However, most infected people show no symptoms or only mild infections. In some cases the disease has been found to reduce productivity in infected adults and decrease growth and school performance in infected children. Treatment in infected regions has resulted in an increase in the health of the population, suggesting that the treatment methods are effective.

In 2001 WHO's decision-making body, the World Health Assembly, passed a resolution calling for the widespread use of anthelmintic drugs to combat schistosomiasis and other parasitic worm infections. A year later, in 2002, the Bill & Melinda Gates Foundation granted Imperial College London £20 million to establish the Schistosomiasis Control Initiative, which aims to provide drug treatment for people suffering from the illness in sub-Saharan Africa. The Schistosomiasis Control Initiative was credited with helping to drive down the price of praziquantel by more than 90 percent by encouraging production of a generic version of the drug.

Such initiatives to use preventive drug administration on a mass scale have helped combat schistosomiasis in the developing world. WHO reported dramatic improvements in certain regions as a result of an increase in treatment administration. Despite such progress various observers have called for more to be done to combat schistosomiasis due to the severe impact it has on the health of people and economies in the developing world. In a 2017 article for the *Lancet Infectious Diseases*, Nathan C. Lo and coauthors estimated that, without improvements in the prevention and treatment of the infection, "the population of sub-Saharan Africa will probably lose 2.3 million disability-adjusted life-years and US$3.5 billion of economic productivity every year, which is comparable to recent acute epidemics, including the 2014 Ebola and 2015 Zika epidemics."

The urgency of the problem and the limitations of drug therapies, which are costly and only partially effective during each treatment, led several leading observers to call for greater emphasis on eliminating transmission of *Schistosoma*. In a 2017 article for *PLOS Neglected Tropical Diseases*, Charles H. King stated that, while it is important to pursue preventive drug treatment in as broad a population as possible, health officials' emphasis should be on the "the elimination of *Schistosoma* transmission using combined drug, snail control, behavior change, and WaSH [water, sanitation, and hygiene] interventions."

Experts have also advocated for the development of a schistosomiasis vaccine. In 2008 the Sabin Vaccine Institute initiated the Schistosomiasis Vaccine Initiative, which ended in 2017. According to the institute, "Studies performed in populations living in schistosomiasis-endemic areas found that people who hadn't been infected with schistosomiasis in the last ten years—and who are therefore likely immune from the disease—were the only ones that exhibited an immune response" against an antigen termed Sm-TSP-2, indicating "an immune response against this antigen may be associated with protection against schistosomiasis." Clinical trials for the vaccine were ongoing as of 2017 in the *S. mansoni*-endemic area of Americaninhas, Brazil.

Another significant impact of schistosomiasis on human health is the likely link between urinary schistosomiasis infection and bladder cancer. In a number of infected regions, including Africa, a significant correlation exists between the occurrence of bladder cancer in patients also showing urinary schistosomiasis.

See Also *Cancer and Infectious Disease; Economic Development and Disease; Immigration and Infectious Disease; Immune Response to Infection; Parasitic Diseases; Swimmer's Ear and Swimmer's Itch (Cercarial Dermatitis); Travel and Infectious Disease; Waterborne Disease; World Health Organization (WHO)*

BIBLIOGRAPHY

Books

Jamieson, Barrie G. M., ed. *Schistosoma: Biology, Pathology, and Control.* Boca Raton, FL: CRC, 2016.

Secor, W. Evan, and Daniel G. Colley, eds. *Schistosomiasis.* New York: Springer, 2005.

Vercruysse, Jozef. "Schistosomiasis." In *Merck Veterinary Manual.* 11th ed. Whitehouse Station, NJ: Merck, 2016. This article can also be found online at https://www.merckvetmanual.com/circulatory-system/blood-parasites/schistosomiasis (accessed January 12, 2018).

Periodicals

Chitsulo, L., et al. "The Global Status of Schistosomiasis and Its Control." *Acta Tropica* 77, no. 1 (October 2000): 41–51. This article can also be found online at http://www.sciencedirect.com/science/article/pii/S0001706X00001224 (accessed January 12, 2018).

King, Charles H. "The Evolving Schistosomiasis Agenda 2007–2017: Why We Are Moving beyond Morbidity Control toward Elimination of Transmission." *PLOS Neglected Tropical Diseases* 11, no. 4 (2017): e0005517. This article can also be found online at https://doi.org/10.1371/journal.pntd.0005517 (accessed January 12, 2018).

Lo, Nathan C., et al. "A Call to Strengthen the Global Strategy against Schistosomiasis and Soil-Transmitted Helminthiasis: The Time Is Now." *Lancet Infectious Diseases* 17, no. 2 (2017): e64–e69.

Websites

"Schistosomiasis." Centers for Disease Control and Prevention, November 7, 2012. https://www.cdc.gov/parasites/schistosomiasis/index.html (accessed January 12, 2018).

"Schistosomiasis." Sabin Vaccine Institute. http://www.sabin.org/programs/schistosomiasis (accessed January 12, 2018).

"Schistosomiasis." World Health Organization, October 2017. http://www.who.int/mediacentre/factsheets/fs115/en/ (accessed January 12, 2018).

"Schistosomiasis (Bilharzia)." National Health Service, June 1, 2016. https://www.nhs.uk/conditions/schistosomiasis/ (accessed January 12, 2018).

"Schistosomiasis Control Initiative." Imperial College London. http://www.imperial.ac.uk/schistosomiasis-control-initiative/ (accessed January 12, 2018).

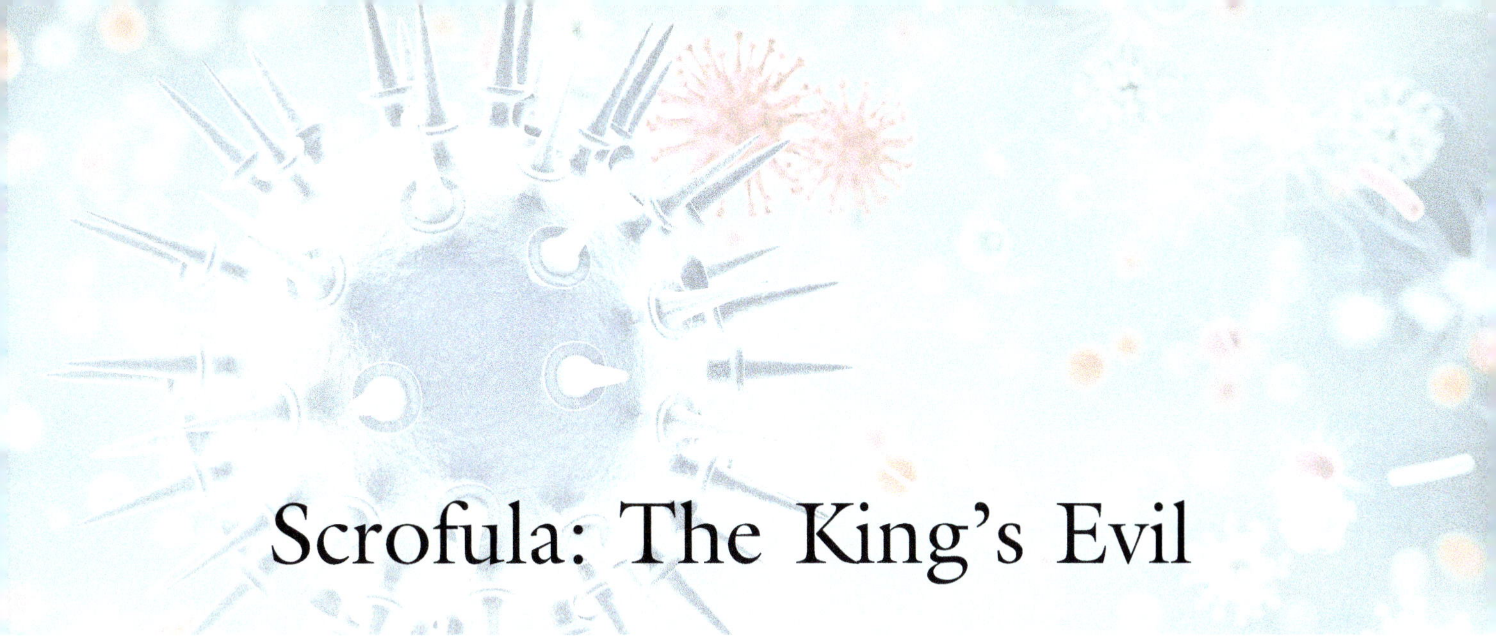

Scrofula: The King's Evil

Introduction

Scrofula is a form of extrapulmonary (outside the lungs) tuberculosis, a bacterial infection of *Mycobacterium tuberculosis.*

Disease History, Characteristics, and Transmission

The disease has a long and interesting history, first mentioned by Greek historian Herodotus (c.484 BCE?–c.430 BCE) in 400 BCE, who recommended that sufferers be quarantined. Scrofula has also had a long association with royalty. It became known as the King's Evil as early as 491 CE and was thought to be cured by the "king's touch." French monarchs claimed the ability to heal the disease from the time of Clovis I (c.466–511) in 481 CE through Louis XVI (1754–1793), who was beheaded in 1793, as did English kings beginning with Edward the Confessor (1042–1066) and ending with the Hanoverian dynasty in the 18th century.

Since antiquity monarchs claimed a quasi-divine status, often asserting that the royal family had a divine right to rule. Various ceremonies of royal courts may have led to the association of royalty with magical powers of healing. Perhaps because the lesions appeared and reappeared, people who were "touched" may have experienced an illusion of cure.

Politics also played a role in kings claiming they could heal scrofula. When the legitimacy of royal power was threatened—for instance, among early Norman kings who ruled England by conquest—"healing ceremonies" became predominant. Usually during these rituals, the physician would hold the head of the patient as the king would pronounce, "The king touches you, and God cures you," making the sign of the cross touching forehead to chin and cheek to cheek. After the ceremony French kings would distribute alms, and in England the king would cross the sore of the sick person with a stamp of gold called an angel, worth ten shillings. The angel had a hole bored through it for a ribbon to be drawn, so the sufferer could wear it around his or her neck.

Other cures included snails pounded to a paste and applied to the sores, the moist paste thought to be equivalent to the watery enlargement of the lymph nodes. The cure was effected by sympathetic medicine, or a "like-cures-like" form of healing.

The true reason why scrofula was contracted was not known until the late 19th century. Because scrofula seemed to affect whole families, it was assumed that it was a hereditary rather than an infectious disease. One of the common

WORDS TO KNOW

ANTIBIOTIC RESISTANCE The ability of bacteria to resist the actions of antibiotic drugs.

BROAD-SPECTRUM ANTIBIOTICS Drugs that kill a wide range of bacteria rather than just those from a specific family. For example, amoxicillin is a broad-spectrum antibiotic that is used against many common illnesses such as ear infections.

ENDEMIC Present in a particular area or among a particular group of people.

LESION The tissue disruption or the loss of function caused by a particular disease process.

QUARANTINE The practice of separating people who have been exposed to an infectious agent but have not yet developed symptoms from the general population. This can be done voluntarily or involuntarily by the authority of states and the federal Centers for Disease Control and Prevention.

PRESCIENTIFIC PRACTICE AND BELIEF

Samuel Johnson, an 18th-century author who wrote the first comprehensive English dictionary, suffered from scrofula as a child and proudly wore an angel around his neck his entire life.

ways it spreads is through infected milk—either from an infected mother's or wet nurse's breast milk or through contaminated cow's milk fed to infants or children. Before Koch's postulates of disease or pasteurization of milk in the 1880s, there was little understanding of the connection between bacteria and illness. During the mid- to late 19th century in the United States, clean and inexpensive milk was also difficult to get; milk was often watered down, chalk or dye could be added to whiten dirty milk, and "swill milk" (produced by cows fed distillery waste) was common. These cows often carried bovine tuberculosis, and milk bottles were not sterilized. It was also not until regulations about food safety were standardized, milk was regularly pasteurized, and dairy cleanliness maintained that scrofula ceased to be a health threat in industrialized nations.

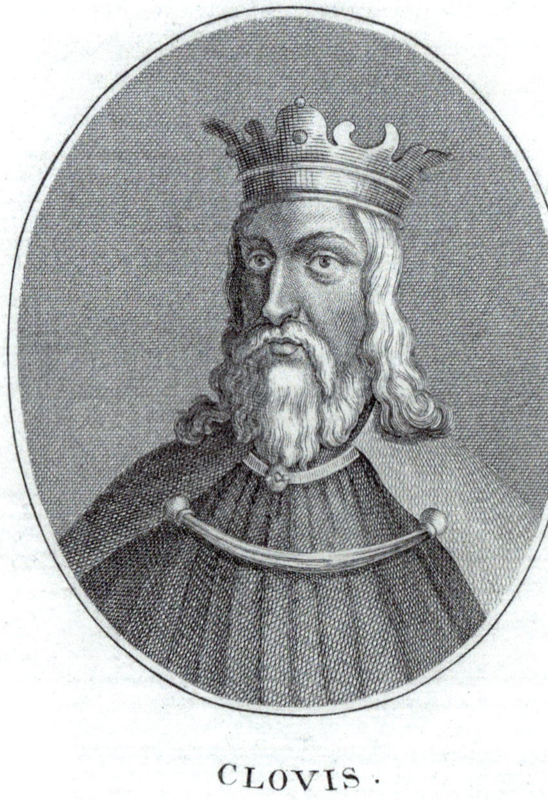

In 1st-century Europe scrofula was known as "the King's Evil" and thought to be cured by "the king's touch." Clovis I was the first king to claim to be able to cure the disease. *© Print Collector/ Getty Images*

The term scrofula comes from the Latin *scrofulae*, or a breeding sow, as pigs were thought to be susceptible to the disease and the glandular swellings on the neck were compared to little pigs. In 1852 the journal *Scientific American* endorsed the view held by some physicians that there was a connection between eating pork flesh and the disease.

In reality, scrofula results in an inflammation of the lymph glands and an enlargement of the lymph nodes in the neck. The nodes often ulcerate, causing draining sores, and the sufferer also has fevers, chills, sweats, and sometimes weight loss. Lesions often subside and then reappear as the disease takes its course and spreads through the skin, mucous membranes, bones, and joints.

The disease can be contracted either through person-to-person contact, contaminated milk, or even household objects that come into contact with the mouth.

Scope and Distribution

Though in developed countries scrofula is now quite rare, lowered immune function resulting from HIV infection increases the risk of contracting the disease. As antibiotic resistance to tuberculosis has increased, scrofula has been making its reappearance, particularly in underdeveloped countries.

Treatment and Prevention

Though the king's touch is no longer considered effective, new challenges have arisen in the treatment of scrofula.

Treatment is largely through broad-spectrum antibiotics in a nine- to twelve-month course, and recovery is usually complete, though there can be scarring around the lymph nodes.

Other treatments include short-course chemotherapy for tuberculosis patients and increased detection protocols. In severe cases surgery is done to remove the infected lymph nodes, but surgery alone tends to have disappointing results, as it does not remove the underlying infection and it can cause scarring.

Impacts and Issues

Since 1985 scrofula has made a comeback in the United States largely due to immigration from endemic countries, rising rates of HIV infection, antibiotic resistance, and the abandonment of aggressive tuberculosis screening and control programs.

In sub-Saharan Africa, and increasingly in Asia and South America, scrofula is also posing a threat, particularly as a form of HIV-related tuberculosis. In its TB/IV Clinical Manual, the World Health Organization reports that growing rates of HIV infections increase demands on programs to control tuberculosis, and there is more tuberculosis recurrence in AIDS patients.

SEE ALSO *Tuberculosis*

BIBLIOGRAPHY

Books

Bloch, Marc. *The Royal Touch: Sacred Monarchy and Scrofula in England and France.* Translated by J. E. Anderson. London: Routledge and Kegan Paul, 1973.

Bynum, Helen. *Spitting Blood: The History of Tuberculosis.* Oxford, UK: Oxford University Press, 2012.

Harries, Anthony, Dermot Maher, and Stephen Graham. "Introduction." In *TB/HIV: A Clinical Manual*, 21. Geneva: World Health Organization, 2004. This introduction can also be found online at http://apps.who.int/iris/bitstream/10665/42830/1/9241546344.pdf (accessed November 6, 2017).

Wolf, Jacqueline H. *Don't Kill Your Baby: Public Health and the Decline of Breastfeeding in the 19th and 20th Centuries.* Columbus: Ohio University Press, 2001.

Periodicals

Barlow, Frank. "The King's Evil." *English Historical Review* 95, no. 374 (January 1980): 3–27.

Lomax, Elisabeth. "Hereditary of Acquired Disease?: Early Nineteenth Century Debates on the Cause of Infantile Scrofula and Tuberculosis." *Journal of the History of Medicine and Allied Sciences* (October 1977): 356–374.

"Scrofula and Pork." *Scientific American* 8, no. 7 (October 1852): 54.

Wheeler, Susan. "Henry IV of France Touching for Scrofula by Pierre Firens." *Journal of the History of Medicine and Allied Sciences* 58 (2003): 79–81.

Websites

Lewis, Michael R. "Scrofula." Medscape. https://emedicine.medscape.com/article/858234-overview (accessed November 6, 2017).

Anna Marie E. Roos

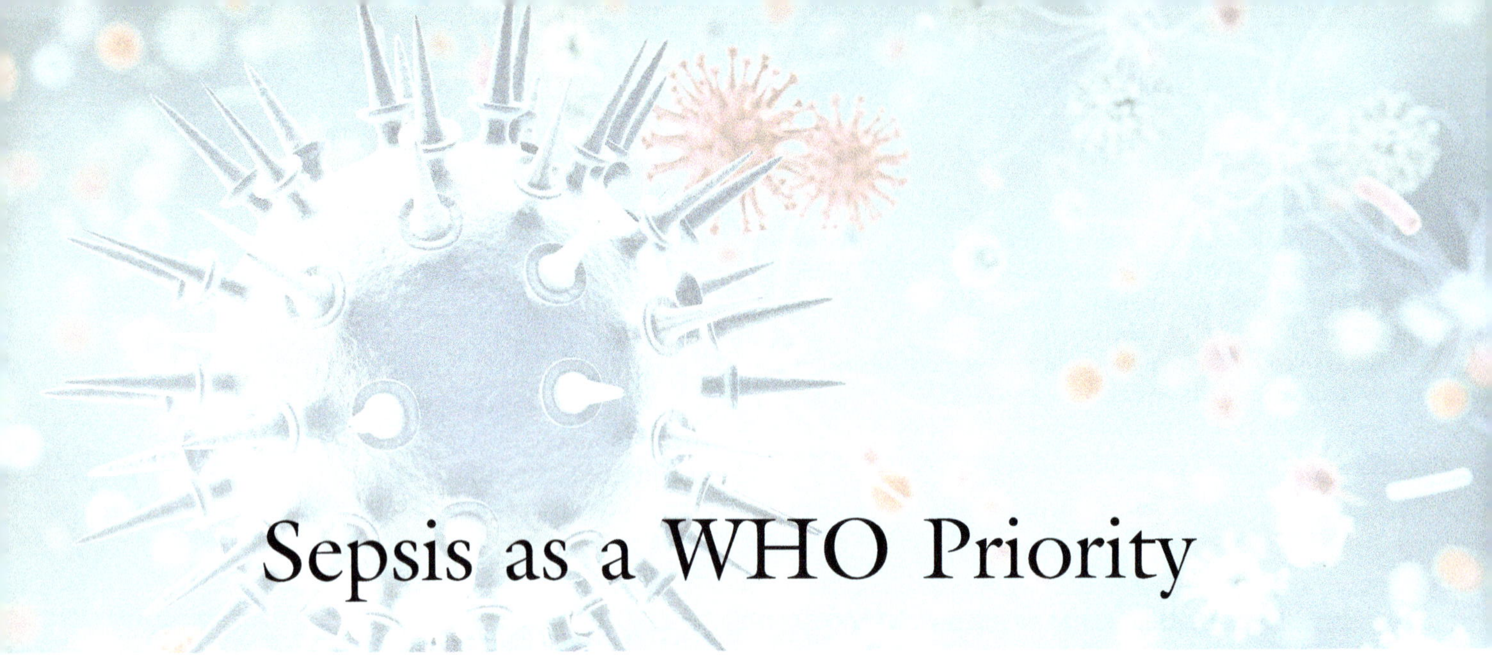

Sepsis as a WHO Priority

■ Introduction

Sepsis, also known as blood poisoning, is a serious condition in which the body's response to infection causes extreme complications, often leading to multiple organ failure and death. Sepsis is fatal if not promptly treated. Because symptoms of sepsis are similar to those of influenza, many patients delay seeking medical intervention.

In 2018 the World Health Organization (WHO) estimated that about 30 million people were affected by sepsis each year, leading to 6 million deaths. However, because data from low- and middle-income countries are scarce, many researchers believe that these numbers are grossly underestimated. According to the US Centers for Disease Control and Prevention (CDC), there are approximately 1.5 million cases of sepsis each year in the United States and approximately 250,000 deaths.

Realizing the enormity of sepsis-related fatality, WHO and the World Health Assembly (WHA) declared sepsis a global health priority by adopting a resolution on May 26, 2017, to "improve, prevent, diagnose and manage" sepsis.

■ History and Scientific Foundations

Sepsis affects patients of all age groups, although 49 percent of the affected population is between the ages of 65 and 84. Also, infants, individuals with compromised immunity, and those suffering from chronic ailments are more susceptible to sepsis.

Although long recognized in the medical community, sepsis has not been well or uniformly defined. To bring clarity, the 2012 sepsis guidelines by R. Phillip Dellinger et al. defined sepsis as "the presence (probable or documented) of infection together with systemic manifestations of infection." In 2016 Mervyn Singer et al. redefined sepsis as "a life-threatening organ dysfunction caused by a dysregulated host response to infection." These terms are key to identifying and treating the disease.

Deaths due to sepsis often go unnoticed, as they are generally attributed to the underlying infection. Therefore, the WHA established proper accounting and reporting of sepsis deaths as one of the steps in its 2017 resolution on sepsis. In addition, because awareness of sepsis is poor among patients, the WHA resolved to create awareness about sepsis and its symptoms through communication and national surveys. The WHA also proposed prevention and control of infection as key factors for limiting sepsis. In developing countries this requires overall improvement in hygiene, access to clean water, sanitation, vaccination, and clean environments for childbirth.

■ Applications and Research

An initiative led by the Global Sepsis Alliance brought together clinicians from 70 countries in 2017. The consensus resulted in the resolution to adopt sepsis as a global priority by the WHA and WHO. By recognizing sepsis as a WHO priority, WHO's governing body urges that the member states of the United Nations (UN) work toward implementing adequate measures to limit its health burden. Toward this goal, WHO also proposes to document the global impact and consequences of sepsis by the end of 2018. In addition, it will support the 194 UN member states in efforts to reduce the burden of sepsis. Furthermore, WHO will collaborate with other UN organizations and report on the implementation of various processes to the WHA by 2020.

Because sepsis is most often a result of infection, quickly recognizing and treating the condition is the key to saving lives. Consequently, health care providers must be adequately trained to identify and prevent sepsis in a timely manner. Because early identification is key, patients, relatives, and health care providers should be trained to ask whether the infection could be sepsis. The WHO initiative will work on educating health care teams and the patient population so they are better prepared for the timely identification, prevention, and treatment of sepsis.

Impacts and Issues

Sepsis is a major cause for concern in developed countries where community-based or health care–acquired infections have reached high rates. For example, in the United States, 50 percent of all hospital-acquired deaths are associated with sepsis, leading to an economic burden of about $24 billion annually. It is projected that this number will increase as the aging population grows. Globally, it is estimated that 1 in 10 patients hospitalized may contract sepsis, thus making it the most common condition among developed, developing, and poor countries.

Apart from creating awareness about hygiene and access to clean water and sanitation, the WHA and WHO recognize the need for research and development to combat antimicrobial resistance, as many microbial infections, left unattended, lead to sepsis.

The WHA has suggested action plans that include governmental interventions in developing strategies involving health care workers and patient advocacy groups. It also emphasizes the need to establish specific guidelines for sepsis awareness and management that will educate health care providers for emergency response.

WHO set aside $4.6 million toward implementing the resolution. It envisaged that the recognition of sepsis as a WHO priority and setting specific goals to address the threat of sepsis are major steps toward controlling the condition and saving millions of lives globally.

WORDS TO KNOW

ANTIMICROBIAL Slows the growth of bacteria or is able to kill bacteria. Antimicrobial materials include antibiotics (which can be used inside the body) and disinfectants (which can only be used outside the body).

IMMUNOCOMPROMISED Having an immune system with reduced ability to recognize and respond to the presence of foreign material.

PRIMARY SOURCE

Excerpt from Global Sepsis Alliance Press Release

SOURCE: *"Misdiagnosed Sepsis Now a Global Health Priority for World Health Organization." The George Institute, May 29, 2017. https://www.georgeinstitute.org.au/media-releases/misdiagnosed-sepsis-now-a-global-health-priority-for-world-health-organization (accessed February 28, 2018).*

INTRODUCTION: *Sepsis kills an estimated 6 million people each year and has an economic impact of tens of billions of dollars. The following excerpt from a Global Sepsis Alliance Press release outlines the key points of the joint World Health Assembly (WHA) and World Health Organization (WHO) resolution making sepsis a global priority and reducing its global burden.*

May 26, 2017

The adopted Resolution on Sepsis states:

1. Each year, sepsis causes approximately six million deaths worldwide, most of which are preventable.
2. Sepsis is a syndromic response to infection and the final common pathway to death from most infectious diseases.
3. Sepsis represents the most vital indication for the responsible use of effective antimicrobials for human health.
4. The UN Member States urgently need to implement and promote measures for prevention; such as clean childbirth practices, infection prevention practices in surgery, improvements in sanitation, nutrition and delivery of clean water.
5. Many vaccine-preventable diseases are a major contributor to sepsis in children and adults; national immunization programs are needed urgently.
6. Sepsis is an emergency that requires time-critical actions, improved training of health care professionals and laypeople.
7. UN Member States are required to promote research aimed at innovative means of diagnosing and treating sepsis across all ages, including research for new antimicrobial and other novel medicines/interventions, rapid diagnostic tests, and vaccines.
8. Public awareness needs to be raised and encouraged, for example by using the term 'sepsis' when communicating with patients, relatives, and other parties, or by supporting World Sepsis Day, every year on September 13.
9. Integrated approaches to the prevention and clinical management of sepsis are urgently needed, including access to appropriate health care for survivors.
10. The International Classification of Diseases (ICD) system needs to be applied and improved

to establish the prevalence and profile of sepsis and the development of specific epidemiologic surveillance systems.

SEE ALSO *CDC (Centers for Disease Control and Prevention); World Health Organization (WHO)*

BIBLIOGRAPHY

Books

Bastarache, Julie A., and Eric J. Seeley, eds. *Sepsis.* Philadelphia: Elsevier, 2016.

Periodicals

Dellinger, R. Phillip, et al. "Surviving Sepsis Campaign: International Guidelines for Management of Severe Sepsis and Septic Shock: 2012." *Critical Care Medicine* 41, no. 2 (February 2013): 580–637. This article can also be found online at https://www.sccm.org/Documents/SSC-Guidelines.pdf (accessed February 28, 2018).

Fleischmann, C., et al. "Assessment of Global Incidence and Mortality of Hospital-Treated Sepsis: Current Estimates and Limitations." *American Journal of Respiratory and Critical Care Medicine* 193, no. 3 (February 2016): 259–272.

Plevin, Rebecca, and Rachael Callcut. "Update in Sepsis Guidelines: What Is Really New?" *Trauma Surgery & Acute Care Open* 2, no. 1 (2017): e000088. This article can also be found online at http://tsaco.bmj.com/content/2/1/e000088 (accessed February 28, 2018).

Reinhart, Konrad, et al. "Recognizing Sepsis as a Global Health Priority: A WHO Resolution." *New England Journal of Medicine* 377 (August 3, 2017): 414–417. This article can also be found online at http://www.nejm.org/doi/full/10.1056/NEJMp1707170 (accessed February 28, 2018).

Singer, Mervyn, et al. "The Third International Consensus Definitions for Sepsis and Septic Shock (Sepsis-3)." *Journal of the American Medical Association* 315 (2016): 801–810. This article can also be found online at https://www.ncbi.nlm.nih.gov/pmc/articles/PMC4968574/ (accessed February 28, 2018).

Websites

"Sepsis." World Health Organization. http://www.who.int/sepsis/en/ (accessed February 28, 2018).

"Sepsis: Basic Information." Centers for Disease Control and Prevention, January 23, 2018 .https://www.cdc.gov/sepsis/basic/index.html (accessed February 28, 2018).

"WHA Adopts Resolution on Sepsis." Global Sepsis Alliance, May 26, 2017. https://www.global-sepsis-alliance.org/news/2017/5/26/wha-adopts-resolution-on-sepsis (accessed February 28, 2018).

Kausalya Santhanam

Severe Fever with Thrombocytopenia Syndrome

Introduction

Severe fever with thrombocytopenia syndrome (SFTS) is a potentially fatal emerging infectious disease caused by a virus known as severe fever with thrombocytopenia syndrome virus (SFTSV). SFTS was first reported in 2009 in China. As of early 2018, the disease had spread within Asia. While the understanding of SFTS is incomplete, researchers believe SFTSV is transmitted by ticks or through contact with the breath or blood of an infected person. Those who contract SFTS experience a wide range of symptoms, including diarrhea, vomiting, abdominal pain, fever, and headache. While many infections are resolved without treatment, the fatality rate of SFTS ranges from 6 percent in some areas up to 30 percent in others, with an average rate of 12 percent. Physicians typically treat SFTS with antibiotics, though their effectiveness varies depending on a range of factors. Because SFTS is a newly identified syndrome, much remains to be discovered about its characteristics, treatment, and prevention.

Disease History, Characteristics, and Transmission

The first reports of what is now known as SFTS occurred in China in 2009, when patients in rural Hubei

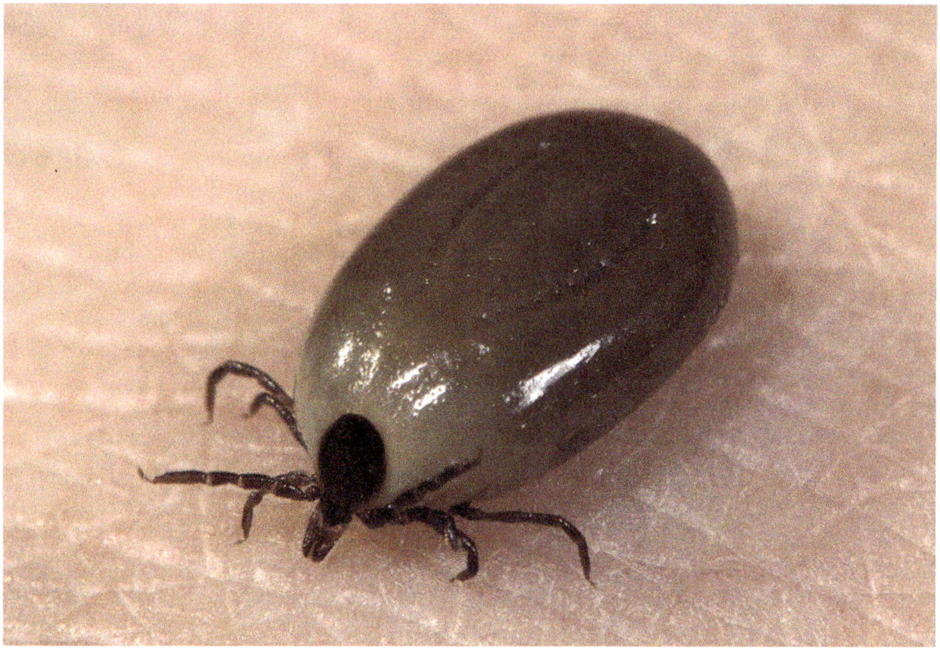

Ticks from the genus ixodes are vectors of severe fever with thrombocytopenia syndrome, an emerging infectious disease identified in South Korea, Japan, and China beginning in 2013. *© Scott Camazine/ Science Source*

WORDS TO KNOW

ANTIBIOTIC A drug, such as penicillin, used to fight infections caused by bacteria. Antibiotics act only on bacteria and are not effective against viruses.

BLOODBORNE PATHOGENS Disease-causing agents carried or transported in the blood. Bloodborne infections are those in which the infectious agent is transmitted from one person to another via contaminated blood.

EMERGING INFECTIOUS DISEASE A new infectious disease such as severe acute respiratory syndrome (SARS) or West Nile virus, as well as a previously known disease such as malaria, tuberculosis, or bacterial pneumonia that is appearing in a new form that is resistant to drug treatments.

ENDEMIC Present in a particular area or among a particular group of people.

OUTBREAK The appearance of new cases of a disease in numbers greater than the established incidence rate or the appearance of even one case of an emergent or rare disease in an area.

STRAIN A subclass or a specific genetic variation of an organism.

TICK Any blood-sucking parasitic insect of suborder *Ixodides*, superfamily *Ixodoidea*. Ticks can transmit a number of diseases, including Lyme disease and Rocky Mountain spotted fever.

and Henan provinces were stricken with an unusual illness that caused them to experience fevers and gastrointestinal issues and that was fatal for approximately 30 percent of them. As physicians looked at these patients' blood, they noticed a decrease in both platelets (thrombocytes) and white blood cells. Though doctors initially suspected the patients may have come down with anaplasmosis, a tick-borne disease, they were unable to detect signs of the bacteria that cause this disease, *Anaplasma phagocytophilum*. Continued investigation and surveillance over the next year led to the discovery of a new virus that was identified as the cause of the outbreak.

Researchers learned that SFTSV is a type of *Bunyaviridae*, a family of viruses that is transmitted by rodents and arthropods, including ticks and mosquitoes, and that causes such diseases as Crimean-Congo hemorrhagic fever and Rift Valley fever. Most specifically, SFTSV is categorized in the genera *Phlebovirus*. As researchers investigated the circumstances that led to patient infection with SFTSV, they found that both ticks and mosquitoes were present in the patients' homes, providing evidence that SFTS was transmitted like other *Bunyaviridae*. After the results of this initial surveillance and study of SFTS were published in the *New England Journal of Medicine* in 2011, further research helped expand on the understanding of the syndrome.

SFTSV is transmitted primarily via ticks, which transfer the virus to humans when they bite. In addition, the virus can be transmitted from one person to another through direct contact with an infected person's blood. Evidence suggests that infected people can also spread the virus in aerosolized form, simply by breathing; however, this had not been definitively proven as of early 2018.

Scope and Distribution

According to the authors of a 2017 article in *PloS ONE* titled "The Changing Epidemiological Characteristics of Severe Fever with Thrombocytopenia Syndrome in China, 2011–2016," 5,360 cases of SFTS were confirmed in China between 2011 and 2016, with reported cases increasing each year during this and the number of counties with cases nearly doubling from 98 to 167. Detailed tracking of SFTS in China is enabled by the China Information System for Disease Control and Prevention's guideline that physicians report cases within 24 hours of diagnosis. While China reports the majority of SFTS cases worldwide, SFTSV infections have also been reported in Japan and South Korea. In 2009 a North Korean working in the United Arab Emirates was diagnosed with SFTS, though he likely contracted the virus in his home country. Heartland virus, a condition similar to SFTS, has also been discovered in the United States.

Some evidence suggests that older people are more susceptible to SFTS and to fatality as a result of infection, but other studies have contradicted this finding. Research also indicates that people with either a low or high body mass index are more likely to die as a result of infection. In addition, research shows that infections typically occur between April and October, likely due to the effect of weather on ticks that carry the virus.

Treatment and Prevention

Treatment of SFTS typically involves the use of antibiotics, though different studies have reached conflicting conclusions on whether such treatment is effective. The antiviral favipiravir, which is typically used to treat influenza, has shown signs of helping combat SFTS, but this has not been confirmed. There is no known means of preventing SFTSV infection. However, people can re-

HEARTLAND VIRUS

In 2009 on a farm in Missouri, a 57-year-old man found and removed a small tick that had burrowed in his abdomen. Four days later he was hospitalized with a fever, diarrhea, and nausea, among other symptoms. For the next 10 days, he remained in the hospital, where his blood tested negative for a number of known tick-borne infections, influenzas, and other conditions. The same year, in the same part of Missouri, a 67-year-old man who had received numerous tick bites was hospitalized after experiencing similar symptoms. He also tested negative for a range of pathogens.

After studying the blood of both patients, researchers discovered that the cause of the illness was the same: a previously unknown strain of phlebovirus. As Laura K. McMullan and her coauthors noted in their 2012 article announcing the discovery of the virus, there are more than 70 strains of phlebovirus, but the newly discovered strain was one of only two to be transmitted by ticks rather than by mosquitoes or sand flies. The other tick-borne phlebovirus, severe fever with thrombocytopenia syndrome virus, also was first discovered in 2009 in China.

McMullan and her coauthors named this new strain Heartland virus. While evidence suggests the virus is spread by a specific kind of tick called the Lone Star tick, little is definitively known about how the virus is transmitted or how it can be treated or prevented. The urgency of finding answers about Heartland virus has increased as reported incidences of it have spread through the midwestern and southern United States since the first known cases occurred. As of July 2017, cases had been reported in Kansas, Oklahoma, Arkansas, Illinois, Kentucky, Tennessee, Georgia, and Missouri.

duce the likelihood of contracting SFTS by avoiding ticks as well as taking precautions when they come in contact with a patient who has a confirmed or suspected case of the syndrome.

Impacts and Issues

Because it is a newly identified disease, much study of SFTS remains to be done. Foremost among the aims of researchers is understanding how to better treat and prevent infection to contain this emerging disease as much as possible. As part of this effort, scientists have conducted research into factors that increase the risk of infection and the risk of death from infection. However, this research has sometimes been contradictory, indicating that more study is required. In addition, observers have pressed for greater education about the disease in endemic areas, for improved reporting of the disease, and for efforts to reduce populations of potential SFTSV-carrying ticks.

See Also *Crimean-Congo Hemorrhagic Fever; Mosquito-Borne Diseases; Rift Valley Fever; Tick-Borne Diseases*

BIBLIOGRAPHY

Books

Ergönül, Önder, Füsun Can, Lawrence Madoff, and Murat Akova, eds. *Emerging Infectious Diseases: Clinical Case Studies.* Waltham, MA: Academic Press, 2014.

Periodicals

Kato, Hirofumi, et al. "Epidemiological and Clinical Features of Severe Fever with Thrombocytopenia Syndrome in Japan, 2013–2014." *PLOS ONE* 11, 10 (2016). This article can also be found online at https://doi.org/10.1371/journal.pone.0165207 (accessed March 1, 2018).

Liu, Yan, et al. "The Pathogenesis of Severe Fever with Thrombocytopenia Syndrome Virus Infection in Alpha/Beta Interferon Knockout Mice: Insights into the Pathologic Mechanisms of a New Viral Hemorrhagic Fever." *Journal of Virology* 88, no. 3 (2014): 1781–1786. This article can also be found online at https://www.ncbi.nlm.nih.gov/pmc/articles/PMC3911604/ (accessed March 1, 2018).

McMullan, Laura K., et al. "A New Phlebovirus Associated with Severe Febrile Illness in Missouri." *New England Journal of Medicine* 367, 9 (2012): 834–841. http://www.nejm.org/doi/full/10.1056/NEJMoa1203378 (accessed March 5, 2018).

Park, Sun-Whan, et al. "Severe Fever with Thrombocytopenia Syndrome Virus, South Korea, 2013." *Emerging Infectious Diseases* 20, no. 11 (2014). This article can also be found online at https://wwwnc.cdc.gov/eid/article/20/11/14-0888_article (accessed March 1, 2018).

Sun, Jimin, et al. "Factors Associated with Severe Fever with Thrombocytopenia Syndrome Infection and Fatal Outcome." *Scientific Reports* 6 (2016). This article can also be found online at https://www.nature.com/articles/srep33175 (accessed March 1, 2018).

Wang, Mengmei, Jinjing Zuo, and Ke Hu. "Identification of Severe Fever with Thrombocytopenia Syndrome Virus in Ticks Collected from Patients." *International Journal of Infectious Diseases* 29 (2014): 82–83. This article can also be found online at https://www.sciencedirect.com/science/article/pii/S1201971214016464 (accessed March 1, 2018).

Yu, Xue-Jie, et al. "Fever with Thrombocytopenia Associated with a Novel Bunyavirus in China." *New England Journal of Medicine* 364, 16 (2011): 1523–1532. This article can also be found online at http://www.nejm.org/doi/full/10.1056/NEJMoa1010095 (accessed March 2, 2018).

Websites

"Heartland Virus." Centers for Disease Control and Prevention. https://www.cdc.gov/heartland-virus/index.html (accessed March 2, 2018).

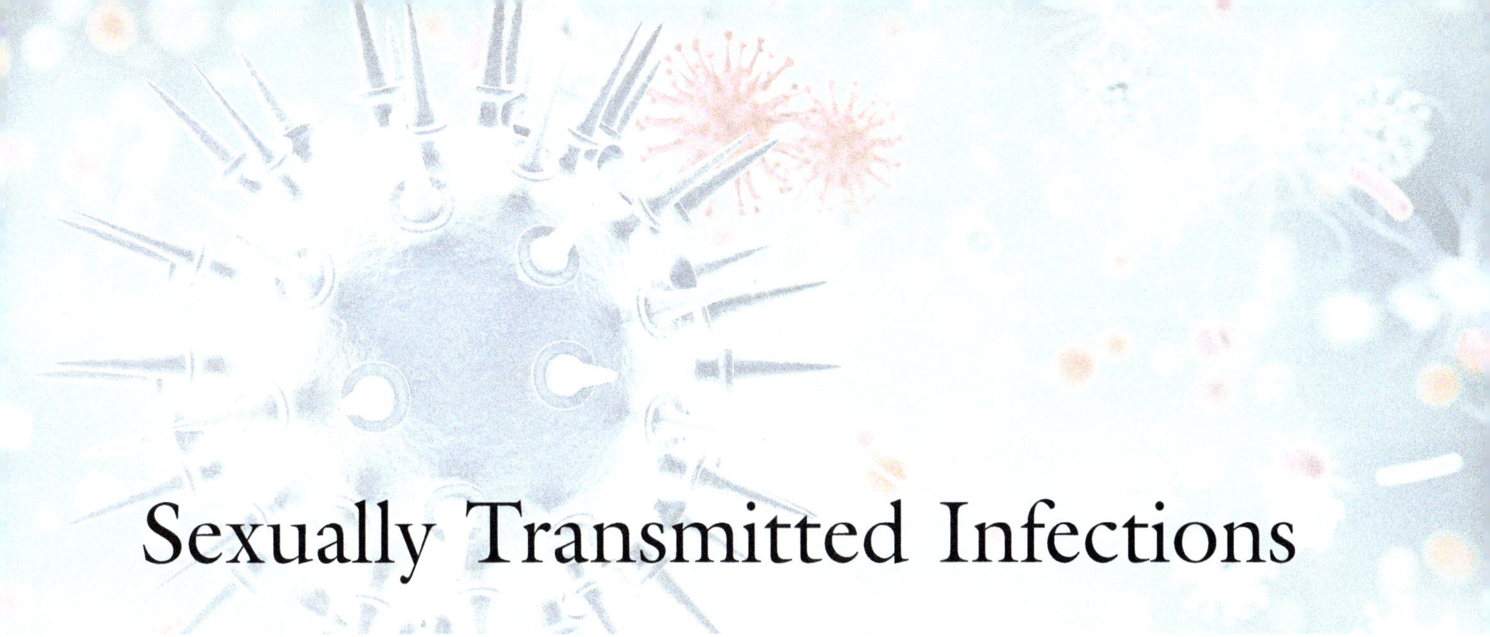

Sexually Transmitted Infections

Introduction

Sexually transmitted infections (STIs), also called sexually transmitted diseases (STDs), are communicable diseases transmitted through intimate sexual contact. STIs include human immunodeficiency virus (HIV)/acquired immunodeficiency syndrome (AIDS), *Chlamydia*, syphilis, human papillomavirus (HPV) infection, genital herpes, and gonorrhea. STIs are caused by different microbes and have varied symptoms and health consequences. People with STIs often do not realize they are infected and may pass the disease onto others through sexual contact. Moreover, having one STI can put people at greater risk of contracting another. For instance, people with syphilis are more likely to become infected with human immunodeficiency virus (HIV).

The stigma attached to visiting a sexual health clinic has declined since the 20th century. But there is still a need for greater awareness of STI risk factors and strategies for prevention. Prevention of STIs is challenging because it involves people's sexual behavior, including whether they choose to use condoms, be selective about their sexual partners, or even abstain from sex.

Sexually transmitted infections cause a serious burden globally. In addition to their immediate impacts on patient

WORDS TO KNOW

ANTIBODIES Proteins found in the blood that help fight against foreign substances called antigens. Antigens, which are usually proteins or polysaccharides, stimulate the immune system to produce antibodies, or Y-shaped immunoglobulins. The antibodies inactivate the antigen and help remove it from the body. While antigens can be the source of infections from pathogenic bacteria and viruses, organic molecules detrimental to the body from internal or environmental sources also act as antigens. Genetic engineering and the use of various mutational mechanisms allow the construction of a vast array of antibodies (each with a unique genetic sequence).

CHANCRE A sore that occurs in the first stage of syphilis at the place where the infection entered the body.

HARM-REDUCTION STRATEGY In public health, a public policy scheme for reducing the amount of harm caused by a substance such as alcohol or tobacco. The phrase may refer to any medical strategy directed at reducing the harm caused by a disease, substance, or toxic medication.

LYMPHADENOPATHY Any disease of the lymph nodes, or the glandlike bodies that filter the clear intercellular fluid called lymph to remove impurities.

NOTIFIABLE DISEASE A disease that the law requires be reported to health officials when diagnosed. Also called a reportable disease.

OPPORTUNISTIC INFECTION An infection that occurs in people whose immune systems are diminished or are not functioning normally. Such infections are opportunistic insofar as the infectious agents take advantage of their host's compromised immune system and invade to cause disease.

PURULENT Any part of the body that contains or releases pus. Pus is a fluid produced by inflamed, infected tissues and is made up of white blood cells, fragments of dead cells, and a liquid containing various proteins.

health, they can put patients at risk for infertility and opportunistic infections such as HIV. Globally, STIs result in morbidity and mortality, affecting the quality of life as well as the sexual and reproductive health of adults and adolescents. STIs range from bacterial infections that are readily treatable to viral infections that have no treatment, such as HIV, which make it difficult for health care workers to educate the affected population globally. Emerging pathogens such as the Zika and Ebola viruses can be transmitted sexually, further complicating the task of managing STIs.

■ Disease History, Characteristics, and Transmission

STIs were once known as venereal diseases (VDs). The term *venereal* derives from Venus, the goddess of love. STIs are a diverse group of conditions. Some, such as HIV/AIDS and syphilis, can be life threatening. Others, such as *Chlamydia* infection, can lead to infertility. HPV can lead to cervical cancer. Some STIs, such as thrush and nonspecific urethritis (infection of the urethra), are not usually medically serious but can cause a great deal of discomfort. The symptoms of STIs vary but often include itching, swelling, or redness around the vagina or penis and unusual discharge or pains in the lower abdomen.

HIV/AIDS

HIV attacks the immune system, rendering the infected person susceptible to opportunistic infections such as *Pneumocystis jirovecii* pneumonia, *Candida*, cytomegalovirus, and a host of other microbial infections that are otherwise harmless in a healthy person. A rare skin cancer called Kaposi's sarcoma may also occur during the later stages of HIV/AIDS.

HIV is spread through blood, semen, vaginal fluids, and breast milk. For infection to occur, fluids from an infected individual must come into contact with a mucous membrane or damaged tissue. It can also enter the bloodstream directly through the use of a syringe that has been previously used by an infected individual. The first stage of HIV/AIDS lasts from first exposure to the appearance of antibodies in the person's blood, which may take up to three months. Some people display symptoms such as fever, sore throat, or headache soon after they have been infected with HIV. This is a sign of the immune system fighting the infection. Sometimes the dentist is the first person to discover symptoms of HIV infection because dental problems, such as sore or bleeding gums, mouth sores, and yeast or fungal infections, are quite common.

After this first stage, HIV infection enters a second, silent phase with few, if any, symptoms. This stage can last as long as 15 years. The immune system is keeping the infection in check, but the person is still infectious to others through sexual contact or other contact with infected

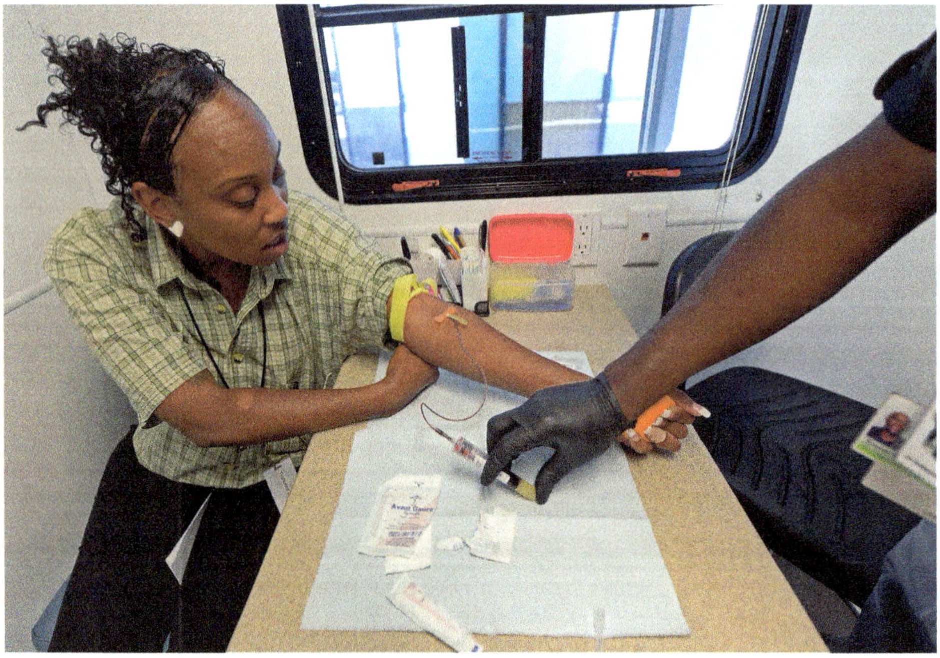

A woman is tested for HIV and other sexually transmitted diseases in a mobile clinic during a 2013 health fair in Los Angeles, California. *© Kevork Djansezian/Getty Images*

blood. In the third stage the immune system begins to show the signs of damage done by HIV. A common symptom at this time is swollen lymph glands, or lymphadenopathy.

In the final stage, which is classified as AIDS, the virus becomes more active than before, and there are many symptoms such as malaise (a general feeling of being unwell), night sweats, weight loss, and diarrhea. This is when opportunistic infections set in and Kaposi's sarcoma takes hold. In its final stages, AIDS may also affect the brain, causing a gradual deterioration in mental faculties called dementia.

ECONOMIC IMPACTS

Sexually transmitted diseases (STIs) are a major public health challenge in the United States. Although there have been advances in prevention, diagnosis, and treatment, the health and economic burdens of these infections remain high. A 2013 study found that in 2008 there were 19.7 million new infections, with an estimated total lifetime direct medical cost of $15.6 billion. The lifetime cost of new HIV infections alone was estimated at $12.6 billion.

Chlamydia

Chlamydia trachomatis infection is probably the most common STI caused by bacteria. It is transmitted through vaginal, oral, or anal intercourse. When *C. trachomatis* infects the genital tract, it often produces no symptoms, although women may report a burning sensation on urination and a vaginal discharge. Men may experience a discharge from the penis, as well as itching and a burning sensation. When left untreated, women run the risk of developing pelvic inflammatory disease (PID), a chronic condition that is often accompanied by severe abdominal pain and fever, long-lasting pelvic pain, and infertility. It is also linked to gonorrhea.

Gonorrhea

Gonorrhea is a bacterial STI caused by infection with *Neisseria gonorrhoeae*. It is spread through vaginal, oral, or anal intercourse and can be passed to an infant from an infected mother during childbirth. Gonorrhea infection causes urethritis (inflammation of the lining of the urethra) among men and cervicitis (inflammation of the cervix) in women. In men the first symptom of gonorrhea is usually painful urination, followed by a thick, purulent (pus-containing) discharge from the urethra. However, many men have no symptoms.

In women painful urination is also the first symptom of gonorrhea. This is followed by a vaginal discharge and, sometimes, bleeding. The symptoms in women are so vague that they may be mistaken for symptoms of a vaginal or urinary infection. In men complications of gonorrhea include inflammation of the epididymis (the coiled tube leading sperm from the testicles), which can lead to infertility. Gonorrhea in women can lead to salpingitis, which is inflammation of the fallopian tubes. It is also a leading cause of pelvic inflammatory disease.

Syphilis

Syphilis is caused by the bacterium *Treponema pallidum* and progresses through an infectious stage and a noninfectious stage over many years. The infectious stage lasts for a few months, during which there may be few symptoms. The noninfectious stage, which follows if syphilis is not treated early on, may also be without symptoms, or it may be accompanied by major heart or neurological damage.

Infectious syphilis starts with the appearance of a single sore, known as a chancre, either on or inside the genitals or elsewhere on the body, such as on the eyelid or lip. Those affected may be completely unaware of the presence of the chancre, which lasts for three to six weeks and heals without treatment but is infectious in case of sexual contacts.

Skin rash and mucous membrane lesions are the key symptoms of the secondary stage of syphilis. Sometimes the rash from secondary syphilis is so faint as to be unnoticeable. There may be other symptoms such as fever, swollen glands, weight loss, headaches, loss of appetite, and fatigue. However, this stage also resolves within a few weeks without any treatment.

Latent or tertiary syphilis is untreated disease after the primary and secondary stages. It has no obvious symptoms and may or may not be infectious. Complications, which may occur many years after the original infection, can affect the brain and the heart. A pregnant woman with syphilis might pass the disease onto her unborn child. Congenital syphilis can lead to stillbirth, death shortly after birth, physical deformity, or neurological problems.

Other STIs

Genital herpes, often known solely as herpes, is caused by the herpes simplex virus (HSV) and may cause no symptoms, remaining undiagnosed for a long time. HSV-2 is generally associated with most cases of genital herpes, whereas HSV-1 causes the condition only occasionally. Possible symptoms of HSV infection include itchiness, burning, and pain in the genital area, pain when passing urine, and the presence of small, fluid-filled blisters developing into sores. People with herpes have an increased risk of becoming infected with HIV, and pregnant women may pass the infection onto their babies during childbirth.

According to the CDC, human papillomavirus is the most common STI, affecting 79 million Americans as of November 2017. It causes both genital warts and cervical cancer. It is most commonly spread through vaginal or anal intercourse, but it can also be spread through oral sex. While HPV infection often causes no symptoms, it sometimes triggers benign tumors known as papillomas, or warts on the hands and feet or in the genital area. Most HPV infections clear up on their own, but they are also capable of causing cancers in the cervix and, more rarely, in the vagina, vulva, penis, and anus.

Other STIs include nonspecific urethritis, which affects men and causes discomfort in the urethra, the tube leading from the bladder to the tip of the penis. A discharge from the urethra is also common. Trichomoniasis is caused by the bacterium *Trichomonas vaginalis* and may have no symptoms or may produce a yellow or green discharge from the vagina and be accompanied by soreness. Men usually act as carriers of trichomoniasis and often do not show symptoms. Thrush is a yeast infection of the vagina or penis, which can result in intense itching and a thick, white discharge. Finally, both pubic lice and scabies are passed on by close contact, including sexual contact, and may cause intense itching.

STIs are generally transmitted through intimate sexual contact with another person. This can occur through unprotected vaginal, oral, or anal sex or by having genital contact with an infected partner. The relative risks of various kinds of sexual activity tend to vary with the disease. For instance, the risk of contracting gonorrhea and syphilis through oral sex appears to be greater than that of contracting HIV.

The risk of becoming infected with HIV is elevated by having another STI, as many STIs can involve breaks in the skin in the genital area, making it easier for the virus to enter the body. Nonulcerative STIs such as trichomoniasis may increase HIV risk through increasing the number of white blood cells that can be infected by the virus.

Scope and Distribution

Most major public health organizations, such as the US Centers for Disease Control and Prevention (CDC), the World Health Organization (WHO), and the UK Health Protection Agency (HPA), collect data on STIs to plan policy and educate and inform the population of the risks.

WHO reports that more than 1 million people contract STIs each day, with about 499 million new cases around the world each year. People between the ages of 15 and 49 are the most susceptible. In 2016 WHO recorded 131 million cases of *Chlamydia trachomatis*, 78 million cases of gonorrhea, 6 million cases of syphilis, 142 million cases of *Trichomonas vaginalis*, 536 million cases of HSV-2, and 291 million cases of HPV. Five million HIV infections were also reported in 2016.

In the United States alone, 20 million cases of STIs are reported each year, primarily affecting people between 15 and 24 years of age. Although many STIs are notifiable diseases, meaning that state health departments mandate their reporting, many cases go unreported. HPV and genital herpes, which are probably extremely common, are not reported at all. In 2017 the CDC reported increased numbers of gonorrhea and syphilis cases in the United States.

Treatment and Prevention

STIs caused by bacteria, such as chlamydia, gonorrhea, and syphilis, and protozoa, such as trichomoniasis, are easily curable with a single dose of antibiotics. In the case of STIs caused by viruses, such as genital herpes and AIDS, antiviral drugs can be used to modulate the course of the disease.

Antiviral drugs are used to treat genital herpes, although they cannot cure the infection. Genital warts eventually disappear without treatment, although some people may choose to have them removed using liquid nitrogen or caustic agents. HIV/AIDS is treatable with antiretroviral drugs, which stop the virus from reproducing. As with herpes, these drugs do not cure the disease.

Informing current and past sexual partners of a positive diagnosis of STI so they can also be diagnosed and treated is key to reducing the risk of spreading the infection and of reinfection. A sexual health clinic normally counsels patients in many aspects of dealing with the disease, including helping their sexual partners seek timely intervention.

Among those who are sexually active, practicing safer sex is the most effective way of preventing STIs. This involves men using a condom for each occasion of penetrative sex. There is no guarantee that a prospective partner is free of STIs. The more sexual partners a person has, the greater the chance of exposure to infection, even with the use of condoms, which do not provide 100 percent effective protection. Monogamous sex with a healthy partner is a behavioral choice that may afford the highest level of protection from STIs. Health care workers advising in this area attempt to exercise sensitivity and avoid judging patients' behaviors while providing them with the information they need to reduce the risk of contracting an STI.

In the United States there are approved vaccines for prevention against HPV. Gardasil® is used for the prevention of cancers in both males (ages 9 to 21) and females (ages 9 to 26). Cervarix® is used only in females for prevention of cervical cancer.

Impacts and Issues

An increasing concern for researchers is the emergence of multidrug-resistant strains of bacteria. Some strains of gonorrhea in particular are showing susceptibility to even the class of antibiotics considered the last line of treatment. In the United States, the CDC is working to monitor the emergence of antibiotic-resistant strains and to develop new treatment options. Drug-resistant strains of chlamydia and syphilis are emerging in other areas of the world. In 2017 WHO warned that the problem is growing.

The increase in STIs in the United States and elsewhere can partly be attributed to an increase in awareness of the issue, better diagnostic techniques, and an increase in the number of sexual health clinics carrying out tests. Other reasons include earlier age of first sexual activity, sexual practices with multiple partners, and increased mobility of groups such as tourists, immigrants, and armed forces, who may be more likely to have partners outside of a primary relationship.

There are ongoing efforts to educate and control STIs all over the world. The Global Health Sector Strategy on STIs, 2016–2021, offers a plan for reducing new STI cases, improving sexual health, and promoting the well-being of people around the globe. Most importantly the strategy promotes quality STI services including identifying the underlying causes of STI epidemics and providing access to effective prevention and treatments.

Many STIs, including gonorrhea, chlamydia, and syphilis, are symptomless. Those affected may be unaware of the infection and continue infecting their sexual partners. There is also the risk of damage to the reproductive system that goes unnoticed, such as in the case of *Chlamydia* infection. These factors increase the need for screenings to identify infection early in order to prevent complications and transmission of the disease to others.

Vaccines are being developed for STIs caused by viral infections. In case of HSV-2 infections, which are responsible for more than 50 percent of HIV cases, vaccines can play a key role in prevention of primary infection. The availability of vaccines against HPV infection has considerably reduced the burden of HPV in developed countries. However, the accessibility, availability, and affordability of these vaccines are concerns in low-income countries.

SEE ALSO *AIDS (Acquired Immunodeficiency Syndrome);* Chlamydia *Infection; Gonorrhea; Herpes Simplex 2 Virus; HIV; HPV (Human Papillomavirus) Infection; Syphilis*

BIBLIOGRAPHY

Books

Beigi, Richard H., ed. *Sexually Transmitted Diseases.* Chichester, UK: John Wiley, 2012.

Marr, Lisa. *Sexually Transmitted Diseases: A Physician Tells You What You Need to Know.* 2nd ed. Baltimore, MD: Johns Hopkins University Press, 2007.

Whiteside, Alan. *HIV & AIDS: A Very Short Introduction.* 2nd ed. Oxford, UK: Oxford University Press, 2016.

Periodicals

Freeman, E. E., et al. "Herpes Simplex Virus 2 Infection Increases HIV Acquisition in Men and Women: Systematic Review and Meta-Analysis of Longitudinal Studies." *AIDS* 20 (2006): 73–83.

Heijne, J. C., et al. "Uptake of Regular Chlamydia Testing by U.S. Women: A Longitudinal Study." *American Journal of Preventive Medicine* 39 (2010): 243–250.

Low, Nicola, Nathalie Broutet, and Richard Turner. "A Collection on the Prevention, Diagnosis, and Treatment of Sexually Transmitted Infections," *PLOS Medicine* 14, no. 6 (2017): e1002333.

Owusu-Edusei, Kwame, Jr., et al. "The Estimated Direct Medical Cost of Sexually Transmitted Infections in the United States, 2008." *Sexually Transmitted Diseases* 40, no. 3 (March 2013): 197–201.

Websites

"Global Health Sector Strategy on Sexually Transmitted Infections 2016–2021: Towards Ending STIs." World Health Organization, June 2016. http://apps.who.int/iris/bitstream/10665/246296/1/WHO-RHR-16.09-eng.pdf?ua=1 (accessed March 6, 2018).

"Report on Global Sexually Transmitted Infection Surveillance 2013." World Health Organization, June 2014. http://apps.who.int/iris/bitstream/10665/112922/1/9789241507400_eng.pdf?ua=1 (accessed March 6, 2018).

"Sexually Transmitted Infections (STIs)." World Health Organization, August 2016. http://www.who.int/mediacentre/factsheets/fs110/en/ (accessed March 7, 2018).

"2016 Sexually Transmitted Diseases Surveillance." Centers for Disease Control and Prevention, January 2018. https://www.cdc.gov/std/stats16/default.htm (accessed March 7, 2018).

Susan Aldridge
Kausalya Santhanam

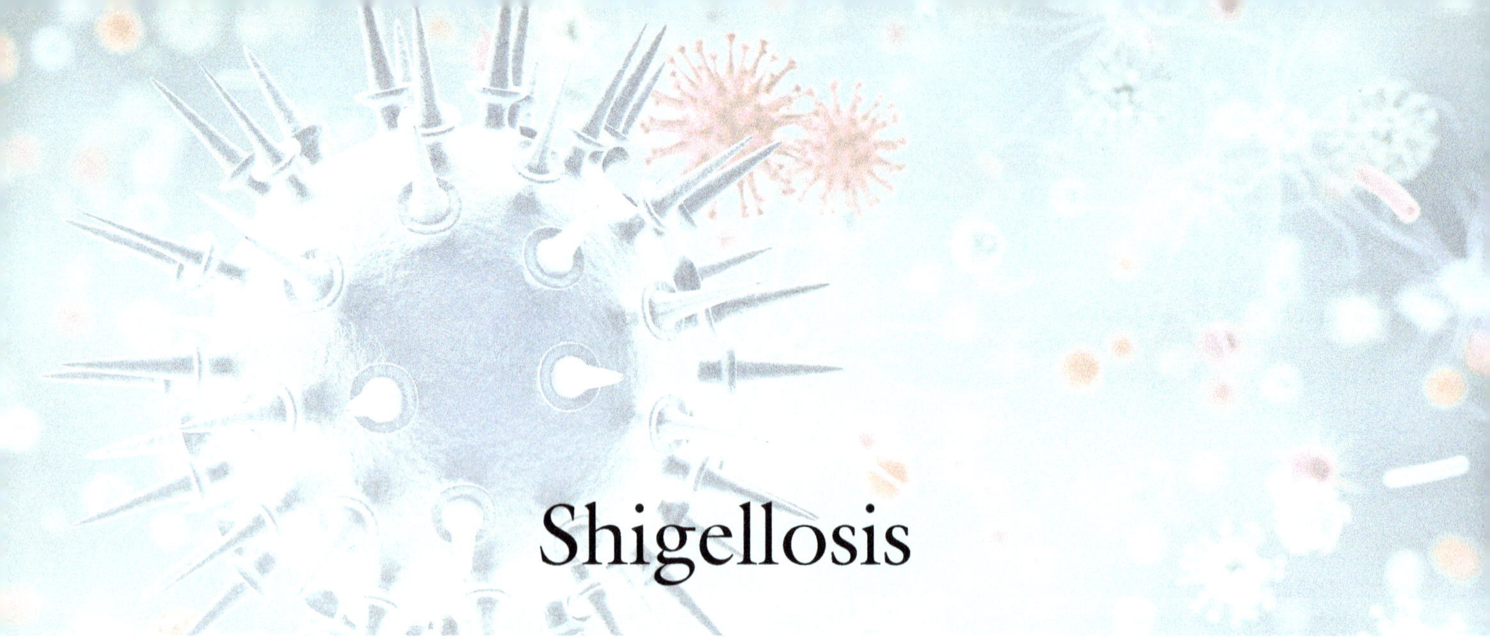

Shigellosis

Introduction

Shigellosis is an infection of the gastrointestinal tract that arises when a person is infected with bacteria in the genus *Shigella*. These bacteria are transmitted among a human population when people ingest food or drink contaminated with fecal matter from an infected person. To a lesser extent the disease is also spread by sexual contact. Following a one- to two-day incubation period, most patients experience nausea, diarrhea, fever, and stomach cramps. Whereas most people recover from shigellosis within a week without treatment, severe cases require antibiotics in order to recover.

Shigellosis occurs worldwide and is very infectious. It is most prevalent in developing nations in which epidemics often occur. Anyone can get shigellosis, but it is more common among people with poor hygiene, such as young children, as well as people living or traveling through areas with dense living conditions and poor sanitation. Because there is no vaccine against shigellosis, prevention is achieved through improving sanitation and hygiene, washing hands prior to handling food, washing food prior to eating, and boiling drinking water.

Shigellosis can become a major issue during emergency situations, such as mass evacuations when many people temporarily live together in poor conditions. There is also potential for *Shigella* bacteria to be used for biological warfare.

Disease History, Characteristics, and Transmission

Shigellosis is a gastrointestinal infection caused by bacteria from the genus *Shigella*. There are four species of *Shigella*: *S. dysenteriae, S. flexneri, S. boydii*, and *S. sonnei*. *Shigella* infect humans and other primates. Bacteria from this genus were first identified by Japanese scientist Kiyoshi Shiga (1871–1957) in 1897 after he isolated *S. dysenteriae*, which was causing the gastrointestinal disease dysentery, in infected people.

Shigellosis is usually transmitted via the fecal-oral route. Inadequate handwashing after using the toilet or changing a baby's diaper, followed by food or water handling, leads to contamination of food and drink. This is a common method for person-to-person transmission of the *Shigella* bacteria. Flies are also a source of transmission, as they travel between infected fecal matter and food or drink.

WORDS TO KNOW

BIOLOGICAL WEAPON A weapon that contains or disperses a biological toxin, a disease-causing microorganism, or another biological agent intended to harm or kill plants, animals, or humans.

DYSENTERY An infectious disease that has ravaged armies, refugee camps, and prisoner-of-war camps throughout history. The disease still is a major problem in developing countries with primitive sanitary facilities.

FECAL-ORAL TRANSMISSION The spread of disease through the transmission of minute particles of fecal material from one organism to the mouth of another organism. This can occur by drinking contaminated water, by eating food exposed to animal or human feces (such as by watering plants with unclean water), or by being exposed to the poor hygiene practices of those preparing food.

REITER'S SYNDROME Named after German doctor Hans Reiter (1881–1969), a form of arthritis (joint inflammation) that appears in response to bacterial infection in some other part of the body. Also called Reiter syndrome, Reiter disease, or reactive arthritis.

Food and water may also become contaminated when vegetables are grown in soil containing sewage or when people defecate in bodies of water.

Shigellosis leads to the development of gastrointestinal symptoms, such as dysentery. Symptoms include diarrhea, fever, stomach cramps, and nausea. Symptoms generally begin a day or two after the bacteria are contracted. Although recovery is common in most cases, infection with *S. flexneri* may result in long-term problems such as arthritis, eye irritation, and painful urination. This is known as Reiter's syndrome and may continue for months to years.

Scope and Distribution

Shigellosis occurs worldwide. It is particularly common in countries with inadequate sanitation systems. Furthermore, *S. dysenteriae* type 1, although rare in the United States, is a major health concern for many developing countries. In the United States and other developed countries, the most common forms of *Shigella* is *S. sonnei*. The Centers for Disease Control and Prevention (CDC) estimates that there are 80 million to 165 million cases of shigellosis each year around the world and

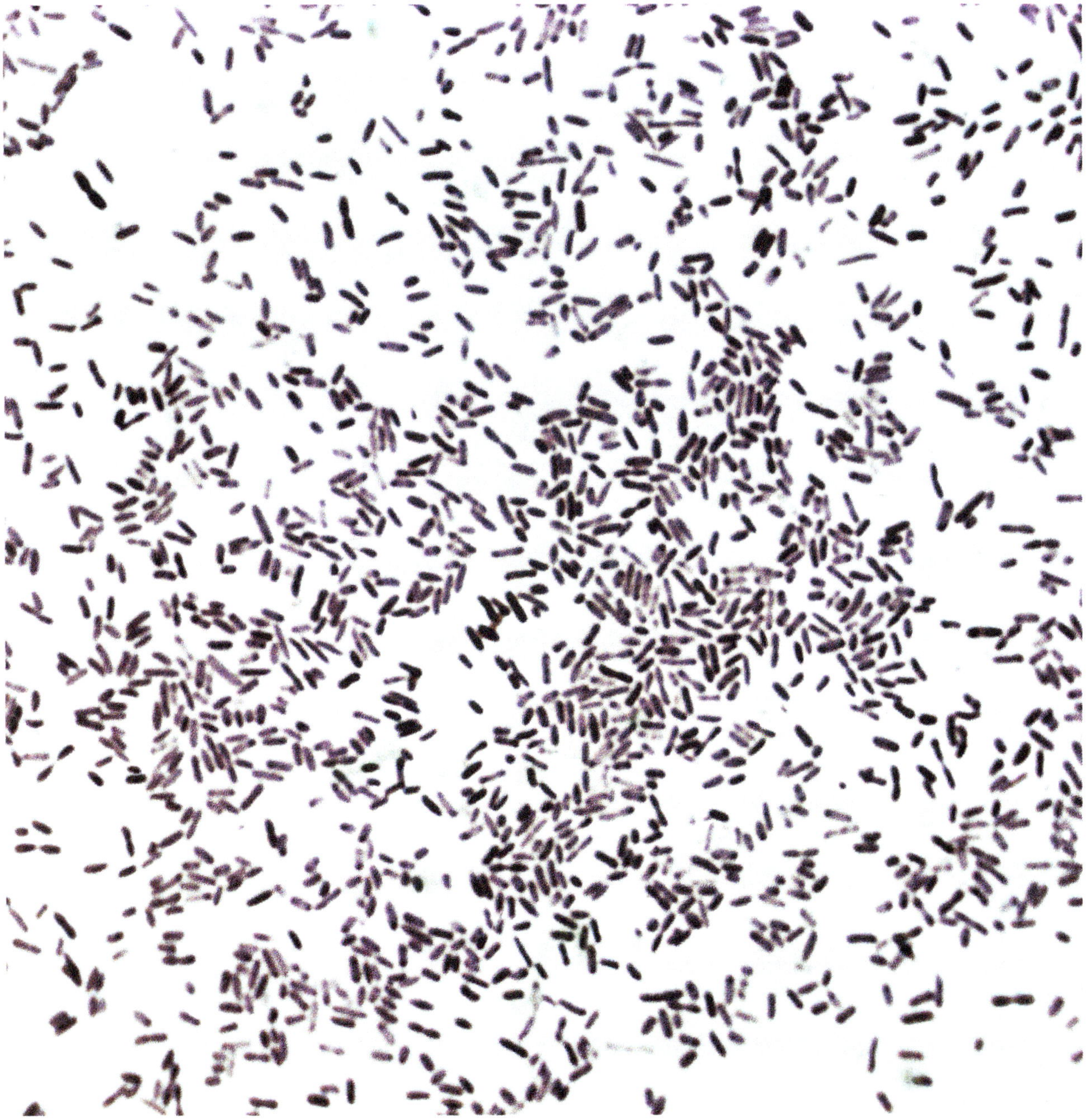

Shigella dysenteriae bacteria is one of the four bacteria in the genus *Shigella* that cause the gastrointestinal infection shigellosis in humans.

that about 600,000 people who are sickened with the bacteria die. The annual number of cases of shigellosis in the United States is around 500,000.

Although anyone is capable of contracting shigellosis, some people are more susceptible than others. This includes toddlers, who usually are not fully toilet trained. In addition, childcare facilities provide a setting in which the bacteria can spread through a number of children in a short period. Foreign travelers are also more susceptible to infection if they travel through regions in which the disease is prevalent and sanitation methods are poor. Men who have sex with men and immunocompromised people are also at greater risk of contracting the disease, as are people living in crowded conditions or institutions, such as prisons.

The transmission of shigellosis is enhanced in conditions of poor sanitation and close human contact. These conditions are common in developing countries where funding for sanitation may be lacking and residents may not be educated about the need for hygiene. In addition, these conditions are common in emergency situations, such as after a hurricane or earthquake, when many people are housed together temporarily.

Treatment and Prevention

Shigellosis is a bacterial disease and may be treated with antibiotics. However, mild cases of shigellosis do not require antibiotics because full recovery usually occurs within a week. People suffering from severe infections, or those who have a compromised immune system that prevents them from fighting the infection themselves, usually require a course of antibiotics. The most common antibiotics used are ciprofloxacin and azithromycin. However, *Shigella* bacteria have begun to develop resistance to antibiotics, which may reduce the effectiveness of treatment.

Other treatments are aimed at the symptoms of the infection. These may include administering fluids to prevent or reverse dehydration and medicines to reduce temperature and prevent convulsions. Antidiarrheal agents are not recommended by the CDC because they are likely to make the illness worse. Bismuth subsalicylate, which is sold under the brand name Pepto-Bismol in the United States, may alleviate some symptoms.

While research on the development of a vaccine against shigellosis has been underway since 1940, no vaccine was available as of 2018. As a result, preventative measures center on avoiding ingestion of *Shigella* bacteria. In developed countries, in which sanitation is usually good and water is clean, prevention is best achieved through handwashing and improving personal hygiene. However, in developing countries, in which sanitation is often poor and clean water is not readily available, improvements in sanitation methods and increased availability of clean water are necessary to prevent communitywide spread of the bacteria. In addition, people with shigellosis can best prevent spreading the disease to others by washing their hands after going to the toilet, avoiding preparing food for others or swimming in public areas, and practicing safe sex.

Impacts and Issues

Shigellosis is common in developing countries due to poor sanitation and, in some cases, overcrowding. However, situations such as this can arise in developed nations when natural disasters cause mass evacuation of people, including during hurricanes, tornadoes, and floods. Often mass evacuations result in a large number of people living in close quarters. Because these living quarters are often temporary and are usually not made to house large numbers of people, sanitation standards tend to be lower than normal. The combination of high-density living with poor sanitation increases the risk of shigellosis within the population.

Another potential issue concerning *Shigella* bacteria is its use as a biological weapon. *Shigella* has been considered a potential agent of biological warfare since at least 1932, when the Japanese investigated its potential. Biological warfare involves using pathogens or toxins to cause mass death and disease among humans, animals, or plants during war. Biological terrorism is similar, except the pathogens and toxins are used for terrorist purposes. In addition to *Shigella*, other bacterial agents, such as *Salmonella* and *Escherichia coli*, are considered potential biological threats. *Shigella* can potentially be spread via a community's water supply, which could cause many cases of shigellosis.

In the developed world, shigellosis outbreaks are uncommon but not unheard of. In 2014, for example, almost 200 people in the San Francisco, California, area were infected with *Shigella* after eating infected food at a restaurant. There is increasing concern that some *Shigella* species transmitted between men who have sex with men are becoming resistant to antibiotics.

PRIMARY SOURCE

Residents of Flint, Mich., Are Still Afraid of the City's Water

SOURCE: *Andrews, Travis M. "Residents of Flint, Mich., Are Still Afraid of the City's Water."* Washington Post *(October 4, 2016). This article can also be found online at https://www.washingtonpost.com/news/morning-mix/wp/2016/10/04/flint-residents-too-scared-of-the-water-to-wash-its-making-them-sick/?utm_term=.c549ee11b881 (accessed February 9, 2018).*

INTRODUCTION: *The following article describes the shigellosis outbreak that occurred in Flint, Michigan, in 2016. It appears that the shigellosis outbreak was a result of poor hygiene. Some residents were afraid that by washing their hands with city water, they would expose themselves to lead-tainted water. In 2015 Flint city water was shown to have "elevated lead levels," which was particularly dangerous for children.*

That fear, caused by the 2015 findings of elevated lead levels in the town's water supply, had led many of the town's residents to forgo some basic hygiene, such as washing their hands or bathing with water—even though the federal government has deemed the water safe when using a water filter.

"People aren't bathing because they're scared," Jim Henry, Genesee County's environmental health supervisor, told CNN. "Some people have mentioned that they're not going to expose their children to the water again."

As a result, the city is facing another outbreak: This time of Shigellosis, an infectious disease caused by the bacteria *Shigella*. The main way to prevent the infection is by washing one's hands, according to the Centers for Disease Control and Prevention.

Symptoms include bloody diarrhea, malaise, abdominal pain and tenesmus—constantly feeling the need to evacuate one's bowels, even with an empty colon.

It is, according to the CDC, "very contagious" and resistant to many "first-line drugs," the most common antibiotics.

"It's very easy to transmit person to person, or through food. If people aren't washing their hands, it runs through the whole county," Henry told CNN.

The disease is fairly common in America—about 500,000 cases appear in the country each year—but incidents in Genesee County, home to Flint, have more than tripled in the past calendar year, according to MLive.com.

Since October 2015, 84 cases of the disease have appeared in Flint, a city that normally experiences 20 instances each year, according to CNN.

In response, the Genesee County Health Department has issued three advisories since May 2016, warning of the disease and urging residents to wash their hands.

The water crisis that led to this outbreak began in April 2014, when the city of Flint began drawing water from the Flint River to save money. Previously, it had shared Detroit's water supply.

A short 18 months later, though, "researchers discovered that the proportion of children with above-average lead levels in their blood had doubled," *The Washington Post* reported.

The city switched back to Detroit's water supply, but it was too late—the water from the Flint River had proved corrosive to the lead pipes, and lead levels in water still remain unsafe. Residents have been forced to drink bottled or filtered water for more than a year now, as *The Post* noted.

As a result, residents are averse to using tap water for much of anything, even when their taps are outfitted with the proper filters.

Take 35-year-old mother of four Bobbie Nicks, who was interviewed by the *Detroit Free Press* in July while nervously watching her children swim in an above-ground pool. Her family uses bottled water to drink, cook and brush their teeth, even though they have filters installed in their home.

But she let her kids swim because she didn't want to steal their childhood.

"We have to find a good balance of letting kids be kids and not dealing with what we have to deal with as parents—of being scared of the water," Nicks told the paper.

Some parents, despite the warnings of health officials like Jim Henry, won't let their children near water in any capacity, which Henry claimed is one of the catalyzing factors in the current Shigellosis outbreak.

Henry told CNN that people of Flint, many of whom still must use filtered and bottled water due to damaged water pipes, use baby wipes—available free of charge at various sites around the city—instead.

Delano Whidbee, a Flint resident with two young daughters, is one such parent. His household has lead filters on the shower and faucets, making them safe to use, but he still refuses to bathe his girls in the water.

"With the kids, we use baby wipes," he told CNN.

Henry said that's a problem.

"Baby wipes are not effective, they're not chlorinated, it doesn't kill the bacteria and it doesn't replace handwashing," Henry said. "People have changed their behavior regarding personal hygiene. They're scared."

Speaking with MLive.com, Suzanna Cupal, public health division director for the Genesee County Health Department, stressed the importance of properly washing hands—for at least 20 seconds using soap and water, taking care to clean under the fingernails—to prevent further outbreak.

It's the latest issue arising from the water disaster, which led to six current and former Michigan state employees to be charged with criminal activity in association with the crisis. It has also led to cries for the resignation of Michigan's Republican Gov. Rick Snyder, who has called the disaster his Hurricane Katrina. Most importantly, it has left a city of nearly 100,000 without safe tap water for more than a year.

See Also *Antibiotic Resistance; Bacterial Disease; Bioterrorism; Childhood-Associated Infectious Diseases, Immunization Impacts; Cohorted Communities and Infectious Disease; Dysentery;* Salmonella *Infection (Salmonellosis)*

BIBLIOGRAPHY

Books

Bowen, Anna. "Shigellosis." In *CDC Yellow Book 2018: Health Information for International Travel*, edited by Gary W. Brunette et al. New York: Oxford University Press, 2017. This article can also be found online at https://wwwnc.cdc.gov/travel/yellowbook/2018/infectious-diseases-related-to-travel/shigellosis (accessed February 8, 2018).

Periodicals

Baker, Kate S., et al. "Intercontinental Dissemination of Azithromycin-Resistant Shigellosis through Sexual Transmission: A Cross-Sectional Study." *Lancet* 15, no. 8 (August 2015): 913–921. This article can also be found online at https://www.sciencedirect.com/science/article/pii/S147330991500002X (accessed February 7, 2018).

Kotloff, Karen L., et al. "Shigellosis." *Lancet* (forthcoming). This article can also be found online at https://www.sciencedirect.com/science/article/pii/S0140673617332968 (accessed February 7, 2018).

Mani, Satchin, Thomas Wierzba, and Richard I. Walker. "Status of Vaccine Research and Development for *Shigella*." *Vaccine* 34, no. 26 (June 3, 2016): 2887–2894. This article can also be found online at https://www.sciencedirect.com/science/article/pii/S0264410X16002863 (accessed February 8, 2018).

Simms, I., et al. "Intensified Shigellosis Epidemic Associated with Sexual Transmission in Men Who Have Sex with Men—*Shigella flexneri* and *S. sonnei* in England, 2004 to End of February 2015." *Eurosurveillance* 20, no. 15 (April 16, 2015). This article can also be found online at http://www.eurosurveillance.org/content/10.2807/1560-7917.ES2015.20.15.21097 (accessed February 7, 2018).

Websites

"Shigella." World Health Organization. http://www.who.int/immunization/topics/shigella/en/ (accessed February 7, 2018).

"*Shigella*—Shigellosis." Centers for Disease Control and Prevention, January 17, 2018. https://www.cdc.gov/shigella/ (accessed February 7, 2018).

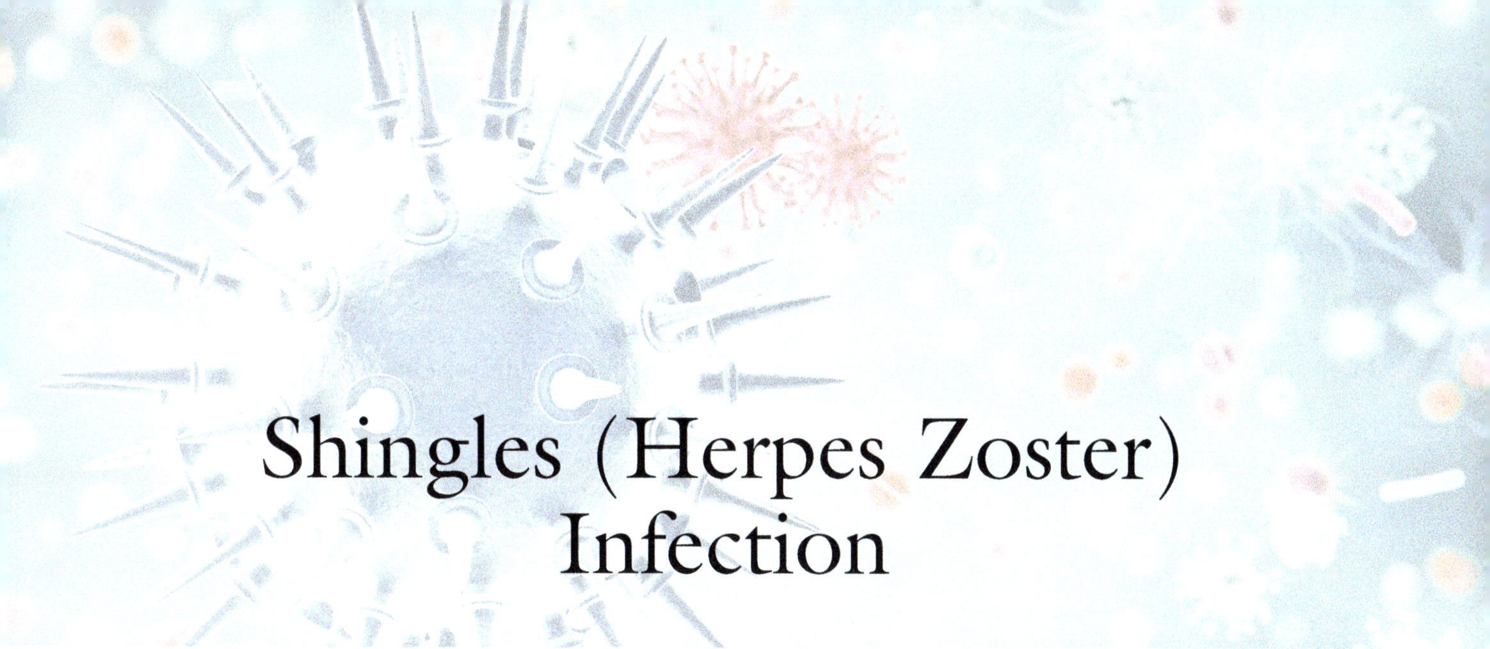

Shingles (Herpes Zoster) Infection

Introduction

Shingles is a disease that arises when the varicella-zoster virus (VZV), which causes chickenpox when it initially infects a human, reactivates after lying dormant in nerve cells. Shingles develops first as localized pain, after which a rash, composed of fluid-filled blisters, forms. Fever, headache, chills, and a general feeling of sickness often accompany the pain. The rash develops within a few days, and it may take several weeks for the blisters to break open and crust over. A person is infectious until the rash crusts over. Some cases of shingles result in serious complications, the most common being postherpetic neuralgia, a type of nerve pain.

Treatment for shingles involves oral administration of an antiviral treatment. In addition, the symptoms and any complications are treated. Treatment for postherpetic neuralgia is aimed primarily at controlling the pain, typically with analgesics.

Shingles is a worldwide disease but is most common in older adults, usually those aged 50 or older. Immunocompromised people are also at a greater risk of developing shingles. According to the Centers for Disease Control and Prevention (CDC), nearly a third of Americans will develop shingles at some time in their life, with risk increasing with age. As a result, two vaccines have been approved for use in the United States, and both are aimed at preventing shingles in the more vulnerable group of patients who are age 60 and older.

Disease History, Characteristics, and Transmission

Shingles, which is also known as herpes zoster, is caused by a virus known as varicella-zoster virus (VZV). This virus also causes chickenpox. Shingles arises in people who have already had chickenpox because the virus remains in the body. Usually, VZV remains dormant in the body. It settles in nerve roots and, when activated, causes the development of shingles.

While shingles cannot be passed directly from one person to another, the varicella-zoster virus can be transmitted (via airborne respiratory droplets or fluid from rash blisters) from a person with shingles to a person who has never contracted chickenpox. If this occurs, the exposed person would initially develop chickenpox rather than shingles, although shingles would eventually arise after a period of dormancy. Only when the rash crusts over does the infected person stop being contagious. This typically occurs within 7 to 10 days of infection. However, it can take two to four weeks for a rash to clear up completely.

WORDS TO KNOW

CHICKENPOX A common and extremely infectious childhood disease that can also affect adults. Also called varicella disease and sometimes spelled chicken pox, it produces an itchy, blistery rash that typically lasts about a week and is sometimes accompanied by a fever.

IMMUNOCOMPROMISED A reduction in the ability of the immune system to recognize and respond to the presence of foreign material.

POSTHERPETIC NEURALGIA Neuralgia is pain arising in a nerve that is not the result of any injury. Postherpetic neuralgia is neuralgia experienced after infection with a herpesvirus, namely *Herpes simplex* or *Herpes zoster*.

VARICELLA-ZOSTER VIRUS (VZV) A member of the alpha herpes virus group. It is the cause of both chickenpox (also known as varicella) and shingles (herpes zoster).

Shingles is characterized by the development of pain, itching, or tingling in a region on the body where a rash will develop a few days later. This pain is often accompanied by fever, headache, chills, or an upset stomach, making patients feel unwell. The rash develops blisters filled with fluid. These blisters break open and crust over. Infection normally lasts four to five weeks, and in most individuals the skin then heals and recovery is complete.

Some cases of shingles develop serious complications, however. Skin may be damaged due to scratching of the rash, and some cases of skin damage result in scarring. Deafness and blindness also can occur when the virus spreads to nerves within the ear or eye regions. This may be temporary but in some cases is permanent. Brain inflammation (encephalitis) and death may also occur in rare cases. More commonly pain may occur following recovery from the rash. Approximately 20 percent of people with shingles develop this pain, known as postherpetic neuralgia. The pain is often severe and most likely is caused by nerve damage.

Scope and Distribution

Varicella-zoster virus occurs worldwide and causes the development of both chickenpox and shingles. Within the United States, the CDC reports an estimated 1 million cases of shingles annually. Anyone who has had chickenpox, and thus retains VZV, can potentially develop shingles. However, approximately half of shingles cases occur in people older than 50 years of age. While children and adults under age 50 do develop shingles, the risk of developing shingles increases with age.

Shingles is also more likely to develop in people who are immunocompromised. People with medical conditions, such as cancer or human immunodeficiency virus (HIV), and those taking immunosuppressive drugs have a compromised immune system that is less able to fight off infections. Therefore, these individuals are more likely to develop shingles.

While the majority of shingles patients recover fully after an infection, the CDC reports that a fifth of US patients suffer from postherpetic neuralgia, which can lead to pain, itching, numbness, and skin sensitivity that persists after the rash has cleared. Some severe shingles cases can also affect vision.

Treatment and Prevention

Treatment is available for shingles, and recovery is more likely the sooner treatment is administered. Shingles is treated using antiviral medications that are administered orally. These include acyclovir, famciclovir, and valacyclovir. Treatment does not cure the viral disease. Instead, it acts to hinder the progression of the disease throughout the nerves.

To treat the symptoms of shingles (in particular, the pain from the rash), pain-relieving medications, such as ibuprofen, naproxen, indomethacin, and nonsteroidal anti-inflammatory drugs, are administered. For more intense pain, stronger analgesics, such as codeine or oxycodone, may be prescribed.

Treatment for postherpetic neuralgia varies. The treatments tend to focus on treating the pain. Some treatments include patches that release the pain-relieving medication

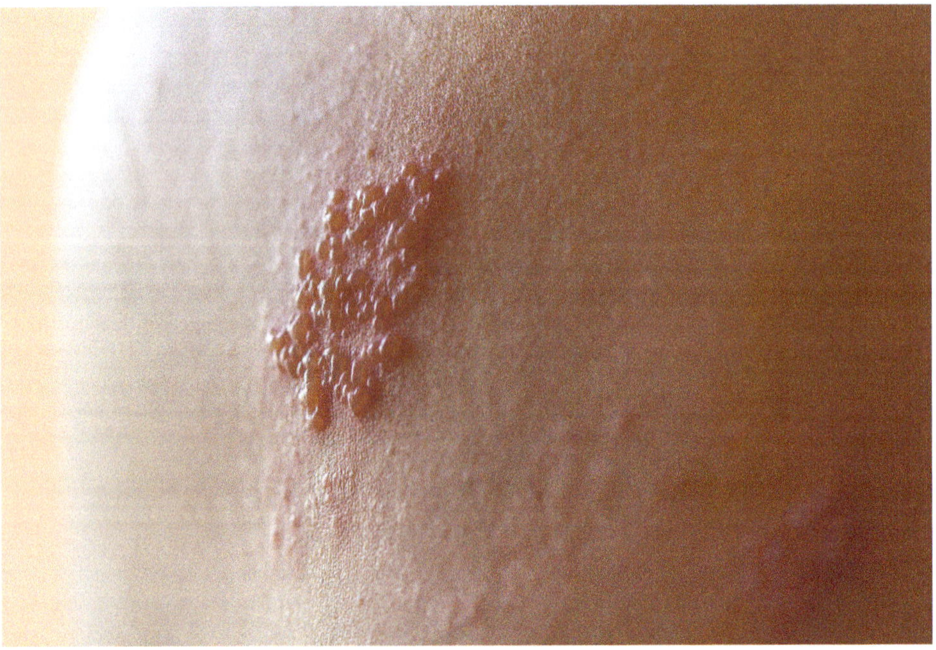

A patient with a shingles (herpes zoster) rash on his back. © *SneSivan/Shutterstock.com*

lidocaine directly into the affected area; analgesics, which have sedating properties; opioids, which control pain; and antidepressants, which help patients tolerate severe pain. Some patients also receive electrical nerve stimulation or have the affected nerve cells blocked. However, the pain experienced often differs from patient to patient, and treatments that work for one patient do not necessarily work for another.

The spread of VZV from shingles patients to previously noninfected people can be prevented by covering the rash, avoiding touching the rash, and washing hands often to prevent contaminating items with fluid from the rash. Once the rash crusts over, the virus is no longer contagious.

A vaccine has been developed that causes people to develop immunity to VZV. The CDC recommends children who have not contracted chickenpox receive this vaccine, with a first dose administered between 12 and 15 months and a second administered between ages four and six years. Those who did not receive the VZV vaccine as young children and who have not developed chickenpox can still get the vaccine. Administration of this vaccine has been found to decrease the number of people developing chickenpox, and it is thought to lessen the risk of the virus remaining dormant and possibly reactivating as shingles.

In 2006 the US Food and Drug Administration (FDA) licensed a new vaccine, Zostavax, designed specifically to prevent shingles and postherpetic neuralgia in people who had already contracted chickenpox. Zostavax has proven effective at reducing the risk of shingles by approximately half and of postherpetic neuralgia by two-thirds. In 2017 the FDA approved a second shingles vaccine, Shingrix. While Shingrix is more expensive than Zostavax and requires two doses, it is also more effective, reducing the risk of shingles infection by 90 percent. In 2017 the CDC's Advisory Committee on Immunization Practices recommended Shingrix for all patients age 50 or older and recommended that those who have received the Zostavax vaccine be revaccinated with Shingrix.

■ Impacts and Issues

Shingles usually affects older people, and, in 20 percent of cases, the patient develops postherpetic neuralgia. Postherpetic neuralgia is nerve pain that lasts for three months or more. The pain can vary from mild to severe, and patients may experience burning, stabbing, or gnawing sensations. This side effect of the varicella-zoster virus is a serious issue for a number of reasons. The pain experienced by people with shingles can often be persistent and debilitating. Furthermore, the treatments used for nerve pain tend to work for some people yet have no effect for other people, making pain management difficult. The number of people in the United States suffering from postherpetic neuralgia is significant, and, although some may be relieved of the pain in a few months, many suffer severe pain for years following recovery from shingles.

Shingles can also be a dangerous disease when it infects the immunocompromised. People with medical conditions such as cancer or HIV or those who have received organ transplants have weakened immune systems and are less capable of fighting off the disease. Therefore, more serious complications, including postherpetic neuralgia, meningitis, and even death, are more likely in these persons if they contract shingles. Furthermore, vaccination is not a viable option, as even small doses of the virus may cause complications for these people. Therefore, avoidance of the virus (or rapid treatment) is vital for patients who are immunocompromised to prevent serious complications.

PRIMARY SOURCE

'This is a game-changer': New Shingles Vaccine Dramatically Improves Protection

SOURCE: *Picard, André. "'This is a game-changer': New Shingles Vaccine Dramatically Improves Protection."* Globe and Mail *(January 1, 2018). This article can also be found online at https://www.theglobeandmail.com/news/national/this-is-a-game-changer-new-shingles-vaccine-dramatically-improves-protection/article37470885/ (accessed January 25, 2018).*

INTRODUCTION: *This article from the* Globe and Mail *(Toronto, Ontario) describes the breakthrough that Shingrix, a shingles vaccine introduced in 2017, represents for older patients.*

"It was like being wrapped in flaming barbed wire."

That's how Erin Bell, a 48-year-old nutritionist from Peterborough, Ont., describes having shingles.

She got shingles at age 42 and the itchy, unsightly blisters that stretched across her torso faded away relatively quickly, but the nerve pain lasted for more than four months.

"The pain was undeniable and unrelenting," she says.

Joan Robicheau, a 61-year-old Montreal teacher, agrees.

Her case of shingles appeared when she was 50 and started with a sharp jaw pain—which she initially thought was a toothache—but, within hours, she was hospitalized and placed in isolation.

At the time, Ms. Robicheau was recovering from CLL, a form of leukemia, and there was a fear the virus could ravage her immune system and be deadly.

"I was in constant pain for four months, and the pain continued for at least two years," she says. "It took over my whole being."

It is a pain many know all too well.

More than 130,000 Canadians are diagnosed with shingles each year—most of them seniors.

Anyone who has had chickenpox—which is about 90 per cent of people born before 1995—can develop shingles later in life, and about one-third do. The varicella zoster virus lies dormant for years, or decades, and erupts for reasons that are unclear, usually after age 50.

The pustules on the skin are bad enough, but one in eight of those afflicted with shingles suffer post-herpetic neuralgia, the medical term for lingering and sometimes debilitating nerve pain. The virus can also destroy nerves, causing blindness or deafness and, in rare cases, lead to grave infections such as meningitis and flesh-eating disease. Shingles also increases the risk of heart attack and stroke.

Yet, the misery that befalls so many is largely preventable.

There has been a moderately effective vaccine to prevent shingles on the market for more than a decade.

And now there is a new vaccine that dramatically improves protection—showing itself to be up to 97 per cent effective in large clinical studies.

"This is a game-changer," says Dr. Iris Gorfinkel, a Toronto physician.

The new vaccine, called Shingrix, will be available in Canada in January.

If you can afford it, get it, Dr. Gorfinkel says. "Everyone over 50 should get this vaccine, no question."

But Shingrix is relatively pricey—a $244 list price, plus dispensing fees and vaccination fees that some providers charge.

(By comparison, Zostavax, another shingles vaccine, has a list price of $177.)

The new vaccine also requires two shots, two to six months apart, compared with one for the competitor. And, unless physicians systematically stock the product, consumers will have to purchase the vaccine and carry it to the doctor's office for injection—except in provinces such as British Columbia that allow pharmacists to administer vaccines.

When—or if—provincial health plans will cover the cost of new shingles vaccines has yet to be determined, although some private plans will likely provide coverage, as they do now for the old vaccine.

Currently, only one province, Ontario, provides Zostavax at no charge, but only for people aged 65–70. Uptake has been good, with more than 60 per cent of those eligible getting the vaccine; but in other age groups, the uptake is less than 30 per cent, likely because of the cost barrier.

"What a public health system pays for is complicated," says Dr. Allison McGeer, director of infection control at Mount Sinai Hospital in Toronto. It depends not only on the effectiveness of the vaccine, but on cost-effectiveness, recommendations from expert bodies, on available budgets, on priorities, and on politics.

What is unquestionable, though, is that the new shingles vaccine is remarkably effective.

"Generally speaking, vaccines don't work as well in older populations. The standard explanation is that our immune system weakens over time," Dr. McGeer says. "But in this case, it works better than anyone ever imagined it could."

In a massive clinical trial of 37,000 patients, the Shingrix vaccine produced eye-popping results, especially when compared with data on Zostavax, the only other shingles vaccine on the market:

- In healthy adults aged 50–59, Shingrix reduced the likelihood of shingles by 97 per cent, compared with 70 per cent for Zostavax;
- In the 60–69 age group, it was 97 per cent versus 64 per cent;
- In the 70–79 age group, Shingrix was 91 per cent effective, compared with 41 per cent for Zostavax;
- In the over-80s, it was Shingrix was five times more effective—91 per cent versus 18 per cent for Zostavax.

The data are noteworthy for a couple of reasons. While the protection afforded by Zostavax appears to fade over time, that does not seem to be the case with Shingrix. (However, researchers caution that the latter has only been studied for four years, while the former has been around for more than a decade.)

More important is how well the new vaccine works in older adults. Almost half of people over the age of 80 will be stricken by shingles and they are significantly more likely to suffer neuralgia.

Until now, there was really nothing they could do to prevent the infection.

See Also *AIDS (Acquired Immunodeficiency Syndrome); Cancer and Infectious Disease; Chickenpox (Varicella); HIV; Vaccines and Vaccine Development; Viral Disease*

BIBLIOGRAPHY

Books

Plum, Jennifer. *Everything You Need to Know about Chicken Pox and Shingles.* New York: Rosen, 2001.

Siegel, Mary-Ellen, and Gray Williams. *Shingles: New Hope for an Old Disease.* Lanham, MD: M. Evans 2008.

Periodicals

Ansaldi, Filippo, et al. "Real-World Effectiveness and Safety of a Live-Attenuated Herpes Zoster Vaccine: A Comprehensive Review." *Advances in Therapy* 33 (2016): 1094–1104. This article can also be found online at https://www.ncbi.nlm.nih.gov/pmc/articles/PMC4939147/ (accessed January 24, 2018).

Bakalar, Nicholas. "New Shingles Vaccine Is Cost Effective." *New York Times* (January 4, 2018). This article can also be found online at https://www.nytimes.com/2018/01/04/well/live/new-shingles-vaccine-is-cost-effective.html?mtrref=undefined (accessed January 24, 2018).

Kimberlin, David W., and Richard J. Whitley. "Varicella-Zoster Vaccine for the Prevention of Herpes Zoster." *New England Journal of Medicine* 356 (March 29, 2007): 1338–1343.

Websites

"Chicken Pox (Varicella)." Centers for Disease Control and Prevention, July 1, 2016. https://www.cdc.gov/chickenpox/index.html (accessed January 24, 2018).

"Shingles." American Academy of Dermatology Association. https://www.aad.org/public/diseases/contagious-skin-diseases/shingles (accessed January 24, 2018).

"Shingles (Herpes Zoster)." Centers for Disease Control and Prevention, October 17, 2017. https://www.cdc.gov/shingles/index.html (accessed January 24, 2018).

"Varicella." World Health Organization, April 4, 2015. http://www.who.int/immunization/diseases/varicella/en/ (accessed January 24, 2018).

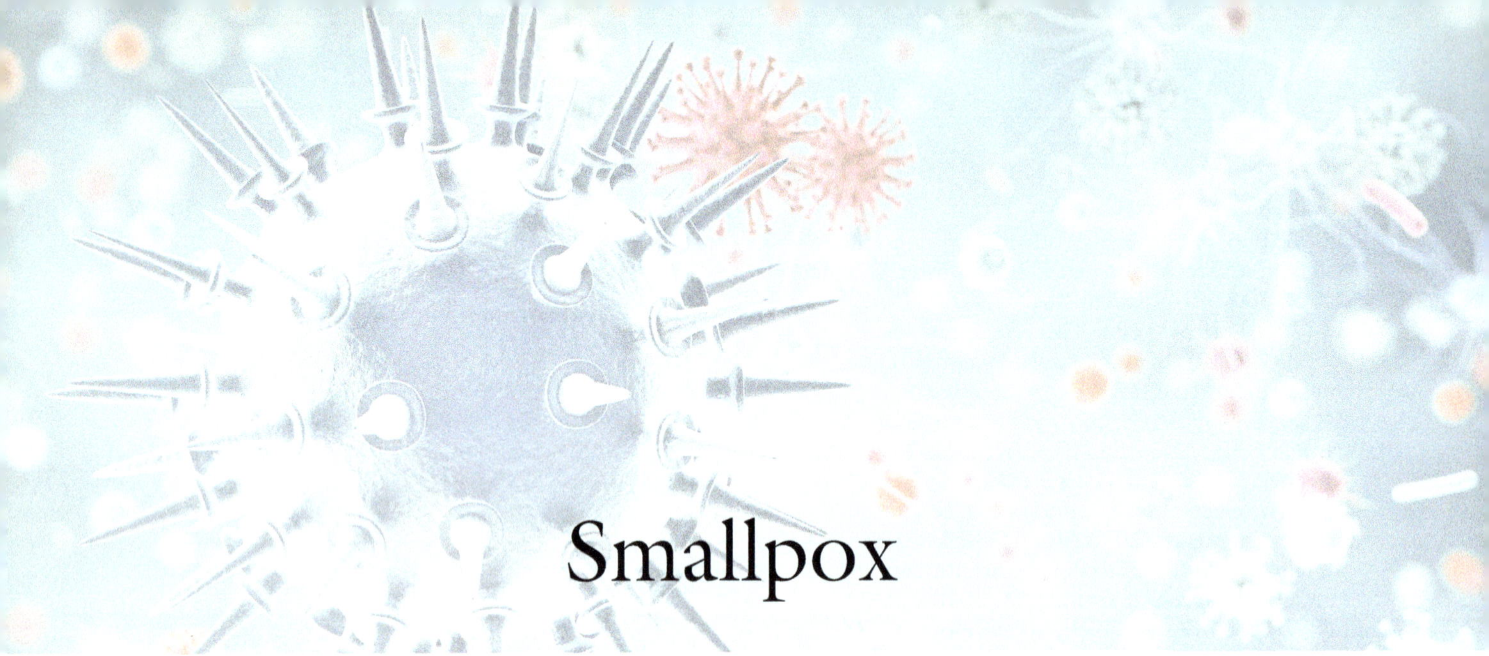

Smallpox

Introduction

Smallpox is an infectious disease caused by a virus. It was eradicated by 1980 thanks to a global vaccination program, but as of 2018 stocks of variola virus were still held by at least two governments, those of the United States and the Russian Federation. The smallpox virus, also called the variola virus or simply variola, is most often spread by ingestion of virus particles in saliva, either through direct contact or by inhaling droplets dispersed in the air by coughing. When ingested, the virus first infects the tissues of the throat and nasal cavities, followed by the blood and lymph nodes. About 12 days after infection, a variety of flu-like symptoms appear, including fever. Pustules (pus-filled lumps) develop on the skin and are painful at first, then itchy.

The deadlier of variola's two varieties, *variola major*, kills about 30 percent of the people it infects. Between 65 and 80 percent of those who survive the disease are disfigured by pitted scars (pockmarks). Some survivors are also blinded by scarring of the retina. Before a vaccine was developed, smallpox was one of the most common causes of blindness worldwide.

WORDS TO KNOW

ERADICATION The process of destroying or eliminating a microorganism or disease.

PRODROME A symptom indicating the disease's onset; it may also be called a prodroma. For example, painful swallowing is often a prodrome of infection with a cold virus.

VARIOLATION The premodern practice of deliberately infecting a person with smallpox to make them immune to a more serious form of the disease. It was dangerous but conferred immunity on survivors.

Disease History, Characteristics, and Transmission

History

The evolutionary origin of the variola (smallpox) virus, a member of the genus *Orthopoxvirus*, family Poxviridae, is still obscure. Variola was traditionally thought to have emerged as a virus in rodents, first infecting humans in Africa about 12,000 years ago. However, a 2016 study of mummified remains in Lithuania dating from the mid-17th century suggests that the strain of the virus most deadly to humans may not have emerged until the mid- to late 1500s, when the first major outbreaks were recorded. The oldest historical reference to a disease resembling smallpox is in a Chinese document dating to the 4th century. The name *variola*, from the Latin for "spotted," dates to the 6th century. The term *smallpox* dates to the 1400s, when it was used to distinguish smallpox from syphilis (the "great pox").

North and South America were free of smallpox until European explorers arrived in the late 1400s. The disease soon spread to the Native American population, which had a much higher mortality rate than the Old World population, probably because there had been no history of natural selection for resistance to the disease. Some historians estimate that 90 percent of the population of the New World was killed by smallpox. For example, the Aztec population in South America fell from 25 million in 1519 to only 3 million in 1569. Smallpox was not originally spread deliberately by the Europeans, although in the French and Indian wars of the mid-1700s, British military forces gave smallpox-infected blankets to Indians who were cooperating with the French, one of the earliest recorded efforts at biological warfare.

In 1796 English physician Edward Jenner (1749–1823) showed that inoculating a person with pus from a cowpox lesion could prevent smallpox. Inoculation had been discovered before. The earliest known use of smallpox inoculation dates to about 1000 BCE, in India. But the idea of inoculation with the harmless cowpox virus had not yet been put forward in Europe by somebody with the professional and class standing to establish it as a known medical fact.

At the time of Jenner's work, smallpox was killing about 400,000 people a year in Europe and millions worldwide. The practice of variolation had already been used to fight smallpox for some decades in Europe and for centuries in Asia. Variolation involved infecting a healthy person with smallpox from a mild case of the disease, either by inserting smallpox scab material into the nostrils or by rubbing it onto a scratch on the skin. People inoculated in this way were far less likely to die from the more severe form of smallpox than were uninoculated people. However, there was still a significant death rate from smallpox contracted through variolation, between 1 and 2 percent.

Jenner's method of inoculation with cowpox virus was much safer. Although his views were not accepted for a few years, they did catch on. More than 100,000 inhabitants of Britain had been vaccinated with cowpox by 1800, and the British Parliament passed the Vaccination Act in 1840 to make vaccination of infants mandatory and to outlaw variolation. Mandatory smallpox vaccination of children soon became the standard in industrialized countries.

So successful was vaccination that the disease was eradicated from prosperous countries. The last case of smallpox in the United States occurred in 1949. At that time smallpox was still infecting about 50 million people every year worldwide, about 30 percent of whom died. Thanks to vaccination, the number of infections dropped to about 15 million per year by 1967. That year the World Health Organization (WHO) started a program to eliminate smallpox completely, known as the WHO Intensified Smallpox Eradication Program. In 1972 the United States began phasing out mandatory vaccination of schoolchildren. In 1977 the last natural case of smallpox was seen in Somalia, and in 1980 WHO declared that the eradication campaign had been a success. Smallpox had become the first, and as of 2018 was still the only, major infectious disease affecting human populations to be completely eradicated.

Characteristics

Smallpox occurs in two forms, variola major and variola minor. Both cause similar symptoms, but variola minor is fatal only about 1 to 2 percent of the time, compared to 30 percent or higher for variola major. These two varieties of variola have been recognized for centuries, even before the viral nature of the disease was understood. The two varieties of virus are similar enough that immunity to one confers immunity to the other. Variolation with scabs or pus from mild smallpox cases, which is an ancient method of immunizing people against smallpox, usually involved infecting people with variola minor to grant them immunity from variola major with a fairly low risk of death from the treatment.

The variola virus is most often caught by inhalation of saliva droplets coughed out by a person who already has the disease. Virus particles lodge in the nasal cavities or throat and infect those tissues first, then grow in the lymph nodes nearest the site of infection. Lymph nodes are small, bean-shaped organs that filter lymph, a clear fluid that is drained from tissues through the system of lymphatic vessels and then returned to the blood. The patient has no symptoms during this phase of the disease. After three or four days, virus particles spread through the bloodstream to the bone marrow, spleen, and other parts of the lymphatic system, where they multiply.

The smallpox virus, like all viruses, multiplies by tricking body cells into manufacturing more virus particles, using genetic material supplied by the virus. More smallpox virus particles appear in the blood 8 to 10 days after infection. During these initial phases, known as the incubation period, the patient feels healthy and cannot infect other persons. About 12 to 14 days after infection, with a range of 7 to 17 days, the incubation period ends and the next phase of the illness begins. This phase is known as the prodrome, prodromal stage, or pre-eruptive stage. In this stage symptoms appear but do not yet include the skin eruptions or lesions that make the patient capable of spreading the infection. Prodromal symptoms may include fever and may last two to four days. After the prodromal stage, the disease can show four distinct courses or clinical presentations, known as ordinary smallpox, modified smallpox, flat smallpox, and hemorrhagic smallpox.

Ordinary Smallpox Ordinary smallpox accounts for about 90 percent of cases. After the prodromal stage, the fever may drop, and the patient may feel less sick. The smallpox rash appears as small red spots (lesions) on the tongue, on the inside of the mouth, and at the back of the throat (on the pharynx). The mouth and throat lesions grow, releasing billions of virus particles into the saliva that may then be transmitted to other people. The lesions in the throat trigger coughing, which tends to spread the disease.

About 24 hours after the appearance of the mouth and throat rash, a rash appears on the skin, first on the face and limbs and then on the trunk. The rashes become lumpier and fill with fluid. In about a week the lumps, now filled with pus and called pustules, have become round, raised, and hard to the touch, like beads under the skin. Generally, the more severe the rash, the greater the chance the patient will die. In another week the fluid in the pustules has been absorbed and a crust or scab begins to form over them. Finally, a week later, the crusts fall off, leaving bleached skin and indented scars. At this point the patient has ceased to be infectious.

Modified Smallpox Modified smallpox is a milder form of the disease that sometimes occurs in people who have been vaccinated. The fever does not return after the prodromal phase, and the rash appears more quickly but produces fewer and smaller lesions. This form of the disease is almost never fatal.

Flat Smallpox In flat smallpox, the raised lesions or pustules of ordinary smallpox do not develop on the skin. This form of the disease has been observed in a study in India to occur about 5 to 10 percent of the time, usually in children. The prodromal stage is more severe in flat smallpox, and so is the rash on the tongue and at the back of the throat. The skin lesions appear slowly and are flatter than in ordinary smallpox. This form of the disease is usually fatal.

Hemorrhagic Smallpox Hemorrhagic smallpox occurs about 2 percent of the time in India. It is called "hemorrhagic" because to hemorrhage means to bleed. Patients with this form of smallpox bleed, sometimes only a few days into the course of the disease, from the eyes, gums, mouth, and skin lesions. Death usually occurs about a week after the onset of symptoms, before the skin rash has had a chance to develop.

Transmission

Variola virus is quite virulent, or easy to spread from one person to another. Only a small number of virus particles need be taken into the body to cause the disease. Virus concentrations in the saliva and mucus are highest during the first week of symptomatic illness, after the prodromal stage. During this time the patient is most infectious. However, the patient remains infectious until all crusts have separated from the healing pustules on the skin. Virus particles can be transmitted through the air or by direct contact with the patient or materials he or she has touched. They do not enter through the skin but may be transferred to the mucous membranes of the mouth, eyes, or nose by hand contact.

Scope and Distribution

Smallpox infection no longer occurs naturally. As of 2018 the only stocks of the virus known to exist are held by the governments of Russia and the United States.

Treatment and Prevention

Because smallpox is caused by a virus, it cannot be treated using antibiotics, which kill only bacteria. As of early 2018, the US Food and Drug Administration (FDA) had not approved any antiviral drug for the treatment of smallpox. However, two antivirals have been stockpiled by the US government for emergency treatment of a smallpox outbreak. In May 2011 the US government ordered 1.7 million doses of ST-246, also known as tecovirimat or TPOXX, which has been shown to be effective against a range of *Orthopoxvirus* diseases,

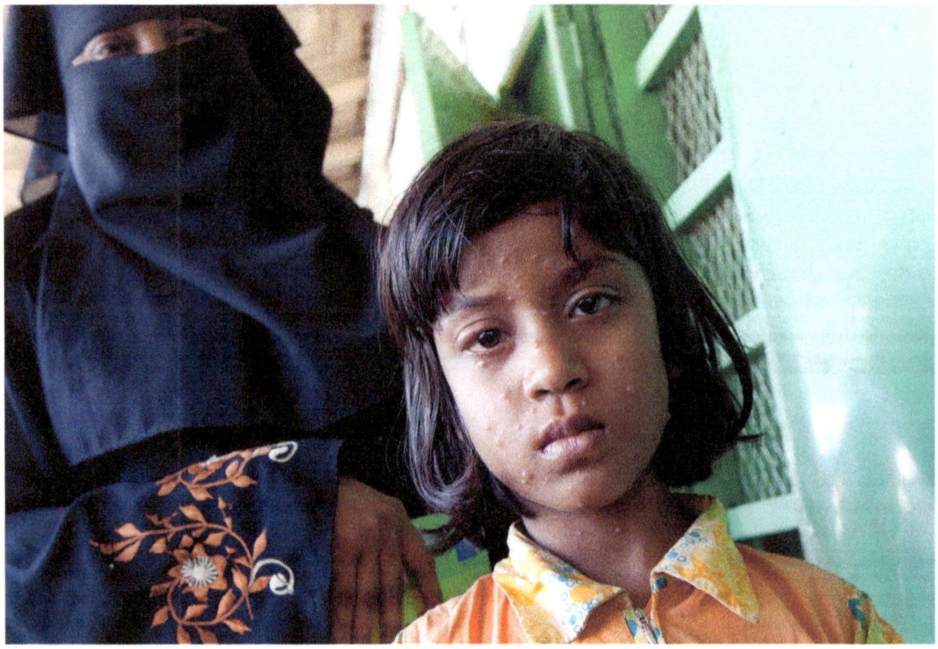

A refugee child of the Rohingya Muslim ethnic community showing signs of smallpox infection. Crowded living conditions in refugee camps, such as the one in which this child was living in Bangladesh, can lead to the spread of infectious diseases such as smallpox. © *Thierry Falise/LightRocket/Getty Images*

including smallpox. The FDA placed the drug on fast-track status, and in February 2016 the drug entered clinical safety trials with human subjects. Another 1.7 million doses of the antiviral brincidofovir were purchased for stockpiling by the US Biomedical Advanced Research and Development Authority in September 2015. A similar drug, cidofovir, had been considered for emergency defense against smallpox but had a number of potentially severe side effects in humans that were largely eliminated in brincidofovir. The FDA fast-tracked brincidofovir in 2011, and on November 18, 2016, the European Medicines Agency approved the drug for the treatment of smallpox.

Smallpox is considered to be eradicated, so there is no routine practice for containment of the disease. However, there is legitimate concern that the virus might be obtained and weaponized, so guidelines for prevention and care are widely distributed in the event of an outbreak. The main method of preventing transmission of smallpox is to avoid having other people ingest the virus. To this end, all people having contact with a smallpox patient should wear fitted breathing masks and disposable gloves, gowns, and shoes. Breathing masks prevent the inhalation of virus particles.

Where high-technology medical settings are available, a smallpox patient should be isolated in a room with negative pressure—that is, one where the air circulation system draws air into the room and filters it before pumping it out rather than allowing it to escape. This is because smallpox transmission can be caused by conveying the virus in tiny, airborne particles. Air that has contacted a smallpox patient must be assumed to be potentially carrying the disease.

The primary method of preventing smallpox infection is the smallpox vaccine. It is not made using smallpox virus but a live vaccinia virus strain. Smallpox vaccine is no longer available through normal drug channels but is stocked by the US Centers for Disease Control and Prevention (CDC) in the Strategic National Stockpile (SNS), which is widely distributed with supplies controlled by local health departments. The SNS has three kinds of smallpox vaccine. Aventis Pasteur Smallpox Vaccine (APSV) and Imvamune are both considered investigational but may be released for use under appropriate conditions. ACAM2000®, the only licensed smallpox vaccine in the United States, is a replication-competent vaccine, meaning that it does not contain variola virus and cannot cause smallpox but can provide active immunization against the smallpox virus.

Unlike most vaccines, which are injected, smallpox vaccine is administered by means of a bifurcated needle, a thin steel rod, approximately 2.5 inches (6 centimeters) long, with two prongs at one end. The end of the needle is dipped into the vaccine and then repeatedly poked into the patient's skin, perhaps 15 times. The repeated poking may draw blood. The amount of vaccine administered in this way is very small, 0.0025 milliliters, but the effective rate of immunization is 95 to 100 percent.

Smallpox vaccine causes a number of medical complications, but death is rare. It should not be taken by pregnant women because the vaccinia virus can cause fetal vaccinia, an infection of the fetus with the vaccinia virus. This usually causes stillbirth or death of the child soon after birth. The CDC releases the vaccine for people who may be exposed to smallpox or the vaccinia virus, including people who administer the vaccine.

Impacts and Issues

The eradication of smallpox was one of the major public health success stories of the 20th century. This effort demonstrated that international cooperation on important health issues could be achieved. Moreover, it also showed that it is possible to eradicate an infectious disease with an effective vaccination program and that vaccination is a useful preventive method in the fight against infectious diseases. Smallpox stocks still exist, however, and, if released into the environment, could cause an epidemic in an unvaccinated population. As of 2018 a large but unknown percentage of Americans were not immune to smallpox. This uncertainty arises because no one is sure how much immunity is still conferred by immunizations received before 1972.

Smallpox has long been considered a biological weapon. In the mid-1700s British army commanders in what is now Canada gave smallpox-infested blankets to American Indians who were collaborating with the French (the enemies of the British at that time). Systematic bioweapons research by the United States, Japan, the Soviet Union, and other countries began during World War II (1939–1945) but for some years concentrated on bacteria such as anthrax rather than viruses.

In the 1950s American bioweapon developers, concerned that the Soviet Union might be developing smallpox and other viruses as well, began studying techniques for producing freeze-dried smallpox powder that could be efficiently spread over a wide area. In the mid-1960s US Army planners approached the bioweapons labs at Fort Detrick, Maryland, to see whether biological weapons could be used to attack military traffic between North and South Vietnam. Smallpox was considered the best candidate, but the idea was abandoned because, if US use of biological warfare were exposed, North Vietnam might retaliate in kind and the disease might spread to friendly forces. Around this time Soviet agents secretly sampled highly virulent smallpox strains in India for use in the large Soviet bioweapons program. In 1969 US president Richard Nixon (1913–1994) abolished the US biological warfare program and supported an international ban on biological weapons. This was formalized as the 1972 Biological and

Toxic Weapons Convention Treaty, which was eventually signed by the Soviet Union and most of the rest of the countries of the world.

After biological attacks using anthrax occurred in the United States in 2001, the issue of smallpox as a potential agent of biological terror again surfaced. In the United States, researchers, members of the military, key health personnel, and first responders in the community were vaccinated against smallpox so that response to any future threat by the smallpox virus can be prompt. Large reserves of smallpox vaccine are maintained by many countries in the developed world and WHO.

In the 21st century the smallpox virus is only known to exist in two secure repositories, both authorized by WHO. One is at the CDC in the United States, and the other is at the State Research Center of Virology and Biotechnology of the Russian Federation in Siberia. Debate continues over whether the last remaining stocks of smallpox virus should be used for research or destroyed.

PRIMARY SOURCE

CDC Media Statement on Newly Discovered Smallpox Specimens

SOURCE: *"CDC Media Statement on Newly Discovered Smallpox Specimens." US Centers for Disease Control and Prevention, July 8, 2014. https://www.cdc.gov/media/releases/2014/s0708-NIH.html (accessed January 31, 2018).*

INTRODUCTION: *In July 2014 six unsecured vials of the smallpox virus were discovered at a US Food and Drug Administration (FDA) facility in Bethesda, Maryland. The discovery sparked concerns about the care and security of a virus that many fear could be used as a biological weapon. In the following press release, the Centers for Disease Control and Prevention (CDC) responds to the discovery.*

July 8, 2014

On July 1, 2014, the National Institutes of Health (NIH) notified the appropriate regulatory agency, the Division of Select Agents and Toxins (DSAT) of the Centers for Disease Control and Prevention (CDC), that employees discovered vials labeled "variola," commonly known as smallpox, in an unused portion of a storage room in a Food and Drug Administration (FDA) laboratory located on the NIH Bethesda campus.

The laboratory was among those transferred from NIH to FDA in 1972, along with the responsibility for regulating biologic products. The FDA has operated laboratories located on the NIH campus since that time. Scientists discovered the vials while preparing for the laboratory's move to the FDA's main campus.

The vials appear to date from the 1950s. Upon discovery, the vials were immediately secured in a CDC-registered select agent containment laboratory in Bethesda.

There is no evidence that any of the vials labeled variola has been breached, and onsite biosafety personnel have not identified any infectious exposure risk to lab workers or the public.

Late on July 7, the vials were transported safely and securely with the assistance of federal and local law enforcement agencies to CDC's high-containment facility in Atlanta. Overnight PCR testing done by CDC in the BSL-4 lab confirmed the presence of variola virus DNA. Additional testing of the variola samples is under way to determine if the material in the vials is viable (i.e., can grow in tissue culture). This testing could take up to 2 weeks. After completion of this testing, the samples will be destroyed.

By international agreement, there are two official World Health Organization (WHO)-designated repositories for smallpox: CDC in Atlanta, Georgia and the State Research Centre of Virology and Biotechnology (VECTOR) in Novosibirsk, Russia. The WHO oversees the inspection of these smallpox facilities and conducts periodic reviews to certify the repositories for safety and security.

CDC has notified WHO about the discovery, and WHO has been invited to participate in the investigation. If viable smallpox is present, WHO will be invited to witness the destruction of these smallpox materials, as has been the precedent for other cases where smallpox samples have been found outside of the two official repositories.

DSAT, in collaboration with the Federal Bureau of Investigation, is actively investigating the history of how these samples were originally prepared and subsequently stored in the FDA laboratory.

SEE ALSO *Smallpox Eradication and Storage; Viral Disease; World Health Organization (WHO)*

BIBLIOGRAPHY

Books

Henderson, Donald A. *Smallpox: The Death of a Disease.* Amherst, NY: Prometheus, 2009.

Ian, Glynn, and Jenifer Glynn. *Life and Death of Smallpox.* New York: Cambridge University Press, 2004.

Rodriguez, Ana Maria. *Edward Jenner: Conqueror of Smallpox.* Berkeley Heights, NJ: Enslow, 2006.

Williams, Gareth. *Angel of Death: The Story of Smallpox*. Basingstoke, UK: Palgrave Macmillan, 2010.

Periodicals

Duggan, Ana T., et al. "17th Century Variola Virus Reveals the Recent History of Smallpox." *Current Biology* 26, no. 24 (December 2016): 3407–3412. This article can also be found online at https://www.sciencedirect.com/science/article/pii/S0960982216313240 (accessed January 30, 2018).

Foster, Scott A., Scott Parker, and Randall Lanier. "The Role of Brincidofovir in Preparation for a Potential Smallpox Outbreak." *Viruses* 9, no. 11 (2017). This article can also be found online at http://www.mdpi.com/1999-4915/9/11/320 (accessed January 30, 2018).

McNeil, Donald G., Jr. "Wary of Attack with Smallpox, U.S. Buys Up a Costly Drug." *New York Times* (March 12, 2013). This article can also be found online at http://www.nytimes.com/2013/03/13/health/us-stockpiles-smallpox-drug-in-case-of-bioterror-attack.html (accessed January 30, 2018).

Websites

"EU/3/16/1777." European Medicines Agency, December 14, 2016. http://www.ema.europa.eu/ema/index.jsp?curl=pages/medicines/human/orphans/2016/12/human_orphan_001896.jsp&mid=WC0b01ac058001d12b (accessed January 24, 2018).

"Smallpox." Centers for Disease Control and Prevention. https://www.cdc.gov/smallpox/index.html (accessed January 24, 2018).

"Smallpox." World Health Organization. http://www.who.int/csr/disease/smallpox/en/ (accessed January 24, 2018).

Larry Gilman
Sam Uretsky

Smallpox Eradication and Storage

■ Introduction

Smallpox is a disease caused by the smallpox virus, also called the variola virus or simply variola. The World Health Organization (WHO) declared smallpox eradicated in 1980 after a decades-long program of global vaccination. However, specimens of smallpox virus are still held in the United States, Russia, and possibly other countries. Samples of variola deoxyribonucleic acid (DNA) may also be recoverable from old medical samples, such as the century-old smallpox scabs discovered in an envelope tucked in a 19th-century medical textbook in a New Mexico library in 2004.

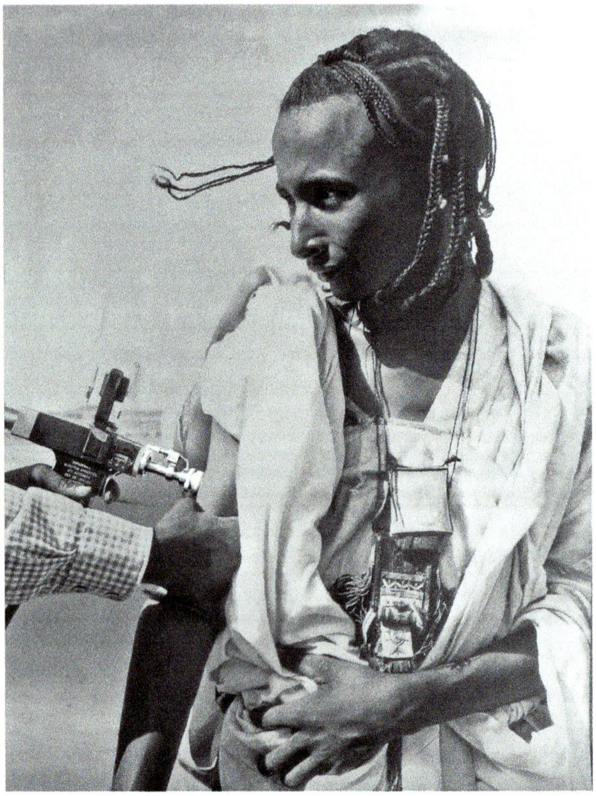

Administration of the smallpox vaccine in Niger in 1969. The World Health Organization declared smallpox eradicated in 1979. *© Smith Collection/Gado/Getty Images*

Since the 1990s there has been ongoing debate about whether remaining stocks of smallpox should be destroyed. Issues include the morality of deliberately causing the extinction of a species and whether continued possession of the virus might someday result in its escape, potentially causing millions of deaths. There is also concern about whether the virus might be used to develop biological weapons and whether keeping the virus intact is necessary as a precaution against its possible use in biological warfare (biowar) or bioterrorism or its accidental or natural rerelease into human populations. WHO has authorized some research with existing variola stocks, but there remains controversy over the continued existence of the virus.

■ History and Scientific Foundations

The eradication of smallpox began with the discovery in 1796 by English physician Edward Jenner (1749–1823) that inoculating a person with pus from a cowpox lesion could prevent smallpox. This fact had been noticed before by a number of people, as had the possibility of inoculation using scabs or pus from people with milder cases of smallpox (variola minor). However, Jenner was the first person with professional standing to discover inoculation with the harmless cowpox virus. This allowed him to publish his findings and make them a standard part of medical knowledge.

Widespread vaccination led to the disappearance of smallpox from industrialized countries. In the United States, for example, the last case was reported in Texas in 1949. From 1967 to 1980, WHO oversaw a global campaign to eliminate smallpox entirely, known as the WHO Intensified Smallpox Eradication Program. The program was declared an official success in May 1980, almost three years after the last case of natural smallpox was seen in 1977 in Somalia.

The eradication strategy had two basic features. First came mass vaccination campaigns in each target country, coordinated with that country's government. The goal was to vaccinate at least 80 percent of the population of each target country. Smallpox vaccination is a simple procedure involving multiple skin punctures in the side of the arm with a two-pronged metal tool resembling a lobster fork. The tool, called a bifurcated needle, is dipped once into a vial containing liquid smallpox vaccine and then repeatedly stuck into the skin over a small area. Earlier, less-convenient methods were displaced by the bifurcated needle procedure during the global eradication campaign.

The smallpox vaccine does not contain smallpox virus but live vaccinia virus. Vaccinia virus almost never causes fatal disease. The reported death rate from smallpox vaccination is approximately one death per 1 million vaccinations. An immune system that has learned to recognize and attack the vaccinia virus will also recognize and attack the variola virus at its first appearance. Smallpox virus may enter the body of an immunized person but is destroyed by the immune system before it can gain a foothold.

The second aspect of the eradication strategy was surveillance and containment. Because a percentage of the population in most countries remained unvaccinated even at the height of the eradication campaign, smallpox still occurred. Surveillance and containment involved monitoring for outbreaks of smallpox and then intensively vaccinating people in the vicinity of the outbreak.

This two-part strategy was successful. Smallpox was eliminated in Brazil in 1971 and in Indonesia in 1972. A few outbreaks in Europe were caused by travelers but were rapidly contained. The last case of the more severe form of smallpox, variola major, occurred in Bangladesh in 1975. The last case of natural smallpox occurred in Somalia in 1977. After several years with no reported cases of the disease, WHO declared smallpox eradicated in 1980. As of 2018 no cases had been reported worldwide in over 40 years.

Following eradication, WHO requested that all laboratories in the world either destroy their smallpox virus stocks or transfer them to one of two reference laboratories, the Institute of Viral Preparations in Moscow, Russia, or the US Centers for Disease Control (CDC) in Atlanta, Georgia. (The CDC's name was changed in 1992 to the Centers for Disease Control and Prevention.) The stocks of the Institute of Viral Preparations were transferred in 1994 to the State Research Center of Virology and Biotechnology of the Russian Federation in Koltsovo, Novosibirsk Oblast, a scientific work settlement within Siberia. The research center later became the WHO Collaborating Centre for Orthopoxvirus Diagnosis and Repository for Variola Virus Strains and DNA.

WORDS TO KNOW

BIFURCATED NEEDLE A needle that has two prongs with a wire suspended between them. The wire is designed to hold a certain amount of vaccine. Development of the bifurcated needle was a major advance in vaccination against smallpox.

BIOSAFETY LEVEL 4 (BSL-4) FACILITY A specially equipped, secured laboratory where scientists study the most dangerous known microbes. BSL-4 labs are designed to contain infectious agents and disease-causing microbes, prevent their dissemination, and protect researchers from exposure.

COWPOX A disease caused by the cowpox or cat pox virus. The virus is a member of the genus *Orthopoxvirus*. Other viruses in this genus include the smallpox and vaccinia viruses. Cowpox is a rare disease and is mostly noteworthy as the basis of the formulation of an injection by Edward Jenner in the 19th century that proved successful in curing smallpox.

VACCINATION Inoculation, or use of vaccines, to prevent specific diseases within humans and animals by producing immunity to such diseases. Vaccination involves the introduction of weakened or dead viruses or microorganisms into the body to create immunity by the production of specific antibodies.

VACCINIA VIRUS A usually harmless virus that is closely related to the virus that causes smallpox, a dangerous disease. Infection with the vaccinia virus confers immunity against smallpox, so vaccinia virus has been used as a vaccine against smallpox.

VARIOLA VIRUS Also known as variola major virus, the virus that causes smallpox. The virus is one of the members of the poxvirus group (family Poxviridae). The virus particle is brick shaped and contains a double strand of deoxyribonucleic acid (DNA). The variola virus is among the most dangerous of all the potential biological weapons.

Under US law smallpox virus may be stored and handled only at biosafety level 4 (BSL-4) facilities. Such a facility consists of a separate building or architecturally isolated section of a building specially equipped for biological isolation. People entering and leaving the facility must take sterilizing showers. Air and sewage leaving the building must pass through special filters to remove any possible disease-carrying particles, and separate air supply and exhaust must be arranged for workers inside the laboratory space. The building must be ventilated so that air flows into the building and toward the part of the building where the most hazardous materials are kept. The building must also remain sealed in the event of a power failure. According to the Federation of American Scientists (FAS), there were 13 operational or planned BSL-4 facilities in the United States as of 2013.

■ Applications and Research

Following eradication, WHO set 1999 as the deadline for the destruction of all variola virus stocks. However, both the United States and Russia failed to carry out this directive, citing the need for further research on the virus. The World Health Assembly (WHA), the governing body of WHO, accepted the continuing existence of the virus and established the Advisory Committee on Variola Virus Research to oversee the study of variola virus until the end of 2002. After that time the virus stocks were to be destroyed.

Some ethicists have raised the question of whether it is permissible to deliberately cause the extinction of any species, even a malignant virus, but this has not been a major concern in the debates over the fate of the variola virus. In 2002 WHA decided, under combined US and Russian pressure, that not enough research had been accomplished and that the deadline for variola destruction would be extended indefinitely.

The goals of variola virus research are said by workers in the field to be a better understanding of the genome of the virus, the proteins produced by the virus, and the precise means by which the virus infects cells to prepare for accidental, natural, or deliberate rerelease of the virus in human populations. The genomes of several dozen varieties of variola virus were completely sequenced by 2007.

In 2004 the Advisory Committee decided to allow the creation of genetically modified varieties of the variola virus, in particular some containing reporter genes (genes that make it easy to identify the presence of the virus, such as genes that encode a protein that glows green when exposed to blue light). In 2005 the Advisory Committee also voted to allow the transfer of variola DNA fragments up to 55 base pairs long between laboratories, the manufacture of gene chips containing smallpox DNA, and the splicing of smallpox genes into other orthopoxviruses.

In December 2010 the WHO Advisory Group of Independent Experts to review the smallpox research programme (AGIES), an independent group of public health experts appointed by WHO, determined that the preservation of the smallpox stocks in the United States and Russia did not fulfill any public health purpose and that new research would not fundamentally benefit the public health.

In July 2014 the US National Institutes of Health notified the CDC's Division of Select Agents and Toxins that six vials of variola virus were found in a US Food and Drug Administration laboratory in Bethesda, Maryland. Testing was subsequently performed on the vials. The analysis concluded that the variola virus DNA was present inside the vials. The containers and their contents were destroyed in February 2015 at the CDC facility under the supervision of WHO officials.

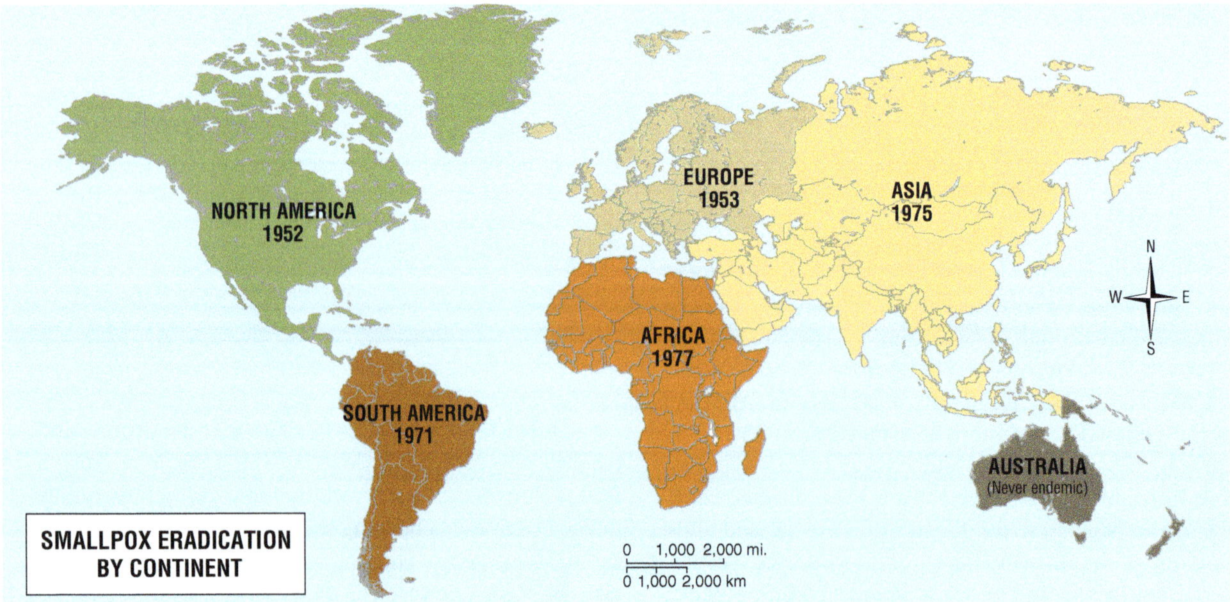

SOURCE: Adapted from "Global Smallpox Eradication." US Centers for Disease Control and Prevention. Available from: https://www.cdc.gov/smallpox/history/history.html

Controversy remains as to whether to destroy or preserve the remaining stores. Some scientists contend that the stocks could be useful in developing new vaccines and for other related matters. Others argue that destruction of the stocks would reduce the risk of a smallpox outbreak in the future.

Impacts and Issues

Research using the surviving smallpox virus stocks remains controversial. WHO's director-general opposed the organization's 2005 decision to allow the transfer of smallpox genes to other viruses, a move also opposed by South Africa, China, the Netherlands, and a number of other countries. Developing countries, which would be more vulnerable to a new smallpox outbreak, are particularly keen on final destruction of virus stocks. Two groups, the Third World Network and the Sunshine Project, mounted campaigns in the early 21st century against continuing smallpox research of this type.

In 2005 the US Congress passed a bill to make it illegal to "produce, engineer, [or] synthesize" the variola virus from scratch. The possibility of from-scratch (also called de novo) manufacture of smallpox virus is not farfetched. Poliovirus was first synthesized from scratch in 2001, starting solely with a record of its genome and without the aid of preexisting ribonucleic acid (RNA), DNA, or living cells. In 2006 Sandia National Laboratories, an arm of the US government, began experiments that involved inserting synthetic (de novo) variola genes into other organisms. Some critics of the continued existence of variola stocks say that, because Sandia's mission has historically been the production of nuclear weapons and the laboratory has no biomedical mission, its research with variola virus genes is inappropriate and signifies deteriorating WHO control over smallpox research.

In January 2007 the WHO Executive Board adopted a draft smallpox resolution to be sent to WHA in May of that year. The resolution asked the director-general of WHO to forbid genetic engineering of the variola virus and called for the topic of setting a definite date for the destruction of variola virus stocks to be placed on the agenda of WHA's 63rd or 64th session, in 2010 or 2011.

As of 2018 smallpox research continued in the United States and in other parts of the world, especially with regard to the development of new diagnostic tests, drugs, and vaccines. As the international threat of terrorism grows, so do prevention activities in case the variola virus is used as a deadly vehicle in an act of bioterrorism. Although it is unlikely such a scenario would arise, public health organizations such as the CDC remain prepared for such an attack. For instance, the CDC stores sufficient quantities of smallpox vaccine at the Strategic National Stockpile to provide adequate protection for everyone in the United States.

SEE ALSO *CDC (Centers for Disease Control and Prevention); Smallpox; Viral Disease; World Health Organization (WHO)*

BIBLIOGRAPHY

Books

Carrell, Jennifer Lee. *The Speckled Monster: A Historical Tale of Battling the Smallpox Epidemic.* New York: Dutton, 2003.

Koplow, David. *Smallpox: The Fight to Eradicate a Global Scourge.* Berkeley: University of California Press, 2004.

Kotar, S. L., and J. E. Gessler. *Smallpox: A History.* Jefferson, NC: McFarland, 2013.

Reinhardt, Bob H. *The End of a Global Pox: America and the Eradication of Smallpox in the Cold War Era.* Chapel Hill: University of North Carolina Press, 2015.

Willrich, Michael. *Pox: An American History.* New York: Penguin, 2011.

Periodicals

Lane, J. Michael, and Gregory A. Poland. "Why Not Destroy the Remaining Smallpox Virus Stocks?" *Vaccine* 29, no. 16 (April 5, 2011): 2823–2824. This article can also be found online at https://www.sciencedirect.com/science/article/pii/S0264410X1100329X?via%3Dihub (accessed January 29, 2018).

Websites

"Advisory Group of Independent Experts to Review the Smallpox Research Programme (AGIES): Comments on the Scientific Review of Variola Virus Research 1999–2010." World Health Organization, December 2010. http://apps.who.int/iris/bitstream/10665/70509/1/WHO_HSE_GAR_BDP_2010.4_eng.pdf (accessed January 29, 2018).

"CDC Media Statement on Newly Discovered Smallpox Specimens." Centers for Disease Control and Prevention, July 8, 2014. https://www.cdc.gov/media/releases/2014/s0708-NIH.html (accessed January 29, 2018).

"FDA Review of the 2014 Discovery of Vials Labeled '*Variola*' and Other Vials Discovered in an FDA-Occupied Building on the NIH Campus." US Food and Drug Administration, December 13, 2016. https://www.fda.gov/downloads/AboutFDA/ReportsManualsForms/Reports/UCM532877.pdf (accessed January 29, 2018).

"Smallpox." Centers for Disease Control and Prevention, July 12, 2017. https://www.cdc.gov/smallpox/index.html (accessed January 29, 2018).

"Smallpox." World Health Organization. http://www.who.int/csr/disease/smallpox/en/ (accessed January 29, 2018).

"Smallpox: Preparedness." Centers for Disease Control and Prevention, December 19, 2016. https://www.cdc.gov/smallpox/bioterrorism/public/preparedness.html (accessed January 29, 2018).

"US BSL Laboratories." Federation of American Scientists, 2013. https://fas.org/programs/bio/research.html (accessed January 29, 2018).

Larry Gilman
William Arthur Atkins

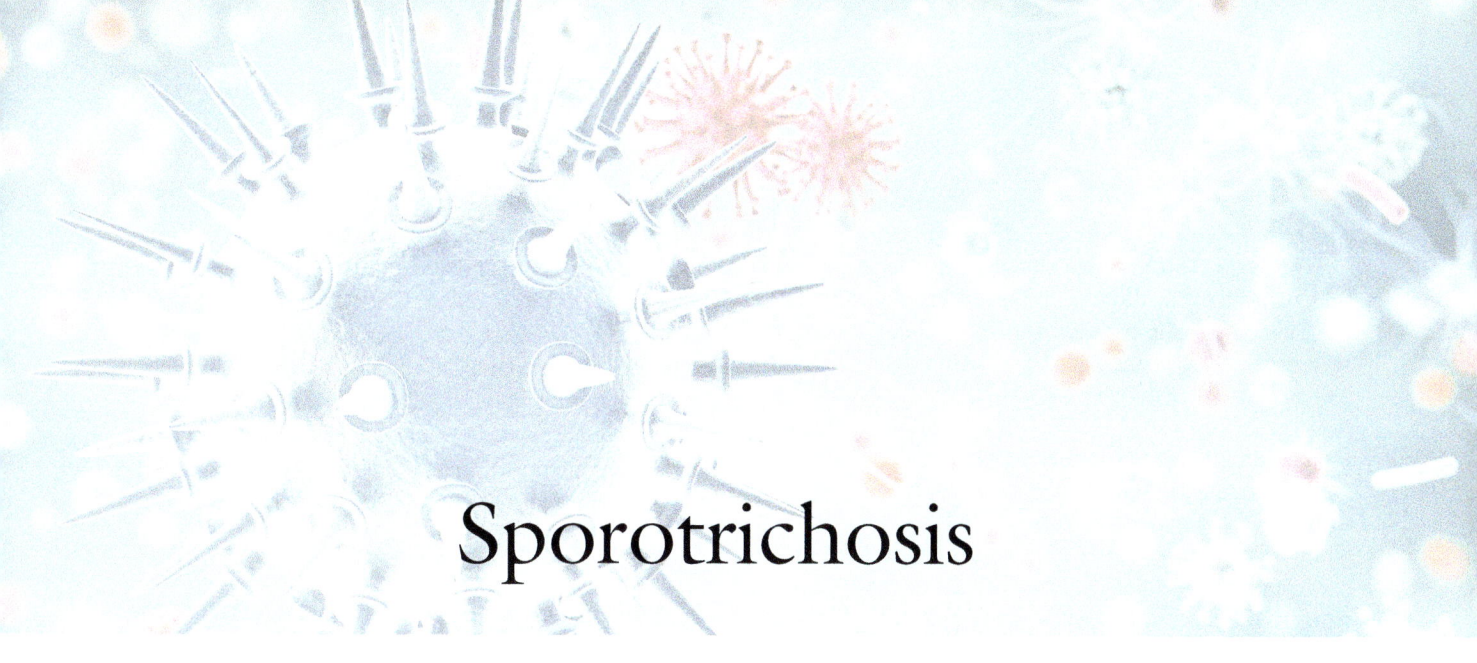

Sporotrichosis

Introduction

Sporotrichosis, also known as rose gardener's or rose thorn disease, is a rare mycotic (fungal) infection that is caused by the fungus *Sporothrix schenckii* complex. Humans most often become infected when they are pricked or scratched by plants that harbor the fungus. The resulting infection is usually a cutaneous (skin) infection involving the formation of ulcerous lesions. However, other forms of sporotrichosis can occur when the fungus is inhaled and include pulmonary sporotrichosis, in which the lungs are infected, and disseminated sporotrichosis, in which the joints, gastrointestinal system, or central nervous system are infected.

Sporotrichosis infection occurs worldwide. Gardeners, florists, and farmers who regularly come in contact with plants harboring the fungus are most at risk of becoming infected.

Sporotrichosis is most commonly treated with antifungal medication. Treatment may be required for months, and in cases that are left untreated, severe skin ulceration can occur. Development of the less common forms of the disease—pulmonary and disseminated sporotrichosis—can lead to serious complications such as meningitis (swelling of the brain) and can be fatal. People with weakened immune systems, such as those with human immunodeficiency virus (HIV) or who have underlying chronic diseases (such as diabetes or alcoholism), are most at risk of these serious complications.

Disease History, Characteristics, and Transmission

The fungus was first identified as the causative agent of sporotrichosis by American physician Benjamin Robinson Schenck (1873–1920) in 1896. For this reason, sporotrichosis is also sometimes known as Schenck's disease. After French physician Charles Lucien de Beurmann (1851–1923) further explained the role of *S. schenckii* in causing disease in 1903, some scientists renamed the organism *Sporotrichum beurmanni.*

After an incubation period of about 1 to 12 weeks from exposure to the fungus, infection with *S. schenckii* causes a small painless nodule (bump), similar to an insect bite, to develop on the skin. This nodule can be red, pink, or purple and tends to be located on the finger, hand, or arm. Eventually a number of similar lesions form, spreading to other regions of the body.

Most sporotrichosis infections are limited to the skin. However, rarely, the fungus may spread through the lymphatic system after it is inhaled to infect the lungs, joints, or central nervous system. This can result in pulmonary sporotrichosis and disseminated sporotrichosis (which includes sporotrichosis meningitis, when the fungus spreads

WORDS TO KNOW

CUTANEOUS Pertaining to the skin.

DISSEMINATED The previous distribution of a disease-causing microorganism over a larger area.

INCUBATION PERIOD The time between exposure to disease-causing virus or bacteria and the appearance of symptoms of the infection. Depending on the microorganism, the incubation time can range from a few hours (an example is food poisoning due to *Salmonella*) to a decade or more (an example is acquired immunodeficiency syndrome, or AIDS).

MYCOTIC Having to do with or caused by a fungus. Any medical condition caused by a fungus is a mycotic condition, also called a mycosis.

to the central nervous system, and osteoarticular sporotrichosis, when the joints are affected). Disseminated sporotrichosis can cause serious complications and can be fatal, particularly for those with sporotrichosis meningitis.

Pulmonary sporotrichosis is more common in middle-aged men who have underlying risk factors such as alcoholism or existing pulmonary issues like chronic obstructive pulmonary disease (COPD). People with pulmonary sporotrichosis are at risk for developing pneumonia.

The fungus is transmitted from plant material such as roses, hay, and sphagnum moss into humans via broken skin. Defensive mechanisms on these plants such as thorns, barbs, and pine needles can cause punctures or cuts in the skin, creating an entry route for transmission of the fungi. It can also be transmitted to humans via bites or scratches from infected animals or through contact with an infected animal, although the latter transmission route is rarer. Sporotrichosis is not spread from person to person.

The fungus can be detected in a high-sensitivity culture, although the culture must be given 10 to 15 days to grow.

Scope and Distribution

Sporotrichosis caused by the *S. schenckii* complex occurs worldwide. The *S. schenckii* complex contains *S. schenckii sensu stricto*, *Sporothrix brasiliensis*, *Sporothrix globosa*, and *Sporothrix luriei*.

Vikram K. Mahajan wrote in a 2014 article for *Dermatology Research and Practice* that "sporotrichosis occurs worldwide with focal areas of hyperendemicity. It is particularly common in tropical/subtropical areas and temperate zones with warm and humid climate." Because sporotrichosis is not required to be reported, worldwide incidence numbers are unknown. Peru and the city of Rio de Janeiro have especially high rates of sporotrichosis.

Treatment and Prevention

The most common form of treatment for sporotrichosis is administration of the antifungal drug itraconazole. Oral administration of a saturated potassium iodide solution is sometimes given when itraconazole is cost-prohibitive, and this treatment is given over a period of about three to six months. Other antifungal drugs such as fluconazole may also be used. When the lesions have become large and filled with fluid, it is sometimes necessary to drain and remove the lesions surgically.

Other forms of sporotrichosis, such as in the lungs, joints, or central nervous system, may also require itraconazole or surgery. An additional treatment sometimes ad-

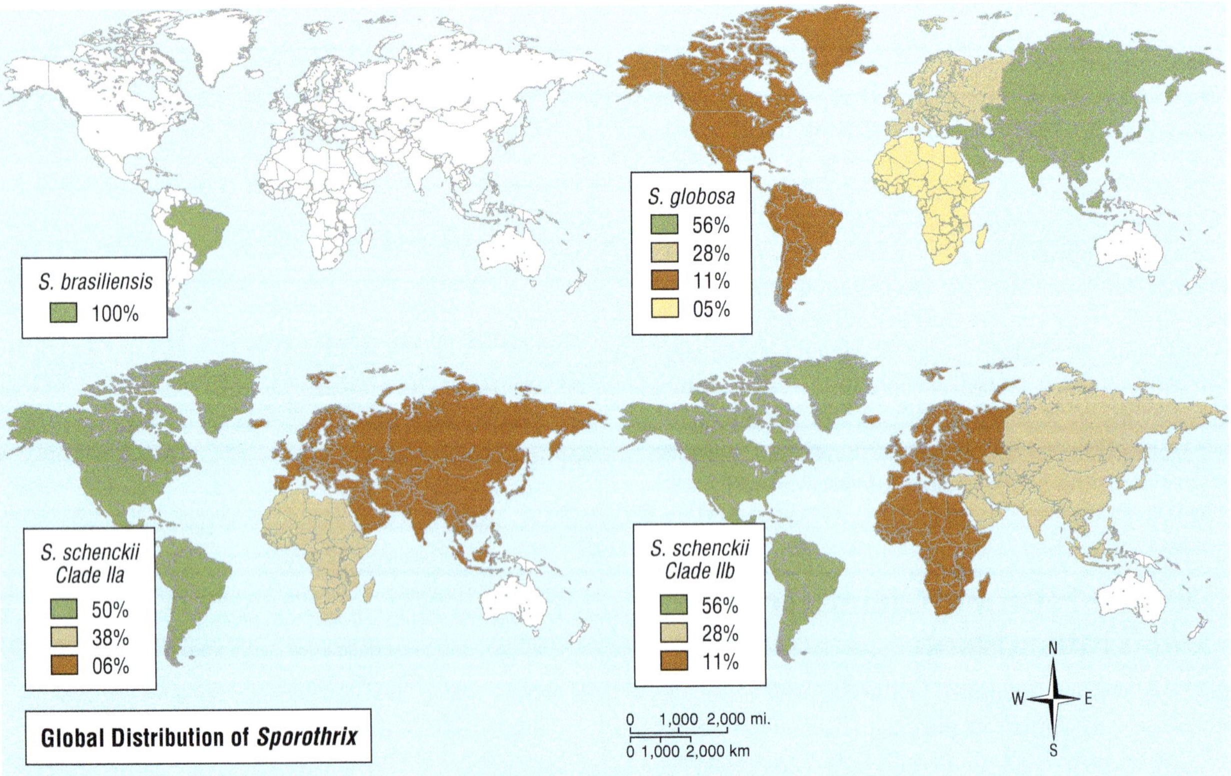

SOURCE: Adapted from "Global distribution of *Sporothrix brasiliensis, S. globosa, S. schenckii* clade IIa, and *S. schenckii* clade IIb."

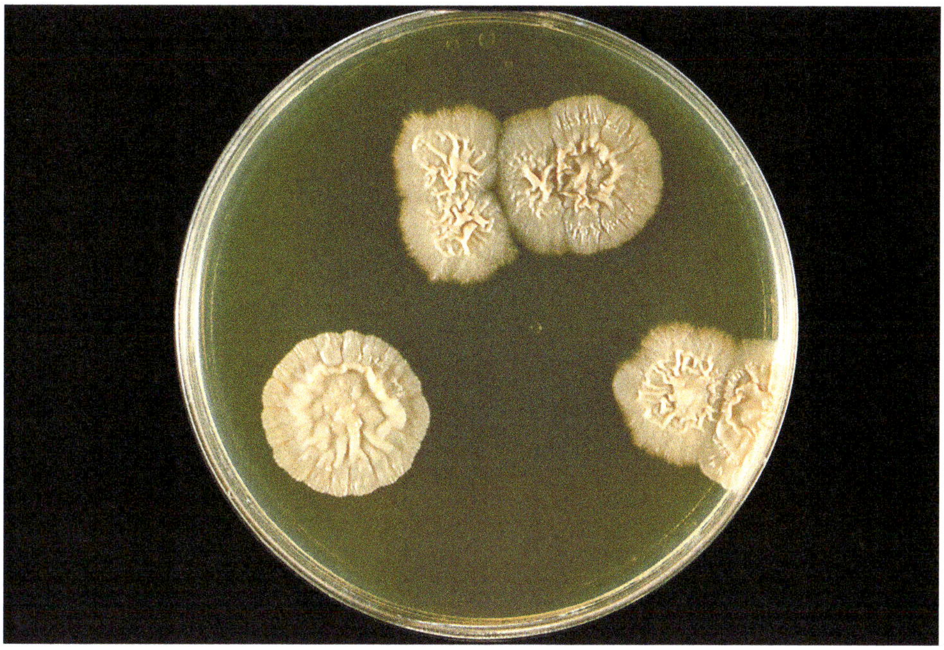

Laboratory culture of *Sporothrix schenckii*, the fungus responsible for the infection Sporotrichosis, also known as rose gardener's disease. © Smith Collection/Gado/Getty Images

ministered in complicated cases involves the antifungal medication amphotericin B.

Wearing protective clothing such as gloves and long sleeves while handling plants may provide protection against infection by *S. schenckii.* In particular, the Centers for Disease Control and Prevention (CDC) recommends workers wear gloves when coming into contact with sphagnum moss due to a number of outbreaks of sporotrichosis associated with this plant. For people living in Rio de Janeiro, where sporotrichosis is endemic in cats, it is advisable to avoid scratches and bites from cats.

Impacts and Issues

Sporotrichosis also occurs in other mammals such as cats and dogs. Pet owners, especially those living on farms, are advised to seek treatment for pets showing nodules. Humans can become infected by coming in contact with the open sores present on animals. Therefore, veterinarians responsible for treating animals infected with sporotrichosis are also at risk of contracting this infection.

S. brasiliensis, a member of the *S. schenckii* complex, has caused outbreaks of sporotrichosis in Rio de Janeiro since 1998. The disease is transmitted from cats to humans. In Brazil, according to *Medical Mycology* in 2015, the group most likely to contract sporotrichosis included "middle-aged women from low socioeconomic background who engage in domestic activities" because of the degree of their exposure "while caring for infected animals at home."

SEE ALSO *AIDS (Acquired Immunodeficiency Syndrome); Immune Response to Infection; Mycotic Disease; Pneumonia; Tuberculosis*

BIBLIOGRAPHY

Books

Carlos, Iracilda Zeppone, ed. *Sporotrichosis: New Developments and Future Prospects.* Cham, Switzerland: Springer, 2015.

Carvalho, Agostinho, ed. *Immunogenetics of Fungal Diseases.* Cham, Switzerland: Springer, 2017.

Homei, Aya, and Michael Worboys. *Fungal Disease in Britain and the United States, 1850–2000: Mycoses and Modernity.* New York: Palgrave Macmillan, 2013.

Periodicals

Barros, Mônica Bastos de Lima, Rodrigo de Almeida Paes, and Armando Oliveira Schubach. "*Sporothrix Schenckii* and Sporotrichosis." *Clinical Microbiology Reviews* 24, no. 4 (2011): 633–654. This article can also be found online at https://www.ncbi.nlm.nih.gov/pmc/articles/PMC3194828/ (accessed January 23, 2018).

Bernardes-Engemann, Andréa Reis, et al. "Validation of a Serodiagnostic Test for Sporotrichosis: A Follow-up Study of Patients Related to the Rio De Janeiro Zoonotic Outbreak." *Medical Mycology* 53, no. 1 (January 1, 2015): 28–33. This article can also be found online at https://academic.oup.com/mmy/article/53/1/28/992696 (accessed January 23, 2018).

Chakrabarti, Arunaloke, et al. "Global Epidemiology of Sporotrichosis." *Medical Mycology* 53, no. 1 (January 1, 2015): 3–14. This article can also be found online at https://academic.oup.com/mmy/article/53/1/3/992886 (accessed January 23, 2018).

Mahajan, Vikram K. "Sporotrichosis: An Overview and Therapeutic Options." *Dermatology Research and Practice* 2014 (2014). This article can also be found online at https://www.hindawi.com/journals/drp/2014/272376/ (accessed January 23, 2018).

Websites

"Sporotrichosis." Centers for Disease Control and Prevention, January 30, 2017. https://www.cdc.gov/fungal/diseases/sporotrichosis/index.html (accessed January 23, 2018).

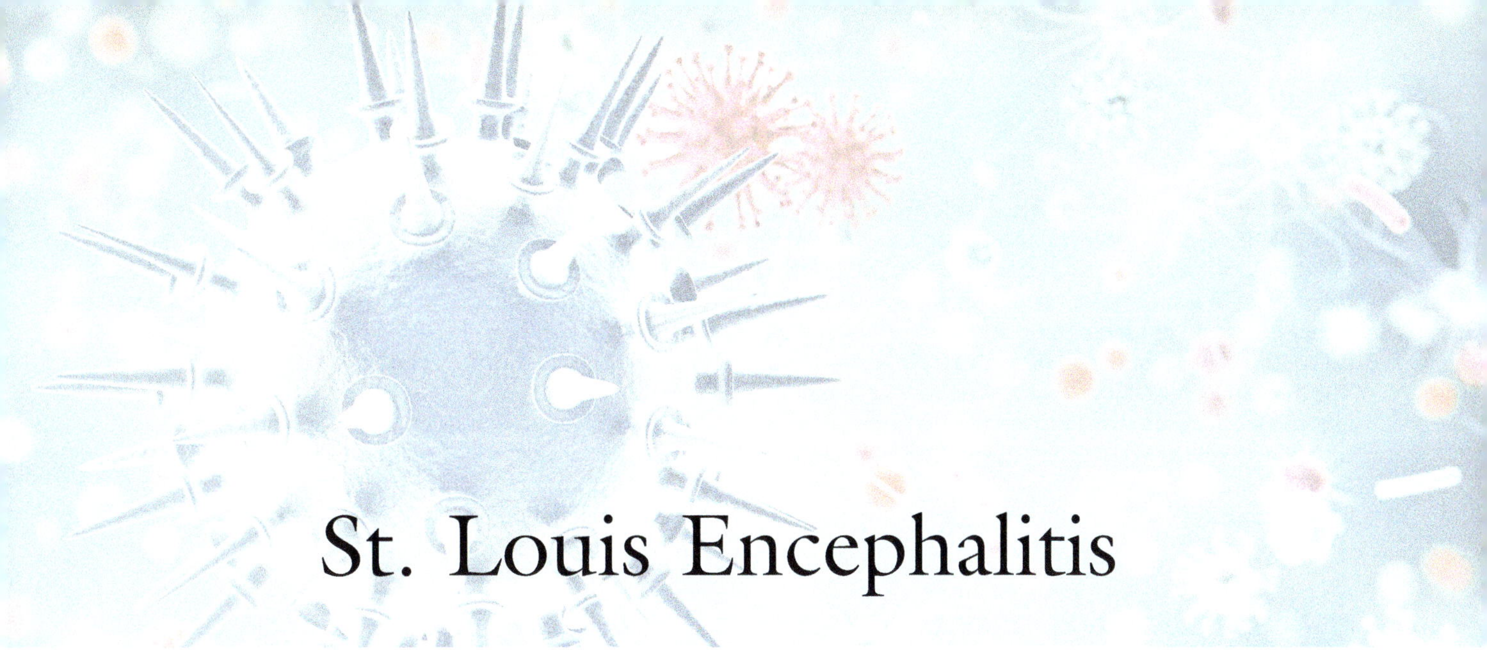

St. Louis Encephalitis

Introduction

St. Louis encephalitis is a serious viral disease that affects the brain and nervous system. The mosquito-borne virus that causes the disease was discovered during an outbreak in St. Louis, Missouri, in 1933, giving the disease its common name: St. Louis encephalitis virus (SLEV). Encephalitis is an inflammation of the brain that can lead to serious symptoms and complications, such as convulsions and paralysis. Contracting the virus does not always lead to encephalitis. Once encephalitis develops, the mortality rate can be as high as 30 percent.

SLEV is an arbovirus—short for arthropod-borne virus. Arboviruses are spread by invertebrates, the most important of which are blood-sucking insects, such as mosquitoes. There is no treatment or vaccine for St. Louis encephalitis and prevention depends on controlling mosquitoes or avoiding their bites. Creating new habitats for mosquitoes through deteriorating urban conditions such as absence of window screens and no access to air conditioners in the summer months encourages the spread of the disease, as does climate change.

Disease History, Characteristics, and Transmission

SLEV is a flavivirus, related to the Japanese encephalitis virus. It is spread by mosquitoes of the *Culex* genus. In temperate areas of the United States, cases tend to occur during late summer and early fall. In the southern states, the infection may occur at any time of the year.

Mild cases of SLEV infection have no symptoms other than fever and headache. An infected person who progresses to St. Louis encephalitis may exhibit a severe headache, high fever, neck stiffness, stupor, disorientation, tremor, convulsions, and paralysis. The affected person may enter a coma. The mortality rate is 5 to 30 percent. It is believed that those who survive the virus will have lifelong immunity to it, preventing reinfection with SLEV in the future.

SLEV is transmitted through the bite of the infected *Culex* mosquito, which serves as the vector by acquiring the virus by feeding on bird hosts such as finches, sparrows, blue jays, doves, and robins. Neither birds nor mos-

WORDS TO KNOW

ANTIBODIES Proteins found in the blood that help fight against foreign substances called antigens. Antigens, which are usually proteins or polysaccharides, stimulate the immune system to produce antibodies, or Y-shaped immunoglobulins. The antibodies inactivate the antigen and help remove it from the body. While antigens can be the source of infections from pathogenic bacteria and viruses, organic molecules detrimental to the body from internal or environmental sources also act as antigens. Genetic engineering and the use of various mutational mechanisms allow the construction of a vast array of antibodies (each with a unique genetic sequence).

ARTHROPOD-BORNE VIRUS A virus caused by one of a phylum of organisms characterized by exoskeletons and segmented bodies.

ENCEPHALITIS A type of acute brain inflammation, most often due to infection by a virus.

HOST An organism that serves as the habitat for a parasite or possibly for a symbiont. A host may provide nutrition to the parasite or symbiont, or it may simply provide a place in which to live.

VECTOR Any agent that carries and transmits parasites and diseases. Also, an organism or a chemical used to transport a gene into a new host cell.

quitoes become ill by being infected with the virus. There are no confirmed cases of person-to-person transmission of the virus; however, in 2015 the virus was detected in the recipient of a kidney transplant in Arizona. Because the kidney donor did not test positive for the virus, researchers believe that it was transmitted through a blood transfusion. The case has led to calls for greater scrutiny of transfusions in settings where the virus is known to be present. This situation is similar to another related, disease-causing, mosquito-borne flavivirus, West Nile virus, which can also be transmitted by blood transfusions.

Scope and Distribution

St. Louis encephalitis occurs in North, Central, and South America and in the Caribbean, although it is mainly a public health problem in the United States. The disease peaked in the second half of the 20th century when 4,478 cases were reported between 1964 and 1998. Outbreaks have occurred in Mississippi, the western states, and Florida. In the Midwest between 1974 and 1977, there were 2,500 cases in 35 states. Outbreaks have been smaller since then. For example, during an outbreak in New Orleans, Louisiana, in 1999, just 20 cases were reported. The virus reemerged on the West Coast in 2015. In Arizona, there were 23 confirmed cases between July and October 2015, resulting in one death. During the Arizona outbreak, mosquito populations in California tested positive for SLEV for the first time since 2002. No human cases were confirmed in California in 2015; however, in 2016 there was one confirmed death from St. Louis encephalitis in the state.

Those living in low-income and crowded conditions are especially at risk of St. Louis encephalitis. Those working outdoors in certain areas, where they may come into contact with infectious mosquitoes, are also at risk. Elderly people who contract SLEV are more likely to develop encephalitis than are younger people.

Treatment and Prevention

There is no treatment for St. Louis encephalitis and no vaccine. The disease is diagnosed by identifying antibodies in the blood or spinal fluid of symptomatic individuals. Symptoms of the disease will be treated as necessary, with the most severe cases requiring hospitalization, intravenous fluid therapy, and respiratory support.

Prevention relies on public health measures to control mosquitoes. People in areas where there have been cases should avoid going out during dusk and dark, when the

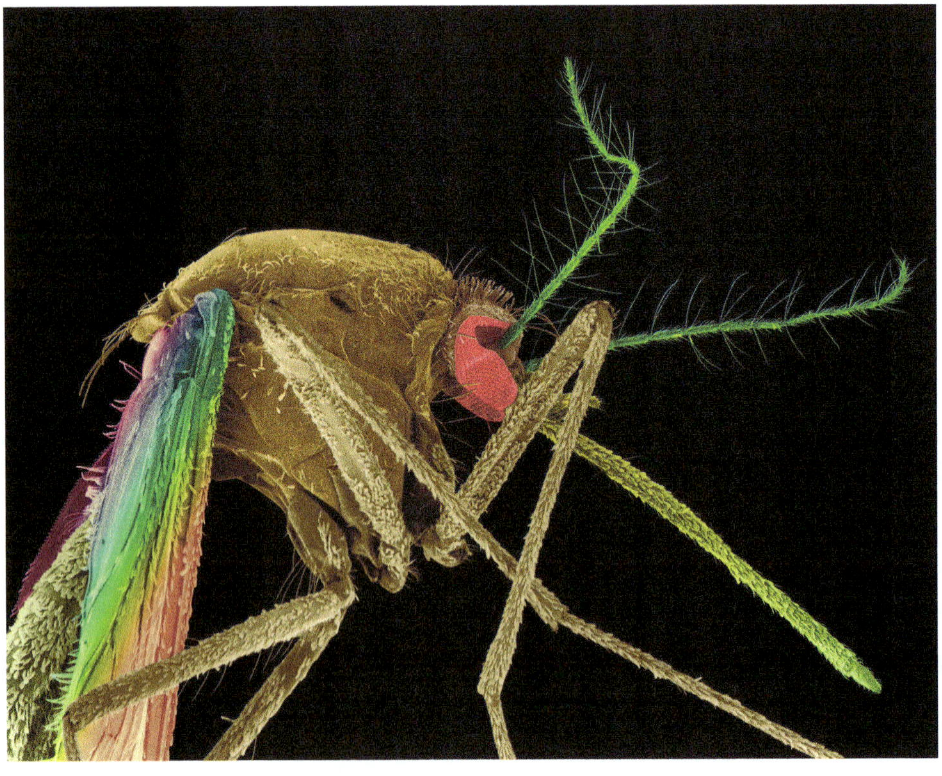

Culex quinquefasciatus, commonly known as the southern house mosquito, is one species of mosquito that can carry St. Louis encephalitis. The *culex* genus is quite diverse, containing over 1,000 species of mosquito. © Dennis Kunkel Microscopy/Science Source

US Cases of St. Louis Encephalitis (2007–2016)

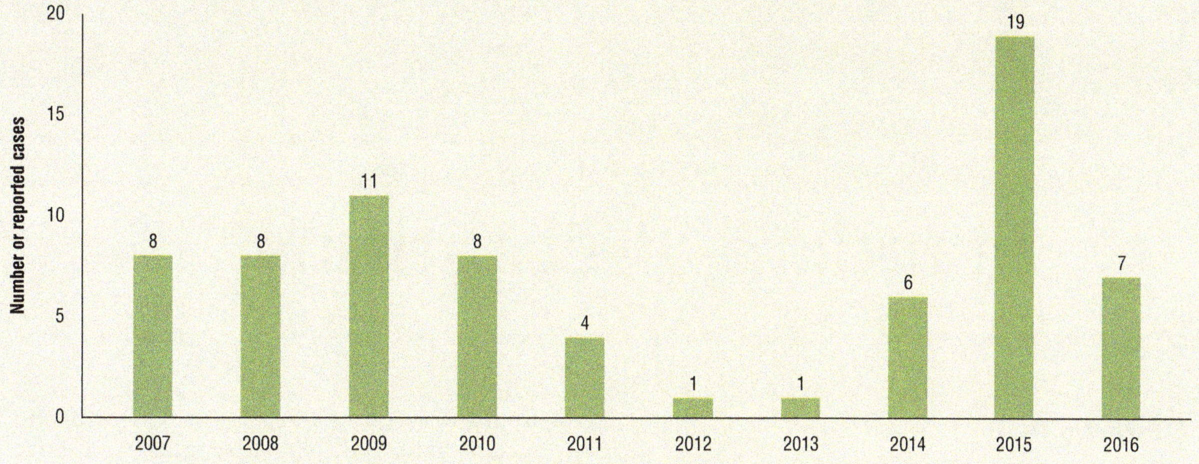

SOURCE: Adapted from "Saint Louis Encephalitis: Epidemiology & Geographical Distribution." Centers for Disease Control and Prevention. November 8, 2017. Available from: https://www.cdc.gov/sle/technical/epi.html

mosquitoes are most active. Properly placed window screens or closing off open windows and relying on air conditioning to cool houses in the summer months is recommended to avoid SLE infection. It is important to cover up with long pants and long-sleeved tops to avoid bites and to use mosquito repellent. The Centers for Disease Control and Prevention recommends using a repellent that contains DEET, picaridin, IR3535, or oil of lemon eucalyptus. Because mosquitos breed in standing water, it is important to empty water from outdoor containers and wading pools.

Impacts and Issues

There is potential for further epidemics of St. Louis encephalitis in the United States because mosquitoes will always create new habitats given the right conditions. In urban areas, conditions such as poor waste disposal may allow new breeding sites for mosquitoes to develop. A major concern is whether global warming will create new favorable habitats for the *Culex* mosquitoes that are the vector for the transmission of St. Louis encephalitis.

Because there is no effective treatment or vaccine for St. Louis encephalitis, and the disease could increase in the coming years, more research is needed. There is potential for a better understanding of the mosquito life cycle, especially with respect to its overwintering, and for better control of this vector. Research leading to development of a vaccine and an antiviral treatment for the disease is also desirable. On a global level, St. Louis encephalitis is currently rare, but it is a disease that could increase in importance if global warming expands its range.

SEE ALSO *Eastern Equine Encephalitis; Encephalitis; Japanese Encephalitis; Mosquito-borne Diseases*

BIBLIOGRAPHY

Books

Mackenzie, J. S., A. D. T. Barrett, and V. Deubel, eds. *Japanese Encephalitis and West Nile Viruses.* New York: Springer, 2013.

Periodicals

Altman, Lawrence K. "After a Phone Tip, Medical Detectives Track Down a Killer." *New York Times* (September 9, 1999). This article can also be found online at http://www.nytimes.com/1999/09/09/nyregion/after-a-phone-tip-medical-detectives-track-down-a-killer.html (accessed November 9, 2017).

White, Gregory S., et al. "Reemergence of St. Louis Encephalitis Virus, California, 2015." *Emerging Infectious Diseases* 22, no. 1 (December 2016): 2185–2188. This article can also be found online at https://wwwnc.cdc.gov/eid/article/22/12/pdfs/16-0805.pdf (accessed November 10, 2017).

Websites

"Saint Louis Encephalitis." Centers for Disease Control and Prevention. https://www.cdc.gov/sle/ (accessed November 9, 2017).

"St. Louis Encephalitis." Vector Disease Control International. http://www.vdci.net/vector-borne-diseases/st-louis-encephalitis-education-and-mosquito-management-to-protect-public-health (accessed November 9, 2017).

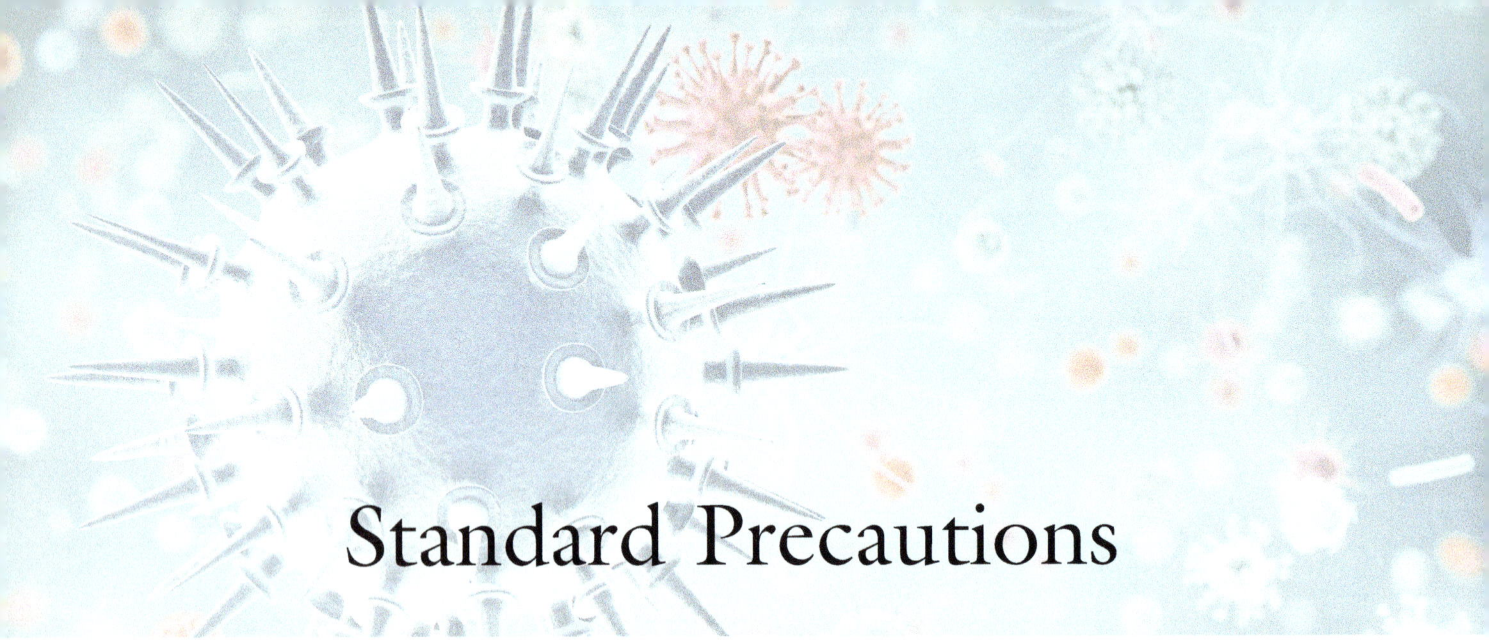

Standard Precautions

Introduction

Standard precautions are precautions that have been put into effect by the US Centers for Disease Control and Prevention (CDC) aimed at reducing the risk of transfer of disease-causing viruses or bacteria (pathogens) from the blood or other moist regions of the body, such as mucous membranes and damaged skin, that can harbor pathogens. Essentially, standard precautions involve good hygiene. This includes proper handwashing and, in a hospital, other practices, such as the proper use of protective equipment, environmental controls, and handling of used linen.

WORDS TO KNOW

AUTOCLAVE A device designed to kill microorganisms on solid items and in liquids by exposure to steam at a high pressure.

HYGIENE Health practices that minimize the spread of infectious microorganisms between people or between other living things and people. Inanimate objects and surfaces such as contaminated cutlery or a cutting board may be a secondary part of this process.

PATHOGEN A disease-causing agent, such as a bacterium, a virus, a fungus, or another microorganism.

PRIONS Proteins that are infectious. Indeed, the name *prion* is derived from "proteinaceous infectious particles." The discovery of prions and confirmation of their infectious nature overturned a central dogma that infections were caused only by intact organisms, particularly microorganisms such as bacteria, fungi, parasites, or viruses. Because prions lack genetic material, the prevailing attitude was that a protein could not cause disease.

UNIVERSAL PRECAUTION An infection-control strategy in which all human blood and other material is assumed to be potentially infectious, specifically with organisms such as human immunodeficiency virus (HIV) and hepatitis B virus. The precautions are aimed at preventing contact with blood or other materials.

History and Scientific Foundations

The standard precaution criteria established by the CDC in 1996 were an extension of guidelines known as universal precautions. Universal precautions were recommended by the CDC in 1987 following the recognition that acquired immunodeficiency syndrome (AIDS) could be contracted by the transfer of blood that was contaminated with the human immunodeficiency virus (HIV).

Universal precautions applied to people known or suspected of having a blood-borne infection. Standard precautions are wider in their scope and apply to all bodily fluids (except sweat) of all patients, whether or not they are recognized as having an infection.

Applications and Research

Handwashing

One of the fundamental standard precautions is handwashing. Hands must be washed after direct contact with a patient's blood or other body fluids or after contact with items, such as fluid-soaked linens, regardless of whether gloves have been worn. This ensures that pathogens that may have contacted the skin through tears or imperfections in a glove are killed.

Handwashing should be done immediately after contact with a patient and before moving on to another patient. Handwashing may also need to be done during the time spent with one patient if different tasks are performed—for example, after probing inside the mouth and before examining other parts of the body.

For routine handwashing the use of ordinary household soap is acceptable, because the soap's ingredients and the friction from rubbing the hands together for a sufficient length of time (at least 30 seconds) will produce the desired antimicrobial effect. However, an alcohol solution is being used increasingly in hospital wards. This is because the alcohol solution is effective more quickly, an important consideration in the time-constrained day of health care providers. In addition, washing the hands with soap many times every day can be harsh on skin, even to the point of causing breaks in the skin that can become infected.

Gloves

Health care providers should wear gloves when coming into contact with blood and other body fluids. Fresh gloves must be worn for each patient, otherwise the gloves can become a route of patient-to-patient transfer of microbes. Similar to handwashing guidelines, gloves should be worn and removed immediately before and after contact with a patient and need to be disposed of in a designated container.

Gown

A hospital gown worn over clothing protects against splashing or spraying of blood and other body fluids. The choice of a gown depends to a large extent on the infection to which a person might be exposed. For example, a gown made of plastic or other water-repellent material should be used when dealing with an infection suspected of being severe, such as Ebola. A gown that becomes soaked with Ebola virus–laden blood could result in the transfer of the virus to the health care provider. In other, less risky, cases, cotton gowns can be appropriate.

A gown should be removed as soon as possible after seeing a patient and always before moving to another patient. Because the removal of a gown involves the hands, handwashing should be done only after a gown is removed and put in a designated container.

Patient-Care Equipment

Equipment that becomes contaminated with blood or another body fluid must be decontaminated before reuse. Equipment that is meant for one-time use must be disposed of properly after that use and should never be reused. Needles and other sharp objects must be disposed of after use in rigid containers to minimize the chances of accidental injury during their disposal.

Environmental Control

Microorganisms can stick to surfaces and in some cases can remain capable of causing an infection for hours. If a contaminated surface is touched by someone, the infectious microbes can be transferred to that person or someone else that person contacts. Thus, an important

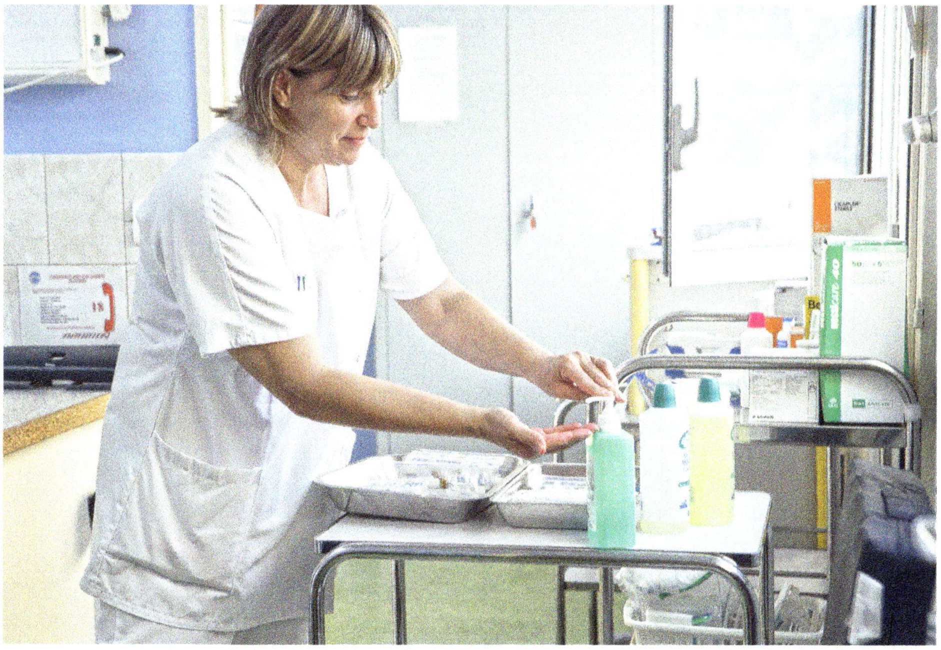

Health care workers use alcohol-based sanitary solutions as a standard precaution against spreading infections. © *Jean-Paul Chassenet/Science Source*

standard precaution is the disinfection of surfaces such as beds, bedrails, toilets and toilet assist rails, and equipment near a patient's bed. The disinfection needs to be done at regular intervals with an approved disinfectant, and all disinfections should be recorded on paper or electronically.

Linens

Soiled bedding needs to be cleaned to completely remove blood and body fluids. It should be washed in hot water to kill living bacteria that may have clung to the fabric. Another standard precaution involving linens relates to the transport of the linens from the bedside to the hospital laundry. Soiled linens should be transported in a closed and waterproof container to lessen the chances that microbes could leak out or become airborne.

■ Impacts and Issues

Standard precautions are an efficient way of minimizing the chances of the transfer of infectious microorganisms from patient to patient and from patients to health care providers. However, diligence is required and, as of 2017, ensuring compliance remained a challenge. Studies continue to document handwashing compliance of less than 50 percent of health care providers, particularly physicians, after finishing with one patient and before seeing another patient. The common explanation is a lack of time. To increase compliance with handwashing, some hospitals have installed alcohol-based handwashing stations at patients' bedsides. The pressure of being caught in noncompliance with handwashing precautions can be a powerful incentive to practice proper hygiene.

The need for standard precautions pertaining to equipment is highlighted by the observation that infectious proteins called prions can remain capable of causing disease even when surgical instruments have been sterilized using the combination of chemicals, high pressure, and high heat known as autoclaving. The World Health Organization has recommended that surgery on patients suspected of having a prion-related disease should be done using disposable instruments or instruments should be incinerated before being used again.

See Also *Airborne Precautions; Handwashing; Isolation and Quarantine; Personal Protective Equipment*

BIBLIOGRAPHY

Books

Pittet, Didier, John M. Boyce, and Benedetta Allegranzi, eds. *Hand Hygiene: A Handbook for Medical Professionals.* New York: Wiley, 2017.

Weston, Debbie, Alison Burgess, and Sue Roberts. *Infection Prevention and Control at a Glance.* New York: Wiley, 2016.

Periodicals

Weinberg, Geoffrey A. "Respiratory Syncytial Mortality among Young Children." *Lancet Global Health* 5 (October 2017): e951–e952.

Websites

"Infection Control." Centers for Disease Control and Prevention. https://www.cdc.gov/infectioncontrol/index.html (accessed November 21, 2017).

"Infection Prevention and Control." World Health Organization. http://who.int/infection-prevention/en/ (accessed November 21, 2017).

Brian Hoyle

Staphylococcus aureus Infections

Introduction

Staphylococcus aureus is a bacterium that colonizes, or normally inhabits, the surface of the skin and, in about 25 percent of humans, the inside of the nose. In a healthy person the bacterium is usually not a health concern. However, if a person's skin is damaged by a cut or a burn, or if *S. aureus* gains access to areas inside the body, infection can result.

S. aureus is the most common cause of staph infections. (Other species of *Staphylococcus* can also cause infections.) *S. aureus* can cause a number of life-threatening infections. The development and spread of resistance to many antibiotics has made *S. aureus* one of the top priorities in the infection-control programs of hospitals all over the world.

Other life-threatening infections can occur in susceptible people. These infections are referred to as opportunistic infections because they normally do not occur in healthy people.

Staphylococcal food poisoning can also occur.

Disease History, Characteristics, and Transmission

S. aureus is a spherical-shaped bacterium. It is Gram-positive, meaning that it consists of a membrane layer made up mainly of lipids and proteins and a thick, strong network, or peptidoglycan. (Gram-negative bacteria have two membrane layers and a thin peptido-

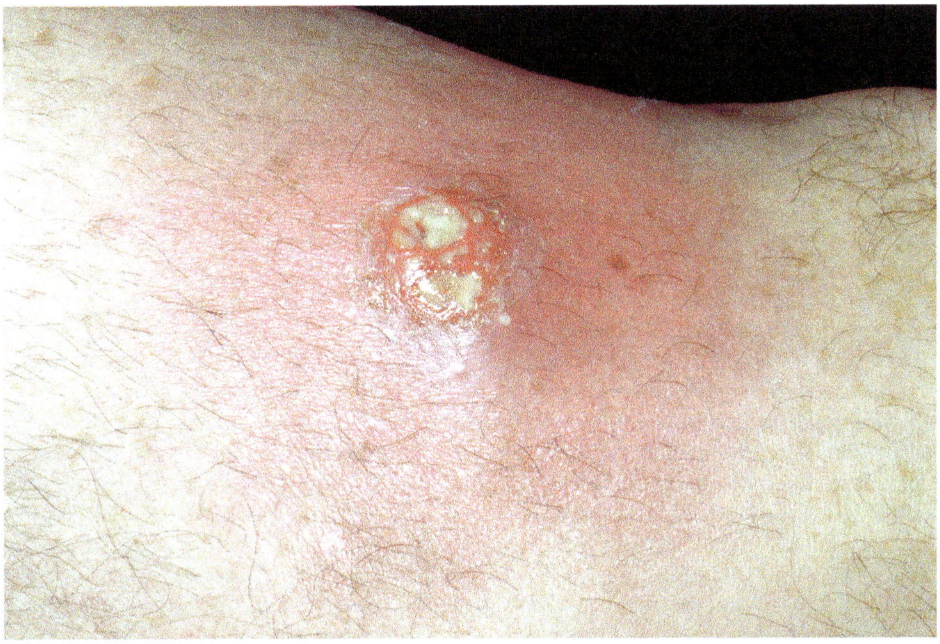

Skin infections caused by the bacterium *Staphylococcus aureus* are commonly called staph infections.

WORDS TO KNOW

ANTIBIOTIC RESISTANCE The ability of bacteria to resist the actions of antibiotic drugs.

COLONIZE To persist and grow at a given location.

IMMUNOCOMPROMISED Having an immune system with reduced ability to recognize and respond to the presence of foreign material.

OPPORTUNISTIC INFECTION An infection that occurs in people whose immune systems are diminished or are not functioning normally. Such infections are opportunistic insofar as the infectious agents take advantage of their hosts' compromised immune systems and invade to cause disease.

RESISTANT ORGANISM An organism that has developed the ability to counter something trying to harm it. Within infectious diseases, the organism, such as a bacterium, has developed a resistance to drugs, such as antibiotics.

SELECTION PRESSURE The influence of various factors on the evolution of an organism. An example is the overuse of antibiotics, which provides a selection pressure for the development of antibiotic resistance in bacteria.

glycan.) The design of the bacterium makes it environmentally hardy, which enables it to live in microscopic depressions on the surface of the skin. The bacterium also thrives in the warm and moist atmosphere inside the nose.

S. aureus typically grows and divides to form microscopic clusters that appear grapelike. When grown on a solid food source that contains blood, the visible mounds of bacteria (colonies) that develop tend to be golden in color (*aureus* means "gold" in Latin). These characteristics aid in the identification of the organism. Other tests of biochemical activity, such the ability of the bacterium to clot blood, are also used in identification.

If the normal barrier of the skin's surface is breached—by a cut or a burn, for example—or if a person is immunocompromised and so is less capable of fighting off invading microorganisms, *S. aureus* can rapidly cause infections. These range from skin infections that are relatively minor, such as boils and pimples, to life-threatening infections of the skin in infants (scalded skin syndrome), the lungs (pneumonia), the lining of certain nerves (meningitis), the heart valves (endocarditis), and, in the case of toxic shock syndrome, the blood (septicemia). Heart-related infections are associated with the implantation of devices designed to assist proper heart function. The devices can become contaminated before being implanted if they are handled by bare hands that have not been washed properly. This transfers *S. aureus* from the skin to the plastic surface of the device, where the bacteria can adhere and grow.

The association of *S. aureus* and infections has been known since 1880, when the bacterium was isolated from wounds. The environmental hardiness of the bacterium is one important factor in its ability to cause infection. If present on a moist surface, such as a towel, the bacteria can remain alive and capable of causing infection for hours. Even more importantly, skin-to-skin contact can easily spread *S. aureus* from one person to another. The ability of the bacterium to invade host tissue is one cause of infection. Toxins can also be produced when *S. aureus* gets into a wound or when the bacterium contaminates food.

■ Scope and Distribution

S. aureus infections can occur anywhere in the world and are very common. Even in a developed country such as the United States with high-quality medical care, more than 500,000 people are hospitalized with *S. aureus* infections every year. The bacterium is one of the main causes of nosocomial (hospital-acquired) infections. The bacterium is also a concern in agriculture because it is the cause of mastitis, a disease in cattle.

Until the beginning of the 21st century, methicillin-resistant *Staphylococcus aureus* (MRSA) was almost exclusively found in hospitals, because the tremendous antibiotic use in hospitals provided a powerful selection pressure—that is, an environment where only the most resilient bacteria could survive. In 2017 MRSA became the leading cause of health care–associated infections in the United States and was also a major problem globally. In addition, the infection has become established outside of hospitals. This form of the bacterium is designated as community-associated MRSA (CA-MRSA). The USA300 type of MRSA is becoming a primary source of infections that require hospitalization.

■ Treatment and Prevention

Despite the antibiotic resistance of some types of *S. aureus*, infections still usually respond to treatment with antibiotics. Completing the full course of antibiotic treatment is important. Some patients may stop taking antibiotics before the course of treatment is completed because they begin to feel better. This is unwise, as the infection may not yet be eliminated. Surviving *S. aureus* can cause the illness to recur, and these survivors may even become resistant to the antibiotic(s) being used in the treatment.

The search continues for new antibiotics that will be effective against MRSA. In 2017 the most common treatment for people at home involved an oral combination of two antibiotics (trimethoprim and sulfamethoxazole), clindamycin, minocycline, or doxycline. Patients in hospitals are usually treated intravenously because it is important to rapidly achieve a level of antibiotic in the bloodstream that is effective in killing the bacteria.

Another potential treatment option is phage therapy. The word *phage* is short for *bacteriophage*, which is a virus that specifically infects and forms new phage particles inside of a bacterium. The phage-bacterium association is specific. A certain type of phage infects a certain type of bacterium. In doing so the phage ultimately destroys the bacterial cell. Scientists are experimenting with a phage that targets MRSA. If this technique proves successful, it would be a powerful treatment because resistance to a phage does not typically develop. As of 2017 phage therapy remained in the research stage.

Impacts and Issues

The impacts of *S. aureus* infections are enormous, in terms of both the number of serious illnesses and deaths caused and the financial cost of caring for these patients. In a nationwide analysis of hospitalized patients in 2001, patients with *S. aureus* were found to average three times the length of hospital stay, three times the total charges, and three times the risk of death while in the hospital than hospitalized patients without *S. aureus* infection.

Furthermore, the development of antibiotic resistance by the bacterium is ominous, as strains that are resistant to almost all antibiotics exist. At the time of the commercial introduction of the first antibiotic, penicillin, in 1943, antibiotic resistance among *S. aureus* isolated from infections was unknown. Only seven years later, approximately 40 percent of all isolates were resistant to penicillin. By 1960 80 percent of hospital isolates of *S. aureus* were penicillin-resistant.

SEE ALSO *Antibiotic Resistance; Bacterial Disease; MRSA; Toxic Shock*

BIBLIOGRAPHY

Books

Dodd, Christine, and Tim G. Aldsworth. *Foodborne Illnesses.* 3rd ed. New York: Academic Press, 2017.

Kon, Kateryna. *Antibiotic Resistance: Mechanisms and New Antimicrobial Approaches.* Edited by Mahendra Rai. New York: Academic Press, 2016.

Periodicals

Klein, Eili Y., et al. "Trends in Methicillin-Resistant *Staphylococcus aureus* Hospitalizations in the United States, 2010–2014." *Clinical Infectious Diseases* 65 (November 2017): 1921–1923.

Websites

"Infection Control." Centers for Disease Control and Prevention. https://www.cdc.gov/infectioncontrol/index.html (accessed November 21, 2017).

"Infection Prevention and Control." World Health Organization. http://who.int/infection-prevention/en/ (accessed November 21, 2017).

Brian Hoyle

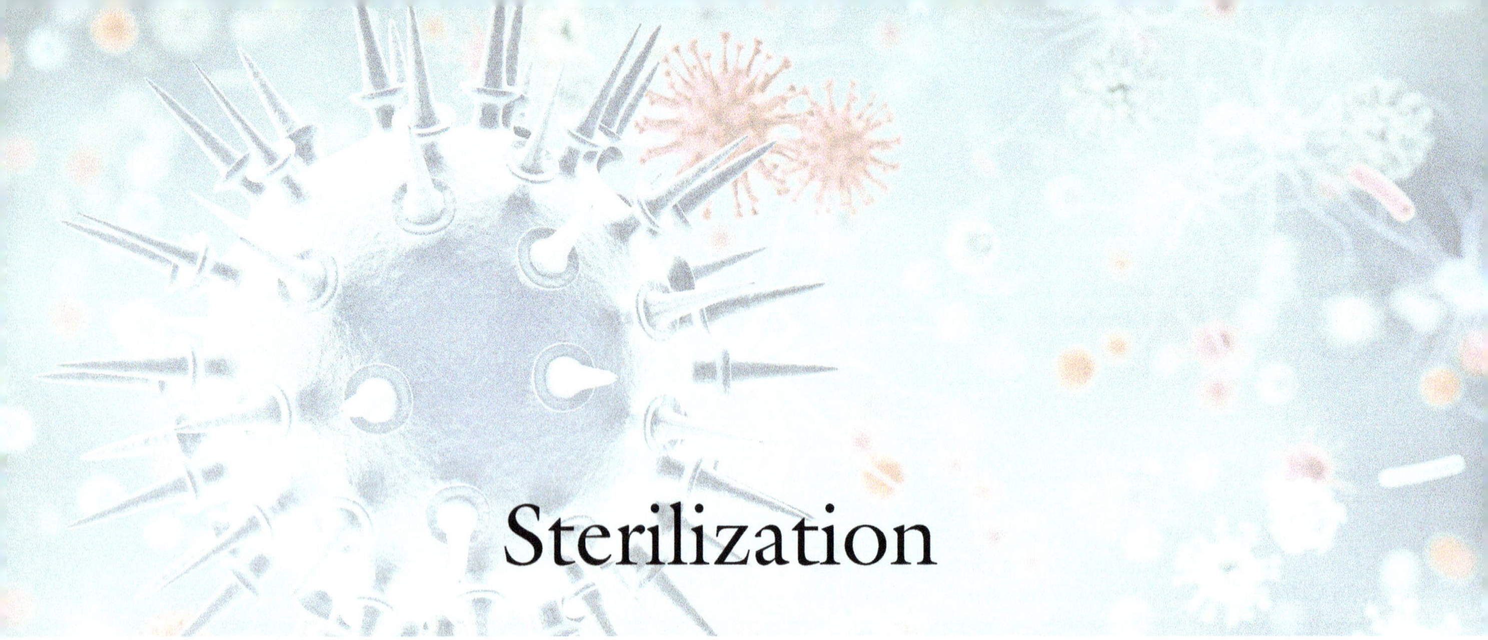

Sterilization

Introduction

Sterilization refers to processes that eliminate microorganisms from surfaces, the interior of equipment, foods, and liquids. A catheter is one example of a device whose surface must be completely sterilized before it is inserted in a person to deliver food or medicine. A cardiac pacemaker is another example of a device whose surface must be sterilized before it is implanted inside the body to control the heart rate. A common example of a liquid requiring sterilization is the liquid-based nutrient medium used to grow bacteria in a laboratory.

Sterilization is intended to eliminate living microorganisms such as bacteria, fungi, and protozoa, along with nonliving microbes such as viruses that, given the appropriate host, can cause disease.

There are various methods of sterilization depending on the aim of the procedure. For example, surgical instruments are sterilized to guarantee the absence of pathogens, while most laboratory growth media used for experimentation is sterilized to guarantee the absence of bacteria. Pharmaceutical medications also need to be free of all potential disease-causing agents.

WORDS TO KNOW

AUTOCLAVE A device designed to kill microorganisms on solid items and in liquids by exposure to steam at a high pressure.

BIOINDICATOR A living organism whose status in an ecosystem offers an idea of the health of its environment.

PATHOGEN A disease-causing agent, such as a bacterium, a virus, a fungus, or another microorganism.

PRIONS Proteins that are infectious. Indeed, the name *prion* is derived from "proteinaceous infectious particles." The discovery of prions and confirmation of their infectious nature overturned a central dogma that infections were caused only by intact organisms, particularly microorganisms such as bacteria, fungi, parasites, or viruses. Because prions lack genetic material, the prevailing attitude was that a protein could not cause disease.

History and Scientific Foundations

Heat has been used to sterilize objects for millennia. Until the late 1800s, the flame of a fire was used. In the 21st century the most common method of heat sterilization employs high temperature and pressure above atmospheric pressure. The combination of temperature and pressure most efficiently heats an object or a volume of liquid; exposure of the samples for a certain period of time has proved sufficient to kill even hardy microorganisms.

An autoclave is the most common instrument used for heat sterilization. Autoclaves range in size from small units that easily fit on the benchtop of a laboratory to large units that have the volume of an average kitchen refrigerator. An autoclave uses steam to sterilize the objects placed inside it. Typically the steam is pumped into the autoclave chamber at a temperature of 250°F (121°C) and a pressure that is 15 pounds per square inch (psi) above atmospheric pressure. These conditions of temperature and pressure are maintained for at least 15 minutes (larger loads or greater volumes of liquid can be held longer). Then the steam is released from the chamber in a controlled and safe manner. The chamber can be opened when it has returned to atmospheric pressure.

As a control over the process, indicator tape can be applied to the objects being autoclaved. Bands form on the tape when the proper conditions of temperature, pressure, and time have been attained. This helps the operator judge whether sterilization has been successful. To be even more certain, solutions that contain bacterial spores of *Bacillus stearothermophilus* can be included with the load being sterilized. Bacterial spores are resistant to the killing action of heat. If the liquid containing the spores is incubated in a suitable liquid growth source and the medium remains clear, it indicates that sterilization was successful. In addition to the use of this bioindicator, many autoclaves record the temperature profile of each sterilization cycle, allowing the user to visually monitor whether the appropriate conditions were achieved.

Monitoring of autoclave performance is important. If, for example, too many items are autoclaved at once, the overcrowded conditions may not allow the steam to effectively penetrate the entire load, which can result in inadequate sterilization.

Although autoclaving is an effective method of sterilization with many applications, it is not foolproof. For instance, research has shown that prions can remain potent following autoclaving of surgical instruments. Even the combination of autoclaving with chemicals has proven ineffective against prion contamination. The World Health Organization has recommended that surgery on patients suspected of having a prion-related disease be performed with disposable instruments or that the instruments used be incinerated after the surgery is completed.

There are other methods of sterilization. Some metal objects can be surface-sterilized by holding them over an open flame. This is a common way of sterilizing an inoculating loop, which is a loop of metal used to transfer microorganisms from one place to another during experiments. Burning trash that contains medical waste is another way of sterilizing the residual ash. This ash can then be safely disposed of. Medical incinerators must be specially designed to retain the vapor given off because infectious material can potentially be carried into the air during incineration. A common method for sterilizing drinking water is boiling. Boiling kills most bacteria and inactivates most viruses. However, agents such as prions and some spore-forming bacteria can survive boiling for 15 minutes. However, in most situations, boiling is better than not treating water at all.

Objects such as plastic, optical equipment, and electrical circuits that cannot stand heat can be sterilized using the chemical ethylene oxide. This chemical is applied as a gas in a specialized machine. Another sporeforming bacterium, *Bacillus subtilus*, is used to monitor the success of ethylene oxide sterilization.

Ozone is another chemical sterilizer. Drinking water can be sterilized using ozone. A diluted solution of bleach (sodium hypochlorite) is an especially useful sterilizing agent for work surfaces. Other chemical sterilizers include glutaraldehyde and hydrogen peroxide.

Applications and Research

Sterilization is a necessity of everyday life in research, health care, and even the supermarket. Ongoing investigations seek to develop chemicals that sterilize more efficiently and quickly while also being safe to use.

Impacts and Issues

Without the ability to sterilize growth media, many scientific experiments could not be accomplished, as it would be impossible to know if the results were due to the organism being studied or a contaminant. In addition, surgeries would have a poor survival rate, as was the case in the days before sterilization techniques were routinely employed.

While important, the quest for sterilization can go too far. One example is the marketing of surface-sterilizing products designed for use in the kitchen and bathroom. Bacteria that are not killed by these products, which contain the chemical triclosan, have the potential to become resis-

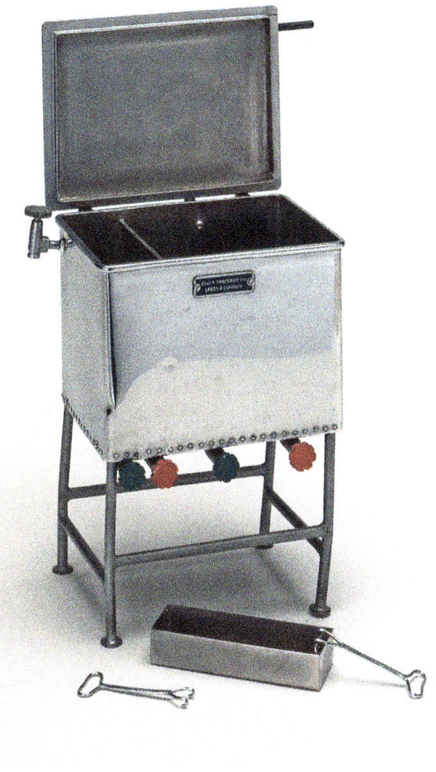

Invented in the 1880s, the autoclave sterilizes medical instruments with high pressure and super-heated steam. © Science & Society Picture Library/Getty Images

BACTERIA SPORES SPUR STERILIZATION RESEARCH

The discovery of bacteria that are resistant to sterilization could potentially contaminate experiments and environments studied by the National Aeronautics and Space Administrations (NASA) and other space agency probes. One species was tentatively named *B. odysseensis* after being isolated from the surfaces of the Mars *Odyssey* spacecraft following routine sterilization. The method of spore formation is suspected of having a role in resistance of spore-forming bacteria to sterilization.

Earth-bound benefits of such research offer hope of improved methods of sterilization and prevention of unintentional contamination.

tant to that chemical, which can make these bacteria a more serious concern than before they developed this resistance.

In 2016 the Food and Drug Administration (FDA) announced a ban on the sale of household soaps that contain triclosan, a decision that took effect in September 2017. The ban does not apply to all products. While triclosan has been eliminated from soap products sold in the United States, one brand of toothpaste (Colgate Total), which contains triclosan, is still allowed to be sold, with the FDA deciding it is safe for use. Furthermore, triclosan-containing products that are not examined by the FDA remain for sale. These include toys such as building blocks, pool-safety products like water wings, and scissors.

In 2015 the European Union also banned the use of triclosan in disinfectants, algaecide products, and some types of preservatives. However, other countries, including Canada, Australia, and Japan, have permitted the sale of these products.

See Also *Disinfection; Infection Control and Asepsis; Sanitation*

BIBLIOGRAPHY

Books

Amer, Fatma. *Hospital Infection Control, Part 1.* 3rd ed. Saarbrücken, Germany: Noor, 2017.

Buchanan, Charles M. *Antisepsis and Antiseptics (Classic Reprint). Joseph Lister and the Story of Antiseptics.* London: Forgotten Books, 2017.

McDonnell, Gerald E. *Antisepsis, Disinfection, and Sterilization.* 2nd ed. Washington DC: ASM, 2017.

Periodicals

Carey, Daniel E., and Patrick J. McNamara. "The Impact of Triclosan on the Spread of Antibiotic Resistance in the Environment." *Frontiers in Microbiology* (January 15, 2015). This article can also be found online at https://www.frontiersin.org/articles/10.3389/fmicb.2014.00780/full (accessed November 16, 2017).

Halden, Rol U. "On the Need and Speed of Regulating Triclosan and Triclocarban in the United States." *Environmental Science and Technology* 48 (April 2014): 3603–3611.

Websites

Hartmann, Erica. "Banned Antimicrobial Chemicals Found in Many Household Products." CNN. Last modified January 25, 2017. http://www.cnn.com/2017/01/25/health/triclosan-household-items-partner/index.html (accessed November 17, 2017).

Jet Propulsion Laboratory, NASA. https://www.jpl.nasa.gov/ (accessed March 17, 2018).

Brian Hoyle

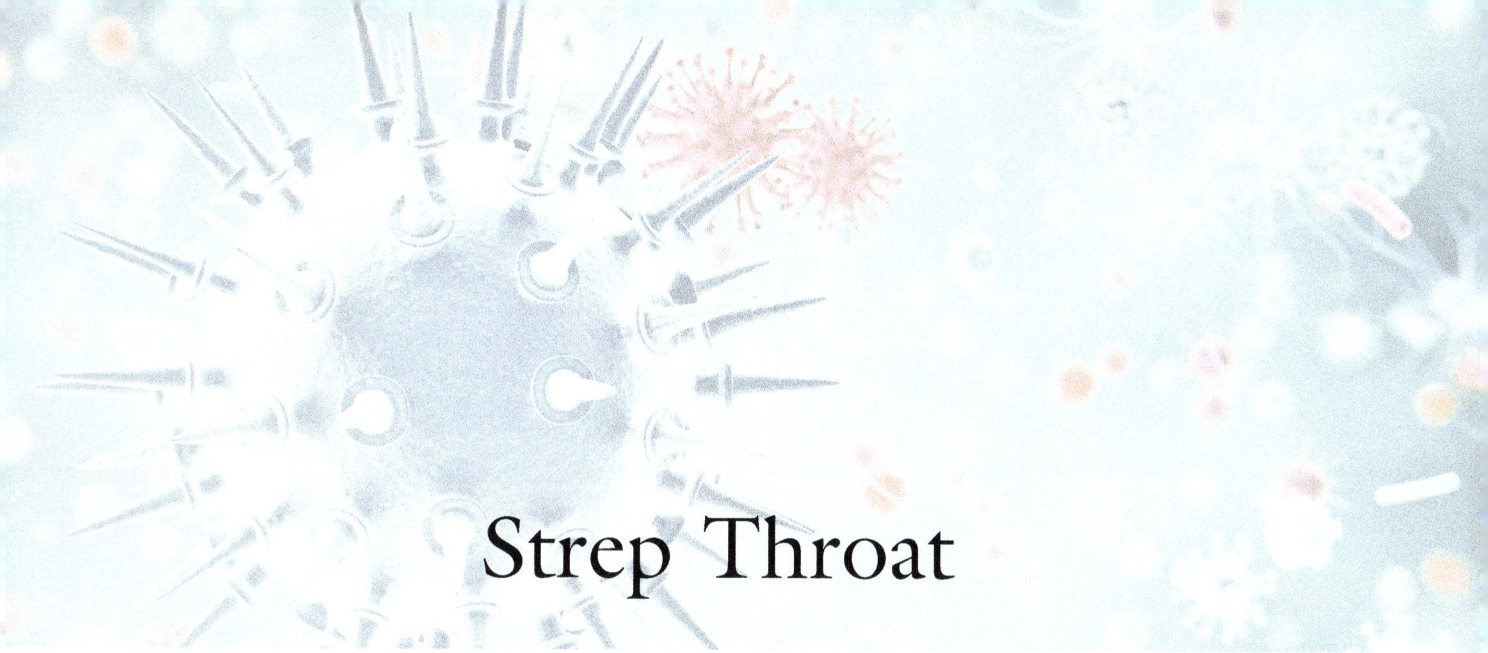

Strep Throat

Introduction

A sore throat is one of the most common symptoms for which people see the doctor. It often precedes a cold, flu, or other respiratory infection. Most sore throats are caused by viral infection. Strep throat, or Streptococcal pharyngitis, is not a virus. It is a bacterial throat infection. *Strep* is short for *Streptococcus pyogenes*, the causative agent. Most people carry *S. pyogenes* in their throat and on their skin, and it normally causes no problems.

Strep throat is considered a mild infection, although it can be very painful. Left untreated, it can sometimes lead to serious complications, such as rheumatic fever. Strep throat responds promptly to antibiotic treatment, which will also prevent the infection from spreading to others. The majority of sore throats will not respond to antibiotics because they are caused by viruses. That is why strep throat should be properly diagnosed whenever possible to prevent the unnecessary use of antibiotics.

Disease History, Characteristics, and Transmission

The *S. pyogenes* bacterium belongs to a large group of bacteria called the *streptococci*, which occur in characteristic long chains. They are subdivided according to the antigen proteins they bear on their surfaces. *S. pyogenes* is, therefore, sometimes called group A streptococcus (GAS) because it carries the A antigen. A certain amount of GAS is found on the skin of most people without causing illness. This is known as colonization. Besides strep throat, GAS can also cause impetigo (a skin infection) and scarlet fever. Some strains of GAS are also responsible for necrotizing fasciitis, which involves the soft tissue under the skin, and toxic shock syndrome, both of which are potentially fatal.

The symptoms of strep throat include throat pain and difficulty swallowing, headache, fever, and swollen glands. The tonsils might be red and swollen with white patches and streaks of pus. Strep throat is distinguished from other conditions, such as tonsillitis or viral throat infection, by testing a throat swab for the presence of GAS.

Possible complications of strep throat include rheumatic fever and kidney inflammation. These may set in weeks after the first symptoms of the throat infection. Rheumatic fever may be indicated by joint pain or rash. The urine may become dark if the kidneys are infected. Rheumatic fever is potentially serious, as it can lead to permanent damage of the heart valves with impairment of heart function. Other possible complications include tonsillitis, scarlet fever, sinus infection, and ear infection.

GAS is highly contagious, and strep throat is spread through coughing, sneezing, and contact with objects, such as kitchen utensils and bathroom items, that have been used by an infected person (fomites). The infection

WORDS TO KNOW

ANTIBIOTIC RESISTANCE The ability of bacteria to resist the actions of antibiotic drugs.

COLONIZATION The process of occupation and increase in number of microorganisms at a specific site.

FOMITE An object or a surface to which infectious microorganisms such as bacteria or viruses can adhere and be transmitted. Papers, clothing, dishes, and other objects can all act as fomites. Transmission is often by touch.

SOCIAL AND PERSONAL RESPONSIBILITY

According to the US Centers for Disease Control and Prevention (CDC), "the best way to keep from getting or spreading strep throat is to wash your hands often, especially after coughing or sneezing and before preparing foods or eating. To practice good hygiene you should:

- Cover your mouth and nose with a tissue when you cough or sneeze
- Put your used tissue in the waste basket
- Cough or sneeze into your upper sleeve or elbow, not your hands, if you don't have a tissue
- Wash your hands often with soap and water for at least 20 seconds
- Use an alcohol-based hand rub if soap and water are not available

You should also wash glasses, utensils, and plates after someone who is sick uses them. After they have been washed, these items are safe for others to use."

often spreads rapidly through family members, schools, and childcare centers—anywhere, in fact, that people come into close contact.

Scope and Distribution

Strep throat is most common among children ages five to 15, although it can affect people of any age. It is most often seen in late winter and spring. In the United States, the risk of complications from strep throat is low.

Treatment and Prevention

Strep throat is usually treated with an antibiotic, such as penicillin or amoxicillin. Studies have shown that treatment with newer-generation antibiotics for a shorter period of time is just as effective as treatment with penicillin (an older-generation antibiotic) for a longer duration. For those with penicillin allergies, other antibiotics, such as cephalexin, should be prescribed.

Antibiotic treatment reduces the severity and duration of symptoms and stops the infection from passing to others. Symptoms will start to clear within a day or two of starting antibiotics. It is important to finish the whole course of prescribed antibiotics. Stopping medication early will increase the risk of complications and encourage the growth of resistant organisms.

Rest, plenty of water, and soothing foods will also help relieve the pain of strep throat, as will gargling with salt water. Acetaminophen and ibuprofen may be prescribed for pain and fever. Aspirin is not recommended for young

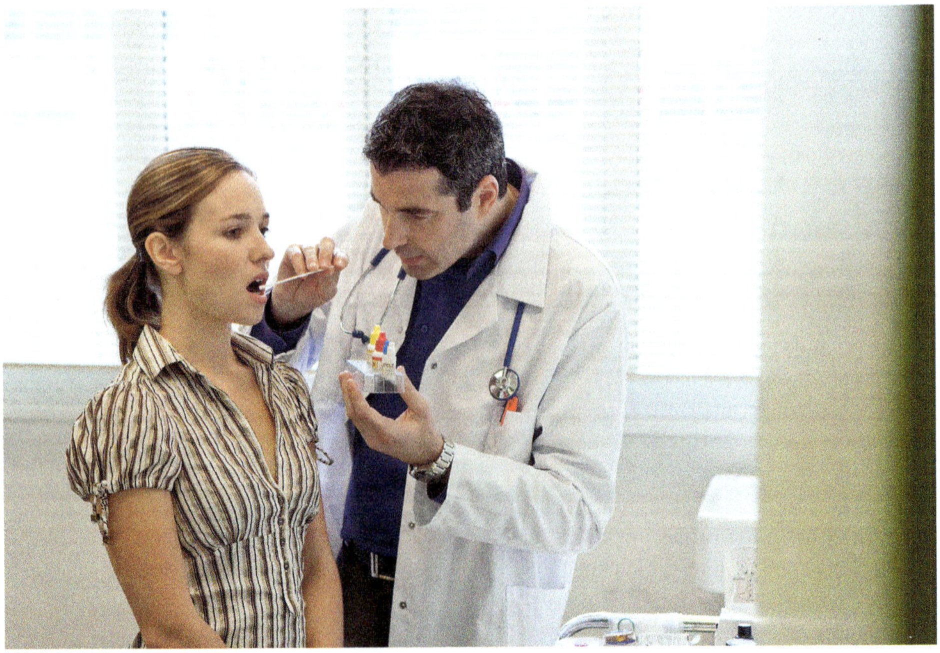

A physician swabs a patient's throat to test for strep throat. © *BSIP/UIG/Getty Images*

children with strep throat because it can contribute to the development of Reye's syndrome, a potentially life-threatening illness.

As with many infections, the best way to prevent strep throat is by practicing good personal hygiene, including covering the mouth and nose when coughing or sneezing and washing the hands frequently and thoroughly. For a child with recurrent strep throat, removal of the tonsils (tonsillectomy) may be helpful.

■ Impacts and Issues

Accurate diagnosis of the cause of a sore throat is important. Viral infections should not be treated with antibiotics. Not only will the infection not respond, but the inappropriate prescription of antibiotics has been linked to antibiotic resistance, which is a growing public health problem. Strep throat can be diagnosed with rapid tests for GAS antigen or deoxyribonucleic acid (DNA), along with confirmation that the patient has strep throat symptoms. Courses of antibiotics prescribed for strep throat should always be completed because stopping early also encourages antibiotic resistance.

SEE ALSO *Antibiotic Resistance; Bacterial Disease; Impetigo; Necrotizing Fasciitis; Scarlet Fever; Toxic Shock*

BIBLIOGRAPHY

Books

Sanyahumbi, Amy Sims, et al. "Global Disease Burden of Group A Streptococcus." In *Streptococcus Pyogenes: Basic Biology to Clinical Manifestations*, edited by Joseph J. Ferretti, Dennis L. Stevens, and Vincent A. Fischetti. Oklahoma City: University of Oklahoma Health Sciences Center, 2016.

Periodicals

Altamimi, Saleh, et al. "Short-Term Late-Generation Antibiotics versus Longer Term Penicillin for Acute Streptococcal Pharyngitis in Children." *Cochrane Database of Systematic Reviews* 8 (2012). This article can also be found online at http://onlinelibrary.wiley.com/wol1/doi/10.1002/14651858.CD004872.pub3/abstract (accessed January 25, 2018).

"Kids' Tonsillectomies Make More Sense for Sleep Apnea Than for Strep Throat." *Washington Post* (January 20, 2017). This article can also be found online at https://www.washingtonpost.com/national/health-science/tonsillectomies-may-not-be-wise-for-stopping-throat-infections/2017/01/20/6655bbf6-ddb7-11e6-ad42-f3375f271c9c_story.html?utm_term=.40825a7e9193 (accessed January 25, 2018).

Shulman, Stanford T., et al. "Clinical Practice Guideline for the Diagnosis and Management of Group A Streptococcal Pharyngitis: 2012 Update by the Infectious Diseases Society of America." *Clinical Infectious Diseases* 55, no. 10 (November 15, 2012): e86–e102. This article can also be found online at https://academic.oup.com/cid/article/55/10/e86/321183 (accessed January 25, 2018).

Walker, Mark J., et al. "Disease Manifestations and Pathogenic Mechanisms of Group A *Streptococcus*." *Clinical Microbiology Reviews* 27, no. 2 (April 1, 2014): 264–301. This article can also be found online at http://cmr.asm.org/content/27/2/264.full (accessed January 25, 2018).

Websites

"Group A Streptococcal (GAS) Disease." Centers for Disease Control and Prevention, September 16, 2016. https://www.cdc.gov/groupastrep/ (accessed January 25, 2018).

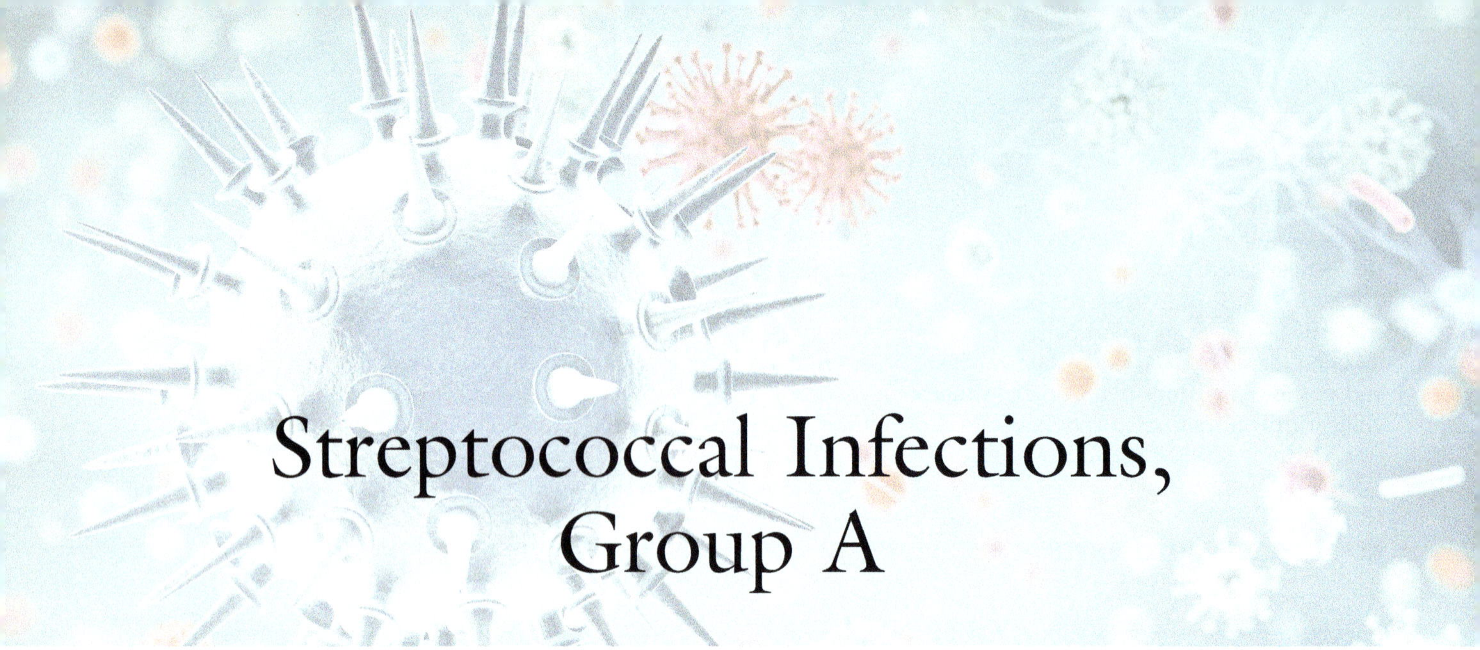

Streptococcal Infections, Group A

Introduction

Group A *Streptococcus* bacteria (also called group A streptococci or GAS) can cause many diseases. *Streptococcus pyogenes* (pie-AHJ-uh-neez) is the group A *Streptococcus* species that causes most disease in humans and is often treated as synonymous with GAS, though there are also non–*S. pyogenes* group A streptococci.

Among the diseases caused by GAS are scarlet fever, strep throat, toxic shock syndrome, and impetigo. GAS diseases were often life threatening before the discovery and mass production of antibiotics. In the 21st century, GAS diseases unduly burden low-resource settings. Untreated GAS infections threaten health by triggering autoimmune diseases, including glomerulonephritis and rheumatic fever. The latter is life threatening, killing about 1 percent of people with the disease worldwide, according to a 2013 article published in *Global Heart.*

Some invasive GAS infections that attack the lungs, blood, or deep muscle and fat tissue are life threatening. The World Health Organization (WHO) estimated in 2005 (the last year data was available) that there were 663,000 cases of invasive GAS infections that resulted in 163,000 deaths. Invasive GAS illnesses have much higher mortality rates than noninvasive GAS infections. Necrotizing fasciitis (also called flesh-eating disease) and streptococcal toxic shock syndrome (STSS) are two of the least common but most severe and aggressive forms of invasive GAS. Approximately 20 percent of patients with necrotizing fasciitis die, while STSS has a mortality rate of over 50 percent.

In the developed world, most routine GAS infections are treated with antibiotics, but resistance to earlier-developed antibiotics is an increasing problem. In the developing world, untreated GAS and its resultant autoimmune diseases are still a widespread problem.

WORDS TO KNOW

GLOMERULONEPHRITIS Inflammation of the kidneys. Mostly glomerulonephritis affects the glomeruli, the small capsules in the kidney where blood flowing through capillaries transfers body wastes to urine.

IMPETIGO A very localized bacterial infection of the skin. It tends to afflict primarily children but can occur in people of any age. Impetigo caused by the bacteria *Staphylococcus aureus* (or staph) affects children of all ages, while impetigo caused by the bacteria called group A streptococci (*Streptococcus pyogenes* or strep) are most common in children ages two to five years.

PUERPERAL FEVER A bacterial infection present in the blood (septicemia) that follows childbirth. The Latin word *puer*, meaning "boy" or "child," is the root of this term. Puerperal fever was much more common before the advent of modern aseptic practices, but infections still occur. Louis Pasteur showed that puerperal fever is most often caused by *Streptococcus* bacteria, which is now treated with antibiotics.

Disease History, Characteristics, and Transmission

Streptococci bacteria were first described by German-Austrian physician Christian Theodor Billroth (1829–1894), who found *Streptococcus pyogenes* growing in infected wounds (the word *pyogenes* is from the Greek for "pus-forming"). *S. pyogenes* was actually named by German physician Michael Joseph Rossbach (1842–1894) in 1884 but was not termed a group A *Streptococcus* until the 1930s, when American scientist Rebecca Lancefield (1895–1981) classed the *Streptococci* into the alphabetically labeled groups that are still called Lancefield groups. Lancefield also established that a protein embedded in the cell wall of group A *Streptococci*, M protein, is crucial to their power to cause disease. There are over 120 varieties of *S. pyogenes*, distinguished by their varying M proteins.

The *Streptococci* are Gram-positive bacteria that tend to grow in chains or pairs. They are classed into two basic groups based on their ability to break down blood cells under laboratory conditions, a process called hemolysis (*hemo* meaning "blood," and *lysis* meaning "breakup"). The beta-hemolytic *Streptococci* break up blood cells completely, creating clear areas around bacteria colonies growing on blood agar in petri dishes. (Petri dishes are small, round, shallow dishes used commonly in laboratories to grow microorganisms. Agar is a form of jelly derived from seaweed or algae, chemically a sugar. Blood agar is agar mixed with blood cells, usually from horses or sheep.)

Further division of the beta-hemolytic *Streptococci* into the Lancefield groups A to T is based on the chemical makeup of the cell wall. The group A *Streptococci*, of which *S. pyogenes* is the most important, are globular and about 0.6 to 1 millimeter in diameter. These bacteria primarily invade human epithelial cells, which constitute the skin and line the respiratory and digestive tracts.

Strep throat is an infection of the throat with *S. pyogenes*. About 18 or 20 days after the end of a strep throat infection, acute rheumatic fever may occur. The primary symptom of rheumatic fever is pain in the joints. Inflammation of the heart may also occur, causing permanent damage to one or more heart valves. Post-streptococcal glomerulonephritis—inflammation of the kidney—may also develop about 10 days after a GAS infection.

Transmission of *S. pyogenes* is via direct contact with mucus, saliva, and open sores or through airborne saliva droplets released by sneezing or coughing.

Severe, invasive GAS infections are rare among otherwise healthy individuals. Invasive GAS infections are most likely to occur in people with diabetes or weakened immune systems or in patients with recent trauma or surgical wounds.

Scope and Distribution

The only known reservoir for *S. pyogenes* is human beings. A minority of the human population carries *S. pyogenes* bacteria, usually in their upper respiratory tract, without any sign of infection. According to the authors of a 2014 study published in the journal of the Pediatric Infectious Diseases Society, "Overall, asymptomatic carriage of GAS is common, especially among school-aged children. The rate of carriage depends highly on the methods of the study, particularly how carriers are defined."

This bacterium is one of the most common causes of bacterial infection in human beings, and in many developed nations it is the most common cause of bacterial infection of the upper respiratory tract for all age groups.

In the 18th and 19th centuries, scarlet fever was a major killer, and, until antibiotics were available to treat GAS infections, rheumatic fever (usually following strep throat) was a widespread childhood disease. In addition, puerperal fever was common in maternity wards, where sanitation was poor (the role of bacteria in causing infec-

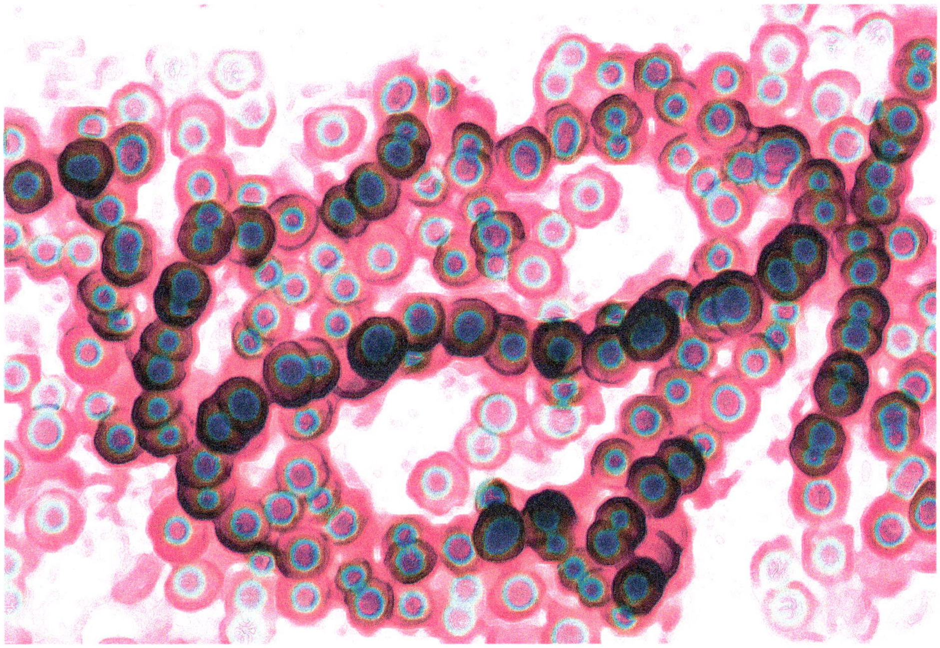

The bacterium *Streptococcus pyogenes* under a microscope. *S. pyogenes* is the strain of group A *Streptococcus* bacteria most likely to cause diseases in humans, including scarlet fever, strep throat, toxic shock syndrome, and impetigo. © BSIP/UIG/Getty Images

TRENDS AND STATISTICS

Streptococcal pharyngitis (strep throat) is one of the most common childhood illnesses worldwide. It is far less common in adults.

In 2016 the US Centers for Disease Control and Prevention (CDC) stated that:

- Four to six of every 20 children with a sore throat have strep throat.
- Only one to three of every 20 adults with a sore throat have strep throat.

tion was not yet known) and *S. pyogenes* was transmitted by doctors' unwashed hands. During childbirth *S. pyogenes* would often infect the mother's bloodstream through tears in the vaginal wall or the skin of the genital area. This commonly resulted in death rates in maternity wards of about 10 to 25 percent, with occasional epidemics leading to much higher death rates. In the early 21st century, puerperal fever is rare in industrialized countries because of standardized medical hygiene and prevalent antibiotics.

Treatment and Prevention

There was no GAS vaccine as of 2017. There have been ongoing efforts to develop one.

Each group A streptococcal infection has its own treatment regimen. They all require antibiotics. Strep throat, for example, is usually treated with penicillin and amoxicillin. Invasive GAS infections are usually treated with a combination of penicillin and clindamycin because penicillin alone may not be as effective.

Prevention of GAS infections consists primarily of handwashing, sterilization in health care environments, and avoiding contact with infected persons. Antibiotics can also play a role in prevention. The CDC states, "Treating an infected person with an antibiotic for 24 hours or longer generally eliminates their ability to transmit the bacteria. Thus, people with group A strep pharyngitis should stay home from work, school, or daycare until afebrile and until at least 24 hours after starting appropriate antibiotic therapy."

Impacts and Issues

WHO estimates that puerperal sepsis, infection of women giving birth, by GAS accounts for about 11 percent of maternal deaths globally, according to a study published in 2014 in *Lancet Global Health*. Most of these deaths occur in developing countries where sterile conditions and antibiotics are more rare. Indeed, the burden of GAS is carried largely by developing nations, not developed ones.

Failure of penicillin to eradicate GAS from the throat has been reported. In these cases antibiotics other than penicillin should be added to standard treatment regimens for strep throat and other GAS infections. Treating resistant infections requires more powerful and recently developed antibiotics. However, many physicians worry that prescribing newer, more powerful antibiotics as a first course of treatment may encourage further antibiotic resistance in GAS infections.

See Also *Impetigo; Necrotizing Fasciitis; Puerperal Fever; Scarlet Fever; Streptococcal Infections, Group B*

BIBLIOGRAPHY

Books

Sanyahumbi, Amy Sims, et al. "Global Disease Burden of Group A *Streptococcus*." In Streptococcus Pyogenes: *Basic Biology to Clinical Manifestations*, edited by Joseph J. Ferretti, Dennis L. Stevens, and Vincent A. Fischetti. Oklahoma City: University of Oklahoma Health Sciences Center, 2016.

Smith, Tara C., and Hilary Babcock. Streptococcus *(Group A)*. 2nd ed. New York: Chelsea House, 2010.

Periodicals

DeMuri, Gregory P., and Ellen R. Wald. "The Group A Streptococcal Carrier State Reviewed: Still an Enigma." *Journal of the Pediatric Infectious Diseases Society* 3, no. 4 (December 1, 2014): 336–342. This article can also be found online at https://academic.oup.com/jpids/article/3/4/336/909914 (accessed January 31, 2018).

Khamnuan, Patcharin, et al. "Necrotizing Fasciitis: Risk Factors of Mortality." *Risk Management Healthcare Policy* 8 (2015): 1–7. This article can also be found online at https://www.ncbi.nlm.nih.gov/pmc/articles/PMC4337692/ (accessed January 31, 2018).

Rac, Hana, et al. "Successful Treatment of Necrotizing Fasciitis and Streptococcal Toxic Shock Syndrome with the Addition of Linezolid." *Case Reports in Infectious Diseases* (2017). This article can also be found online at https://www.hindawi.com/journals/criid/2017/5720708/ (accessed January 31, 2018).

Say, Lale, et al. "Global Causes of Maternal Death: A WHO Systematic Analysis." *Lancet Global Health* 2, no. 6 (June 2014): e323–e333. This article can also be found online at http://www.thelancet.com/journals/langlo/article/PIIS2214-109X(14)70227-X/fulltext (accessed January 31, 2018).

Walker, Mark J., et al. "Disease Manifestations and Pathogenic Mechanisms of Group A *Streptococcus*." *Clinical Microbiology Reviews* 27, no. 2 (April 1, 2014). This article can also be found online at http://cmr.asm.org/content/27/2/264.full (accessed January 29, 2018).

Zacharioudaki, Maria E., and Emmanouil Galanakis. "Management of Children with Persistent Group A Streptococcal Carriage." *Expert Review of Anti-infective Therapy* 15, no. 8 (2017): 787–795. This article can also be found online at http://www.tandfonline.com/doi/abs/10.1080/14787210.2017.1358612 (accessed January 31, 2018).

Zühlke, Liesl J., and Andrew C. Steer. "Estimates of the Global Burden of Rheumatic Heart Disease." *Global Heart* 8, no. 3 (September 2013): 189–195. This article can also be found online at https://www.sciencedirect.com/science/article/pii/S2211816013001142 (accessed January 30, 2018).

Websites

"The Current Evidence for the Burden of Group A Streptococcal Diseases." Department of Child and Adolescent Health and Development, World Health Organization. http://apps.who.int/iris/bitstream/10665/69063/1/WHO_FCH_CAH_05.07.pdf?ua=1&ua=1 (accessed January 30, 2018).

"Group A Streptococcal (GAS) Disease." Centers for Disease Control and Prevention, September 16, 2016. https://www.cdc.gov/groupastrep/ (accessed January 29, 2018).

"Streptococcal Toxic Shock Syndrome (STSS) (*Streptococcus pyogenes*) 2010 Case Definition." Centers for Disease Control and Prevention, 2010. https://wwwn.cdc.gov/nndss/conditions/streptococcal-toxic-shock-syndrome/case-definition/2010/ (accessed January 31, 2018).

Streptococcal Infections, Group B

Introduction

Group B *Streptococcus* bacteria, primarily the species *Streptococcus agalactiae*, are a major cause of sickness and death among newborns worldwide. The bacteria affect other age groups to lesser extents, with the rate of serious group B strep disease increasing with age. Group B *Streptococcus* illnesses are also known as group B strep (GBS), beta strep, or group B *Streptococci*.

GBS infection increases risks to both the mother and the fetus before birth. In the newborn infection can cause pneumonia (fluid in the lungs) and sepsis (an infection of the bloodstream) within the first week after birth. The late-onset form of the disease occurs from 7 to 90 days after birth, usually causing meningitis, which is inflammation of the meninges (the tough membranes that surround the brain and spinal cord). Pneumonia, sepsis, and meningitis can all be fatal.

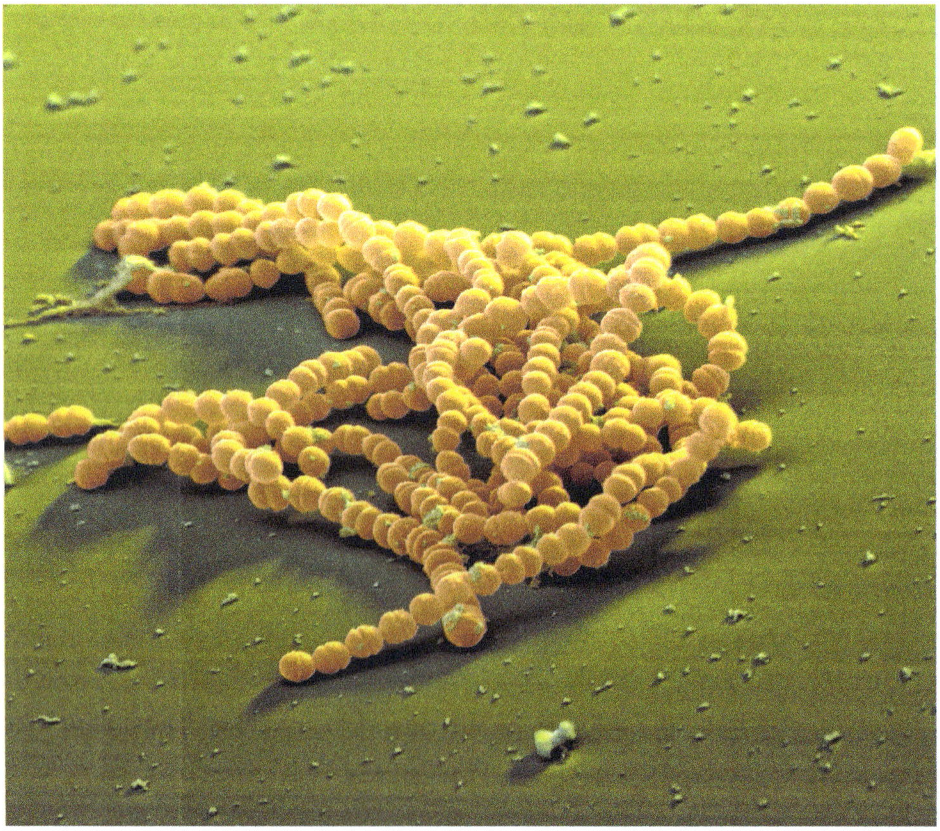

Streptococcus agalactiae bacteria, the species of group B *Streptococcus* (GBS) most likely to cause illnesses among humans, viewed under a scanning electron micrograph. GBS infections are particularly dangerous to pregnant women and newborns. © *Eye of Science/Science Source*

GBS infection can be treated with antibiotics. No vaccine is available, although late-stage trials were under way as of early 2018.

Disease History, Characteristics, and Transmission

Streptococci, which are Gram-positive bacteria that tend to grow in chains or pairs, were first described in 1874 by Christian Theodor Billroth (1829–1894). Around 1903 Hugo Schottmuller (1867–1936) distinguished between alpha-hemolytic and beta-hemolytic *Streptococci*. Beta-hemolytic *Streptococci*, which include almost all group A and many group B *Streptococci*, are distinguished by their ability to completely break up blood cells when grown in the laboratory, a process called hemolysis (*hemo* means "blood," and *lysis* means "breakup"). Hemolysis creates clear areas around colonies of beta-hemolytic bacteria growing in petri dishes on blood agar, a jellylike substance derived from seaweed or algae and usually mixed with sheep's blood.

GBS in pregnant mothers is associated with preterm birth and stillbirth, especially in developing countries and in low-resource settings. GBS is most often noted for causing sepsis, pneumonia, and meningitis in newborns, with a high fatality rate.

GBS is also known to cause infections in adults with preexisting conditions such as cancer, obesity, and diabetes. In adults GBS can manifest as a soft-tissue infection, pneumonia, meningitis, bloodstream infections, or infections of the bones or joints. People age 65 and older are at greatest risk from these invasive GBS infections.

GBS is usually transmitted by direct contact. Newborns may contract the bacteria during labor and delivery by mothers who are vaginally or anally colonized with the bacteria. Alternatively, fetuses may contract the bacteria from their mothers during development, before birth. This can lead to miscarriage or premature birth and increases the risk of cerebral palsy.

WORDS TO KNOW

BACTEREMIA This condition occurs when bacteria enter the bloodstream through, for example, a wound or an infection or through a surgical procedure or injection. Bacteremia may cause no symptoms and resolve without treatment, or it may produce fever and other symptoms of infection. In some cases, bacteremia leads to septic shock, a potentially life-threatening condition.

COLONIZATION The process of occupation and increase in number of microorganisms at a specific site.

HEMOLYSIS The destruction of blood cells, an abnormal rate of which may lead to lowered levels of these cells. For example, hemolytic anemia is caused by destruction of red blood cells at a rate faster than they can be produced.

MENINGITIS An inflammation of the meninges, the three layers of protective membranes that line the spinal cord and the brain. Meningitis can occur when there is an infection near the brain or spinal cord, such as a respiratory infection in the sinuses, the mastoids, or the cavities around the ear. Disease organisms can also travel to the meninges through the bloodstream. The first signs may be a severe headache and neck stiffness followed by fever, vomiting, a rash, and then convulsions leading to loss of consciousness. Meningitis generally involves two types: nonbacterial meningitis, or aseptic meningitis, and bacterial meningitis, or purulent meningitis.

SEPSIS A bacterial infection in the bloodstream or body tissues. Sepsis is a very broad term covering the presence of many types of microscopic disease-causing organisms. It is also called bacteremia. Closely related terms include septicemia and septic syndrome.

Scope and Distribution

Like group A *Streptococci*, GBS is common in human populations. About one in four women have GBS in their vagina or rectum, according to the US Centers for Disease Control and Prevention (CDC). It is particularly significant as a cause of infection in newborns, causing death in 4 to 6 percent of babies with GBS.

Treatment and Prevention

Although GBS can be treated with antibiotics, infection can spread quickly, and symptoms can be difficult to diagnose in newborns. Intravenous administration of antibiotics, usually penicillin, to the mother during delivery can prevent infection in newborns. However, mothers in low-resource settings may not be tested for GBS and may not have access to antibiotics during labor.

As of 2017 there was no vaccine, but late-stage research was under way. That year the pharmaceutical company Pfizer began clinical human trials of a vaccine given to pregnant mothers to immunize their children against GBS.

Impacts and Issues

In the United States in the 1970s, there were 7,500 GBS infections in newborns per year. The death rate for

GBS infection was as high as 50 percent. In the 1980s it was found that giving antibiotics to women who tested positive for GBS and were therefore at risk of transmitting the bacteria to their babies greatly reduced the rate of early-onset (first week of life) disease. As a result, the CDC issued guidelines in 1996 recommending vaginal and rectal screening between the 35th and 37th weeks of pregnancy to identify women with GBS. Women who test positive are offered antibiotics during labor.

According to a 2016 study published in *Infectious Diseases*, rates of GBS bloodstream infections (BSI) such as bacteremia and sepsis in people age 60 or older in Australia, Canada, Denmark, Sweden, Finland, and the United Kingdom doubled between 2000 and 2010. Authors of the study noted that, "while marked variability in the incidence of GBS BSI was observed among these regions, it was consistently found that rates increased among older adults, especially in association with diabetes. The burden of this infection may be expected to continue to increase in ageing populations worldwide."

PRIMARY SOURCE

Inflammation Affects Fetal Cardiac Gene Expression and May Be Linked to Adult Heart Disease

SOURCE: *"Inflammation Affects Fetal Cardiac Gene Expression and May Be Linked to Adult Heart Disease."* Genetic Engineering and Biotechnology News, *January 23, 2018. https://www.genengnews.com/gen-news-highlights/inflammation-affects-fetal-cardiac-gene-expression-and-may-be-linked-to-adult-heart-disease/81255410 (accessed January 25, 2018).*

INTRODUCTION: *The following article describes a 2018 study that shows that babies who are exposed to GBS in the uterus and are born prematurely may be at a greater risk for developing heart disease as an adult.*

It has often been suggested that things we are exposed to in early childhood go on to affect us as adults, often at a subconscious level. Yet now, a new study led by researchers at the University of Washington School of Medicine in Seattle shows that, in preterm animal models, inflammation due to infection can disrupt the activity of genes that are crucial for normal development of the heart. Moreover, the altered gene activity may be linked to adult-onset cardiac disease.

"This study connects the dots between preterm birth and heart disease in adult life by defining the gene networks disrupted by infection and inflammation that program normal heart development," explained lead study investigator Kristina Adams Waldorf, M.D., a professor of obstetrics and gynecology at the University of Washington School of Medicine who specializes in maternal and fetal infections. "When I was in training, we talked to women in preterm labor about the risk to their infants of lung and brain injury. We now know that long-term health risks of a preterm birth extend beyond the developing lungs and brain to involve vision, hearing, kidney, and even heart function."

Findings from the new study were published online recently in the *American Journal of Obstetrics & Gynecology.*

In the current study, the investigators looked at the heart tissue from fetal pigtail macaque monkeys whose mothers' uteruses had been infected with bacteria, namely group B *Streptococcus* and *Escherichia coli.* These often cause infections in human mothers and trigger preterm birth. The investigators compared gene expression patterns from fetal heart tissues infected with bacteria to normal heart tissues. The animals were chosen because macaques are considered one of the closest animal models to human pregnancy. They also are ideal for the development of vaccines and treatments to protect pregnant women from bacterial infections.

"This study is the first to show that the gene program for heart development in preterm babies is interrupted in preterm babies exposed to fetal infection and inflammation, which may lead to incomplete heart development," noted study co-author Timothy Mitchell, M.D., an obstetrician specializing in high-risk pregnancies and a former UW Medicine fellow in maternal and fetal medicine. "This incomplete development, in turn, may lead to the higher risk of abnormal heart rhythms and heart failure seen when preterm babies reach adulthood."

The infections in the current study were severe, a scenario that is typical of early preterm births, which occur in approximately 2% of all U.S. births. Infection triggered a marked inflammatory response in the fetus. Inflammation was also present in the heart tissues and characterized by elevations in inflammatory proteins, like interleukin-6 and interleukin-8.

Many of the genes with altered expression—*NPPA*, *MYH6*, and *ACE2*—have known functions in heart development or are linked to heart disease. For example, the gene *NPPA*, which encodes natriuretic peptide A, is essential for the formation and expansion of the walls of the heart.

Interestingly, the researchers also found significant alteration in the expression of gene networks involved in heart and blood vessel formation, including the movement and migration of cells, growth of smooth and cardiac muscle, and the migration of endothelial cells that line the inside of the heart and blood vessels.

"These findings suggest that many pathways related to fetal heart development may be impacted by inflammation and infection," remarked Dr. Mitchell.

"We are only beginning to understand the health risks that infection and inflammation pose to the developing fetus, particularly in the setting of an early preterm birth," added study co-author Lakshmi Rajagopal, Ph.D., an associate professor of pediatrics at the University of Washington School of Medicine and expert on newborn infectious diseases at Seattle Children's Research Institute and UW Medicine. "We need a better understanding of how bacteria invade the uterus to cause preterm birth so that we can develop therapies to prevent fetal infections. Ultimately, we must also develop an effective vaccine for group B *Streptococcus* to protect pregnant women and their fetuses."

"Future research should investigate whether combining antibiotics to treat the infection and anti-inflammatory drugs can lessen inflammation and damage to the fetal heart," concluded Dr. Adams Waldorf. "If we can better understand how to prevent infections that cause preterm birth, we can protect fetuses and enhance their long-term health into adulthood."

SEE ALSO *Streptococcal Infections, Group A*

BIBLIOGRAPHY

Books

Bennett, John E., Raphael Dolin, and Martin J. Blaser. *Mandell, Douglas, and Bennett's Principles and Practice of Infectious Diseases.* 8th ed. Philadelphia: Elsevier/Saunders, 2015.

Periodicals

Ballard, Mark S, et al. "The Changing Epidemiology of Group B *Streptococcus* Bloodstream Infection: A Multi-National Population-Based Assessment." *Infectious Diseases* 48, no. 5 (2016): 386–391. This article can also be found online at http://www.tandfonline.com/doi/abs/10.3109/23744235.2015.1131330 (accessed January 23, 2018).

Bianchi-Jassir, Fiorella, et al. "Preterm Birth Associated with Group B *Streptococcus* Maternal Colonization Worldwide: Systematic Review and Meta-Analyses." *Clinical Infectious Diseases* 65, no. 2 (November 6, 2017): S133–S142. This article can also be found online at https://academic.oup.com/cid/article/65/suppl_2/S133/4589591 (accessed January 23, 2018).

Seale, Anna C, et al. "Stillbirth with Group B *Streptococcus* Disease Worldwide: Systematic Review and Meta-Analyses." *Clinical Infectious Diseases* 65, no. 2 (November 6, 2017): S125–S132. This article can also be found online at https://academic.oup.com/cid/article/65/suppl_2/S125/4589583 (accessed January 23, 2018).

Websites

"Group B Strep (GBS)." Centers for Disease Control and Prevention (CDC), May 23, 2016. https://www.cdc.gov/groupbstrep/about/index.html (accessed January 23, 2018).

"Group B Strep Infection: GBS." American Pregnancy Association, March 2, 2017. http://americanpregnancy.org/pregnancy-complications/group-b-strep-infection/ (accessed January 23, 2018).

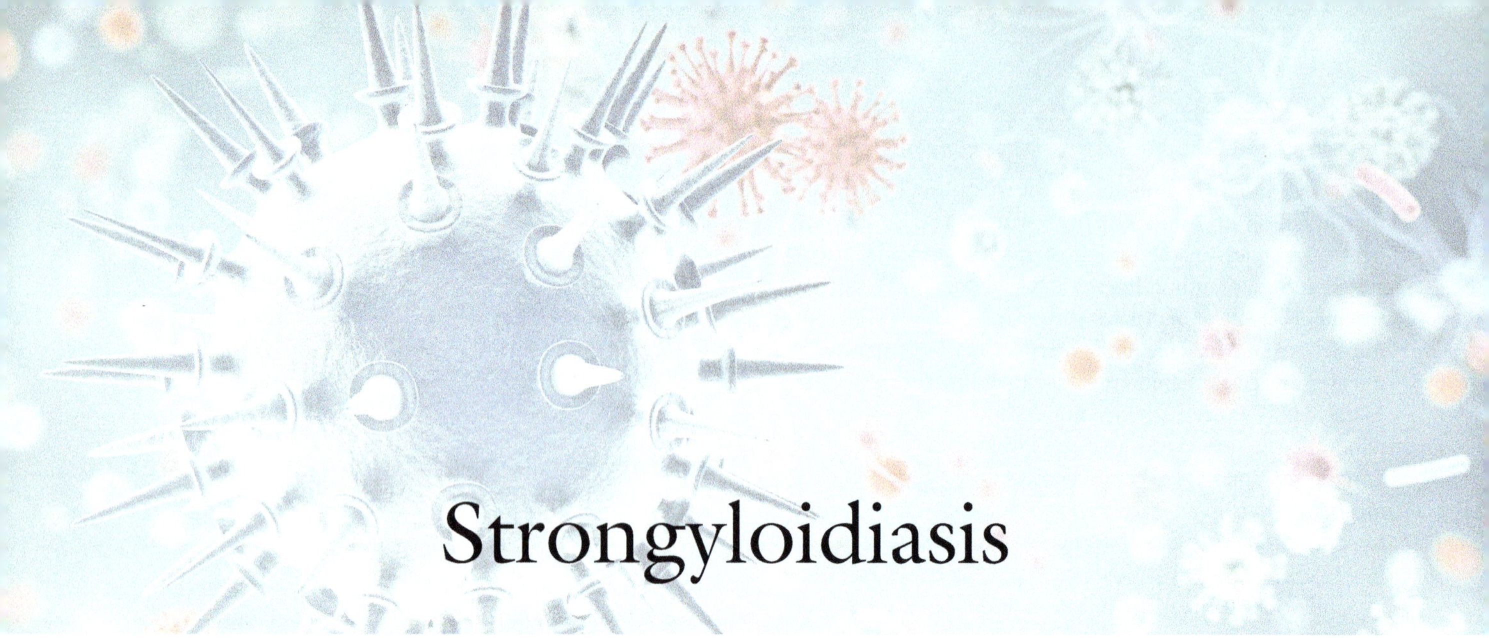

Strongyloidiasis

Introduction

Strongyloidiasis is an infection with a parasitic nematode (roundworm) known as *Strongyloides stercoralis.* It occurs in tropical and subtropical areas, as well as in the southern part of the United States. *S. stercoralis* has a complex life cycle involving infection through the skin by the larvae, which travel to the intestine, where they reproduce, causing chronic infection in the original host. They can also pass onto new hosts and cause further infections.

In people with compromised immunity, such as organ transplant recipients, strongyloidiasis can cause a hyperinfection involving the intestines and the rest of the body. The condition can also be difficult to diagnose because the symptoms are varied and nonspecific. However, the parasitic worms can be eliminated by drug treatment. All patients at risk of hyperinfection should be treated, and those about to undergo an organ transplant ought to be screened for the infection.

WORDS TO KNOW

AUTOINFECTION Reinfection of the body by a disease organism already in the body, such as eggs left by a parasitic worm.

HOST An organism that serves as the habitat for a parasite or possibly for a symbiont. A host may provide nutrition to the parasite or symbiont, or it may simply provide a place in which to live.

HYPERINFECTION An infection that is caused by a very high number of disease-causing microorganisms. The infection results from an abnormality in the immune system that allows the infecting cells to grow and divide more easily than would normally be possible.

IMMUNOCOMPROMISED A reduction of the ability of the immune system to recognize and respond to the presence of foreign material.

ROUNDWORM Also known as nematodes; a type of helminth characterized by long, cylindrical bodies. Roundworm infections are diseases of the digestive tract and other organ systems that are caused by roundworms. Roundworm infections are widespread throughout the world, and humans acquire most types of roundworm infection from contaminated food or by touching the mouth with unwashed hands that have come in contact with the parasite larva. The severity of infection varies considerably from person to person. Children are more likely to have heavy infestations and are also more likely to suffer from malabsorption and malnutrition than adults.

Disease History, Characteristics, and Transmission

S. stercoralis has a more complicated life cycle than other parasitic worms, which means it can set up a high burden of persistent infection in a human host, especially one who has weakened immunity. Where the burden of parasites is low, the individual may have no, or merely intermittent, symptoms.

S. stercoralis larvae are very small. The largest are only the size of a grain of sand or mustard seed. Transmission of strongyloidiasis starts when larvae in contaminated soil penetrate the skin of the human host and are transported through blood to the lungs. Here, they first penetrate the alveoli (tiny air sacs through which gases are exchanged between the lung surface and the blood). From there, the larvae travel up to the throat area and are swallowed, reaching the small intestine.

In the small intestine, the larvae become female adult worms. These lay eggs via parthenogenesis (without involvement of a male worm). The resulting larvae may pass through the stool, returning to the environment to repeat the cycle and infect other hosts. They can also cause autoinfection, in which the larvae continue to develop and penetrate the mucosal surface of the intestine or the skin of the anal area. They then repeat the previous infection cycle —skin, lungs, and intestine—thereby massively increasing the parasitic burden on the host.

Patients with a significant burden of parasites can develop symptoms in multiple areas of the body. Skin symptoms include dermatitis and irritation, while the lung stage may involve dry cough, wheezing, fever, shortness of breath, and even coughing up blood. Parasites in the intestine will cause bloating, swelling, flatulence, indigestion, and diarrhea.

Hyperinfection, or disseminated strongyloidiasis, may cause blood poisoning, peritonitis (inflammation of the lining of the abdominal cavity), neurological complications, and liver problems.

Strongyloidiasis can be life threatening for patients with chronic illnesses or compromised immune systems. Those at greatest risk include patients with leukemia or lymphoma, patients taking steroids for immunosuppression, and patients infected with human T-cell leukemia virus type 1 (HTLV-1). Recipients of organ transplants are also at high risk of life-threatening complications if infected. For this reason, people being assessed for an organ transplant ought to be screened for infection and treated before surgery.

Scope and Distribution

S. stercoralis infection is found in humid tropical and subtropical areas where the larvae can survive in the soil. Cases have also been found in temperate areas, including the southeastern part of the United States. The infection is more frequently found in rural areas, institutional settings, and among immigrants from the developing world. In the United States, cases have occurred in military personnel returning from service in tropical areas, immigrants from countries where the parasite is endemic, and occasionally in Appalachia.

Those with reduced immunity, including patients with leukemia, organ transplant recipients, or those receiving steroids, seem to be at higher risk of strongyloidiasis. However, human immunodeficiency virus (HIV)/acquired immunodeficiency syndrome (AIDS) does not seem to be a risk factor, despite the patient's immunocompromised status. In the Caribbean and Japan, an association between strongyloidiasis and human T-cell leukemia has been found.

Treatment and Prevention

The symptoms of strongyloidiasis are easily confused with other medical conditions, such as irritable bowel syndrome. Diagnosis depends on identifying the *S. stercoralis* larvae within either a stool or a duodenal fluid sample (taken from the small intestine). The condition is less commonly diagnosed through a blood test.

S. stercoralis infection can be treated successfully by ivermectin. In areas of the world where *S. stercoralis* is endemic, prevention efforts rely on proper disposal of sewage. Wearing shoes when walking on contaminated soil can also help prevent infection, although this preventive measure is not available to many residents of areas where the parasite is endemic.

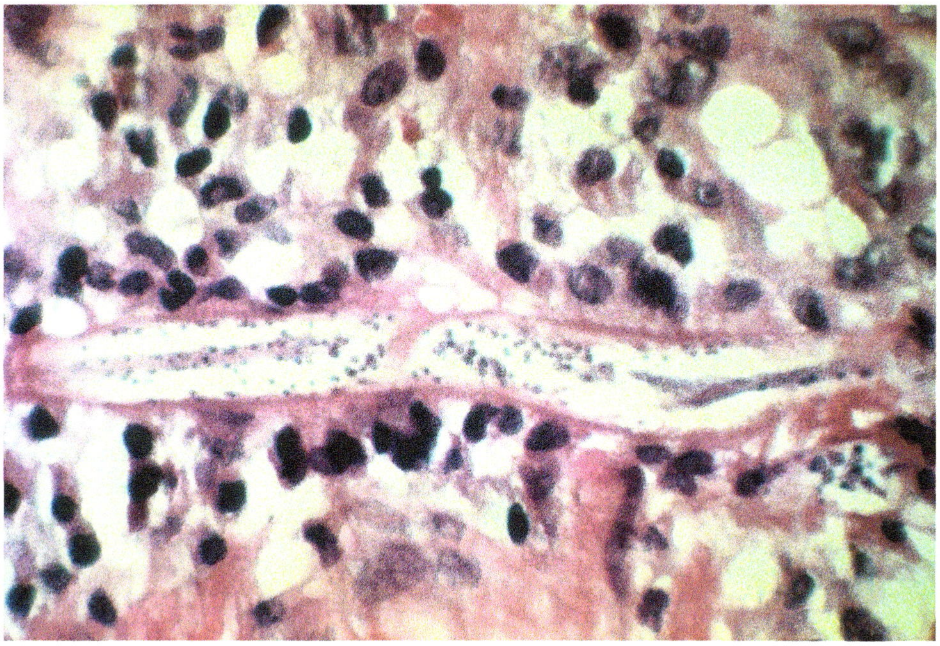

A micrograph showing *Strongyloidiasis stercoralis*, the parasite that causes strongyloidiasis. © Smith Collection/Gado/Getty Images

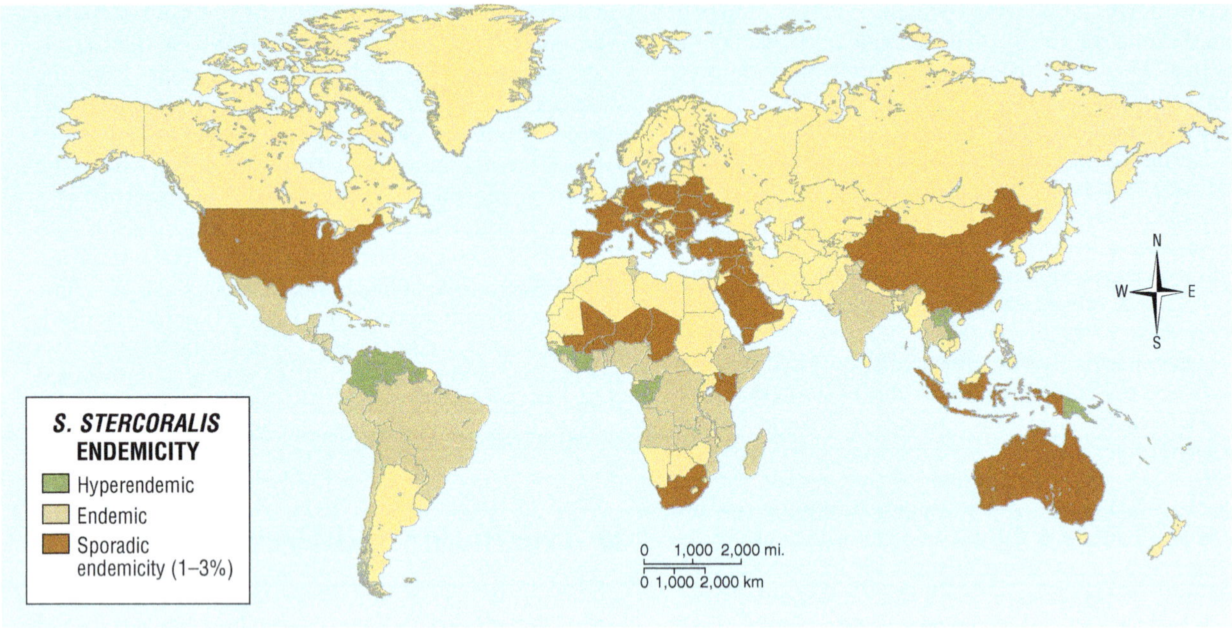

Rare cases of person-to-person transmission of strongyloidiasis have occurred in institutional settings such as long-term care facilities and childcare centers. In these settings, attention to sanitation, including proper hygiene and disposal of fecal matter, can prevent the spread of infection.

Impacts and Issues

Although infection with *S. stercoralis* may not cause symptoms, the nature of the parasite's life cycle means that some patients may be at risk of life-threatening complications. The path the larvae take through the body mean that there are many and varied symptoms, which can cause confusion with other conditions. Careful diagnosis of the condition is essential so the parasite can be eradicated before the infection spreads throughout the body in those whose immunity is compromised.

Global efforts to eliminate strongyloidiasis have focused on mass administration of ivermectin in areas where *S. stercoralis* is endemic. According to the journal *PLOS Neglected Tropical Diseases* in 2015, a mass administration program initiated in an area of Ecuador in the early 1990s resulted in a reduction of the prevalence of *S. stercoralis* in tested children. Serological (blood) testing showed a decrease from 6.8 percent of tested children in 1990 to 1.3 percent in 2013.

See Also *Parasitic Diseases; Tropical Infectious Diseases*

BIBLIOGRAPHY

Books

Crompton, D. W. T., and Lorenzo Savioli. *Handbook of Helminthiasis for Public Health.* New York: CRC, 2006.

Rollinson, D., and J. R. Stothard, eds. *Advances in Parasitology.* New York: Elsevier, 2015.

Periodicals

Anselmi, Mariella, et al. "Mass Administration of Ivermectin for the Elimination of Onchocerciasis Significantly Reduced and Maintained Low the Prevalence of *Strongyloides Stercoralis* in Esmeraldas, Ecuador." *PLOS Neglected Tropical Diseases* 9, no. 11 (November 5, 2015). This article can also be found online at https://doi.org/10.1371/journal.pntd.0004150 (accessed January 29, 2018).

Websites

"Strongyloidiasis." World Health Organization. http://www.who.int/intestinal_worms/epidemiology/strongyloidiasis/en/ (accessed January 12, 2018).

"Strongyloidiasis Infection FAQs." Centers for Disease Control and Prevention, July 10, 2014. https://www.cdc.gov/parasites/strongyloides/gen_info/faqs.html (accessed January 12, 2018).

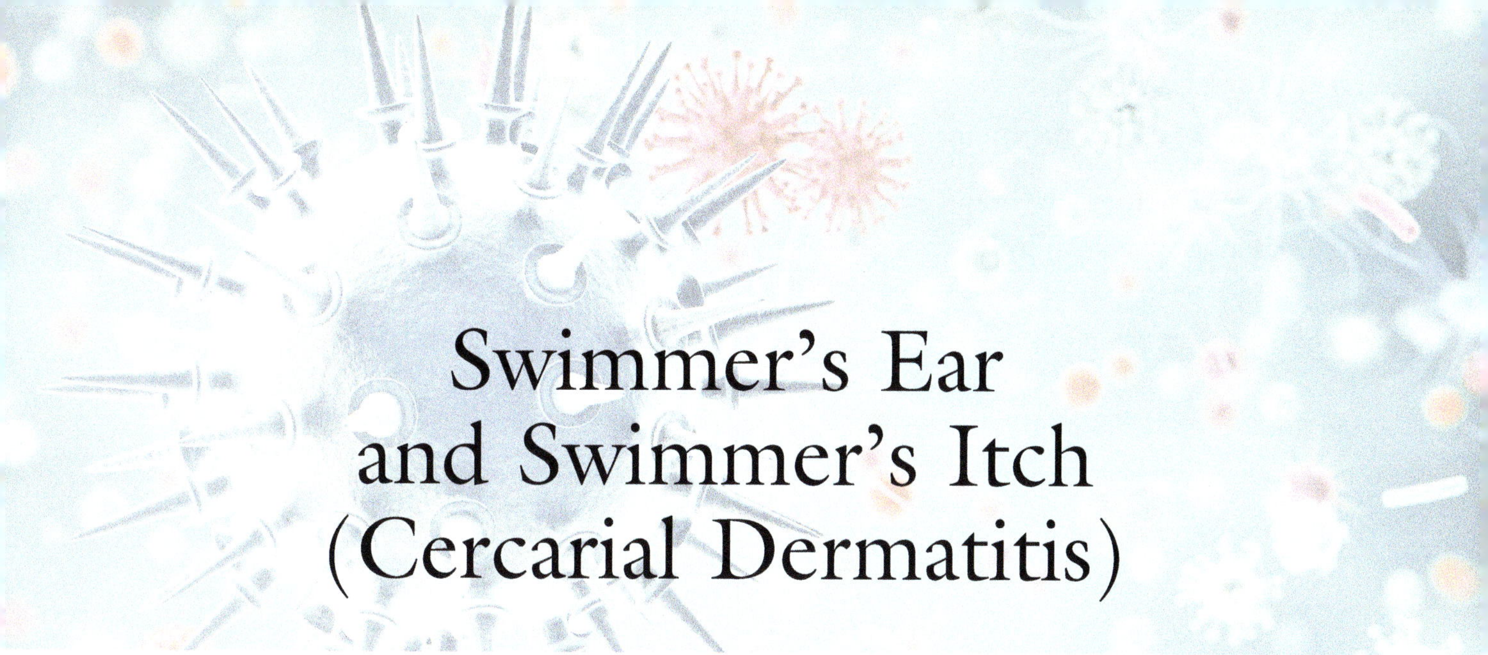

Swimmer's Ear and Swimmer's Itch (Cercarial Dermatitis)

Introduction

Swimmer's ear (otitis externa) is an infection of the ear canal. Swimmer's itch (cercarial dermatitis) is an allergic reaction to various types of microscopic waterborne parasites infecting human skin.

Many types of fungi or bacteria can infect the ear canal (the hollow, cylindrical opening that allows sounds to enter the eardrum). Swimmer's ear, sometimes also called duck itch or clam digger's itch in the United States and various other names around the world, is a distinctly different infection caused by parasitic schistosomes (small flukes that live in blood) that infect snails and vertebrates. Most schistosomes infect waterfowl. The parasites are discharged from infected snails and vertebrates into fresh water (often slow-moving ponds and lakes). The parasites then burrow into the skin of swimming humans, causing an allergic reaction, including itch and rash.

These schistosomes cannot become long-term parasites in humans. They only cause mild itchy spots, which later can become raised bumps that are much itchier. The parasites die within a few hours, and the symptoms disappear.

Disease History, Characteristics, and Transmission

Swimmer's ear occurs frequently in children because they usually spend more time swimming than adults. It can also occur in environments with high humidity or anytime a break in the skin occurs within the ear canal. Thus, any extended exposure to moisture in the ear often irritates the ear canal, which allows fungi or bacteria to enter. People often get swimmer's ear when they have skin conditions affecting the ear canal, such as eczema or seborrheic dermatitis, a condition that causes red, scaly patches on the skin. Swimmers who frequently or aggressively scratch or clean the ear canal, or insert objects such as cotton swabs into the ear canal, are also at greater risk for contracting swimmer's ear.

Trichobilharzia and *Gigantobilharzia* are two genera of schistosome that commonly cause swimmer's itch. These schistosomes infect waterfowl, such as ducks and geese, and aquatic mammals, such as beavers. The parasites lay eggs that are then transferred in the feces of infected birds or mammals. The eggs, if dropped into water, hatch and release larvae that can infect humans.

Schistosomatium douthitti is a species of schistosome that infects snails. It first infects a nonhuman vertebrate, such as a waterfowl or mammal, and completes its life cycle

WORDS TO KNOW

MALIGNANT A general term for cells that can dislodge from a tumor and invade and destroy other tissues and organs.

PARASITE An organism that lives in or on a host organism and that gets its nourishment from that host. The parasite usually gains all the benefits of this relationship, while the host may suffer from various diseases and discomforts or show no signs of the infection. The life cycle of a typical parasite usually includes several developmental stages and morphological changes as the parasite lives and moves through the environment and one or more hosts. Parasites that remain on a host's body surface to feed are called ectoparasites, whereas those that live inside a host's body are called endoparasites. Parasitism is a highly successful biological adaptation. There are more known parasitic species than nonparasitic ones. Parasites affect almost all forms of life, including most all animals, plants, and even bacteria.

SCHISTOSOMES Blood flukes.

THE EXTERNAL EAR

The external ear consists of the flesh and cartilage structure on either side of the head known as the auricle or pinna, and the hole into the head. The auricle helps focus the incoming sound waves. The hole leads into the auditory canal, a roughly cylinder-shaped, small-diameter canal about 1 inch (2.5 centimeters) long. Toward the inner end the canal widens slightly and ends at the eardrum. The ear canal can be thought of as a tube with a resonating column of air inside it, having open and closed ends, like an organ pipe.

The ear canal enhances sound vibrations that enter from the outside. The canal typically resonates, or vibrates, at frequencies that the ear hears most sharply. The vibration increases the wavelength of the sound waves traveling down the canal. The amplified waves eventually contact the eardrum, which is positioned at the end of the canal and marks the boundary between the outer ear and the middle ear.

The eardrum is a membrane that is capable of vibration. When sound waves reach the eardrum, the vibrational energy is converted to mechanical vibrations in the solid materials of the middle ear. These solid materials are three bones: the malleus, incus, and stapes. The bones form a system of linked levers that are driven by the eardrum. The outer malleus pushes on the incus, which in turn pushes on the stapes. This further amplifies the sound vibrations, typically two- or threefold. Tiny muscles are positioned around the bones to dampen the mechanical vibrations if they become too pronounced. These muscles are a form of safety device, restricting movement of one or more of the bones. They protect against the creation of too great a vibration from a very loud sound.

within these hosts. However, humans can become indirectly infected when coming into contact with infected waters or shorelines.

Symptoms of swimmer's ear include fever, skin inflammation inside the ear canal, temporarily reduced hearing (caused by swollen tissue), and itchiness. More severe symptoms include reddening and swelling of the outer ear, enlarged and tender lymph nodes around the ear, and yellowish drainage. Sharp pain often affects the earlobe or other external parts. In severe cases the skin infection spreads to the face and salivary gland in the cheek. Eating can become painful. According to the Nemours Foundation, swimmer's ear is not contagious.

Swimmer's itch has symptoms that occur from minutes to days after contact. Common symptoms include mildly itchy areas on the skin, which can become more itchy and redder after a few hours. There is also a tingling or burning sensation in the infected areas. Later small blisters can appear. Itching usually stops within a week, and other symptoms gradually disappear. According to the US Centers for Disease Control and Prevention (CDC), swimmer's itch cannot be spread from person to person.

Scope and Distribution

Swimmer's ear is found in all temperate climates of the world where water is available for swimming.

Swimmer's itch occurs throughout the world. The parasites causing the infection are more frequently found around lakes or other such bodies of slow-moving fresh and salt water. Inshore waters, rather than open waters, are more likely to contain schistosomes. They commonly infect humans during the hotter months of the year and often infect humans who wade or swim close to shore or in shallow water.

Treatment and Prevention

Swimmer's ear is diagnosed following an examination of the ear canal and eardrum. In some cases, particularly

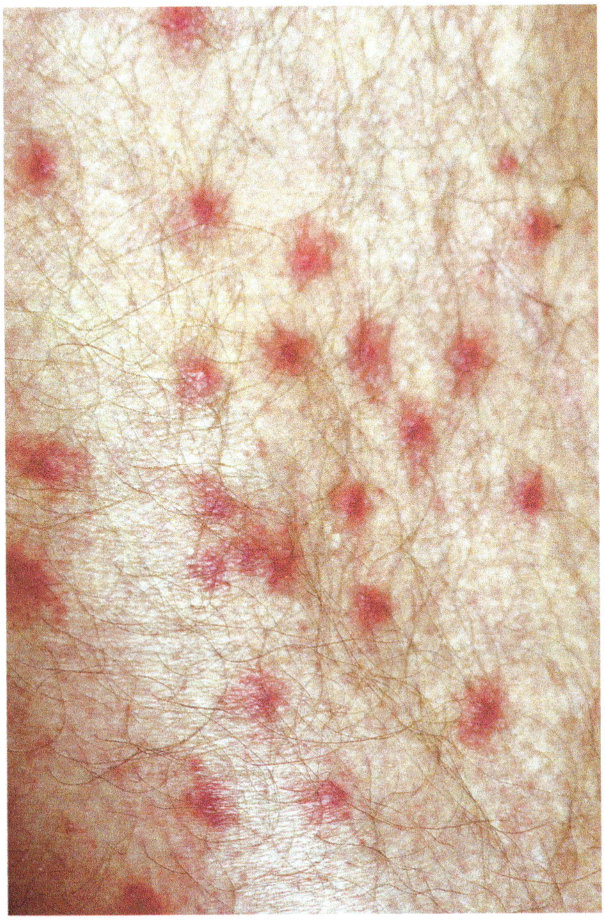

Cercarial dermatitis, commonly known as swimmer's itch, exhibited on a patient's leg. The rash is the result of an allergic reaction to infection by the parasitic flatworm *Schistosomatidae*. © Scimat/ Science Source

when the infection does not respond to treatment, a sample of discharge from the ear may be tested to identify the microorganism involved. Doctors will generally clean the ear to remove flaking skin, ear wax, and debris at the time of the diagnosis. Treatment of swimmer's ear includes antibiotic ear drops. Such drops are usually used several times a day for 10 to 14 days. Care should be taken because improper use can irritate or damage membranes located past the ear canal. In severe cases doctors may prescribe oral antibiotics to treat the infection. Ear drops containing quinolone antibiotics are useful for stopping fluid discharge and combating bacterial infection. A corticosteroid is used to prevent inflammation, itching, and swelling. Treatment usually will cure the problem within 7 to 10 days.

Swimmer's ear can be prevented by drying ears with a towel. Battery-powered ear dryers may also be used. Another method of removing water from the ears is to tilt the head to the side so that excess water runs out. Doctors may recommend earplugs while swimming. However, the earplugs should be professionally fitted because they can irritate the ear canal if used improperly. Until the infection clears up, doctors recommend against swimming. During treatment it is also important to avoid getting water in the ear while bathing.

Swimmer's itch can usually be treated at home. The American Osteopathic College of Dermatology (AOCD) recommends treating the condition with an antihistamine cream or a mild corticosteroid cream. Both may be purchased as over-the-counter medicines. During treatment it is important to avoid scratching affected areas to avoid infection. If symptoms continue longer than three days, the AOCD recommends a visit to a dermatologist.

Prevention of swimmer's itch usually involves the long-term removal of the schistosome hosts. For instance, various control agents such as copper sulfate have been used to eliminate snail populations around lakes. The application of the insect repellant DEET (N,N-diethyl-meta-toluamide) to the body can help to repel schistosomes. Swimmers should avoid swimming in water tied to cases of swimmer's itch. Avoiding marshy areas where snails are common is another preventative measure.

■ Impacts and Issues

People with diabetes or immune system disorders should get medical assistance immediately when affected with swimmer's ear. They are more likely to suffer severe symptoms including malignant otitis externa, which is a rare form of otitis externa. Rather than staying on the surface of the outer ear, this disease can move into the bony structures of the ear and may permanently destroy them.

Because marine pollution is increasing around the world, especially in developed and developing countries, more incidents of swimmer's itch are occurring. In addition, global warming is creating conditions favorable to expanded populations of waterborne parasites. Many people have more leisure time and may choose to spend this time around water. More people are also moving to areas containing slow-moving bodies of water, such as lakes and estuaries. The rate of swimmer's itch increases both with the amount of time spent in infected waters and with the level of pollution in waters where swimming is done.

SEE ALSO *Ear Infections (Otitis Media); Waterborne Disease*

BIBLIOGRAPHY

Books

Preciado, Diego, ed. *Otitis Media: State of the Art Concepts and Treatment.* New York: Springer, 2015.

Wilhelm, Klaus-Peter, Hongho Zhai, and Howard I. Maibach. *Dermatotoxicology.* 8th ed. New York: CRC, 2012.

Periodicals

Brant, Sara V., et al. "Cercarial Dermatitis Transmitted by Exotic Marine Snail." *Emerging Infectious Diseases* 16, no. 9 (September 2010): 1357–1365.

Websites

"Cercarial Dermatitis (Also Known as Swimmer's Itch)." Centers for Disease Control and Prevention, January 10, 2012. https://www.cdc.gov/parasites/swimmersitch/index.html (accessed November 14, 2017).

"Swimmer's Ear." American Academy of Otolaryngology. http://www.entnet.org/content/swimmers-ear (accessed November 15, 2017).

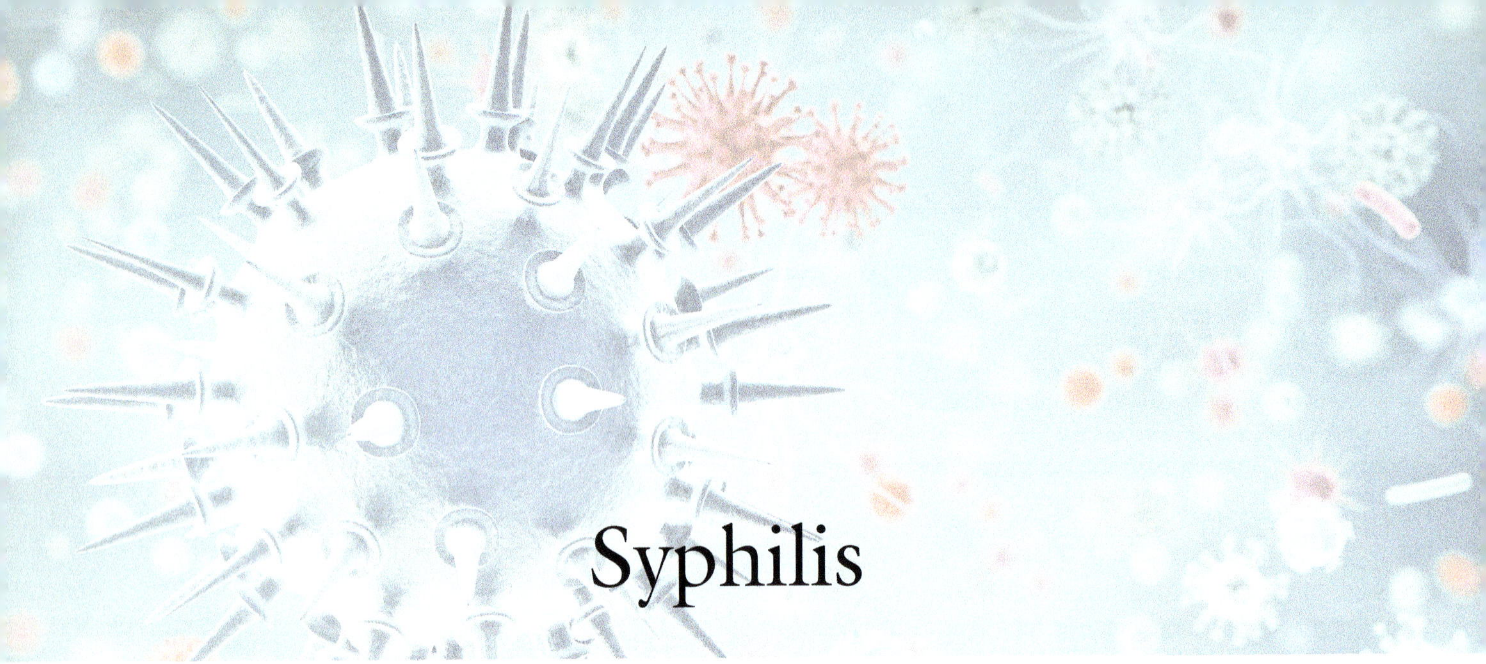

Syphilis

Introduction

Syphilis, caused by the bacterium *Treponema pallidum*, is one of the world's most significant sexually transmitted infections (STIs). An estimated 5.6 million new infections occur each year in people ages 15 to 49 worldwide. Syphilis is very infectious. Most cases are caused by sexual contact. Many people with syphilis may not be aware that they have the disease.

A deceptive condition, syphilis starts with a single, painless sore usually on the genitals. The sore may not even be detected, but untreated it may progress over a period of years to potentially fatal complications such as heart damage, dementia, and paralysis.

The advent of the antibiotic penicillin in the late 1940s led to a dramatic decrease in the number of cases. However, syphilis has been on the increase in the 21st century in the United States and in other countries, so there is a great need to treat the disease at an early stage and to educate people about the risks.

WORDS TO KNOW

ANTIBIOTIC A drug, such as penicillin, used to fight infections caused by bacteria. Antibiotics act only on bacteria and are not effective against viruses.

CHANCRE A sore that occurs in the first stage of syphilis at the place where the infection entered the body.

SEXUALLY TRANSMITTED INFECTION (STI) Infections that vary in their susceptibility to treatment, their signs and symptoms, and the consequences if they are left untreated. Some are caused by bacteria. These usually can be treated and cured. Others are caused by viruses and can typically be treated but not cured.

VENEREAL DISEASE Diseases that are transmitted by sexual contact. They are named after Venus, the Roman goddess of female sexuality.

Disease History, Characteristics, and Transmission

Syphilis is caused by *T. pallidum*, which belongs to the spirochete class of fine, spiral, and highly motile bacteria. Its incubation time is from 10 to 90 days, and the disease progresses through an infectious and a noninfectious stage. The infectious stage lasts for a few months, when symptoms may cause little or no illness. The noninfectious stage, which follows if syphilis is not treated early on, may also be without symptoms or may be accompanied by cardiovascular or neurological damage.

Infectious syphilis is divided into four stages: primary, secondary, latent (divided into early and late), and tertiary.

The primary stage is characterized by the appearance of a sore, known as a chancre, either on or inside the genitals or elsewhere on the body, such as on the eyelid or lip. There can be more than one chancre. Typically, the chancre is firm, round, small, and painless. It appears at the site of entry of *T. pallidum* into the body. The chancre, which those affected may be completely unaware of, lasts for three to six weeks and heals without treatment. If treatment is not administered, the infection will progress to the secondary stage.

A skin rash and mucous membrane lesions are the prime symptoms of the secondary stage. A nonitching rash develops, either while the chancre is healing or several weeks afterward. This might appear as rough, red or reddish-brown spots on the palms of the hands and the soles of the feet. However, a rash may appear on some other part of the body and resemble that from another disease, especially if the primary stage has not been identified. Sometimes the rash from secondary syphilis is so faint as to be unnoticeable. There may be other symptoms such as fever, swollen glands, weight loss, headaches, loss of appetite, and fatigue. This stage also resolves within a few weeks without any treatment.

Latent syphilis occurs when the disease is untreated in the primary or secondary stage. It has no obvious symptoms and is known as early latent syphilis or late latent syphilis, depending on whether it develops earlier or later than two years after the first infection. This is an arbitrary cutoff time that refers to whether the disease is likely to still be infectious. (The disease is likely not infectious in the late latent stage.)

Around 25 percent of people with latent syphilis develop tertiary syphilis, according to the World Health Organization (WHO). Tertiary syphilis occurs around 10 to 30 years after infection. The symptoms of tertiary syphilis may include cardiovascular syphilis, gummatous syphilis, neurosyphilis, and oracular syphilis. Both neurosyphilis and oracular syphilis are not limited to the tertiary stage.

Cardiovascular syphilis affects the aorta, the main vessel leaving the heart to supply the rest of the body with oxygenated blood. The disease leads to aneurysm (a weakness in the artery), which may lead to a potentially fatal rupture. Gummatous syphilis leads to the presence of sores on the skin and mucous membranes many years after the primary infection.

Neurosyphilis affects the brain and nervous system. It can occur at any stage of syphilis and is not limited to the tertiary stage. Neurosyphilis produces early symptoms such as personality change, tremor, and impaired memory, often followed by paralysis, delusions, and seizures. Another form of neurosyphilis, *tabes dorsalis*, is accompanied by sharp pains in the legs and an absence of normal reflexes. The meningovascular type of neurosyphilis is an inflammation of the covering of the brain, and headache is usually a major symptom. Neurosyphilis may not have any symptoms, but evidence of infection can still be found in the cerebrospinal fluid. Oracular syphilis, which can occur at any syphilis stage and is not limited to the tertiary stage, affects the eyes and can cause vision problems and blindness.

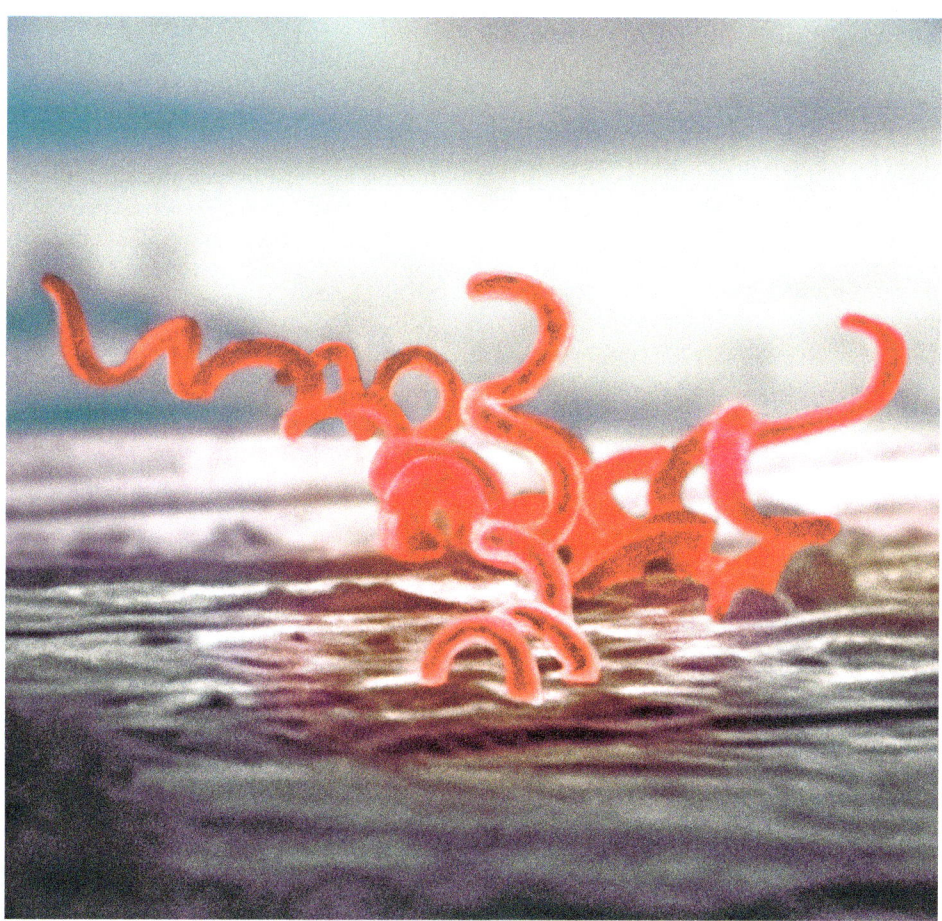

The spiral-shaped bacterium *Treponema pallidum* viewed under an electron microscope. *T. pallidum* causes syphilis, a highly infectious sexually transmitted disease. *© CDC/SCIENCE PHOTO LIBRARY/ Getty Images*

A pregnant woman with syphilis might pass the disease on to her unborn child. Congenital syphilis leads to miscarriage, stillbirth, preterm birth, death shortly after birth, physical deformity, or neurological problems. All pregnant women should be tested for syphilis. Increasing awareness of the dangers of syphilis can decrease the risk of all these complications by treating cases at the earliest possible stage with antibiotics.

Transmission of syphilis is by direct contact with a chancre, which usually occurs through sexual contact (vaginal sex, anal sex, and oral sex). Because the sore may be inside the body, such as on the cervix, it is possible that neither person will realize the danger of infection. It is also possible to become reinfected with syphilis at some later stage. Unlike with some other infectious diseases, one infection does not confer lifelong immunity. A person with syphilis can transmit it to a sexual partner during the primary, secondary, or early latent stage of the disease but not during the late latent stage or tertiary stage.

Scope and Distribution

There were approximately 18 million people around the world with syphilis in 2012, according to the WHO. Syphilis is a global disease but is most prevalent in Africa and in developing countries where access to health care may be limited. Prevalence of syphilis was lowest in Europe and Southeast Asia, according to the authors of a 2015 study published in *PLOS One*. The authors of this study noted that rates of syphilis in women were connected with country wealth: "For syphilis in women, the infection with the most robust available data, the prevalence of infection decreased as average country income increased."

According to the US Centers for Disease Control and Prevention (CDC), where data on syphilis infection is collected, the disease fell to an all-time low in 2000 but has been increasing since then. Accordingly, in the United States, there were 36,958 reported cases of syphilis (all stages) in 2006, 49,915 cases in 2012, and 88,042 cases in 2016. Between 2002 and 2014, the rates of congenital syphilis were the lowest they had ever been in the United States, ranging from 8.2 to 11.7 per 100,000 births. But in 2015 and 2016, the rate of congenital syphilis increased. In 2015 the rate was 12.6, and in 2016 the rate was 15.7.

Treatment and Prevention

Penicillin, specifically benzathine penicillin G, is the mainstay of treatment for syphilis. Because other penicillin injections are less effective in treating syphilis, only benzathine penicillin G should be used. Doxycycline and tetracycline are alternatives for those who are allergic to penicillin. Early cases can be treated by a single injection, but the more the disease progresses, the longer the duration of treatment must be. Regardless, the treatment is effective.

The only way to completely prevent the disease is to have no sexual contact. Having monogamous sexual contact with a partner who has tested negative for syphilis is also a good way to avoid infection. Correct use of latex condoms may help prevent the transmission of the disease between men and between men and women. Sores from syphilis, however, may not be covered by the condom. Reducing the number of sexual partners can also be helpful in preventing syphilis. Avoiding anonymous sex is also a recommended prevention strategy.

If a person discovers he or she has syphilis and are infectious, sex should be avoided until after treatment is completed. The person should also inform those with whom he or has had sex during the infectious stage of the disease because they might be infected as well and should seek prompt treatment.

Impacts and Issues

During World War I (1914–1918), many involved nations launched public campaigns to combat the spread of STIs (then commonly called venereal disease, or VD) that often rose dramatically during and immediately after wartime. Posters and pamphlets warned soldiers of contracting venereal disease from prostitutes and transmitting venereal disease to wives back home. Syphilis was the focus of most anti-VD campaigns because it was then the most devastating and difficult to treat venereal disease. Anti-VD, and especially antisyphilis, campaigns were again launched during World War II (1939–1945). But the advent of antibiotics shifted the focus to wartime rationing and conservation, saving precious antibiotics for those most in need by reducing the risk of exposure to VD.

Incidence of syphilis in the United States reached a historic low in 2000. Since then overall rates have increased. However, the rate of syphilis among African American women began declining in 2008. Much of the increase in syphilis cases occurred among men who have sex with men (MSM), who account for over half of all new cases. The CDC reported in 2014 and 2015 that 0.6 percent of all people infected with syphilis developed oracular syphilis, a serious complication. In 2014 and 2015, there were 388 known cases of oracular syphilis in eight monitored regions in the United States. Of these cases, 93 percent were in MSM.

About 50 to 70 percent of MSM have both syphilis and human immunodeficiency virus (HIV), which, left untreated, can lead to acquired immunodeficiency syndrome (AIDS), according to the CDC. The presence of a chancre makes it easier for HIV to enter the body. Studies have shown that the risk of HIV transmission is two to five times higher among those who already have syphilis. The symptoms of HIV and syphilis tend to overlap, which may confuse the diagnosis. It is recommended that anyone diagnosed with syphilis have an HIV test. Those who are HIV positive should be tested for syphilis so treatment can be given as soon as possible. Sex with many different people, sex with anonymous people, and sex without appropriate use of latex condoms are risk factors for contracting both syphilis and HIV.

PRIMARY SOURCE

President William Jefferson Clinton's Apology on Behalf of the United States of America

SOURCE: *Clinton, William J. "U.S. Public Health Service Syphilis Study at Tuskegee: Presidential Apology." News release, May 16, 1997. https://www.cdc.gov/tuskegee/clintonp.htm.*

INTRODUCTION: *The Tuskegee Syphilis Study (1932–1972) documented the effects of untreated syphilis in approximately 400 African Americans living near Tuskegee, Alabama. Most of the subjects of the study were poor and had scant access to health care. Many were illiterate or had little formal education. The study was kept secret for almost four decades, with minimal concern for the welfare of participants. Individuals who volunteered for the study were told they would receive free meals and medical care for their "bad blood." The families of participants who died were eligible to receive $35 for funeral expenses. When the Tuskegee Syphilis Study began in 1932, antibiotic penicillin had been discovered but was not yet commonly available for medical use. Standard treatments for syphilis were neither effective or safe. Many involved toxic substances that damaged the liver, kidneys, and nervous system.*

The originators of the Tuskegee Syphilis Study claimed it might be more beneficial for patients to receive no treatment at all than to be subjected to the syphilis remedies then available. However, the study continued long after penicillin became commonly available after World War II (1939–1945), and patients were denied antibiotics or information about antibiotic treatments. Participants were never fully informed that they had syphilis or that treatment was available. Throughout the course of the study, participants were subjected to repeated injections of nonmedicinal solution, routine examinations, and medical testing. Many participants suffered painful symptoms for many years. Many died from complications related to untreated syphilis. The experiment terminated abruptly in 1972 after information about the Tuskegee Study was leaked to the press.

In the aftermath of the Tuskegee Experiment revelations, calls for government investigations, reparations, and apologies were met with congressional hearings. The Henderson Act of 1943 had required that all forms of venereal disease be documented and treated. The US Surgeon General sent letters of commendation to men enrolled in the study on its 25th anniversary in 1957. The study violated the 1964 World Health Organization Declaration of Helsinki, in which informed consent is required. All of these events pointed to a level of government involvement and neglect that led the National Association for the Advancement of Colored People (NAACP) to file a 1973 class action that resulted in a financial settlement.

In 1997 US president Bill Clinton (1946–) issued an apology on behalf of the United States to the survivors and the family members of the people victimized by the experiment. When President Clinton issued his apology, only eight of the 399 study participants who had syphilis were still alive.

The East Room

2:26 P.M. EDT.

THE PRESIDENT: Ladies and gentlemen, on Sunday, Mr. Shaw will celebrate his 95th birthday. I would like to recognize the other survivors who are here today and their families: Mr. Charlie Pollard is here. Mr. Carter Howard. Mr. Fred Simmons. Mr. Simmons just took his first airplane ride, and he reckons he's about 110 years old, so I think it's time for him to take a chance or two. I'm glad he did. And Mr. Frederick Moss, thank you, sir.

I would also like to ask three family representatives who are here—Sam Doner is represented by his daughter, Gwendolyn Cox. Thank you, Gwendolyn. Ernest Hendon, who is watching in Tuskegee, is represented by his brother, North Hendon. Thank you, sir, for being here. And George Key is represented by his grandson, Christopher Monroe. Thank you, Chris.

I also acknowledge the families, community leaders, teachers and students watching today by satellite from Tuskegee. The White House is the people's house; we are glad to have all of you here today. I thank Dr. David Satcher for his role in this. I thank Congresswoman Waters and Congressman Hilliard, Congressman Stokes, the entire Congressional Black Caucus. Dr. Satcher, members of the Cabinet who are here, Secretary Herman, Secretary Slater, members of the Cabinet who are here, Secretary Herman, Secretary Slater. A great friend of freedom, Fred Gray, thank you for fighting this long battle all these long years.

The eight men who are survivors of the syphilis study at Tuskegee are a living link to a time not so very long ago that many Americans would prefer not to remember, but we dare not forget. It was a time when our nation failed to live up to its ideals, when our nation broke the trust with our people that is the very foundation of our democracy. It is not only in remembering that shameful past that we can make amends and repair our nation, but it is in remembering that past that we can build a better present and a better future. And without remembering it, we cannot make amends and we cannot go forward.

So today America does remember the hundreds of men used in research without their knowledge and consent. We remember them and their family members. Men who were poor and African American, without resources and with few alternatives, they believed they had found hope when they were offered free medical care by the United States Public Health Service.

They were betrayed.

Medical people are supposed to help when we need care but even once a cure was discovered, they were denied help, and they were lied to by their government. Our government is supposed to protect the rights of its citizens; their rights were trampled upon. Forty years, hundreds of men betrayed, along with their wives and children, along with the community in Macon County, Alabama, the City of Tuskegee, the fine university there, and the larger African American community.

The United States government did something that was wrong—deeply, profoundly, morally wrong. It was an outrage to our commitment to integrity and equality for all our citizens.

To the survivors, to the wives and family members, the children and the grandchildren, I say what you know: No power on Earth can give you back the lives lost, the pain suffered, the years of internal torment and anguish. What was done cannot be undone. But we can end the silence. We can stop turning our heads away. We can look at you in the eye and finally say on behalf of the American people, what the United States government did was shameful, and I am sorry.

The American people are sorry—for the loss, for the years of hurt. You did nothing wrong, but you were grievously wronged. I apologize and I am sorry that this apology has been so long in coming.

To Macon County, to Tuskegee, to the doctors who have been wrongly associated with the events there, you have our apology, as well. To our African American citizens, I am sorry that your federal government orchestrated a study so clearly racist. That can never be allowed to happen again. It is against everything our country stands for and what we must stand against is what it was.

So let us resolve to hold forever in our hearts and minds the memory of a time not long ago in Macon County, Alabama, so that we can always see how adrift we can become when the rights of any citizens are neglected, ignored and betrayed. And let us resolve here and now to move forward together.

The legacy of the study at Tuskegee has reached far and deep, in ways that hurt our progress and divide our nation. We cannot be one America when a whole segment of our nation has no trust in America. An apology is the first step, and we take it with a commitment to rebuild that broken trust. We can begin by making sure there is never again another episode like this one. We need to do more to ensure that medical research practices are sound and ethical, and that researchers work more closely with communities.

Today I would like to announce several steps to help us achieve these goals. First, we will help to build that lasting memorial at Tuskegee. The school founded by Booker T. Washington, distinguished by the renowned scientist George Washington Carver and so many others who advanced the health and well-being of African Americans and all Americans, is a fitting site. The Department of Health and Human Services will award a planning grant so the school can pursue establishing a center for bioethics in research and health care. The center will serve as a museum of the study and support efforts to address its legacy and strengthen bioethics training.

Second, we commit to increase our community involvement so that we may begin restoring lost trust. The study at Tuskegee served to sow distrust of our medical institutions, especially where research is involved. Since the study was halted, abuses have been checked by making informed consent and local review mandatory in federally-funded and mandated research.

Still, 25 years later, many medical studies have little African American participation and African American organ donors are few. This impedes efforts to conduct promising research and to provide the best health care to all our people, including African Americans. So today, I'm directing the Secretary of Health and Human Services, Donna Shalala, to issue a report in 180 days about how we can best involve communities, especially minority communities, in research and health care. You must—every American group must be involved in medical research in ways that are positive. We have put the curse behind us; now we must bring the benefits to all Americans.

Third, we commit to strengthen researchers' training in bioethics. We are constantly working on making breakthroughs in protecting the health of our people and in vanquishing diseases. But all our people must be assured that their rights and dignity will be respected as new drugs, treatments and therapies are tested and used. So I am directing Secretary Shalala to work in partnership with higher education to prepare training materials for medical researchers. They will be available in a year. They will help researchers build on core ethical principles of respect for individuals, justice and informed consent, and advise them on how to use these principles effectively in diverse populations.

Fourth, to increase and broaden our understanding of ethical issues and clinical research, we commit to providing postgraduate fellowships to train bioethicists especially among African Americans and other minority groups. HHS will offer these fellowships beginning in September of 1998 to promising students enrolled in bioethics graduate programs.

And, finally, by executive order I am also today extending the charter of the National Bioethics Advisory Commission to October of 1999. The need for this commission is clear. We must be able to call on the thoughtful, collective wisdom of experts and community representatives to find ways to further strengthen our protections for subjects in human research.

We face a challenge in our time. Science and technology are rapidly changing our lives with the promise of making us much healthier, much more productive and more prosperous. But with these changes we must work harder to see that as we advance we don't leave behind our conscience. No ground is gained and, indeed, much is lost if we lose our moral bearings in the name of progress.

The people who ran the study at Tuskegee diminished the stature of man by abandoning the most basic ethical precepts. They forgot their pledge to heal and repair. They had the power to heal the survivors and all the others and they did not. Today, all we can do is apologize. But you have the power, for only you—Mr. Shaw, the others who are here, the family members who are with us in Tuskegee—only you have the power to forgive. Your presence here shows us that you have chosen a better path than your government did so long ago. You have not withheld the power to forgive. I hope today and tomorrow every American will remember your lesson and live by it.

Thank you, and God bless you.

See Also *AIDS (Acquired Immunodeficiency Syndrome); HIV; Sexually Transmitted Infections*

BIBLIOGRAPHY

Books

Bennett, John E., Raphael Dolin, and Martin J. Blaser. *Mandell, Douglas, and Bennett's Principles and Practice of Infectious Diseases.* 8th ed. Philadelphia: Elsevier/Saunders, 2015.

Periodicals

Newman, Lori, et al. "Global Estimates of Syphilis in Pregnancy and Associated Adverse Outcomes: Analysis of Multinational Antenatal Surveillance Data." *PLOS Medicine* (February 26, 2013). This article can also be found online at http://journals.plos.org/plosmedicine/article?id=10.1371/journal.pmed.1001396 (accessed February 16, 2018).

Newman, Lori, et al. "Global Estimates of the Prevalence and Incidence of Four Curable Sexually Transmitted Infections in 2012 Based on Systematic Review and Global Reporting." *PLOS One* 10, no. 12 (2015): e0143304. This article can also be found online at https://www.ncbi.nlm.nih.gov/pmc/articles/PMC4672879/ (accessed February 16, 2018).

Gomez, Gabriela B., et al. "Untreated Maternal Syphilis and Adverse Outcomes of Pregnancy: A Systematic Review and Meta-Analysis." *Bulletin of the World Health Organization* 91 (2013): 217–226. This article can also be found online at https://www.scielosp.org/pdf/bwho/v91n3/a13v94n3.pdf (accessed February 16, 2018).

Oliver, Sara E, et al. "Ocular Syphilis—Eight Jurisdictions, United States, 2014–2015." *Morbidity and Mortality Weekly Report* 65, no. 43 (November 4, 2016): 1185–1188. This article can also be found online at https://www.cdc.gov/mmwr/volumes/65/wr/mm6543a2.htm (accessed February 16, 2018).

Patton, Monica E., et al. "Primary and Secondary Syphilis—United States, 2005–2013." *Morbidity and Mortality Weekly Report* 63, no. 18 (May 9, 2014): 402–406. This article can also be found online at https://www.cdc.gov/mmwr/preview/mmwrhtml/mm6318a4.htm (accessed February 16, 2018).

Websites

Bolan, Gail. "Syphilis and HIV: A Dangerous Duo Affecting Gay and Bisexual Men." HIV.gov, December 13, 2012. https://www.hiv.gov/blog/syphilis-and-hiv-a-dangerous-duo-affecting-gay-and-bisexual-men (accessed February 16, 2018).

"Clinical Advisory: Ocular Syphilis in the United States." Centers for Disease Control and Prevention, March 24, 2016. https://www.cdc.gov/std/syphilis/clinicaladvisoryos2015.htm (accessed February 16, 2018).

"Syphilis." Centers for Disease Control and Prevention, November 30, 2017. https://www.cdc.gov/std/syphilis/default.htm (accessed February 15, 2018).

"WHO Guidelines for the Treatment of *Treponema pallidum* (Syphilis)." World Health Organization, 2016. http://apps.who.int/iris/bitstream/10665/249572/1/9789241549806-eng.pdf?ua=1 (accessed February 15, 2018).

Susan Aldridge
Claire Skinner

Taeniasis (*Taenia* Infection)

Introduction

Taenia infection, or taeniasis, is an infection of the digestive tract caused by parasitic flatworms, generally called cestodes or tapeworms. It is caused by species within the *Taenia* genus that infect carnivores (flesh-eating animals). Taeniasis is acquired when humans (definitive hosts) eat raw or undercooked meat from infected animals (intermediate hosts).

Cows and other ruminants carry the tapeworm species *Taenia saginata*. Pigs, dogs, cats, and sheep harbor the species *Taenia solium*. When humans acquire taeniasis from cows, the tapeworm is commonly called beef tapeworm. When it is from pigs, it is called pig tapeworm. In addition, *Taenia multiceps* infects hares, rabbits, and squirrels while only rarely infecting humans.

Disease History, Characteristics, and Transmission

When humans eat infected meat from an intermediate host, tapeworm larvae hatch and develop inside the intestines. *T. saginata* matures to a length of 13 to 26 feet (4 to 8 meters). *T. solium* reaches adulthood at a length of 3 to 7 feet (1 to 2 meters). Both tapeworms

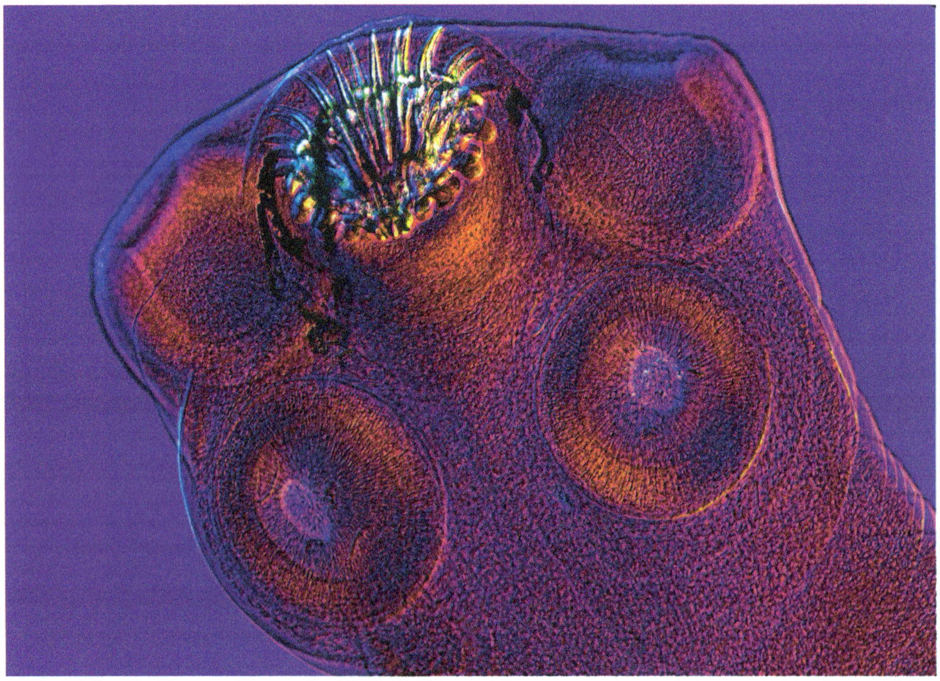

A light micrograph of *Taenia solium*, also known as a pig tapeworm, with suckers and hooks used to attach to the digestive tract of its host. Consumption of undercooked pork can transmit the parasite to humans and lead to taeniasis. © *Michael J. Klein, M.D./Getty Images*

WORDS TO KNOW

CHEMOTHERAPY The treatment of a disease, infection, or condition with chemicals that have a specific effect on its cause, such as a microorganism or cancer cell. The first modern therapeutic chemical was derived from a synthetic dye. Sulfonamide drugs developed in the 1930s, penicillin and other antibiotics developed in the 1940s, hormones developed in the 1950s, and later drugs that interfere with cancer cell metabolism and reproduction have all been part of the chemotherapeutic arsenal.

ERADICATION The process of destroying or eliminating a microorganism or disease.

HOST An organism that serves as the habitat for a parasite or possibly for a symbiont. A host may provide nutrition to the parasite or symbiont, or it may simply provide a place in which to live.

PARASITE An organism that lives in or on a host organism and gets its nourishment from the host. The parasite usually gains all the benefits of this relationship, whereas the host may suffer from various diseases and discomforts or show no signs of the infection. The life cycle of a typical parasite usually includes several developmental stages and morphological changes as the parasite lives and moves through the environment and one or more hosts. Parasites that remain on a host's body surface to feed are called ectoparasites, whereas those that live inside a host's body are called endoparasites. Parasitism is a highly successful biological adaptation. There are more known parasitic species than nonparasitic ones, and parasites affect just about every form of life, including most all animals, plants, and even bacteria.

RUMINANTS Cud-chewing animals with a four-chambered stomach and even-toed hooves.

SEIZURE A sudden disruption of the brain's normal electrical activity accompanied by altered consciousness or other neurological and behavioral abnormalities. Epilepsy is a condition characterized by recurrent seizures that may include repetitive muscle jerking called convulsions. Seizures are traditionally divided into two major categories: generalized seizures and focal seizures. Within each major category, however, there are many different types of seizures. Generalized seizures come about due to abnormal neuronal activity on both sides of the brain, whereas focal seizures, also named partial seizures, occur in only one part of the brain.

TAPEWORM Parasitic flatworms of class *Cestoidea*, phylum *Platyhelminthes*, that live inside the intestine. Tapeworms have no digestive system but absorb predigested nutrients directly from their surroundings.

can be found as an adult in the human intestines and as larvae in muscles and other tissues of cattle and other ruminants (in the case of *T. saginata*) and pigs, dogs, cats, and sheep (in the case of *T. solium*). Adult tapeworms can stay inside their hosts for many years. The eggs are passed into the soil from human feces and are eaten by intermediate hosts. The eggs hatch and larvae enter tissues of the animal host, where the larvae enclose themselves in cysts. When humans eat infected animal flesh, they also eat the cysts.

Tapeworms are long, segmented worms with each segment able to produce eggs. Each segment can detach from the worm and pass through the feces or it can crawl on its own through the anus. The worms do not have an intestinal tract, so they must obtain their nourishment through their integument (outer covering). The structure of an adult consists of a head, neck, and segmented body that contain both male and female reproductive features. The head attaches to the mucous lining of the intestine.

Humans infected with *T. solium* can become infected again when eggs are ingested from human hands after coming in contact with the anal area. These infected individuals can infect other humans through improper food handling and other unsanitary means. These humans are considered intermediate hosts. The larvae will travel to various tissues of organs within the human host. Thus, *T. solium* are tapeworms that can infect humans as intermediate and definitive hosts.

Taenia infection does not usually cause any symptoms. However, sometimes there can be minor gastrointestinal pain, weight loss, and persistent ill feelings. The infection is usually recognized when the infected person passes tapeworm segments in the stool, especially if the segment is moving.

■ Scope and Distribution

Taenia infection is found worldwide. In the United States *T. saginata* is found in less than 1 percent of cattle because cattle are thoroughly treated for tapeworms. *T. solium* is also rare in the United States, but it is becoming more frequent as immigrants come in increasing numbers from areas infected with the parasite.

T. saginata is found most often in Latin America, Central Asia, Africa, and the Middle East. It is also found somewhat in Europe, South Asia, Japan, and the Philippines. *T. solium* is found mostly in Latin America, Africa, the Slavic countries of central and southern Europe, Southeast Asia, India, and China.

According to the US Centers for Disease Control and Prevention (CDC), *T. solium* is found more often than *T. saginata* in underdeveloped areas because people live close to pigs and often eat undercooked pork.

T. solium causes an estimated 28,000 deaths per year and leads to 2.7 million disability-adjusted life years lost annually, according to Anna L. Okello and Lian Francesca Thomas in a 2017 article for *Risk Management and Healthcare Policy*. Data on the effects of other strains of *Taenia* is less reliable and more uncertain.

Treatment and Prevention

Taenia infection is diagnosed with a stool sample. Tapeworm eggs can be found with a medical examination. Segments of worms can also be readily seen in feces after they are passed from the body. An infected person is treated with oral antiparasitic worm medications. Usually one dose of niclosamide (Niclocide®) is used, and sometimes either praziquantel (Biltricide®) or albendazole (Albenza®, Eskazole®, or Zentel®) is given. After the treatment is complete, tapeworm infection is normally eliminated. Reinfection is possible if more cysts are ingested.

Any complications are usually from an infected person reinfecting him- or herself with tapeworm eggs. In rare cases worms may cause blockage of the intestines and obstruct the bowels, resulting in a medical emergency.

Taenia infection is prevented in the United States and other industrial countries with strict federal laws governing the feeding and inspection of domesticated animals slaughtered for food. According to the CDC, taeniasis has been largely eliminated in the United States. In addition, fully cooking meat destroys any tapeworm larvae that may be present and any infection they may carry. Anyone infected with tapeworms can prevent infecting him- or herself again by practicing good hygiene, especially by thorough handwashing after using the toilet.

Impacts and Issues

T. saginata infection can cause obstruction of the appendix (a small outgrowth of the intestines), pancreatic duct (a carrier of pancreatic juices), and biliary duct (a transporter of bile).

Infections involving *T. solium* can cause debilitating complications to the central nervous system and skeletal muscles. Under many conditions a neurologic examination

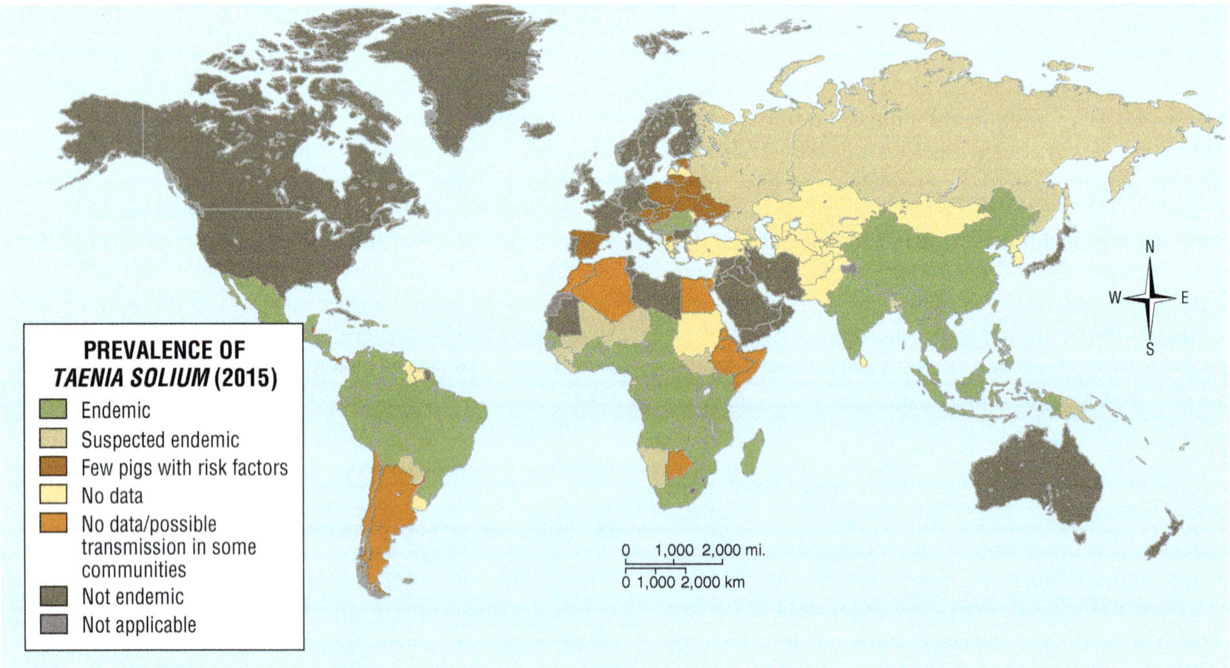

SOURCE: Adapted from "Endemicity of *Taenia solium*, 2015." World Health Organization. Available from: http://www.who.int/taeniasis/Endemicity_Taenia_Solium_2015.jpg?ua=1

comes back normal, making it difficult to diagnose the infection. Other complications that can set in include meningitis (inflammation of the meninges), dementia (deterioration of memory functions), and hydrocephalus (increased fluid around the brain).

Larvae can also migrate from the intestines to other tissues of the body. If larvae migrate to the brain, they can cause neurological problems that are generally called cysticercosis. Seizure can occur when the brain is affected, along with earlier signs of vomiting, confusion, visual changes, and headaches.

Several international health organizations, including the World Health Organization (WHO), have identified taeniasis as potentially eradicable, meaning that health officials hope to eliminate the disease in humans by focusing on hygiene education, improved sanitation, and preventative vaccinations for carrier animals. In South America and parts of Asia and Africa, efforts to control *T. solium* employ aggressive campaigns of chemotherapy (using drugs or chemicals that are toxic to sources of diseases within the body) to reduce the number of human carriers.

In late 2017 delegates representing 13 countries signed the Chengdu Declaration for Action, which called for a global collaborative network to combat taeniasis, cysticercosis, and echinococcosis (a related disease caused by parasitic tapeworms). According to a WHO release about the declaration, "Part of the public health interventions to prevent and control these risks requires consideration of powerful interventions in animals, food and the environment that break the cycle of transmission. In addition, conditions must be created to provide early diagnosis and management of people infected with these parasites."

SEE ALSO *Helminth Disease; Parasitic Diseases; Tapeworm Infections*

BIBLIOGRAPHY

Books

Maule, Aaron G., and Nikki J. Marks, eds. *Parasitic Flatworms: Molecular Biology, Biochemistry, Immunology and Physiology.* Wallingford, UK: CABI, 2006.

Singh G., and S. Prabhakar, eds. *Taenia Solium Cysticercosis: From Basic to Clinical Science.* Chandigarh, India: CABI, 2002.

Periodicals

Ng-Nguyen, Dinh, Mark A. Stevenson, and Rebecca J. Traub. "A Systematic Review of Taeniasis, Cysticercosis and Trichinellosis in Vietnam." *Parasites & Vectors* 10 (March 2017): 150.

Okello, Anna L., and Lian Francesca Thomas. "Human Taeniasis: Current Insights into Prevention and Management Strategies in Endemic Countries." *Risk Management and Healthcare Policy* 10 (April 2017): 107–116.

Yanagida, Tetsuya, et al. "Taeniasis and Cysticercosis Due to *Taenia solium* in Japan." *Parasites & Vectors* 5 (January 2012): 18.

Websites

"Chengdu Declaration on Cestode Infections Calls for Global Collaboration into Research and Control." World Health Organization, December 13, 2017. http://www.who.int/neglected_diseases/news/Chengdu_Declaration_on_cestode_infections_calls/en/ (accessed January 10, 2018).

"Taeniasis." Centers for Disease Control and Prevention, January 10, 2013. https://www.cdc.gov/parasites/taeniasis/index.html (accessed January 10, 2018).

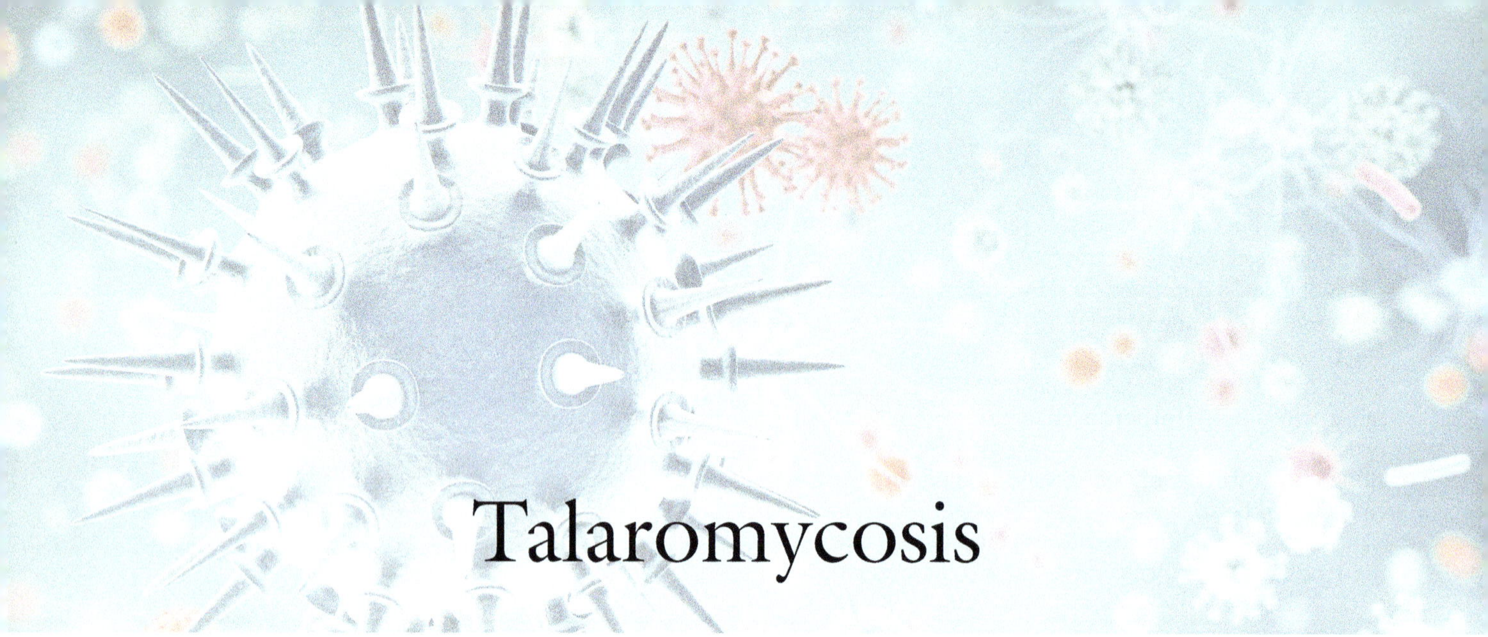

Talaromycosis

Introduction

Talaromycosis is a life-threatening opportunistic infection caused by the fungus *Talaromyces marneffei*. Formerly, the fungus was named *Penicillium marneffei*, and the disease was known as penicillinosis. But the names were changed after the fungus was reclassified to the genus *Talaromyces* in 2015. Once thought a rare disease, talaromycosis is among the three most common opportunistic infections, along with tuberculosis and cryptococcosis, in patients suffering from acquired immunodeficiency syndrome (AIDS) in some parts of Southeast Asia. Talaromycosis is also considered a growing threat to individuals whose immune system has been compromised by other conditions.

WORDS TO KNOW

ANTIRETROVIRAL (ARV) THERAPY A form of drug therapy that prevents the reproduction of a type of virus called a retrovirus. Human immunodeficiency virus (HIV), which causes acquired immunodeficiency syndrome (AIDS), is a retrovirus. ARV drugs are used to treat HIV infections and keep the virus in check, but they cannot prevent or cure the infection.

ENDEMIC Present in a particular area or among a particular group of people.

MORTALITY The condition of being susceptible to death. The term *mortality* comes from the Latin word *mors*, which means "death." Mortality can also refer to the rate of deaths caused by an illness or injury (e.g., "Rabies has a high mortality rate").

RESERVOIR The animal or organism in which a virus or parasite normally resides.

VECTOR Any agent that carries and transmits parasites and diseases. Also, an organism or a chemical used to transport a gene into a new host cell.

Disease History, Characteristics, and Transmission

T. marneffei is endemic to Southeast Asia and southern China. It was first isolated in 1956 from bamboo rats in Vietnam. The first human case was recorded in 1959 when researcher Gabriel Segretain (1913–2008) accidentally injected the fungus into his finger, resulting in small lesions at the site of the infection and swollen lymph nodes.

The fungus grows like a mold at room temperature and transforms into a yeastlike form at 37°C (98.6°F). The mold form, also known as the mycelial form, grows in a branched, ribbonlike structure and forms a grayish-white woolly structure after two to three days in culture. The mold produces a characteristic red pigment that may spread into the culture medium. The yeast form is responsible for the spread of talaromycosis throughout white blood cells and can be isolated from clinical samples.

In individuals with healthy immune function, talaromycosis manifests as a localized infection resembling the symptoms of tuberculosis, including fever, weight loss, cough, or anemia. In individuals with weak immunity, such as AIDS patients, the infection is typically spread throughout the body via the bloodstream. The clinical symptoms of the systemic form of the disease include lymphadenopathy (swollen lymph nodes), hepatosplenomegaly (enlargement of the liver and spleen), prolonged fever, weight loss, fatigue, anorexia, anemia, persistent cough, micronodular pulmonary infiltrates (small nodules in the lungs) or other lung diseases, clam-like skin lesions, abscesses or subcutaneous nodules, and leukocytosis (an increase in the number of white blood cells). Seventy percent of systemic cases present skin lesions found on the face, chest, and extremities. Oral lesions in the form of ulcers with yellow discharge are also common.

The exact route of human infection is not known, but it is presumed that humans acquire infection through inhalation of fungal spores from soil. The spores are embedded in macrophages (white blood cells) in the lung and subsequently spread throughout the body, resulting in systemic infection. Although bamboo rats act as a reservoir, they are not considered a significant vector due to their limited contact with humans, though infection through consumption of infected rat meat has been recorded. As of 2018 there was no reported incidence of human-to-human infection. After entering the body, the fungus proliferates inside the macrophages and spreads throughout the body, leading to infection of the liver, lymph nodes, bone marrow, and spleen.

Infected individuals with a healthy immune system may remain asymptomatic for long periods, whereas those with a weakened immune system typically exhibit symptoms within weeks of exposure.

Scope and Distribution

Talaromycosis is endemic in Southeast Asia, particularly northern Thailand, as well as Vietnam, Hong Kong, southern China, India, and Japan. The disease has also been reported in AIDS patients in Europe, Australia, and the United States who had recently traveled to or migrated from endemic areas.

Exposure to soil, especially during the rainy season, is considered a risk factor for talaromycosis. Prior to the 1980s, there were few recorded cases of natural human infections. However, with the rapid spread of the HIV/AIDS pandemic in the late 20th century, the number of cases increased dramatically in the 1980s and 1990s. The introduction of antiretroviral therapy (ART) has helped to decrease the incidence of talaromycosis among HIV/AIDS patients in the 21st century, but the emergence of other immunosuppressive diseases, along with improved diagnostics, has resulted in an increased recognition of the disease among individuals who are HIV negative.

Treatment and Prevention

Specific diagnosis of talaromycosis can be difficult, particularly outside of endemic areas, due to the similarity of symptoms to those of tuberculosis and a variety of fungal infections. Diagnosis is made by histology and culture of *T. marneffei* from clinical samples such as skin scrapings or lymph node biopsies.

Untreated talaromycosis may lead to death, usually due to liver failure caused by toxins released by the fungus into the bloodstream. The mortality rate is believed to be about 75 percent for untreated cases and around 20 percent with treatment. Antifungal agents such as ketoconazole, itraconazole, miconazole, flucytosine, and amphotericin B are effective treatment options against *T. marneffei*. Newer treatment options include antifungal agents known as azoles, including posaconazole, ravucon-

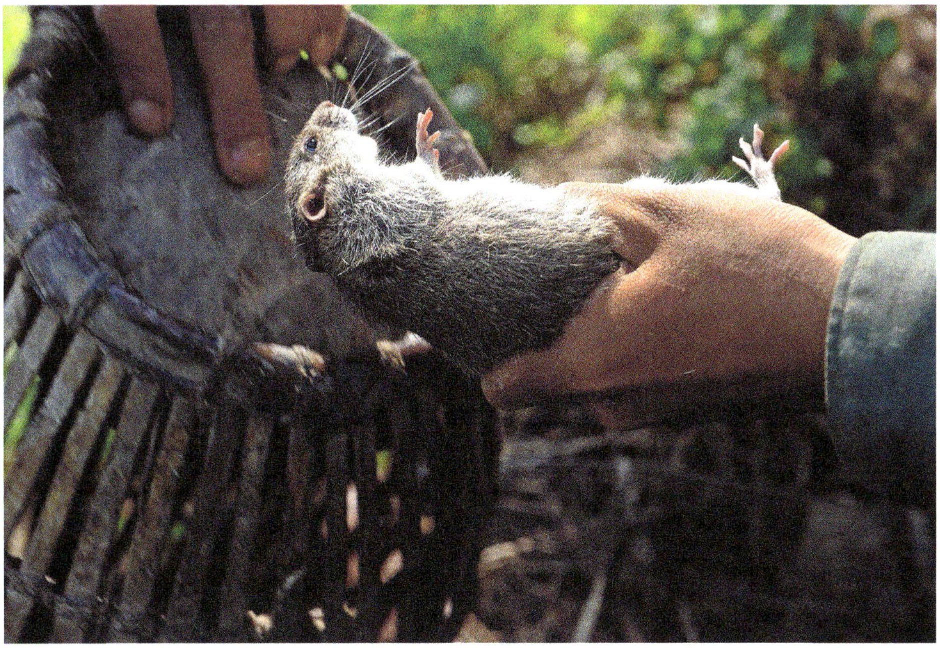

Pencilliosis is fungal infection that bamboo rats pass to immune-compromised patients in Southeast Asia. *© HOANG DINH NAM/AFP/Getty Images*

Reported Cases of *Talaromyces marneffei* Infection in Non-HIV-Infected Adults

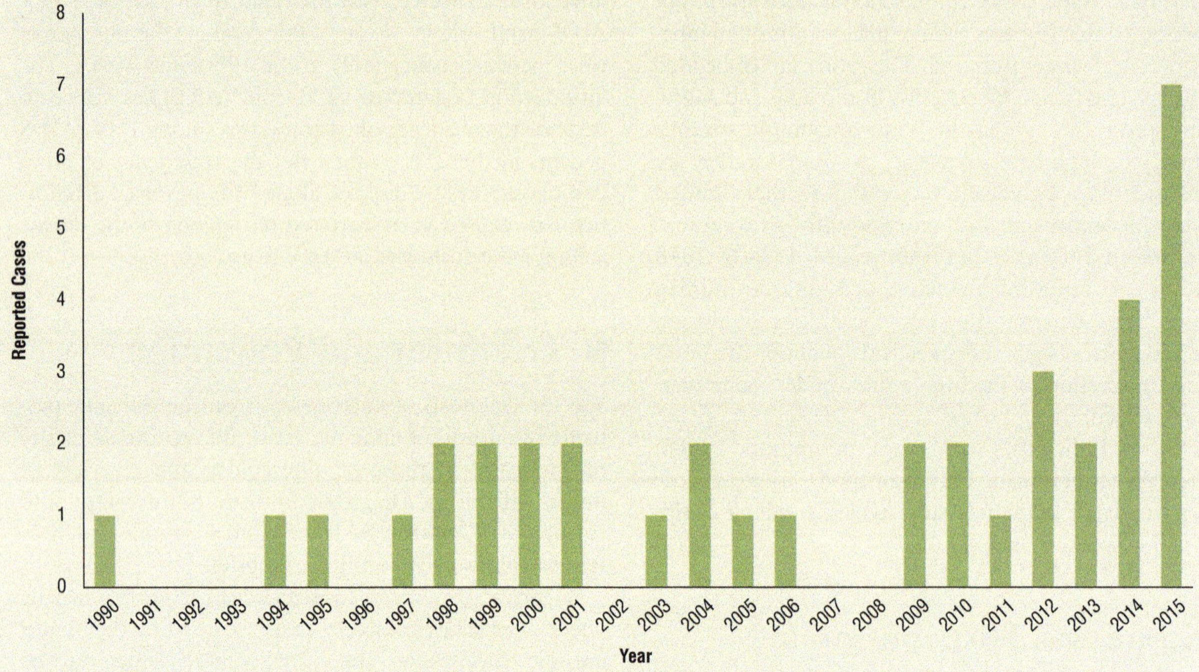

SOURCE: Adapted from Chan, Jasper F. W., et al. "*Talaromyces (Penicillium) marneffei* Infection in Non-HIV-Infected Patients." *Emerging Microbes & Infections* 5 (2016). Available from: https://www.nature.com/articles/emi201618

azole, and voriconazole. Patients can be monitored for efficacy of the drug by routine liver function tests. Maintenance therapy with itraconazole is often required, as relapse of the infection is common.

Impacts and Issues

The World Health Organization has listed talaromycosis as an opportunistic infection in HIV-infected patients, especially in Southeast Asia and southern China. Although research on the disease has been largely focused on its effects on individuals with HIV/AIDS, studies have shown a decline in infections among HIV/AIDS patients due to increased use of ART and an increase in infections among HIV-negative patients. Fatality rates have also been shown to be somewhat higher in HIV-negative patients, though this is thought to be due to delayed diagnosis and treatment of populations thought to be less at risk of the disease.

The changing epidemiology of talaromycosis requires new research in at-risk populations, as well as further development of diagnostic tests. Health care providers in endemic areas must become more aware of the signs and symptoms of the disease to improve response times and patient outcomes.

See Also *AIDS Acquired Immunodeficiency Syndrome); HIV; Opportunistic Infection*

BIBLIOGRAPHY

Books

Chander, Jagdish. "Talaromycosis." In *Textbook of Medical Mycology*, 506–523. New Delhi: Jaypee Brothers Medical, 2018.

O'Connor, Louise, and Barry Glynn, eds. *Fungal Diagnostics: Methods and Protocols*. New York: Humana, 2013.

Periodicals

Chan, Jasper F. W., et al. "*Talaromyces* (*Penicillium*) *marneffei* Infection in Non-HIV-Infected Patients." *Emerging Microbes & Infections* 5, no. 3 (2016): e19. This article can also be found online at https://www.nature.com/articles/emi201618 (accessed February 21, 2018).

Cooper, Chester R., and Nongnuch Vanittanakom. "Insights into the Pathogenecity of *Penicillium marneffei*." *Future Microbiology* 3, no. 1 (2008): 43–55. This article can also be found online at https://www.futuremedicine.com/doi/abs/10.2217/17460913.3.1.43?rfr_dat=cr_pub%3Dpubmed&url_ver=Z39.88-2003&rfr_id=ori%3Arid%3Acrossref.org&journalCode=fmb (accessed February 21, 2018).

Larsson, Mattias, et al. "Clinical Characteristics and Outcome of *Penicillium marneffei* Infection among HIV-Infected Patients in Northern Vietnam." *AIDS Research and Therapy* 9, no. 1 (2012): 24. This article can also be found online at https://aidsrestherapy.biomedcentral.com/articles/10.1186/1742-6405-9-24 (accessed February 21, 2018).

Websites

"Penicilliosis and HIV." HIV InSite. http://hivinsite.ucsf.edu/InSite?page=kb-00&doc=kb-05-02-07 (accessed February 21, 2018).

"Talaromycosis (Formerly Penicilliosis)." Centers for Disease Control and Prevention, September 26, 2017. https://www.cdc.gov/fungal/diseases/other/talaromycosis.html#four (accessed February 21, 2018).

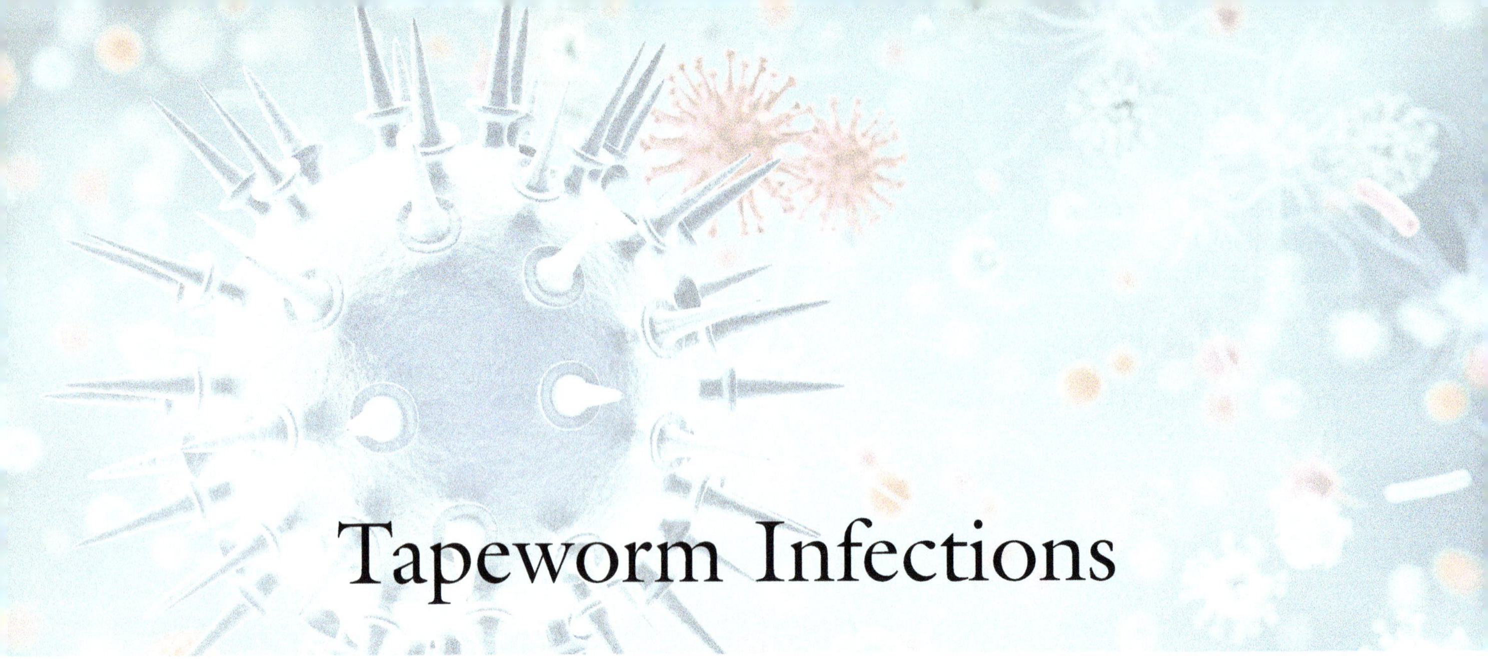

Tapeworm Infections

■ Introduction

Tapeworms, or cestodes, are parasitic animals. Humans become infected with tapeworms when they either ingest meat containing encysted tapeworms (tapeworms enclosed in cysts) or when they ingest tapeworm eggs. In the first case, humans act as primary hosts. In the second case, humans act as intermediate hosts.

While tapeworm infections tend to be asymptomatic, some symptoms may appear, including abdominal pain. However, if a human is an intermediate host (i.e., infected with eggs), more serious complications can arise. Cysts formed by the larvae in human tissues can cause damage, including damage to vital organs such as the brain. Treatment for all tapeworm infections involves antiparasitic medications, such as praziquantel, and is usually effective.

Tapeworm infections occur worldwide but are more prevalent in developing countries with poor sanitation conditions or in areas where humans live close to infected livestock.

WORDS TO KNOW

CESTODE A class of worms characterized by flat, segmented bodies, commonly known as tapeworms.

INTERMEDIATE HOST An organism infected by a parasite while the parasite is in a developmental, not sexually mature, form.

PRIMARY HOST An organism that provides food and shelter for a parasite while allowing it to become sexually mature. A secondary host, by contrast, is one occupied by a parasite during the larval or asexual stages of its life cycle.

■ Disease History, Characteristics, and Transmission

Tapeworms are parasitic flatworms belonging to the class Cestoda. The life cycle of a tapeworm generally involves a primary host and an intermediate host. The life cycle begins when a tapeworm egg is passed from a primary host into soil or water. An intermediate host ingests the egg, and the larvae hatch, enter tissues, and form cysts. A primary host then ingests cysts when they consume the flesh of the intermediate host. These cysts develop into adults, which sexually reproduce in the host's intestines.

In most cases humans become infected with tapeworms after eating undercooked or raw meat or fish containing tapeworm cysts and serve as primary hosts. These worms migrate to the intestines, where they reproduce. The most common tapeworms that infect humans in this manner are *Taenia solium* (pork tapeworm), which is present in pigs; *Taenia saginata* (beef tapeworm), which is present in cattle; *Diphyllobothrium* species, which are present in freshwater fishes; *Hymenolepis* species (dwarf tapeworms), which are found in rodents and insects; and *Diphyllobothrium caninum* (flea tapeworm), which is present in cat and dog fleas. In general, tapeworm infections in primary hosts tend to be asymptomatic. However, possible symptoms include abdominal pain, nausea, diarrhea, stools containing mucus, and the passing of tapeworm segments, or proglottids. The fecal matter of these infected individuals is infectious, as it contains tapeworm eggs.

In some cases humans are intermediate hosts—that is, they ingest the tapeworm eggs. This occurs with *T. solium* if humans swallow food or water that contains contaminated human fecal matter. The eggs in the contaminated food or water hatch in the body, and the larvae migrate to tissues within the body and form cysts. It also occurs when humans accidentally swallow insects containing the larvae of *Hymenolepis* species.

A serious risk associated with an infestation of *T. solium* is that of developing the tissue infection cysticercosis. This occurs when the eggs are ingested and the larvae form cysts within tissues. The most serious form of this infection, neurocysticercosis, involves cysts that form in the central nervous system. This can cause neurological problems and seizures. In severe cases permanent brain damage or death may occur. Of the tapeworm infections, *T. solium* causes the most serious health problems if left untreated.

■ Scope and Distribution

Tapeworm infections occur worldwide. However, certain species are only present, or are more prevalent, in certain regions. Such species are less common in Europe, North America, Australia, and New Zealand, although they do exist. In the United States, only a few tapeworms commonly cause infection: *T. saginata*, *T. solium*, and *T. diphyllobothrium*. Infection resulting from *T. saginata*, although common worldwide, has less than 1 percent prevalence in the United States because most US cattle are uninfected. *T. saginata* infections are most common in Latin America and Africa, and, to a lesser extent, Asia.

T. solium is common in Latin America, Africa, and Asia. Cysticercosis, which occurs when humans are infected by the larval form of *T. solium* tapeworms, is endemic in almost all Latin American countries. Infection from *Diphyllobothrium* species is most common in Northern Hemisphere countries. The most frequently diagnosed tapeworm, *Hymenolepis nana* (dwarf tapeworm), occurs globally but is most common in the Mediterranean, Indian subcontinent, and South America. Children in these areas, who are most affected, have infection rates of up to 20 percent. Infections resulting from *T. solium*, *Diphyllobothrium*, and *H. nana* tapeworms are commonly found in regions with poor hygiene and sanitation methods.

Tapeworm Life Cycle

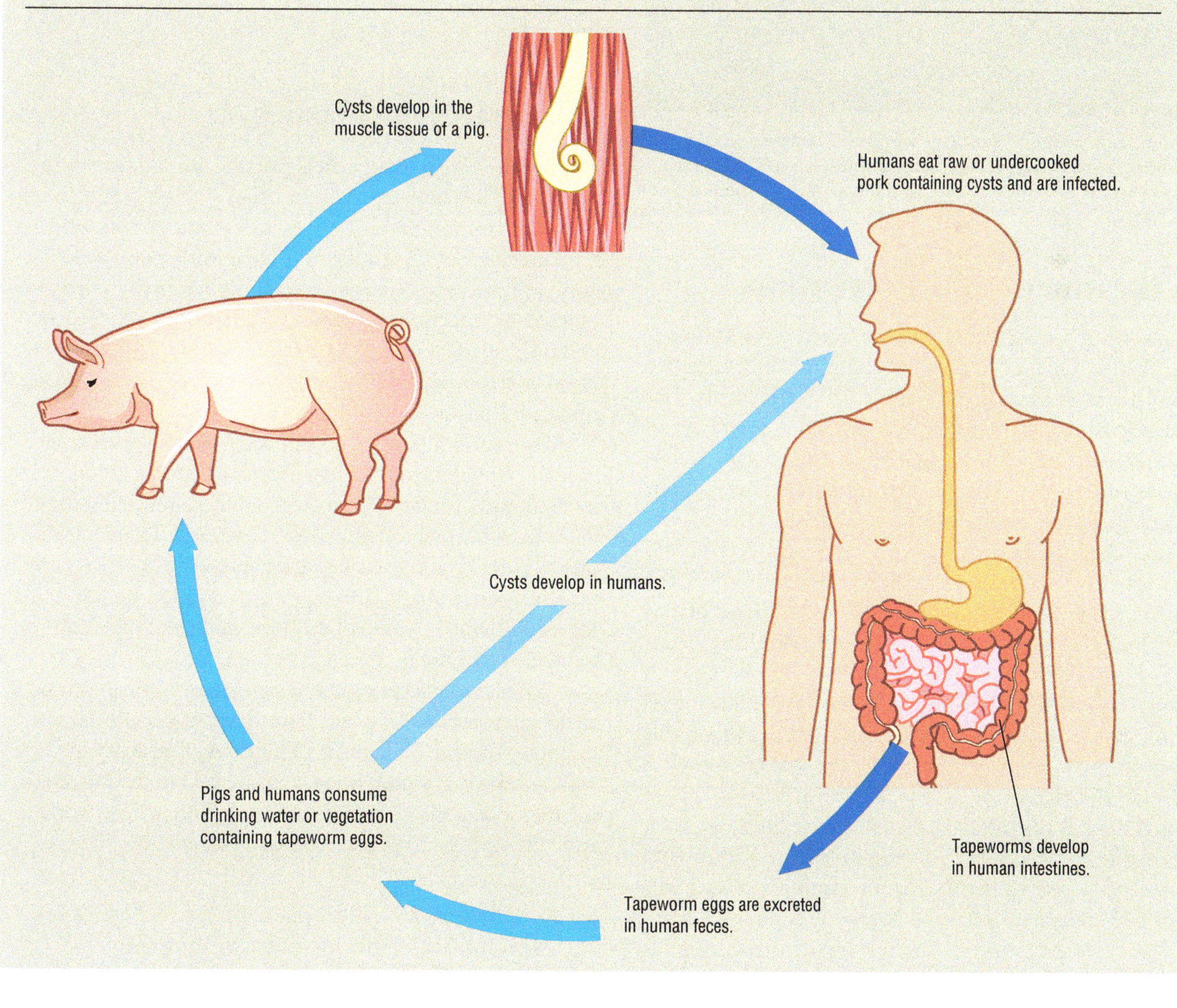

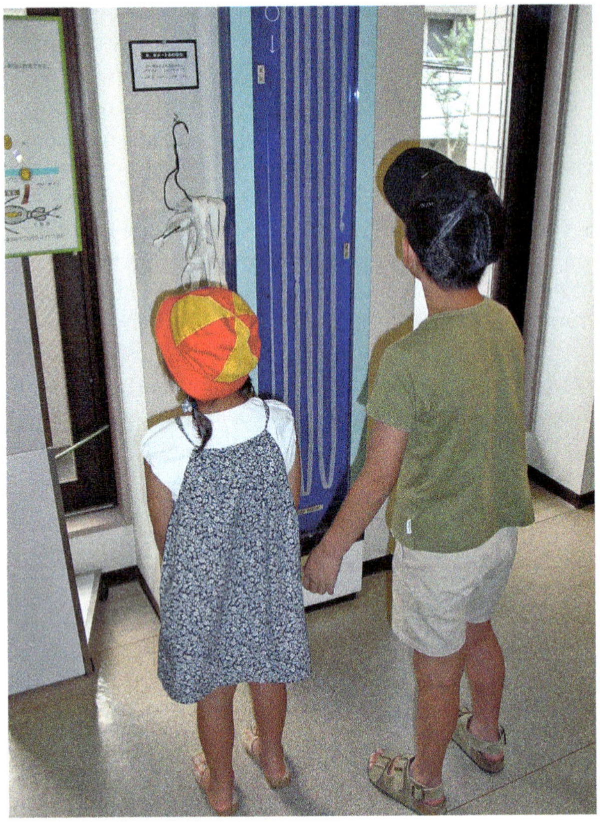

Children look at the longest tapeworm ever removed from a human being at the Meguro Parasiological Museum in Tokyo, Japan. The tapeworm measures 26 feet (8 meters). © Barry Cronin/Newsmakers/Getty Images

Treatment and Prevention

Tapeworm infections are usually treated with antiparasitic drugs. One of the most common and effective medications is praziquantel. This drug effectively kills adult tapeworms. There are a few mild side effects of praziquantel, but they are generally short-lived. Albendazole is an alternative to praziquantel, with similar effects. Another alternative to praziquantal is niclosamide, which is used to treat infections by *Taenia* and *Diphyllobothrium* tapeworms; it is not available in the United States for human usage. The side effects of this drug include nausea, abdominal pain, vomiting, diarrhea, light-headedness, and skin rash. In the case of neurocysticercosis, in which tapeworm larvae form cysts in the central nervous system, early treatment of this infection can minimize damage to the system and thus decrease the risk of neurological complications. These treatments kill the adult tapeworms, not the eggs, so it is possible for a patient to remain infected following treatment. A visit to the doctor three months after treatment is therefore necessary to check for continued infection and to determine whether further treatment is needed.

There are no vaccinations to prevent tapeworm infections in humans. The best method of prevention is to avoid becoming contaminated through good sanitation and appropriate handling of meat. For tapeworms found in meats, cooking the meat above a temperature of 150°F (66°C) for whole cuts or 160°F (71°C) for ground meats or freezing it for 24 hours kills the tapeworms. Cooking fish to 145°F (63°C) or freezing it at −4°F (−20°C) or cooler for seven days is recommended. In addition, ensuring that livestock are dewormed decreases the risk that they are infected and likely to pass on an infection to humans.

Food and water may be contaminated with infected fecal matter, particularly in regions with poor hygiene and sanitation. Therefore, washing raw food or thoroughly cooking it helps to ensure parasites are removed. In addition, boiling or filtering drinking water decreases the chance of ingesting parasites from the water. Good personal hygiene, such as washing hands with soap and water prior to handling food, and rigorous sanitation practices, especially where human waste is involved, also decrease the likelihood that parasites will be transmitted among a human population.

Impacts and Issues

Tapeworms are a major health issue for a number of countries. Because tapeworms usually originate in livestock or contaminated human feces, regions in which humans live near livestock and areas with poor hygiene and sanitation standards have a higher prevalence of tapeworm infections. Tapeworm infections tend to be endemic in developing countries, where sanitation is poor due to a lack of funding and medical treatment is often unavailable.

Tapeworm infections do still occur in developed countries for a number of reasons. Travel and immigration can be a source of tapeworm infection when infected people interact with noninfected people, potentially spreading the tapeworms. In addition, because tapeworm infections are usually asymptomatic, the tapeworm may go undetected for years before treatment is given and the tapeworm is removed from the body.

Tapeworm infections that occur when a human is used as an intermediate host can have devastating effects. For example, around 30 percent of all cases of epilepsy in the regions where *T. solium* is endemic are caused by untreated neurocysticercosis. Approximately 28,000 people worldwide die each year from *T. solium* infections.

See Also *Endemicity; Foodborne Disease and Food Safety; Handwashing; Parasitic Diseases; Sanitation; Taeniasis (*Taenia *Infection)*

BIBLIOGRAPHY

Books

Goater, Timothy M., Cameron P. Goater, and Gerald W. Esch. *Parasitism: The Diversity and Ecology of Animal Parasites.* 2nd ed. Cambridge, UK: Cambridge University Press, 2014.

Grove, David I. *Tapeworms, Lice, and Prions: A Compendium of Unpleasant Infections.* Oxford, UK: Oxford University Press, 2014.

Lamb, Tracey J., ed. *Immunity to Parasitic Infections.* Chichester, UK: Wiley-Blackwell, 2012.

Periodicals

Devleesschauwer, Brecht, et al. "Taenia Solium in Europe: Still Endemic?" *Acta Tropica* 165 (2017): 96–99.

Okello, Anna L., and Lian Francesca Thomas. "Human Taeniasis: Current Insights into Prevention and Management Strategies in Endemic Countries." *Risk Management and Healthcare Policy* 10 (2017): 107–116.

Websites

"Parasites—Hymenolepis." Centers for Disease Control and Prevention, January 10, 2012. https://www.cdc.gov/parasites/hymenolepis/ (accessed January 23, 2018).

"Tapeworm Infestation." Medscape, September 11, 2017. https://emedicine.medscape.com/article/786292-overview (accessed January 23, 2018).

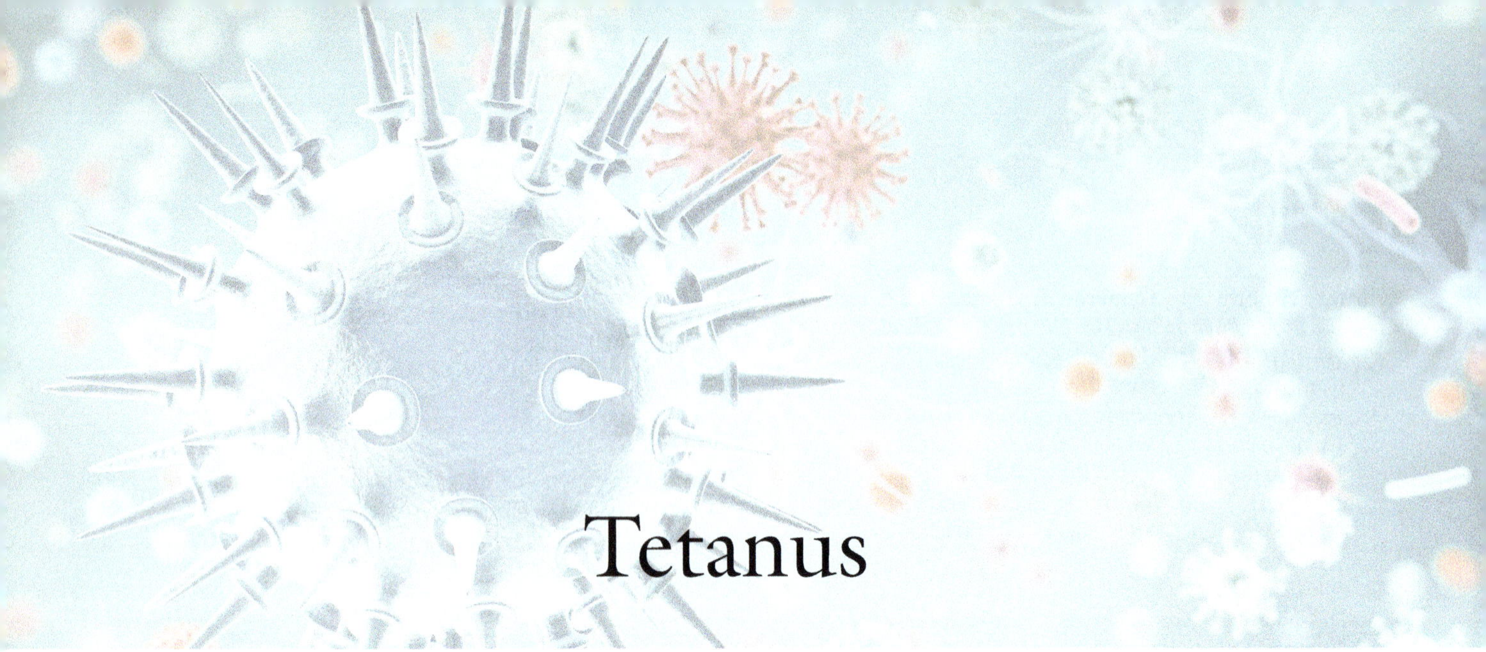

Tetanus

Introduction

Tetanus is a serious but easily prevented acute neurological disease that affects the muscles and nerves of the human body. The bacterium *Clostridium tetani* causes the disease, typically through any injury to the skin that becomes contaminated, such as a burn, crushing injury, cut, gangrene, or wound. Tetanus can also come about from the use of nonsterile needles for intravenous drugs, body piercing, and tattooing. Tetanus can be classified as local (muscle contraction in one local area) or cephalic (found in the middle ear). Newborn babies can also get neonatal tetanus, a special type of tetanus, when they are born in unsanitary conditions.

However, most tetanus is generalized tetanus, which descends from the head down through the body. Once in the human body, the bacteria produce a neurotoxin called tetanospasmin. The neurotoxin causes contraction and rigidity of the skeletal muscles. According to the US Centers for Disease Control and Prevention (CDC), tetanus cannot be spread from human to human. Thus, it is not contagious.

Disease History, Characteristics, and Transmission

Tetanus has been medically reported as far back as the 5th century BCE. According to the CDC, the first passively transferred antitoxin was developed in 1897. In 1924 the first tetanus toxoid was developed.

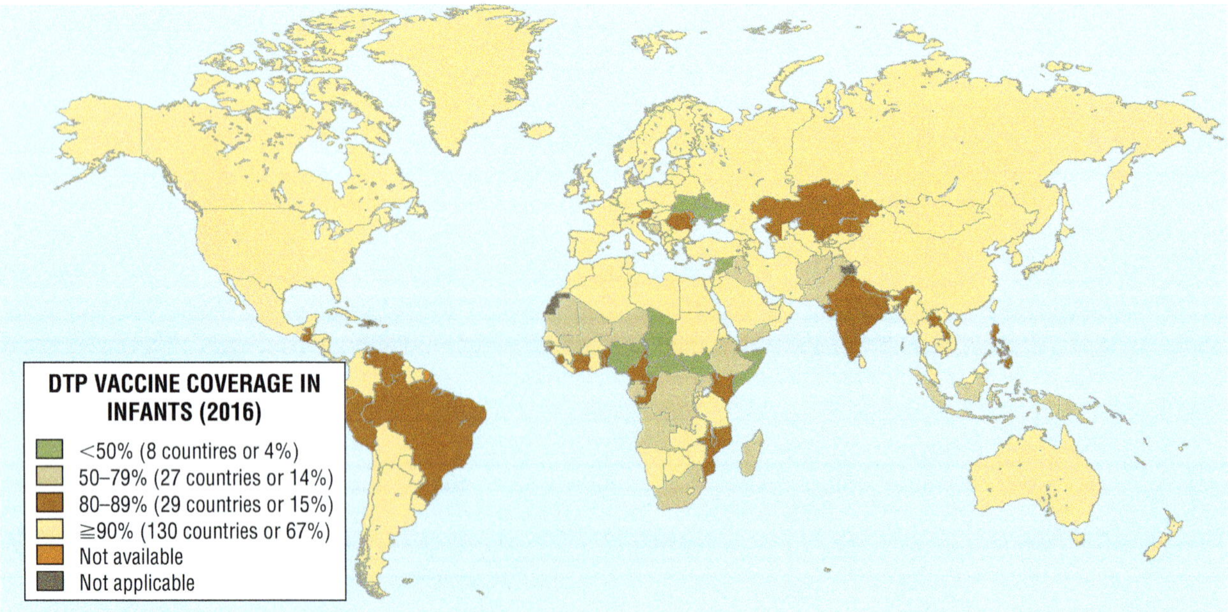

SOURCE: Adapted from "Immunization Coverage with DTP3 Vaccines in Infants (from <50%), 2016." World Health Organization/United Nations Children's Fund. Available from: http://www.who.int/immunization/monitoring_surveillance/burden/vpd/surveillance_type/passive/big_dtp3_map_global_coverage.jpg?ua=1

C. tetani is widely found in soil and in the intestines and feces of such animals as cattle, chickens, cats and dogs, guinea pigs, horses, rats, and sheep. Manure-treated soils also may contain large amounts of the bacteria. Cases of tetanus in the United States are usually from a cut or deep wound that has been contaminated with feces, saliva, or soil.

The puncture of the skin with a rusty nail, for instance, is typically seen as a source of tetanus. However, rust does not cause tetanus. Instead, the rust may harbor *C. tetani* on its surface, and the puncture caused by the nail can allow the bacteria to enter the body.

The first sign of tetanus is usually in the nerves that control the muscles near the wound where the bacteria entered the body. Later, as the bacteria have had time to travel through the bloodstream and lymph system, other nerves become adversely affected. The widely spreading bacteria soon produce general muscle spasms. Without treatment, tetanus can cause death to humans.

The incubation period for tetanus is 2 to 21 days. Symptoms often begin around the seventh or eighth day. Initial symptoms include muscle spasms in the jaw (known as trismus). These spasms give tetanus its more common name, lockjaw. Later, swallowing may become difficult, and stiffness or pain may occur in the muscles of the shoulders, neck, and back. Eventually, spasms may spread throughout the muscles of the upper arms, thighs, and abdomen. Other symptoms include fever, sweating, high blood pressure, and rapid heart rate. Symptoms generally begin to subside after about 17 days. Spasms may continue for three to four weeks. A complete recovery may take months.

WORDS TO KNOW

ANTITOXIN An antidote to a toxin that neutralizes the toxin's poisonous effects.

INCUBATION PERIOD The time between exposure to a disease-causing virus or bacteria and the appearance of symptoms of the infection. Depending on the microorganism, the incubation time can range from a few hours, such as with food poisoning due to *Salmonella*, to a decade or more, such as with acquired immunodeficiency syndrome (AIDS).

NEUROTOXIN A poison that interferes with nerve function, usually by affecting the flow of ions through the cell membrane.

TOXIN A poison produced by a living organism.

TOXOID A bacterial toxin that has been altered chemically to make it incapable of causing damage but still capable of stimulating an immune response. Toxoids are used to stimulate antibody production, which is protective in the event of exposure to the active toxin.

TRISMUS The medical term for lockjaw, a condition often associated with tetanus, which is an infection by the *Clostridium tetani* bacillus. In trismus or lockjaw, the major muscles of the jaw contract involuntarily.

Scope and Distribution

Tetanus is relatively rare in the United States and other countries with comprehensive tetanus vaccination programs to prevent and immunize their citizens when compared to countries without such programs. Most cases of tetanus occur in densely populated areas with

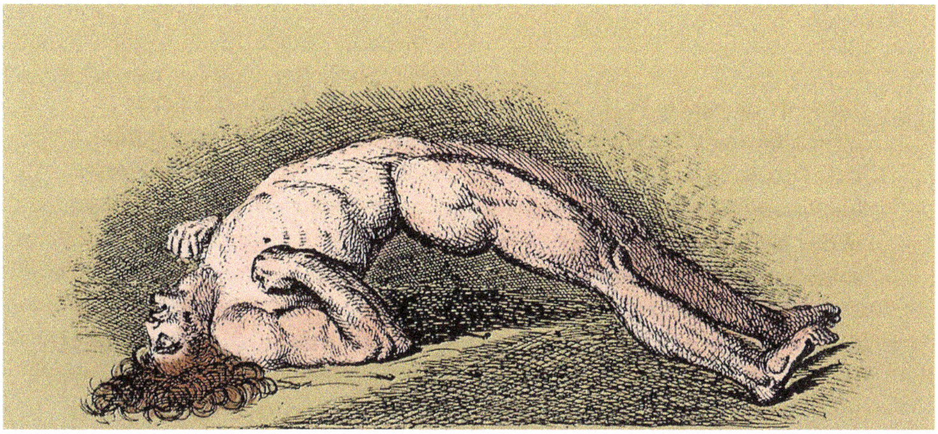

Tetanospasmin, the neurotoxin produced by *Clostridium tetani* bacteria, causes contraction and rigidity of the skeletal muscles. Illustrated here is a man suffering from opisthotonus ("the backward spasm") and lockjaw, two infamous symptoms caused by tetanospasmin. *© New York Public Library/Science Source*

hot, humid climates and rich organic soils. According to the CDC, 197 cases were reported in the United States between 2009 and 2015. Sixteen of these cases resulted in fatalities.

Since the introduction of the tetanus vaccine, tetanus has been on the decline. World Health Organization (WHO) global figures for 2016 noted 13,502 cases worldwide, a sharp decline from approximately 118,000 cases in 1980. Between the advent of statistical reporting established in 1947 and 2017, deaths declined 99 percent in the United States. This trend was in part due to the advent of the tetanus vaccine and use of tetanus antitoxin for wound management. However, despite the availability of immunization, tetanus remains a health concern. Lack of vaccine utilization and an improper dosing regimen continue to be the most common risk factors associated with this health problem. Ongoing surveillance by the National Notifiable Diseases Surveillance System continues to monitor prevalence, incidence, and regions most susceptible to the condition. Twenty-nine cases and two deaths were reported through the system in 2015. People most susceptible to death from tetanus are unvaccinated persons, young children, and those over the age of 60.

Treatment and Prevention

Tetanus is diagnosed only by clinical signs and symptoms. There is no laboratory confirmation for the bacteria. It is treated with a tetanus booster (for children still receiving their series of tetanus shots) or an injection of tetanus antitoxin, such as tetanus immune globulin (TIG), to neutralize any toxin released by the bacteria. Intravenous immune globulin (IVIG) can be given if TIG is unavailable. Metronidazole can be given to control bacteria. The wound should be cleaned, and all dead or infected skin should be removed. Severe cases of tetanus should be treated in the intensive care unit of a hospital. Medicines to control breathing and prevent muscle spasms are usually given.

Tetanus is prevented with a routine tetanus immunization. Children in the United States and other countries usually receive an injection that combines diphtheria and tetanus toxoids with pertussis vaccine. This immunization protects children from diphtheria (throat and respiratory infection), tetanus, and pertussis (whooping cough). The latest version is called the diphtheria and tetanus toxoids and acellular pertussis (DTaP) vaccine. The DTaP vaccine generally consists of a series of five shots in the arm or thigh given to children at 2 months, 4 months, 8 months, 15 to 18 months, and 4 to 6 years of age. The Mayo Clinic recommends that adolescents get a booster shot between the ages of 11 and 18. Thereafter, a vaccination should be given every 10 years.

Impacts and Issues

Although tetanus is rare, it is still a serious illness. It is considered an international health problem because so many people around the world are still unvaccinated or inadequately vaccinated. It is especially serious in children. As a result, children are often treated in intensive care units of hospitals after contracting tetanus. The child being treated in such situations will usually be given antibiotics to kill bacteria and TIG to neutralize the toxins. Medicines may be given to control muscle spasms. Other medicines may need to be given to support life functions for cases involving pneumonia and other respiratory problems.

Adults may also have complications including spasms of the vocal cords, spasms of the respiratory muscles, and fractures of the spine and longer bones of the body. Various treatment methods have been tried in such serious cases. However, no medical consensus has yet been reached as to the best method to use.

Even though tetanus can be prevented and treated, many countries do not immunize their citizens against tetanus. Many underdeveloped and developing countries continue to ignore the problem. Newborn babies are especially at risk in such countries. Their umbilical cords are likely to become infected due to unhygienic conditions during and following birth.

See Also *Bacterial Disease; CDC (Centers for Disease Control and Prevention); Diphtheria*

BIBLIOGRAPHY

Books

Bennett, John E., Raphael Dolin., and Martin J. Blaser. *Mandell, Douglas, and Bennett's Infectious Disease Essentials.* Philadelphia: Elsevier, 2016.

Bennett, John E., Raphael Dolin., and Martin J. Blaser. *Mandell, Douglas, and Bennett's Principles and Practice of Infectious Diseases.* 8th ed. Philadelphia: Elsevier, 2014.

Hamborsky, Jennifer, Andrew Kroeger, and Skip Wolfe, eds. *Epidemiology and Prevention of Vaccine-Preventable Diseases.* 13th ed. Atlanta: Centers for Disease Control and Prevention, 2015.

Holst, Otto., ed. *Microbial Toxins: Methods and Protocols.* 2nd ed. New York: Humana, 2017.

Murray, Patrick R., Ken S. Rosenthal, and Michael A. Pfaller. *Medical Microbiology.* Philadelphia: Elsevier, 2015.

Wilson, Walter R., and Merle A. Sande. *Current Diagnosis and Treatment in Infectious Diseases.* New York: McGraw Hill, 2014.

Periodicals

Advisory Committee on Immunization Practices, Centers for Disease Control and Prevention. "Preventing Tetanus, Diphtheria, and Pertussis among Adolescents: Use of Tetanus Toxoid, Reduced Diphtheria Toxoid and Acellular Pertussis Vaccines." *Morbidity and Mortality Weekly Report* 55 (February 23, 2006): 1–34. This article can also be found online at http://www.cdc.gov/mmwr/preview/mmwrhtml/rr55e223a1.htm (accessed December 9, 2017).

Advisory Committee on Immunization Practices, Centers for Disease Control and Prevention. "Preventing Tetanus, Diphtheria, and Pertussis among Adults: Use of Tetanus Toxoid, Reduced Diphtheria Toxoid and Acellular Pertussis Vaccines." *Morbidity and Mortality Weekly Report* 55 (December 15, 2006): 1–33. This article can also be found online at http://www.cdc.gov/mmwr/preview/mmwrhtml/rr5517a1.htm (accessed December 9, 2017).

Koepke, Ruth., et al. "Estimating the Effectiveness of Tetanus-Diphtheria-Acellular Pertussis Vaccine (Tdap) for Preventing Pertussis: Evidence of Rapidly Waning Immunity and Difference in Effectiveness by Tdap Brand." *Journal of Infectious Diseases* 210, no. 6 (September 15, 2014): 942–953.

Miller, Taylor, Patrick Olivieri, and Elizabeth Singer. "The Utility of Tdap in the Emergency Department." *American Journal of Emergency Medicine* 35, no. 9 (September 2017): 1348–1349.

Websites

"Tetanus." Centers for Disease Control and Prevention, April 14, 2017. https://www.cdc.gov/tetanus/index.html (accessed December 9, 2017).

"Tetanus." Mayo Clinic, August 8, 2017. https://www.mayoclinic.org/diseases-conditions/tetanus/symptoms-causes/syc-20351625 (accessed December 9, 2017).

"Tetanus Vaccination." Centers for Disease Control and Prevention, November 28, 2017. https://www.cdc.gov/vaccines/vpd/tetanus/index.html (accessed December 9, 2017).

Laurie J. Cataldo

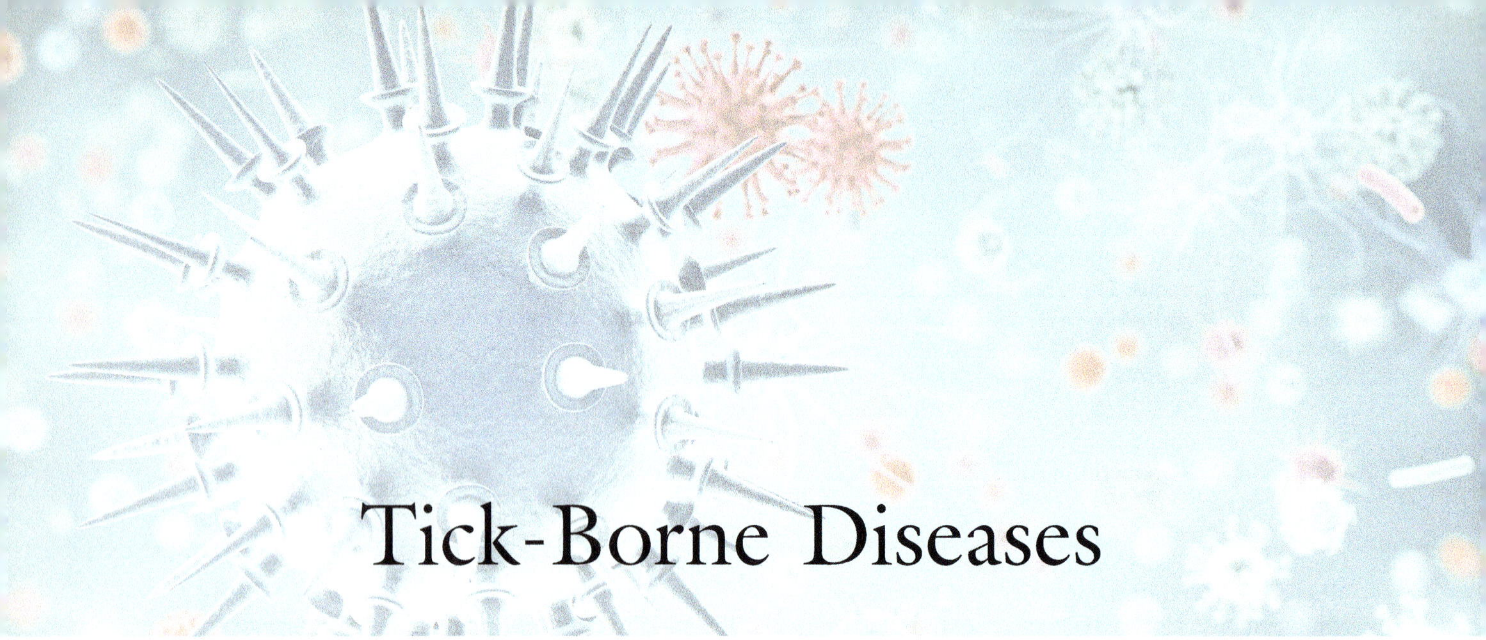

Tick-Borne Diseases

Introduction

Ticks are small arthropods from the class Arachnida. They are external parasites that feed on the blood of vertebrates, birds, and occasionally reptiles or amphibians. There are two major families of ticks found throughout the world: soft and hard ticks. A third family consists of a single species, *Nuttalliella namaqua*, and is found in sub-Saharan Africa.

The life cycle of ticks consists of four developmental stages. The female tick lays eggs. After 40 to 60 days, six-legged larvae appear. These larvae then change to eight-legged nymphs, which later transform into adults. Before each change ticks require a blood meal. It can take ticks up to three years to complete their life cycle. Although ticks are active throughout the year, most human transmissions occur in the spring and summer months.

Ticks are present worldwide and can cause and transmit numerous diseases. Their prime hosts are animals, with humans being accidental bite victims. Out of the 850 species of ticks, only a few are known to bite people and transmit diseases. Different infections are carried by different species of ticks. Species vary between continents and countries.

WORDS TO KNOW

ARACHNID An arthropod that belongs to class Arachnida, such as a spider or scorpion. Arachnids have eight legs, which differentiates them from six-legged insects.

ARTHROPOD A member of the largest single animal phylum, consisting of organisms with segmented bodies, jointed legs or wings, and exoskeletons.

PERMETHRIN A synthetic chemical used as insecticide. It is commonly used for insect control and can be found on food, crops, livestock, pets, and clothing. It affects the nervous system of the insects, resulting in death if consumed or touched by them. Humans and pets are more resistant to the effects but should still avoid consuming food covered with it, touching it, or breathing it.

RESERVOIR The animal or organism in which a virus or parasite normally resides.

VECTOR Any agent that carries and transmits parasites and diseases. Also, an organism or a chemical used to transport a gene into a new host cell.

Disease History, Characteristics, and Transmission

Diseases caused by ticks can be grouped into four categories: transmitted infections, allergic reactions to tick saliva, tick-derived red-meat allergies, and tick-induced paralysis. Transmitted infections can be viral, bacterial, or protozoan in origin. While feeding on infected animals, ticks ingest pathogens and then transmit them through saliva into the human bloodstream. Upon feeding, a tick will increase its size and become much more visible on a body. Once feeding is complete, the tick falls off the host.

Attachment to a host requires direct contact of the tick to a host, as ticks cannot fly or jump. Most frequently this contact happens when an animal host or a human host brushes against grass, leaves, or bushes with ticks on them. Once attached, ticks wander to find a feeding spot. Their preferred spots have thin skin cover and good blood supply, such as the arms or legs.

General symptoms of tick-borne infection are flu-like symptoms, including fever, chills, muscle aches, fatigue, and headache. Some infections produce a characteristic rash, which can help in diagnosing the disease. These are Lyme disease, southern tick-associated rash illness (STARI), Rocky Mountain spotted fever (RMSF), and tularemia. Lyme disease and STARI produce a rash that looks like a

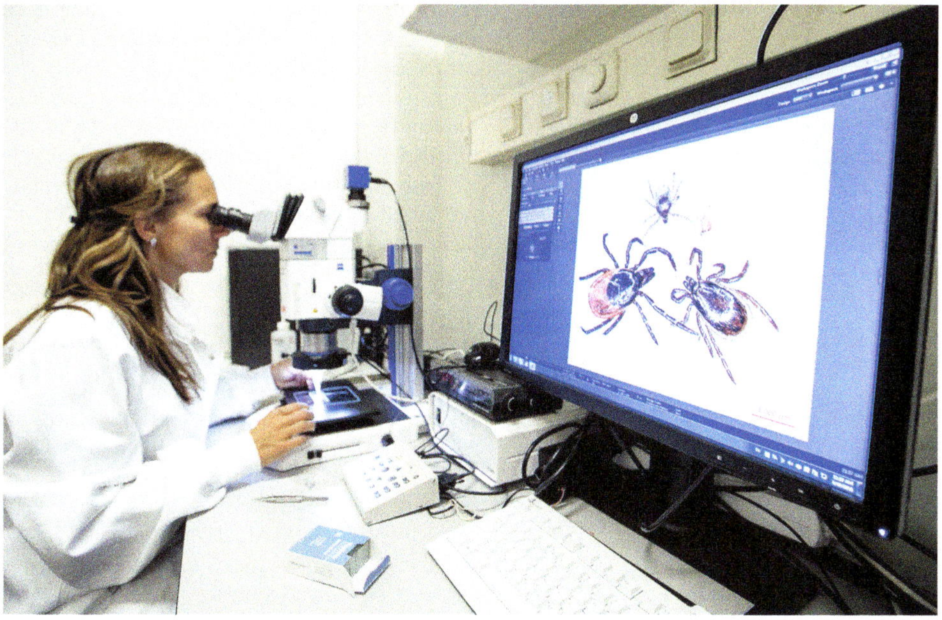

A researcher at the Dutch National Institute for Public Health and the Environment studies the tick-borne encephalitis (TBE) virus in 2016. The virus affects the central nervous system. © ROBIN VAN LONKHUIJSEN/AFP/Getty Images

target or bull's-eye. The difference between these two infections is lack of neurological symptoms in STARI. RMSF produces a rash in 90 percent of people. It starts with pink, nonitchy spots on the wrists, forearms, or ankles before spreading to the torso. A red rash develops six days after onset of symptoms.

In rare cases ticks can cause paralysis by secreting toxin in their saliva. This is easily treated by removing the tick. The allergic reaction can vary from mild with a local reaction to severe, which can lead to anaphylaxis. In case of a severe reaction, often due to disturbing the tick, it is important to kill the tick before removal. Another rare outcome of a tick bite is a red-meat allergy, which can be very severe and lead to anaphylactic shock.

Scope and Distribution

The major protozoan disease transmitted by ticks is babesiosis, caused by the parasite *Babesia spp.* infecting red blood cells. It is found in North America, Europe, Asia, and Australia. Vectors for the disease are the *Dermacentor* and *Ixodes* ticks, including *Ixodes ricinus* and *Ixodes scapularis.* The main reservoirs of *Babesia* are cattle, deer, and rodents.

Some of the bacterial infections are widespread and are present in the Americas, Europe, Asia, Africa, and Australia. These include:

- Lyme disease caused by *Borrelia burgdorferi*
- Relapsing fever caused by various *Borrelia* species
- Spotted fever Rickettsioses caused by rickettsia bacteria
- Anaplasmosis caused by *Anaplasma phagocytophilum*
- Ehrlichiosis caused by *Ehrlichia chaffeensis*

Others, such as Q fever and tularemia, have a narrower distribution. Q fever, caused by *Coxiella burnetii*, is associated with tick transmission in Australia. However, cases of the disease have been reported in the United States, Thailand, Japan, China, and Africa. Tularemia is caused by the bacteria *Francisella tularensis* and is widespread in the United States, with small outbreaks in Asia and northern Europe.

Some viral diseases are less widespread than others. Three viruses spread by ticks only in North America are Bourbon virus, Heartland virus, and Colorado tick fever (CTF), which is caused by CTF virus. All of these viruses cause fever, fatigue, headache, and body aches. Others, such as Crimean-Congo hemorrhagic fever (CCHF), tick-borne encephalitis (TBEV), and Powassan virus, are found on at least two continents.

Tick transmission of CCHF virus occurs in Asia, Africa, and Europe. This is an emerging disease in Europe with no vaccine or treatment. Fatality rates can reach 40 percent in some places. There is also no vaccine or treatment for Powassan virus, which is a tick-borne disease primarily found in North America and eastern Russia. This virus is capable of inducing encephalitis, with 10 percent of cases being fatal. In contrast, there is an effective vaccine against TBE virus found across Europe and northern Asia.

The species of ticks involved in transmission of diseases across the world vary with geographical location. In North America the most common ticks are American dog tick (*Dermacentor variabilis*), black-legged tick (*Ixodes scapularis*), brown dog tick (*Rhipicephalus sanguineus*), Gulf Coast tick (*Amblyomma maculatum*), lone star tick (*Amblyomma americanum*), Rocky Mountain wood tick (*Dermacentor andersoni*), and western black-legged tick (*Ixodes pacificus*). European ticks of special interest are *Ixodes ricinus, Hyalomma marginatum*, and *Ornithodoros* ticks (soft ticks). In Australia there are three known vectors: paralysis tick (*Ixodes holocyclus*), kangaroo tick (*Amblyomma triguttatum*), and southern reptile tick (*Bothriocroton hydrosauri*).

Treatment and Prevention

Prevention of tick bites is the best way to avoid any of the diseases spread by them. This can be achieved by dressing appropriately when working or hiking in tall grass, forest, or bush. Clothes should be light in color and should include a hat, long pants tucked into shoes or socks, a long-sleeve shirt, and enclosed shoes. Using insect repellent is also advised, as is use of permethrin-treated clothing. Bushy and high grass areas are best avoided when hiking. Ticks are most active during the spring and summer months, between April and September in the northern hemisphere and between August and February in the southern hemisphere.

Following exposure in a region infested with ticks, it is important to check whether any ticks have attached themselves to clothing, backpacks, pets, or other items. Clothing may need heat treatment to ensure that any potential ticks are removed. This can be done by washing them in hot water or drying them in a tumble dryer for 60 minutes on high heat or 90 minutes on low heat. It is important to remember that ticks are very small and hard to see on dark, hairy, or furry surfaces.

Taking a shower or bath should help to wash them away or expose their location. It is best to use a mirror or have someone else check difficult-to-see parts of the body, such as the back or neck. Pets should be checked using a fine-toothed comb or flea comb.

If a tick has attached to a human, it should be removed as soon as possible. Fine tweezers may be used to grab the tick close to the skin and then pull it slowly, in a steady motion, directly upward. If the tick breaks, the remaining part may be removed with tweezers. The wound should be cleaned with alcohol, iodine, or soap and water. If the tick is still alive, it should be submerged in alcohol, sealed in a plastic bag or container, or flushed down the toilet. It should not be crushed between the fingers. If a rash or other reaction develops, whether immediately or within weeks, a doctor should be consulted.

Carrying an epinephrine injector is recommended for people who know they have an allergy to tick saliva and serves as a means to kill an attached tick. In such people killing the tick is more important than removing it. Removal should be performed by medical staff in a safe environment to ensure anaphylactic reaction does not occur. Products recommended for killing ticks include ether-containing aerosol sprays.

Protozoan and bacterial infections, such as from *Babesia*, can be treated with antibiotics and quinine. Viral infections are treated symptomatically by reducing fever or pain. At least one viral infection, tick-borne encephalitis, can be prevented by a vaccine. It is advisable to talk to a doctor before heading into an area infected by ticks transmitting TBEV.

Impacts and Issues

Prevention of tick bites is extremely important, as not all of the diseases transmitted can be treated. None of the viral infections can be effectively treated, and only one can be prevented by vaccination. While in most cases infected individuals recover within days, there is risk of fatal complications such as encephalitis or persistence of chronic symptoms, as with Lyme disease.

Lyme disease is one of the most widespread and common tick-borne infections in the northern hemisphere. The typical rash may not develop in up to 50 percent of patients. Those individuals are at high risk of remaining untreated. If untreated, borreliosis or Lyme disease can result in side paralysis, joint pain, headache, neck stiffness, and even heart complications. The symptoms can last for months after the initial bite.

According to the US Centers for Disease Control and Prevention (CDC), as of 2013 there were up to 300,000 suspected cases of Lyme disease each year in the United States and more than 65,000 each year in Europe. The number of cases steadily increased in the following years, making Lyme disease an epidemiologically important illness. According to the CDC, as of 2015 Lyme disease was the sixth-most common notifiable disease in the United States, making it one of the top public health priorities. The main concern in Europe and North America is the incomplete recovery of those with late diagnosis. This can affect their quality of life and ability to work, and the problem is growing with more cases every year.

PRIMARY SOURCE

What You Know about Ticks May Be Just Wrong Enough!

SOURCE: *Mather, Thomas. "What You Know about Ticks May Be Just Wrong Enough!" University of Rhode Island TickEncounter Resource Center, December 3, 2017. http://www.tickencounter.org/tick_notes/just_wrong_enough (accessed March 1, 2018).*

INTRODUCTION: *Ticks and tick-borne disease received a lot of media attention in 2017. In this excerpt from a blog post from the University of Rhode Island's TickEncounter Resource Center, "Tick Guy" Thomas Mather, a professor of public health entomology at the university, addresses misinformation about ticks that many people believe is true.*

December 3, 2017

It seems that almost everyone knows something about TICKS, and that *should* be a good thing. We live in a "more ticks in more places world," and it seems like almost every other month scientists find yet another disease-causing germ in some type of tick. Besides, ticks are disgusting.

But the more we hear people telling us their tick stories, the more we're realizing that much of the information that a majority of people "know" about ticks is just wrong enough to leave them at risk. Often it means that they're not taking appropriate TickSmart precautions to keep themselves, their family, and their pets from getting a tick bite—or worse—one of those dangerous tickborne diseases.

Maybe you're already thinking—'What do you mean, "just wrong enough"?' Maybe you've read all the precautions on popular Lyme disease websites, or any number of well-intentioned books or pamphlets. But here's where we plug the importance of especially leaning in on the information that comes from public health entomologists—scientists with specific training about ticks, who are familiar with the difference between anecdote and empirical data, between what may make sense to a person and what makes "sense" to the tick. Someone with an empathetic open mind but tempered by dispassionate scientific reasoning. First-hand knowledge, not re-hashed and subject to misinterpretation. Like Joe Friday, "just the facts, m'am."

I was recently asked by a Baltimore newscaster to explain this "just wrong enough" thesis. So, I asked for him to tell me two things he knew about ticks; no lie, here's what he said:

1. "Ticks jump out of trees to get on you and suck your blood;" and
2. "Ticks die when it turns cold, so then we're not a risk."

Hoping that my response didn't sound too rude, I replied, "Hmmm ... but you'd be just wrong enough and likely still be at risk for a tick bite."

I went on to explain, that if ticks did jump out of trees —which, by the way, every tick biologist knows that they don't—you'd likely think it was most important to protect your head; you'd try to avoid walking under trees; your tick checks would focus on your head, potentially neglecting to check where the ticks more likely would be.

But instead, if what you knew was that ticks don't have eyes ... can't jump ... don't have sophisticated sensing equipment that can triangulate host speed and the effect of wind ... that if they missed their target they would then have to dust themselves off and crawl back up that tree to try again, which would be a huge drain of energy for an already hungry tick ... that they need high humidity just to survive and because of that they hang out close to the ground where humidity is higher ... and that all ticks crawl upward from the point where they latch on. If that's what you knew about ticks, then you'd be more likely to wear tick repellent shoes and pants, check for tiny ticks below the belt, and maybe, just maybe tuck your shirt in to keep the ticks on the outside of your clothing longer. That would be TickSmart!

And, oh BTW, if you're ever sitting under a tree and a "tick" falls on you, please look closely to see if it has 6 legs or 8. If you're not sure, take a picture and send it to Tickspotters. More than likely, it's going to be a 6-legged weevil or aphid, harmless bugs—not a tick but just a tock look-alike.

What about ticks dying when it turns cold? If they did, then where would the next year's crop of ticks come from? In truth, some types of ticks like American dog ticks do cease their host-seeking activity in August as the day length gets shorter leading towards colder weather. But die? Every tick biologist knows that each type of tick and life-stage of tick has its own season of activity. Ticks have adapted over eons to survive and even thrive under the conditions typically found in their season of activity. Tick seasons have been like they are for a long while and are not likely to change anytime soon, so it's TickSmart to know what types of ticks are active at different times of the year where you live—we've got an app for that, too.

And it turns out that just when the weather turns cold, when we get our first killing frost up in the northeastern states, that is indeed peak season for the adult stage blacklegged tick vectors of Lyme disease in the east and south. And head's up West Coast: December is when adult stage western blacklegged ticks appear, too. If it gets too cold for these ticks to move their little leg muscles, then they can't latch on or crawl up. But they're not dead (thanks perhaps to some antifreeze proteins they produce). Just a little bit of warmth, and they are ready for action. In the southeastern states, they're ready for action pretty much all winter long.

See Also *Babesiosis; Crimean-Congo Hemorrhagic Fever; Encephalitis; Lyme Disease; Notifiable Diseases; Q Fever; Relapsing Fever; Rickettsial Disease; Rocky Mountain Spotted Fever; Tularemia*

BIBLIOGRAPHY

Books

Nuttall, Patricia A., and M. Labuda. "Saliva-Assisted Transmission of Tick-Borne Pathogens." In *Ticks: Biology, Disease and Control*, edited by Alan S. Bowman and Patricia A. Nuttall, 205–219. New York: Cambridge University Press, 2008.

Periodicals

Mansfield, K. L., et al. "Tick-Borne Encephalitis Virus: A Review of an Emerging Zoonosis." *Journal of General Virology* 90 (2009): 1781–1794.

Pfeffer, Martin, and Gerhard Dobler. "Emergence of Zoonotic Arboviruses by Animal Trade and Migration." *Parasites and Vectors* 3 (2010): 35–49. This article can also be found online at https://parasitesandvectors.biomedcentral.com/articles/10.1186/1756-3305-3-35 (accessed February 25, 2018)

Shapiro, E. D. "Clinical Practice: Lyme Disease." *New England Journal of Medicine* 370, no. 18 (May 2014): 1724–1731.

Stone, B., et al. "Brave New Worlds: The Expanding Universe of Lyme Disease." *Vector Borne and Zoonotic Diseases* 17, no. 9 (2017): 619–629.

Van Nunen, S., et al. "The Association between *Ixodes holocyclus* Tick Bite Reactions and Red Meat Allergy." *Internal Medicine Journal* 39, no. S5 (2007): A132.

Websites

"Life Cycle of Hard Ticks That Spread Disease." Centers for Disease Control and Prevention, April 20, 2017. https://www.cdc.gov/ticks/life_cycle_and_hosts.html (accessed February 25, 2018).

"Q Fever: Epidemiology and Statistics." Centers for Disease Control and Prevention, December 26, 2017. https://www.cdc.gov/qfever/stats/index.html (accessed February 25, 2018).

"Tick Allergy." Australasian Society of Clinical Immunology and Allergy, 2016. https://allergy.org.au/images/pcc/ASCIA_PCC_Tick_allergy_2016.pdf (accessed February 25, 2018).

"Tick-Borne Diseases." European Centre for Disease Prevention and Control, 2018. https://ecdc.europa.eu/en/tick-borne-diseases (accessed February 25, 2018).

"Tickborne Diseases of the United States: A Reference Manual for Health Care Providers." Centers for Disease Control and Prevention, 2017. https://www.cdc.gov/lyme/resources/TickborneDiseases.pdf (accessed February 25, 2018).

"Ticks." Centers for Disease Control and Prevention, May 22, 2017. https://www.cdc.gov/ticks/index.html (accessed February 25, 2018).

"Ticks and Tick-Borne Diseases Protecting Yourself." Australian Association of Bush Regenerators, May 2, 2014. http://aabr.org.au/site/wp-content/uploads/2013/12/AABR-Ticks-and-tick-borne-diseases-protecting-yourself1.pdf (accessed February 25, 2018).

"Why Is CDC Concerned about Lyme Disease?" Centers for Disease Control and Prevention, December 1, 2017. https://www.cdc.gov/lyme/why-is-cdc-concerned-about-lyme-disease.html (accessed February 25, 2018).

Agnes Caruso

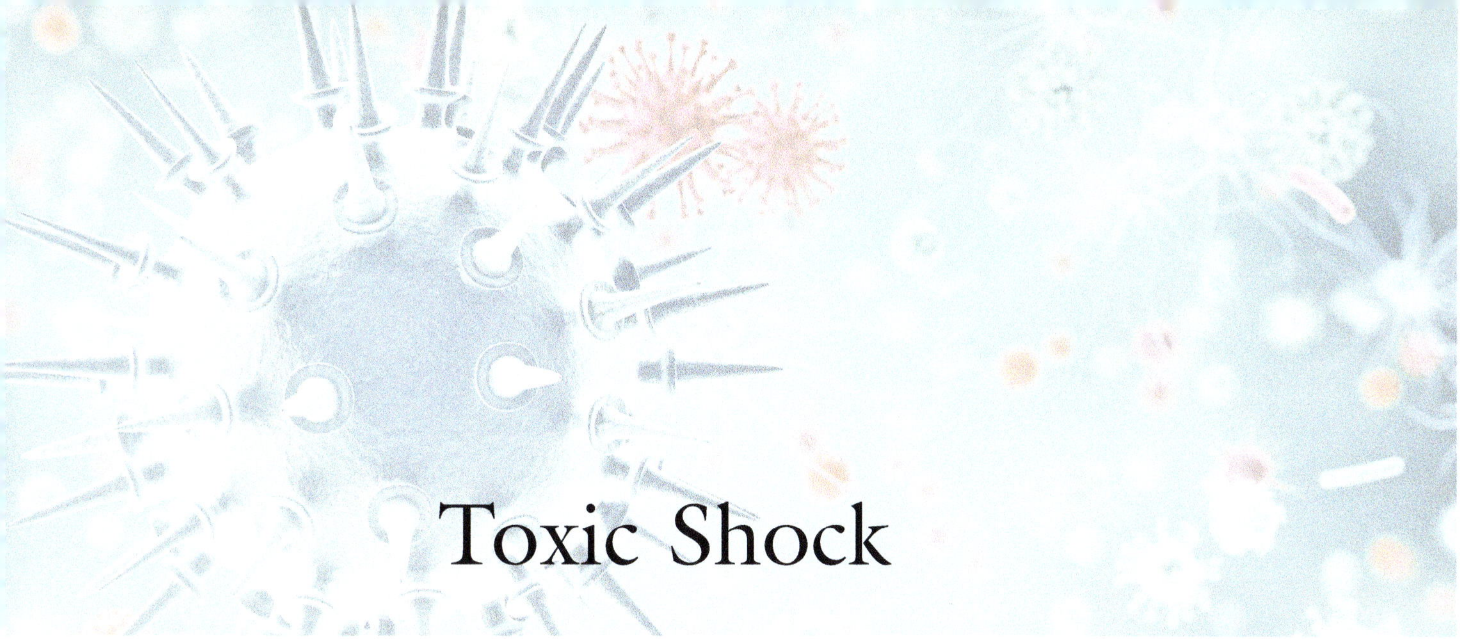

Toxic Shock

Introduction

Toxic shock syndrome (TSS) is a potentially fatal form of blood poisoning that is usually associated with a toxin-producing strain of the bacterium *Staphylococcus aureus.* It has been associated with the use of certain high-absorbency tampons during menstruation but may also arise after surgery and as a consequence of severe burns.

In any form of shock, the circulation is impaired, blood pressure falls dramatically, and body organs begin to fail. Burns, severe blood loss, traumatic injury, and infections can cause shock, but in toxic shock the bacterial toxin is the underlying cause. Intensive care with rehydration and monitoring of vital functions such as respiration and blood pressure are necessary to treat a patient in shock.

Toxic shock syndrome is a rare condition, and in its early stages may be confused with other illnesses. Prompt and accurate diagnosis of TSS is essential.

Disease History, Characteristics, and Transmission

Most cases of toxic shock are caused by exposure to a toxin-producing strain of *S. aureus*, a normally harmless bacterium. According to a report by CNN, about 50 percent of the population may intermittently carry *S. aureus*, and about 20 percent may carry it all the time. Some strains produce toxins that can cause toxic shock. The most common of these is known as toxic shock syndrome toxin, but others have been identified. The toxin invades the blood through a "focus" of infection, such as a postoperative wound or a tampon used during menstruation. A few cases of toxic shock have been linked to group A streptococcus or *Streptococcus pyogenes*, which also causes scarlet fever and necrotizing fasciitis, a deep-tissue infection known as "flesh-eating disease."

Symptoms of toxic shock come on suddenly and include high fever, a sunburn-like rash, diarrhea, vomiting, fainting, dizziness, and confusion. There is a dramatic fall in blood pressure, which can lead to multi-organ failure affecting the liver, kidneys, heart, and brain. According to the *Washington Post*, the fatality rate of toxic shock is 5 to 15 percent due to *S. aureus* but jumps to 30 to 70 percent for streptococcal TSS. It can mimic other conditions, such as severe flu, in its earlier stages. One or two weeks after the illness, the skin on the palms and soles may start to peel. Long-term complications of toxic shock include memory loss, decreased ability to concentrate, and emotional instability.

Scope and Distribution

Toxic shock is rare, but the risk of TSS is greater among young people. About half of all TSS cases are associated with women using tampons, and the rest result from localized infections, usually following burns, boils, insect bites, or surgery.

WORDS TO KNOW

SHOCK A medical emergency in which the organs and tissues of the body are not receiving an adequate flow of blood. This condition deprives the organs and tissues of oxygen (carried in the blood) and allows the buildup of waste products. Shock can result in serious damage or even death.

TOXIC Something that is poisonous and that can cause illness or death.

TOXIN A poison produced by a living organism.

TRENDS AND STATISTICS

According to the National Center for Biotechnology Information, US National Library of Medicine, "The incidence of TSS is estimated to be around 0.8 to 3.4 per 100,000 in the United States. The incidence tends to be higher in the winter and is more prevalent in developing countries."

Treatment and Prevention

Antibiotics can reduce the risk of recurrence of toxic shock but cannot always modify the course of the illness. Clindamycin, usually in combination with another antibiotic, is often recommended, as it reduces the rate of production of toxin from *S. aureus.* Foreign bodies associated with the infection, such as a tampon, must be removed, and infected wounds should be cleaned.

Intensive care is generally needed to treat shock. The circulation and supply of oxygen to affected organs must be restored with rehydration therapy. Blood pressure, respiration, and other vital functions must be monitored constantly.

Women can avoid TSS associated with tampons by using a tampon with the lowest possible absorbency and changing them every four to six hours. In addition, women can avoid TSS associated with menstrual cups, menstrual sponges, and diaphragms by removing them regularly.

Impacts and Issues

Toxic shock is a rare condition and may not be readily recognized. The symptoms accompanying TSS, such as fever or rash, occur in many other illnesses. However, multi-organ failure can occur rapidly once the *S. aureus* toxin has entered the bloodstream, at which point the patient's life may be in danger. Therefore, prompt medical attention is needed whenever there is a rapid onset of fever and other symptoms.

In 1980 an outbreak of TSS occurred among women who used a certain tampon brand. Researchers traced most cases to use of the Rely superabsorbent tampon designed to be used over several hours or even days, though there were cases in women who used other superabsorbent brands. From March 1980 to March 1981, almost 1,000 US women were diagnosed with TSS. Forty women died. When Rely and similar superabsorbent tampons were taken off the market, incidence of TSS dropped dramatically the following year. However, researchers noted that fewer women used any tampons immediately following the TSS outbreak. More modern tampons are designed to be

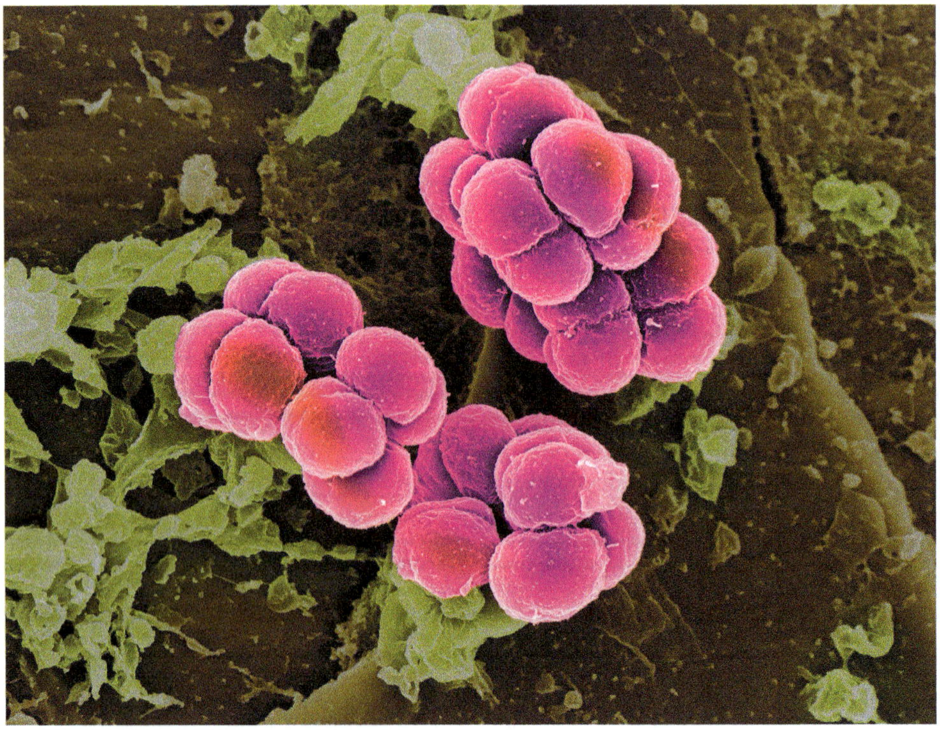

Staphylococcus aureus, the bacterium responsible for toxic shock syndrome, on a nasal hair under an electron microscope. *© Dr. Stanley Flegler/Visuals Unlimited, Inc./Getty Images*

changed more frequently, and women are encouraged to use tampons of varying absorbencies to match their menstrual flow. Tampons are also now packaged and sold with informative literature about TSS and TSS prevention.

Discussion of toxic shock syndrome was revived in English-language media in 2015 when American model Lauren Wasser developed TSS from a tampon. She became gravely ill and needed to have a leg amputated to survive. Wasser had the remaining leg amputated in 2018 to reduce lingering pain in the appendage. Since recovering from TSS, she has worked to educate women about tampon safety.

A possible drug to combat TSS is undergoing animal trials. Injection of a specific peptide called AB103 has been shown to reduce death rates of rats and mice infected with *Staphylococcus aureus* and group A *Streptococcal pyogenes*. The effect of AB103 in humans with such infections is still unknown as of early 2018.

See Also Staphylococcus aureus *Infections; Streptococcal Infections, Group A*

BIBLIOGRAPHY

Books

Stone, C. Keith, and Roger Humphries. *Current Diagnosis and Treatment: Emergency Medicine.* New York: McGraw-Hill Education, 2017.

Periodicals

Burnham, Jason P., and Marin H. Kollef. "Understanding Toxic Shock Syndrome." *Intensive Care Medicine* 41, no. 9 (September 2015): 1707–1710.

Cowart, Leigh. "Women Are Still Getting Toxic Shock Syndrome, and No One Quite Knows Why." *Washington Post* (March 21, 2016). This article can also be found online at https://www.washingtonpost.com/news/speaking-of-science/wp/2016/03/21/women-are-still-getting-toxic-shock-syndrome-and-no-one-quite-knows-why/?utm_term=.eccd5e2bcc05 (accessed January 17, 2018).

Fetters, Ashley. "The Tampon: A History." *Atlantic* (June 1, 2015). This article can also be found online at https://www.theatlantic.com/health/archive/2015/06/history-of-the-tampon/394334/ (accessed January 17, 2018).

Websites

Morgan, Kate. "Use Tampons? Don't Panic about Toxic Shock Syndrome." CNN, December 22, 2017. http://www.cnn.com/2017/12/22/health/toxic-shock-syndrome-partner/index.html (accessed January 17, 2018).

Ross, Adam, and Hugh W. Shoff. "Toxic Shock Syndrome." National Center for Biotechnology Information, US National Library of Medicine, October 6, 2017. https://www.ncbi.nlm.nih.gov/books/NBK459345/ (accessed January 17, 2018).

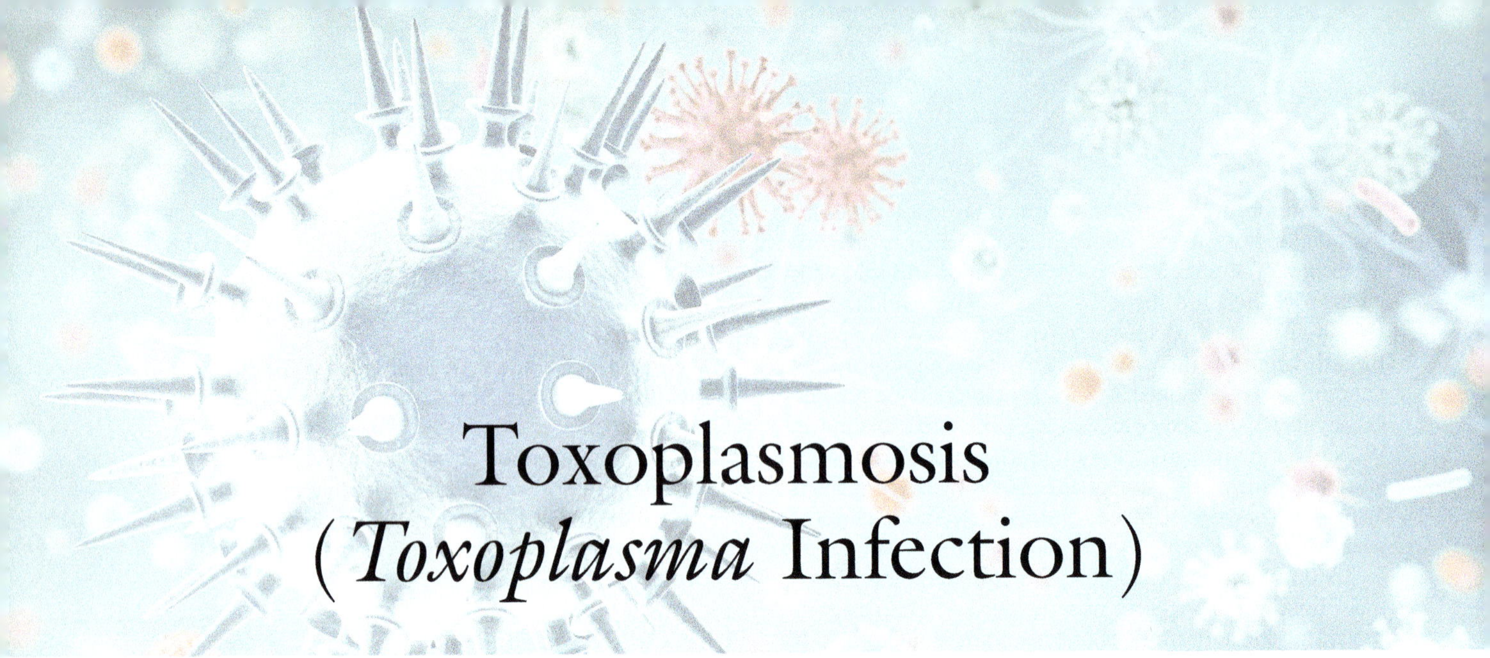

Toxoplasmosis (*Toxoplasma* Infection)

Introduction

Toxoplasmosis (TOX-o-plaz-MO-sis) refers to an infection caused by a protozoan, a type of microorganism. The protozoan responsible for the infection is *Toxoplasma gondii.* The infection is part of a parasitic association between *T. gondii* and a human host. The microbe benefits from the association, but the host does not. In the case of toxoplasmosis, the infection enables the protozoan to complete its life cycle.

Toxoplasmosis, or toxo, is a serious concern in people whose immune systems are not functioning properly, such as those with acquired immunodeficiency syndrome (AIDS). For those with AIDS, toxoplasmosis can be lethal.

WORDS TO KNOW

ENCEPHALITIS A type of acute brain inflammation, most often due to infection by a virus.

OOCYST A spore phase of certain infectious organisms that can survive for a long time outside the organism and therefore continue to cause infection and resist treatment.

PROTOZOA Single-celled animal-like microscopic organisms that live by taking in food rather than making it by photosynthesis and must live in the presence of water. (Singular: protozoan.) Protozoa are a diverse group of single-celled organisms, with more than 50,000 different types represented. The vast majority are microscopic, many measuring less than 0.005 of an inch (0.13 millimeters), but some, such as the freshwater *Spirostomun,* may reach 0.17 inches (4.3 millimeters) in length, large enough to enable it to be seen with the naked eye.

ZOONOSES Diseases of microbiological origin that can be transmitted from animals to people. The causes of the diseases can be bacteria, viruses, parasites, and fungi.

Disease History, Characteristics, and Transmission

Toxoplasmosis is an example of a zoonotic disease, a disease passed from animals to humans. The animal most responsible for the spread of toxoplasmosis is the cat. The US Centers for Disease Control and Prevention (CDC) estimated that as of 2017 approximately 30 percent of domestic cats in the United States harbored *T. gondii.* Cats can acquire the protozoan by eating infected rodents. Other animals can carry the protozoan, including cattle, sheep, or other livestock, which poses an increased risk to farmers, ranchers, veterinarians, and others who come in contact with farm animals.

T. gondii has a life cycle that involves two forms of the organism. The actively growing and dividing form causes the disease. This is not typically the form of the organism that first enters the body, however. Rather, a person ingests the form known as an oocyst. A smaller and hardier form of *T. gondii* that is analogous to a bacterial spore, an oocyst is designed to survive environmental conditions that would otherwise kill the growing protozoan. When ingested, the oocyst can convert to the growing form in the less hostile conditions of the intestinal tract.

Oocysts are shed in the feces of cats and other animals. People can ingest the oocysts after stroking a cat's fur (on which oocysts can stick, although this route is rare), by handling a cat's litter box and not properly washing their hands before hand-to-mouth contact, by eating produce that was irrigated with oocyst-contaminated water, or by eating undercooked meat that contains the protozoan. Eating undercooked meat is the most common route of infection.

Following the regeneration of the *T. gondii* oocysts into the growing form, the symptoms of toxoplasmosis are produced. These include a fever that comes and goes, swollen lymph nodes, generalized muscle pain, and fatigue. For

EFFECTIVE RULES AND REGULATIONS FOR KEEPING A CAT

The Centers for Disease Control and Prevention (CDC); the National Center for HIV/AIDS, Viral Hepatitis, STD, and TB Prevention (NCHHSTP); and the Division of HIV/AIDS Prevention (DHAP) state that even people at risk for a severe infection (e.g., those with a weakened immune system or who are pregnant) may still keep cats as pets if at-risk persons follow safety precautions as shown below to avoid being exposed to *Toxoplasma*. People at risk should consult with their personal health care provider for full details.

- Have someone who is healthy and not pregnant change your cat's litter box daily. If this is not possible, wear gloves and clean the litter box every day because the parasite found in cat feces needs one or more days after being passed to become infectious. Wash your hands well with soap and water afterward.
- Keep your cat indoors to prevent it from hunting. Feed your cat dry or canned cat food rather than allowing it to have access to wild birds and rodents or to eat food scraps. A cat can become infected by eating infected prey or by eating raw or undercooked meat infected with the parasite. Do not bring a new cat into your house that might have spent time out of doors or might have been fed raw meat.
- Feed your cat only cat food or cook all meat thoroughly before giving it to your cat.
- Do not give your cat raw or undercooked meat.
- If you adopt or buy a cat, get one that is healthy and at least one year old.
- Avoid stray cats and kittens. They are more likely than other cats to be infected.
- Your veterinarian can answer any other questions you may have regarding your cat and risk for toxoplasmosis.

those who recover fairly rapidly, protection from a future infection is guaranteed for life. For others, toxoplasmosis can persist as a chronic infection. Chronic toxoplasmosis can cause retinochoroiditis, an inflammation of the eyes. This condition can cause jaundice, a yellowing of the skin and the whites of the eyes. More seriously, inflammation of the brain, or encephalitis, can produce numbness, severe headaches, impaired vision or blindness, and convulsions.

Toxoplasmosis is not readily spread from person to person. An exception is the spread from mother to fetus

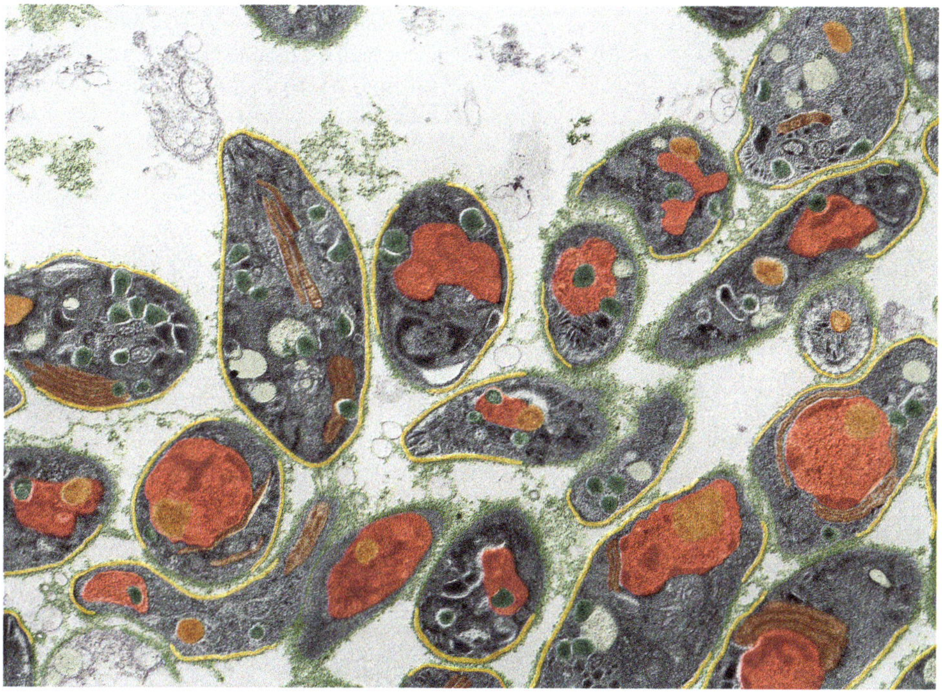

Toxoplasma gondii is a parasitic protozoa. Human consumption of *T. gondii* oocytes can result in toxoplasmosis. The infection is a serious threat to pregnant women and to people whose immune systems do not function properly, such as AIDS patients. *© Eye of Science/Science Source*

that can occur during pregnancy. As of 2017 approximately 6 out of every 1,000 pregnant women acquire the infection; about half of these women pass the infection to the fetus. In the United States over 3,000 cases of congenital toxoplasmosis occur each year. In newborns, toxoplasmosis can be rapidly lethal. Other newborns will retain the infection and display symptoms months or years later.

Scope and Distribution

Toxoplasmosis is global in distribution and its incidence is common. In 2017 the CDC reported that approximately 11 percent of the US population six years and older has been infected with *Toxoplasma*, whereas up to 95 percent of populations in various places worldwide have been infected.

Treatment and Prevention

As with many other microbial diseases, good personal hygiene, including handwashing, is an important preventive measure. Pregnant women should not handle cat litter. Common-sense food-handling precautions, such as washing cutting boards after use, help minimize the risk of transferring meat-borne *T. gondii*.

Medication can be prescribed for pregnant women and those with AIDS to kill the protozoan, even those residing in the brain. Other medications prevent the protozoan from acquiring vitamin B, which is vital for its survival.

Impacts and Issues

For most people who become infected with *T. gondii*, there is little danger, as they have the immune system capability to fight off the infection. However, for people with a malfunctioning immune system, toxoplasmosis is a serious, even lethal, disease. People with AIDS, infants, the elderly, and those whose immune systems have been deliberately impaired to avoid rejection of a transplant are at risk.

SEE ALSO *Parasitic Diseases; Zoonoses*

BIBLIOGRAPHY

Books

Akyar, Isin, ed. *Toxoplasmosis.* London: InTechOpen, 2017.

Ribeiro, Janete N. *Human Toxoplasmosis: Clinical Data and Microbiology.* Rio de Janeiro: Luiz Galileu Spoladore, 2016.

Periodicals

McAuley, James B. "Congenital Toxoplasmosis." *Journal of the Pediatric Infectious Diseases Society* 3, no. S1 (September 2014): S30–S35.

Torgerson, Paul R., and Pierpaolo Mastroiacovo. "The Global Burden of Toxoplasmosis: A Systematic Review." *Bulletin of the World Health Organization* 91 (May 2013): 501–508.

Websites

Guerina, Nicholas, and Lucila Marquez. "Congenital Toxoplasmosis: Clinical Features and Diagnosis." UpToDate. http://www.uptodate.com/contents/congenital-toxoplasmosis-clinical-features-and-diagnosis (accessed on November 22, 2017).

"Parasites: Toxoplasmosis (Toxoplasma Infection)." Centers for Disease Control and Prevention. https://www.cdc.gov/parasites/toxoplasmosis/index.html (accessed on November 22, 2017).

Brian Hoyle

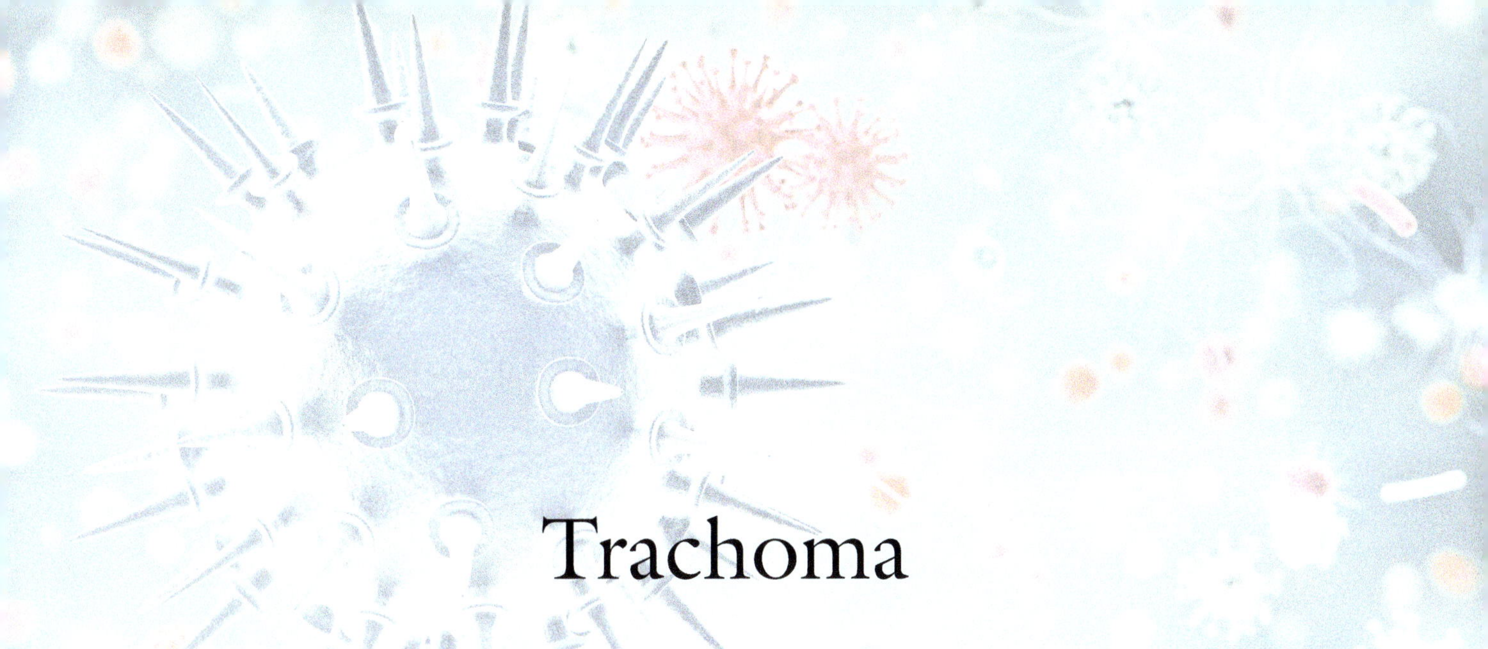

Trachoma

Introduction

Trachoma, also called granular conjunctivitis and Egyptian ophthalmia, is a contagious bacterial disease of the eye caused by the bacterium *Chlamydia trachomatis.* Flies become infected when they lay eggs on human feces lying in soil. The infection occurs when a host fly, infected with the bacterium, bites a human. A fly can also become a host and harbor the bacteria when it makes direct contact with eye, nose, or throat secretions from an infected person. The bacterium can also be carried directly to humans from contaminated hands by fomites (objects contaminated with infective material) such as clothing. The disease is reported as one of the leading infectious causes of blindness.

Disease History, Characteristics, and Transmission

The International Trachoma Initiative (ITI) states that trachoma is one of the oldest infectious diseases known to humankind and was reported as far back as ancient Egypt. General improvements in public health and sanitation have eliminated trachoma from most industrialized nations such as those in North America and Europe. However, it continues to infect people at high rates in developing countries around the world.

An incubation period of about 5 to 12 days occurs before the eye becomes inflamed. Then additional symptoms occur, including pus discharge, eyelid swelling, eye tearing, and light sensitivity. Within a few weeks more symptoms begin to appear, including chronic swelling (such as swelling of lymph nodes in front of the ears), eye blisters, cornea clouding, and cornea scarring. Extensive damage to the cornea can eventually lead to blindness.

Scope and Distribution

According to the World Health Organization (WHO), about 2.2 million people are visually impaired because of trachoma and about 21 million people suffer active symptoms. An estimated 1.2 million people were blind from trachoma as of 2017. It causes 1.4 percent of the blindness occurring throughout the world.

Trachoma is hyperendemic in 41 countries. According to WHO, "Overall, Africa remains the most affected continent, and the one with the most intensive control efforts." Trachoma occurs most commonly among populations living in overcrowded conditions and with limited contact to clean water and health care facilities. Children and women who take care of children are most susceptible to trachoma. Children between the ages of three and five are most at risk among all groups of children, according to WHO.

WORDS TO KNOW

FOMITE An object or a surface to which an infectious microorganism such as bacteria or viruses can adhere and be transmitted. Transmission is often by touch.

HOST An organism that serves as the habitat for a parasite or possibly for a symbiont. A host may provide nutrition to the parasite or symbiont, or it may simply provide a place in which to live.

HYPERENDEMIC Endemic (commonly present) in all age groups of a population. A related term is *holoendemic*, meaning a disease that is present more in children than in adults.

MORBIDITY A term that comes from the Latin word *morbus*, which means sick. In medicine it refers not just to the state of being ill but also to the severity of the illness. A serious disease is said to have a high morbidity.

DISEASE ELIMINATION EFFORTS

In 1996 the World Health Organization (WHO) began a campaign to eliminate trachoma by 2020 known as the WHO Alliance for the Global Elimination of Trachoma by the Year 2020 (GET2020). WHO stated that "GET2020 is a partnership which supports country implementation of the SAFE strategy and the strengthening of national capacity through epidemiological assessment, monitoring, surveillance, project evaluation and resource mobilization." Significant reduction of trachoma in affected countries has occurred since 1996. As of July 1, 2017, 10 countries reported to WHO that they had virtually eliminated trachoma, including Cambodia, China, Gambia, Ghana, Islamic Republic of Iran, Lao People's Democratic Republic, Mexico, Morocco, Myanmar, and Oman.

When infected early in life, the person may not notice the degradation in sight until adulthood.

In wealthy, industrialized countries, trachoma is rare, although it can occur in populations living in extreme poverty and crowdedness, as well as those with poor hygienic conditions.

Treatment and Prevention

According to the National Library of Medicine (NLM) of the National Institutes of Health (NIH), symptoms start as an apparent irritation near the eye known as conjunctivitis (pink eye). Soon, hard pimples or granular outgrowths appear on the inner surface of the eyelids, and inflammation occurs on its membrane.

If left untreated, scar tissue develops on the inside of the eyelid. Such scarring in children is usually not noticeable until they are adults. Formation of scarring eventually forces the eyelid to curve inward and the eyelashes to scrape the eye. Severe infection of the cornea can occur later. This activity can cause eye ulcers, which further cause scarring and vision problems. Eventually, slow and painful blindness develops over many years.

In the early stage of the infection, trachoma responds well to oral or topical antibiotics such as azithromycin, doxycycline, and erythromycin. Officials from NLM/NIH report that people who receive early treatment for trachoma before scarring and lid deformities occur have an excellent chance of being cured. WHO recommends using oral eye ointments such as azithromycin and tetracycline to control trachoma.

According to WHO, relief from trachoma can be attained by following the SAFE strategy: surgery, antibiotics, facial cleanliness, and environmental improvement. Surgery can be performed to correct advanced problems related to the disease. Early treatment with antibiotics can prevent

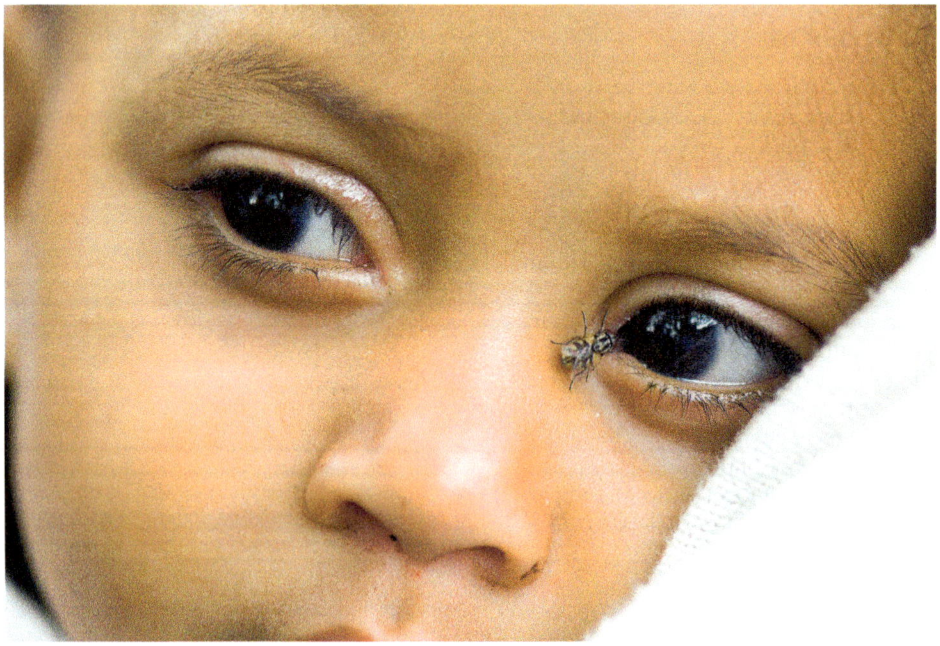

A female *Musca sorbens* fly lands on the eye of a small child in Ethiopia. Bites from infected *Musca sorbens* flies spread trachoma, one of the leading infectious causes of blindness. *© Louise Gubb/Corbis/Getty Images*

long-term complications. Good hygiene such as washing of the face should be consistently and thoroughly practiced to reduce transmission. Access to clean water and improved sanitation facilities (especially the safe disposal of human and animal feces) also help greatly to reduce the occurrence and severity of the disease.

In addition, regular eye examinations can pinpoint abnormal redness on the white areas of the eyes, scarring on the inside of the upper eyelid, and improper blood vessel growth on the corneas. Laboratory tests, especially the polymerase chain reaction (PCR) technique, are used to identify the bacterium that causes trachoma. Such tests, however, are usually too costly for use in the poorest areas of the world where trachoma occurs the most.

Impacts and Issues

The infection often results in significant morbidity, striking people during their productive working years. According to WHO, women are two to four times more likely to become blind after becoming infected with trachoma than men. Often they cannot take care of themselves and their children when infected by the disease, especially when they are blinded. Consequently, WHO reported that about $2.9 billion to $5.3 billion is lost worldwide annually in human productivity because of trachoma.

Common complications of trachoma include scarring of the conjunctiva (membrane under the eyes) and cornea, eyelid abnormalities, turned-in eyelashes, vision reductions, and, in severe cases, blindness. The prognosis for each individual depends on the severity of the disease, the treatment used to combat it, and the number of times the eyes are reinfected. People with trachoma who are treated with the proper drugs and in the early stage of the infection are much more likely to fully recover. Severe symptoms can often be eliminated, but eyesight, once lost, cannot be regained.

From 2012 to 2016, the international nonprofit organization Sightsavers implemented the Global Trachoma Mapping Project (GTMP), which examined approximately 2.6 million people for trachoma in 29 countries to find out where trachoma was the most endemic. Knowing where trachoma affects people the most allows organizations like WHO to better target their trachoma elimination efforts.

Meanwhile, between 2014 and 2016, there was a 63 percent increase in the number of people receiving trachoma treatment worldwide, according to WHO in 2017. Treatment included antibiotic regimens and surgery. This increase in treatment is largely due to the donation of antibiotics (azithromycin) from the pharmaceutical company Pfizer.

SEE ALSO *Antibacterial Drugs; Bacterial Disease; Chlamydia Infection; Handwashing*

BIBLIOGRAPHY

Books

Taylor, Hugh R. *Trachoma: A Blinding Scourge from the Bronze Age to the Twenty-First Century.* East Melbourne, Australia: Centre for Eye Research Australia, 2008.

Periodicals

Stocks, Meredith E., et al. "Effect of Water, Sanitation, and Hygiene on the Prevention of Trachoma: A Systematic Review and Meta-Analysis." *PLOS Medicine* (February 25, 2014). This article can also be found online at http://journals.plos.org/plosmedicine/article?id=10.1371/journal.pmed.1001605 (accessed January 18, 2018).

West, Sheila K., et al. "The 'F' in SAFE: Reliability of Assessing Clean Faces for Trachoma Control in the Field." *PLOS Neglected Tropical Diseases* (November 30, 2017). This article can also be found online at http://journals.plos.org/plosntds/article?id=10.1371/journal.pntd.0006019 (accessed January 18, 2018).

Websites

"About Trachoma." International Trachoma Initiative. 2017. http://www.trachoma.org/about-trachoma (accessed January 18, 2018).

"85 Million People Treated for Trachoma through Expanded Access to Medicine." World Health Organization. July 13, 2017. http://www.who.int/neglected_diseases/news/85_million_people_treated_for_trachoma/en/ (accessed January 18, 2018).

"Trachoma." National Library of Medicine, National Institutes of Health. December 21, 2017. http://www.nlm.nih.gov/medlineplus/ency/article/001486.htm (accessed January 18, 2018).

"Trachoma: Epidemiological Situation." World Health Organization. http://www.who.int/trachoma/epidemiology/en/ (accessed February 10, 2018).

"Trachoma." World Health Organization. July 2017. http://www.who.int/mediacentre/factsheets/fs382/en/ (accessed January 18, 2018).

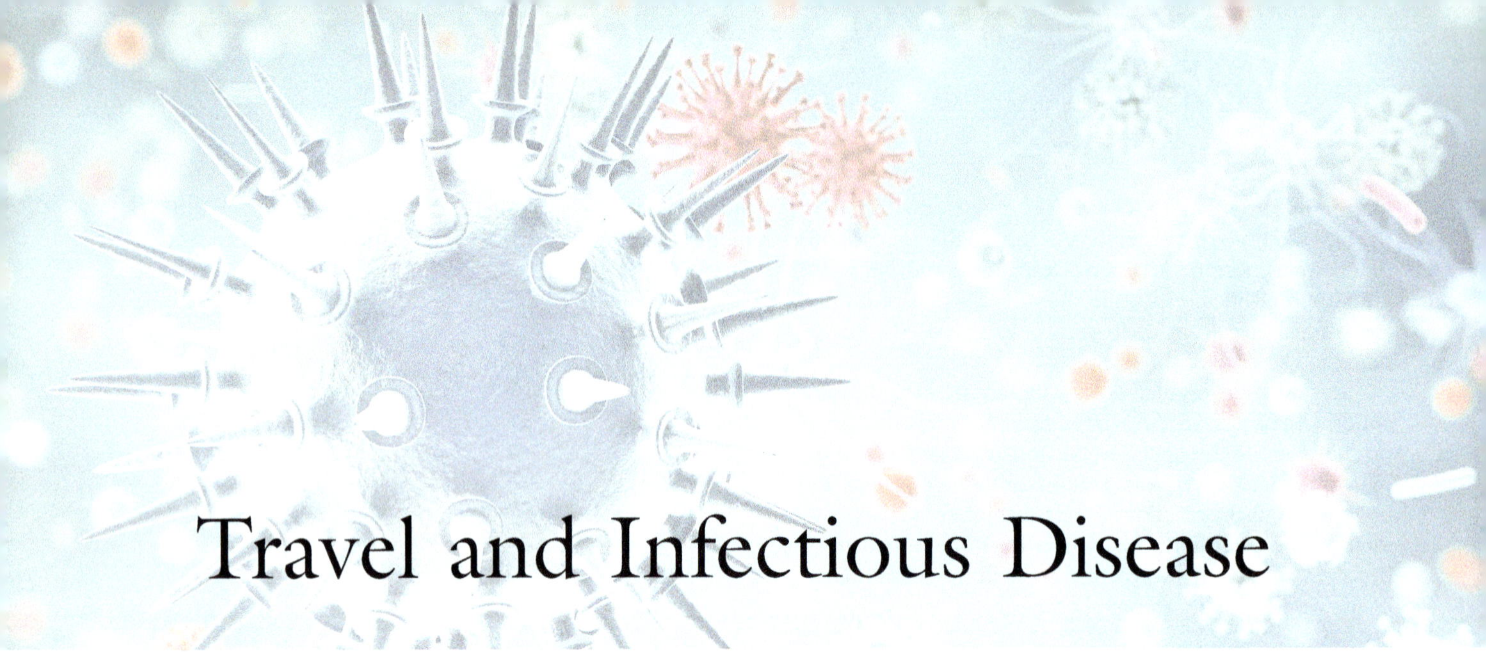

Travel and Infectious Disease

Introduction

Travel-related infection has had a significant impact on world history. The Black Death (plague), which began in Europe during the 14th century, was caused by bacteria that infected rat fleas introduced into Italy by ships. The "great pox" that affected Europe during the 16th century was caused by a new disease introduced by travelers from Africa or possibly South America. The disease eventually evolved into modern-day syphilis. Another pox disease that traveled in the opposite direction was instrumental in decimating Indian tribes in the New World during later years. In similar fashion, liver fluke and river blindness were introduced into Latin America as diseases of slaves from Africa but went on to adopt themselves to the local ecology, residing in insects or snails.

History and Scientific Foundations

The spread of major diseases across geographical borders became commonplace in the 20th century as a result of widespread immigration, world conflict, and air travel. Previously, diseases characterized by an incubation period measured in days would appear and run its course (or kill the infected person) long before the human host could arrive in a far-off country by horse or schooner. Ebola outbreaks in Africa in the early 1990s prompted concerns around the world that an infected person might travel abroad and unwittingly infect the population there. This is because the Ebola virus can remain in a human host for up to 21 days before onset of symptoms, whereas a flight from Africa to another continent is only a matter of hours.

Many infectious diseases are limited to specific regions, or even specific countries, because they require a particular environment, such as specific plants, animals, insects, or climatic factors, to propagate and survive. Other diseases are quite capable of adapting to new countries if introduced by humans or their activities. Examples in recent years have included West Nile virus, which arrived in the United States in 1999 and quickly entered a favorable ecological environment consisting of compatible insects (mosquitoes) and birds (primarily crows). Acquired immunodeficiency syndrome (AIDS), which scientists suspect evolved into a human disease in Africa during the 1950s, exploded onto the world stage largely because of air travel, intravenous drug use, and sexual practices.

On February 21, 2003, Liu Jianlun, a 64-year-old Chinese physician from Zhongshan Hospital, traveled to Hong Kong to attend a family wedding despite the fact that he had a fever. Epidemiologists subsequently determined that he passed on the SARS virus to other guests at the Metropole Hotel, including an American businessman en route to Hanoi, three women from Singapore, two Canadians, and a Hong Kong resident. Liu was later determined to have been a "superspreader," or a person capable of infecting unusually high numbers of contacts. Liu's travel to Hong Kong and the subsequent travel of those he infected allowed SARS to spread from China to the infected travelers' destinations. One of the Canadians infected in Hong Kong, Kwan Sui-Chu, returned to Toronto, Ontario, and died in a Toronto hospital on March 5, 2003. Because there were no alerts from China about the SARS outbreak, Canadian officials did not initially suspect that Kwan had

WORDS TO KNOW

HOST An organism that serves as the habitat for a parasite or possibly for a symbiont. A host may provide nutrition to the parasite or symbiont or simply a place in which to live.

PROPHYLAXIS Pre-exposure treatment (e.g., immunizations) to prevent the onset or recurrence of a disease.

VECTOR Any agent that carries and transmits parasites and diseases. Also, an organism or chemical used to transport a gene into a new host cell.

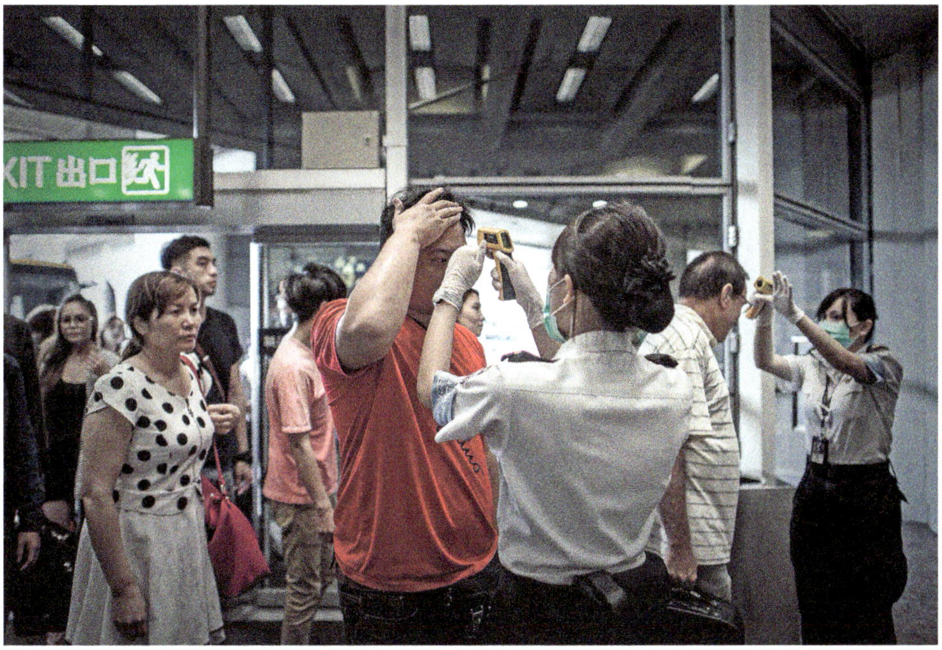

Health inspectors check the temperature of passengers arriving at Hong Kong International Airport in June 2015 amid an outbreak of Middle East respiratory syndrome (MERS) in nearby South Korea. © *PHILIPPE LOPEZ/AFP/Getty Images*

been infected with a highly contagious virus until Kwan's son and five health care workers showed similar symptoms. By mid-April 2003 Canada had reported more than 130 SARS cases and 15 fatalities.

During the Ebola outbreak in Africa between 2014 and 2016, more than 15,000 people were infected and over 11,300 were killed. The disease was spread to the United States by individuals who were in the region of the infection and traveled to the United States before being diagnosed. Although the spread of the disease in the United States was limited to two health care workers, it highlighted the potential for an infectious disease to spread rapidly. If hospital staff had not quickly identified the infection as Ebola, the situation could have been much worse. As a result, many medical facilities began routinely asking all patients about their recent travel history.

■ Impacts and Issues

Each year billions of travelers cross international boundaries. The majority do not seek medical advice and remain well. The most common medical problem is traveler's diarrhea, which in some countries affects as many as 40 percent of tourists. In malaria-prone regions, the chance of contracting malaria during a one-month tour varies from less than one per 1,000 in Southeast Asia to more than 1 percent in sub-Saharan Africa. Many travelers are exposed to venereal disease, and a few acquire AIDS. Tourists in rare instances can also acquire exotic or even life-threatening diseases such as yellow fever and African sleeping sickness.

SEE ALSO *AIDS: Origin of the Modern Pandemic; Dysentery; Globalization and Infectious Disease; Plague, Early History; Plague, Modern History; Tropical Infectious Diseases*

BIBLIOGRAPHY

Books

Bayry, Jagadeesh. *Emerging and Re-emerging Infectious Diseases of Livestock*. New York: Springer, 2017.

Pulcini, Céline, and Onder Ergonul. *Antimicrobial Stewardship*. Vol. 2 of *Developments in Emerging and Existing Infectious Disease*. New York: Academic Press, 2017.

Shah, Sonia. *Pandemic: Tracking Contagions, from Cholera to Ebola and Beyond*. New York: Picador, 2017.

Periodicals

Collier, Beth-Ann, et al. "Clinical Development of a Recombinant Ebola Vaccine in the Midst of an Unprecedented Epidemic." *Vaccine* 35 (2017): 4465–4469.

Websites

"NIAID Emerging Infectious Diseases/Pathogens." National Institute of Allergy and Infectious Diseases. https://www.niaid.nih.gov/research/emerging-infectious-diseases-pathogens (accessed November 15, 2017).

Stephen A. Berger
Brian Hoyle

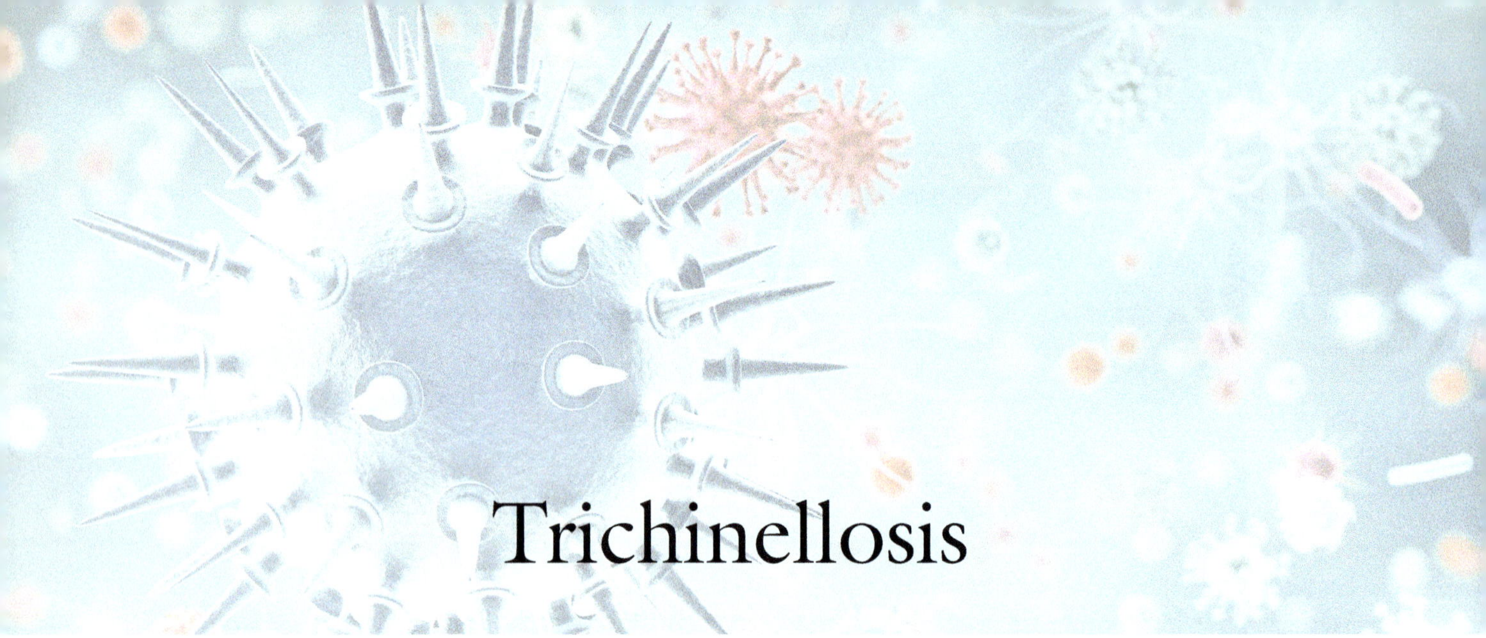

Trichinellosis

Introduction

Trichinellosis (TRICK-a-NELL-o-sis), also known as trichinosis or trichiniasis, is an infection caused by a roundworm of the genus *Trichinella*, usually the species *Trichinella spiralis.* The infection is contracted by eating meat (usually pork, but also the meat of wild game) that contains live helminth (parasitic worm) cysts. These cysts are the larvae or young of the worm, which are curled up inside tiny protective capsules. The cysts hatch in the small intestine and breed a new generation of larval worms, which then infect various body tissues. Thorough cooking destroys the larvae and renders infected meat safe to eat.

Trichinellosis is rare in most of the world, although it is fairly common in Eastern Europe and continues to increase in frequency in other areas. Eating undercooked pork is the most common path of trichinellosis infection worldwide; in North America, eating wild game is the most common path of infection. Death from the infection is rare.

WORDS TO KNOW

ANTHELMINTIC Medicines that rid the body of parasitic worms.

DORMANT Inactive, but still alive. A resting state.

ENCYSTED LARVAE Larvae that are not actively growing and dividing and that are more resistant to environmental conditions.

HELMINTH A representative of various phyla of wormlike animals.

Disease History, Characteristics, and Transmission

British physician Sir James Paget (1814–1899) discovered the worm that causes trichinellosis in 1835 while still a medical student. However, he did not know how humans became infected with the worm. In 1846 American parasitologist Joseph Leidy (1823–1891) discovered the parasite in pork. His early results were misreported in 1851 in Europe, another region where trichinellosis is common, as being descriptions of *Trichinella affinis*, which does not infect humans. In 1853 and 1856 Leidy again published accounts of finding *T. spiralis* in pork and reported that thorough cooking destroyed the parasite and made the meat safe to eat. Despite these later publications, European application of his results was delayed for decades by the original error.

In the early 21st century, some experts believe trichinellosis should be categorized as a reemerging disease because it is increasingly being reported in previously unaffected areas.

When meat containing encysted larvae is eaten, the larvae are liberated by the digestive process. They develop into adults in the small intestine, mate, and produce offspring. These adult worms are eventually excreted. The new larvae drill through the wall of the intestine and enter the bloodstream, which conveys them to destinations throughout the body, including the muscles, eyes, lungs, and brain. The larvae encyst themselves in muscle and become dormant. Because humans with the disease are usually not eaten by other animals or people, that is usually the end of the disease cycle in human beings. If the encysted larvae are in the muscle of any animal that might be eaten by human beings or other carnivores, the life cycle can continue.

Abdominal symptoms appear a day or two after infection and include nausea, diarrhea, vomiting, and abdominal pain. Other symptoms may appear two to four weeks after infection and include headaches, fevers and chills, muscle and joint pain, itching, diarrhea, rash, and swelling of the eyes. The later-stage symptoms are caused by the larvae encysting in the muscles and the body's immune response to their presence. Not all cases of infection, even in humans, produce noticeable symptoms.

Scope and Distribution

Trichinellosis occurs worldwide in the 21st century but is found mostly in Eastern Europe, Southeast Asia, and Latin America. Infection rates have declined significantly since the mid-20th century in places such as North America and Western Europe as a result of stronger regulations on the treatment and slaughter of commercial pork. According to the European Centre for Disease Prevention and Control (ECDC), 384 cases of trichinellosis were reported in the 28 countries of the European Union (EU) in 2014 (320 of which were confirmed). Among the confirmed cases, 88 percent were attributed to Romania and Bulgaria, with most linked to consumption of wild boar meat.

In North America the primary source of trichinellosis infection is wild game, with only 13 cases per year being reported in the United States in both 2014 and 2015, down from an average of 20 cases reported to the US Centers for Disease Control and Prevention (CDC) each year from 2008 to 2010. Outbreaks of trichinellosis have occurred among Inuit in Alaska who consume raw or undercooked walrus, including two outbreaks from July 2016 to May 2017 in which 10 total cases were identified. Almost all mammals can be infected by one or more species of *Trichinella*, but humans are more likely than most other species to develop symptoms.

Pork and bear meat are primary sources of *T. spiralis* infection in humans. Beaver, opossums, rats, walruses, and whales can also carry the parasite. Infected animals remain asymptomatic. Humans can experience gastrointestinal symptoms one to two days after consuming raw or undercooked meat from an infected animal, followed by "classic" trichinellosis symptoms such as muscle pain, fever, swelling of the face, and fatigue within two weeks (potentially last-

EFFECTIVE RULES AND REGULATIONS

The US Centers for Disease Control and Prevention (CDC) states that trichinellosis "infection is now relatively rare. During 2008–2012, 15 cases were reported per year on average." The CDC further asserted that "the number of cases decreased beginning in the mid-20th century because of legislation prohibiting the feeding of raw-meat garbage to hogs, commercial and home freezing of pork, and the public awareness of the danger of eating raw or undercooked pork products. Cases are less commonly associated with pork products and more often associated with eating raw or undercooked wild game meats."

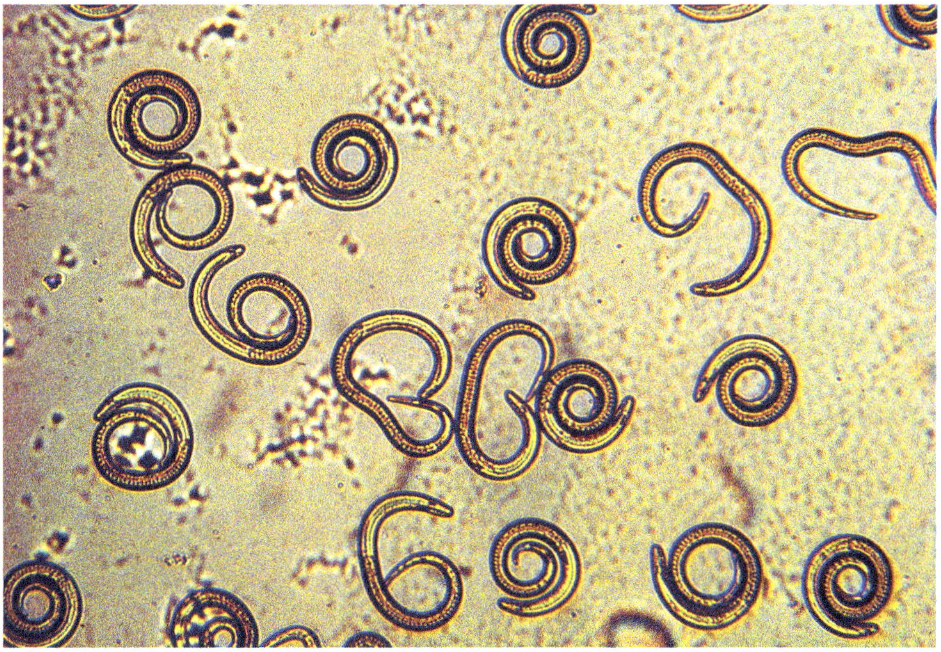

Trichinella spiralis, the parasite most commonly responsible for trichenellosis infections in humans, is viewed under a light micrograph. © Dickson Despommier/Science Source ing up to eight weeks), according to the CDC. Though rare, death can occur in severe cases. Severity depends on the number of parasites ingested. Although trichinellosis is found in some grain-fed pigs, swine fed on garbage containing infected meat scraps are the primary source of human trichinellosis.

Treatment and Prevention

Diagnosis is confirmed by observing the adult worms in a stool sample or by finding larvae in a muscle biopsy (a small piece of muscle tissue removed for laboratory testing). Treatment is supportive (intended to sustain the strength and condition of a patient), except during the intestinal phase of the infection when several drugs can be given to kill the worms in the intestine. These anthelmintic drugs include mebendazole and tiabendazole. No drug exists that can kill the encysted larvae, which may persist alive in the tissue, though inactive, for many years.

Trichinellosis can be prevented by eating only thoroughly cooked meats. Laws have been passed in both the United States and Europe forbidding feeding garbage-containing raw meat to hogs. To prevent trichinellosis, the CDC recommends cooking commercial pork to a temperature of 145°F (63°C) and all wild game to a temperature of 160°F (71°C) before eating, or freezing pork less than 6 inches (15 centimeters) thick for 20 days at 5°F (–15°C). Freezing, however, does not reliably kill larvae in wild game, nor does microwaving, drying, or smoking wild or commercial meat.

Impacts and Issues

The economic impact of trichinellosis is high because measures taken to reduce its presence in the food supply can be expensive. In the EU the domestic pig control program designed to minimize trichinellosis can cost as much as $500 million per year. In China large herds of infected pigs are occasionally destroyed, which can be a severe hardship for uninsured farmers. Because control programs have been so effective at reducing the prevalence of *Trichinella* in commercial pig farms, many developed countries have begun shifting their testing and prevention efforts toward wild game populations.

In the early 21st century, an increase in trichinellosis cases related to travel prompted many countries to adopt stricter bans on the importation of pork and game products by travelers to some regions. Many popular tourist destinations, such as Argentina, Croatia, Mexico, Romania, Serbia, and Laos, have endemic problems with trichinellosis. In 2016 three cases of trichinellosis were reported by travelers who had consumed polar bear meat in Greenland. In 2014 an outbreak of 16 cases in France was attributed to wild boar meat imported from Spain. Many nations now include trichinellosis in traveler health warnings.

See Also *Parasitic Diseases; Zoonoses*

BIBLIOGRAPHY

Books

Despommier, Dickson D., et al. *Parasitic Diseases*, 6th ed. New York: Parasites without Borders, 2017. This book can also be found online at http://www.parasiteswithoutborders.com/parasitic-diseases-6th-edition/ (accessed January 12, 2018).

Periodicals

Devleesschauwer, Brecht, et al. "The Low Global Burden of Trichinellosis: Evidence and Implications." *International Journal for Parasitology* 45 (2015): 95–99. This article can also be found online at http://www.cbra.be/publications/Devleesschauwer2015.pdf (accessed January 11, 2018).

Rostami, Ali, et al. "Meat Sources of Infection for Outbreaks of Human Trichinellosis." *Food Microbiology* 64 (June 2017): 65–71.

Websites

"Parasites—Trichinellosis (also known as Trichinosis)." Centers for Disease Control and Prevention, August 8, 2012. http://www.cdc.gov/ncidod/dpd/parasites/trichinosis/factsht_trichinosis.htm (accessed January 12, 2018).

Springer, Yuri P., et al. "Two Outbreaks of Trichinellosis Linked to Consumption of Walrus Meat —Alaska, 2016–2017." Centers for Disease Control and Prevention, July 7, 2017. https://www.cdc.gov/mmwr/volumes/66/wr/mm6626a3.htm (accessed January 25, 2018).

"Trichinellosis." European Center for Disease Prevention and Control. https://ecdc.europa.eu/en/trichinellosis (accessed January 11, 2018).

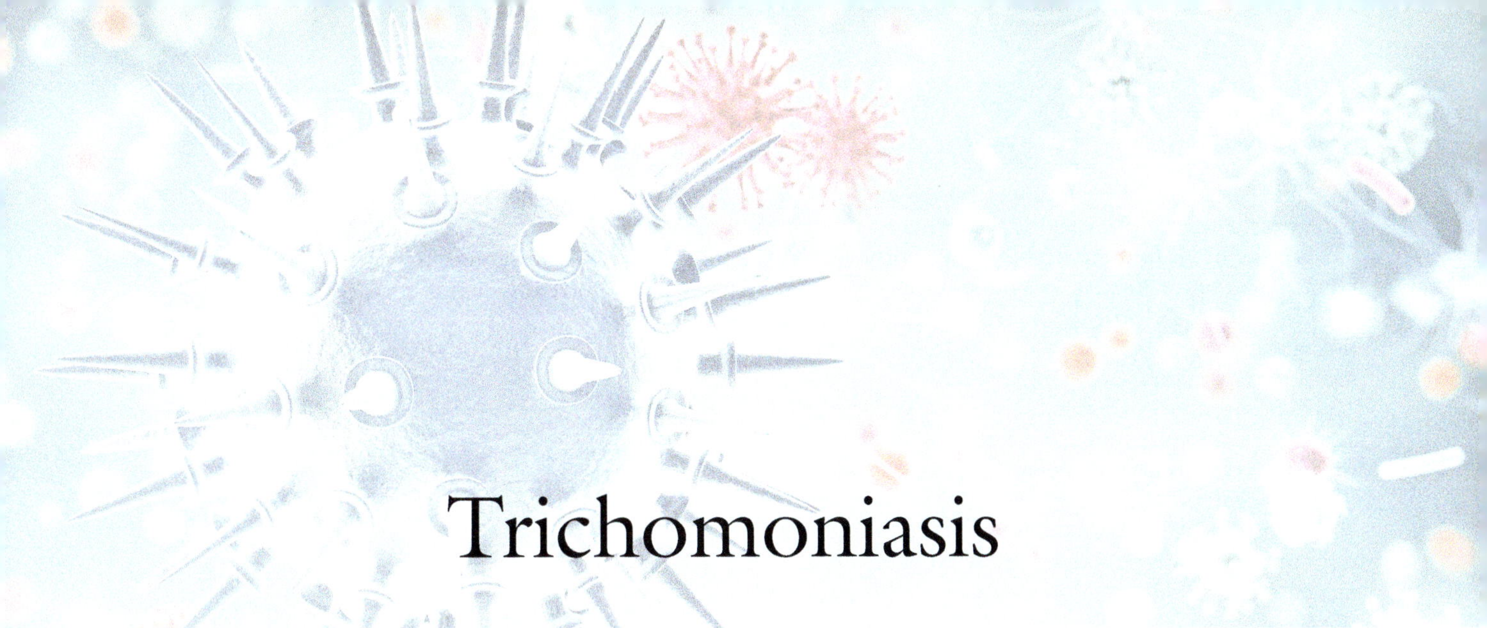

Trichomoniasis

Introduction

Trichomoniasis, also called *Trichomonas* infection, is a sexually transmitted infection of the urogenital system (relating to urinary and reproductive organs) of humans. It is caused by one-celled parasitic microbes of the species *Trichomonas vaginalis*. The *T. vaginalis* parasite has a round body with four flagella (tails) and a jerky motility that gives it a distinctive appearance and behavior that is easily identifiable under a microscope. The species, sometimes referred to as "trich," is classified within the order Trichomonadida and genus *Trichomonas*. It is likely the most common disease transmitted sexually between humans that is not a virus.

The World Health Organization (WHO) estimates that 8.1 percent of all women and 1 percent of men have trichomoniasis, but these percentages might be underestimated. Most of the people affected with the disease are age 20 to 45. The highest incidence of trichomoniasis occurs within women who have multiple sexual partners at the same time. The Centers for Disease Control and Prevention (CDC) estimates that more than 3.7 million people have trichomoniasis in the United States.

Disease History, Characteristics, and Transmission

Trichomonas bacteria are present in pre-ejaculate fluid, semen, and vaginal fluids. Infection is transmitted through certain sex acts. The primary modes of transmission are vaginal intercourse, genital-to-genital contact, and touching genitals with infected fluid on the hands. *Trichomonas* can live for up to 24 hours on moist surfaces such as bathing suits and hot tubs. However, such environments rarely contribute to transmission of the infection. It is not known to be transmitted through anal sex or oral sex.

Only about 30 percent of people with trichomoniasis have symptoms. If symptoms do occur, most do not show up until 5 to 28 days after being infected, according to the CDC. To complicate matters, people with trichomoniasis may mistake their symptoms for other common urogenital infections, such as urinary tract infections (UTIs).

Trich occurs more often in women than in men. In women it may be found in the vagina, urethra, or cervix. It

WORDS TO KNOW

FLAGELLUM A hairlike structure in a cell that serves as an organ of locomotion.

PATHOGEN A disease-causing agent, such as a bacterium, a virus, a fungus, or another microorganism.

PROTOZOA Single-celled, animal-like microscopic organisms that live by taking in food rather than making it by photosynthesis and must live in the presence of water. (Singular: protozoan.) Protozoa are a diverse group of single-celled organisms, with more than 50,000 different types represented. The vast majority are microscopic, many measuring less than 5 one-thousandth of an inch (or 0.005 millimeters), but some, such as the freshwater Spirostomun, may reach 0.17 inches (3 millimeters) in length, large enough to be seen with the naked eye.

SEXUALLY TRANSMITTED INFECTION (STI) Infections that vary in their susceptibility to treatment, their signs and symptoms, and the consequences if they are left untreated. Some are caused by bacteria. These usually can be treated and cured. Others are caused by viruses and can typically be treated but not cured.

can cause burning, itching, and abnormal vaginal discharge. It may make urination uncomfortable or make a woman feel like she needs to urinate more often. Trichomoniasis can make sex uncomfortable for both men and women.

If left untreated, trichomoniasis can cause cervicitis (inflammation of the cervix) or contribute to the development of pelvic inflammatory disease (PID).

In men trichomoniasis may occur in the prostate gland and urethra. Although there are usually no symptoms in men, if they do occur, they are usually described as itching of the genital area, a burning feeling while urinating or ejaculating, and fluid discharge from the urethra. In rare cases men can develop epididymitis or prostatitis (inflammation of the epididymis or prostate).

Scope and Distribution

Trichomoniasis occurs worldwide. There are no international surveillance programs of the disease. This makes it difficult for researchers to assess the full scope and distribution of the disease.

In the United States, trichomoniasis is more predominant among African American women. Patricia Kissinger wrote in a 2015 article for *BMC Infectious Diseases* that "African American women have rates that are ten times higher than white women, constituting a remarkable health disparity." In addition, incarcerated people in the United States are more likely to have trichomoniasis than the general population.

Kissinger also noted a relationship between the disease and certain risk factors, such as "increased age, incarceration, intravenous drug use, commercial sex work and the presence of bacteria vaginosis."

Treatment and Prevention

The infection can be diagnosed in women by studying fluid discharge from the vagina with a Pap smear. Such an examination under a microscope reveals the parasites. In the 2000s and 2010s, newer, more sensitive tests for *Trichomonas* were developed. Nucleic acid probe technique tests are the most sensitive tests and can detect *Trichomonas* present in a sample 95 to 100 percent of the time.

The infection is more difficult to diagnose in men. More often than not, it is first diagnosed in a female sexual partner. However, men can be diagnosed through continued symptoms of burning or itching in the genital area, even with treatment for chlamydia or gonorrhea, two other sexually transmitted infections. Specimens for examination under a microscope are often collected from the urethra.

For people without human immunodeficiency virus (HIV), antibiotics such as metronidazole and tinidazole are usually taken orally in a single dose for treatment. People with HIV usually take lower doses each day for seven days. Antibiotics should be prescribed to the infected individual's sexual partner too. Sex should be avoided until the disease

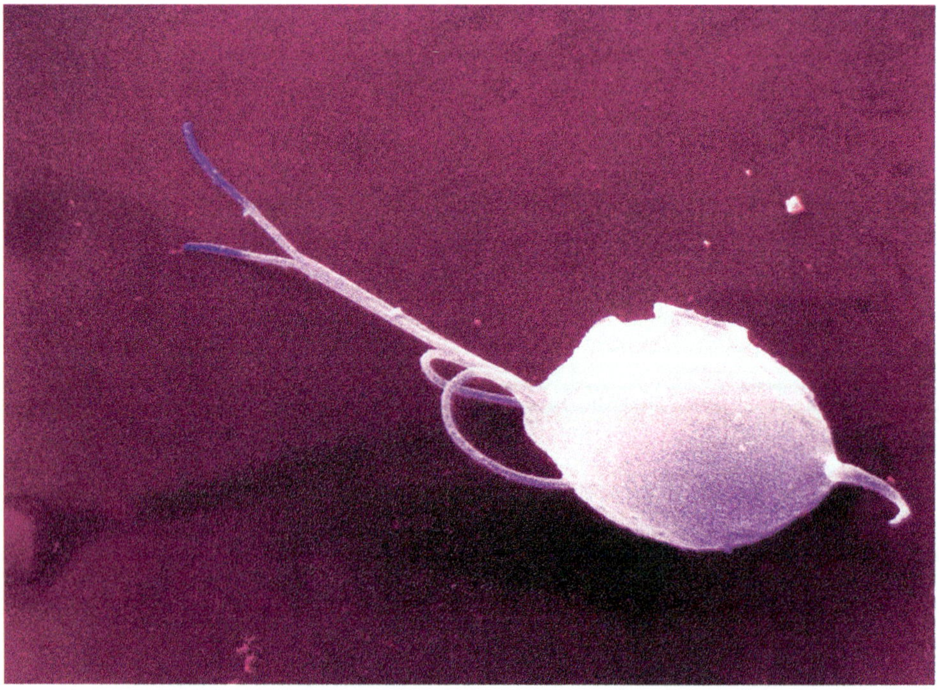

The parasite *Trichomonas vaginalis*, with its distinctive round body and four flagella (tails), is viewed under an electron microscope. *T. vaginalis* causes the sexually transmitted disease trichomoniasis. © *BSIP/UIG/Getty Images*

is cured. Women should be retested for *Trichomonas* three months after treatment because there is a 7 to 10 percent chance of treatment failure.

For sexually active people, the risk of contracting the disease can be reduced through proper use of latex condoms during sex and by having only one partner at a time. The disease can be prevented through abstaining from sex. There is evidence that men who are circumcised may be less likely to contract trichomoniasis. There is no vaccine.

The prognosis for trichomoniasis is excellent if treated properly with antibiotics. Complications can happen, however, if proper treatment is not given in a timely manner.

■ Impacts and Issues

Having trichomoniasis can double to triple the risk of contracting HIV. According to the CDC, just over 50 percent of women with HIV also have trichomoniasis. Treating trichomoniasis is beneficial for people with HIV because it reduces the HIV viral load in the urogenital tract.

Although extremely rare, pregnant women who are infected can also give the infection to their baby during the delivery process. Symptoms in pregnant females also often include preterm labor and birth of babies, as well as babies with low birth weights.

Infection in young children can be an indication of sexual abuse. These children are treated for the infection, and, if sexual abuse is suspected, additional investigations are conducted.

PRIMARY SOURCE

Treating ADHD with Medication May Lower the Risk of Sexually Transmitted Infections.

SOURCE: *Frye, Devon. "Treating ADHD with Medication May Lower the Risk of Sexually Transmitted Infections."* ADDitude, *January 4, 2018. https://www.additudemag.com/adhd-medication-sexually-transmitted-infection-risk/ (accessed January 23, 2018).*

INTRODUCTION: *In the following article, the author summarizes the findings from a recent study demonstrating that, if adolescent and young adult men treat their attention-deficit/hyperactivity disorder (ADHD) with medication, they are less likely to contract sexually transmitted infections (STIs), including trichomoniasis. The researchers believe that medicating men with ADHD reduces the likelihood that they will engage in "risky behaviors," such as unsafe sex. Treating adolescent and young women with ADHD medication, however, did not lower their likelihood of contracting STDs.*

Adolescents and adults with ADHD have a heightened risk of engaging in unsafe sexual behaviors—and they are more likely to contract sexually transmitted infections (STIs) as a result. According to a large new study, however, the use of ADHD medications may help to mitigate that STI risk—at least in male subjects.

A cohort of 89,490 Taiwanese adolescents and young adults—17,898 of whom had been diagnosed with ADHD—were culled from the Taiwan National Health Insurance Research Database, which contains healthcare data for 99 percent of the population of Taiwan. The ADHD subjects were each matched with a control subject of the same age and gender who had not been diagnosed with ADHD. The researchers tracked subjects' diagnosis and treatment rates for the most common STIs, including HIV, syphilis, genital warts, gonorrhea, chlamydial infection, and trichomoniasis, as well as their use of ADHD medication and the presence of comorbid conditions.

Confirming past studies, the researchers found that the ADHD group had a much higher rate of STIs than did the control group (1.2 percent vs. 0.4 percent)—and its members typically contracted the diseases at a younger age.

Males with ADHD who managed their symptoms with medication, however, demonstrated a significantly lower risk of developing an STI—30 percent less for individuals with short-term medication use, and 40 percent less for individuals with long-term medication use. On the other hand, female subjects who used medication demonstrated no similar decrease in risk, and were also more likely to have comorbid substance abuse disorders alongside STIs.

Still, the researchers said, the study adds to the growing body of evidence that ADHD medication can help manage some patients' propensity for dangerous or unhealthy behavior.

"Increasing evidence supports an association between ADHD and various health-risk behaviors, such as risky driving, substance abuse, and risky sexual behaviors," said lead author Mu-Hong Chen, M.D., of the College of Medicine at National Yang-Ming University. "Clinical psychiatrists [should] focus on the occurrence of risky sexual behaviors and the risk of STIs among patients with ADHD, and emphasize that treatment with ADHD medications may be a protective factor for prevention of STIs.""

SEE ALSO *Antibiotic Resistance; Gonorrhea; HIV; Parasitic Diseases; Sexually Transmitted Diseases*

BIBLIOGRAPHY

Books

Bennett, John E., Raphael Dolin, and Martin J. Blaser. *Mandell, Douglas, and Bennett's Principles and Practice of Infectious Diseases.* Philadelphia: Elsevier/Saunders, 2015.

Berger, Stephen. *Trichomoniasis: Global Status.* Los Angeles: GIDEON Informatics, 2017.

Sweet, Richard L., and Ronald S. Gibbs. *Infectious Diseases of the Female Genital Tract.* Philadelphia: Wolters Kluwer, 2015.

Periodicals

Kenyon, C., et al. "Incident *Trichomonas vaginalis* Is Associated with Partnership Concurrency: A Longitudinal Cohort Study." *Sexually Transmitted Infections* 93, no. 2 (2017). This article can also be found online at http://sti.bmj.com/content/93/Suppl_2/A109.1 (accessed January 22, 2018).

Kissinger, Patricia. "*Trichomonas vaginalis*: A Review of Epidemiologic, Clinical and Treatment Issues." *BMC Infectious Diseases* 15, no. 307 (August 5, 2015). This article can also be found online at https://bmcinfectdis.biomedcentral.com/articles/10.1186/s12879-015-1055-0 (accessed January 22, 2018).

Meites, Elissa, et al. "A Review of Evidence-Based Care of Symptomatic Trichomoniasis and Asymptomatic *Trichomonas vaginalis* Infections." *Clinical Infectious Diseases* 61, no. 8 (December 15, 2015). This article can also be found online at https://academic.oup.com/cid/article/61/suppl_8/S837/344844 (accessed January 22, 2018).

Silver, Bronywn J., et al. "*Trichomonas vaginalis* as a Cause of Perinatal Morbidity: A Systematic Review and Meta-Analysis." *Sexually Transmitted Diseases* 41, no. 6 (June 2014): 369–376. This article can also be found online at https://journals.lww.com/stdjournal/Abstract/2014/06000/Trichomonas_vaginalis_as_a_Cause_of_Perinatal.5.aspx (accessed January 22, 2018).

Websites

"Trichomoniasis—CDC Fact Sheet." Centers of Disease Control and Prevention, July 14, 2017. https://www.cdc.gov/std/trichomonas/stdfact-trichomoniasis.htm (accessed January 22, 2018).

"Trichomoniasis." Office on Women's Health, US Department of Health and Human Services, June 12, 2017. https://www.womenshealth.gov/a-z-topics/trichomoniasis (accessed January 22, 2018).

"2015 Sexually Transmitted Diseases Treatment Guidelines: Trichomoniasis." Centers for Disease Control and Prevention, August 12, 2016. https://www.cdc.gov/std/tg2015/trichomoniasis.htm (accessed January 22, 2018).

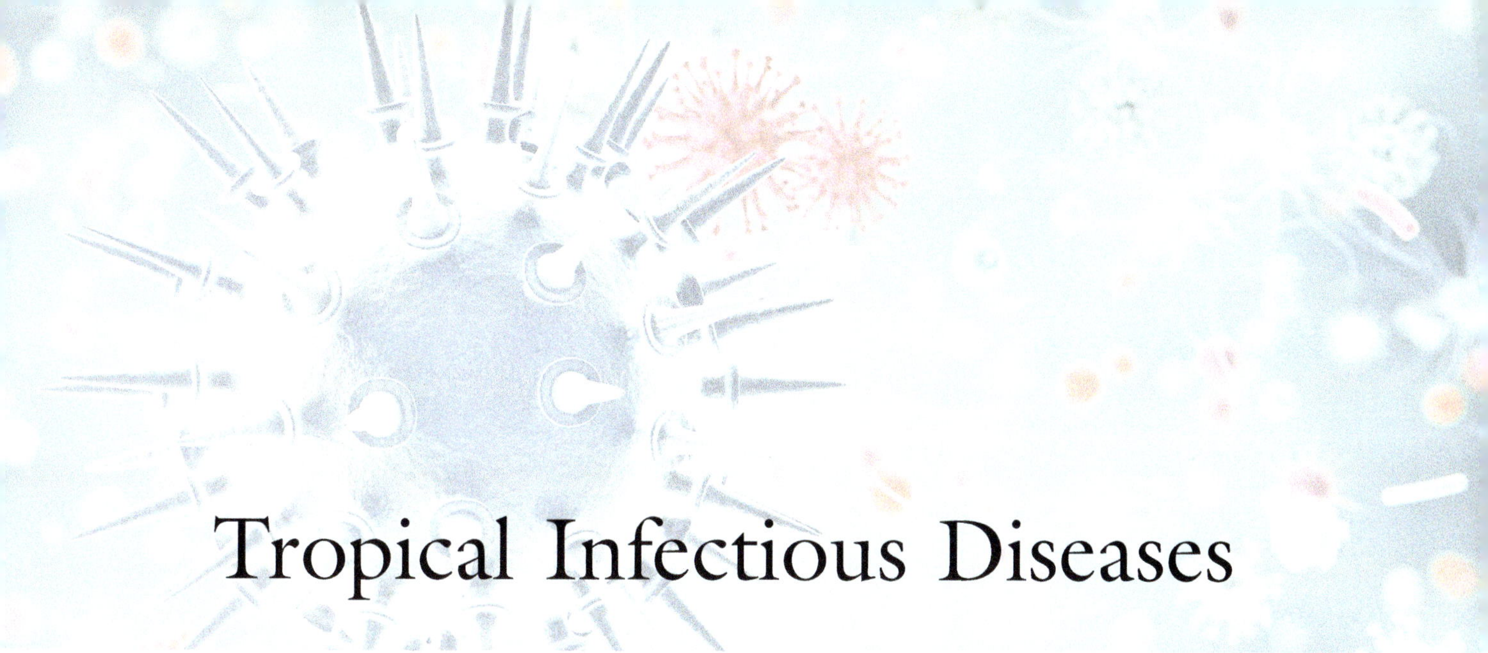

Tropical Infectious Diseases

Introduction

The warm, humid climate of the tropics can, in itself, encourage diseases that are rare or uncommon in the West, such as those borne by mosquitoes or flies. Conditions of poverty and poor sanitation are also common in tropical regions, such as sub-Saharan Africa, which encourages the spread of these diseases, even when there is a known cure for them.

Compared to heart disease, cancer, or other lifestyle diseases (diseases characterized by daily habits, such as bad food habits, physical inactivity, incorrect body posture, and disturbed biological clock), tropical diseases are neglected in terms of research and development aimed at prevention and cure. The World Health Organization (WHO) estimates that one in six of the world's population suffers from one of the many neglected tropical diseases, including leprosy, sleeping sickness, or elephantiasis. Control of some tropical diseases has been successful in the past. WHO and its collaborators seek to fight tropical infectious disease by improving both surveillance and drug delivery.

Disease History, Characteristics, and Transmission

Malaria, which is caused by the protozoan parasite Plasmodium, and the viral infection dengue are perhaps the

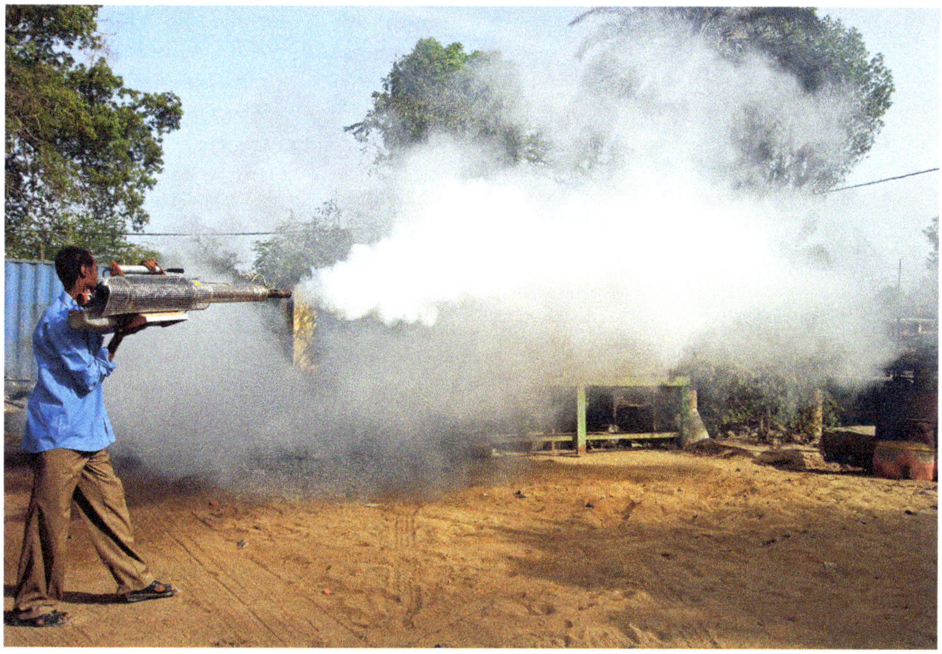

A public health worker sprays insecticide near Djibouti City to fight the spread of malaria. Many tropical infectious diseases, including malaria and yellow fever, are transmitted by mosquitoes, which thrive in warm, humid environments. *© Stephanie Rabemiafara/Art in All of Us/Getty Images*

WORDS TO KNOW

CUTANEOUS Pertaining to the skin.

NEGLECTED TROPICAL DISEASE Many tropical diseases are considered to be neglected because, despite their prevalence in developing areas, new vaccines and treatments are not being created for them. Malaria was once considered a neglected tropical disease, but recently a great deal of research and money has been devoted to its treatment and cure.

PARASITE An organism that lives in or on a host organism and that gets its nourishment from that host. The parasite usually gains all the benefits of this relationship, while the host may suffer from various diseases and discomforts or show no signs of the infection. The life cycle of a typical parasite usually includes several developmental stages and morphological changes as the parasite lives and moves through the environment and one or more hosts. Parasites that remain on a host's body surface to feed are called ectoparasites, while those that live inside a host's body are called endoparasites. Parasitism is a highly successful biological adaptation. There are more known parasitic species than nonparasitic ones, and parasites affect just about every form of life, including most all animals, plants, and even bacteria.

RESERVOIR The animal or organism in which a virus or parasite normally resides.

VECTOR Any agent that carries and transmits parasites and diseases. Also, an organism or a chemical used to transport a gene into a new host cell.

VISCERAL Pertaining to the viscera. The viscera are the large organs contained in the main cavities of the body, especially the thorax and abdomen, including the lungs, stomach, intestines, kidneys, or liver.

best known of the tropical infectious diseases. Another significant mosquito-borne disease is yellow fever, which is caused by a flavivirus spread by certain *Aedes* and *Haemogogus* mosquito species. The name is derived from the jaundice that often accompanies the late or toxic form of the disease, which has a 50 percent fatality rate. Lymphatic filariasis, or elephantiasis, is also spread by mosquitoes, the infective agent being the microscopic parasitic worms *Wuchereria bancrofti*, *Brugia malayi*, and *Brugia timori*. These lodge in the lymphatic system, causing immense and disfiguring swelling of the arms, legs, genitals, vulva, and breast, which may be accompanied by internal damage to the kidneys and lymphatic system.

Leishmaniasis, another common tropical disease, is spread by the bite of sandflies infected with parasites of various *Leishmania* species; there are two types of leishmaniasis: visceral and cutaneous. Untreated, visceral leishmaniasis is fatal in 95 percent of cases. It typically causes extensive internal organ damage after an initial phase of fever, night sweats, and weight loss. The cutaneous form causes a long-term rash, which sometimes leads to internal tissue damage and accompanying secondary bacterial infection, which is potentially fatal.

African trypanosomiasis, or sleeping sickness, is spread by tsetse flies that carry protozoa of the *trypanosome* genus. More than 90 percent of cases are caused by *T. brucei gambiense*; the rest are caused by *T. brucei rhodesiense*. The former has a slower onset than the latter. At first the trypanosomes multiply in subcutaneous tissues, blood, and lymph, then they cross the blood-brain barrier to infect the central nervous system. Left untreated, sleeping sickness will prove fatal.

There are many tropical infectious diseases that require an insect vector. Leprosy has been a feared and stigmatizing disease since antiquity. In the 21st century, however, leprosy is easily treatable and need not be debilitating. Untreated, it may lead to permanent damage and disfigurement to skin, nerves, limbs, and eyes. Leprosy is caused by the bacillus bacterium *Mycobacterium leprae*, which is related to the bacterium that causes tuberculosis (TB). It is spread by droplets from the nose and mouth from untreated cases, although it is not highly infectious.

Yaws, chikungunya, rabies, lymphatic filariasis, taeniasis (also called cysticercosis), dracunculiasis, leprosy, Buruli ulcer, onchocerciasis (also known as river blindness), and schistosomiasis are included on a list of neglected tropical diseases released by WHO. Yaws is a chronic infection that affects mainly skin, bone, and cartilage. The causative agent is the bacterium *Treponema pertenue*, and humans are the only reservoir. Another less-known condition is Buruli ulcer disease, which is caused by the bacterium *Mycobacterium ulcerans*, which is also related to the TB bacterium. The infection leads to destruction of the skin and soft tissue, with the formation of large ulcers on the arms and legs. The disease is not only disfiguring but can also cause disability through restriction in joint movement. Similarly, taeniasis is an intestinal infection caused by tapeworms *Taenia solium* (most common), *T. asiatica*, and *T. saginata*. Humans acquire the infection by ingesting tapeworm larval cysts (cysticerci) after consuming undercooked infected pork or by ingesting water or food contaminated with the tapeworm eggs. The cysts lodge in different parts of the body, and, upon entering the central nervous system, they cause neurological symptoms, including epileptic seizures and death in some cases.

There are many other tropical infectious diseases, varying widely in their cause, symptoms, and health consequences. Tropical diseases remain a serious health threat because many people in tropical disease–prone areas do not have access to existing treatment. Furthermore, medical research has not yet discovered effective therapies, mainly due to the development of drug resistance in pathogens.

Scope and Distribution

According to WHO's World Malaria Report 2017, malaria affected up to 216 million people worldwide in 2016 and caused an estimated 445,000 deaths. The majority of malarial deaths occur in the African region. WHO collects data on many infectious tropical diseases but warns that such diseases are underreported and their effects likely underestimated.

There are an estimated 170,000 cases of yellow fever each year, causing 30,000 to 60,000 deaths. Yellow fever is reported in 47 countries, including Africa, Central America, and South America. Meanwhile, millions of people in 36 different countries in sub-Saharan Africa are at risk of sleeping sickness, although only a small proportion of the countries are under constant surveillance and medical monitoring.

Leishmaniasis is widely distributed around the Mediterranean, tropical Africa, South America, and in East and Central Asia, with an estimated 700,000 to 1 million new cases per year. The disease is associated with weak immune system, malnutrition, and population displacement.

According to WHO, 856 million people in 52 countries were at risk of lymphatic filariasis in 2017, with at least 36 million affected with the disease, primarily in India, Africa, Southeast Asia, the Pacific, and the Americas. Leprosy is still a public health problem. According to WHO, there were 216,108 cases from 145 countries registered around the globe in 2016. There had been some success in controlling yaws up until the 1970s. However, the control campaign has slowed due to lack of knowledge of yaws among medical providers, increasingly mobile populations, and a lack of proper communication by the affected countries. As of 2012 WHO has renewed its effort to eradicate yaws globally.

Buruli ulcer is found in at least 33 countries in Africa, South America, and the western Pacific. It most commonly affects children ages 15 and younger. According to WHO, there has been a decline in the number of cases since 2010, and the reported number of cases from 13 countries in 2015 was 2,037.

Treatment and Prevention

There is an effective vaccine but no treatment for yellow fever. Sleeping sickness can be treated with benznidazole and nifurtimox if given soon after the onset of infection. Lymphatic filariasis can be cured by treatment with the antiparasitic drugs albendazole or ivermectin. There are a number of drugs that can treat leishmaniasis, but many have severe side effects.

INITIATIVES TO CONTROL NEGLECTED TROPICAL DISEASES

There have been a multitude of programs aimed at preventing or controlling tropical diseases in affected countries. Many of these have yielded positive and encouraging results.

Preventive therapy with a combination of medicines repeated annually for at least five years is key to eliminating lymphatic filariasis. According to a 2017 fact sheet by the World Health Organization (WHO), due to successful implementation, 6.7 billion people have been delivered medication since 2000, and 499 million no longer require preventive chemotherapy.

Mass drug administration has also been effective in combating dracunculiasis (guinea-worm disease), trachoma, onchocerciasis (also known as river blindness), and leprosy. Dracunculiasis has almost been eradicated, with only 25 cases reported in 2016.

In addition to WHO, organizations such as the Global Fund to Fight AIDS, Tuberculosis and Malaria (GFATM); the US President's Emergency Plan for AIDS Relief (PEPFAR); and the Bill & Melinda Gates Foundation are continually working in the area of neglected tropical diseases.

Leprosy usually responds to treatment with a combination therapy consisting of rifampicin, clofazimine, and dapsone. Yaws is curable with a single oral dose of the antibiotic azithromycin.

Many tropical diseases, such as malaria, dengue, chikungunya, lymphatic filariasis, Chagas, and leishmaniasis, need sound vector control programs as prevention strategies. Focus is also toward early detection and effective management of the diseases to prevent progression to disabilities and death.

Impacts and Issues

Tropical infectious diseases have a serious impact on many millions of people, particularly in Africa and Latin America, causing death, disability, loss of economic productivity, and impaired quality of life. There are many approaches to keeping these diseases under control or eliminating them. Where the disease is well understood and a cure or vaccine is available, surveillance, monitoring, and effective distribution are key to targeting supplies where they are needed. Public-private partnerships, between WHO and drug companies, for instance, can be valuable.

Tropical infectious diseases should also be higher up the agenda when it comes to basic and applied research.

There is still an urgent need, for instance, to understand the life cycle of the malaria parasite better in the search for a vaccine. Understanding the pathways of the disease-causing microorganisms at the genome level may aid in designing novel drugs for treating the diseases.

Tropical infectious diseases remain a significant global health threat. More than 1 billion people are affected by neglected tropical diseases. These diseases are called "neglected" because they have been essentially eliminated from developed nations but are endemic to some of the world's most underdeveloped nations and marginalized communities. Neglected tropical diseases flourish in tropical and subtropical regions, especially those with poor sanitation systems, contaminated drinking water, lack of adequate health care, and endemic disease-carrying insect problems.

WHO and other organizations have reenergized research into tropical diseases. Several neglected tropical diseases can be treated with drugs that cost as little as 2 cents per dose. International health organizations have focused on educating health officials and training community volunteers to administer and distribute therapeutic drugs. Improved sanitation and hygiene programs, increased access to clean drinking water, and use of insecticides, traps, and mosquito netting have helped to reduce the incidence of these diseases. However, treatments for some neglected tropical diseases remain expensive, outdated, and toxic or dangerous if administered incorrectly. Development of vaccines and cheaper, more effective, and safer drugs are vital to combating them.

Some scientists predict that global climate change may result in the reemergence of tropical diseases. Warmer temperatures and increased surface water may increase the habitat of disease vectors such as insects. Some assert that tropical diseases will become more common, more widespread, and increasingly virulent.

SEE ALSO *African Sleeping Sickness; Buruli (Bairnsdale) Ulcer; Chikungunya; Climate Change and Infectious Disease; Dengue and Dengue Hemorrhagic Fever; Developing Nations and Drug Delivery; Dracunculiasis; Filariasis; Host and Vector; Leishmaniasis; Leprosy (Hansen's Disease); Malaria; Mosquito-Borne Diseases; Rabies; River Blindness (Onchocerciasis); Taeniasis (*Taenia *Infection); Tapeworm Infection; Tuberculosis; Yaws; Yellow Fever*

BIBLIOGRAPHY

Books

Guerrant, Richard L., David H. Walker, and Peter F. Weller. *Tropical Infectious Diseases: Principles, Pathogens and Practice.* Philadelphia: Elsevier Health Sciences, 2011.

Hotez, P. J. "The Neglected Tropical Diseases and the Neglected Infections of Poverty." In *The Causes and Impacts of Neglected Tropical and Zoonotic Diseases: Opportunities for Integrated Invention Strategies.* Washington, DC: National Academies Press, 2011.

Periodicals

Hotez, Peter J. "Tropical Diseases: The New Plague of Poverty." *New York Times* (August 19, 2012): SR4. This article can also be found online at http://www.nytimes.com/2012/08/19/opinion/sunday/tropical-diseases-the-new-plague-of-poverty.html (accessed January 30, 2018).

McNeil, Donald G., Jr. "Fight against Tropical Diseases Is Framed as Efficient." *New York Times* (July 28, 2015): D5. This article can also be found online at https://www.nytimes.com/2015/07/28/health/fight-against-tropical-diseases-is-framed-as-efficient.html (accessed January 30, 2018).

Websites

"Buruli Ulcer." World Health Organization, February 2017. http://www.who.int/mediacentre/factsheets/fs199/en/ (accessed January 30, 2018).

"Leprosy." World Health Organization, January 2018. http://www.who.int/mediacentre/factsheets/fs101/en/ (accessed January 30, 2018).

"Fact Sheets: Neglected Tropical Diseases." World Health Organization. http://www.who.int/topics/tropical_diseases/factsheets/neglected/en/ (accessed January 20, 2018).

"Fact Sheets: Tropical Diseases." World Health Organization. http://www.who.int/topics/tropical_diseases/factsheets/en/ (accessed January 19, 2018).

"World Malaria Report 2017." World Health Organization, 2017. http://apps.who.int/iris/bitstream/10665/259492/1/9789241565523-eng.pdf?ua=1 (accessed January 30, 2018).

"Yellow Fever. Fact Sheet." World Health Organization, May 2016. http://www.who.int/mediacentre/factsheets/fs100/en (accessed January 19, 2018).

Susan Aldridge
Kausalya Santhanam

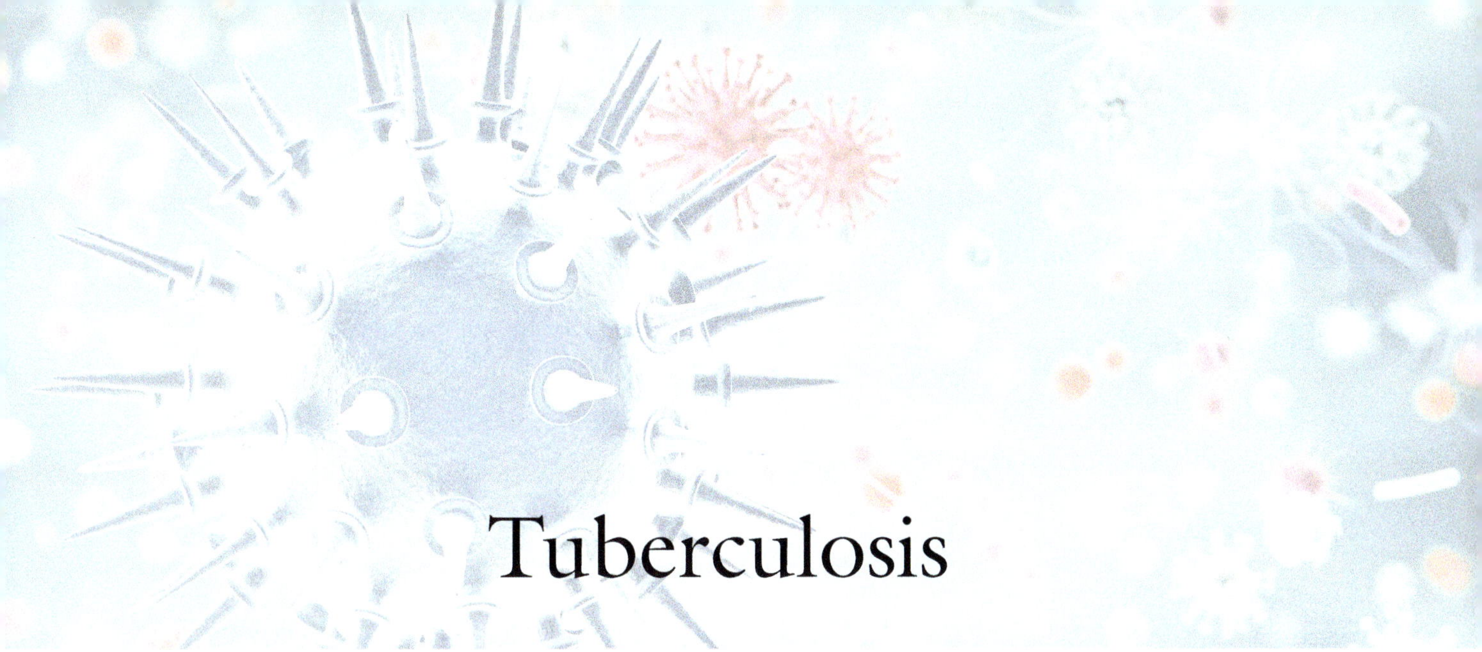

Tuberculosis

Introduction

Tuberculosis, often known as TB, is a disease caused by infection with the bacterium *Mycobacterium tuberculosis.* A few other types of mycobacterium can cause a tuberculosis-like illness but are only rarely encountered. Most commonly, the infection affects the lungs. However, along with the pulmonary form of tuberculosis, the infection can become extrapulmonary, affecting other parts of the body, including the central nervous system, kidneys, joints, spine, and skin.

In a tuberculosis infection, symptoms may be absent initially. In about 10 percent of those who are infected, latent tuberculosis, which cannot be spread from person to person, becomes active and more serious, killing up to 50 percent of those who are infected. The presence of the latent form of tuberculosis is especially dangerous in people whose immune systems are not functioning properly, such as those with acquired immunodeficiency syndrome (AIDS).

Disease History, Characteristics, and Transmission

Tuberculosis is an ancient disease. In about 400 BCE Greek physician Hippocrates (460–377 BCE) described a disease that is thought to have been tuberculosis. Then the disease was called phthisis, a name derived from the Greek word meaning "to waste away." This description was apt because the hallmark features of tuberculosis are weight loss and physical deterioration that occur over the often-considerable length of time that the infection persists. In the 19th century the characteristic physical wasting associated with the disease led to its popular name: consumption.

A fragment of *M. tuberculosis* DNA was found in lung tissue from the remains of an Egyptian mummy. Testing by researchers from the University of Birmingham in the United Kingdom determined that the female had died at about 50 years of age around 600 BCE. It has been argued that diseases like tuberculosis were unknown in South America until being introduced by European explorers in the 16th century. However, this may not be true, as preserved remains of people with tuberculosis-like lung damage have been dated to hundreds of years before the time of explorer Christopher Columbus (1451–1506). (There is no evidence that the Viking explorations, which predate Columbus, took them south of the equator.) It seems likely that tuberculosis may have been globally common even centuries ago.

The name *tuberculosis* was coined in 1839 by Johann Lukas Schonlein (1793–1864). At that time the pathogen responsible for the disease had not been discovered. *M. tuberculosis* was finally identified in 1882 by Robert Koch (1843–1910), one of the pioneers of the study of bacteria (bacteriology). In 1890 Koch reported on the extraction of a bacterial protein from dead bacteria recovered from tuberculosis infections. The protein, *tuberculin*, is still important as a means of detecting the presence of the bacteria.

With the discovery and use of X-rays at the end of the 19th century, the presence of the lung infection that is a consequence of the growth of *M. tuberculosis* was revealed. On X-ray images the masses of bacteria that develop appear as more opaque regions in the lungs. Lung infection with *M. tuberculosis* results from inhaling droplets of moisture that contain the bacteria. Most commonly this occurs when someone who has the infection expels droplets from their lungs by coughing. The droplets, which tend to be 0.5 to 5 microns in diameter (a micron is one-millionth of a meter), can contain more than 40,000 living *M. tuberculosis* bacteria. *M. tuberculosis* also can be transmitted in milk that has not been pasteurized to kill the bacteria.

Symptoms of this form of tuberculosis, or active tuberculosis, include a feeling of tiredness, loss of weight, a fever that tends to occur during sleep, chills, and a cough that persists for weeks. The coughing can dislodge and expel sputum, mucus that may be tinged with blood, as the infection can damage cells lining the lungs. In some people the infection can spread beyond the lungs to other parts of

WORDS TO KNOW

ACTIVE INFECTION An infection that is currently producing symptoms or in which the infective agent is multiplying rapidly. By contrast, a latent infection is one in which the infective agent is present but not causing symptoms or damage to the body or reproducing at a significant rate.

AIRBORNE PRECAUTIONS Procedures designed to reduce the chance that certain disease-causing (pathogenic) microorganisms will be transmitted through the air.

AIRBORNE TRANSMISSION The ability of a disease-causing (pathogenic) microorganism to be spread through the air by droplets expelled during sneezing or coughing.

ANTIBIOTIC RESISTANCE The ability of bacteria to resist the actions of antibiotic drugs.

LATENT INFECTION An infection already established in the body but not yet causing symptoms or having ceased to cause symptoms after an active period.

the body. If not treated this extrapulmonary tuberculosis is fatal in about 20 percent of the cases. The extrapulmonary form cannot be spread from person to person.

Scope and Distribution

TB is a common disease with a global distribution. While present in every country, it can be especially prevalent in regions where health care is substandard and poverty affects the overall health of the inhabitants. Traditionally this has been a more significant problem in underdeveloped and developing countries.

TB is one of the top 10 diseases globally in terms of the number of people infected. According to the World Health Organization (WHO), 10.4 million people became infected and 1.7 million died in 2016. More than 95 percent of the deaths were in low- and middle-income nations. In the United States in 2016, 9,272 new cases of TB were reported by the Centers for Disease Control and Prevention (CDC), a 3.6 percent decrease from 2015 and the lowest number of annual cases in the United States on record.

Some people are at increased risk for contracting tuberculosis. These include children, whose immune systems are not fully developed, and elderly people, whose immune function may have deteriorated. The immune system can also deteriorate due to diseases (for example, acquired immunodeficiency syndrome [AIDS]), poor nutrition, and the physical consequences of chronic alcohol or drug abuse. In addition, immune function may be deliberately suppressed in transplant patients to help minimize the chance of rejection of the transplanted organ. Health care providers may also be at risk of contracting tuberculosis, because they are exposed more frequently to people with the infection. Other risk factors include diabetes, various cancers, kidney disease, and abnormally low body weight.

Treatment and Prevention

The diagnosis of tuberculosis relies on recognition of the symptoms and detection of the infection. The presence of the lung infection can be visualized using a chest X-ray. *M. tuberculosis* also can be detected, either by obtaining sputum samples and growing the organism or by isolating protein components of the bacterium. The latter test can be faster, as the bacterium can be difficult to grow in laboratory conditions. For example, the length of time needed for *M. tuberculosis* to grow and divide in the nutritionally rich conditions of a laboratory culture dish can be 16 to 20 hours, which is far longer than the 15 to 20 minutes required by the common intestinal bacterium *Escherichia coli.* Thus, identification of the tuberculosis bacterium by laboratory culturing can take days.

A well-known test for tuberculosis is the skin test. In this test the tuberculin protein from *M. tuberculosis* is injected just under the skin of the forearm. The development of redness and swelling at the injection site within several days indicates that the person has at least been exposed to the infection.

The QuantiFERON-TB Gold (QFT) test is also approved for use in the diagnosis of *M. tuberculosis* infection. The test detects the release of a compound called interferon-gamma from blood cells in those who have tuberculosis. The test has been approved as a replacement for the skin test and as a means of confirming the results of the skin test. Both tests reveal TB infections but do not indicate whether a symptom-free (latent) infection is present.

In the past the treatment of tuberculosis was associated with images of hospital wards filled with bedridden patients or images of people slowly recovering from the infection while at sanatoriums located in the countryside. Even into the 1960s sanatoriums that were located in areas with clean, dry air were a popular part of treatment for tuberculosis.

Sanatoriums did aid recovery, but their usefulness was supplanted during the 1960s by the introduction of antibiotics that were effective against *M. tuberculosis.* The antibiotic treatment needs to be carried out for up to six months to be effective, in part because of the slow growth of the bacteria (many antibiotics are effective only on bacteria that are growing). It can be tempting to stop taking the antibiotics before the end of the prescribed period of treatment, as the patient begins to feel better after only a few weeks.

But, as with other bacterial infections, discontinuing treatment prematurely is dangerous because it can allow surviving bacteria to reestablish the infection. In fact, the surviving bacteria may be resistant to the antibiotics used, making treatment more difficult and more expensive.

The first few decades of the antibiotic therapy were resoundingly successful. More than 90 percent of tuberculosis infections were cured. However, in the early years of the 21st century, resistance to the antibiotics emerged and became more prevalent.

A tuberculosis vaccine does exist. It was developed during World War I (1914–1918) by French scientists Albert Calmette (1863–1933) and Camille Guerin (1872–1961) and was first used in 1921. The vaccine uses a live but weakened strain of the bacterium *Mycobacterium bovis.* Bacillus Calmette-Guerin (BCG) is still the only vaccine for tuberculosis, although researchers are continuing to investigate new vaccine candidates.

As of 2017 the vaccine was not recommended for use in the United States by the CDC. This is due to a combination of factors: the relatively low number of cases of the disease in the United States, the vaccine's 80 percent success rate, and the risks associated with the use of live bacteria in a vaccine. Health care providers and others at higher risk to acquire the infection are vaccinated, however, as are people who have the multidrug-resistant form of tuberculosis (MDR-TB). People who come to the United States from areas of the world where tuberculosis is prevalent are required to be examined for the presence of the active and latent forms of the infection and to be treated if necessary.

Efforts to develop new tuberculosis vaccines are ongoing. Several vaccine candidates have been developed using recombinant genetic techniques. They are not yet available for general use.

Impacts and Issues

Throughout history tuberculosis has been a threat to health and life. For example, in the mid-19th century, about 25 percent of all deaths were due to tuberculosis. The devastation caused to families and the economic consequences of the loss of so many wage earners were immense. At that time the disease was especially prevalent in children, adolescents, and young adults, and whole generations were affected.

This situation changed during the 1940s with the introduction of antibiotics that were effective against *M. tuberculosis.* There was a steep drop in the number of cases of tuberculosis worldwide. This fueled optimism that the disease had been controlled. But, as with other bacterial diseases that were initially suppressed by antibiotic therapy, this optimism was premature. Several factors have fueled the return of tuberculosis, including the increasing incidence of immunosuppressive diseases (primarily AIDS), the impact of the growing gap in health care between the richer and poorer nations, and the emergence of a type of tuberculosis infection that is resistant to multiple antibiotics.

In other countries, including the United States, tuberculosis is less common and is mainly found in cities among the poor and homeless. In the United States a program called Directly Observed Therapy (DOT) is being used by

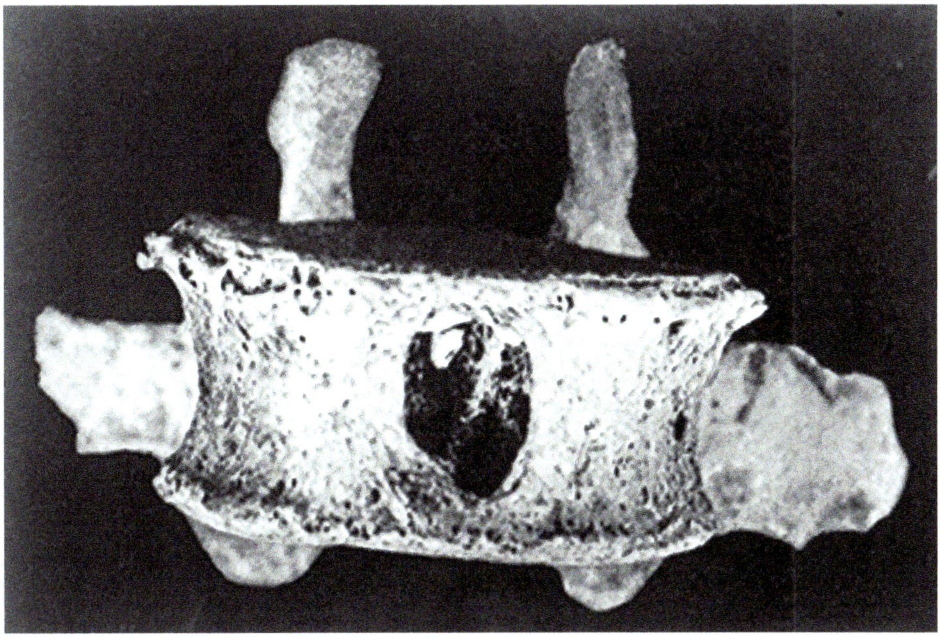

This vertebra from an Egyptian mummy shows signs of tubercular decay. Archaeological evidence like this suggests that tuberculosis has plagued humankind for thousands of years. © Wellcome Images/Science Source

some states to help deal with the rising prevalence of tuberculosis. The program, which focuses on the poor and homeless in cities such as New York, involves direct meetings between the patient and a health care provider and the delivery of every scheduled dose of tuberculosis medication by that health care provider.

In 1990 there were 7,537,000 tuberculosis cases worldwide, according to WHO, with approximately 30,000 of those cases reported in the United States. The 14,097 reported cases in the United States in 2005 represented a 47 percent decline from 1990. However, in some states and among certain ethnic groups, the prevalence of tuberculosis is still increasing. Furthermore, the situation elsewhere in the world is bleak. WHO estimated that in 2016 10.4 million people globally contracted TB and 1.7 million died from the infection. More than 95 percent of the deaths occurred in low- and middle-income countries.

In May 2007 a CDC investigation of a suspected case of extremely drug-resistant tuberculosis (XDR-TB) made news headlines around the world and heightened public awareness of XDR-TB. The case involved a US citizen that the CDC publicly asserted had a "potentially infectious XDR-TB who traveled to and from Europe on commercial flights between May 12 and May 24 [2007], and then re-entered the United States at the Canada-U.S. border via automobile."

Because of the international travel implications, for the first time in more than 40 years the CDC issued a federal isolation order under authority of the US Public Health Service Act. Such orders are rare because state and local health departments usually order isolation. In fact, in early June 2007 Denver's public health department issued an order that the patient be detained for treatment at the Denver-area hospital where he had ultimately been transferred for treatment, so the federal order was lifted.

Although the patient was asymptomatic and physicians later stated that he did not appear to be highly infectious, the case came under intense media scrutiny. As of late 2017, many issues existed concerning the facts and timeline of events related to the case, including the investigation of how the patient may have initially contracted the disease and the events surrounding the response by a number of health and security agencies to his infection and subsequent travel. Intense media coverage was also fueled by initial disinformation about the nature of transmission, with reports failing to specify that transmission of the bacterium responsible usually takes prolonged contact.

In 2017 MDR-TB was a global health threat. There were an estimated 600,000 new cases globally in 2016, according to WHO. Efforts to prevent the spread of the infections, such as the more controlled use of antibiotics, had a positive effect. Globally the incidence of MDR-TB was decreasing by about 2 percent each year. The decline will have to be greater to meet the targets of WHO's End TB Strategy, which was adopted in 2014 and seeks a 35 percent reduction in the number of TB deaths globally by 2020 and a 75 percent reduction by 2025.

The resurgence of tuberculosis has resulted in part from the increasing prevalence of immunodeficiency diseases but also from a lack of attention to the control of tuberculosis. As with diseases such as polio, the early success in combating the disease led to complacency regarding control programs, with the result that the disease rebounded.

The emergence of antibiotic-resistant forms of *M. tuberculosis* is especially troubling. From 2000 to 2004, according to the CDC, 20 percent of tuberculosis cases in the United States were resistant to commonly used antibiotics, and approximately 2 percent were resistant to the more potent and more expensive drugs employed as a next step. MDR-TB includes strains of tuberculosis that are resistant to at least two first-line drugs, isoniazid and rifampicin, used to treat TB.

According to WHO, XDR-TB is another emerging threat. The disease is initially latent. When symptoms appear and treatment is initiated, the resistance of the infection to virtually all antibiotics makes XDR-TB extremely difficult to treat.

WHO reported that, by the end of 2015, XDR-TB cases had been reported in 117 countries worldwide. However, as of 2017 identified XDR-TB was still uncommon in the United States and globally.

PRIMARY SOURCE

The Patients' Charter for Tuberculosis Care

SOURCE: *"The Patients' Charter for Tuberculosis Care." World Care Council. 2006. http://www.who.int/tb/publications/2006/istc_charter.pdf (accessed December 12, 2017).*

INTRODUCTION: *The World Care Council (WCC), based in France, is a nongovernmental organization dedicated to mobilizing public and private forces together worldwide in the fight against AIDS, malaria, and tuberculosis. The Patients' Charter for Tuberculosis Care, developed by the WCC, aims to empower people with tuberculosis by describing their rights and responsibilities regarding the disease. WCC intends for the charter to become the catalyst for effective collaboration between health providers, authorities, and persons with TB. The charter is the first global patient-powered standard for care.*

The Patients' Charter outlines the Rights and Responsibilities of People with Tuberculosis. It empowers people with the disease and their communities through this knowledge. Initiated and developed by patients from around the world, the Charter makes the relationship with health care providers a mutually beneficial one. The Charter sets out the ways in which patients, the community, health providers, both private and public, and governments can work as partners in a positive and open relationship with a view to improving tuberculosis care and enhancing the effectiveness of the health care process. It allows for all parties to be held more accountable to each other, fostering mutual interaction and a 'positive partnership'. Developed in tandem with the International Standards for Tuberculosis Care to promote a 'patient-centered' approach, the Charter bears in mind the principles on health and human rights of the United Nations, UNESCO, WHO, Council of Europe, as well as other local and national charters and conventions. The Patients' Charter for Tuberculosis Care practices the principle of Greater Involvement of People with TB. This affirms that the empowerment of people with the disease is the catalyst for effective collaboration with health providers and authorities, and is essential to victory in the fight to stop TB. The Patients' Charter, the first global 'patient-powered' standard for care, is a cooperative tool, forged from common cause, for the entire TB Community.

PATIENTS' RIGHTS

You have the right to:

Care

- The right to free and equitable access to tuberculosis care, from diagnosis through treatment completion, regardless of resources, race, gender, age, language, legal status, religious beliefs, sexual orientation, culture, or having another illness.
- The right to receive medical advice and treatment which fully meets the new International Standards for Tuberculosis Care, centering on patient needs, including those with MDR-TB or TB-HIV coinfections, and preventive treatment for young children and others considered to be at high risk.
- The right to benefit from proactive health sector community outreach, education, and prevention campaigns as part of comprehensive care programs.

Dignity

- The right to be treated with respect and dignity, including the delivery of services without stigma, prejudice, or discrimination by health providers and authorities.
- The right to quality health care in a dignified environment with moral support from family, friends, and the community.

Information

- The right to information about what health care services are available for tuberculosis, and what responsibilities, engagements, and direct or indirect costs are involved.
- The right to receive a timely, concise, and clear description of the medical condition, with diagnosis, prognosis (an opinion as to the likely future course of the illness), and treatment proposed, with communication of common risks and appropriate alternatives.
- The right to know the names and dosages of any medication or intervention to be prescribed, its normal actions and potential side-effects, and its possible impact on other conditions or treatments.
- The right of access to medical information which relates to the patient's condition and treatment, and a copy of the medical record if requested by the patient or a person authorized by the patient.
- The right to meet, share experiences with peers and other patients, and to voluntary counseling at any time from diagnosis through treatment completion.

Choice

- The right to a second medical opinion, with access to previous medical records.
- The right to accept or refuse surgical interventions if chemotherapy is possible, and to be informed of the likely medical and statutory consequences within the context of a communicable disease.
- The right to choose whether or not to take part in research programs without compromising care.

Confidence

- The right to have personal privacy, dignity, religious beliefs, and culture respected.
- The right to have information relating to the medical condition kept confidential and released to other authorities contingent upon the patient's consent.

Justice

- The right to make a complaint through channels provided for this purpose by the health authority, and to have any complaint dealt with promptly and fairly.
- The right to appeal to a higher authority if the above is not respected, and to be informed in writing of the outcome.

Organization

- The right to join, or to establish, organizations of people with or affected by tuberculosis, and to seek support for the development of these clubs and community-based associations through the health providers, authorities, and civil society.

- The right to participate as 'stakeholders' in the development, implementation, monitoring, and evaluation of TB policies and programs with local, national, and international health authorities.

Security

- The right to job security after diagnosis or appropriate rehabilitation upon completion of treatment.
- The right to nutritional security or food supplements if needed to meet treatment requirements.

PATIENTS' RESPONSIBILITIES

You have the responsibility to:

Share Information

- The responsibility to provide the health care giver as much information as possible about present health, past illnesses, any allergies, and any other relevant details.
- The responsibility to provide information to the health provider about contacts with immediate family, friends, and others who may be vulnerable to tuberculosis or may have been infected by contact.

Follow Treatment

- The responsibility to follow the prescribed and agreed treatment plan and to conscientiously comply with the instructions given to protect the patient's health, and that of others.
- The responsibility to inform the health provider of any difficulties or problems with following treatment, or if any part of the treatment is not clearly understood.

Contribute to Community Health

- The responsibility to contribute to community well-being by encouraging others to seek medical advice if they exhibit the symptoms of tuberculosis.
- The responsibility to show consideration for the rights of other patients and health care providers, understanding that this is the dignified basis and respectful foundation of the TB Community.

Show Solidarity

- The moral responsibility of showing solidarity with other patients, marching together towards cure.
- The moral responsibility to share information and knowledge gained during treatment and to pass this expertise to others in the community, making empowerment contagious.
- The moral responsibility to join in efforts to make the community tuberculosis free.

World Care Council

SEE ALSO *Airborne Precautions; Antibiotic Resistance; Developing Nations and Drug Delivery; Re-emerging Infectious Diseases; Resistant Organisms*

BIBLIOGRAPHY

Books

Murphy, Jim, and Alison Blank. *Invincible Microbe: Tuberculosis and the Never-Ending Search for a Cure.* New York: HMH, 2015.

Schlossberg, David. *Tuberculosis and Nontuberculosis Mycobacterial Infections.* Washington, DC: ASM, 2017.

Periodicals

Abubakar, Ibrahim, Chris Griffiths, and Peter Ormerod. "GUIDELINES: Diagnosis of Active and Latent Tuberculosis: Summary of NICE Guidance." *BMJ: British Medical Journal* 345, no. 7881 (November 2012): 45–47.

Brighenti, Susanna, and Jan Andersson. "Local Immune Responses in Human Tuberculosis: Learning from the Site of Infection?" *Journal of Infectious Diseases* 205, no. 2. (May 2012): S316–S324

Websites

"Tuberculosis (TB)." Centers for Disease Control and Prevention. https://www.cdc.gov/tb/default.htm (accessed November 22, 2017).

"Tuberculosis." World Health Organization. http://www.who.int/mediacentre/factsheets/fs104/en/ (accessed November 22, 2017).

Brian Hoyle

Tularemia

Introduction

Tularemia, also known as rabbit fever, deerfly fever, and lemming fever, is a bacterial zoonotic disease that is endemic throughout the United States. The bacterium *Francisella tularensis* is one of the most highly infectious bacteria and therefore poses a significant threat to humans. The bacteria that causes tularemia has also been considered a potential bioterrorism agent.

Francisella tularensis naturally colonizes in many species of small animals. Transmission of the disease to humans is via vectors such as ticks and mosquitoes, contact with infected animals, or ingestion of contaminated soil, water, or food. Symptoms present after a short incubation and may include fever, nausea, headache, diarrhea, and joint and muscle pain. The infection can spread to the lungs, liver, and lymphatic system. In a little less than 2 percent of cases, tularemia is fatal.

Treatment with antibiotics is usually effective and readily available. Prevention may be achieved through the use of insect repellents, avoidance of contact with infected animals, and the maintenance of uncontaminated food and water sources.

Disease History, Characteristics, and Transmission

Tularemia was first described in Japan in 1837 but gained its name from Tulare County, California, where

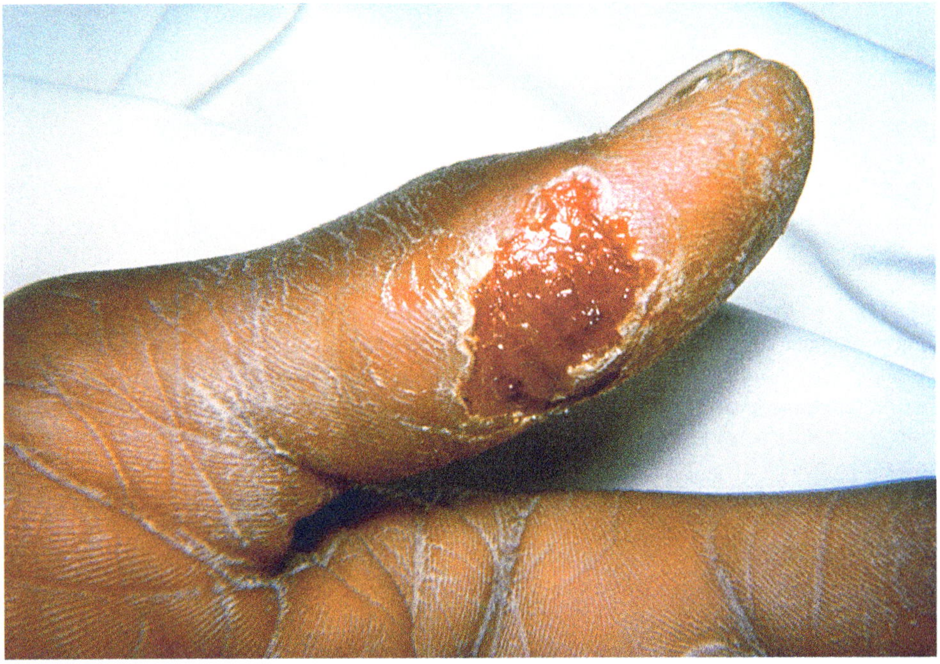

A thumb with a skin ulcer characteristic of tularemia. © *Smith Collection/Gado/Getty Images*

WORDS TO KNOW

AEROSOL Particles of liquid or solid dispersed as a suspension in gas.

ARTHROPOD A member of the largest single animal phylum, consisting of organisms with segmented bodies, jointed legs or wings, and exoskeletons.

COLONIZE To persist and grow at a given location.

ENDEMIC Present in a particular area or among a particular group of people.

FULMINANT INFECTION An infection that appears suddenly and whose symptoms are immediately severe.

HOST An organism that serves as the habitat for a parasite or possibly for a symbiont. A host may provide nutrition to the parasite or symbiont, or it may simply provide a place in which to live.

INOCULUM A substance such as a virus, a bacterial toxin, or a viral or bacterial component that is added to the body to stimulate the immune system, which then provides protection from an infection by the particular microorganism.

RESERVOIR The animal or organism in which the virus or parasite normally resides.

VECTOR Any agent that carries and transmits parasites and diseases. Also, an organism or a chemical used to transport a gene into a new host cell.

VIRULENCE The ability of a disease organism to cause disease. A more virulent organism is more infective and liable to produce more serious disease.

ZOONOTIC A disease that can be transmitted between animals and humans. Examples of zoonotic diseases are anthrax, plague, and Q fever.

a plague-like illness arose among squirrels in 1911. The causative agent, *Francisella tularensis*, is considered to be among the most infectious bacteria known, and, if left untreated, infection may prove fatal. Prior to the invention of antibiotics, the fatality rate was 5 to 15 percent, according to the Centers for Disease Control and Prevention (CDC). In severe cases of the disease, the fatality rate was anywhere from 30 to 60 percent.

Symptoms of tularemia usually appear within 3 to 5 days of exposure but can take up to 21 days in some cases. Presentation includes a sudden fever, chills, headache, diarrhea, muscle aches, joint pain, dry cough, and progressive weakness. Disease caused by tularemia can vary in severity and presentation according to virulence of the infecting organism, dose, and site of inoculums (where the bacteria enters the body). Symptoms can include ulcers on the skin or mouth, swollen, painful lymph glands, and a sore throat. Some people with tularemia also become susceptible to pneumonia and develop chest pain and bloody sputum (mucus from the lungs) and have breathing complications.

Only a small number of the bacteria are required for tularemia disease to fulminate (appear suddenly and intensely); the infection is established when particles invade white blood cells and subsequently attack the immune system following multiplication. The major target organs are the lymph nodes, lungs, spleen, liver, and kidneys. While the inoculation may be focal, the disease will often become disseminated and cause problems throughout the body. The disease is fatal in around 2 percent of cases, with the most common cause of death being failure of the respiratory system or multiple organs.

Many small animals, including rodents, rabbits, and hares, provide natural reservoirs for the bacteria. Transmission of the infection to humans may occur through vectors such as ticks, biting flies, and mosquitoes. Humans may also contract the disease by handling infected animals or by ingesting contaminated water, soil, or food. Inhalation is also a significant form of transmission, but person-to-person transmission has not been established.

Scope and Distribution

The *F. tularensis* bacterium is endemic throughout North America and in parts of Europe and Asia. Cases of tularemia have been reported in every US state except Hawaii, with the majority occurring in south-central states. The widely present nature of the bacteria may be attributed to the fact that *F. tularensis* is found in diverse hosts and habitats, and it can survive for weeks at low temperatures in water, moist soil, hay, straw, and decaying animal carcasses.

People at a higher risk of contracting tularemia include hunters and trappers engaging in the skinning of potentially infected animals. Activities that lead to the aerosolization (dispersion into the air) of the bacteria can also increase the likelihood of infection, with lawn mowing the most common example of such an activity.

Cases of tularemia occur most commonly in the United States between May and September, when they are largely attributed to transmission by infected ticks or deer flies. This is in contrast to the historical incidence of tularemia, which was previously considered a winter disease contracted mostly from infected rabbits.

The incidence of tularemia has dropped significantly in the United States, from several thousand cases per year in the 1950s to around 200 per year beginning in the 1990s. The fatality rate in the United States has also declined and is relatively low, at less than 2 percent. This is most likely due to the current availability of antimicrobial therapies. Tularemia occurs more often among males than females; it is also more prevalent among children between the ages of 5 and 9 and among men aged 59 to 65.

Treatment and Prevention

Treatment of tularemia is generally effective with antibiotics, usually streptomycin or gentamicin. Due to the nature of the infection, treatment should be continued for 10 to 21 days to ensure complete recovery. Long-term immunity will usually follow recovery from tularemia, but reinfection is possible, and repeated cases have been reported.

As of 2017 a vaccine against the disease was unavailable to the public, although efforts were ongoing to develop one. Postexposure vaccination is not considered a viable public health strategy due to the three- to five-day incubation period of the disease, as well as the time necessary for immunity to develop.

Preventive measures should be adopted by people working in endemic areas. These should include the use of insect repellent on skin and clothing to minimize the chance of insect bites and effective handwashing using antibacterial soap for people handling animal carcasses. The general public can also minimize infection by thoroughly cooking animal meat and ensuring the safety of water sources.

Impacts and Issues

Tularemia is identified as a Category A agent by the CDC, meaning that it is considered a high risk to society and poses a potential threat to national security. The extremely low infectious dose required by the *F. tularensis* bacteria, in addition to the possible aerosol nature of transmission, makes tularemia potentially hazardous in large populations.

It is for these reasons that tularemia has been previously considered a viable option as a biological warfare agent. During World War II (1939–1945), Japanese researchers investigated this avenue. In the 1950s and 1960s, the United States developed weapons to deliver aerosolized *F. tularensis* organisms. These were destroyed in 1973. The World Health Organization released a statement in 1969 that estimated that the successful release of 110 pounds (50 kilograms) of the virulent bacteria over a metropolitan area housing 5 million people in a developed country would result in 250,000 cases of illness, including 19,000 fatalities. Although it was removed from the list of nationally notifiable diseases in 1994, it was reinstated in 2000 due to its potential for use as a biological weapon. As of 2017 this impact is still recognized, and the CDC acts to ensure the rapid availability of substantial amounts of available antibiotics effective against the bacteria that causes tularemia.

TERRORISM AND BIOLOGICAL WARFARE

The Division of Vector-Borne Diseases at the Centers for Disease Control and Prevention (CDC) states that "*Francisella tularensis* is very infectious. A small number (10–50 or so organisms) can cause disease. If *F. tularensis* were used as a weapon, the bacteria would likely be made airborne for exposure by inhalation. People who inhale an infectious aerosol would generally experience severe respiratory illness, including life-threatening pneumonia and systemic infection, if they are not treated. The bacteria that cause tularemia occur widely in nature and could be isolated and grown in quantity in a laboratory, although manufacturing an effective aerosol weapon would require considerable sophistication."

A part of the CDC program for bioterrorism preparedness and response, the CDC states that as part of its preparations the CDC (or partners in the preparedness program) is "stockpiling antibiotics to treat infected people; coordinating a nationwide program where states share information about tularemia; [and] creating new education tools and programs for health professionals, the public, and the media."

SEE ALSO *Antibacterial Drugs; Bacterial Disease; Bioterrorism; CDC (Centers for Disease Control and Prevention); Vaccines and Vaccine Development; World Health Organization (WHO); Zoonoses*

BIBLIOGRAPHY

Books

Bennett, John E., Raphael Dolin, and Martin J. Blaser. *Mandell, Douglas, and Bennett's Principles and Practice of Infectious Diseases.* 8th ed. Philadelphia: Elsevier/Saunders, 2015.

Periodicals

Nelson, Christina, et al. "Tularemia—United States, 2001–2010." *Morbidity and Mortality Weekly Report* 62, no. 47 (November 29, 2013): 963–966. This article can also be found online at https://www.ncbi.nlm.nih.gov/pmc/articles/PMC4585636/ (accessed February 9, 2018).

Weber, Ingrid B., et al. "Clinical Recognition and Management of Tularemia in Missouri: A Retrospective Records Review of 121 Cases." *Clinical Infectious Diseases* 55, no. 10 (November 15, 2012): 1283–1290. This article can also be found online at https://academic.oup.com/cid/article/55/10/1283/323868 (accessed February 9, 2018).

Websites

"Emergency Preparedness and Response: Tularemia." Centers for Disease Control and Prevention, November 18, 2015. https://emergency.cdc.gov/agent/tularemia/index.asp (accessed February 9, 2018).

"Tularemia." Centers for Disease Control and Prevention, September 27, 2016. https://www.cdc.gov/tularemia/ (accessed February 9, 2018).

"WHO Guidelines on Tularaemia." World Health Organization, 2007. http://www.who.int/csr/resources/publications/WHO_CDS_EPR_2007_7.pdf?ua=1 (accessed February 9, 2018).

Tony Hawas
Claire Skinner

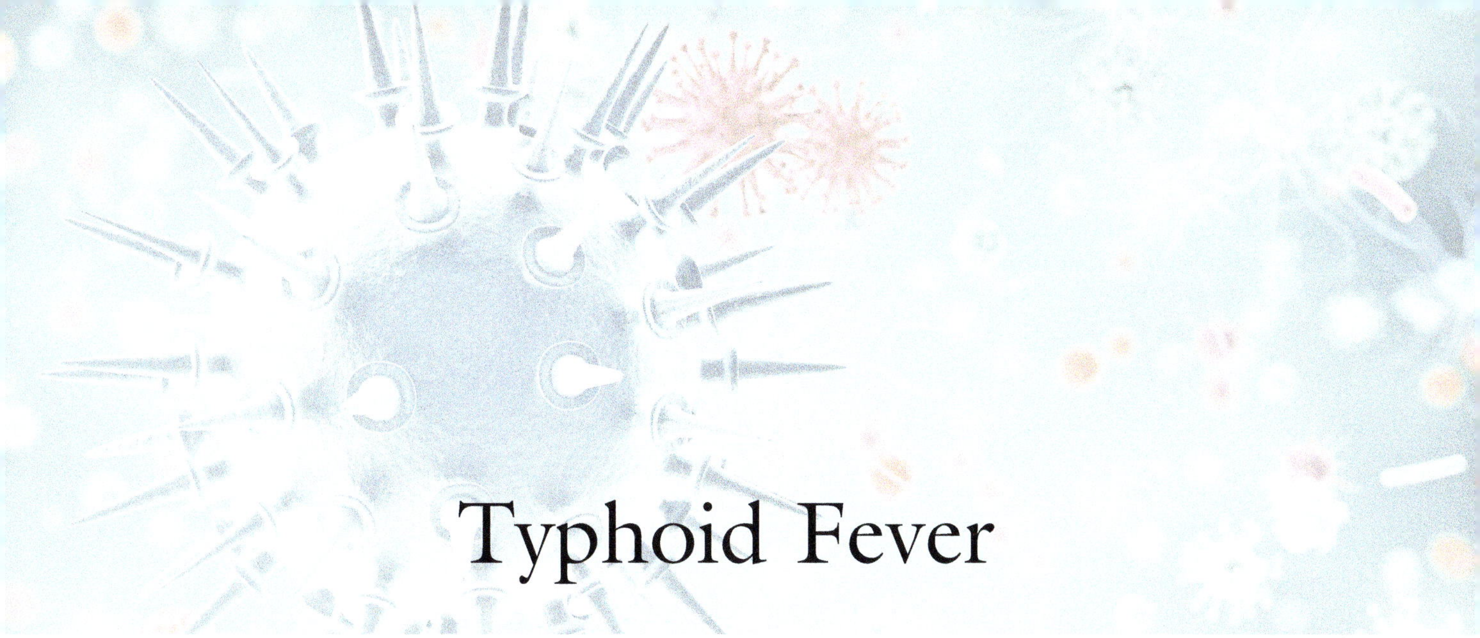

Typhoid Fever

Introduction

Typhoid fever, sometimes also known as enteric fever, is a potentially life-threatening infection caused by the bacterium *Salmonella typhi*. It is rare in the United States and other Western countries, and most cases in these areas have been acquired when traveling abroad. The disease is spread by contaminated food and water.

People who have had typhoid fever may be infectious for many months after they have recovered. One of the most famous carriers of typhoid fever was Mary Mallon, commonly known by the nickname "Typhoid Mary." An asymptomatic carrier of *S. typhi*, she worked as a cook for a family in New York City between 1901 and 1915. She infected 53 people with typhoid, and three of the people she infected died. Typhoid is treatable with antibiotics but can have a fatality rate of up to 30 percent if it goes untreated. There are also several types of vaccines that travelers can use to protect themselves in areas where typhoid is endemic. However, protection afforded by the vaccines is not lifelong, and those who may be exposed may need to have a booster dose.

Disease History, Characteristics, and Transmission

Typhoid fever is caused by the bacterium *S. typhi*, which infects the blood and the intestines. Paratyphoid fever is a milder condition caused by related species of *Salmonella*. The two are sometimes referred to as enteric fever because of the site of infection. *Salmonella* species also cause food poisoning and only infect humans. There is no animal reservoir. At one time typhoid was confused with typhus because of the similarity between the symptoms. However, it is now known that the causes and pathology of the two diseases are very different.

The symptoms of typhoid include high fever, chills, cough, muscle pain, weakness, stomach pain, headache, and a rash made up of flat, rose-colored spots. Diarrhea is a less common symptom of typhoid fever even though it is a gastrointestinal disease. Constipation and loss of appetite are also observed. Sometimes there are mental changes, known as typhoid psychosis. A characteristic feature of typhoid psychosis is plucking at the bedclothes if the patient is confined to bed.

Typhoid fever is diagnosed by identification of *S. typhi* in blood or in stool samples. Left untreated, fever may persist for many months, leading to potentially fatal complications. For instance, the mucosal walls of the intestine may weaken, allowing the infection to spread into the bowel. Typhoid fever has a 1 percent fatality rate in the United States, assuming prompt treatment with antibiotics. Without treatment the death rate rises to about 10 percent. In parts of Africa and Asia, where the disease is far more common, mortality rates from typhoid may approach 30 percent.

Typhoid fever is spread through food and water contaminated by people with typhoid shedding *S. typhi*. About

WORDS TO KNOW

ENDEMIC Present in a particular area or among a particular group of people.

MULTIDRUG RESISTANCE A phenomenon that occurs when an infective agent loses its sensitivity against two or more of the drugs that are used against it.

TYPHUS A disease caused by various species of *Rickettsia*, characterized by a fever, rash, and delirium. Insects such as lice and chiggers transmit typhus. Two forms of typhus, epidemic disease and scrub typhus, are fatal if untreated.

1 to 4 percent of typhoid cases become chronic carriers, meaning they continue to shed *S. typhi* in their urine and feces for more than a year after recovery. Typhoid is also transmitted by water into which contaminated sewage has been discharged.

Scope and Distribution

Typhoid has long been a feared human disease. According to the World Health Organization (WHO), as of 2014 there were around 21 million cases of typhoid fever each year, approximately 220,000 of which were fatal. Typhoid fever is endemic in the Indian subcontinent and in parts of Asia, Africa, and Central and South America. In some of these places, typhoid is one of the top five causes of death. The peak age for contracting typhoid in countries where it is endemic is between 5 and 19 years, although it can affect people of either sex at any age.

In the United States around 400 cases of typhoid fever are reported each year, 70 percent of which are contracted during travel to areas where it is endemic. In England and Wales, there are 150 to 200 cases of typhoid annually, again mainly in returning travelers. People have been known to develop typhoid after less than one week's stay in an endemic country. The disease has been all but eliminated from developed nations, although sporadic cases such as those mentioned above still arise.

Treatment and Prevention

Typhoid fever has been treated with antibiotics, with chloramphenicol, ampicillin, trimethoprim-sulfamethoxazole, and ciprofloxacin being common choices. However, a major concern is the emergence of multidrug-resistant strains of *S. typhi* in parts of Asia and South America. Therefore, the choice of antibiotic should be guided by local knowledge of which drugs will be effective against the strain of *S. typhi* involved in the infection.

There are two vaccines commonly used to prevent typhoid. One is an inactivated (killed) vaccine administered as a shot. The other is a live, attenuated (weakened) vaccine that is taken orally. Both are about 75 percent effective. Travelers should consult their national public health authority as to whether they need to be vaccinated against typhoid if they are going to a country where the disease is endemic. People who take the inactivated typhoid vaccine need only one shot, which should be taken at least two weeks prior to visiting an area where typhoid is endemic. Boosters are required every two years. People taking the oral vaccine require four doses, given every other day. The last dose should be given at least one week before travel to allow the vaccine time to work.

A major problem with these vaccines, however, is that neither is licensed for use in children under the age of two, even though children are typically most at risk of contracting typhoid fever. In January 2018 WHO approved the use of a new vaccine type, known as a Vi conjugate vac-

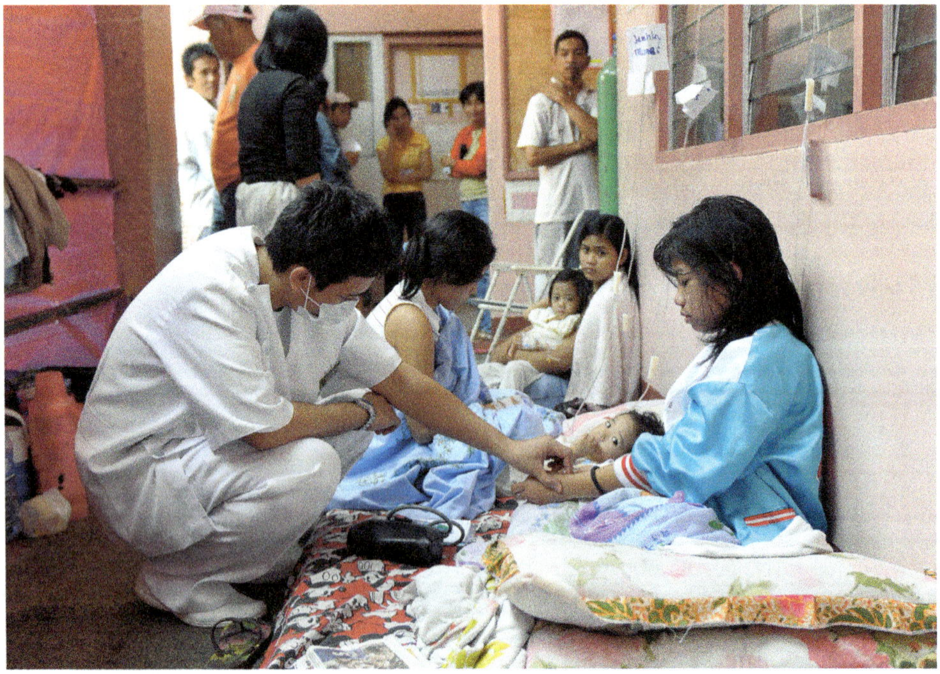

A health care worker assesses a typhoid fever patient at a hospital in the Filipino city of Calamba in 2008. That year a typhoid fever outbreak in the city infected approximately 2,400 people. *© JAY DIRECTO/AFP/ Getty Images*

TYPHOID MARY

Mary Mallon, a known carrier of typhoid, refused to stop behaving in ways that risked spreading the disease and forced the government to jail her to protect the public health. The first person in North America to be identified as a healthy typhoid carrier, Mallon was an Irish-born cook who worked for wealthy New Yorkers. In 1906 she was employed in the rented summer home of banker Charles Henry Warren in Oyster Bay, Long Island, when typhoid fever struck six people in the household of 11. The owners of the rental house hired investigators to determine the source of the epidemic. The detectives traced 47 cases of typhoid and three deaths to Mallon.

A contagious bacterial disease, typhoid bacteria remain in the intestine, liver, and bile ducts until they are transmitted via urine and feces. Victims suffer fever, chills, headaches, malaise, severe cramping, and diarrhea or constipation. The symptoms often continue for over a month. While sick, people with typhoid weaken and became susceptible to complications such as dehydration or intestinal bleeding.

As a single, working-class woman, Mallon needed to work in order to support herself. She was reputedly an excellent cook but was unaware of the germ theory of disease and of the simple measures (such as handwashing) necessary to prevent spreading disease. Investigators discovered that 30 percent of the bacteria excreted by Mallon in her urine were the bacteria that cause typhoid.

In March 1907 New York City health officials literally dragged Mallon kicking and screaming into a city ambulance. They deposited her in a small cottage on North Brother Island that formed part of the grounds of an isolation hospital. Although she was released for brief periods, Mallon, who had been offered employment as a laundress, persisted in cooking, and she infected additional people. As a result, she was returned to the isolation hospital, where she died in 1938 at the age of 69, after spending 26 years in her island prison.

cine, which could be given to children as young as six months. The vaccine, developed in India and licensed for use there since 2013, has been shown to prevent around 50 percent of infections and has been hailed as a potential breakthrough in the fight against the disease.

Taking care to avoid risky food or drink is as important as being vaccinated in protecting against typhoid fever. All drinking water should either be bottled or boiled rapidly for one minute. Ice should be avoided in case it was made from contaminated water. Travelers in countries where there is typhoid should eat food that is thoroughly cooked and is still hot and steaming. Raw vegetables and fruits should be avoided unless they can be peeled, in which case hands should be carefully washed first. Many travelers get sick with typhoid and other gastrointestinal illnesses by eating food they bought from street vendors.

People who have had typhoid fever ought to assume they have carrier status unless a series of stool samples analyses for *S. typhi* proves negative for the bacterium. Therefore, they should not prepare or serve food and should take extra care with personal hygiene.

■ Impacts and Issues

Typhoid continues to be a problem worldwide because of poor sanitation, which forces people into frequent contact with contaminated water and food. Inadequate sewage disposal continues to be an issue in many places, placing populations at risk of a number of diseases, including typhoid fever.

The higher mortality rates from typhoid fever seen in many developing countries can be attributed to a weak or nonexistent health care infrastructure, which does not provide ready access to the antibiotics that could cure the disease. War and natural disasters, such as earthquakes, disrupt clean water supplies, which is why typhoid has often accompanied such disasters, both in the early 21st century and throughout the course of history.

For example, WHO reported a significant outbreak of typhoid fever in Kinshasa in the Democratic Republic of the Congo involving a total of 13,400 cases by mid-December 2004. The fatality rate from the outbreak was 22 percent (134 deaths), mainly due to peritonitis, a severe inflammation of the lining of the abdominal cavity. Poor sanitation and lack of access to clean drinking water had been reported in the affected areas. The number of cases increased to over 42,000 through the early months of 2005, while the death toll mounted to 214. The medical charity Médecins sans Frontières Belgium (Doctors without Borders Belgium) helped to provide clean water, which, along with other control measures such as health education, began to bring the outbreak under control.

Likewise, in February 2015 the Ministry of Health of Uganda received reports of a strange illness that had resulted in one fatality and left 30 others with headaches, severe abdominal pain, and high fever. By June 2015 there were more than 10,000 suspected cases of typhoid fever in the area. The source of the outbreak was traced to drinking water and street vendor juices contaminated with *S. typhi.*

Although typhoid fever is thought to be easily treatable, researchers have become increasingly concerned with the rapid emergence of drug-resistant strains of the disease. A 2015 study, for example, found that the presence of the multidrug-resistant typhoid strain H58 in Malawi increased from around 7 percent of all infections between 1998 and 2010 to 97 percent in 2014. Another study from 2015 found H58 in samples from 21 out of 63 countries primarily in Africa and Asia. Experts have suggested that the bacterium had acquired resistance to many commonly used antibiotics over time due to widespread and often unnecessary use of the drugs and have stressed prevention efforts as a key to limiting the need for such treatments. WHO's approval of conjugate vaccines for children in 2018 has been touted as a positive step toward limiting antibiotic use in areas facing high rates of typhoid.

SEE ALSO *Travel and Infectious Disease; War and Infectious Disease*

BIBLIOGRAPHY

Books

Adler, Richard, and Elise Mara. *Typhoid Fever: A History.* Jefferson, NC: McFarland, 2016.

Grove, David I. *Tapeworms, Lice, and Prions: A Compendium of Unpleasant Infections.* Oxford, UK: Oxford University Press, 2014.

Periodicals

Feasey, Nicholas A., et al. "Rapid Emergence of Multidrug Resistant, H58-Lineage *Salmonella* Typhi in Blantyre, Malawi." *PLOS Neglected Tropical Diseases* 9, no. 4 (2015): e0003748. This article can also be found online at http://journals.plos.org/plosntds/article?id=10.1371/journal.pntd.0003748 (accessed January 29, 2018).

Kabwama, Steven Ndugwa, et al. "A Large and Persistent Outbreak of Typhoid Fever Caused by Consuming Contaminated Water and Street-Vended Beverages: Kampala, Uganda, January–June 2015." *BMC Public Health* 17, no. 23 (October 2017). This article can also be found online at https://bmcpublichealth.biomedcentral.com/articles/10.1186/s12889-016-4002-0 (accessed January 29, 2018).

Marineli, Filio, et al. "Mary Mallon (1869–1938) and the History of Typhoid Fever." *Annals of Gastroenterology* 26, no. 2 (2013): 132–134. This article can also be found online at https://www.ncbi.nlm.nih.gov/pmc/articles/PMC3959940/ (accessed January 29, 2018).

Mogasale, Vittal, et al. "Burden of Typhoid Fever in Low-Income and Middle-Income Countries: A Systematic, Literature-Based Update with Risk-Factor Adjustment." *Lancet Global Health* 2, no. 10 (October 2014): 570–580. This article can also be found online at http://www.thelancet.com/journals/langlo/article/PIIS2214-109X(14)70301-8/fulltext (accessed January 29, 2018).

Wong, Vanessa K., et al. "Phylogeographical Analysis of the Dominant Multidrug-Resistant H58 Clade of *Salmonella* Typhi Identifies Inter- and Intracontinental Transmission Events." *Nature Genetics* 47, no. 6 (June 2015): 632–639. This article can also be found online at https://www.nature.com/articles/ng.3281 (accessed January 29, 2018).

Websites

Berkley, Seth. "A New Vaccine against Typhoid Fever Will Also Help Fight Antimicrobial Resistance." STAT, November 30, 2017. https://www.statnews.com/2017/11/30/typhoid-fever-antimicrobial-resistance/ (accessed January 29, 2018).

"Typhoid." World Health Organization, April 13, 2015. http://www.who.int/immunization/diseases/typhoid/en/ (accessed January 29, 2018).

"Typhoid Fever." Centers for Disease Control and Prevention, July 18, 2016. https://www.cdc.gov/typhoid-fever/index.html (accessed January 29, 2018)

Susan Aldridge
Sam Uretsky

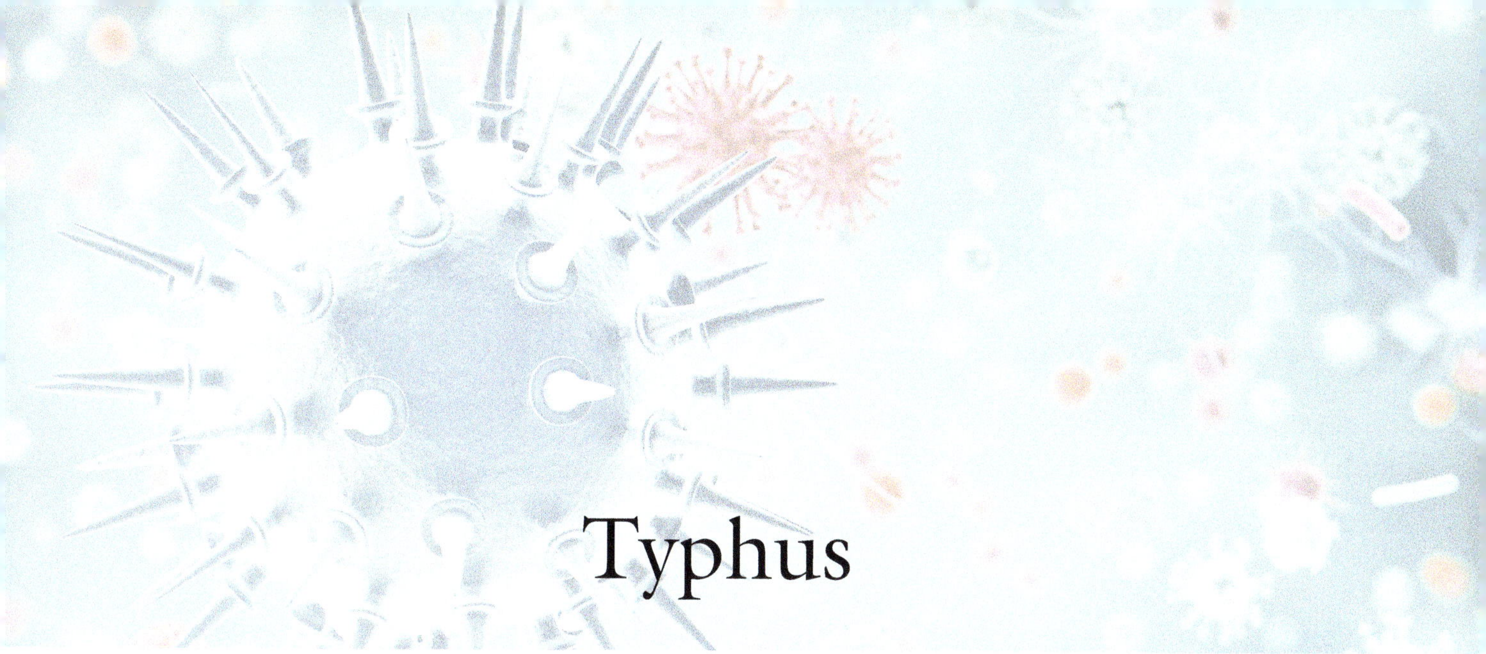

Typhus

Introduction

Typhus is a group of diseases caused by bacteria belonging to the *Rickettsiae* genus. They are spread by ticks and small insects and are found in specific geographical locations around the world. Typhus has caused millions of deaths over the course of human history, being particularly common under conditions of war, famine, and mass migration.

There are four main types of typhus. Epidemic typhus is spread by lice and tends to occur in conditions of overcrowding and poor hygiene. The spotted fevers (sometimes also known as tick-borne typhus), including Rocky Mountain spotted fever, are a group of tick- and mite-borne rickettsial diseases found in parts of the United States, Africa, India, Australia, and the Mediterranean. Endemic flea-borne typhus is spread by rats and occurs in rodent-infested environments such as garbage dumps and markets. Scrub typhus is spread by mites and is found in parts of Southeast Asia. Typhus is a potentially fatal disease, with prevention depending on control of its insect vectors.

Disease History, Characteristics, and Transmission

Typhus was confused with typhoid fever until the 1830s, when it was shown to be a separate disease, although the similarity between the two names persists. The *Rickettsiae*, which are the causative agents of the various forms of typhus, get their name from Howard Taylor Ricketts (1871–1910), an American pathologist who discovered them and who also died from typhus. They are Gram-negative cocci or bacilli, having an oval shape or existing as chains. Gram-negative refers to the way in which the bacteria react with Gram stain, which is used to prepare samples for microscopy.

The specific *Rickettsiae* associated with the different types of typhus have been identified. Therefore, *R. prowazekii* is the agent of epidemic louse-born typhus, and *R. rickettsii, R. conorii, R. africae, R. japonica, R. australis,* and several other species are involved in tick-borne typhus, each organism being found in a different geographical area. Endemic flea-borne typhus is associated with *R. mooseri*, and *R. tsutugamusi* is the agent of scrub typhus.

The incubation time of typhus is 12 to 15 days. The bacteria enter the bloodstream and can spread throughout the body. They invade the endothelial cells, which line the inner walls of the small veins, arteries, and capillaries and make them swell. This can cause thrombosis, or blood clotting, and small characteristic nodules made up of white blood cells and platelets may develop in the blood.

The early symptoms of all kinds of typhus are nonspecific and may range from mild to severe, consisting of fever, headache, an extensive rash, and perhaps mental confusion. Symptoms persist for about two weeks, but several months may pass before complete recovery occurs. A characteristic eschar, or thick, blackened scab, is seen at the site of the vector bite in scrub typhus and some of the spotted fevers. It is not uncommon for typhus to be improperly diagnosed.

Epidemic typhus may cause a high fever, headache, chills, confusion, and limb pain, progressing to agitation, coma, and other complications. Photophobia, which is an aversion to light, vomiting, and a rash that starts on the trunk can also occur. Epidemic typhus is a far more severe condition than endemic typhus, whose symptoms are milder but similar.

Rocky Mountain spotted fever causes headache, fever, abdominal pain, and a rash that begins on the hands and feet and spreads to the rest of the body. The other spotted fevers cause similar symptoms but with some regional variations. For example, African tick-bite fever is not usually associated with a rash, and its symptoms are similar to those of North Asian tick typhus. Scrub typhus causes breathing difficulties, cough, fever, headache, sweating, swollen glands, a swelling at the site of the bite, and a rash starting on the trunk.

Rickettsiae may damage blood vessels, causing clotting and even gangrene, the death of tissue at the extremities of the body because of oxygen deprivation. This can lead to

WORDS TO KNOW

ARTHROPOD A member of the largest single animal phylum, consisting of organisms with segmented bodies, jointed legs or wings, and exoskeletons.

ENDEMIC Present in a particular area or among a particular group of people.

ESCHAR Any scab or crust forming on the skin as a result of a burn or disease. Scabs from cuts or scrapes are not eschars.

HOST An organism that serves as the habitat for a parasite or possibly for a symbiont. A host may provide nutrition to the parasite or symbiont, or it may simply provide a place in which to live.

MACULOPAPULAR A macule is any discolored skin spot that is flush or level with the surrounding skin surface; a papule is a small, solid bump on the skin. A maculopapular skin disturbance is one that combines macules and papules.

PROPHYLAXIS Pre-exposure treatment (e.g., immunizations) to prevent the onset or recurrence of a disease.

RESERVOIR The animal or organism in which a virus or parasite normally resides.

VECTOR Any agent that carries and transmits parasites and diseases. Also, an organism or a chemical used to transport a gene into a new host cell.

the loss of limbs or fingers and toes. The infection can also cause organ failure. Other complications may occur, depending on the type of typhus involved. For instance, tick-borne typhus may result in liver and kidney failure, while brain damage and coma can occur with scrub typhus.

Typhus is usually more severe in adults than in children. The introduction of antibiotics has reduced overall mortality rates to between 3 and 4 percent. Untreated, the mortality rate of epidemic typhus, which is the most serious form of the disease, ranges from 5 to 40 percent; in healthy individuals, the mortality rate is around 20 percent but can be as high as 60 percent in elderly, malnourished, or debilitated individuals. Mortality from treated endemic typhus is about 1 to 4 percent, and is less than 1 percent for scrub typhus.

Those who survive endemic typhus generally have lifelong immunity to another attack but may relapse many years later with a milder form called Brill-Zinsser disease. This occurs because the *Rickettsiae* may linger even after antibiotic treatment, especially if this has been incomplete or the person is malnourished. People surviving other forms of typhus generally have long-term or lifelong immunity from further attacks.

Transmission of typhus is from an animal or human host infected with *Rickettsiae* through an arthropod (flea, tick, mite) vector. In epidemic, louse-borne typhus, the bacteria pass—usually under crowded, unhygienic conditions—from one person to another via the body (clothing) louse, which thrives on worn, unwashed clothing. Head and pubic lice do not usually act as vectors for *Rickettsiae.*

The *Rickettsiae* live in the digestive tract of the louse and are shed in its feces. Transmission usually occurs when the louse bites a human for a blood meal, defecating as it eats. The bite itches, and scratching it crushes the louse and releases the bacteria from contaminated louse feces into the bloodstream. *Rickettsia* can survive for many months in dust containing dried louse feces and may be transmitted in this form through the eyes or mouth.

Endemic typhus, sometimes called murine typhus, is carried by the flea *Xenopsylla cheopsis*, with rats, mice, opossums, raccoons, and skunks acting as the animal reservoirs. In tick-borne typhus, including the spotted fevers, rodents, dogs, cats, opossums, and hares act as animal reservoirs in various locations, with the vectors usually being ticks. However, rickettsial pox, which occurs in Russia, South Africa, and Korea, is carried by mites and *R. felis* infection (similar to endemic typhus) is spread by cat and dog fleas in parts of Europe and South America. Finally, scrub typhus is spread by mite bites.

■ Scope and Distribution

Typhus is a disease that has killed millions over the course of human history and is particularly prevalent under conditions of war, famine, and natural disaster where hygiene is poor and overcrowding and malnutrition are common. First described in the 15th century, typhus has been known as famine fever, ship fever, camp fever, and gaol (jail) fever, names that reflect the conditions under which it is most commonly found. It arrived in Europe in 1489 with soldiers who had been fighting in Cyprus. An outbreak between 1557 and 1559 killed around 10 percent of the English population.

In the 19th century typhus ravaged French leader Napoleon's (1769–1821) troops on their Moscow campaign and hit Ireland between 1816 and 1819 and again during the famine of the 1840s. London experienced a serious typhus epidemic in the 1840s during a time of railway construction and building trade strikes that led to dislocation and deprivation in the city, and the disease began to claim more lives than smallpox.

During World War I (1914–1918), typhus caused 150,000 deaths in Serbia in 1915. The epidemic was eventually brought under control by a British sanitary team. Between 1918 and 1922, epidemic louse-borne typhus caused 30 million cases and 3 million deaths in Eastern Europe and Russia. This epidemic was triggered by war and revolution, food and fuel shortages, and economic collapse and was spread by the railways that enabled mass movement of people.

A famous victim of typhus was the teenage diarist of World War II (1939–1945) Anne Frank, who died of typhus in the Bergen-Belsen concentration camp in 1945. Frank was just one victim in an epidemic that had a mortality of around 50 percent, killing almost 35,000 of the inhabitants of the camp.

In 1997 the World Health Organization (WHO) reported an outbreak of nearly 24,000 cases of epidemic typhus in Burundi, the largest outbreak in 50 years. The epidemic began with 216 cases occurring in a prison in Ngozi, ideal conditions for contracting the disease, and then spread to the malnourished residents of refugee camps in the central highlands. WHO joined local teams in investigating the focal points of the outbreak, handing out doses of antibiotics to get the epidemic under control.

Epidemic typhus now occurs mainly in northeastern and central Africa. It is rare in most developed countries and would generally only be seen in communities and populations where body louse infestations are common, such as in refugee and prisoner populations during wars or famine.

The southern flying squirrel (*Glaucomys volans*) is known to carry *R. prowazekii*. Between 1976 and 2009, there were 45 reported cases of epidemic typhus in individuals with no history of lice infestation who had had contact with flying squirrels and their nests. Therefore, campers and wildlife workers could be at risk of typhus if they come into contact with squirrels or their nests, which are typically made in houses or in tree holes. The insect vector in such cases is the flying squirrel louse or flea, although it is also possible that the affected individuals were exposed to *R. prowazekii* through contact with louse feces.

Epidemic typhus in the 21st century occurs sporadically in cool, mountainous regions of Africa, Asia, and Central and South America, especially during the colder months when louse-infested clothing may not be washed frequently. Travelers who do not come into contact with either lice or people with lice are not at risk in areas where epidemic typhus occurs. However, health care workers and military personnel who do have such contact may be at risk of contracting typhus.

Tick-borne typhus occurs in many places throughout the world, including the eastern United States, Brazil, the Mediterranean basin, the African veldt, India, and Australia. For instance, Rocky Mountain spotted fever occurs in Mexico, Central America, and South America, while tick-borne disease caused by *R. slovaca* is found in Europe. The spring and summer months are the peak times for transmission of tick-borne typhus. Travelers taking part in outdoor activities such as camping or hiking could be at risk of acquiring tick-borne typhus if they do not take adequate precautions against tick bites.

Endemic flea-borne typhus causes sporadic cases in locations worldwide where humans and rodents live close together, such as in markets and garbage dumps. Flea-infested rats are found all year-round in humid tropical climates and are more common in the warmer winter months in temperate regions. In the United States cases have occurred in Southern California and southern Texas, more commonly among adults. A 2017 study in *Emerging Infectious Diseases* reported a total of 1,762 cases of endemic typhus in Texas between 2003 and 2013 and noted that the average number of cases per year doubled from the time period 2003–2007 (102 cases per year) to 2008–2013 (209 cases per year), though the reason for the apparent increase in cases was unclear. In November 2017 the Texas Department of State Health Services announced that there were over 400 cases reported in 2017 and urged health care providers to be aware of the symptoms and available treatments.

Travelers to places where there are rat-infested buildings and homes, especially by rivers and coastal port regions, could be at risk of contracting endemic typhus. Other animals, such as feral cats and opossums, may carry the flea vectors of the disease, and contact with them should be avoided in endemic countries.

Scrub typhus is acquired from the bite of larval mites living on waist-high Imperata grass that grows in previously cleared jungle around villages and in plantations. It occurs in Southeast Asia, the Indian subcontinent, Sri Lanka and other Indian Ocean islands, Papua New Guinea, and North Queensland in Australia. No cases have occurred in the United States except among travelers coming back from endemic areas. The incidence of scrub typhus worldwide is unknown because its rather nonspecific symptoms make it difficult to diagnose and there is a lack of diagnostic lab facilities in many parts of the world where it is endemic.

■ Treatment and Prevention

In 1948 the antibiotic chloramphenicol was introduced for the treatment of scrub typhus. Tetracycline and doxycycline later became alternative drugs. The type of antibiotic treatment for all forms of typhus is similar.

According to the US National Library of Medicine in November 2016, tetracycline, doxycycline, and chloramphenicol are the preferred drugs for treatment of typhus. A 2017 review of studies of antibiotic treatment of typhus published in *Transactions of the Royal Society of Tropical Medicine and Hygiene* compared these drugs with azithromycin and the less frequently used antibiotics roxithromycin, telithromycin, levofloxacin, and rifampicin. The authors concluded that, of the commonly used antibiotics, azithromycin offered the best combination of favorable results and low frequency of adverse effects. However, they noted that "the preferred choice of antibiotics for each patient depends on the adverse effect profile, personal circumstances (e.g., age, pregnancy), cost and local prescription guidelines." In contrast, a Chinese study published in 2017 in the journal *Medicine* observed that the advantages of azithromycin were sufficient to make it the drug of first choice for treatment of scrub typhus.

Some antibiotic-resistant cases of scrub typhus have been reported. In areas where this is the case, first-line treatment with rifampicin or ciprofloxacin might be recommended.

Lab tests are important to determine the cause of the disease, but treatment is usually begun before the results of these are available to prevent complications. Treatment usually continues for up to three days after the fever has cleared.

There is no vaccine against typhus. Where there is epidemic typhus, mass prophylaxis with doxycycline is often necessary, as was accomplished in the Burundi outbreak. When prophylaxis is used, the protocol must be rigidly followed. In a 2016 report from an Australian military post published in *Microbes and Infection*, 36 percent of the population developed infections due to failure to follow the prophylactic regimen.

Long-term prevention efforts depend on controlling the insect vector and the animal reservoirs of *Rickettsia.* For louse-borne typhus, clean clothes, dusted with 1 percent malathion or 1 percent permethrin insecticide, helps protect against the disease. Tickborne typhus can be prevented by the use of DEET (N,N-diethyl-meta-toluamide) or permethrin. Finally, prevention of scrub typhus is aided by clearing jungle grass within or near affected villages. Travelers should protect themselves with boots and long trousers and cover their clothing with DEET or permethrin. Prophylactic doxycycline may also be useful for those who must travel through high-risk areas.

According to WHO, insect carriers transmit up to 17 percent of infectious diseases. The organization has developed a plan for global vector control, calling on all countries to improve surveillance and provide coordination and integration across sectors and diseases. This plan encourages nations to work together to reduce the problem of insect carriers across borders and is aimed not only at typhus but at all infectious diseases carried by insects.

Travelers are generally not at high risk of developing typhus via exposure to an infected person, except in cases of epidemic typhus. However, people traveling to any of the many countries where typhus is endemic should seek advice from their health care provider about precautions. In general, covering the body to avoid tick and flea bites and frequent washing and changing of clothes will help prevent typhus. Insecticides also have an important role to play in keeping the vectors under control.

■ Impacts and Issues

Typhus has long been one of the great human killers. It remains a threat in many parts of the world where the relevant animal reservoirs and disease vectors are not adequately controlled and where sanitation and the health infrastructure are poor. War, famine, and mass migration have created epidemics of typhus in the past and will likely continue to do so, especially in the absence of an effective vaccine against the disease.

The advent of antibiotic treatment has greatly reduced the death toll from typhus, where it is available. However, there have been reports of strains of *Rickettsiae* that are becoming resistant to the drug of choice, doxycycline. Small clinical trials conducted in areas of drug resistance have suggested that rifampicin and azithromycin may be effective alternative treatments. But, in case resistance against these drugs also emerges, researchers are focusing on developing a wider range of treatments for all types of typhus.

PRIMARY SOURCE

How Charles Nicolle of the Pasteur Institute Discovered that Epidemic Typhus Is Transmitted by Lice: Reminiscences from My Years at the Pasteur Institute in Paris

SOURCE: *Gross, Ludwick. "How Charles Nicolle of the Pasteur Institute Discovered That Epidemic Typhus Is Transmitted by Lice: Reminiscences from My Years at the Pasteur Institute in Paris."* Proceedings of the National Academy of Sciences of the United States of America *93 (October 1996): 10539–10540.*

INTRODUCTION: *Ludwick Gross (1904–1999) was a physician and medical researcher who pioneered the study of viruses as a possible cause of human cancers. After earning his medical degree in 1929 in his native Poland, Gross began a long association with the Pasteur Institute in Paris, where he met Charles Nicolle (1866–1936), the scientist who unraveled the mystery of how epidemic typhus is transmitted. Gross recounts Nicolle and the significance of his typhus research in the following excerpted memoir.*

Until the first decade of this century, our information about epidemic, i.e., exanthematic typhus was rather scarce. We knew only that there existed a very dangerous, easily communicable disease, which decimated populations during wars, hunger, or flood, spreading with great speed and affecting large numbers of people. After World War I, 20–30 million people died in Eastern Europe from this disease, and an additional several million died during and after World War II. Crowding, the scarcity of clean clothes, and dirt were the principal factors enabling the spread of typhus. The disease causes high fever and maculopapular [small, red, raised] eruptions of the skin. Typhus is similar to a disease that occurs in the Rocky Mountains in the United States and is transmitted by ticks.

The fact that epidemic typhus is transmitted by lice was discovered by Dr. Charles Nicolle; a discovery for which he received the Nobel Prize in 1928. I met Dr. Nicolle in 1934 at the Pasteur Institute in Paris during my years as a guest investigator. I spoke to him several times in the corridor adjoining my laboratory. At my invitation he came to visit. He was a tall man, distinguished looking, impeccably dressed, lean, and slightly stooped, with dry skin and sparkling eyes. He was 68 years old at that time. It was difficult to talk with him because he was hard of hearing. In spite of his listening device, with its batteries and wires, which he was carrying, one had to almost shout to be understood. He was, like many Frenchmen, very polite and attentive. He agreed, at my request, to spend some time in my laboratory at the Pasteur Institute, and talk about his discovery.

Before long, still a few years before World War II, he came to my laboratory. He arrived wearing a shirt with a starched collar and starched cuffs, and sat himself comfortably in a large chair. He told the following story.

"I was delegated, some 30 years ago," recalled Dr. Nicolle, "to become director of the Pasteur Institute in Tunis, and decided to do something about typhus, which was decimating the local population. The first step was to try to transmit the disease to experimental animals. I injected guinea pigs with blood from patients with typhus and observed that, at least in some of these animals, the injection produced only high temperature. I realized, nevertheless, that even though some of them did not develop fever, they still carried the causative agent. This way we learned that typhus could exist, at least in some species, without any symptoms, except now and then, only fever. The most important point, however, was to discover how it was transmitted from man to man under natural life conditions. I learned this by accident. Tunis was full of typhus patients; the hospital was full and the number of new patients increased every day. Not only was every bed occupied and waiting rooms filled, but patients were waiting in front of the hospital, on the streets, to be admitted. At that point I made the crucial observation," said Dr. Nicolle, "that patients infected others out on the street, and also that their clothing was infectious; service personnel at the hospital and also in the laundry room became infected. The moment the patients were admitted to the hospital, however, after they had a hot bath and were dressed in hospital clothing, they ceased to be infectious. There was no longer fear of disease transmission in a hospital room full of patients. This observation was so simple and uncomplicated that it could have been made not necessarily by a physician, but by an administrator without professional medical training. I determined that there must therefore exist a transmitting vector, in the clothing and underwear of the patients. I anticipated," said Dr. Nicolle, "that most probably lice could be responsible for the transmission of typhus from man to man."

Dr. Nicolle continued his story.

"At the end of June, 1909, I asked Dr. Emile Roux, who was at that time Director of the Pasteur Institute in Paris, for a few chimpanzees. My request was granted, and the chimpanzees arrived promptly. I injected one chimpanzee with blood from a patient suffering from typhus. After several days, I collected from the injected chimpanzee a few lice, and transferred them to another chimpanzee; before long, after about 10 days, this animal developed typhus. I repeated this experiment, with similar results. It was now obvious that typhus was transmitted by lice. That was in September 1909. The first step in the search for typhus control was accomplished. Lice were demonstrated to be the transmitting vectors. The Tunisian government now began intensive measures to limit the typhus epidemic with attempts to combat infestation by lice.

The initial step had been accomplished, but great difficulties were ahead. Typhus is very infectious and many laboratory workers engaged in research on the typhus epidemic became infected accidentally, in the course of their laboratory work, and some of them died of the disease."

See Also *Arthropod-Borne Disease; Lice Infestation (Pediculosis); Rickettsial Disease; Rocky Mountain Spotted Fever*

BIBLIOGRAPHY

Books

Hechemy, Karim E., ed. *Rickettsiology and Rickettsial Diseases: Fifth International Conference.* Boston: Blackwell, 2009.

Pelis, Kim. *Charles Nicolle, Pasteur's Imperial Missionary: Typhus and Tunisia.* Rochester, NY: University of Rochester, 2006.

Periodicals

Cowan, George. "Rickettsial Diseases: The Typhus Group of Fevers—a Review." *Postgraduate Medical Journal* 76 (May 2000): 269–272.

Harris, Patrick N. A., et al. "An Outbreak of Scrub Typhus in Military Personnel Despite Protocols for Antibiotic Prophylaxis: Doxycycline Resistance Excluded by a Quantitative PCR-based Susceptibility Assay." *Microbes and Infection* 18, no. 6 (June 2016): 406–411.

Lee, Szu-Chia, et al. "Comparative Effectiveness of Azithromycin for Treating Scrub Typhus: A PRISMA-Compliant Systematic Review and Meta-Analysis." *Medicine* 96, no. 36 (September 2017). This article can also be found online at https://journals.lww.com/md-journal/Fulltext/2017/09080/Comparative_effectiveness_of_azithromycin_for.37.aspx (accessed January 23, 2018).

Murray, Kristy O., et al. "Typhus Group Rickettsiosis, Texas, USA, 2003–2013." *Emerging Infectious Diseases* 23, no. 4 (April 2017): 645–648. This article can also be found online at https://wwwnc.cdc.gov/eid/article/23/4/16-0958_article (accessed January 23, 2018).

Prusinski, Melissa A. et al. "Sylvatic Typhus Associated with Flying Squirrels (*Glaucomys volans*) in New York State, United States. *Vector-Borne and Zoonotic Diseases* 14.4 (2014): 1–5. This article can also be found online at https://www.researchgate.net/publication/261290069_Sylvatic_Typhus_Associated_with_Flying_Squirrels_Glaucomys_volans_in_New_York_State_United_States.

Wee, Ian, Adeline Lo, and Chaturaka Rodrigo. "Drug Treatment of Scrub Typhus: A Systematic Review and Meta-Analysis of Controlled Clinical Trials." *Transactions of the Royal Society of Tropical Medicine and Hygiene* 111, no. 8 (December 2017): 336–344.

Websites

"Health Alert: Increased Flea-Borne (Murine) Typhus Activity in Texas." Texas State Department of Health Services, November 30, 2017. http://www.dshs.texas.gov/news/releases/2017/HealthAlert-11302017.aspx (accessed January 22, 2018).

"Typhus." National Library of Medicine. https://medlineplus.gov/ency/article/001363.htm (accessed January 21, 2018)

"Typhus Fevers." Centers for Disease Control and Prevention, March 7, 2017. https://www.cdc.gov/typhus/ (accessed January 22, 2018).

Susan Aldridge
Sam Uretsky

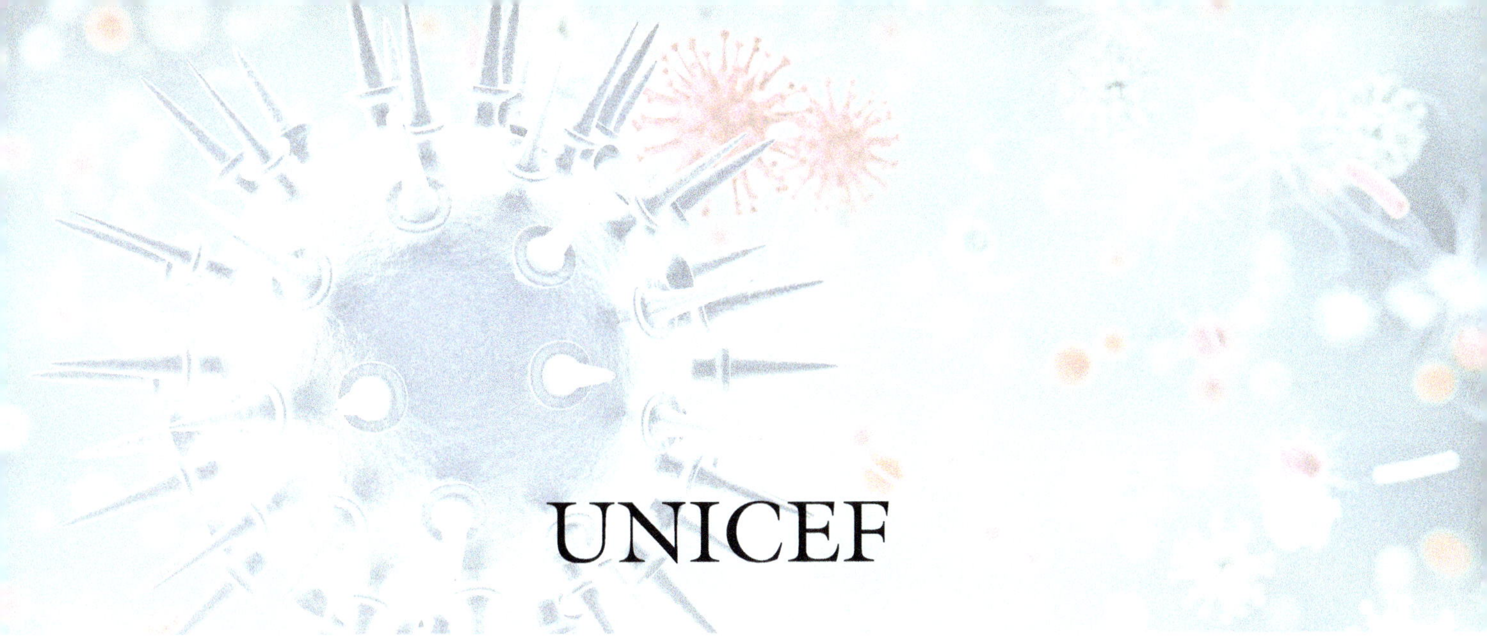

UNICEF

Introduction

Founded by the United Nations (UN), the United Nations Children's Fund (UNICEF, retained from its original name, United Nations International Children's Emergency Fund) is an organization responsible for providing humanitarian assistance to children and their mothers in developing countries, all without discrimination or with regard to political affiliation. Its services promote the development of community groups for the well-being of local children. UNICEF is a member of the United Nations Development Group, a group of UN agencies dedicated to improving the overall effectiveness of the United Nations.

UNICEF, which is headquartered in New York City, participates in efforts to improve children's rights in more than 190 developing and transitional countries and territories. With 200 offices located in partner countries, UNICEF works with governmental and nongovernmental organizations (NGOs) around the world to counter the devastating effects that abuse, discrimination, disease, exploitation, neglect, poverty, and violence have on children. UNICEF strongly believes in the following statement found on its website: "All children have a right to survive, thrive and fulfill their potential—to the benefit of a better world."

History and Scientific Foundations

The UN General Assembly founded UNICEF on December 11, 1946, to furnish clothing, food, health care (including immunizations and medicines), and other necessities to European children adversely affected by World War II (1939–1945). Its original name was the United Nations International Children's Emergency Fund. The founder of UNICEF is widely viewed to have been the Polish physician Ludwik Witold Rajchman (1881–1965), who also served as the organization's first chairperson. The UN expanded its charter in 1950 to help relieve wider hardships and sufferings being inflicted on children, especially those outside of Europe, such as children in China and the Middle East. The expansion helped make UNICEF responsible for children's welfare in more than 150 developing countries.

UNICEF became a permanent part of the United Nations in 1953, when its name was modified to the United Nations Children's Fund. Its well-known acronym, UNICEF, remained the same. The organization's first major activity during this period was a global campaign to eliminate the infectious disease yaws, which at the time affected millions of children. A disfiguring tropical disease of the bones, joints, and skin, yaws is caused by the bacterium *Treponema pertenue*. With the help of penicillin, the incidence of yaws among children was reduced.

In 1959 UNICEF became guided by the UN's Declaration of the Rights of the Child, which made it easier to establish international standards for children's rights to education, health care, nutrition, protection, and shelter.

The Nobel Peace Prize was awarded to UNICEF in 1965 for "the promotion of brotherhood among nations." UNICEF highlighted the rights of children in 1979—naming it the UN International Year of the Child. Though controversial at the time, UNICEF began providing aid for family planning in 1967, specifically to promote the health of the mother and child.

During the 1980s UNICEF adopted the International Code of Marketing of Breast-milk Substitutes (to promote breast milk use); launched Child Survival and Development Revolution (founded on low-cost techniques applied to breastfeeding, child development, and immunization); and adopted the Convention on the Rights of the Child (which became a global human rights treaty).

In the 1990s UNICEF sponsored the World Summit for Children, whose goal is to improve children's education, health, and nutrition. It also emphasized the harmful influence that armed conflicts have on children. In the early 21st century, UNICEF sponsored the Global Move-

WORDS TO KNOW

ACQUIRED IMMUNODEFICIENCY SYNDROME (AIDS) A disease of the immune system caused by the human immunodeficiency virus (HIV). It is characterized by destruction of a particular type of white blood cell and increased susceptibility to infection and other diseases.

IMMUNODEFICIENCY When part of the body's immune system is missing or defective, thus impairing the body's ability to fight infections. As a result, a person with an immunodeficiency disorder will have frequent infections that are generally more severe and last longer than usual.

NEGLECTED TROPICAL DISEASE Many tropical diseases are considered to be neglected because, despite their prevalence in developing areas, new vaccines and treatments are not being created for them. Malaria was once considered a neglected tropical disease, but a great deal of research and money was then devoted to its treatment and cure.

NONGOVERNMENTAL ORGANIZATION (NGO) A voluntary organization that is not part of any government; often organized to address a specific issue or perform a humanitarian function.

NUTRITIONAL SUPPLEMENTS Nutritional supplements are substances necessary to health, such as calcium or protein, that are taken in concentrated form to compensate for dietary insufficiency, poor absorption, unusually high demand for that nutrient, or other reasons.

SANITATION Sanitation is the use of hygienic recycling and disposal measures that prevent disease and promote health through sewage disposal, solid waste disposal, waste material recycling, and food processing and preparation.

ment for Children and organized a historic Special Session of the UN General Assembly that was dedicated to children's rights.

Although UNICEF primarily focuses its work in the countries least able to take care of the basic needs of their children, the organization maintains a clear presence within the United States. In 2014 UNICEF began the program UNICEF Kid Power, which provides information to American children about how others their age live around the world. As these children learn more about their world, they earn points, which are then converted to nutritious food given to the world's malnourished children.

Trick-or-Treat for UNICEF, which started in 1950, remains a popular fundraiser for the organization. Children in countries such as Canada and the United States collect money for UNICEF while out celebrating and trick-or-treating. UNICEF calls the activity "Scary Good Fun." Contributions help needy children affected by recent emergencies, both domestically in North America and in foreign countries.

In 2016 UNICEF dispensed about $3.6 billion worth of services and supplies to children all over the globe. These essentials consist of emergency structures, equipment, and materials to help in the diagnosis of infectious diseases and water treatment facilities to provide clean and safe water, along with a multitude of other items. The UNICEF mission statement remains: "We work for the survival, protection and development of children worldwide through fundraising, advocacy and education."

UNICEF is supported solely by contributions from corporations, foundations, governments, NGOs, and private individuals. For instance, as of July 2016, the Bill & Melinda Gates Foundation had contributed more than $100 million to UNICEF. The 36 national committees created by UNICEF are the primary means by which funds are raised. New York City–based UNICEF USA, one of these committees, states that out of every dollar donated through fundraising efforts, 88 cents goes to helping children, while 9 cents is spent on fundraising expenses and 3 cents on administration costs. This percentage (88 percent going directly to children), along with its accountability and transparency scores, earned UNICEF USA the second-highest Charity Navigator ranking, as of July 2017.

■ Applications and Research

The United Nations Economic and Social Council (ECOSOC) is the parent organization to UNICEF. In 2000 the United Nations set for itself the Millennium Development Goals (MDGs). Six of the eight goals are directly related to children and have been adopted by UNICEF for its own goals: poverty and hunger; universal primary education; gender equality and empowerment of women; child mortality; maternal health; and HIV/AIDS, malaria, and other diseases.

UNICEF upholds the United Nations Convention on the Rights of the Child (UNCRC), which was first approved on November 20, 1989, and became effective the next year on September 2, after the human rights treaty was ratified by a minimum-required number of countries. The Committee on the Rights of the Child (CRC), based on the UNCRC, is an international convention, consisting of 18 independent experts, that establishes the cultural, economic, political, and social rights of children and monitors the implementation of the UNCRC.

UNICEF also participates in the Global Movement for Children (GMC), an international effort of thousands of organizations dedicated to building a better world for children by ensuring that violations of their rights do not occur. Begun in April 2001, GMC's international campaign is generally defined by its slogan, "Say Yes for Children," and is guided by the following issues: (1) children on the move and child trafficking, (2) children and AIDS, (3) child survival, (4) girls' education, and (5) violence against children.

Impacts and Issues

UNICEF works to counter diseases dangerous to children around the world by providing information, services, and products such as educational programs, immunizations, and nutritional supplements. For example, its Immunization Plus program has made significant improvements in children's health with respect to infectious diseases over the last several decades. UNICEF says the "plus" in Immunization Plus is "about using the vehicle of immunization to deliver other life-saving services for children." One important extra service is the delivery and distribution of vitamin A supplements in countries where it is widely deficient in diets. At least 100 billion children under the age of five suffer from vitamin A deficiency. A coalition of governments and UN agencies work closely with UNICEF to provide vitamin A supplements to children twice a year as part of the Vitamin A Global Initiative, which was initiated in 1997.

Despite its efforts, UNICEF estimates that roughly 2 million children still die from diseases that are preventable with inexpensive vaccines. For instance, malaria is primarily found in countries of the sub-Saharan Africa. Though there is no vaccine for the disease, it can be inexpensively controlled though insect repellant and mosquito nets and effectively treated with antimalarial drugs. Through the Roll Back Malaria program, UNICEF is working with the World Health Organization (WHO), the United Nations Development Programme (UNDP), and the World Bank to prevent malaria from happening and to quicken recovery times when it does.

In addition, UNICEF partners with public and private organizations in the Global Alliance for Vaccines and Immunization (Gavi, sometimes also called the Vaccine Alliance). Created in January 2000 and headquartered in Geneva, Switzerland, Gavi is an international organization whose mission is to provide new and underused vaccines to poor children of the world. The organization was made possible with a five-year, $750 million pledge from the Bill & Melinda Gates Foundation.

UNICEF is also especially concerned with children who are targets of abuse, exploitation, and violence. Millions of children are exposed to or suffer cyberbullying/bullying, sexual/nonsexual abuse and exploitation, and violence each day. UNICEF's child protection programs work to counter such practices as childhood marriages, child labor, female genital mutilation, sexual exploitation, slave trafficking, and more. For instance, the United Nations Population Fund (UNFPA)–UNICEF Global Programme to Accelerate Action to End Child Marriage is helping to emphasize the right of girls to delay marriage past childhood. In the 2010s approximately 750 million girls and women were married in childhood. The program is especially geared toward helping adolescent females from the ages of 10 to 19 who live in the countries of Bangladesh, Burkina Faso, Ethiopia, Ghana, India, Mozambique, Nepal, Niger, Sierra Leone, Uganda, Yemen, and Zambia.

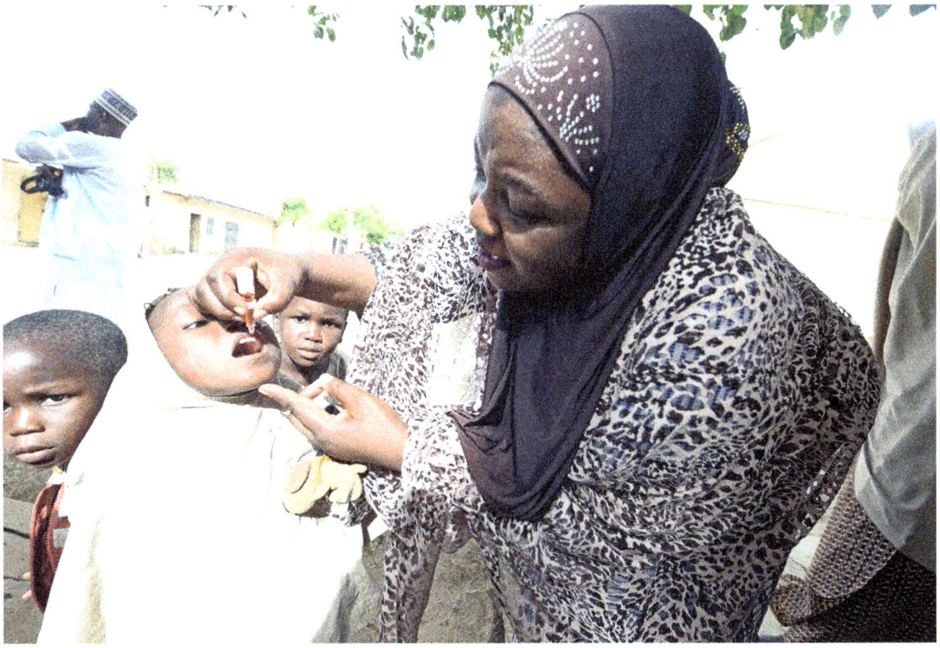

A UNICEF health consultant vaccinates a child against polio in Nigeria in 2017. *© PIUS UTOMI EKPEI/AFP/Getty Images*

In September 2000 the Millennium Declaration was established at the UN Millennium Summit in New York City. Many global statistics from the time concerned children, hunger, poverty, and diseases and became driving forces for the declaration. For example, nearly 600 million children lived on less than one US dollar a day; over 500 million did not have access to sanitation facilities; around 15 million had one or both parents die from HIV/AIDS; and more than 10 million died of hunger and preventable diseases each year.

During this time UNICEF personnel continue to work to break the connection between poverty, hunger, and diseases among children. Poverty contributes to hunger and malnutrition in children, which leads to increased incidences of diseases that, in turn, are a leading factor of children's deaths under five years of age in developing countries.

The goals of the Millennium Declaration stated that, by the year 2015, it would reduce by 50 percent the proportion of people living on less than one US dollar per day and the proportion of people who suffer from hunger. The *Millennium Development Goals Report 2015* stated, "Although significant achievements have been made on many of the MDG targets worldwide, progress has been uneven across regions and countries, leaving significant gaps." The report added, "Millions of people are being left behind, especially the poorest and those disadvantaged because of their sex, age, disability, ethnicity or geographic location. Targeted efforts will be needed to reach the most vulnerable people."

Even though many of the goals of the Millennium Declaration have not been attained as of January 2018, UNICEF continues to dedicate itself to reducing hunger and poverty in children throughout developing countries. (As of 2016 the MDGs have been superseded by SDGs, or Sustainable Development Goals.) Immunization for infectious diseases remains one of the critical factors in UNICEF's work. As a result, UNICEF has become an international leader in providing vaccines to children. Into the 2010s and beyond, UNICEF will continue to purchase and distribute vaccines to children in developing countries. It will also carry on its work to create and maintain local health systems and to improve at-home childcare.

Based on its *State of the World's Children 2016* report, UNICEF declared that "the lives and futures of millions of children are in jeopardy." The report continued, "But around the world, millions of children are trapped in an intergenerational cycle of disadvantage that endangers their futures–and the future of their societies." However, the world has a choice: "Invest in the most excluded children now or risk a more divided and unfair world." The report stated that, unless the world reverses the course of these disadvantaged children by the year 2030, 167 million children will live in "extreme poverty," 69 million under the age of five "will die" between 2016 and 2030, and 60 million children of primary school age will "be out of school." As it has for so many decades, UNICEF continues to tackle this and other challenges to help children around the world.

See Also *Childhood-Associated Infectious Diseases, Immunization Impacts; Developing Nations and Drug Delivery; ; Tropical Infectious Diseases; United Nations Millennium Goals and Infectious Disease; Vaccines and Vaccine Development*

BIBLIOGRAPHY

Books

Kek, Peggy, and Penny Whitworth, eds. *Singapore and UNICEF: Working for Children.* Hackensack, NJ: World Scientific, 2016.

Maddocks, Steven. *UNICEF.* Chicago: Raintree, 2004.

Szente, Judit. *Assisting Young Children Caught in Disasters: Multidisciplinary Perspectives and Interventions.* New York: Springer, 2017.

UNICEF. *1946–2006: Sixty Years for Children.* New York: UNICEF, 2006.

Widmer, Jocelyn. *Investing in Young Children for Peaceful Societies.* Washington, DC: National Academies, 2016.

Websites

"Child Protection." UNICEF. https://www.unicef.org/protection/ (accessed January 16, 2018).

"Declaration of the Rights of the Child." UNICEF. https://www.unicef.org/malaysia/1959-Declaration-of-the-Rights-of-the-Child.pdf (accessed January 16, 2018).

"ECOSOC." United Nations Economic and Social Council. https://www.un.org/ecosoc/ (accessed January 16, 2018).

"Millennium Development Goals." UNICEF. https://www.unicef.org/mdg/ (accessed January 16, 2018).

"The Millennium Development Goals Report 2015." UNICEF. http://www.un.org/millenniumgoals/2015_MDG_Report/pdf/MDG%202015%20rev%20(July%201).pdf (accessed January 16, 2018).

"The Nobel Peace Prize 1965." Nobelprize.org. http://nobelprize.org/nobel_prizes/peace/laureates/1965/ (accessed January 16, 2018).

"A Promise to Children." UNICEF. http://www.unicef.org/wsc/ (accessed January 16, 2018).

"The State of the World's Children 2016." UNICEF. https://www.unicef.org/sowc2016/ (accessed January 16, 2018).

"UNICEF." UNICEF. https://www.unicef.org/ (accessed January 16, 2018).

William Arthur Atkins

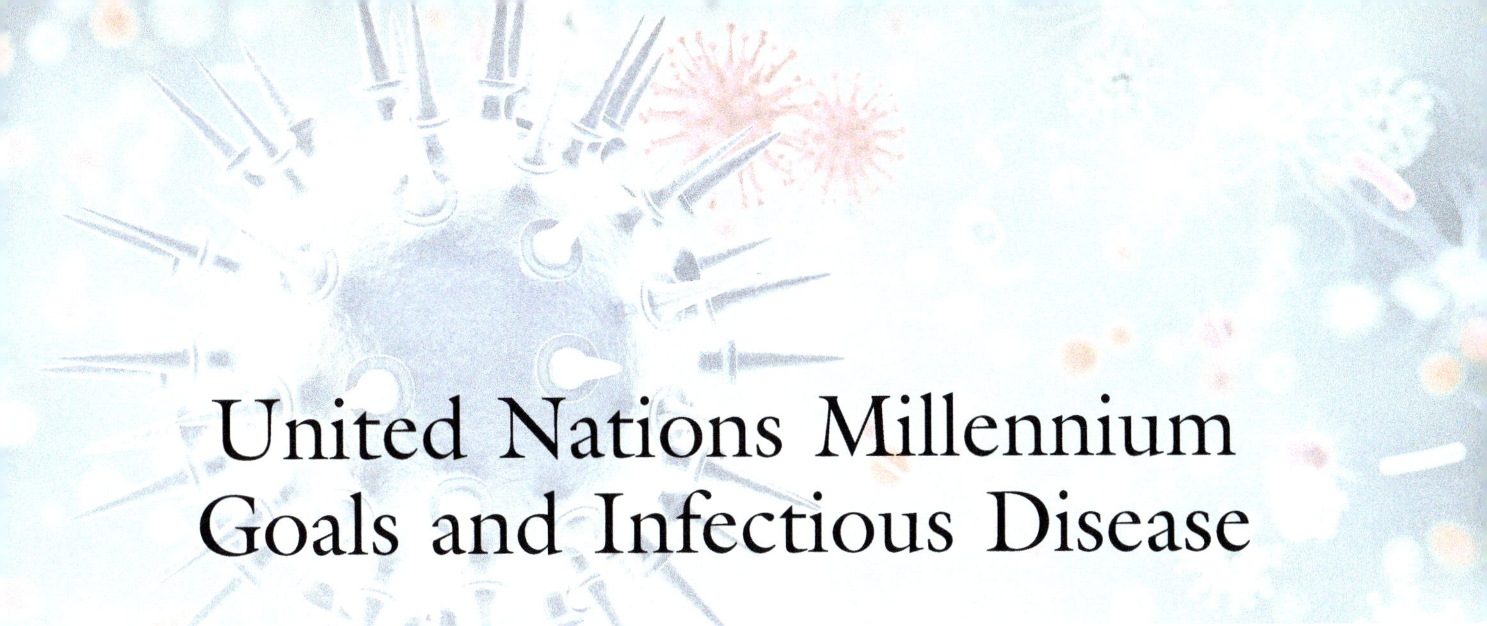

United Nations Millennium Goals and Infectious Disease

Introduction

In 2000 the United Nations (UN) adopted a series of goals designed to improve the lives of people throughout the world by reducing poverty, hunger, disease, and maternal and infant mortality; providing better education for children and equal opportunities for women; and moving toward a healthier environment. According to the UN, these eight Millennium Development Goals (MDGs) provide "a framework for countries around the world for development, as well as time-bound targets by which progress can be measured." Several of these goals were specifically aimed to reduce the incidence and prevalence of infectious disease, most notably human immunodeficiency virus (HIV), malaria, and tuberculosis, as well as prevent infectious disease, especially measles, among children.

The MDGs pertaining to the global control of infectious disease include "reduce child mortality," a major part of which is reducing childhood deaths from measles through vaccination programs. Another is "combat HIV/AIDS [acquired immunodeficiency syndrome], malaria and other diseases," in part by providing international aid to developing nations through prevention and treatment measures known to be effective. Although substantial progress in achieving health-related targets has been achieved in some countries, others affected by high levels of AIDS, economic crisis, or war are falling behind.

Significant progress toward the goal of reducing mortality for children under age five has been achieved. In 2013 about 6 million children under age five died worldwide compared with 12.7 million in 1990. During that time the mortality rate for children under age five declined by 49 percent, from 90 deaths per 1,000 live births to 46. The rate of decline accelerated in the early 21st century, increasing from 1.2 percent per year in 1990–1995 to 4.0 percent in 2005–2013. Nevertheless, the world did not achieve the MDG target of a two-thirds reduction in 1990 mortality levels by 2015.

Higher levels of immunization coverage are being achieved in many countries. By 2013 66 percent of UN member states had reached at least 90 percent coverage, with global measles immunization coverage reaching 84 percent among children aged 12 to 23 months. Measles deaths decreased by approximately 74 percent between 2000 and 2013.

The fifth MDG, "improve maternal health," targeted a reduction of the maternal mortality ratio by 75 percent. Although there was a significant reduction in maternal deaths between 1995 and 2013, the decline was less than half of what was required to meet the MGD target. The UN cited the need for more high-quality reproductive health care and prenatal interventions. There was a substantial increase in preventing or postponing childbearing using contraception, which also affected the maternal death rate.

The proportion of women receiving prenatal care at least once during pregnancy was about 83 percent for the period 2007–2014, but the proportion receiving the recommended number of four care visits was much lower.

WORDS TO KNOW

ENDEMIC Present in a particular area or among a particular group of people.

IMMUNOCOMPROMISED Having an immune system with reduced ability to recognize and respond to the presence of foreign material.

INCIDENCE The number of new cases of a disease or injury that occur in a population during a specified period.

PANDEMIC An epidemic that occurs in more than one country or population simultaneously. *Pandemic* means "all the people."

Progress toward reducing neonatal and maternal deaths has been hampered in certain regions, such as the WHO African Region, by the low proportion (51 percent) of births attended by skilled personnel, although the proportion is above 90 percent in three out of the six WHO regions.

The goal of combating HIV/AIDS, malaria, and other diseases has three subgoals. According to WHO, efforts toward target 6A, halting the spread of HIV/AIDS and beginning to reverse it by 2015, have produced some significant results. New HIV infections were reduced by about 40 percent between 2000 and 2013. However, an estimated 35 million people worldwide were still living with HIV in 2013. That year 15 countries accounted for 75 percent of the new infections, and almost 1 percent of adults aged 15 to 49 were living with HIV.

Work toward target 6B, "achieve, by 2010, universal access to treatment for HIV/AIDS for all those who need it," has also shown progress. By June 2014 the number of people receiving antiretroviral treatment (ART) increased from 800,000 in 2003 to 13.6 million in 2014. In developing nations the number of new people receiving ART rose by almost 2 million individuals. This treatment prevented nearly 8 million deaths from AIDS between 1995 and 2013 and was delivered to more than 12 million people in these countries in 2014.

Progress toward target 6C, "have halted by 2015 and begun to reverse the incidence of malaria and other major diseases," has also been substantial. The increase in malaria treatment led to a 58 percent decline in malaria mortality rates worldwide between 2000 and 2015. Malaria interventions prevented more than 6 million deaths, mostly in children in sub-Saharan Africa younger than five years of age. Increased funding of insecticide-treated nets has expanded the number of children protected from malaria-carrying mosquitoes at night. Tuberculosis prevention efforts have also borne fruit, having saved about 37 million lives between 2000 and 2013.

History and Policy Response

HIV/AIDS

Since the 1980s more than 78 million people have been infected with HIV, 35 million of whom have died of illnesses associated with AIDS. This death toll among adults in their sexual and occupational prime has resulted in the orphaning of 15 million children and economic devastation, which has in turn exacerbated poverty and hunger. During the global HIV epidemic, approximately 17 million children have lost one or both parents due to AIDS. Nine out of 10 of these children

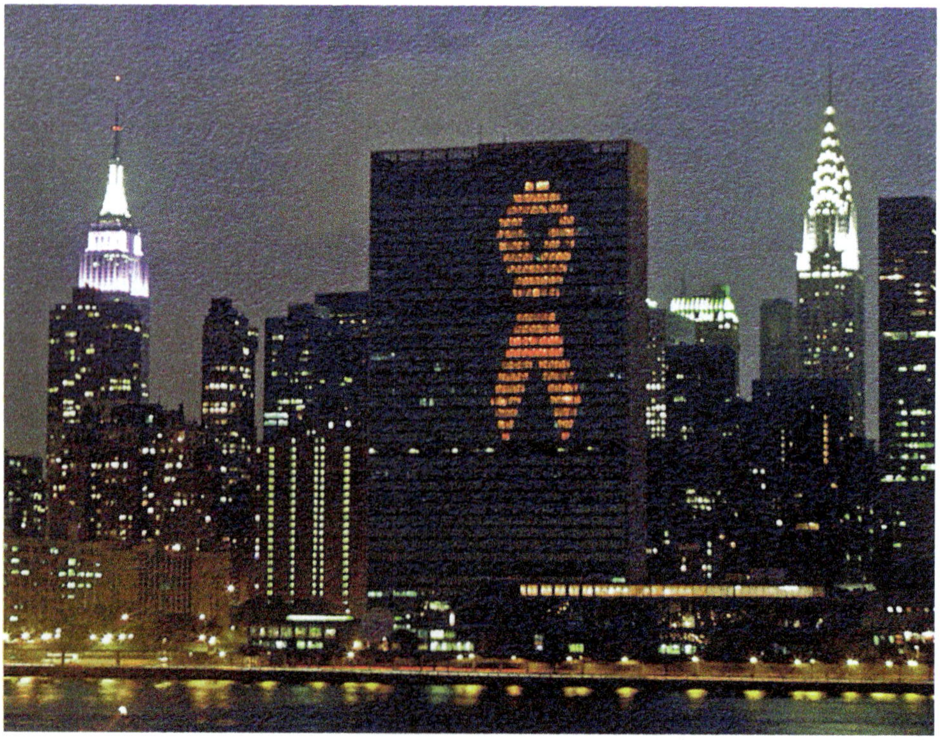

The United Nations (UN) Secretariat Building in New York City is lit up with a red AIDS ribbon in June 2001 to draw attention to the General Assembly Special Session on HIV/AIDS that month. Among the UN goals were halting the spread of HIV/AIDS by 2015 and providing universal access to HIV/AIDS treatment by 2010. © DOUG KANTER/AFP/Getty Images live in sub-Saharan Africa. Although there has been some decline in the global prevalence of HIV among adults and an increase in access to treatment, the plight of children affected by or vulnerable to HIV remains tragic.

HIV/AIDS has become the leading cause of death among adults ages 15 to 59 and has afflicted both genders equally worldwide. It has taken most of these 35 years for the world community to mount a strong and concerted response to the epidemic, signified by the adoption of the Declaration of Commitment on HIV/AIDS in June 2001. A major component of this response has been the establishment of the Global Fund to Fight AIDS, Tuberculosis and Malaria in 2002 to provide low- and middle-income nations with financial aid to help control the epidemic. In addition, the prices of some AIDS medicines have been significantly reduced. In 2003 the World Health Organization (WHO) and the Joint United Nations Programme on HIV/AIDS (UNAIDS) launched the 3 by 5 Initiative, helping to substantially increase the number of people receiving antiretroviral treatment.

Programs that promote behavioral changes, such as reducing the number of sexual partners, using condoms, and avoiding sharing needles, and those that improve access to antiretroviral treatment have started to reduce the rates of both new infection with HIV/AIDS and mortality among those who are infected. Between 2010 and 2015, rates of new infection declined 6 percent. Notably, infection rates among children fell by approximately half during this period.

Antiretroviral treatments have both improved the quality of life of those who are infected and extended their life span. As a result, while infection rates decline, the total number of people living with HIV/AIDS has increased. As of late 2015, approximately 36.7 million people globally were infected with HIV. In 2015 some 1.8 million people became infected with HIV and an estimated 1 million died from AIDS. While work remains to be done to combat HIV/AIDS, the international community has been able to stop and even reverse the long-term trend of rising HIV/AIDS infection and mortality rates. In so doing the UN met one of its major MDGs.

While progress has been made to combat HIV/AIDS throughout the world, East Africa and southern Africa continue to be disproportionately affected by the epidemic. With 19.4 million people living with HIV as of 2016, the region accounted for more than half of all people with the virus and more than 40 percent of new infections, despite having only 6 percent of the world's total population. However, access to diagnosis and treatment has improved greatly. In 2016 three-quarters of HIV-infected people in the region knew they had the virus, and nearly 80 percent of those who knew they were being treated. In addition, nearly half of HIV-positive people in the region had suppressed the virus through treatment.

Malaria

A greater awareness of the heavy toll exacted by malaria has been matched by a greater commitment to contain the disease. Increased funding coming from the World Bank's Global Fund to Fight AIDS, Tuberculosis and Malaria, along with the US President's Malaria Initiative and the Bill & Melinda Gates Foundation, among others, is expected to encourage important malaria control interventions, particularly the use of insecticide-treated nets and improved access to effective antimalarial drugs. Although the sale of insecticide-treated mosquito nets has increased, mostly among urban-dwellers, poor rural communities in endemic areas remain extremely vulnerable to malaria.

Tuberculosis

Between 2000 and 2015, global efforts to combat tuberculosis helped dramatically reduce deaths from the disease. Over this 15-year span, the mortality rate dropped 37 percent, saving approximately 53 million lives. Despite this progress tuberculosis still killed about 1.7 million people per year worldwide as of 2016. Of the approximately 10.4 million new cases in 2016, more than 90 percent occurred in low- and middle-income countries, and 10 percent occurred among people infected with HIV. The persistence of tuberculosis led the UN's World Health Assembly (WHA) to adopt a new strategy for reducing cases of tuberculosis by 90 percent between 2015 and 2035. To achieve this ambitious goal, new vaccines will have to be developed.

Measles

One major aspect of the MDGs concerning child mortality includes reducing measles deaths through immunization. Measles vaccination of children is one of the most cost-effective public health interventions on record. However, the disease killed nearly half a million children in 2004 and left many others blind or deaf. Most unvaccinated children live in China, the Democratic Republic of the Congo, India, Indonesia, Nigeria, or Pakistan. However, considerable progress in measles immunization has been achieved in Latin America, the Caribbean, and sub-Saharan Africa. According to the MDG report, sub-Saharan Africa achieved the largest reduction in measles deaths of any region, with a decrease of nearly 60 percent between 1999 and 2004.

Impacts and Issues

Of the four diseases mentioned in the MDG report (HIV/AIDS, malaria, tuberculosis, and measles), HIV/AIDS presents the greatest long-term challenge from both a technical and policy standpoint. To a large extent, malaria, tuberculosis, and measles require more as-

WHO AND GLOBAL HEALTH GOALS

In 2015 the World Health Organization (WHO), the primary health agency of the United Nations (UN), released a report titled *Health in 2015: From MDGs to SDGs*. In it WHO sought to move beyond the Millennium Development Goals (MDGs) that it had announced in 2000 and to set new Sustainable Development Goals (SDGs) that would drive global health policy over the next 15 years.

According to WHO, the 17 SDGs outlined in the 2015 report sought to integrate economic, social, and environmental policies as a means of creating improved health care outcomes for all people. Among the highly ambitious goals were calls to "end poverty in all its forms everywhere," to "ensure sustainable consumption and production patterns," and to "take urgent action to combat climate change and its impact." While only one goal ("Ensure healthy lives and promote well-being for all at all ages") pertained directly to health, the report explained that "progress in health is dependent on economic, social and environmental progress."

Despite the broad scope of the SDGs, the report's authors noted the importance of tracking progress toward meeting these goals by monitoring specific criteria such as life expectancy and deaths before age 70. The authors also noted the utility of a measure of health life expectancy, which would capture not only how long people live but also how long they live without a disability.

siduous application of existing therapies and prevention methods, as well as the prevention of resistant strains. Although the fight against HIV/AIDS will require all of these measures, it will also require the development of new treatments and vaccines. The AIDS pandemic has helped fuel current malaria and tuberculosis epidemics due to coinfection. Therefore, containing the HIV/AIDS epidemic is the paramount public health challenge worldwide.

In response to the call from the UN General Assembly to increase efforts to combat the AIDS pandemic, UNAIDS and its cosponsors developed a program in 2006 that aimed to help countries move toward universal access to antiretroviral treatment by 2010. In 2007 UNAIDS issued a report on these efforts titled *Towards Universal Access*, which includes practical recommendations on setting and supporting national priorities, including:

- Ensuring predictable and sustainable financing
- Strengthening human resources and systems
- Removing the barriers to ensure affordable commodities
- Protecting the AIDS-related human rights of people living with HIV, women, children, and people in vulnerable groups
- Setting targets and accountability mechanisms

In a 2011 report, UNAIDS noted the "extraordinary progress" that had been made toward achieving these goals: "The global incidence of HIV infection has stabilized and begun to decline in many countries with generalized epidemics. The number of people receiving antiretroviral therapy continues to increase, with 6.65 million people getting treatment at the end of 2010." In addition, the report noted that nearly of half of HIV-positive pregnant women were receiving antiretroviral regimens designed to prevent transmission to their infants.

Progress in the fight against HIV/AIDS has continued. A 2015 UNAIDS report stated that the world had again made "extraordinary progress" against HIV, cutting the new infection rate by more than a third since 2000 and preventing nearly 8 million deaths. Work during that time to improve access to antiretrovirals and other drugs that can maintain health and prevent infecting others has had dramatic effects on the AIDS pandemic.

Education regarding how HIV is spread and the distribution of condoms were estimated to have saved 50 million lives between 1995 and 2013. About 15 million people were on antiretroviral therapy as of 2015. New HIV infections had fallen by 35 percent, and AIDS deaths had dropped by 41 percent since 2000. According to UNAIDS, "the global response to HIV has averted 30 million new HIV infections and 7.8 million AIDS-related deaths since 2000.... Had the world stood back to watch the epidemic unfold, the annual number of new HIV infections is likely to have risen to around 6 million by 2014."

As of early 2018, the UN was continuing to pursue ambitious goals for stopping HIV's spread and improving access to treatment for the 36.9 million people who remained infected with HIV. The UN set the following goals for 2020: for 90 percent of people living with HIV to know their status, for 90 percent of those who know their status to receive treatment, for 90 percent of those being treated to be virally suppressed, and for there to be under half a million new infections per year.

Political leaders worldwide agree that the HIV/AIDS epidemic requires an extraordinary response. To bring the pandemic under control, the health care community must work more closely and openly with populations affected most by HIV/AIDS, including men who have sex with men, sex workers, and injecting drug users. Moving from short-term emergency responses to a longer-term response that recognizes the uniqueness of AIDS and is incorporated into national development planning and execution will be necessary. Ultimately, however, eradicating AIDS will require a vaccine against infection and a cure for those who contract the virus, neither of which had been developed as of 2018.

SEE ALSO *AIDS (Acquired Immunodeficiency Syndrome); Antiviral Drugs; Developing Nations and Drug Delivery; Malaria; Médecins Sans Frontières (Doctors Without Borders); Measles (Rubeola); Mosquito-Borne Disease; Puerperal Fever; Reemerging Infectious Diseases; Tuberculosis; Vector-Borne Disease; War and Infectious Disease*

BIBLIOGRAPHY

Websites

"Extraordinary Progress against AIDS." NBC News, July 14, 2015. https://www.nbcnews.com/health/health-news/extraordinary-progress-against-aids-report-n391861 (accessed March 6, 2018.)

"Health in 2015: From MDGs to SDGs." World Health Organization, 2015. http://apps.who.int/iris/bitstream/10665/200009/1/9789241565110_eng.pdf?ua=1 (accessed March 9, 2018).

"Millennium Development Goals (MDGs)." World Health Organization, May 2015. http://www.who.int/mediacentre/factsheets/fs290/en/ (accessed March 6, 2018).

"The Millennium Development Goals Report 2006." United Nations, 2006. http://unstats.un.org/unsd/mdg/Resources/Static/Products/Progress2006/MDGReport2006.pdf (accessed March 6, 2018).

"Progress towards the Millennium Development Goals, 1990–2005." United Nations, 2005. http://mdgs.un.org/unsd/mdg/Host.aspx?Content=Products/Progress2005.htm (accessed March 6, 2018).

"Report of the Secretary-General on the Work of the Organization." United Nations, 2006. http://mdgs.un.org/unsd/mdg/Resources/Static/Products/SGReports/61_1/a_61_1_e.pdf (accessed March 6, 2018).

Kenneth T. LaPensee

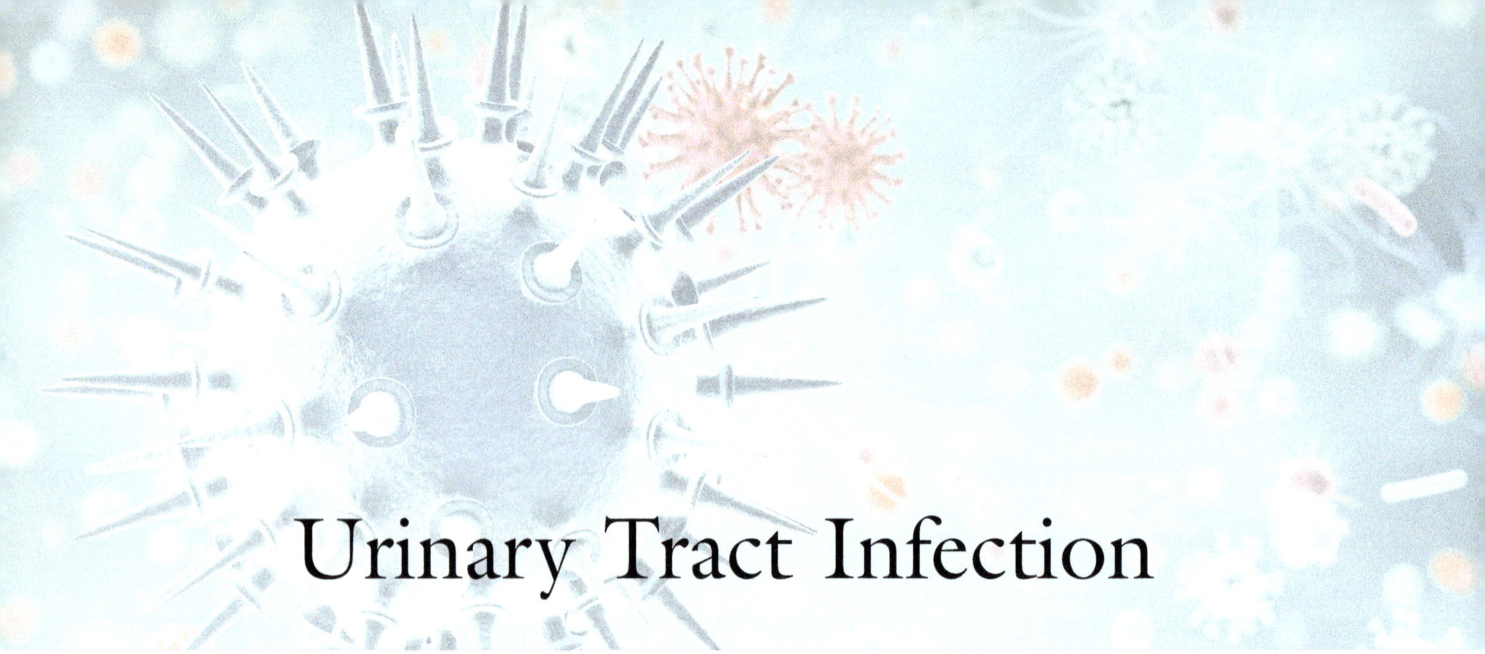

Urinary Tract Infection

■ Introduction

The urinary tract is the system that produces, stores, and excretes urine. Its purpose is to remove undesirable compounds and some of the waste products of body processes. The human urinary tract is composed of a pair of kidneys that filter waste from blood, two tubes (ureters) that connect the kidneys to a storage bag called the urinary bladder, a pair of sphincter muscles that help control urine flow, and the exit channel (urethra).

WORDS TO KNOW

BIOFILM A biofilm is a population of microorganisms that forms following the adhesion of bacteria, algae, yeast, or fungi to a surface. These surface growths can be found in natural settings, such as on rocks in streams, and in infections, such as those that occur on catheters. Microorganisms can colonize living and inert natural and synthetic surfaces.

PYELONEPHRITIS Inflammation caused by bacterial infection of the kidney and associated blood vessels.

RESISTANT ORGANISM An organism that has developed the ability to counter something trying to harm it. Within infectious diseases, the organism, such as a bacterium, has developed a resistance to drugs, such as antibiotics.

SEPSIS A bacterial infection in the bloodstream or body tissues. This is a very broad term covering the presence of many types of microscopic disease-causing organisms. Sepsis is also called *bacteremia*. Closely related terms include *septicemia* and *septic syndrome*.

An infection involving all or a portion of the urinary system is a urinary tract infection (UTI). The infection may remain confined to the urinary system—common sites of infection are the urethra and the bladder—but the kidney(s) can also become infected. Alternatively, a UTI can infrequently spread elsewhere in the body via the circulatory system. Infections of the urinary tract are the second most common type of infection in the human body.

■ Disease History, Characteristics, and Transmission

Although some people with a UTI do not display symptoms (asymptomatic), most men and women with a UTI display a range of characteristic symptoms, including urgent and frequent urination, a burning feeling when urinating, frequent urination but only in small amounts, urine that is cloudy and strong-smelling instead of clear yellow and relatively odorless, and blood in the urine (hematuria).

Pyelonephritis is an infection of the kidney. This usually occurs after the bladder has been infected, and the infection grows up the inner wall of the ureters that connect the bladder with each kidney. A kidney infection is accompanied by a high fever and flank pain. An infection of the bladder, or *cystitis*, is associated with abdominal discomfort, frequent and painful urination, and strong-smelling urine. Urethritis, an infection of the urethra, is associated with the burning sensation upon urination.

UTIs begin when bacteria enter the urethra from the outside world. This can occur if the external region around the urethra is touched by hands that have not been properly washed, or it can occur accidently during a bowel movement. Females are more prone to this accidental contact because the anus is nearer to the urethra in females than it is in males. The typical contaminating bacterium is *Escherichia coli*, which is a normal resident of the gastrointestinal tract and so is present in feces.

Another way of contracting an infection is through sexual activity. In women, the pathogens typically involved are the herpes simplex virus and the bacterium *Chlamydia trachomatis*, which are normal causes of sexually transmitted disease. In men, *C. trachomatis* and *Neisseria gonorrhoeae* (the bacterium that causes gonorrhea) are typically involved.

Scope and Distribution

While they occur both in males and females, UTIs are almost a fact of life for some women. The chances that a woman will have a bladder infection during her lifetime is about 50 percent. Physicians are not sure why women have more urinary infections than men, but one factor may be anatomical: a woman's urethra is short, allowing bacteria to access the bladder quickly. In addition, a woman's urethra opens near sources of bacteria from the anus and vagina. Postmenopausal women tend to be more infection-prone because hormonal changes make the urinary tract walls thinner and more susceptible to infection. Both men and women who are sexually active with multiple partners also tend to have more UTIs.

Another factor that contributes to the development of a UTI is the presence of an obstruction in the urinary tract. In men this can be an enlarged prostate. Other conditions that can predispose a person to UTIs include kidney stones, diabetes, and diseases or drugs that impair the function of the immune system. In addition, extended use of a catheter (tube) to help drain the bladder can increase the risk of a UTI. Epidemiologists estimate that a catheterized patient in a hospital has a 3 to 7 percent greater chance of developing a UTI for each day that the same catheter is in place. This is because bacteria readily adhere to catheter material and form biofilms, colonies of bacteria that adhere to tissue, which can then migrate upward to the bladder.

Treatment and Prevention

UTIs are often treated using antibiotics, especially if they cause troublesome symptoms. These infections can be minimized by drinking plenty of water, which prevents urine from stagnating. Cranberry juice is also beneficial for some people because a compound in the juice can outcompete bacteria for a specific attachment site on the bladder wall. In addition, wiping from front to back after a bowel movement lessens the chance that bacteria in feces will be accidentally deposited at the end of the urethra.

UTIs that involve bacteria resistance to several antibiotics can sometimes be treated using the drug fosfomycin.

Impacts and Issues

The majority of UTIs can be treated successfully, and the patient suffers no lasting ill effects. However, kidney infections can be a serious complication of an untreated UTI. In addition, a chronic or complicated UTI in a pregnant woman increases the risk of premature birth or lower-than-average birth weight, which can pose risks for the newborn.

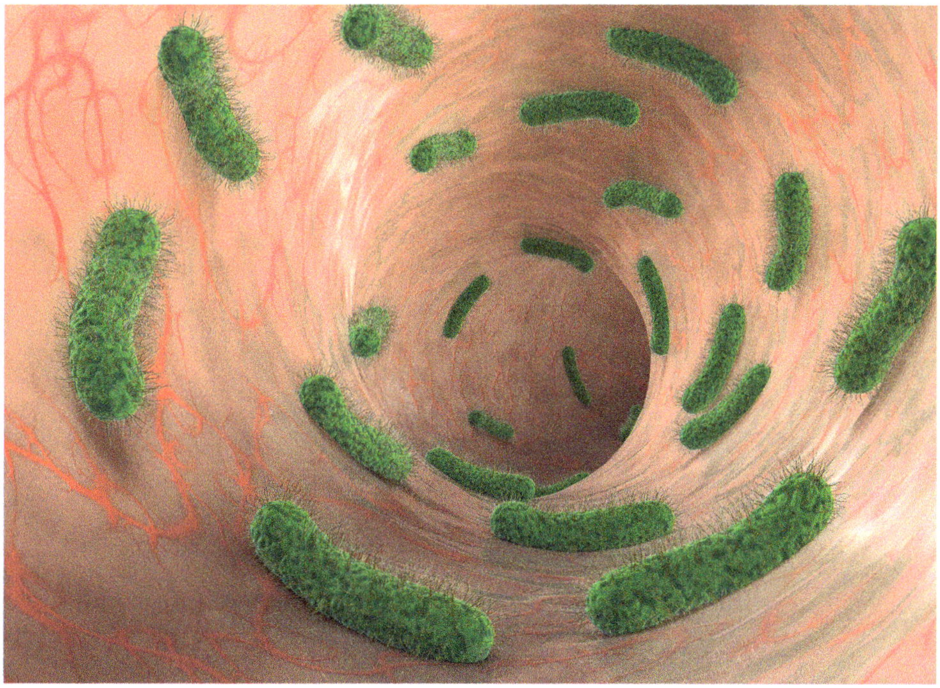

Urinary tract infections occur when bacteria enter the body through the urethra. They occur in both men and women but are more common in women. *© David Mack/Science Source*

OPERATION SEA SPRAY

The US Army conducted a study from 1951 to 1952, "Operation Sea Spray," to study wind currents that might carry biological weapons. As part of the project design, balloons were filled with *Serratia marcescens* (then thought to be harmless) and exploded over San Francisco. Shortly thereafter, there was a corresponding dramatic increase in reported pneumonia and UTIs. In the week following the test, 11 people visited the Stanford University Hospital for treatment of UTIs that turned out to be caused by *S. marcescens*. This was surprising because the organism had been selected for the aerial testing based on the knowledge that it was benign. One person who was recovering from prostate surgery died of the UTI.

UTIs caused by bacteria that are resistant to two or more antibiotics are of special concern, as they can be hard to treat. A 2016 study indicated the value of fosfomycin in treating these infections. The drug can be taken orally rather than having to be injected, so treatment is convenient. The possible drawback is that patients must be vigilant in maintaining the treatment schedule. Another drug that is proving to be worthwhile, especially in the treatment of elderly people with UTIs, is methenamine hippurate. This drug was first developed more than 60 years ago but has been repurposed for use with UTIs.

UTIs are of special concern for persons who have spinal cord injuries or who are immobile. If the muscles responsible for emptying the urinary bladder are paralyzed, repeated catheterizations or the placement of indwelling catheters are necessary to empty the bladder of urine, and recurrent UTIs often develop. Pyelonephritis and sepsis (infection in the blood) are more common complications of UTI in these groups, and such patients sometimes receive prolonged antibiotic therapy.

Even if a UTI is asymptomatic, it is important to finish the entire course of the prescribed antibiotic. Failure to do this can contribute to specific and overall antibiotic resistance. UTIs are sometimes caused by bacteria that grow as biofilms. When enclosed in a biofilm, bacteria can be resistant to antibiotics and may not be killed if antibiotic use is stopped prematurely. Moreover, the surviving bacteria, which may have been exposed to a sublethal dose of an antibiotic, may develop resistance to the drug. When the UTI recurs as the bacterial numbers subsequently rebound, the antibiotic may no longer be effective against the pathogen.

SEE ALSO *Bacterial Disease; Chlamydia Infection; Resistant Organisms*

BIBLIOGRAPHY

Books

Mulvey, Matthew A., David J. Klumpp, and Ann E. Stapleton. *Urinary Tract Infections: Molecular Pathogenesis and Clinical Management.* Washington, DC: ASM, 2017.

Periodicals

McAllister, Rebecca, and Janice Allwood. "Recurrent Multidrug Resistant Urinary Tract Infections in Geriatric Patients." *Federal Practitioner* 31, no. 7 (July 2014): 32–35.

Nicolle, Lindsay E. "Catheter Associated Urinary Tract Infections." *Antimicrobial Resistance and Infection Control* 3 (2014): 23.

Websites

"Urinary Tract Infection (UTI)." Mayo Clinic. https://www.mayoclinic.org/diseases-conditions/urinary-tract-infection/symptoms-causes/syc-20353447 (accessed November 22, 2017).

"Your Guide to Urinary Tract Infections (UTIs)." WebMD. https://www.webmd.com/women/guide/your-guide-urinary-tract-infections#1 (accessed November 22, 2017).

Brian Hoyle

USAMRIID (United States Army Medical Research Institute of Infectious Diseases)

Introduction

USAMRIID is an acronym for the United States Army Medical Research Institute of Infectious Diseases. The facility is operated by the US Department of Defense (DoD) and serves as the country's principal laboratory for research into the medical aspects of biological warfare. Its mission is "to provide leading edge medical capabilities to deter and defend against current and emerging biological threat agents." Specifically, the facility aims to develop vaccines for infectious diseases, other treatments such as drugs, and tests to detect and identify disease-causing microorganisms.

The USAMRIID is part of the US biological defense program, also known as the National Biodefense Strategy. Called the "birthplace of medical biodefense," the USAMRIID plays an essential role in the defense of the country with respect to biological terrorism and biological warfare. Adding to its importance, the USAMRIID is the only DoD laboratory that has attained a biosafety level 4 (BSL-4) certification, which is the highest level attainable for biosafety.

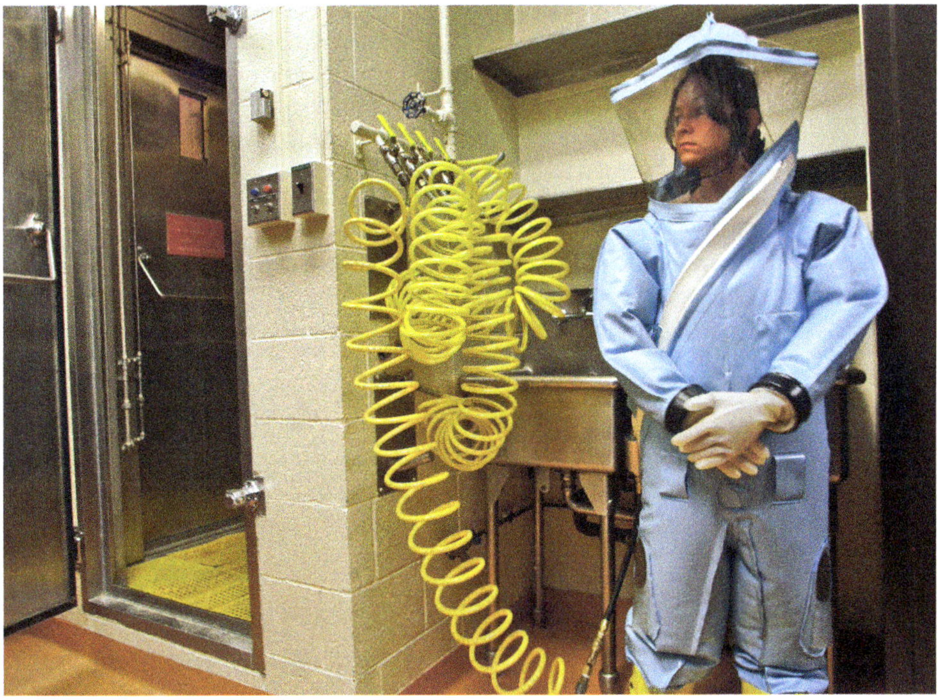

Sgt. Michelle Bergantino demonstrates the use of a bio-containment suit during an event at a USAMRIID facility at Fort Detrick in Frederick, Maryland, in 2005. *© Bill O'Leary/The Washington Post/Getty Images*

History and Scientific Foundations

The US Office of the Surgeon General of the Army established the USAMRIID on January 27, 1969. The facility replaced the United States Army Medical Unit (USAMU), which had been operating at Fort Detrick, Maryland, since 1956. The USAMU had a mandate to conduct research into the offensive use of biological and chemical weapons. This research was stopped by US president Richard Nixon (1913–1994) in 1969. In 1971 and 1972 the stockpiled biological weapons were ordered destroyed.

The defensive research that the USAMU had been conducting, such as vaccine development, was continued by the USAMRIID. In 1971 the facility was reassigned to the US Army Medical Research and Development Command. The USAMRIID contains a BSL-4 facility (the highest level of safety and security controls), a BSL-3 area, and a BSL-2 area. It is one of the largest high-level containment facilities in the United States.

Work within the BSL-4 facility necessitates the wearing of positive-pressure suits ("space suits") and the breathing of filtered air, whereas activities within the BSL-3 area are performed in scrub suits. Showers are required of all personnel upon leaving. Activities within the BSL-2 area are performed with laboratory coats and under the use of basic precautions. All BSL activities are guided by the manual *Biosafety in Microbiological and Biomedical Laboratories* (BMBL).

The USAMRIID BSL-4 patient ward may house people who have been infected during a disease outbreak or researchers who have been accidentally exposed to an infectious microbe. This ward was used in 1982 to care for two researchers from the US Centers for Disease Control (CDC; its name was changed to the Centers for Disease Control and Prevention in 1992, with its acronym remaining the same) who were exposed to rat blood contaminated with the Lassa virus, which causes Lassa fever, a type of viral hemorrhagic fever, also called Lassa hemorrhagic fever (LHF). The two researchers, along with three others thought to have been exposed to the virus, remained in the containment ward until they were determined to be free of infection.

Equipment is also available that allows the BSL-4 conditions to be mimicked in the field. Thus, an infected person can be isolated at the site of an outbreak and transported back to Fort Detrick for medical treatment and study of the infection.

In 2009 construction of a new advanced-technology, high-security USAMRIID facility was begun next to the existing building to expand the capabilities of the organization. As of February 2018, the facility remained under construction after a fire during construction in August 2013 caused $10 million in damage and delayed completion of the facility.

WORDS TO KNOW

BIOLOGICAL WARFARE As defined by the United Nations, the use of any living organism, such as a bacterium or virus, or an infective component, such as a toxin, to cause disease or death in humans, animals, or plants. In contrast to bioterrorism, biological warfare is defined as the state-sanctioned use of biological weapons on an opposing military force or civilian population.

BIOSAFETY LEVEL 4 (BSL-4) FACILITY A specialized biosafety laboratory that deals with dangerous or exotic infectious agents or biohazards that are considered high risks for spreading life-threatening diseases, either because the disease is spread through aerosols or because there is no therapy or vaccine to counter the disease.

HEMORRHAGIC FEVER A high fever caused by viral infection combined with copious (a high volume of) bleeding due to the formation of tiny blood clots throughout the bloodstream. These blood clots, also called microthrombi, deplete platelets and fibrinogen in the bloodstream. When bleeding begins, the factors needed for the clotting of the blood are scarce. Thus, uncontrolled bleeding (hemorrhage) ensues.

MIMICKING In biology, imitating another organism, often for evolutionary advantage. A disease that resembles another (for whatever reason) is sometimes said to have mimicked the other. Pathomimicry is the faking of symptoms by a patient, also called malingering.

OUTBREAK The appearance of new cases of a disease in numbers greater than the established incidence rate, or the appearance of even one case of an emergent or rare disease in an area.

SEQUENCING Finding the order of chemical bases in a section of DNA.

STRAIN A subclass or a specific genetic variation of an organism.

Applications and Research

As of 2018 the research staff at the USAMRIID numbered about 750 people, including civilians, military personnel, and contract employees. The facility had about 200 doctoral-level scientists, including biochemists, immunologists, physicians, microbiologists, molecular biologists, virologists, pathologists, and veterinarians. Among the technical and scientific support staff who assist the researchers are laboratory technicians who have volunteered to be test subjects during clinical trials of vaccines and drugs. Other support personnel include those working in security, regulatory affairs, personnel and administration, and other such positions.

USAMRIID scientists can rapidly identify infectious microorganisms. Vaccines are in various stages of development for several microbes, including the anthrax bacterium and the Ebola and Marburg viruses. In 2016 a team of USAMRIID researchers used data stored at their facility to perform a full genome reconstruction and analysis of the Ebola virus Kikwit R4368 and its 2014 replacement, R4415. Their study chronicles the history and genomic characteristics of the viruses, and their conclusions help to deepen understanding of the various populations of Ebola viruses and their possible disease outcomes.

Researchers and support staff can also respond to disease outbreaks. On short notice, teams can journey to the site of the infection to begin an investigation. This response is often conducted in conjunction with CDC personnel. USAMRIID teams can also respond to combat situations. A portable laboratory to treat biological warfare casualties can be quickly set up near a battlefield.

One well-known USAMRIID response occurred in 1989, when an outbreak of an Ebola virus occurred at a primate holding facility in nearby Reston, Virginia. Some personnel became infected with the virus, which was later determined to be a different variety from that which causes hemorrhagic Ebola fever in humans. The virus, known as *Reston ebolavirus*, was subsequently called by such names as Reston Ebola virus (REBOV) and Ebola virus Reston (EBOV-R). In 2010 it was renamed Reston virus (RESTV). The USAMRIID response was subsequently detailed in best-selling books such as *The Hot Zone* (1994) by Richard Preston and popular movies such as *Outbreak* (1995) and *Carriers* (1998), which were broadly based on Preston's book.

In 2014 USAMRIID supported relief efforts in West Africa during an outbreak of Ebola virus disease. One of their functions was to train US military troops on the proper way to wear equipment to protect themselves from the deadly virus. The facility has played an important role in several military campaigns, serving as the medical support staging area for vaccines, drugs, and medical equipment.

Each year USAMRIID personnel train US soldiers on how to handle biological warfare or terrorism. Such preparedness helped American forces near the end of the Gulf War (code-named Operations Desert Shield and Desert Storm), which lasted from August 1990 to February 1991. At the time a biological threat against American soldiers was deemed likely.

LABORATORY SAFETY

Laboratories are rated according to a four-level system indicating the types of microbes that can safely be studied there. A typical university research lab with no specialized safety features (such as a fume hood, biological safety cabinet, or filtration system for exhausted air) is assigned biosafety level 1 (BSL-1). Progression to a higher level requires more stringent safety and biological controls. A biosafety level 4 (BSL-4) laboratory is the only laboratory that can safely handle microbes such as Ebola virus, *Bacillus anthracis* (the bacterium that causes anthrax), Marburg virus, and hantavirus.

Entry to the BSL-4 area requires passage through several checkpoints and keying in a security code that is issued only after the person has been successfully vaccinated against the microorganism under study. All work in the BSL-4 lab is conducted in a pressurized and ventilated suit. Air for breathing is passed into the suit through a hose and is filtered so as to be free of microorganisms.

USAMRIID was embroiled in the aftermath of the September 11, 2001 (9/11), terrorist attacks on targets in the United States, after several letters containing anthrax spores were sent to various locations in the eastern United States via the US Postal Service. Sequencing of the genetic material from the spores determined that the source of the anthrax was a strain of the microbe that had been developed in the USAMRIID labs in the 1980s. After a four-year investigation by the Federal Bureau of Investigation (FBI) and the Department of Justice (DOJ), deoxyribonucleic acid (DNA) evidence led federal investigators in 2005 to suspect American microbiologist Bruce Edwards Ivins (1946–2008) to have committed the crime.

At the time of the crime, Ivins was working as a senior biodefense researcher at the USAMRIID. Investigators believed that he attempted suicide after he suspected he would be charged for the crime. He died on July 29, 2008, from an overdose of Tylenol and codeine. On February 19, 2010, the investigation was closed after federal prosecutors declared Ivins the only person involved in the attacks. However, a subsequent investigation by the FBI concluded in 2011 that there was insufficient evidence to find whether or not the specific strain of anthrax had come from Ivins's laboratory.

Impacts and Issues

While some of the research conducted at the USAMRIID is classified, other research findings of the resident civilian and military scientists are used to benefit the public. The USAMRIID and its counterpart, the US Army Medical Research Institute of Chemical Diseases (USAMRICD), train military medical personnel each year on biological and chemical defense measures. Furthermore, military and civilian medical professionals attend annual courses and seminars on such topics contained in *USAMRIID's Medical Management of Biological Casualties Handbook*, informally called the USAMRIID Bluebook.

The USAMRIID is mandated to explore the use of the treatments and tests in the battlefield environment. According to the law, the research conducted at the USAMRIID is defensive in nature. Infectious microbes are to be investigated only to develop means of protecting soldiers from the use of the microbes by opposition forces during a conflict.

The infectious disease research expertise at the USAMRIID is also used to develop strategies and training programs related to medical defense against infectious microorganisms. For example, the agency regularly updates and publishes a handbook that details the various medical defenses against biological warfare or terrorism. This handbook is available to the public.

Throughout the history of the USAMRIID, its personnel have performed research, development, testing, and evaluation of many vaccines. They continue to develop new vaccines within clinical trials as part of their important mandate. Some of the vaccines developed include those against the following biological threats:

- Anthrax, which is caused by the bacterium *Bacillus anthracis*
- Botulism, which is caused by the bacterium *Clostridium botulinum*
- Ebola, also known as Ebola virus disease (EVD) and Ebola hemorrhagic fever (EHF), which is caused by Ebola viruses (genus *Ebolavirus*)
- Hantaviruses, also called orthohantaviruses, which are caused by viruses in the Hantaviridae family of the order Bunyavirales
- Marburg virus disease (MVD), formerly known as Marburg hemorrhagic fever, which is caused by two Marburg viruses: Marburg virus (MARV) and Ravn virus (RAVV)
- Plague, which is caused by the bacterium species *Yersinia pestis*
- Ricin toxin, which is a naturally produced lectin contained within the seeds of the castor oil plant (species name *Ricinus communis*)
- Staphylococcal enterotoxin B, also called enterotoxin type B, which is produced by the bacterium *Staphylococcus aureus*

The USAMRIID continues to improve its methods for developing new ways to protect Americans from biological threats. Much of its work is recorded within the Joint Biological Agent Identification and Detection System, which is used throughout the DoD. When a vaccine or other drug is needed on an emergency basis, USAMRIID studies can allow for the immediate use of that medicine, known as Emergency Use Authorization.

See Also *Biological Weapons Convention; Bioterrorism; Ebola; Hemorrhagic Fevers; Lassa Fever; Marburg Hemorrhagic Fever; Vaccines and Vaccine Development; War and Infectious Disease*

BIBLIOGRAPHY

Books

Biosafety in Microbiological and Biomedical Laboratories. 5th ed. Washington, DC: Government Printing Office, 2009. This book can also be found online at https://www.cdc.gov/biosafety/publications/bmbl5/index.htm> (accessed January 31, 2018).

USAMRIID's Medical Management of Biological Casualties Handbook. 8th ed. Fort Detrick, MD: US Army Medical Research Institute of Infectious Diseases, 2014. This book can also be found online at http://www.usamriid.army.mil/education/bluebookpdf/USAMRIID%20BlueBook%208th%20Edition%20-%20Sep%202014.pdf (accessed January 31, 2018).

Periodicals

Carignan, Sylvia. "Fort Detrick's $10 Million Fire." *Frederick News-Post* (March 17, 2014). This article can also be found online at https://www.fredericknewspost.com/news/disasters_and_accidents/fires/fort-detrick-s-million-fire/article_6b0025de-2989–5e29–8005-edc9297cc984.html (accessed January 31, 2018).

Hernandez, Nelson, and Philip Rucker. "Anthrax Case Raises Doubt on Security." *Washington Post* (August 8, 2008): A01. This article can also be found online at http://www.washingtonpost.com/wp-dyn/content/story/2008/08/07/ST2008080703559.html (accessed January 31, 2018).

Kugelman, Jeffrey R., et al. "Informing the Historical Record of Experimental Nonhuman Primate Infections with Ebola Virus: Genomic Characterization of USAMRIID Ebola Virus/H.sapiens-tc/COD/1995/Kikwit-9510621 Challenge Stock 'R4368' and Its Replacement 'R4415.'" *PLOS One* (March 22, 2016). This article can also be found online at http://journals.plos.org/plosone/article?id=10.1371/journal.pone.0150919 (accessed January 31, 2018).

Websites

"About USAMRIID." US Army Medical Research Institute of Infectious Diseases. http://www.usamriid.army.mil/aboutpage.htm (accessed January 31, 2018).

"Recognizing the Biosafety Levels." Centers for Disease Control and Prevention. https://www.cdc.gov/training/quicklearns/biosafety/ (accessed January 31, 2018).

Vanderlinden, Caree. "USAMRIID Supports Ebola Virus Disease Outbreak Response in West Africa." US Army, October 22, 2014. https://www.army.mil/article/136531/usamriid_supports_ebola_virus_disease_outbreak_response_in_west_africa> (accessed January 31, 2018).

Paul Davies
William Arthur Atkins

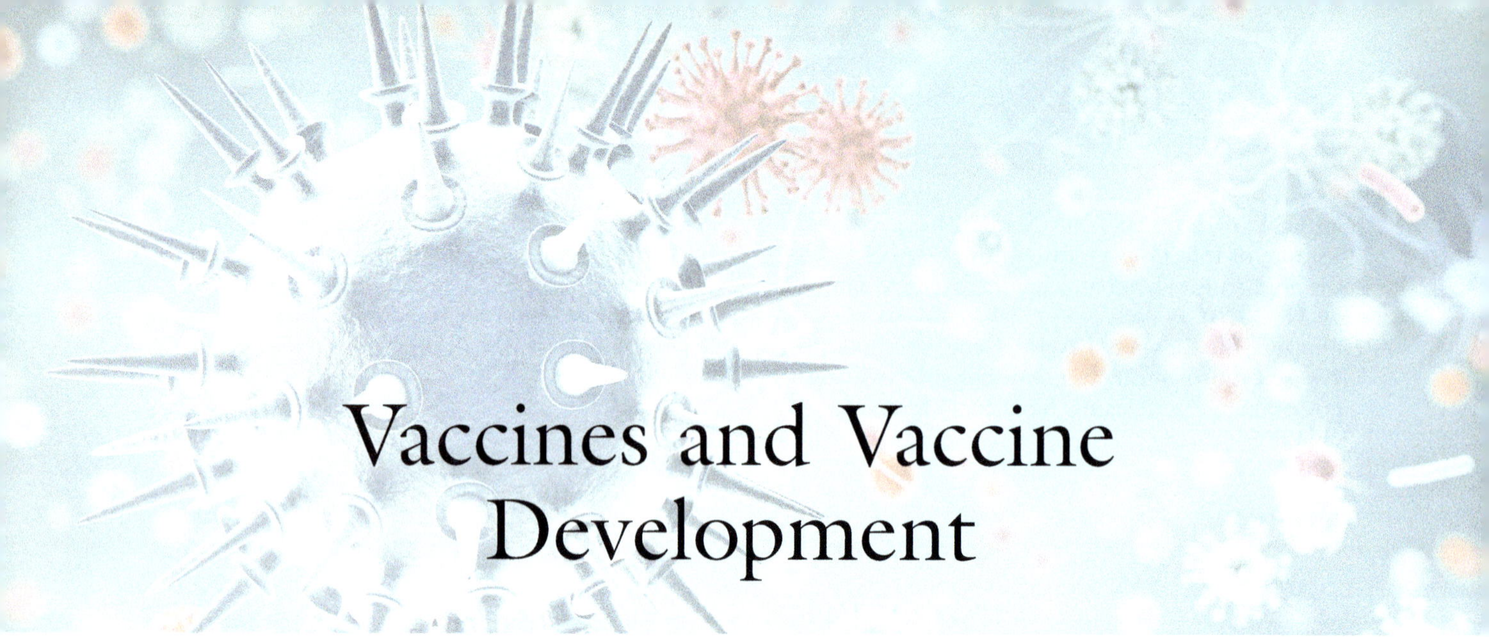

Vaccines and Vaccine Development

Introduction

Vaccines are substances that boost immune response to a specific disease. Vaccines closely resemble the pathogens of the diseases they are intended to counteract. However, they are designed so as not to cause the disease. This means they allow the immune system an opportunity to recognize and combat the pathogen without a high risk of the person becoming sick. Later, when a person contracts the pathogen in its unaltered and more virulent (severe) form, the immune system knows how to fight it more effectively. In some cases vaccines prevent a person from developing the disease in question. In other cases they reduce the virulence of the disease if the person contracts it.

Due to their preventative potential, vaccines have been responsible for great advances in public health since their advent in the late 1700s, greatly decreasing the incidence of once-common diseases that caused millions of deaths, significant public health expenditures, and terrible human suffering. Even diseases that were once universally fatal, such as rabies, are now averted with vaccines. Despite overwhelming evidence of their effectiveness at preventing infections without causing severe side effects, there is a persistent antivaccine movement that claims these agents cause autism and other negative outcomes. However, no scientific studies support the claims of these so-called antivaccinationists.

WORDS TO KNOW

ATTENUATED STRAIN A bacterium or virus that has been weakened. Often used as the basis of a vaccine against the specific disease caused by the bacterium or virus.

GERM THEORY OF DISEASE A fundamental tenet of medicine that states that microorganisms, which are too small to be seen without the aid of a microscope, can invade the body and cause disease.

PATHOGEN A disease-causing agent, such as a bacterium, a virus, a fungus, or another microorganism.

RING VACCINATION The vaccination of all susceptible people in an area surrounding a case of an infectious disease. Because vaccination makes people immune to the disease, the hope is that the disease will not spread from the known case to other people. Ring vaccination was used in eliminating the smallpox virus.

VARIOLATION The premodern practice of deliberately infecting a person with smallpox to make them immune to a more serious form of the disease. It was dangerous but did confer immunity on survivors.

History and Research

The origins of vaccine research can be traced to efforts to prevent smallpox, an extremely serious disease in humans from its first recorded appearances in Europe and China in the 3rd century CE until its eradication in the 1970s. The smallpox virus produced fever and headache, followed by a rash of pustules (small, pus-filled swellings), which give the disease its name. In about 35 percent of cases, such severe damage was done to the skin or internal organs that death occurred. Even when the victims survived, they would often be badly scarred or even blinded.

Efforts to avoid infection with smallpox were early and widespread. Variolation, or intentional infection with smallpox, was prevalent because it was thought to produce a less virulent infection. This method was eventually recognized as ineffective and even dangerous, leading to serious disease and deaths. At the end of the 18th century, Edward Jenner (1749–1823) noticed that many milkmaids who had been infected with the cowpox virus did not contract smallpox. He proved his theory by vaccinating a young boy with cowpox virus and then exposing him to smallpox. The vaccine was further developed into a stable and convenient dehydrated form in the 1950s.

The work of Louis Pasteur (1822–1895) led to the germ theory of disease and the first vaccine for rabies. The 1920s saw an increased number of inoculations for diseases such as diphtheria, pertussis (whooping cough), and tuberculosis, followed later by tetanus, yellow fever, polio, measles, mumps, and rubella. These familiar vaccinations, routinely given to children in the Western world, markedly reduced incidences of these diseases. Expanded vaccination programs led to the goal of disease eradication.

Although as of 2018 the only disease to have been eliminated in natural settings was smallpox, a number of diseases have been eradicated in parts of the world and have been brought under tight control globally. For example, in 2017 there were only 22 reported cases of polio, a contagious disease that can lead to paralysis and meningitis, down from an estimated 350,000 people in 1988. While polio was not officially eradicated as of early 2018, this more than 99 percent decrease in cases suggests it may be eradicated soon.

Impacts and Issues

Despite great improvements in human health due to vaccines, controversy has arisen over the possible unintended effects of vaccines. Some parents have chosen not to vaccinate their young children against disease. Indeed, since vaccines were first developed, different groups have opposed their use. Early arguments were religious in nature, stating that God sent smallpox afflictions as punishment. Thus, to circumvent the disease was to thwart God's will. More recent objections have focused on a purported link between vaccines and serious conditions such as autism.

In 1998 Andrew Wakefield published a study in the *Lancet* that purported to link the measles, mumps, and rubella (MMR) vaccine with the development of bowel disease and autism. His appearance at a press conference fed a media frenzy that caused many concerned parents to reject the MMR vaccine specifically and sometimes vaccines in general. Subsequent reassurances by the medical establishment and politicians were disbelieved by so many parents in the United Kingdom that vaccination rates fell and outbreaks of disease were recorded.

Although Wakefield's hypothesis did not find support in many subsequent studies and was retracted in 2004 by the journal that published it, distrust of the MMR vaccine persisted. In 1999 the US Centers for Disease Control and Prevention (CDC) recommended the removal of the mercury-containing vaccine preservative thimerosal, identified by antivaccinationists as a possible source of contamina-

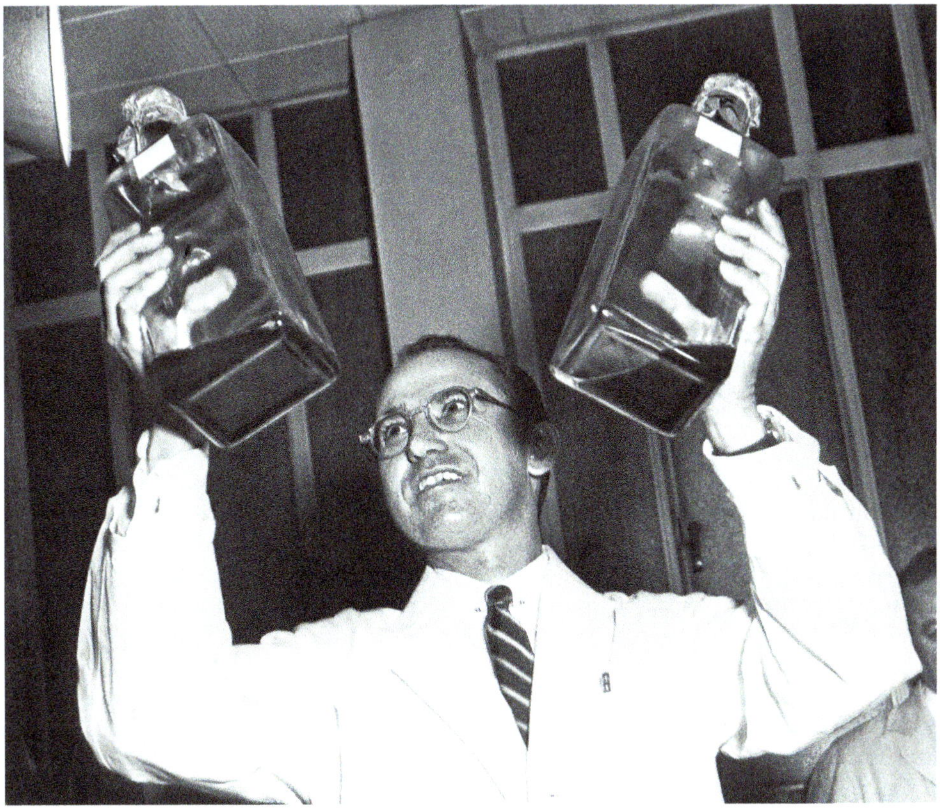

Dr. Jonas Salk holds up containers of the polio vaccine at his laboratory at the University of Pittsburgh. Salk's pioneering vaccine was announced on March 26, 1953. © *Bettmann/Getty Images*

VACCINE TYPES

Vaccines with living, but weakened, viruses are termed *attenuated vaccines*. The attenuated virus does not cause a severe infection. Rather, it presents the body with sufficient challenge to mount and thus "learn" an immune response. The measles, mumps, and rubella (MMR) vaccine is an example of an attenuated vaccine.

Vaccination can also involve the use of dead viruses and bacteria. The antigen, usually a specific molecule that resides on the surface of the cell, is sufficient alone to provoke an immune response that subsequently provides protection against live bacteria or viruses carrying the same surface molecule.

The third type of vaccination uses toxin produced by the living bacterium but not the bacteria themselves. Diphtheria and tetanus vaccines are examples of toxoid vaccines.

The fourth class of vaccine is engineered or uses a chemical compound formed from the fusion of portions of two antigens. The *Haemophilus influenzae* type b (Hib) vaccine is one such biosynthetic vaccine.

tion, as a cautionary measure. However, there was no evidence of thimerosal causing side effects beyond redness and swelling when used in small doses.

Vaccines are not, and have never been, without risk. Localized reactions, such as itching, swelling, pain, or discomfort are common, whereas systemic reactions, such as fever, headache, and malaise, are less so. More seriously, illnesses such as encephalitis, dangerous seizures, unintentional infection with the target pathogen, and even death have occurred. The smallpox vaccine in particular, despite its long history, has been known to be comparatively more dangerous than other vaccines. For this reason only a small number of people with specific occupations have been recommended for pre-exposure vaccination against smallpox, despite the concern about potential bioterrorism attacks with smallpox following the terrorist attacks of September 11, 2001.

Regardless of these concerns, vaccines are still considered an important foundation of public health efforts around the world. The CDC considers it better to prevent a disease than to treat its symptoms. Although many once-fatal diseases can be successfully treated with advanced supportive care and antibiotics, the costs of vaccination are much lower than those of treating infection. The National Institute of Allergy and Infectious Diseases cites a study stating that, for each dollar spent on vaccinating against rubella, eight dollars are saved in costs that would have been spent treating the infection.

Infectious disease outbreaks have created public interest in the quick development of therapeutic vaccines. In the face of epidemics, however, mass vaccination is not always feasible and may present hazards to public health. Ring vaccination, or administering vaccine to populations within and immediately surrounding the outbreak, is an alternative measure used in many outbreaks of infectious disease. Similarly, development of vaccines is a long and complex process that requires extensive research and testing before vaccines become available.

In some cases epidemics provide researchers with a rare opportunity to test new vaccines. For example, in 2015, amid a major Ebola epidemic in West Africa, researchers conducted trials of several Ebola vaccines known as rVSV-ZEBOV, cAd3-EBOZ, and cAd3-EBOZ. All three demonstrated promise in helping prevent infection and perhaps limit future epidemics.

The most promising was rVSV-ZEBOV. While rVSV-ZEBOV had been proven effective in monkeys in earlier studies, little was known about its effectiveness in humans. Researchers administered the vaccine to about half of the 11,841 people selected to participate in a 2015 study in the hard-hit Basse-Guinée region of Guinea. Using ring vaccination, which had helped eradicate smallpox in the 20th century, the study's designers identified all people who were likely in contact with a confirmed Ebola patient over a three-week period. Of these people, half were placed in a control group, and the other half received the vaccine.

According to the authors of the study, which was published in the *Lancet* in 2017, the vaccine was 100 percent effective, with no new cases reported among those who were inoculated, 10 days or more after they received the vaccine. Among those who did not receive the vaccine, there were 23 cases recorded during the study. The *New York Times* called the vaccine a "scientific triumph that will change the way the world fights a terrifying killer," and many observers share this optimism about rVSV-ZEBOV's potential to help prevent future Ebola outbreaks. Nevertheless, the vaccine showed limitations, as evidence suggested that it works against only one of two common Ebola strains.

Despite some limitations and lingering questions, evidence of rVSV-ZEBOV's effectiveness was sufficiently strong that 300,000 doses were produced. In 2017 regulators in the Democratic Republic of the Congo were the first in the world to approve rVSV-ZEBOV for use during an Ebola outbreak in that country. As of early 2018, no other country had approved the vaccine, and research continued into its safety and efficacy.

Researchers have also engaged in an urgent effort to develop a vaccine for Zika virus, which emerged as a major health crisis in Brazil in 2015 due to its association with various birth defects, including microcephaly. The development of a Zika vaccine was hastened by the existence of vaccines against other members of the genus *Flavivirus*. As of December 2017, seven Zika vaccines were undergoing clinical trials, and 40 other vaccine candidates were in earlier stages of development. In an article for the *Journal of Infec-*

tious Diseases, Kaitlyn M. Morabito and Barney S. Graham wrote, "The rapid progress in vaccine development demonstrates the capacity of governments, public health organizations, and the scientific community to respond to pandemic threats when sufficient prior knowledge exists, emergency funding is made available, and interagency cooperation is achieved and serves as a paradigm for preparing for future emerging infectious diseases."

Many different types of vaccines exist, some of which are easier to produce and administer than others. Different types of vaccines produce varying degrees of resistance to disease, some requiring multiple doses or booster shots to remain effective. A great deal of study and preparation are required before work on a vaccine can begin. The life cycle of the pathogen, the way it functions and causes harm in the body, and the response of the immune system must all be examined before the most appropriate course of action can be determined.

Nearly all vaccines are administered with needles and must be kept cold in a freezer or refrigerator before being administered. As public health officials seek to improve access to vaccines, especially in developing countries, they often have difficulty keeping vaccines at the right temperature and enlisting medical personnel who can administer the inoculations properly. This has led to efforts to develop vaccines that can be taken in the form of pills that would require no special storage and less specialized knowledge to administer. In 2018 researchers writing in the *Journal of Clinical Investigation* revealed notable progress in the development of synthetic influenza vaccines that might be able to be contained in a pill form. According to the authors, the "study highlights the power of synthetic biology to expand the horizons of vaccine design and therapeutic delivery." If that potential bears out, it could lead to greater control, and perhaps the eradication, of a greater number of diseases, including those for which a vaccine exists but is not accessible to populations in the developing world.

Some types of vaccines are well understood, produce reliable immune responses, and are easy to produce. Many of these use attenuated (weakened but live) pathogens, whereas others use dead organisms or portions of their proteins or antigens. Vaccines containing live, attenuated pathogens are not always appropriate for patients with weakened immune systems. Likewise, vaccines containing dead pathogens often produce a weak or short-lived immune response. Newer, possibly more effective types of vaccines are being explored, including those that use parts of the pathogen's DNA to cause the body to produce "natural vaccine" on its own. Once a vaccine is developed, it must undergo the usual three phases of clinical trials to establish safety, dosage, and effectiveness, as well as a stringent licensing process and continued monitoring for safety and contamination. The length of this process means that new vaccines cannot always be quickly developed to meet an immediate need.

The risk of an epidemic must also be balanced with the real likelihood of adverse events associated with vaccinating large numbers of people in short periods. If mass vaccinations are required, the timing of the campaign can help the health care system deal with adverse events more successfully. By increasing the length of a vaccination campaign from 2 to 10 days, officials can reduce the number of people who will experience adverse events at the same time, thereby reducing strain on doctors and hospitals. In cases of extreme shortage, vaccines such as smallpox can be diluted to much weaker solutions than their intended strength and still produce immunity in a portion of those vaccinated.

As a public health tool, vaccines are an inexpensive way to prevent serious disease before it develops and spreads. Health officials, individuals, and parents must maintain high levels of compliance to ensure protection against disease outbreak. At the same time, officials must responsibly evaluate the risks of vaccines when faced with the outbreak of dangerous disease.

See Also *Childhood-Associated Infectious Diseases, Immunization Impacts; Influenza, Tracking Seasonal Influences and Virus Mutation; Polio Eradication Campaign; Smallpox; Smallpox Eradication and Storage*

BIBLIOGRAPHY

Books

Plotkin, Stanley A., Walter A. Orenstein, and Paul Offit, eds. *Vaccines.* 5th ed. Philadelphia: Saunders/Elsevier, 2008.

White, Andrew Dickinson. "Theological Opposition to Inoculation, Vaccination, and the Use of Anaesthetics." In *A History of the Warfare of Science with Theology in Christendom.* New York: Routledge, 2017.

Periodicals

Belongia, Edward A., and Allison L. Naleway. "Smallpox Vaccine: The Good, the Bad, and the Ugly." *Clinical Medicine and Research* 1, no. 2 (2003): 87–92.

Daley, Matthew F. "Straight Talk about Vaccination." *Scientific American* (September 1, 2011). This article can also be found online at https://www.scientificamerican.com/article/straight-talk-about-vaccination/ (accessed March 15, 2018).

McNeil, Donald G., Jr. "New Ebola Vaccine Gives 100 Percent Protection." *New York Times* (December 22, 2016). This article can also be found online at https://www.nytimes.com/2016/12/22/health/ebola-vaccine.html (March 19, 2018).

Miles, John J., et al. "Peptide Mimic for Influenza Vaccination Using Nonnatural Combinatorial Chemistry." *Journal of Clinical Investigation* 128 (March 12, 2018): 1–12. This article can also be found online at https://www.jci.org/articles/view/91512 (accessed March 15, 2018).

Morabito, Kaitlyn M., and Barney S. Graham. "Zika Virus Vaccine Development." *Journal of Infectious Diseases* 216, no. S10 (2017): S957–S963.

Websites

McCulloch, J. Huston, and James R. Meginniss. "A Statistical Model of Smallpox Vaccine Dilution." Ohio State University, January 18, 2002. http://www.econ.ohio-state.edu/jhm/dilution.pdf (accessed March 15, 2018).

"Vaccines." US Food and Drug Administration, February 2, 2018. https://www.fda.gov/BiologicsBloodVaccines/Vaccines/ (accessed March 15, 2018).

"Vaccines." World Health Organization. http://www.who.int/topics/vaccines/en/ (accessed March 15, 2018).

"Vaccines and Immunizations." Centers for Disease Control and Prevention, August 14, 2017. http://www.cdc.gov/od/science/iso/concerns/thimerosal.html (accessed March 15, 2018).

Kenneth T. LaPensee

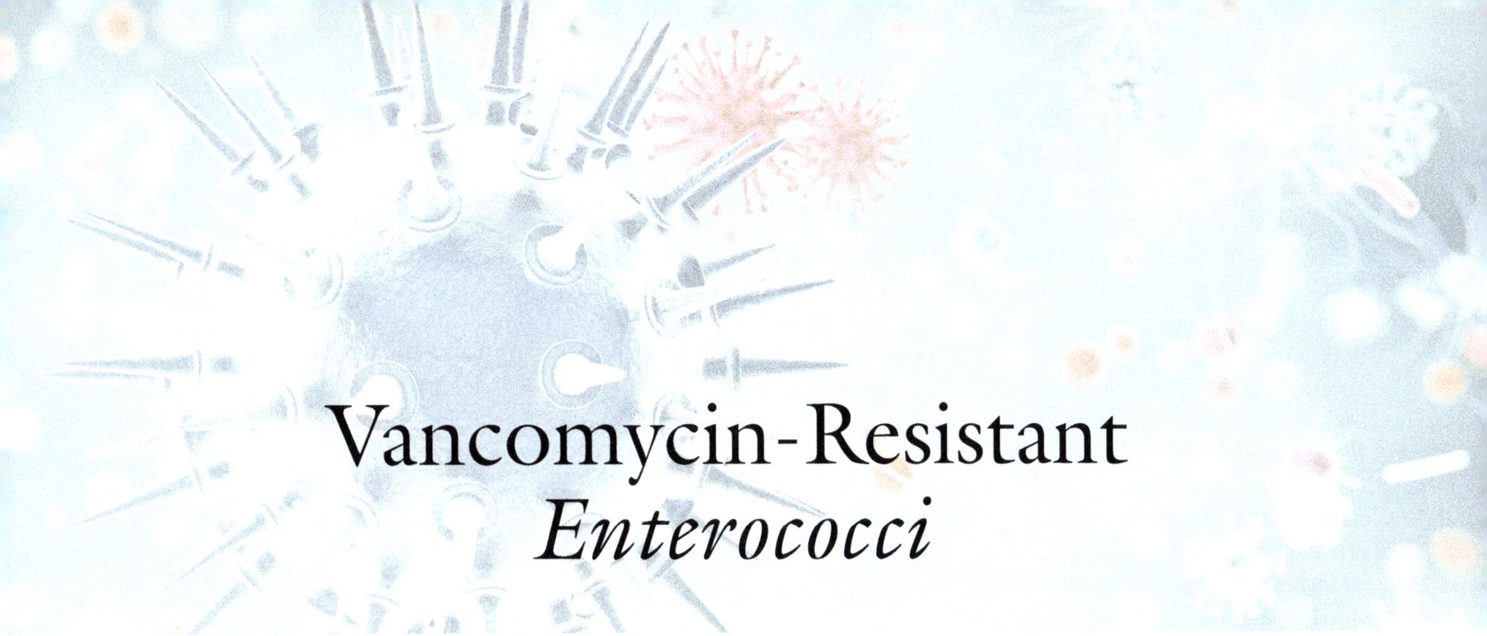

Vancomycin-Resistant *Enterococci*

Introduction

Vancomycin-resistant *Enterococcus* (VRE) is a category of bacteria that is resistant to the antibiotic vancomycin, which is used to treat a broad spectrum of infections. VRE belongs to a group of drug-resistant bacteria that were first reported in 1986, almost 30 years after the vancomycin was introduced. Since these initial reports, organisms that have developed resistance to the drugs designed to kill them have become a rapidly growing threat to global public health.

As of 2017 some 70,000 people died annually as a result of infection with resistant organisms. The rise of drug resistance among microorganisms is tied to the widespread use of antibiotics in humans and animals. In fact, it was the emergence of microorganisms resistant to the antibiotics developed in the early and mid-20th century, such as penicillin, methicillin, and ampicillin, that led to the development of vancomycin. At the time vancomycin was invented, it was often effective when bacterial infections had demonstrated resistance to other drug therapies.

VRE infections are difficult to treat and dangerous to those who are infected, including high fatality rates. Although VRE presents serious problems in treating hospitalized patients, it should be noted that vancomycin is not prescribed outside of hospitals and specialized clinics. Because of this, vancomycin resistance beyond *Enterococci* remains infrequent, and vancomycin continues to be a mainstay of treatment for methicillin-resistant *Staphylococcus aureus* (MRSA).

According to a 2010 study, the prevalence of VRE in Canadian hospitals was 0.5 percent. While this figure is low, it still presents difficulties for clinicians and is life-threatening for patients.

History and Scientific Foundations

Enterococci have been identified as the cause of a number of conditions, including meningitis, urinary tract infections, and endocarditis. But as antibiotic treatments were developed during the 20th century, *Enterococci* demonstrated both "intrinsic resistance to several commonly used antibiotics," as well as an "ability to acquire resistance to all currently available antibiotics, either by mutation or by receipt of foreign genetic material," according to a 2000 article on VRE for *Clinical Microbiology Reviews.* This resistance made *Enterococcus* infections difficult to treat until the introduction of vancomycin in the mid-20th century. Unlike other antibiotics, vancomycin offered one of the only reliable treatment methods for potentially life-threatening infections for more than three decades.

WORDS TO KNOW

COLONIZATION The process of occupation and increase in number of microorganisms at a specific site.

ISOLATION Within the health community, precautions taken in the hospital to prevent the spread of an infectious agent from an infected or colonized patient to susceptible people. Isolation practices are designed to minimize the transmission of infection.

PATHOGEN A disease-causing agent, such as a bacterium, a virus, a fungus, or another microorganism.

PREVALENCE The actual number of cases of disease or injury that exists in a population.

RESISTANT ORGANISM An organism that has developed the ability to counter something trying to harm it. Within infectious diseases, the organism, such as a bacterium, has developed a resistance to drugs, such as antibiotics.

However, the effectiveness of vancomycin was called into question in 1986, when scientists reported the emergence of VRE in England and France. A year later vancomycin-resistant strains of the bacteria were identified in the United States. Research suggests that VRE infections emerge when large amounts of oral vancomycin are taken for an infection and some of the drug's proteins are not absorbed and instead remain in the gastrointestinal tract. This environment leads to colonization with vancomycin-resistant organisms when the antibiotic concentrations in the intestines are high enough to encourage resistant *Enterococci* to grow but not sufficiently high enough to kill these organisms.

Throughout the 1990s there were few, if any, antimicrobial agents to treat VRE infection. In the 21st century, however, newly developed antibiotics have been effective against VRE and other multidrug-resistant organisms. But *Enterococci* continue to develop new forms of resistance, and strains of microorganisms that are resistant to these new agents have emerged. Many of these strains are resistant not only to vancomycin but also to other antibiotics that have been widely used against infections with similar bacteria in hospital settings, a condition known as cross resistance.

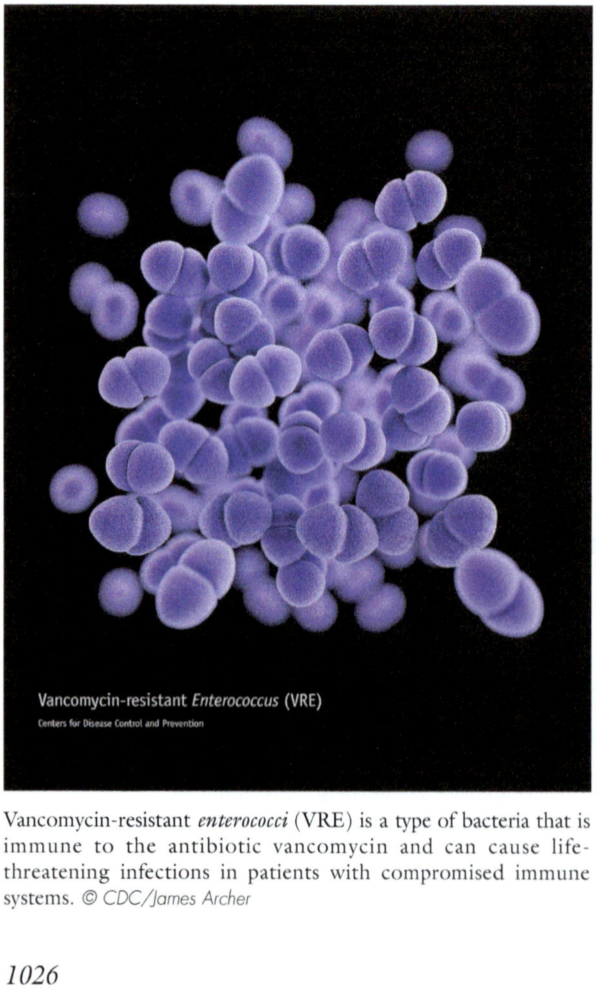

Vancomycin-resistant *enterococci* (VRE) is a type of bacteria that is immune to the antibiotic vancomycin and can cause life-threatening infections in patients with compromised immune systems. *© CDC/James Archer*

The connection between VRE and MRSA is particularly alarming. In one study almost 25 percent of hospitalized people who had growing populations of both bacteria present on their bodies died. Another nearly 35 percent were discharged to other facilities and took with them significant risk of further transmitting the infection to other patients.

Most of the VRE recovered in the United States involves one of two species: *E. faecium* and *E. faecalis.* These *Enterococci* occur naturally in the intestinal tract of all people and are not generally harmful, whether or not they are vancomycin resistant. Most infections resolve without treatment. Nevertheless, infections with these microbes, especially with *E. faecalis*, can be dangerous to immunocompromised people. Such individuals include those receiving chemotherapy for cancer or an organ transplant and those who have weakened immune systems due to a variety of conditions, including acquired immunodeficiency syndrome (AIDS).

From 1990 to 1997, the prevalence of VRE in hospitalized patients with infections arising from *Enterococci* increased from less than 1 percent to about 15 percent. By 1999 VRE accounted for nearly a quarter of all *Enterococcus* infections in hospital intensive care units (ICUs), as reported by the National Nosocomial Infection Surveillance System (NNIS). This figure rose to 28.5 percent in 2003. According to Tristan O'Driscoll and Christopher W. Crank in a 2015 article in *Infection and Drug Resistance*, rates of VRE are highest in the United States, where 35.5 percent of "enterococcal hospital-associated infections were resistant to vancomycin" between 2009 and 2010. VRE is also prevalent in parts of Europe, including in Portugal, Greece, and the United Kingdom, where rates of VRE exceed 20 percent.

■ Applications and Research

VRE can only be contracted through touch. It cannot be passed in aerosolized form via an infected person's breath. VRE is usually contracted in health care settings—in particular, hospitals. Caregivers may unwittingly pass the bacteria between patients. To reduce the likelihood of transmission, public health officials urge caregivers treating patients with VRE to use gloves when coming into contact with bodily fluids and to wash their hands frequently. People with VRE are encouraged to frequently and carefully wash their hands, as well as clean areas likely to become contaminated with these bacteria, such as bathrooms. Health care providers should also be notified when a person contracts VRE so that appropriate sanitary and precautionary measures can be taken to limit the likelihood of the bacteria spreading.

Although VRE is resistant to some drugs, laboratory testing can sometimes identify antibiotics that will be effec-

SUPERBUGS

As public health officials become increasingly concerned about the rise of vancomycin-resistant *Enterococcus* (VRE) and other drug-resistant organisms in the early 21st century, researchers have come to study the ways in which health care settings serve as breeding grounds for new superbugs, or pathogens that are impervious to the effects of antibiotics and other drug therapies. The most concerning of these resistant organisms to emerge is a class of bacteria known as carbapenemase-producing organisms (CPO), carbapenem-resistant enterobacteriaceae (CRE), or carbapenemase-producing enterobacteriaceae (CPE). In a 2013 press release, Tom Frieden, the director of the US Centers for Disease Control and Prevention, deemed these organisms "nightmare bacteria" because they are fatal in about half of cases of bloodstream infection, they can transfer their drug resistance to other bacteria, and they are found primarily in hospitals and other health care settings.

In 2018 Rebecca A. Weingarten and her colleagues published a study of CPOs in hospital wastewater systems in *mBio*. Their findings suggested a "vast, resilient reservoir" of these deadly organisms within the plumbing of the hospitals they studied. According to the authors, "the presence of CPOs in the hospital environment is concerning because of the potential for spread to an immunocompromised or otherwise vulnerable patient population and because of the transmissibility of carbapenemase genes by mobile genetic elements to other bacteria within the hospital and into the community." More optimistically, however, the authors also found the "physical separation of wastewater from patients, combined with proper cleaning practices and active infection control responses, was largely sufficient to prevent transmission to patients, as few clonal isolates were detected in patients and the environment."

tive in combatting infection in a patient. As of 2018 doctors relied on drugs such as linezolid, daptomycin, quinupristin/dalfopristin, and tigecycline to combat infections. In addition, evidence suggests that other drugs, including telavancin, dalbavancin, tedizolid, and oritavancin, might be effective against VREs, though more research is required to confirm their efficacy. Researchers have also found promise in combination therapies that involve the use of more than one of these drugs.

Despite various promising avenues, VRE remains difficult to treat. According to O'Driscoll and Crank, "a lack of randomized controlled trials assessing the efficacy of limited treatment options have made therapy difficult, but new agents, combination therapies, and improved dosing strategies have broadened the practitioner's armamentarium and hold promise for the future treatment of VRE." In general, however, physicians tend to be careful about not overtreating VRE infections due to concerns that VRE will develop new resistances and become increasingly virulent. As a result, doctors typically treat symptomatic VRE infections and not asymptomatic infections.

■ Impacts and Issues

In the United States and around the world, VRE infections present a growing burden of illness with considerable economic impact. In the 21st century, VRE prevalence in the United States has steadily increased. Researchers have documented increased mortality, length of hospital stay, ICU admissions, surgical procedures, and costs for VRE patients.

Public health officials and hospital-based infectious disease specialists and hospital pharmacists have become increasingly concerned with the spread of infection with VRE in hospitals, rehabilitation centers, and nursing homes. The US Centers for Disease Control and Prevention (CDC) reports that concerted efforts involving the isolation of VRE-infected patients, active surveillance, use of waterless hand disinfectant, and staff training have resulted in significant decreases in VRE prevalence.

Hospitals are responding with strategies designed to limit the spread of VRE by limiting the use of vancomycin. Powerful new antibiotics such as piperacillin-tazobactam are often effective against VRE but are expensive and require intravenous administration.

Such anti-VRE strategies can be highly effective across the entire health care system. Some hospitals in the Netherlands and Denmark, for example, proactively isolate all patients considered at risk for VRE until tests show them to be free of multidrug-resistant organisms. This step prevents carriers from passing infections to other patients and hospital workers. The strategy has significantly reduced VRE-related infections in these countries. Also in the European Union, the nontherapeutic use of antibiotics in animals was banned in 2006 to stop the transfer of resistant bacteria from farm animals to people. This prescription was on top of an existing ban on the agricultural use of vancomycin-type drugs in animal feed.

Traditional methods of infection control are not universally considered an adequate response to the antibiotic-resistant infection crisis. Some observers have begun advocating environmental strategies directed at farming practices such as restricting the use of antibiotics in farm animal feed that promote VRE and related cross-resistant strains that multiply in dairy effluent lagoons. Such broad-ranging strategies have a political and economic policy aspect but have not yet been endorsed by the CDC, which continues to emphasize institutional infection control measures. However, as alarm spreads over the increase in antibiotic resistance, more comprehensive, environmentally based, and economy-wide measures may eventually be implemented to preserve the effectiveness of antibiotics as life-saving drugs.

SEE ALSO *Antibiotic Resistance; Contact Precautions; Microbial Evolution; Resistant Organisms*

BIBLIOGRAPHY

Books

Shnayersen, Michael, and Mark J. Plotkin. *The Killers Within: The Deadly Rise of Drug-Resistant Bacteria.* Boston: Little, Brown, 2003.

Periodicals

Cetinkaya, Yesim, Pamela Falk, and C. Glen Mayhall. "Vancomycin-Resistant *Enterococci.*" *Clinical Microbiology Reviews* 13, no. 4 (2000): 686–707. This article can also be found online at https://www.ncbi.nlm.nih.gov/pmc/articles/PMC88957/ (accessed March 7, 2018).

Eliopoulus, George M., and H. S. Gold. "Vancomycin-Resistant *Enterococci*: Mechanisms and Clinical Observations." *Clinical Infectious Diseases* 33, no. 2 (July 2001): 210–219. This article can also be found online at https://doi.org/10.1086/321815 (accessed March 7, 2018).

O'Driscoll, Tristan, and Christopher W. Crank. "Vancomycin-Resistant Enterococcal Infections: Epidemiology, Clinical Manifestations, and Optimal Management." *Infection and Drug Resistance* 8 (2015): 217–230. This article can also be found online at https://www.ncbi.nlm.nih.gov/pmc/articles/PMC4521680/ (accessed March 8, 2018).

Rice, Louis B. "Emergence of Vancomycin-Resistant *Enterococci.*" *Emerging Infectious Diseases* 7, no. 2 (March–April 2001): 183–187. This article can also be found online at https://wwwnc.cdc.gov/eid/article/7/2/70-0183_article (accessed March 8, 2018).

Simor, Andrew E., et al. "Prevalence of Colonization and Infection with Methicillin-Resistant *Staphylococcus aureus* and Vancomycin-Resistant *Enterococcus* and of *Clostridium difficile* Infection in Canadian Hospitals." *Infection Control and Hospital Epidemiology* 34, no. 7 (July 2013): 687–693. This article can also be found online at http://www.jstor.org/stable/10.1086/670998 (accessed March 9, 2018).

Weingarten, Rebecca A. "Genomic Analysis of Hospital Plumbing Reveals Diverse Reservoir of Bacterial Plasmids Conferring Carbapenem Resistance." *mBio* 9, no. 1 (February 2018): e02011–17

Websites

"Vancomycin-Resistant *Enterococcus* (VRE)." New York State Department of Health. http://www.health.state.ny.us/diseases/communicable/vancomycin_resistant_enterococcus/fact_sheet.htm (accessed March 7, 2018).

"Vancomycin-Resistant *Enterococci* (VRE) Overview." National Institute of Allergy and Infectious Diseases, March 9, 2009. https://www.niaid.nih.gov/research/vre-overview (accessed March 7, 2018).

"VRE in Healthcare Settings." Centers for Disease Control and Prevention, May 10, 2011. https://www.cdc.gov/hai/organisms/vre/vre.html (accessed March 7, 2018).

Kenneth T. LaPensee

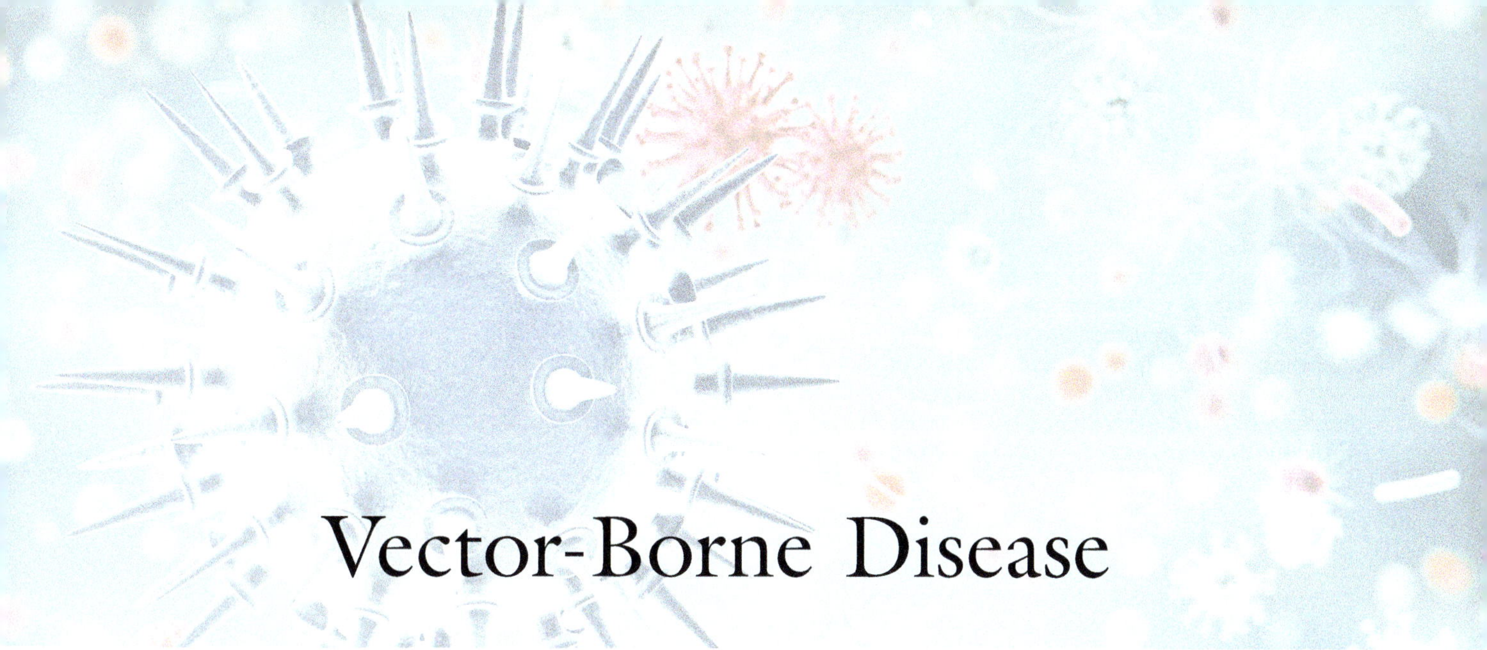

Vector-Borne Disease

Introduction

Vector-borne disease refers to the transmission of a disease that is caused by a microorganism from one organism (the host) to another organism via a third organism (the vector). Put another way, a vector is the means by which microbes can get from their normal place of residence, where they typically cause no harm, to a susceptible organism, in which an infection results.

There are numerous examples of vector-borne diseases that involve a variety of pathogens and vectors, including such well-known maladies as malaria, yellow fever, Lyme disease, plague, and West Nile disease. One vector-borne disease, Zika virus, became prominent in Brazil in the months preceding the 2016 Summer Olympics in Rio de Janeiro.

Disease History, Characteristics, and Transmission

Vector-borne diseases are characterized by the vector-mediated movement of a microorganism (such as a bacterium, virus, or protozoa) from the host to a recipient. The host and recipient can belong to the same species. A well-known example of this is malaria, in which the protozoan that causes the infection is acquired from an infected person by a mosquito during a blood meal and transferred to another human that the mosquito subsequently feeds on. Alternatively, the host and recipient can belong to different species. An example is Western equine encephalitis, in which the host is a bird that is infected by the disease-causing species of arbovirus and the recipient is a horse or a human. As with malaria, the vector is a mosquito.

Dengue hemorrhagic fever is another example of a vector-borne disease. Dengue is caused by a virus in the *Flavivirus* genus. The virus is transmitted from the host to the susceptible person by a species of mosquito called *Aedes aegypti.* Nearly 4 billion people in more than 128 countries were at risk of dengue in 2017, according to the World Health Organization (WHO), with the most at-risk group being those under age five.

Lyme disease is also a vector-borne disease. The disease, which is transmitted from contaminated animals such as deer to humans by the bite of several species of tick, is the most prevalent tick-borne ailment in North America. Lyme disease is caused by a bacterium called *Borrelia burgdorferi.* It is debilitating if not treated promptly and can cause severe fatigue, joint pain, and heart trouble that can persist for years even when the disease is diagnosed and treated.

Still another bacterial vector-borne disease is plague. The disease, which is caused by *Yersinia pestis,* is ancient. Passages found in the Old Testament of the Bible describe the ravages of epidemics of plague. Rodents harbor the bacterium. The vector that transmits the bacterium from rodents to humans is another rat or, more commonly, a flea. Both can feed on an infected rat and subsequently spread the infection to a human whom they bite. There are several types of plague, depending on the site of the infection. Infection of the lungs (pneumonic plague) is almost always fatal within a week if not treated.

WORDS TO KNOW

HOST An organism that serves as the habitat for a parasite or possibly for a symbiont. A host may provide nutrition to the parasite or symbiont, or it may simply provide a place in which to live.

VECTOR Any agent that carries and transmits parasites and diseases. Also, an organism or chemical used to transport a gene into a new host cell.

Another example of a vector-borne disease is yellow fever. Another viral disease caused by a member of the *Flavivirus* genus, the disease is transferred from the host (a type of monkey) to humans via a mosquito. In tropical regions devastating outbreaks of yellow fever have occurred over the past several hundred years. A noteworthy outbreak occurred during the construction of the Panama Canal in the early 20th century. Even in 2013, between 84,000 and 170,000 cases were estimated to have occurred in Africa, according to WHO, with between 29,000 and 60,000 deaths.

In 2016 the vector-borne disease encephalitis caused by Zika virus was emerging. The disease was of particular threat to pregnant women because if a woman is bitten by a mosquito that carries the virus, her fetus is at risk of a variety of birth defects, including brain malformation. The threat of Zika virus was highlighted by the refusal of some athletes to attend the 2016 Summer Olympics held in Rio de Janeiro because of fears of contracting the virus. At the time some regions of South America were experiencing a spike in the number of cases of birth defects attributed to the infection. The number of cases in Brazil subsequently declined from 170,535 cases in 2016 to 7,911 cases in 2017, according to health statistics from Brazil. The cause of the upsurge and decline in cases was not known.

Scope and Distribution

Vector-borne diseases occur worldwide and account for more than 17 percent of all infectious diseases, according to WHO. While some diseases, such as malaria, are concentrated in tropical equatorial regions of the globe, other diseases can occur in more temperate climates. One example of a vector-borne disease found in more temperate regions is the mosquito-borne West Nile disease. The West Nile virus that causes this disease has spread as far north as Canada, where it can be transmitted by mosquitoes during the warmer months of the year and even during the cooler days of spring by mosquitoes that have survived the winter. Cases of the infection first appeared in Canada in 2002. In 2007 the number of annual infections was highest, with 2,215 cases reported by Health Canada. From 2010 to 2016 there were 5, 101, 428, 115, 21, 80, and 104 Canadian cases, respectively.

Treatment and Prevention

Vector-borne diseases can be treated, and even prevented, by interrupting the vector-mediated transmission between the infected host and the susceptible person or animal. Treatment and prevention strategies for malaria focus on the mosquito vector. For example, spraying mosquito breeding grounds with insecticide can be an effective control. The carefully controlled application of dichloro-diphenyl-trichloroethane (DDT), a powerful insecticide used in the 1960s that effectively reduced malaria vectors but also resulted in significant loss of bird populations, is again beginning to be used as a means of mosquito control.

Another efficient and environmentally friendly way of controlling the mosquito-borne spread of malarial protozoa

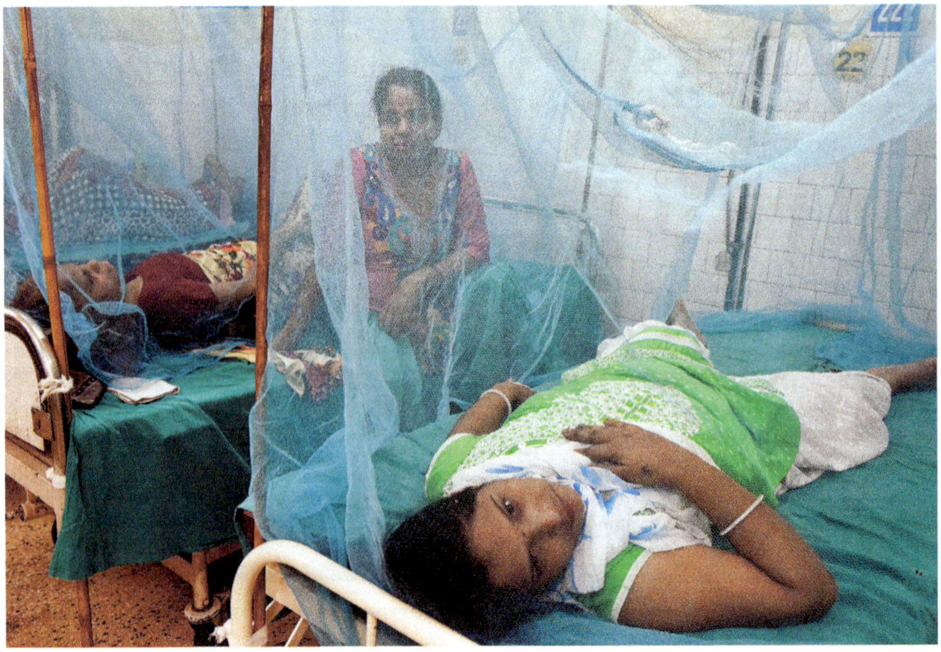

Patients infected with dengue fever and chikungunya rest behind mosquito nets at a hospital in New Delhi, India, in September 2016. Dengue and chikungunya are two prominent vector-borne diseases, infections transmitted to humans by infected insects such as mosquitoes, ticks, and fleas. © *Saumya Khandelwal/Hindustan Times/Getty Images*

is draping beds with insecticide-treated mosquito netting to protect people during sleep. Organizations such as World Vision International have campaigns to supply villages in Africa with bed netting. Similarly, protective clothing with overlapping upper and lower layers minimize the amount of skin that is exposed to a bite from the vector.

Another trial program aimed at preventing malaria involves releasing laboratory-bred infertile male mosquitoes. The program is based on the hypothesis that a greater population of infertile males will decrease the numbers of female mosquitoes due to reduced reproductive success. Because malaria is transmitted by female mosquitoes, fewer female mosquitoes should result in a reduction in the number of cases of malaria. There have been several successful small-scale trials of this program, but the large number of sterile male mosquitoes needed is likely to make this approach impractical for larger-scale implementation.

Other treatment and prevention strategies include vaccine development and the use of genetic material (*morpholino antisense oligonucleotides*) that can outcompete viral genetic material for binding onto cells of the host, blocking a crucial step in the formation of new virus particles.

Impacts and Issues

Vector-borne diseases exact a large toll worldwide. More than 500 million cases of malaria occur each year, according to WHO, with approximately 3 million deaths attributed to the disease. One million of these deaths are children. The disease is particularly prevalent in Africa. WHO estimated that in 2017 more than 2.5 billion people were at risk for malaria. Yellow fever continues to infect hundreds of thousands of people in less-developed tropical countries annually, despite the existence of a vaccine that can provide long-term protection. In Asia a form of encephalitis puts about 3 billion people at risk each year.

The burden of these and other vector-borne diseases have a substantial economic and social impact on areas of the world that are already destitute. In malaria-prone areas, school attendance can be poor, as schoolchildren are either sick, tending to other sick family members, or being pressed into work as parents and older siblings can no longer work due to illness. With a lack of education, hope for a more promising future can diminish, and the economy of a nation can be undermined by the illness of a sizable portion of the workforce.

PRIMARY SOURCE

Treated Bed Nets Shorten the Lifespan Even of Mosquitos That Evolved Resistance

SOURCE: *Vlasits, Anna. "Treated Bed Nets Shorten the Lifespan Even of Mosquitos That Evolved Resistance."* STAT. July 11, 2016. https://www.statnews.com/2016/07/11/mosquitoes-bed-nets-insecticide/ (accessed November 27, 2017).

INTRODUCTION: *Insecticide-treated mosquito nets have become an important weapon in the battle against vector-borne diseases. In the following article from the medical publication STAT, Anna Vlasits explores an unexpected benefit of the nets in fighting insecticide-resistant mosquitoes.*

It sounds like a contradiction, but it's true: Insecticide-treated mosquito nets are effective even against some insecticide-resistant mosquitoes, a new study shows.

WHY IT MATTERS

Mosquito nets treated with insecticides are one of the most effective ways to prevent malaria. The nets work both by preventing people from being bitten and by killing mosquitoes that come in contact with the nets. But the World Health Organization has only approved one class of insecticide to use on the nets, called pyrethroids, and mosquitoes across Africa are evolving resistance to that insecticide.

THE NITTY GRITTY

Researchers led by Hilary Ranson at the Liverpool School of Tropical Medicine in the UK exposed *Anopheles gambiae* mosquitoes in the lab to insecticidal nets or untreated nets and then looked to see how long they lived. In previous research, scientists had only looked at whether the mosquitoes survived for 24 hours after touching a net, calling the ones who survived "insecticide-resistant."

But "whether the mosquitoes live long enough to transmit disease is the really more interesting parameter," said Ransom.

Surprisingly, in data published Monday in *Proceedings of the National Academy of Sciences*, they found that lots of the mosquitoes exposed to insecticides were dying after the first 24 hours. Overall, the supposedly resistant mosquitoes were living about half as long as mosquitoes that weren't exposed to the insecticide.

And that has a big impact on malaria transmission. The researchers calculated that contact with a treated net reduced a resistant insect's likelihood of passing along malaria by two-thirds.

YOU SHOULD KNOW

More-resistant mosquitoes lived longer after contact with the treated net. "I think it still does raise quite a lot of alarm bells for what might happen in the future," Ransom said, if resistance continues to increase.

WHAT THEY'RE SAYING

"This particular study is very interesting and tantalizing, but we need a lot more studies like this" to really know for sure how insecticides affect malaria transmission, said Andrew Read, the director of the Center for Infectious Disease Dynamics at Penn State University. He pointed out that the research was limited to two strains of a single *Anopheles* mosquito; others of the genus also transmit malaria.

Ranson agreed, suggesting that field studies of resistant mosquitoes would be an important next step.

THE BOTTOM LINE

Treated bed nets are still working, despite mosquitoes' growing resistance, but monitoring resistant strains and developing new insecticides will be important going forward.

SEE ALSO *Arthropod-Borne Disease; Bloodborne Pathogens; Host and Vector*

BIBLIOGRAPHY

Books

Bayry, Jagadeesh. *Emerging and Re-emerging Infectious Diseases of Livestock.* New York: Springer, 2017.

Kaslow, Richard A., and Lawrence R. Stanberry. *Viral Infections of Humans: Epidemiology and Control.* New York: Springer, 2014.

Payne, Susan. *Viruses: From Understanding to Investigation.* New York: Academic Press, 2017.

Periodicals

van den Berg, Henk. "Global Status of DDT and Its Alternatives for Use in Vector Control to Prevent Disease." *Environmental Health Perspectives* 117, no. 11 (November 2009): 1656–1663.

Websites

"National Center for Emerging and Zoonotic Infectious Diseases (NCEZID): About the Division of Vector-Borne Diseases." Centers for Disease Control and Prevention. https://www.cdc.gov/ncezid/dvbd/index.html (accessed November 22, 2017).

"Vector-Borne Diseases." World Health Organization. http://www.who.int/mediacentre/factsheets/fs387/en/ (accessed November 22, 2017).

"World Malaria Report 2017." World Health Organization. http://www.who.int/malaria/publications/world_malaria_report/en/ (accessed November 22, 2017).

Brian Hoyle

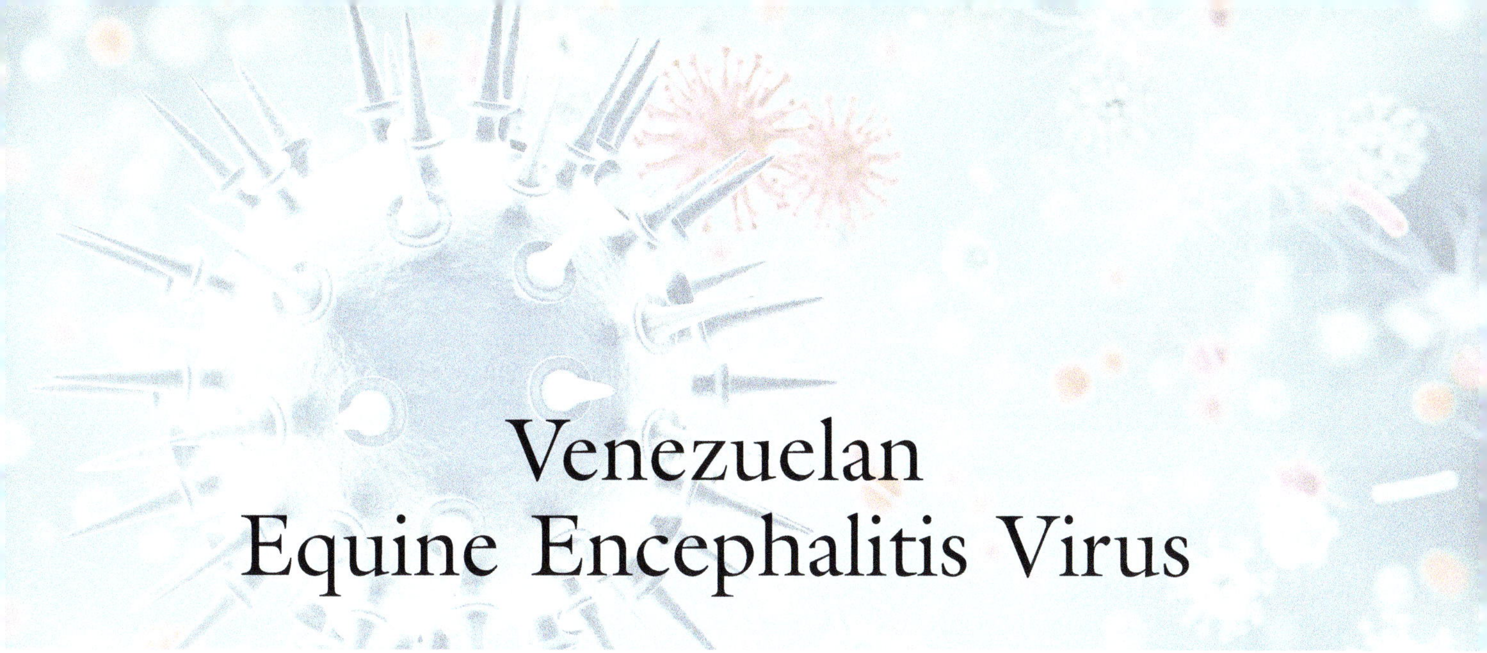

Venezuelan Equine Encephalitis Virus

Introduction

Venezuelan equine encephalitis virus (VEEV) is an arbovirus that belongs to genus *Alphavirus* and family Togaviridae. Alphaviruses found in North, South, and Central America include three encephalitis viruses: Eastern equine encephalitis virus, Western equine encephalitis virus, and VEEV. Out of these VEEV is the most significant human and equine pathogen in the Americas. It has been associated with numerous outbreaks, leading to hundreds of thousands of horse deaths and human infections.

The virion of VEEV is spherical and 70 nanometers in size. In the center of the viral particle is a ribonucleic acid (RNA) genome, surrounded by 240 copies of capsid protein, followed by a viral membrane consisting of 240 copies of envelope proteins E1 and E2. The envelope protein arrangement forms spikes derived from E2 protein, which gives the virus the appearance of a spiky sphere.

There are six subtypes of VEEV: I, II, III, IV, V, and VI. Within subtype I there are five variants: AB, C, D, E, and F. Only two of these subtypes (I-AB and I-C) are associated with large outbreaks, due to their ability to replicate to high levels in horses and other equids. Other sub-

WORDS TO KNOW

ALPHAVIRUS A genus of small, spherical RNA viruses. The genus contains some of the most important human and animal pathogens, such as chikungunya virus; Sindbis virus; Semliki Forest virus; Western, Eastern, and Venezuelan equine encephalitis viruses; and the Ross River virus. Alphaviruses are transmitted by arthropods, in particular mosquitoes.

ARBOVIRUS A virus that is typically spread by blood-sucking insects, most commonly mosquitoes. Over 100 types of arboviruses cause disease in humans. Yellow fever and dengue fever are two examples.

ATTENUATED STRAIN A bacterium or virus that has been weakened. Often used as the basis of a vaccine against the specific disease caused by the bacterium or virus.

CAPSID The protein shell surrounding a virus particle.

ENZOOTIC Affecting animals, naturally present in an environment, and occurring at regular intervals.

EPIZOOTIC The abnormally high occurrence of a specific disease in animals in an area, similar to a human epidemic.

EQUID A mammal of the horse family, such as a horse, donkey, mule, or zebra.

GENOME All of the genetic information for a cell or organism. The complete sequence of genes within a cell or virus.

VECTOR Any agent that carries and transmits parasites and diseases. Also, an organism or a chemical used to transport a gene into a new host cell.

VIRION A mature virus particle consisting of a core of ribonucleic acid (RNA) or deoxyribonucleic acid (DNA) surrounded by a protein coat. This is the form in which a virus exists outside of its host cell.

types were isolated from small vertebrates and mosquitoes and were not found in any large outbreaks. Despite not being able to replicate well in horses, the I-C, I-D, and I-E subtypes can infect humans or other vertebrates.

Disease History, Characteristics, and Transmission

The first observations of VEEV were recorded in 1935, coinciding with an outbreak in Colombia. It took another three years before VEEV was isolated in Venezuela. Since then VEEV has been isolated in outbreaks as far south as Argentina and as far north as the Rocky Mountains in the United States. However, prevalence of the virus is highest in Central America and the northern part of South America.

Major outbreak episodes were recorded on the Pacific coast of Peru in 1942, in Mexico between 1962 and 1964, and in Guatemala in 1969, which then spread north to Texas in 1971. Two years later, in 1973, a last episode involving subtype I-AB was recorded. It was due to a poorly inactivated vaccine used in field immunizations. More recently, in 1995, a disease outbreak started in the northern part of Venezuela and spread to neighboring Colombia. VEEV continued to cause outbreaks, with episodes reported in Ecuador between 2001 and 2003 and in Bolivia between 2005 and 2007.

Mosquitoes transmit VEEV from their salivary glands to a host's blood. There are two transmission cycles of the virus: epizootic and enzootic. Epizootic transmission occurs between equids, such as horses or donkeys, and mosquitoes. Enzootic transmission occurs between small forest rodents and mosquitoes. Humans can be infected in both types of transmission cycles. Other potential targets of infection are domestic animals such as cattle, goats, sheep, pigs, dogs, and chickens. Epizootic transmission is responsible for all the large outbreaks of VEEV on record.

VEEV is transmitted by numerous mosquito species. The main mosquito vectors in epizootic transmission are *Psorophora confinnis*, *Aedes taeniorhynchus*, *Psorophora columbiae*, and *Aedes sollicitans*. However, epizootic strains also have been isolated from the *Culex* genus of mosquitoes. In contrast, enzootic transmission is mainly carried by genus *Culex*, with some *Aedes* and *Psorophora* species. While mosquitoes remain the primary carrier of the virus, there is evidence that VEEV can also be transmitted by aerosols or via direct contact of infectious material with open wounds. As of 2017 direct person-to-person transmission had not been demonstrated.

The incubation time of the infection lasts between one and six days. In humans this is followed by flu-like symptoms such as headaches, muscle pain, fever, fatigue, and pharyngitis. Encephalitis develops only in a minority of cases, on average 4 to 15 percent, within 4 to 10 days after

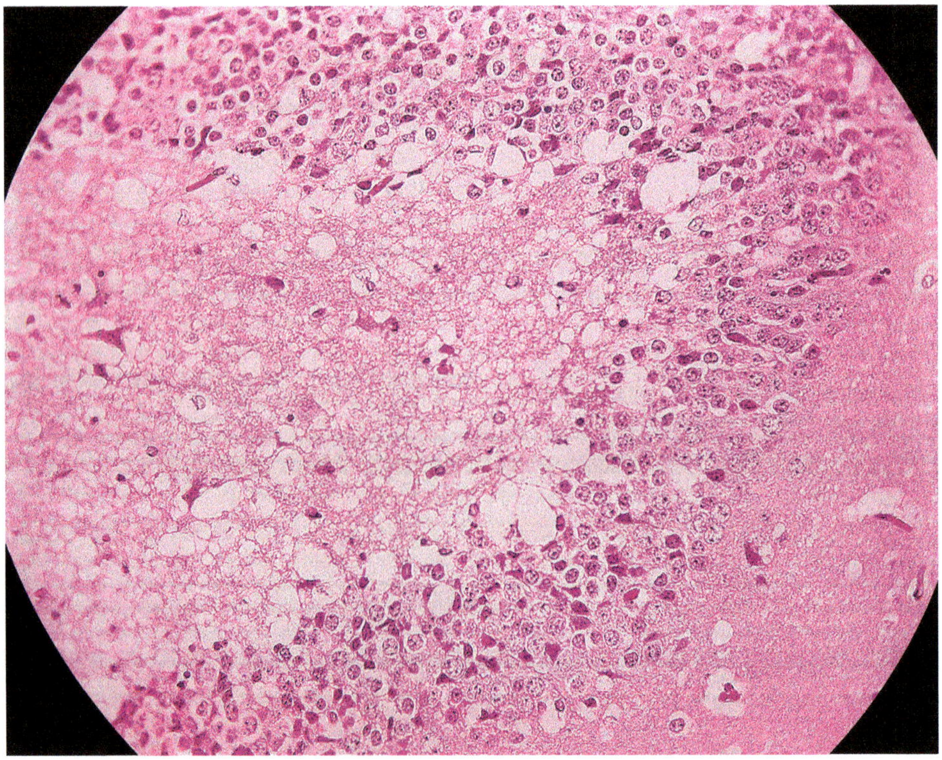

Photomicrograph of mouse brain tissue infected with Venezuelan equine encephalitis and showing significant deterioration of the tissue. Though primarily found in horses and other equine animals, the disease can be spread to humans via mosquito bites. *© Media for Medical/Getty Images*

infection. Symptoms of encephalitis last 3 to 8 days, but a relapse can occur within a week. An infection with VEEV in pregnancy can lead to birth defects or stillbirth. In horses an infection can cause fever, poor feeding, head pressing, circling, incoordination, and blindness. Encephalitis in equids is common and requires euthanizing of sick animals.

Scope and Distribution

Active surveillance of VEEV is critical to better understand the evolution of the virus and for prevention of the next large outbreak. Subtypes I-AB and I-C are genetically very similar to I-D and I-E, making efforts in finding effective prevention strategies difficult. Evidence based on genetic analysis suggests that epizootic strains emerged from enzootic ones, which adds levels of complexity when researching prevention or reduction strategies. Geographical distribution of the virus is limited by mosquito distribution. However, expansion of current vectors to new geographical areas or adaptation of other mosquito species to transmission of epizootic subtypes could change this pattern.

Treatment and Prevention

As there is no treatment for VEEV, research efforts focus on prevention and reduction of viral transmission. Infection control is achieved by controlling mosquito populations in the wild through the elimination of breeding grounds, especially near human settlements. Additionally, insecticides are used to reduce mosquito populations. People working in high-risk areas are advised to use protective clothing and insect repellents.

Another preventative measure is vaccination against VEEV. Early vaccines based on subtype I-AB were a complete failure due to incomplete inactivation of the virus. This was remedied with an introduction of the live attenuated T-83 vaccine. The vaccine was subsequently modified further to create an attenuated and inactivated vaccine known as T-84. Further work on vaccine development produced an attenuated V3526 vaccine. It confirms immunity in horses, rodents, and nonhuman primates. While T-84 vaccine is used for immunization of laboratory staff, neither of the vaccines have been licensed for general human immunization.

The only drawback of the existing vaccines is that they are based on subtype I-AB and offer limited protection against type I-C. There is an ongoing effort to create a better vaccine that can also be used on humans. Additionally, researchers work toward developing an antiviral treatment for VEEV. One idea is to identify inhibitors of viral entry as drug candidates. However, this work is in its early stages.

PREVENTION

The Centers for Disease Control and Prevention recommends the following precautions to prevent contracting Venezuelan equine encephalitis virus in areas where mosquitos are present.

- Use an insect repellent containing DEET, picaridin, or IR3535.
- Wear long sleeves and pants. Using the insecticide permethrin on clothing can provide additional protection against mosquitoes that can last through several washings.
- Use screens on windows and doors. Check screens to make sure there are no holes or tears large enough to allow mosquitos to fit through.
- Empty standing water from buckets, barrels, and flowerpots, and empty wading pools when not in use. This helps eliminate mosquito breeding sites.

Impacts and Issues

There have been several large outbreaks of VEEV, resulting in both human and horse deaths. One of the largest was the 1967 Colombia outbreak, resulting in 220,000 human cases and more than 67,000 horse deaths. The ensuing outbreak reached as far north as Texas and ended with more than 100,000 horse deaths. In 1995 the Venezuelan and Colombian outbreak resulted in up to 100,000 human infections and 300 deaths. Whereas human cases are large in number, fatality rates are generally under 1 percent. Horse infectivity in a susceptible population can be as high as 90 percent, with fatality rates ranging from 10 to 100 percent.

The difficulty in surveillance, detection, and control of the outbreaks is also related to the remote location of some of the sites. In those communities each of the epizootic episodes has effects beyond the immediate health issues. Horses are frequently the only way locals can reach cities. Equids of all kinds, including donkey and mules, are an important part of the South and Central American economy. Significant losses in their numbers affect local transportation, trade, and ability to work, resulting in loss of income. Prevention of the disease becomes extremely important for those communities.

See Also *Eastern Equine Encephalitis; Encephalitis*

BIBLIOGRAPHY

Books

Krauss, Hartmut, et al., eds. *Zoonoses: Infectious Diseases Transmissible from Animals to Humans.* 3rd ed. Washington, DC: ASM, 2003.

Periodicals

Aguilar, Patricia V., et al. "Endemic Venezuelan Equine Encephalitis in Northern Peru." *Emerging Infectious Diseases* 10 (2004): 880–888.

Anishchenko, M., et al. "From the Cover: Venezuelan Encephalitis Emergence Mediated by a Phylogenetically Predicted Viral Mutation." *Proceedings of the National Academy of Sciences of the United States of America* 103 (2006): 4994–4999.

De La Monte, S., et al. "The Systemic Pathology of Venezuelan Equine Encephalitis Virus Infection in Humans." *American Journal of Tropical Medicine and Hygiene* 34 (1985): 194–202.

Fine, D. L., et al. "Venezuelan Equine Encephalitis Virus Vaccine Candidate (V3526) Safety, Immunogenicity and Efficacy in Horses." *Vaccine* 25 (2007): 1868–1876.

Forrester, N. L., et al. "Evolution and Spread of Venezuelan Equine Encephalitis Complex Alphavirus in the Americas" *PLOS Neglected Tropical Diseases* 11 (2017): e0005693.

Navarro, J., et al. "Postepizootic Persistence of Venezuelan Equine Encephalitis Virus, Venezuela." *Emerging Infectious Diseases* 11 (2005): 1907–1915.

Paessler, S., and S. C. Weaver. "Vaccines for Venezuelan Equine Encephalitis." *Vaccine* 27, no. S4 (2009): D80–D85

Shechter, Sharon, et al. "Novel Inhibitors Targeting Venezuelan Equine Encephalitis Virus Capsid Protein Identified Using *In Silico* Structure-Based-Drug-Design." *Scientific Reports* 7, no. 1 (December 2017): 17705.

Torres, Rolando, et al. "Enzootic Mosquito Vector Species at Equine Encephalitis Transmission Foci in the República de Panamá" *PLOS ONE* 12 (2017): e0185491. This article can also be found online at https://doi.org/10.1371/journal.pone.0185491 (accessed February 25, 2018).

Weaver, S., et al. "Venezuelan Equine Encephalitis." *Annual Review of Entomology* 49 (2004): 141–174.

Websites

"Eastern, Western and Venezuelan Equine Encephalomyelitis." Iowa State University Center for Food Security and Public Health, January 2015. http://lib.dr.iastate.edu/cfsph_factsheets/49 (accessed February 25, 2018).

"Venezuelan Equine Encephalitis." World Organisation for Animal Health, April 2013. http://www.oie.int/fileadmin/Home/eng/Animal_Health_in_the_World/docs/pdf/Disease_cards/VEE.pdf (accessed February 25, 2018)

Agnes Caruso

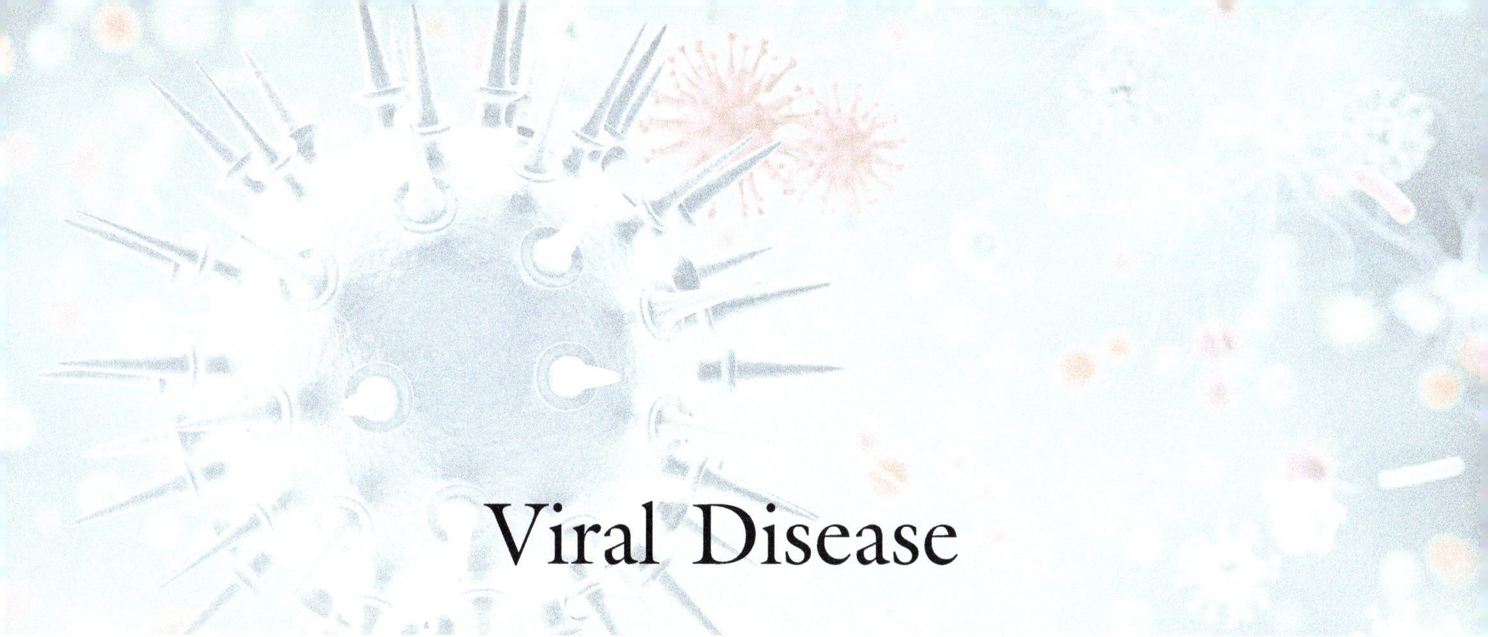

Viral Disease

Introduction

Viruses are microorganisms that do not have the ability to independently produce new copies of themselves. Instead, the intact virus or its payload of deoxyribonucleic acid (DNA) or ribonucleic acid (RNA) must get inside the host cell. Once inside, copies of the genetic material are made at the same time as the host's genetic material is being replicated, using the various constituents of the host's replication machinery.

WORDS TO KNOW

BACTERIOPHAGE A virus that infects bacteria. When a bacteriophage that carries the diphtheria toxin gene infects diphtheria bacteria, the bacteria produce diphtheria toxin.

DEGRADATION (CELLULAR) The destruction of host cell components, such as DNA, by infective agents such as bacteria and viruses.

DEOXYRIBONUCLEIC ACID (DNA) A double-stranded, helical molecule that forms the molecular basis for heredity in most organisms.

ENDOCYTOSIS A process by which host cells allow the entry of outside substances, including viruses, through their cell membranes.

HOST An organism that serves as the habitat for a parasite or possibly for a symbiont. A host may provide nutrition to the parasite or symbiont, or it may simply provide a place in which to live.

LATENT VIRUS Viruses that can incorporate their genetic material into the genetic material of the infected host cell. Because the viral genetic material can then be replicated along with the host material, the virus becomes effectively "silent" with respect to detection by the host. Latent viruses usually contain the information necessary to reverse the latent state. The viral genetic material can leave the host genome to begin the manufacture of new virus particles.

RECEPTOR Protein molecules on a cell's surface that act as a "signal receiver" and allow communication between cells.

REVERSE TRANSCRIPTASE An enzyme that makes it possible for a retrovirus to produce DNA (deoxyribonucleic acid) from RNA (ribonucleic acid).

RIBONUCLEIC ACID (RNA) Any of a group of nucleic acids that carry out several important tasks in the synthesis of proteins. Unlike DNA (deoxyribonucleic acid), it has only a single strand. Nucleic acids are complex molecules that contain a cell's genetic information and the instructions for carrying out cellular processes. In eukaryotic cells, the two nucleic acids, RNA and DNA, work together to direct protein synthesis. Although it is DNA that contains the instructions for directing the synthesis of specific structural and enzymatic proteins, it is actually several types of RNA that carry out the processes required to produce these proteins. These include messenger RNA (mRNA), ribosomal RNA (rRNA), and transfer RNA (tRNA). Further processing of the various RNAs is carried out by another type of RNA called small nuclear RNA (snRNA). The structure of RNA is similar to that of DNA, however, instead of the base thymine, RNA contains the base uracil in its place.

VIRION A mature virus particle consisting of a core of ribonucleic acid (RNA) or deoxyribonucleic acid (DNA) surrounded by a protein coat. This is the form in which a virus exists outside of its host cell.

Typically, the host cell eventually ruptures, releasing the newly made viruses, which in turn initiate another cycle by infecting other host cells. The host suffers because cells are being destroyed.

There are many types of viruses that can cause infections in virtually every living thing, including humans.

Disease History, Characteristics, and Transmission

In general, viral diseases result from the attachment of a virus to the host cell and entry of either the virus particle (virion) or its genetic material into the cell. The attachment of a virion to a host involves the interaction of components of the viral and host cell outer surfaces. Often these components are proteins, but carbohydrates and lipids can be involved. The host component is also known as the receptor. The receptor is not present specifically to allow viral infection. Rather, this host constituent is usually used by the host for some other purpose and is exploited by the virus. The infecting virus has evolved the capability of using this constituent to adhere to the cell surface. As one example, human immunodeficiency virus (HIV), which causes acquired immunodeficiency syndrome (AIDS), uses the host protein CD4 as the receptor. HIV enters only cells, such as white blood cells, that have this receptor. The entry of the virus kills the white blood cell. Because white blood cells are important in the proper functioning of the host's immune system, their gradual destruction by HIV causes the immune system to break down, leaving the infected person vulnerable to a variety of opportunistic infections and maladies, including some types of cancer.

Following the fusion between the virion and the host cell surface, the virion or the viral genetic material enters

How a Virus Works

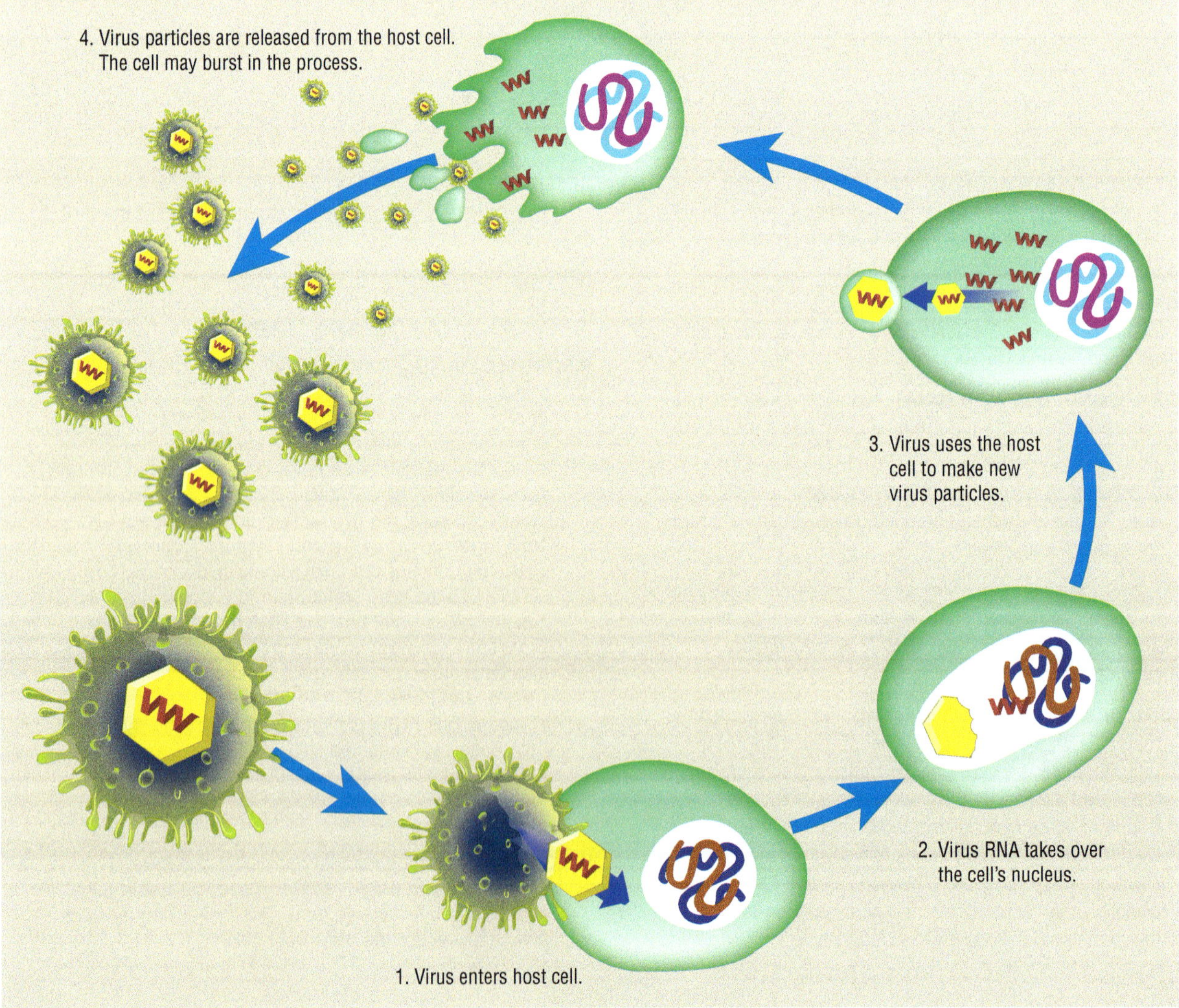

the host cell. This fusion can happen in several different ways. An individual virion can enter the host cell during endocytosis, the folding of a portion of the cell surface around the virion. The folding creates a spherical portion of the host cell's surface (a vesicle) that buds off inside the cell. The virion located inside the vesicle is degraded, releasing its genetic material. For other viruses the viral surface layer melds with the host cell's outer surface, which releases the genetic material inside the host cell. Finally, the viral DNA or RNA can directly enter the host cell, leaving the viral particle stuck to the host cell's surface. An example of this process is the injection of DNA from a bacteriophage into the host cell that it adheres to.

The viral DNA or RNA can then be replicated. In the case of DNA, this replication can occur directly because the host's genetic material is also DNA. RNA-containing viruses, such as retroviruses (e.g., HIV), require an additional step in which the viral RNA is used to make DNA. This is done using reverse transcriptase, a virus-encoded enzyme.

Depending on the virus, the replicated DNA, which is not recognized as foreign by the host's replication machinery, is used to manufacture the proteins that are encoded by the viral genes. The proteins assemble around the copies of replicated genetic material to form the new virus particles that are the hallmark of the viral disease. For other, so-called latent viruses, the replicated genetic material is incorporated into the host's DNA, where it can remain for years until certain conditions—as yet only partially understood—stimulate the viral DNA to excise and begin the production of virus particles. An active infection results. Examples of latent viral infections include AIDS, hepatitis B, Creutzfeld-Jacob disease, and herpes.

■ Scope and Distribution

Viruses are classified into a number of families. The members of a given family share similarities in the type of genetic material and its arrangement (either as a double-strand of DNA or RNA or as a single strand of the genetic material), chemistry, and physical properties, such as viral size and shape. Members of a given family differ in some characteristics from the members of another family, and different families of viruses cause different diseases.

Parvoviruses are members of the family Parvoviridae. These DNA-containing viruses are small. Their genetic material only codes for three or four proteins. Nonetheless, this small protein armada is sufficient to establish an infection. Diseases caused by parvoviruses include fifth disease, a mild illness characterized by a rash that usually occurs in children.

Papovaviruses are members of the family Papovaviridae. These DNA viruses also have a small genome that encodes five to eight proteins. Examples of papovavirus infections include warts, inflammation of the kidney (nephritis) and the urethra (urethritis), and progressive multifocal leukoencephalopathy. The latter is a disease that causes the loss of the brain component myelin. The increasing damage to the transmission of nerve impulses is progressively disabling and can be fatal.

The 88 known adenoviruses are members of the family Adenoviridae. These viruses have a distinctive shape that consists of 20 triangular faces (an icosahedron) with long fibers protruding from 12 regions around the viral surface. Adenoviruses cause the common cold and infections of the liver, bladder (cystitis), eye (keratoconjunctivitis), and gastrointestinal tract (gastroenteritis).

Herpesviruses are members of the family Herpesviridae. These viruses cause latent infections whose symptoms may not appear for years. The eight types of herpesvirus that can be recognized by the immune system cause a variety of infections. These infections include cell damage and the formation of ulcers in the mouth, lips (cold sores), skin, and genitals; keratoconjunctivitis; chickenpox; shingles; two forms of mononucleosis; three types of cancer (Burkitt's lymphoma, oropharyngeal carcinoma, and, in AIDS patients, Kaposi's sarcoma); cytomegalovirus infection (which can be fatal in infants); and inflammation of the brain (encephalitis).

Poxviruses are members of the family Poxviridae. The name of the virus refers to the major characteristic of the diseases caused by poxviruses, namely a raised lesion on the skin (pox). Poxviruses are the largest viruses known and may be an intermediate between viruses and bacteria. However, they are still classified as viruses because they are not capable of independent replication. Diseases caused by poxviruses include smallpox, monkeypox, cowpox, and a type of skin infection. However, not all poxviruses are deadly. The poxvirus vaccinia virus can bestow immunity to smallpox.

Viruses in the families Hepadnaviridae and Coronaviridae cause type B hepatitis and liver cancer and the common cold, respectively.

Picornaviruses are RNA-containing viruses that are members of the family Picornaviridae. They are the smallest of the RNA viruses, coding for only six to nine genes. Infections caused by picornaviruses include polio, meningitis, the common cold, inflammation of the heart (myocarditis), and inflammation of the tissue surrounding the heart (pericarditis).

Calciviruses are members of the family Calciviridae. There are two members of note. The first is the Norwalk virus, which is notorious for causing disease outbreaks on cruise ships and in crowded communal areas, such as university residences. The virus causes a contagious form of gastroenteritis (infection of the gastrointestinal tract) that is characterized by several days of intense diarrhea and vomiting. The second virus is hepatitis E, which is frequently fatal if contracted by pregnant women.

Of the more than 150 known types of reovirus, which belong to the family Reoviridae, two are significant to hu-

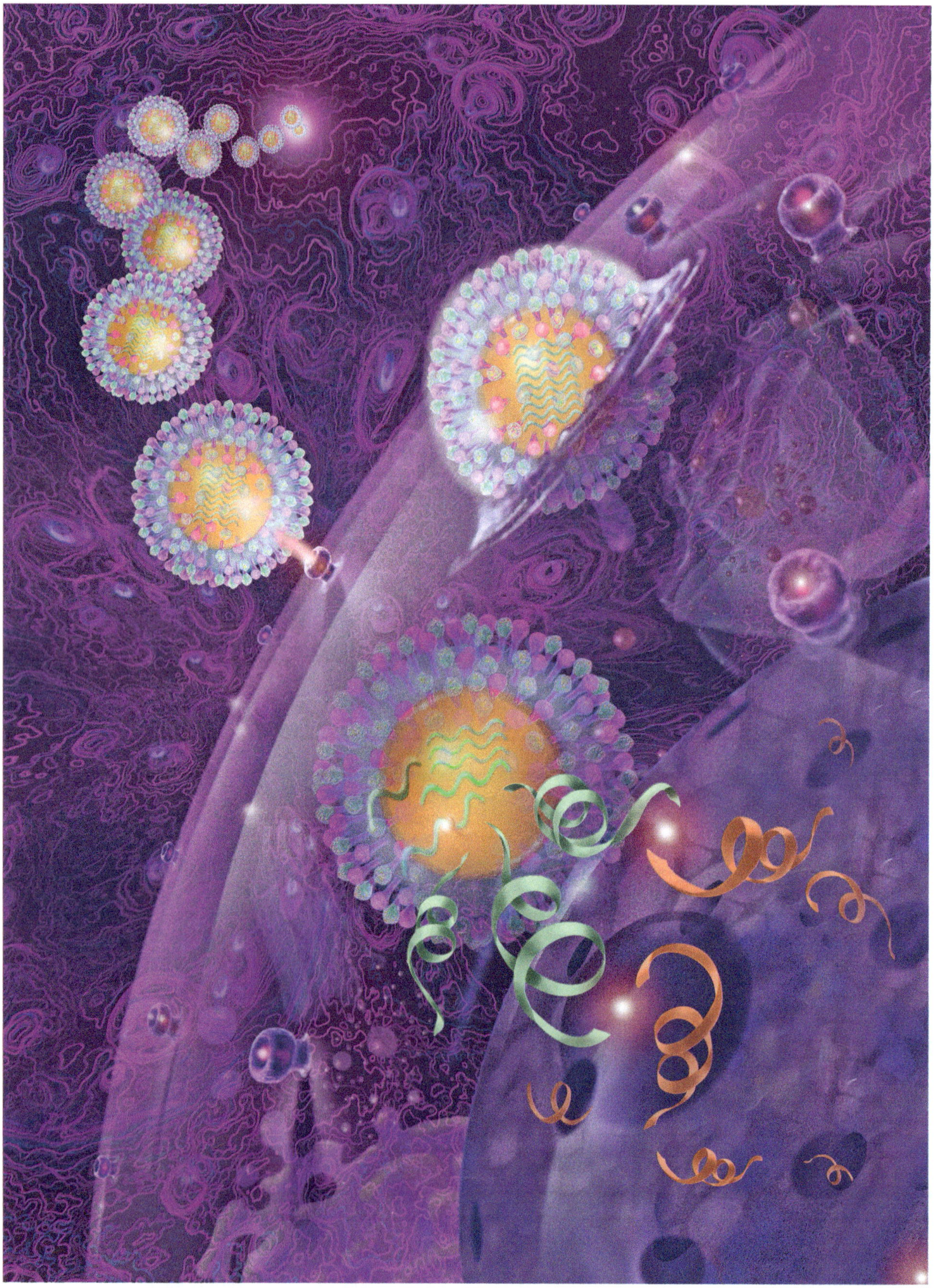

Viruses reproduce by infiltrating host cells and using their replication machinery. There are hundreds of thousands of viruses that can infect mammals. © Jim Dowdalls/Science Source mans, causing encephalitis and, most commonly, diarrhea in infants. The latter infection, which is caused by rotavirus, produces dehydration that is fatal if not treated quickly.

Togaviruses are members of the family Togaviridae. Infections caused by togaviruses include rubella (German measles), various forms of encephalitis, inflammation of joints (arthritis), and skin inflammation.

Flaviviruses are members of the family Flaviviridae. These viruses cause a number of serious human infections that are transmitted by insects, such as mosquitoes. These infections include yellow fever, dengue, West Nile disease, and encephalitis. The latter is caused by Zika virus.

Arenaviruses are members of the family Arenaviridae. The infections caused by arenaviruses are also serious and include hemorrhagic fever and inflammation of the brain and spinal cord or the membranes that cover these regions (lymphocytic choriomeningitis).

Retroviruses, which are members of the family Retroviridae, are given this name because they contain genetic information for the production of the enzyme reverse transcriptase. The enzyme allows the viral RNA to be used to produce DNA. Retroviruses are important human pathogens, causing cancer of the blood (leukemia) and, most significantly, AIDS.

Orthomyxoviruses include several types of influenza virus, including influenza A (H5N1), which is the cause of avian influenza. Avian influenza is one example of an emerging disease, a previously unknown or rare disease that has appeared and is spreading in terms of the number of people infected, in terms of the number of locations of illness outbreaks, or both. Other orthomyxoviruses can cause hemorrhagic fever and, along with bunyaviruses, encephalitis. Another viral class, paramyxovirus, includes the virus that causes measles.

Coronaviruses belongs to the family Coronaviridae. A coronavirus of particular significance causes severe acute respiratory syndrome (SARS) and is another example of an emerging disease.

Finally, filoviruses are members of the family Filoviridae. The two known filoviruses are the Marburg and Ebola viruses, which cause hemorrhagic fevers that can be severe and rapidly lethal. Little is known about the infectious disease processes of these viruses or of their natural hosts because they are so dangerous to work with (a special containment facility called a biosafety level 4 [BSL-4] laboratory is required for research on these microbes) and because illness outbreaks appear sporadically and end quickly.

Treatment and Prevention

Reflecting the diversity of viruses and viral diseases, treatment is variable. One common characteristic is the ineffectiveness of antibiotics because antibiotics are effective against bacteria. Treatment strategies include blocking the attachment of the virus to host cells by occupying the host cell receptor with another molecule, use of a vaccine that has been developed for a particular virus or a similar target of different viruses, and taking medications that assist the immune system in responding to the presence of the infecting virus.

Likewise, prevention strategies vary. Wearing a protective mask to prevent inhalation of viral-contaminated droplets is mandated for health care providers when treating someone known or suspected of having SARS, for example. Protective gowns and gloves can be prudent measures when coming into contact with someone who has a hemorrhagic fever, as splashing or copious loss of blood can occur. Another viral barrier is the condom. Wearing a condom can lessen the risk of transmission of HIV during sexual intercourse. Complete abstinence from sex is the ultimate preventive strategy for sexually transmitted viral disease.

The incidence of viral diseases, such as West Nile virus, that are transmitted by insects can be reduced by eradicating insect breeding grounds and wearing clothing that protects the body from insect bites. Insect repellents are also a helpful preventive measure.

Impacts and Issues

The toll from viral diseases throughout history is incalculable. The death toll from viral gastroenteritis and measles exceeds 2 million each year, according to the World Health Organization (WHO). In the past 40 years, AIDS grew in scope from a handful of cases to over 40 million cases and almost 3 million deaths in 2006. Since then the number of cases has decreased, with WHO reporting 550,100 measles-related deaths in 2016, most of which occurred in developing countries.

The tragedy of many viral diseases is their concentration in poorer regions of the world, where access to health care and personal living conditions are not as good as in developed countries. AIDS, for example, exacts a huge toll in sub-Saharan Africa. It is common to find villages populated mainly by preadolescents and the elderly, with the generations from ages 20 to 60 having been decimated. Aside from the human tragedy, the massive loss of the majority of productive wage earners is economically devastating. Many African nations have been economically crippled, and little relief is foreseen for generations.

Finally, several of the highest-profile emerging diseases are viral diseases. Ebola, avian influenza, and SARS are examples of diseases that have emerged as problems only in the late 20th and early 21st centuries. Of these, avian influenza has been of particular concern because the virus that causes this disease may have developed the ability to spread directly from person to person instead of only spreading from poultry to humans. This evolution combined with the expanding geographical range of the disease has raised concerns that this virus could cause a worldwide epidemic of a serious and frequently lethal form of influenza.

The number of cases of encephalitis caused by the Zika virus has increased significantly since 2000, up from only a handful of cases reported in the 1980s up to that time. If a pregnant woman is bitten by a mosquito that carries the virus, the fetus is at risk of a variety of birth defects, including brain malformation. According to WHO, the following countries reported cases of encephalitis and other fetal malformations believed to be caused by the Zika virus in 2016: Brazil (1,046), Cabo Verde (2), Colombia (7), French Polynesia (8), Martinique (3), and Panama (1). Two other cases, which both originated in Brazil, were detected in the United States and Slovenia. The Zika virus became prominent after some athletes refused to attend the 2016 Summer Olympics in Rio de Janeiro because of fears of contracting the virus, which was circulating at that time in regions of Brazil. The cause of the upsurge and subsequent decline in cases was not known as of 2017.

See Also *AIDS (Acquired Immunodeficiency Syndrome); Antiviral Drugs; Arthropod-Borne Disease; Avian Influenza; B Virus (Cercopithecine herpesvirus 1) Infection; CMV (Cytomegalovirus) Infection; Eastern Equine Encephalitis; Ebola; H5N1 Virus; Hepatitis A; Hepatitis B; Hepatitis C; Hepatitis D; Hepatitis E; Influenza; Influenza, Tracking Seasonal Influences and Virus Mutation;Influenza Pandemic of 1918; Influenza Pandemic of 1957; Measles (Rubeola); Monkeypox; Mononucleosis; Mosquito-Borne Diseases; Mumps; Nipah Virus Encephalitis; Norovirus Infection; Polio (Poliomyelitis); Polio Eradication Campaign; Rabies; Retroviruses; Rotavirus Infection; RSV (Respiratory Syncytial Virus) Infection; SARS (Severe Acute Respiratory Syndrome); St. Louis Encephalitis; West Nile Virus*

BIBLIOGRAPHY

Books

Bayry, Jagadeesh. *Emerging and Re-emerging Infectious Diseases of Livestock.* New York: Springer, 2017.

Quamann, David. *Ebola: The Natural and Human History of a Deadly Virus.* New York: Norton, 2014.

Richards, Paul. *Ebola: How a People's Science Helped End an Epidemic.* London: Zed, 2016.

Shah, Sonia. *Pandemic: Tracking Contagions, from Cholera to Ebola and Beyond.* New York: Picador, 2017.

Periodicals

Kharsany, Ayesha B.M., and Quarraisha A. Karim. "HIV Infection and AIDS in Sub-Saharan Africa: Current Status, Challenges and Opportunities." *Open AIDS Journal* 10 (2016): 34–48.

Sullivan, C., et al. "Using Zebrafish Models of Human Influenza A Virus Infections to Screen Antiviral Drugs and Characterize Host Immune Cell Responses. *Journal of Visualized Experiments* 119 (2017).

Verma, Dinesh, Jacob Thompson, and Sankar Swaminathan. "Spironolactone Blocks Epstein-Barr Virus Production by Inhibiting EBV SM Protein Function." *Proceedings of the National Academy of Sciences* 113 (2016): 3609–3614.

Websites

"Emerging Infectious Diseases/Pathogens." National Institute of Allergy and Infectious Diseases. https://www.niaid.nih.gov/research/emerging-infectious-diseases-pathogens (accessed November 15, 2017).

"Zika Situation Report." World Health Organization. Last modified April 7, 2016. http://www.who.int/emergencies/zika-virus/situation-report/7-april-2016/en/ (accessed December 10, 2017).

Brian Hoyle

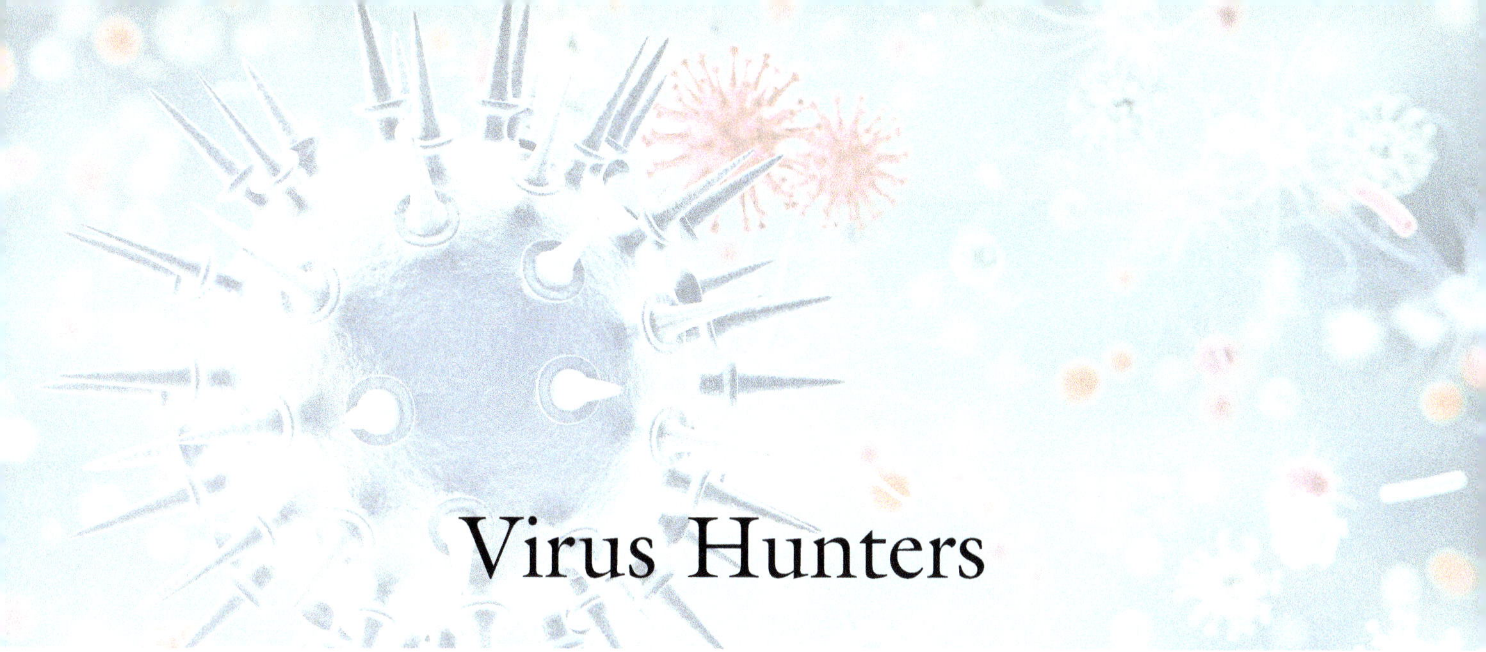

Virus Hunters

Viruses are responsible for some of the deadliest diseases on the planet, including Ebola, yellow fever, smallpox, acquired immunodeficiency syndrome (AIDS), severe acute respiratory syndrome (SARS), polio, and human and bird influenza. The scientists who seek to understand how viruses work, how they are transmitted, and how to stop them from infecting and harming humans are known formally as virologists and colloquially as "virus hunters."

History and Scientific Foundations

Although humans have dealt with the effects of viruses throughout history, it was not until 1892 that Russian scientist Dmitri Ivanovski (1864–1920) first identified a virus, specifically a plant virus that infected tobacco. Soon after, in 1898, a pair of German scientists, Friedrich Loeffler (1852–1915) and Paul Frosch (1860–1928), identified the first animal virus, which caused foot-and-mouth disease in cows. According to Michael B. A. Oldstone's *Viruses, Plagues, and History: Past, Present, and Future* (2010), this pioneering work in virology "provided the basis for defining viruses as subcellular entities that could cause distinct forms of tissue destruction, which became marks of specific diseases."

In 1899 the US Army established the Yellow Fever Commission, which was tasked with identifying the cause of a deadly disease that was infecting soldiers in Cuba. The work of that commission, which included Walter Reed (1851–1902), Carlos Juan Finlay (1833–1915), James Carroll (1854–1907), Aristides Agramonte (1868–1931), and Jesse Williams Lazear (1866–1900), identified a virus as the fever's cause. This discovery of the yellow fever virus marked the first time a human virus was identified. A number of US military physicians and volunteers died in early tests that proved that the virus was transmitted by mosquitoes. This discovery paved the way for control programs led by General William C. Gorgas (1854–1920), which resulted in the eradication of yellow fever from Havana, Cuba, and urban areas of Brazil. It also permitted the completion of the Panama Canal, work on which had been stalled by the huge toll exacted by yellow fever and malaria.

After making the eradication of yellow fever and malaria a top priority in 1915, the Rockefeller Foundation's International Health Division set up laboratories in Africa and South America to study yellow fever at its source. Six of their researchers died of the disease, but their work paid

WORDS TO KNOW

ANTIGEN A substance, usually a protein or polysaccharide, that stimulates the immune system to produce antibodies. While antigens can be the source of infections from pathogenic bacteria and viruses, organic molecules detrimental to the body from internal or environmental sources also act as antigens.

ANTIGENIC SHIFT An abrupt, major genetic change, such as in genes coding for surface proteins of a virus.

DROPLET TRANSMISSION The spread of microorganisms from one space to another (including from person to person) via droplets larger than 5 microns in diameter. Droplets are typically expelled into the air by coughing and sneezing.

NECROPSY Also called an autopsy, a medical examination of a dead body.

PANDEMIC Occurring as an epidemic in more than one country or population simultaneously. The term *pandemic* means "all the people."

STRAIN A subclass or specific genetic variation of an organism.

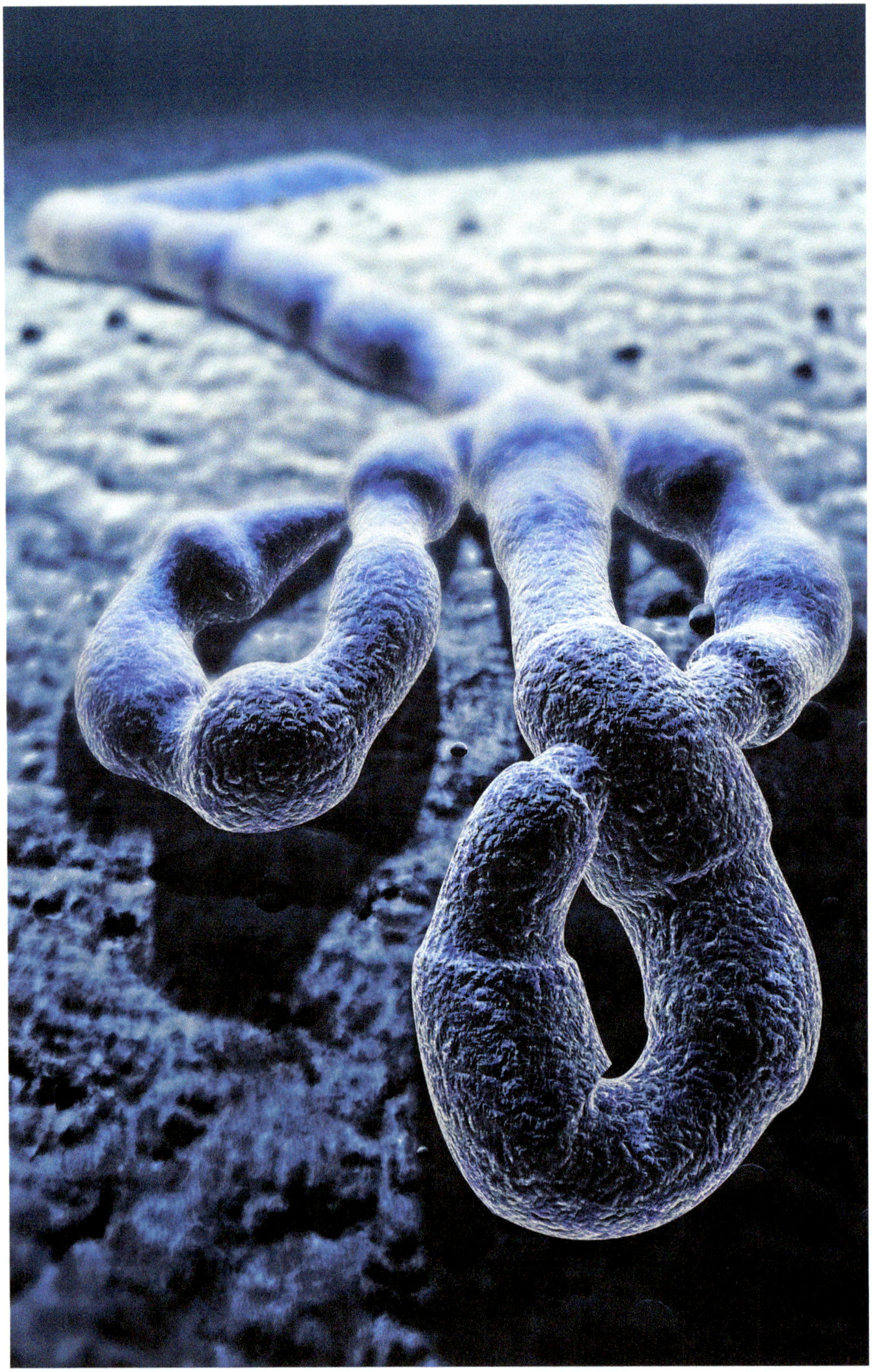

American virus hunter Karl Johnson discovered the Ebola virus, shown here, and other viruses. © 3D4Medical/Science Source off with the isolation of the virus and the development of the 17D yellow fever vaccine, considered one of the safest vaccines ever invented.

The work of the Yellow Fever Commission and the Rockefeller Foundation demonstrated the transformative potential that virologists could exercise by identifying viruses, understanding how they are transmitted, and determining how to reduce infections. In so doing they paved the way for generations of virus hunters. Over the course of the early 20th century, virus hunters working around the world tracked down a number of viral causes of plant, animal, and human disease, including rabies, dengue fever, avian leukemia, polio, measles, and influenza. The discoveries occurred even though it was not until the invention of electron microscopy in the mid-1930s that technology enabled scientists to see the viral agents they identified. In the late 1940s, techniques were developed that allowed researchers to isolate and grow viruses in cell cultures. This radically transformed virology, allowing scientists to study the properties of viruses in the lab and to more efficiently produce vaccines that would prevent infection with those viruses.

As technology, techniques, and knowledge improved, researchers were increasingly called to help identify and eradicate viral outbreaks in developing nations, where public health infrastructure tends to be less robust. For example, when people in San Joaquín, Bolivia, began bleeding to death from a disease no one had seen before in 1963, the Bolivian government requested help from the United States, which dispatched a team from the US National Institutes of Health (NIH) Middle America Research Unit. Heading this unit was physician Karl Johnson, one of the great virus hunters of the end of the 20th century.

In San Joaquín, Johnson and his team sought answers for what was causing *el tifo negro* ("the black typhus"), as it was known locally, or Bolivian hemorrhagic fever, as it would come to be known. One of the first things Johnson's team did was set up a breeding colony of hamsters and a separate infected-animal room. Another lab had a glove box, inside which the hamsters could be inoculated safely with specimens. There was also a thatched hut where the zoologist took the rodents he trapped in the town for processing and where the entomologist combed their fur for ectoparasites, such as ticks and mites, in case these were involved in the transmission of the disease. It was later found that these ectoparasites did not transmit Bolivian hemorrhagic fever. There was also an autopsy room for humans.

Using this improvised laboratory, Johnson and his fellow researchers isolated the virus that was causing the disease ravaging the area. Once the virus had been identified, the next step was to find out where the disease was coming from and how to stop its transmission. Johnson suspected the vector was the wild rodents that seemed to have recently overrun the town, so he set up a system to trap all the rats in half of the infected area. No further cases occurred in that area. As a result, the trapping was extended to the whole town, which stopped the epidemic.

As Johnson and his fellow researchers examined why the outbreak of Bolivian hemorrhagic fever had occurred in San Joaquín, they learned that antimalaria teams had deluged the town with dichlorodiphenyltrichloroethane (DDT) on a control visit. Cats are highly susceptible to DDT, and all the cats in the town had died, allowing the wild rodents from the fields and forest around the town to infiltrate the houses. Some of the rodents were infected with the virus, which they excreted in their urine and droppings inside houses. These excretions dried out in the tropical heat and turned to dust, which, when stirred up by walking through or sweeping the rooms, was inhaled by the inhabitants, giving them the disease. As a result, an intervention to control one fatal disease (malaria) ended up causing another (Bolivian hemorrhagic fever).

Applications and Research

Similar efforts to understand viruses and how they spread has been repeated many times throughout the world in the decades since the identification of Bolivian hemorrhagic fever in 1963. In 1976 a highly deadly disease began to spread through Yambuku, Zaire, in what is now the Democratic Republic of the Congo. After blood samples were sent to a lab in Belgium, doctors using an electron microscope identified a virus that appeared similar to Marburg virus, which was first identified in 1967 and caused a similar kind of fever. To determine whether the virus was Marburg virus or something else, a blood sample was sent to the Centers for Disease Control and Prevention's (CDC) special pathogens lab in Atlanta, Georgia. There Johnson and a team of scientists showed that the disease agent was a member of a new family of viruses, the Filoviridae or "thread viruses," so called because the virus looks like a partially coiled thread under an electron microscope. The scientists named it Ebola virus after a river located near where the disease initially struck.

A team of CDC researchers subsequently dispatched to Yambuku found that the virus was transmitted through the inadequately sterilized needles and syringes being reused on patients. The epidemic was spread in the hospital and then by local burial customs, which demanded that relatives of the deceased remove by hand the viscera of the body. Because this was done without any sterile precautions, the blood of the deceased infected the relatives. When these practices in the hospital and home were stopped, the epidemic ceased.

Ebola virus outbreaks have persisted since the initial epidemic was controlled, creating the need for newer generations of virus hunters to investigate how the disease spreads and how it can be stopped. After a 2014 outbreak, for example, virus hunters traced its origin to a child's encounter with bat droppings in rural Guinea. The researchers stopped the outbreak but only after it had killed more than 11,000 people.

Among the many important 20th-century virus hunters was Robert Shope (1929–2004), who devised various novel techniques for hunting new viruses from his base in Belém, Brazil, along the Amazon River. His lab had a small mammal recapture program with a grid of traps in the forest at the edge of town, where wild rodents and marsupials were trapped daily, weighed, and measured. Their blood was also drawn so their medical history could be followed. The rodents were exposed to forest mosquitoes that transmitted all sorts of viruses to them, which were then isolated from their blood samples. Many of the viruses were new to science.

Other mammals such as bats, sloths, and tree porcupines were also caught and studied, and a series of ingenious mosquito traps baited with monkeys or mice were run daily to provide pools of mosquitoes, which were sorted by species and yielded more such viruses. There were even lab workers who volunteered to go out into the forest at night to catch mosquitoes attempting to bite them. Some of the volunteers were bitten by the mosquitoes, so they came down with jungle fever. The viruses isolated from their blood provided proof that some of these new viruses could cause disease in people who went into the forest to hunt, collect timber, or clear plantations. Shope ultimately left Belém for the Yale Arbovirus Research Unit (YARU), where he studied a variety of arboviruses, or arthropod-borne viruses transmitted by fleas, ticks, mites, and mosquitoes.

Impacts and Issues

Virologists continue to make strides in retrospectively understanding how viruses have been transmitted. Virus hunters in the early 21st century have focused increasingly on finding ways to preempt viral outbreaks before they happen. In 2009 the US Agency for International Development (USAID) launched PREDICT, a massive and searchable database with information about zoonotic pathogens, which account for almost three-quarters of "all new, emerging, or re-emerging diseases affecting humans at the beginning of the 21st century," according to USAID. As Jeffrey Marlow writes in a 2017 *Scientific American* article, the aim of PREDICT is ambitious: "If scientists can detail the places where lethal viruses simmer in wait, the thinking goes, they can head off a swelling pandemic and better manage outbreaks while they are still small and local. Researchers and other outbreak responders could consult this database to begin mapping the source of an emerging disease, for example, and quickly get to work on minimizing transmission and developing potential new vaccines that could save countless lives." The effort to gather the information needed to populate this database has created a new kind of virus hunting, one that has seen researchers spread throughout the world in search of animal viruses that have not yet, but may soon, jump to humans and initiate the next deadly disease outbreak.

See Also *Arthropod-Borne Disease; Ebola; Emerging Infectious Diseases; Epidemiology; Hemorrhagic Fevers; Tropical Infectious Diseases; Vector-Borne Disease*

BIBLIOGRAPHY

Books

McCormick, Joseph B., and Susan Fisher-Hoch. *Level 4: Virus Hunters of the CDC: Tracking Ebola and the World's Deadliest Viruses.* New York: Sterling, 2016.

Oldstone, Michael B. A. *Viruses, Plagues, and History: Past, Present, and Future.* New York: Oxford University Press, 2010.

Periodicals

Marlow, Jeffrey. "The Virus Hunters." *Scientific American* (May 26, 2017). This article can also be found online at https://www.scientificamerican.com/article/the-virus-hunters/ (accessed January 31, 2018).

Morrison, Jim. "Can Virus Hunters Stop the Next Pandemic Before It Happens?" *Smithsonian Magazine* (January 25, 2018). This article can also be found online at https://www.smithsonianmag.com/science-nature/how-to-stop-next-animal-borne-pandemic-180967908/#FW1WmlrbGHJa2jjj.99 (accessed January 31, 2018).

Rogers, Adam. "Ebola Returns, and Central Africa's Virus Hunters Are Ready." *Wired* (May 12, 2017). This article can also be found online at https://www.wired.com/2017/05/ebola-returns-central-africas-virus-hunters-ready/ (accessed January 31, 2018).

Websites

Branswell, Helen. "History Credits This Man with Discovering Ebola on His Own. History Is Wrong." *STAT*, July 14, 2017. https://www.statnews.com/2016/07/14/history-ebola-peter-piot/ (accessed January 31, 2018).

Bresnahan, Samantha. "Virus Hunters Search for the Next Deadly Disease Outbreak." CNN, August 23, 2016. http://www.cnn.com/2016/08/23/health/virus-hunters-bat-cave-south-africa/index.html (accessed December 11, 2017).

"Emerging Pandemic Threats." USAID, May 24, 2016. https://www.usaid.gov/news-information/fact-sheets/emerging-pandemic-threats-program (accessed January 31, 2018).

Jack Woodall
Brian Hoyle

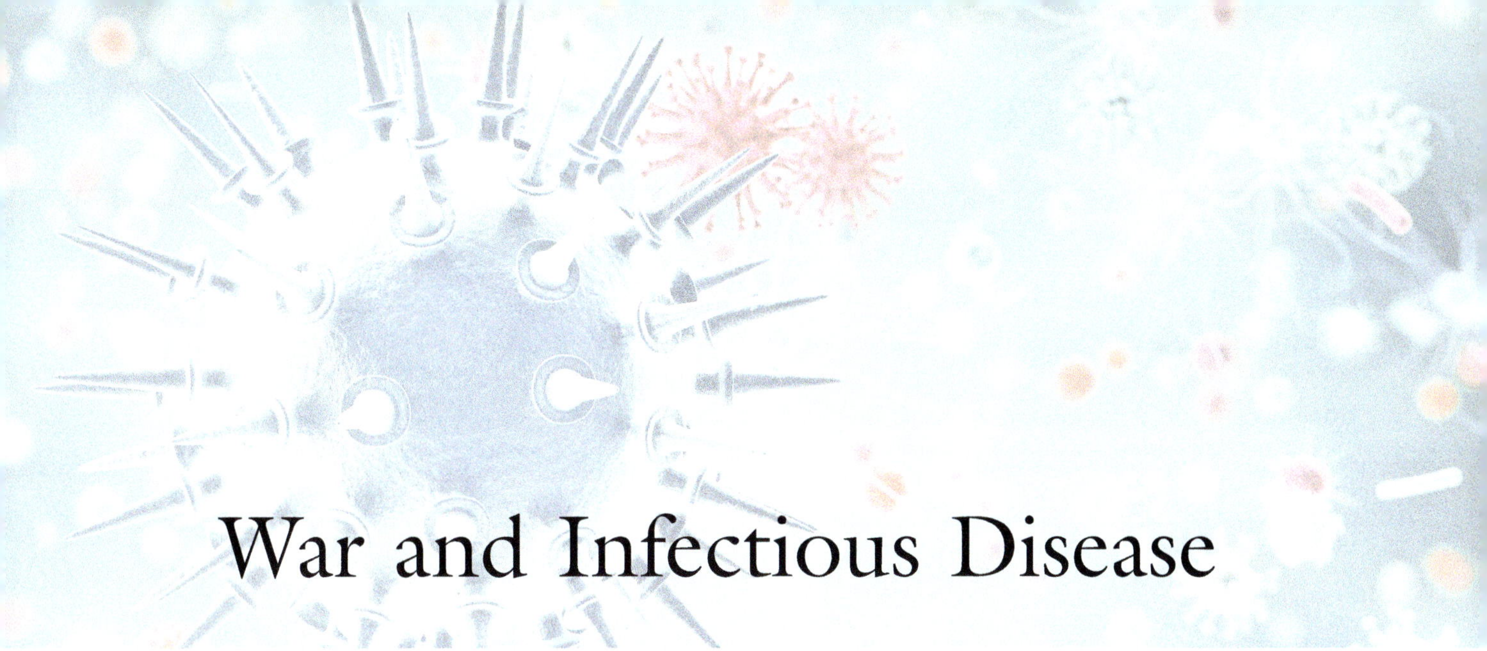

War and Infectious Disease

Introduction

Throughout history epidemics during wartime have sapped and destroyed armies, halted military operations, and brought death and disaster to the civilian populations of the warring factions. The historical occurrence and geographical spread of infectious diseases associated with war raises the question of how the distribution of disease in epidemics is influenced by military operations. Historically, epidemics have been associated with military mobilization and the bringing together of tens and even hundreds of thousands of individuals into close quarters and contact in camps and garrisons. Deployment to parts of the world in which diseases are endemic, emerging, or reemerging expose troops to diseases for which they have no immunity.

History and Scientific Foundations

The 1918 Influenza Pandemic and World War I

Following World War I (1914–1918), the 1918–1919 influenza pandemic, the first known avian influenza pandemic, killed more people than any other outbreak of disease in human history. Estimates of the death toll range from 20 million to 100 million, with 50 million to 100 million being the most likely estimate. Most of the deaths occurred between October and December of 1918.

The origin of the 1918 pandemic, sometimes called the Spanish flu, is still a mystery. Although the virus did not originate in Spain, its exact origins remain in dispute. One hypothesis based on epidemiological research suggests the most likely site of origin was Haskell County, Kansas, an isolated and sparsely populated county in the southwestern corner of the state, in January 1918. Some competing hypotheses are that the pandemic originated in Asia or that it began in British army camps. However, a number of epidemiologists argue that these hypotheses are not as well supported as the theory that the flu spread between US army camps and might have been carried by US troops to Europe. The first known US outbreak of epidemic influenza was identified in epidemiological studies and in lay accounts as having occurred at Camp Funston, now Fort Riley, in Kansas. However, a previously unknown epidemic of influenza occurred in Haskell County, Kansas, 300 miles (483 kilometers) west of Funston.

In late January and early February 1918, a local physician in the county faced an epidemic of influenza of extraordinary suddenness and lethality. Dozens of previously strong and healthy patients were struck down as suddenly "as if they had been shot." They then progressed to pneumonia and died. The local epidemic raged and worsened for several weeks and then disappeared as suddenly as it had emerged. Although influenza was not a reportable disease, the physician warned national public health officials, and this warning was published by the US Public Health Service in its *Public Health Reports*, the precursor to the *Morbidity and Mortality Weekly Report* (*MMWR*). The physician's report was the only reference in that journal to influenza anywhere in the world during the first six months of 1918. It was the first recorded instance in history of an influenza outbreak so violent that a physician warned public health officials, suggesting a new virus was adapting to humans with lethal effect.

During the Haskell County outbreak, local army personnel reported to Funston for training. The virus spread as friends and family visited them at Funston and as the soldiers returned home on leave. The local press recorded several cases between February 26 and March 2 of people from the county who had visited the army base who either fell ill or who had children who were stricken with influenza and pneumonia. The first soldier at the camp reported ill with influenza at sick call on March 4. Within three weeks

WORDS TO KNOW

AEROSOL Particles of liquid or solid dispersed as a suspension in gas.

BIOMODULATOR Short for biologic response modulator, an agent that modifies some characteristic of the immune system, which may help in the fight against infection.

DEBRIDEMENT The medical process of removing dead, damaged, or infected tissue from pressure ulcers, burns, and other wounds to speed healing of the surrounding healthy tissue.

ENDEMIC Present in a particular area or among a particular group of people.

ENTEROPATHOGEN A virus or pathogen that invades the large or small intestine, causing disease.

EXOTOXIN A toxic protein produced during bacterial growth and metabolism and released into the environment.

MATERIEL A French-derived word for equipment, supplies, or hardware.

PROPHYLAXIS Pre-exposure treatment (e.g., immunizations) to prevent the onset or recurrence of a disease.

PYROGENIC A substance that causes fever. The word *pyrogenci* comes from the Greek word *pyr*, meaning "fire."

more than 1,100 soldiers at the camp, which held an average of 56,222 troops, required hospitalization, and thousands more required infirmary treatment. Meanwhile, Funston sent an uninterrupted stream of men to other American locations and to Europe, especially France. On March 18 influenza cases were reported in Camps Forrest and Greenleaf in Georgia. By the end of April, 24 of the 36 main army camps suffered an influenza epidemic. Thirty of the 50 largest cities in the country also had a spike in excess mortality from influenza and pneumonia in April.

Also at the end of April, influenza erupted in France, beginning at Brest, the main port of disembarkation for American troops. After that army operations proved to be the most influential factor in the spread of the epidemic elsewhere in the world. It seems likely that military policy makers either did not appreciate the role of their operations in spreading the epidemic or chose to regard it as an unfortunate but necessary consequence of war. Another lesson from this occurrence has been that a worldwide flu epidemic could emerge anywhere, including a sparsely populated county in the United States, not only in a densely populated region in Asia.

Typhus Fever in World War I

As devastating as the 1918 flu pandemic was for the military and civilian populations alike during the latter part of World War I, it probably did not influence the course of the war and of history as much as the outbreak of typhus fever on the European Eastern Front during World War I. Typhus fever is a louse-borne disease, and the lice that carry typhus fever are common in large aggregations of people who do not bathe or change clothes with any regularity and are forced by circumstances to live in close quarters, which are also the situations that infantry, refugees, and prisoners are likely to encounter. In late November 1914, typhus fever, which had been endemic in Serbia for centuries, began to appear among Serbian refugees fleeing the Austrian attack on Belgrade. Shortly afterward cases were reported from the army and among the prisoners of war but caused little alarm. However, this disease had played a decisive role earlier in European military history, when typhus fever shattered Napoleon's invasion of Russia in 1812, destroying the French army well before it reached Moscow.

The Austrian invasion was soon repulsed, but the devastation of northern Serbia created ripe conditions for the spread of typhus. The first outbreak of cases occurred among Austrian prisoners at Valjevo, followed within a week by outbreaks throughout the rest of the country. The infection traveled with the refugee population, on prisoner-of-war trains, and with moving armies and was rapidly disseminated to all parts of Serbia. At the start of World War I, Serbia numbered some 3 million people. Within six months, one in six Serbians developed typhus fever. More than 200,000 people, including 70,000 Serbian troops and half of the 60,000 Austrian prisoners, died from the disease. The outbreak spread beyond Serbia into Russia, as the famine and dislocation of the Russian revolution destroyed sanitation and social infrastructure, eventually resulting in 20 million cases in that country, half of whom died.

Iraq War, Syrian Civil War, and Yemeni Civil War

In the spring of 2003, 83,000 US marines participated in the opening phase of the Iraq War (2003–2011). A US Navy Preventive Medicine Department laboratory was set up to provide diagnostic support for marine medical units during a period of repositioning in south-central Iraq. Specimen collection boxes were sent to more than 30 primary care medical stations, handling 500 to 900 personnel each. The laboratory had the capability to detect many different disease agents. By far the most common reason for infectious disease sick call visits was gastrointestinal illness. No other symptoms had equivalent impact.

An enteropathogen was detected in 23 percent of stool samples, with norovirus detected in 30 stool samples obtained from 14 different battalion or similar-sized units. Next in frequency were *Shigella flexneri* and *Shigella sonnei*, which were isolated from 26 stool samples (20 percent) obtained from 15 units. Ciprofloxacin was effective in vitro against most bacterial agents, but neither the antibiotics doxycycline (which was taken daily as the antimalarial prophylaxis dose) or trimethoprim-sulfamethoxazole were effective. Otherwise, personnel remained free of infectious illness during this phase of the conflict because other infectious agents were rare or absent.

Ongoing and protracted violence can disrupt the public health system. Around half of children born in Syria during the civil war that began in 2011, for example, had not had their routine immunizations. According to research published in *PLOS Pathogens* in 2014, immunization rates in Syria declined from around 91 percent of the population to 45 percent after the outbreak of the war. Because children were not receiving their vaccinations, there were two outbreaks of polio, a virus that can cause paralysis, one in 2014 and another in 2017.

Meanwhile, a civil war in Yemen that began in 2015 sparked perhaps the worst cholera outbreak in the country's history. The bacteria that causes cholera infected many Yemenis' sources of drinking water. The outbreak was due in part to the disintegration of the public health care system, as well as the lack of access to safe, clean water.

War Wounds

Wound infection control is another important facet of the relationship between war and infectious disease. Prior to contemporary efficient and airborne medevac procedures, military surgeons worked by a rule of thumb: patch up and move on. Even in the 21st century, at frontline dressing stations, no time is wasted on the hopelessly injured. A seriously wounded soldier has to survive the stretcher trip through the field treatment station, hospital station, evacuation hospital, and base hospital, which is sometimes in a different country, before he or she receives thorough surgical care. For example, during the Iraq War, American combatants received definitive treatment in a hospital in Germany. In the military every wound is treated as though it were infected. For example, prior to World War I, tetanus, a great killer in all previous wars, was practically eliminated by routine injections of antitetanic serum to all wounded soldiers.

Penicillin was first tested for military use in the spring of 1943. By autumn doctors were using the antibiotic in combat zones, where it was limited to US and Allied military and patients with life-threatening infections. Flight crews of the 8th Air Force stationed in Britain were the first to directly benefit from the drug. Rationing was necessary, as a single infection could require 2 million or more

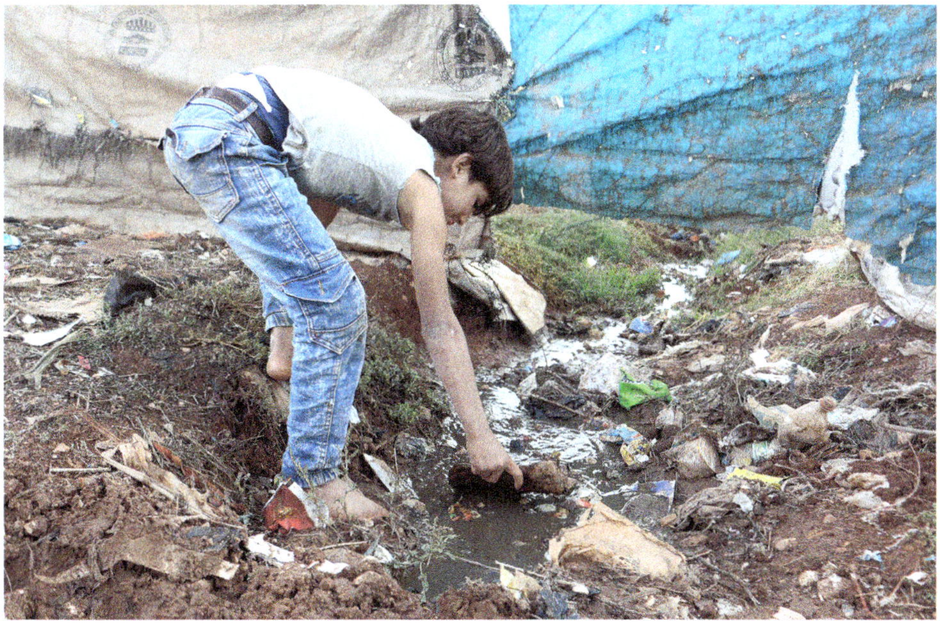

A boy plays in rainwater in a camp for internally displaced persons in Syria in 2017. Beginning in 2012 civil war in Syria displaced millions of people. Many live in camps where crowded conditions and contaminated water leave them vulnerable to disease. © Mohamad al abd Lla/Anadolu Agency/Getty Images units of the drug. During the war the armed forces received 85 percent of the nation's production. With the implementation of successful mass-production techniques, production of units tripled during 1944–1945. Penicillin became the war's wonder drug, and its remarkable medical effects on infectious disease made World War II (1939–1945) different from any previous war.

The mass production of penicillin for military use gave impetus to the widespread use of antibiotics to fight infection on a wide scale in civil society after the war. Contemporary antibiotic-resistant bacterial strains pose an analogous threat to wounded troops. In spite of antibiotic treatment and better antiseptic practices under combat conditions, it is still necessary to debride wounds and amputate seriously damaged limbs under combat situations to prevent gangrene and other runaway infections. In 1914 a French medical officer was the first to use debridement, the surgical excision of necrotic (dead) or infected tissue and the removal of foreign bodies from contaminated wounds to forestall infection. Prior to the introduction of debridement, all but simple incised wounds were treated by surgically opening the wound, removing obvious foreign bodies, and then irrigating with sterile salt solution or oxidizers such as hydrogen peroxide in an attempt to sterilize the lesion. The wound was left open and freely drained or was packed with gauze and immobilized by suitable splints if necessary. Discharge of pus was treated by drainage tubes made of glass or rubber.

War and Public Health Infrastructure Damage

Often the public health impact of war goes unmeasured. Efforts were made to gauge the effects of the Balkan wars in the early 1990s. A public health assessment in Bosnia-Herzegovina and in the areas of Serbia and Montenegro hosting Bosnian refugees in 1993 revealed widespread disruption to basic health services, displacement of more than 1 million Bosnians, severe food shortages in Muslim enclaves, and extensive destruction of public water and sanitation systems. War-related violence was the most important public health risk in that nation. Civilians on all sides of the conflict were intentional targets of physical and sexual violence.

Although the impact of the war on the health status of the population was difficult to document, in central Bosnia perinatal and child mortality rates doubled between 1991 and 1993. The crude death rate in one Muslim enclave between April 1992 and March 1993 was four times the prewar rate. Prevalence rates of severe malnutrition among both adults and children in central Bosnia increased steadily throughout the course of the conflict. Major epidemics of communicable diseases were not reported, even though public health conditions were ripe for such epidemics. The lack of epidemics in this case is scientifically significant to infectious disease studies. It challenges many historical assertions and assumptions about public health in wartime.

■ Impacts and Issues

The intentional release of biological agents is a possibility that has received urgent attention following the anthrax attacks in the United States in 2001. However, the military was engaged in intensive study of biological agents prior to that time. Law enforcement agencies, military planners, public health officials, and clinicians are gaining an increasing awareness of this potential threat. From a military perspective, an important component of the protective pre-exposure resources against this threat is immunization. In addition, certain vaccines are an accepted component of postexposure prophylaxis against potential bioterrorist threat agents. These vaccines might therefore be used to respond to a terrorist attack against civilians.

Biological warfare agents may be classified in several ways. First, they may be classified operationally as lethal or incapacitating agents with or without potential for secondary transmission. Second, they may be classified according to the intended target as antipersonnel, anti-animal, anti-plant, or anti-materiel. Third, they may be classified according to type as replicating pathogens, toxins, or biomodulators. Among the greatest threats are both replicating pathogens (bacteria and viruses) and toxins.

Anthrax

Few infectious agents possess characteristics suitable for effective large-scale employment. However, *Bacillus anthracis* has properties that are ideal for this purpose. It is omnipresent in soil, and the ease with which it can be cultured makes it readily available to armies and terrorists. Its lethality, ability to form tough spores, and affinity for aerosolization (production as a fine mist) combine to make anthrax one of the greatest biological threats. Anthrax was prominent in the biological weapons programs of Iraq and the former Soviet Union. The Japanese Aum Shinrikyo cult also stockpiled it. Consequently, research programs at military laboratories have devoted considerable effort to improving the anthrax vaccines that have been in use for decades.

Plague

One of the earliest recorded attempts at biological warfare was the effort of besieging Tatar warriors in the 14th century to catapult the corpses of their plague victims over the city walls of Kaffa in the Crimea to initiate an epidemic within the city. The Japanese released millions of infected fleas over Manchurian cities, resulting in numerous human plague cases during World War II. During the Vietnam War (1954–1975), plague vaccine was routinely administered to members of the US armed services. Only eight cases of plague were reported among this population, which corresponds to a rate of about one case per million person-years of

PREPARING FOR BIOTERRORISM

Although an anthrax attack on the United States is highly unlikely, the US Centers for Disease Control and Prevention (CDC) has prepared public health departments and health care providers to respond quickly and efficiently to such an attack to minimize morbidity and mortality. As a result, the CDC has engaged in the following activities:

- Providing funds and guidance to help health departments strengthen their abilities to respond to all types of public health incidents and build more resilient communities.
- Providing training in emergency response for the public health workforce and healthcare providers, as well as leaders in the public and private sector.
- Coordinating response activities and providing resources to health departments through the CDC Emergency Operations Center.
- Regulating the possession, use, and transfer of biological agents and toxins that could pose a severe threat to public health and safety through the CDC Select Agent Program.
- Promoting science and practices to strengthen preparedness and response activities.
- Ensuring that the United States has enough laboratories that can quickly conduct tests when anthrax is suspected.
- Working with hospitals, laboratories, emergency response teams, and health care providers to make sure they have the medicine and supplies they would need if an anthrax attack occurred.
- Developing guidance to protect the health and safety of workers who would be responding during an anthrax emergency.

exposure. The success of this vaccine is evident when compared with the 330-fold greater incidence of plague among the unvaccinated South Vietnamese civilian population.

Brucellosis

Brucellosis is considered to be an incapacitating agent likely to produce large numbers of casualties but little mortality. Nevertheless, brucellosis is highly infective. In the 1950s the United States chose the bacteria *Brucella suis* as the first agent to be produced for its biological warfare program. Veterinary vaccines that have significant efficacy against brucellosis have been studied and employed. The vaccination of livestock in combination with the slaughter of infected animals is largely responsible for the declining incidence of human brucellosis. In the United States the decline of human brucellosis cases reported to the US Centers for Disease Control and Prevention (CDC) has paralleled the control of infections due to *Brucella abortus* in cattle.

Tularemia

The bacteria *Francisella tularensis* is sometimes considered a lethal biological warfare agent because high-dose aerosol dissemination could result in a disproportionate number of cases of the pneumonic form of tularemia. *F. tularensis* followed *B. suis* into the US bioweapons program in 1955, and extensive testing of the weaponization potential of the agent was conducted in human volunteers at Fort Detrick. The organism was also thought to have been prominent in the biological arsenal of the Soviet Union. American and Russian collaboration has provided the seed stock for tularemia vaccines currently in use throughout the world.

Q Fever

Coxiella burnetii, the causative agent of Q fever, is a Gram-negative coccobacillus resistant to heat and dryness that grows easily in embryonated chicken eggs and is highly infectious by aerosol. This organism was cultivated by the US bioweapons program as a potential incapacitating agent.

Smallpox

Although endemic smallpox was eradicated throughout the world in 1977, the virus remains a potential biological weapon in the eyes of many military planners. Concerns persist that clandestine stocks of virus may exist outside of the CDC in Atlanta, Georgia, and Koltsovo in Novosibirsk Oblast, Russia, the two repositories of the virus authorized by the World Health Organization.

Botulism

Botulinum toxin (BTX) is a neurotoxin produced by the bacterium *Clostridium botulinum* and related bacterial species. It blocks the release of acetylcholine, a neurotransmitter from endings of axons at the point where they enervate muscles, thus causing flaccid paralysis.

Iraq chose to weaponize botulinum toxin during the Gulf War in 1991, although its usefulness as a weapon might be limited by its instability during storage and modest range upon aerosolization. Nonetheless, when delivered by aerosolization, botulinum toxins would be expected to produce cases of typical clinical botulism. Moreover, terrorists might also use botulinum toxins to sabotage food supplies. No licensed vaccine exists as of 2018.

Staphylococcal Enterotoxin B (SEB) Intoxication

SEB is one of several pyrogenic exotoxins produced by *Staphylococcus aureus* and is considered a viable incapacitating agent by biological warfare planners. Although SEB is a cause of foodborne disease, its use in biological warfare would likely involve aerosolization, with which it would cause a systemic fever accompanied by pulmonary symptoms. As of 2018 no SEB vaccine was available for human use.

Although the US Department of Defense initiated an anthrax immunization campaign throughout the armed forces, it is likely that other anti-biological-warfare vaccines will eventually be employed to protect armed services personnel. In a civilian context, the use of these vaccines is more problematic because the nature of the threat is less well defined. Nonetheless, certain vaccines, such as anthrax and smallpox, may have applicability in the prevention and management of exposed civilian populations.

SEE ALSO *Anthrax; Bioterrorism; Influenza Pandemic of 1918; Plague, Early History; Plague, Modern History; Public Health and Infectious Disease*

BIBLIOGRAPHY

Books

Barry, John M. *The Great Influenza: The Epic Story of the Deadliest Plague in History.* New York: Penguin, 2005.

Krug, Etienne G., et al., eds. *World Report on Violence and Health.* Geneva: World Health Organization, 2002. This report can also be found online at http://www.who.int/violence_injury_prevention/violence/world_report/chapters/en/ (accessed March 8, 2018).

Periodicals

Alawieh, Ali, et al. "Revisiting Leishmaniasis in the Time of War: The Syrian Conflict and the Lebanese Outbreak." *International Journal of Infectious Diseases* 29 (December 2014): 115–119. This article can also be found online at http://www.ijidonline.com/article/S1201-9712(14)01519-7/fulltext (accessed March 8, 2018).

Lyons, Kate. "Yemen's Cholera Outbreak Now the Worst in History as Millionth Case Looms." *Guardian* (October 12, 2017). This article can also be found online at https://www.theguardian.com/global-development/2017/oct/12/yemen-cholera-outbreak-worst-in-history-1-million-cases-by-end-of-year (accessed March 8, 2018).

Sharara, Sima L., and Souha S. Kanj. "War and Infectious Diseases: Challenges of the Syrian Civil War." *PLOS Pathogens* 10, no. 11 (November 13, 2014): e1004438. This article can also be found online at http://journals.plos.org/plospathogens/article?id=10.1371/journal.ppat.1004438 (accessed March 8, 2018).

Thornton, S. A., et al. "Gastroenteritis in US Marines during Operation Iraqi Freedom." *Clinical Infectious Diseases* 40, no. 4 (February 15, 2005): 519–525. This article can also be found online at https://www.ncbi.nlm.nih.gov/pubmed/15712073 (accessed March 8, 2018).

Websites

Alwan, Ala. "The Cost of War." World Health Organization, November 6, 2015. http://www.who.int/mediacentre/commentaries/war-cost/en/ (accessed March 8, 2018).

"Anthrax: What CDC Is Doing to Prepare." Centers for Disease Control and Prevention, September 1, 2015. https://www.cdc.gov/anthrax/bioterrorism/cdc-action.html (accessed March 15, 2018).

"Bioterrorism Agents/Diseases." Centers for Disease Control and Prevention, January 4, 2018. https://emergency.cdc.gov/agent/agentlist.asp (accessed March 8, 2018).

Kenneth T. LaPensee

Water-Borne Disease

Introduction

Water-borne diseases are caused by water that is contaminated with microorganisms. Microbes such as bacteria, viruses, protozoa, and parasites are usually found in the intestinal tracts of humans and other creatures. In most cases of water-borne disease, the water becomes contaminated by feces that carry microbes.

More than 2 billion people worldwide use a source of drinking water that is contaminated with feces, and around 842,000 people die each year from diarrhea caused by unsafe drinking water, poor sanitation, or poor hand hygiene, according to a 2017 report from the World Health Organization (WHO). Indeed, water-borne diseases are the most common cause of disease and death in the world, according to WHO. Although this is largely a problem in developing and underdeveloped countries, developed nations, including the United States, are not immune. Although precise figures for the United States are difficult to obtain because many water-borne illnesses are not reported there, the US Centers for Disease Control and Prevention (CDC) reported 1,261 water-borne illnesses in 2012.

Disease History, Characteristics, and Transmission

Water-borne diseases are caused by a wide range of pathogens, typically bacteria, viruses, parasites, or protozoa. Examples of bacteria that are prominent

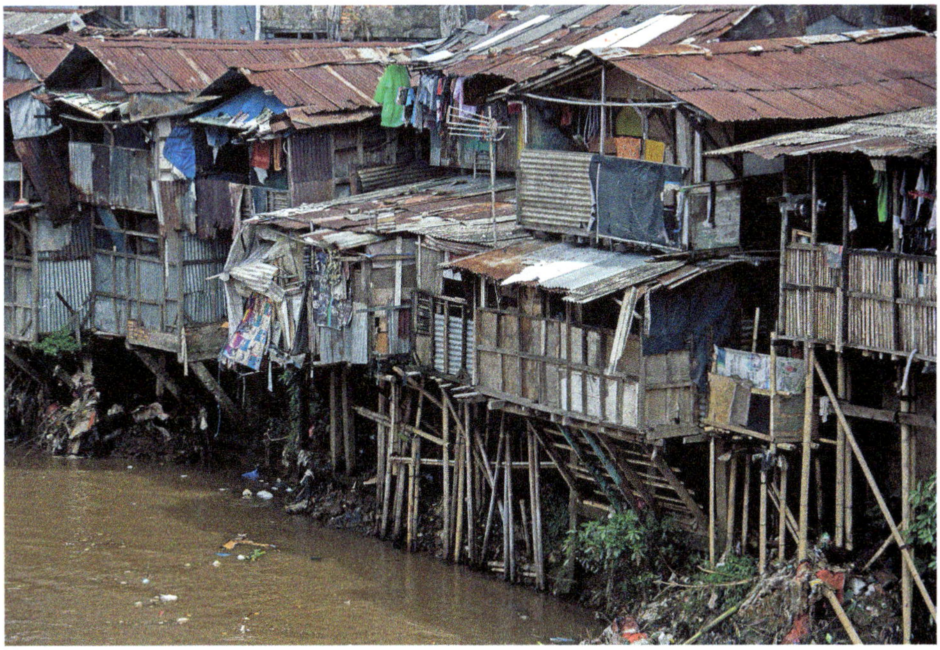

Many people in developing countries get their drinking water from surface water sources such as rivers and lakes. In the Indonesian city of Jakarta, contaminated surface water gives rise to high rates of water-borne disease. *© BAY ISMOYO/AFP/Getty Images*

WORDS TO KNOW

CHLORINATION A chemical process that is used primarily to disinfect drinking water and spills of microorganisms. The active agent in chlorination is the element chlorine or a derivative of chlorine (e.g., chlorine dioxide). Chlorination is a swift and economical means of destroying many, but not all, microorganisms that are a health threat in fluids such as drinking water.

DIARRHEA To most individuals, diarrhea means an increased frequency or decreased consistency of bowel movements. However, the medical definition is more exact than this explanation. In many developed countries, the average number of bowel movements is three per day. However, researchers have found that diarrhea, which is not a disease, is best correlated with an increase in stool weight. Stool weights above 10.5 ounces (300 grams) per day generally indicate diarrhea. This is mainly due to excess water, which normally makes up 60 to 85 percent of fecal matter. Thus, diarrhea is distinguished from diseases that cause only an increase in the number of bowel movements (hyperdefecation) or incontinence (involuntary loss of bowel contents). Physicians classify diarrhea as acute (lasting one to two weeks) or chronic (lasting for more than four weeks). Viral and bacterial infections are the most common causes of acute diarrhea.

FECES Solid waste excreted from a living body.

PATHOGEN A disease-causing agent, such as a bacteria, virus, fungus, or other microorganism.

water-borne pathogenic organisms include *Vibrio cholerae* (the bacteria that cause cholera); various species of *Campylobacter*, *Salmonella*, and *Shigella*; and a type of *Escherichia coli* designated O157:H7.

Drinking or bathing in contaminated freshwater is often the cause of water-borne diseases. Saltwater-borne microbial diseases also exist, and bacteria, viruses, and algae are typically associated with these illnesses. Explosive growth of certain algal species in ocean water can lead to the accumulation of these algae in oysters and other shellfish that feed by filtering water. If people eat the affected shellfish, various diseases can result. Some of these can be serious, producing paralysis and death.

Amebiasis is a common water-borne disease that is caused by the parasite *Entamoeba histolytica*. This parasite is normally found in feces and can cause disease when fecal-contaminated water is consumed. About one in every 10 people who consume *E. histolytica* becomes ill. This translates to millions of people worldwide. The symptoms can be mild (diarrhea, stomachache, and cramping), but some people develop a severe form of amebiasis called amebic dysentery. The destruction of cells lining the intestinal tract produces bloody diarrhea. More rarely the parasite can spread to the liver, lungs, or brain.

Cryptosporidiosis is another water-borne disease caused by a parasite. This illness is caused by parasites of the genus *Cryptosporidium*, especially *C. parvum*. The organism's life cycle consists of a small, inert form and an actively growing form. The inert form can pass through the filters used in water treatment plants and can survive exposure to chlorine. Once inside a person, the resulting infection can persist for months despite treatment.

Once relatively rare, cryptosporidiosis increased in prevalence in the United States beginning in the 1980s as expansion of urban areas brought more people into contact with the animals that naturally harbor the parasite in their intestinal tracts. Symptoms of cryptosporidiosis include dehydration, persistent stomach upset, weight loss, nausea, and vomiting. The parasite can be passed from person to person. As of 2017 cryptosporidiosis remained one of the most common causes of water-borne disease in the United States. In an infamous example, an outbreak in Milwaukee, Wisconsin, in 1993 sickened more than 200,000 people.

Yet another parasite-mediated water-borne disease is cyclosporiasis, which is caused by *Cyclospora cayetanensis.* A hallmark of this infection is sudden, repeated explosive diarrhea. Other symptoms include weight loss, dehydration, stomach upset, and fatigue.

Giardiasis is a disease caused by an intestinal parasite called *Giardia lamblia* (sometimes called *Giardia intestinalis*). As of 2017 this disease also remained one of the most common water-borne human diseases in the United States. In North America it is sometimes known as beaver fever because beavers, among other animals, naturally harbor the parasite in their intestinal tracts. Symptoms of giardiasis include diarrhea, intestinal gas, stomach cramps, upset stomach, and nausea. The lingering intestinal upset of giardiasis can be debilitating.

Scope and Distribution

Water-borne diseases caused by microorganisms occur worldwide. Virtually every country experiences water-borne illnesses, although the diseases tend to be more prevalent in tropical countries where the warmer climate favors the persistence of bacteria and viruses that enter the water from the intestinal tract. Water-borne diseases are especially problematic in developing and underdeveloped nations, where adequate water treatment facilities may be lacking and safe drinking water may be in short supply. For example, there were an estimated 1.3 million to 4 million cases of cholera in 2016, according to WHO, and an estimated 21,000 to 143,000 deaths. A cholera outbreak that began in April 2017 in Yemen had resulted in about 500,000 illnesses and 2,000 deaths by August 2017, according to WHO. Deaths from water-borne diseases are almost always preventable with proper hydration.

Treatment and Prevention

Drinking water can be treated to remove or destroy contaminating microorganisms. Chlorination, one well-known treatment, destroys pathogenic bacteria, nuisance bacteria, parasites, and other organisms. Other treatments include exposure of the water to ultraviolet light (which rearranges the microbes' genetic material so that they cannot reproduce) and ozone, or the passage of water through a filter whose openings are so small that even viruses are removed.

Water-borne diseases that are caused by bacteria, protozoa, and some parasites can be treated using compounds that kill the target organism. For example, antibiotics are effective against bacteria. Viruses are more problematic because antibiotics are not effective.

The best strategy for dealing with water-borne diseases is to avoid getting the infection. Sensible precautions include washing hands after having a bowel movement, avoiding drinking water that has not been treated (if in doubt, do not drink), and abstaining from bathing or swimming in water that is known to be polluted. In many North American and European communities, recreational water is monitored, and notices are posted restricting swimming when the water is determined to be contaminated.

Impacts and Issues

The global impact of water-borne disease is enormous. The CDC estimated that every year there are more than 4 billion episodes of diarrhea due to the consumption of contaminated water and more than 2 million deaths. Most of these deaths occurred among children in developing or underdeveloped countries. WHO estimated that 4,000 children die each day from water-borne diseases. According to the CDC and WHO, more than 2 billion people living in poverty are especially susceptible to water-borne disease, mainly due to contaminated surface water or inadequately treated drinking water.

People whose immune systems are not operating efficiently can develop severe or persistent forms of water-borne diseases, such as cryptosporidiosis. The latter has become a significant threat for people with acquired immunodeficiency syndrome (AIDS) and those who take immunosuppressive drugs to reduce the chance of rejection of a transplanted organ.

The massive loss of life due to water-borne diseases also robs countries of the next generation of citizens and workers. This has serious consequences for the future population and economic strength of these nations. For such nations, water treatment must be a priority.

Nevertheless, the problem of water-borne disease is not confined to the poorer regions of the globe. Even in developed countries, a breakdown of water treatment can lead to disease.

In many countries, drinking water is monitored to ensure that it is free from pathogenic bacteria, viruses, and protozoa. In the United States CDC surveillance programs detect water-borne outbreaks and help direct federal, state, and municipal responses to the outbreaks. Similar efforts in developing and underdeveloped countries have been far less successful, as population increases in these poorer countries have outstripped the economic capability of governments to put in place the necessary water treatment technologies. In 2005 the United Nations set a goal of cutting the number of people without access to safe drinking water by 50 percent by 2015, and by 2010 it had met its goal. As of 2017 91 percent of the population worldwide drank water whose quality had been improved. However, as of 2015 663 million people still lacked access to reliably safe drinking water, according to statistics from the United Nations.

Despite the continuing challenges to providing safe drinking water, the global community has made some progress. Initiatives such as the CDC's Safe Water Program, the United Nations International Decade for Action "Water for Life," and WHO's International Network to Promote Household Water Treatment and Safe Storage have brought simple and relatively inexpensive water treatment methods to rural areas in Africa, Central America, and South America. The CDC has also helped to safeguard water in the United States. For example, a disease called dracunculiasis, which formerly affected almost 4 million

DISEASE IN DEVELOPING NATIONS

Contaminated clean water supplies are often a major factor in the spread of disease. Besides climate, the most common reason for clean water shortages is human activity. Water pollution can occur due to industry or the leaking of septic (waste) water into the water supply system. In either case the water may become dangerous for the health of the people and unusable for industry. Purification of industrial waste is expensive, and sometimes economic interests may conflict with protecting the environment. Many developing countries cannot afford proper water purification because their main concern is survival rather than the quality of the environment. Pollution, however, is a global concern and can affect people in neighboring countries as well.

people each year in African countries, has been almost eliminated. In 2016 only 25 cases of dracunculiasis were reported, according to WHO.

SEE ALSO *Amebiasis; Bacterial Disease;* Campylobacter *Infection; Cholera; Cryptosporidiosis; Cyclosporiasis; Dracunculiasis; Dysentery;* Escherichia coli *O157:H7; Giardiasis; Mosquito-Borne Diseases; Norovirus Infection;* Salmonella *Infection (Salmonellosis); Shigellosis; Viral Disease*

BIBLIOGRAPHY

Books

Bayry, Jagadeesh, ed. *Emerging and Re-emerging Infectious Diseases of Livestock.* New York: Springer, 2017.

Kaslow, Richard A., ed. *Viral Infections of Humans: Epidemiology and Control.* New York: Springer, 2014.

Payne, Susan. *Viruses: From Understanding to Investigation.* New York: Academic Press, 2017.

Periodicals

Dewey-Mattia, Daniel, et al. "Foodborne and Waterborne Disease Outbreaks—United States, 1971–2012." *Morbidity and Mortality Weekly Report* 62, no. 54 (October 23, 2015): 86–89.

Websites

"Drinking-Water." World Health Organization. http://www.who.int/mediacentre/factsheets/fs391/en/ (accessed November 22, 2017).

"Water." United Nations. http://www.un.org/en/sections/issues-depth/water/ (accessed November 22, 2017).

Brian Hoyle

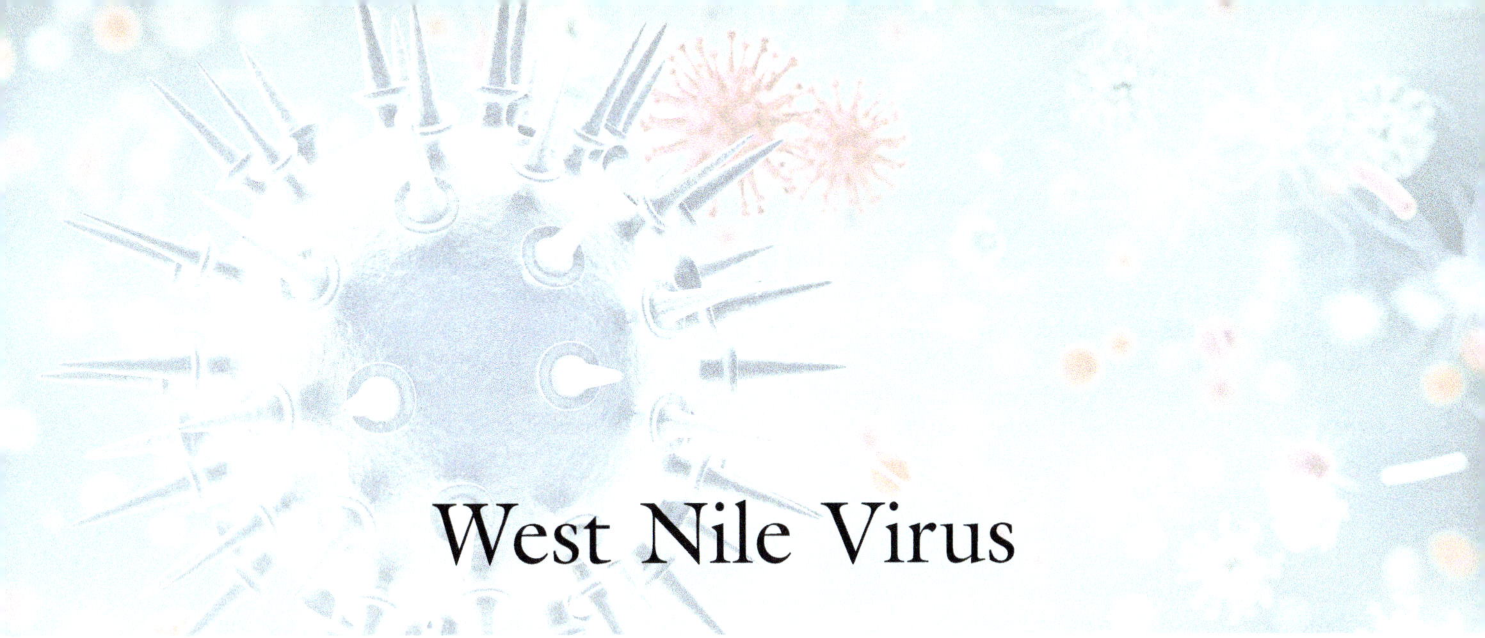

West Nile Virus

■ Introduction

The West Nile virus is a member of the Flaviviridae family. It causes an inflammation of the lining of nerve cells located in the spinal cord (meningitis) and the brain (encephalitis). Originally detected in Africa in the late 1930s, the virus did not spread to North America until 1999. Since that time its North American prevalence and geographical distribution has increased.

■ Disease History, Characteristics, and Transmission

West Nile virus was first isolated in 1937 from a woman in the West Nile District of Uganda. The virus took its name from this location. During the 1950s the ability of the virus to cause meningitis and encephalitis in humans and the resulting health threat of the virus was recognized. A decade later the virus was linked to the development of encephalitis in horses.

Since the 1930s the virus has been detected in humans, animals, and birds in Africa, the Middle East, Eastern Europe, and western Asia, but it did not arrive in North America until the end of the 20th century. Scientists are not certain if West Nile virus spread from Africa to other regions of the world, such as North America, or if the virus was always present in North America, only to be revealed when tests for it were performed. However, the pattern of reported cases in North America is more consistent with the introduction of the virus from overseas and its subsequent spread. Assuming that the virus was, in fact, introduced to the North American continent, the way in which it was transported across the Atlantic Ocean to the East Coast of the United States is still unknown. Bird migration is one theory. Another theory suggests that a mosquito infected with the virus could have arrived in a shipment of goods.

Immediately after its appearance in North America, West Nile became noteworthy. In the summer of 1999, 62

WORDS TO KNOW

ENCEPHALITIS A type of acute brain inflammation, most often due to infection by a virus.

MENINGITIS An inflammation of the meninges, the three layers of protective membranes that line the spinal cord and the brain. Meningitis can occur when there is an infection near the brain or spinal cord, such as a respiratory infection in the sinuses, the mastoids, or the cavities around the ear. Disease organisms can also travel to the meninges through the bloodstream. The first signs may be a severe headache and neck stiffness followed by fever, vomiting, a rash, and then convulsions leading to loss of consciousness. Meningitis generally involves two types: nonbacterial meningitis, or aseptic meningitis, and bacterial meningitis, or purulent meningitis.

RESERVOIR The animal or organism in which a virus or parasite normally resides.

VECTOR Any agent that carries and transmits parasites and diseases. Also, an organism or chemical used to transport a gene into a new host cell.

VECTOR-BORNE DISEASE One in which the pathogenic microorganism is transmitted from an infected individual to another individual by an arthropod or other agent, sometimes with other animals serving as intermediary hosts. The transmission depends on the attributes and requirements of at least three different living organisms: the pathologic agent, either a virus, protozoa, bacteria, or helminth (worm); the vector, commonly arthropods such as ticks or mosquitoes; and the human host.

---

cases of West Nile disease were reported in New York City. Seven people died from the infection. The city experienced another outbreak the following summer, when 21 more cases and two deaths occurred. In the span of 1999 to 2000, the virus was also detected in other states along the coast of the northeastern United States. These early infections generated a great deal of concern because they raised the possibility of a looming epidemic. This proved not to be the case, although the geographical range of the virus began to expand.

West Nile virus is a vector-borne disease, a disease spread from one species to another by a third species. West Nile spreads from infected birds to humans, mainly by mosquitoes (most commonly, the mosquito species *Culex pipiens*). Robins, jays, and crows are the most common avian reservoirs of the virus. As with other mosquito-transmitted diseases, the virus is acquired by a mosquito when it feeds on the blood of an infected animal or bird. The virus remains in the salivary gland of the mosquito and, when the same mosquito subsequently seeks a blood meal from a person, transfer of the virus can occur. The cases in New York City in 1999, and especially in 2000, were probably caused by mosquitoes that survived the cold winter months by seeking refuge in warm and damp pipes, abandoned tunnels, subway tunnels, or other locations such as root cellars, barns, and caves. In the spring the mosquitoes reemerged and a new round of infections began. In addition to humans being affected, many crows died from the viral infection in the springs of 2000 and 2001. Indeed, for those who monitor the appearance of West Nile disease, bird die-offs in the spring can be a signal that the infection is reemerging and that precautions are necessary to avoid human infection.

Research has shown that two populations of *Culex pipiens* exist in Europe. One seeks its blood meal exclusively from humans, and the other seeks it from animals. The chances of a mosquito taking a blood meal from an infected bird and then feeding on a human are low. However, in North America the mosquito population has adapted to feed on both birds and humans, so the probability that a mosquito will seek blood meals from an animal and then from a human is greater. This is probably why West Nile disease has spread so much faster in North America than in Europe.

When the West Nile virus enters a human host via a mosquito bite, the virus replicates in the blood. Then, in a way that is still not clear, the virus is able to cross the blood brain barrier and enter the brain. Normally, passage into the brain is regulated by this efficient blood-brain barrier. The barrier is so efficient that some drugs are unable to cross it, but the barrier is not able to keep the virus out of the brain. Formation of new virus particles in the brain tissue stimulates an immune response that—along with the infection—can cause inflammation of the brain, a serious condition known as encephalitis.

Approximately 80 percent of infected individuals present no symptoms, according to the World Health Organization (WHO). Many individuals, however, can exhibit symptoms of West Nile that include the development of fever, headache, muscle aches throughout the body (particularly in the back), loss of appetite, nausea with vomit-

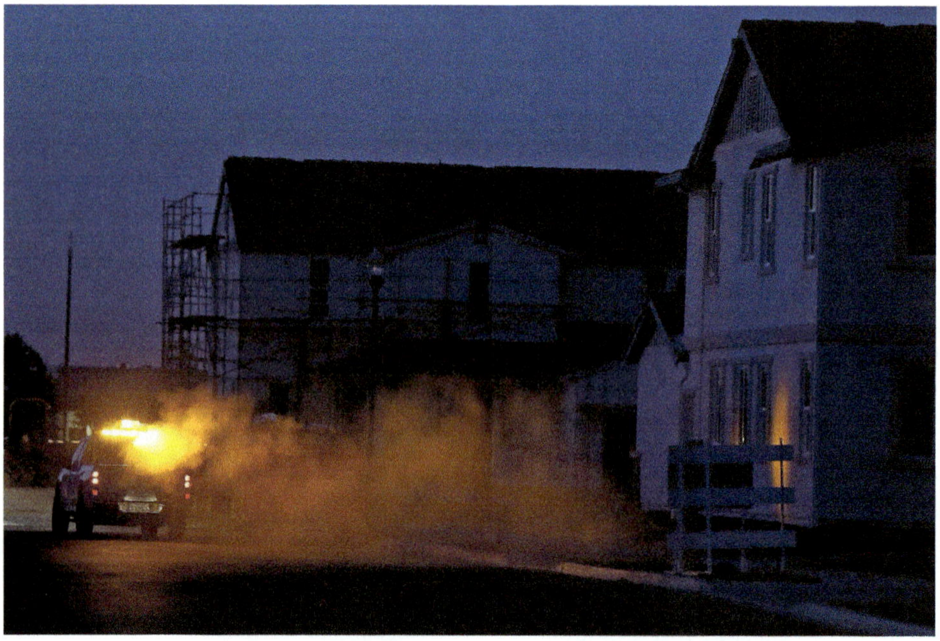

During a 2012 outbreak in California, officials from the Mosquito and Vector Control District sprayed Pyrocide 7396 insecticide to limit the spread of West Nile disease. West Nile has become a significant public safety concern in the United States. *© Justin Sullivan/Getty Images*

ing, diarrhea, swelling of the lymph nodes, and a skin rash. The infection tends to clear within a few weeks with no or mild complications.

According to WHO, in fewer than 1 percent of people who are infected with the virus, the infection becomes more serious. Inflammation of the nerve lining in the brain (encephalitis) and spinal cord (meningitis) develops. When meningitis or encephalitis develops, symptoms include a high fever, severe headache, stiff neck, mental disorientation, uncontrolled muscle spasms, loss of coordination, paralysis, and convulsions. A person can lapse into a coma and die. Survivors can be left with permanent damage, such as paralysis on one side of the body, similar to the paralysis seen in cases of polio. In severe cases the paralysis affects the muscles used for breathing, and mechanical breathing assistance may be necessary.

The prospect that a serious disease can be acquired from a mosquito bite is alarming to many, as mosquitoes are often common during spring and summer in North America and, despite precautions, can be hard to avoid. Fortunately, as of 2017 the incidence of the virus in North American mosquito populations was low. Scientists who have sampled mosquitoes for the presence of the virus have determined that typically only about 1 percent of mosquitoes harbor the virus, even in an area that is a known hotspot of the disease. The risk of a person contracting West Nile disease is small and can be minimized still further by taking some common-sense precautions, such as avoiding mosquito habitats, clearing a yard of pails and other objects like tires that can collect water (which can be breeding sites for mosquitoes), and using mosquito netting to cover the sleeping area in locations where the disease is more common.

A number of factors increase the risk of contracting West Nile disease. The time of year is one factor. In more northern climates, late spring to early fall is the peak season for mosquitoes, and the risk of contracting the disease is higher during those seasons. In southern regions that are warmer year-round, the risk is more constant.

Another risk factor is geography. Certain areas of the United States and Canada have greater mosquito populations than other areas and therefore are areas of higher risk. For example, Texas—which has coastline on the Gulf of Mexico—reported 330 cases of West Nile disease in 2006,

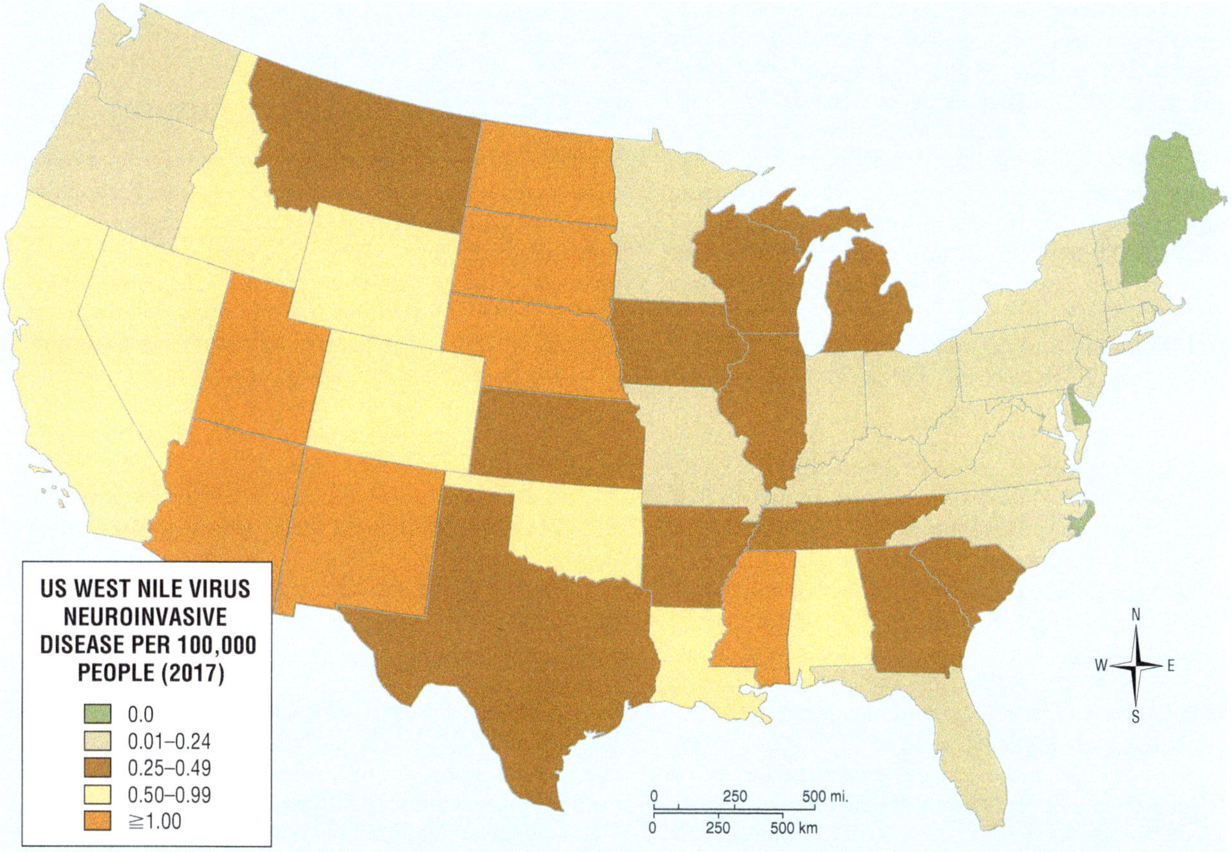

SOURCE: Adapted from "West Nile Virus Neuroinvasive Disease Incidence by State." US Centers for Disease Control and Prevention. 2017. Available from: https://www.cdc.gov/westnile/statsmaps/preliminarymapsdata2017/incidencestate.html

while the drier and more inland state of New Mexico reported only eight cases. Areas that have more stagnant water are more apt to be a breeding ground for mosquitoes.

A third risk factor is occupation. Someone whose job or recreational activities takes them outdoors is more at risk of exposure to mosquitoes than someone who spends more time indoors. Finally, people whose immune systems are not functioning efficiently—such as the elderly, the sick, and transplant patients whose immune systems have been deliberately suppressed—are at higher risk because they are less able to fight a viral infection.

Scope and Distribution

West Nile disease has occurred in Europe, Africa, the Middle East, parts of Asia, and North America. Outbreaks have occurred in all these regions, most recently in the United States and Canada from 1999 to 2003. The geographical distribution of the virus in North America has been steadily increasing since its appearance on the continent in 1999. By the summer of 2001, dead birds that tested positive for the virus were found in Toronto, Ontario (Canada), northern Florida, and Milwaukee, Wisconsin. A year later over 300 cases and at least 14 deaths were reported, and the virus was recovered from dead birds in more western states. By August 2002 West Nile virus was reported in 41 states, and by 2003 only the states of Alaska, Hawaii, Washington, Oregon, and Maine had not reported cases of the disease. This has remained the case through 2017.

The number of cases have been increasing as well. In 2002 4,155 cases and 284 deaths were reported to the US Centers for Disease Control and Prevention (CDC). The next year 9,862 cases and 264 fatalities were reported. About 30 percent of these cases involved meningitis or encephalitis and required extensive hospital care. From 2004 to 2006, 9,758 cases and 380 deaths were reported. During these last three years, the number of cases and deaths increased each year. In 2016, the last full year of reporting, there were 2,149 cases reported to the CDC. California reported 442 cases, followed by Texas with 370.

In Canada the virus was uncovered in dead birds and mosquitoes in the province of Ontario in 2001. The next year 10 deaths occurred among the 416 cases reported to Health Canada, and the disease had spread to the province of Quebec. The number of cases increased to 1,494, and 14 deaths were reported in 2003. By that year the virus had been detected across the country from British Columbia to Nova Scotia and as far north as the Yukon. Thereafter, the number of annual cases has fluctuated, with no trend of increase evident. There were 2,215 cases in 2007, followed by only 36 in 2008. In 2016, the last full year for which data was available, there were 104 cases in Canada.

While birds are involved in the transmission of West Nile disease to people, dogs and cats can also be infected with the virus. This has caused fears that many pet owners could be at risk of the disease. While it does mean that a pet owner could acquire the virus after a mosquito has bitten a cat or dog, there is no evidence of a direct transmission from either animal to people.

Squirrels may also be susceptible to infection with West Nile virus. While there is no evidence that the virus is transmitted to someone from a squirrel or from handling a squirrel carcass, the presence of a dead squirrel could be an indication that West Nile disease is present in an area. Sensible precautions, including the use of gloves when disposing of a squirrel carcass, will prevent infection.

There may also be a genetic component to West Nile virus susceptibility. Researchers have found that an alteration in a gene called *CCR5*, which affects the functioning of T cells (important immune system cells), can produce more serious symptoms of the disease. Several studies have found that the proportion of people possessing the gene mutation is much higher in those with West Nile disease than in the general population. Curiously, the gene mutation helps protect people infected with the human immunodeficiency virus (HIV) from developing acquired immunodeficiency syndrome (AIDS). As of 2017 *CCR5* was still being studied. The accumulating data has affirmed the importance of *CCR5* in the ability of the virus to cause infection. The hope is that this knowledge will be exploited in a strategy that prevents the infection.

Treatment and Prevention

West Nile disease is almost always acquired from a mosquito bite. While some species of ticks can harbor the virus, no tick-borne disease has been reported in a human. Furthermore, West Nile disease is not contagious, as routine person-to-person transmission does not occur. It is possible to transmit West Nile virus via transfusion of virus-contaminated blood, via transplant of a contaminated organ, and via breast milk. Infection of a fetus by its mother prior to birth may also be possible. However, infections that do not involve mosquito bites are considered rare.

In Canada all donated blood is screened year-round. Blood banks in the United States screen donated blood during peak infection periods. In addition, Britain's National Blood Service screens donated blood for the virus if the donor is known to have visited the United States or Canada in the previous month.

While as of 2017 there was still no human vaccine effective against West Nile virus, a vaccine for horses has become available. The vaccine has been used by some zoos to vaccinate birds; however, whether this strategy worked cannot be gauged until the birds are exposed to the virus. The equine vaccine, which contains weakened but intact West Nile virus, has not been studied in humans, and people should not use it. Veterinary vaccines are not subject to the same regulatory approvals as are human vaccines, and their safety for humans cannot be assured.

Prevention of infection focuses on minimizing the opportunity for contact with mosquitoes. Sensible precautions include using insect-repellent sprays or creams that contain DEET (N,N-diethyl-meta-toluamide), wearing protective clothing such as long-sleeve shirts and long pants when outdoors, avoiding areas of stagnant water that can be breeding grounds for mosquitoes, and removing any objects that could contain stagnant water—birdbaths, clogged roof gutters, unused swimming pools, and disused tires—from a backyard. In addition, avoiding outdoor activity during the early morning and evening, when mosquitoes are most active, is a wise precaution.

DEET-containing insect repellents should not be used on infants or young children. For these youngsters and for those who prefer not to be exposed to DEET, the CDC recommends oil of lemon eucalyptus. It is an efficient repellent but does not retain its potency as long as DEET does.

Impacts and Issues

West Nile disease has quickly become a significant public health threat in North America. The possibilities of large outbreaks and the potential seriousness of the infection—1 of every 150 people who contract the disease develops meningitis or encephalitis—has created near panic in the public. Agencies such as the CDC have devoted significant effort to informing people about the disease and publicizing the common-sense preventive measures that can help protect people.

Spraying of mosquito breeding sites is a proven way of reducing the mosquito population. However, those opposed to such spraying are concerned that the possible environmental degradation from the chemical spray is a greater danger than any cases of West Nile that might develop. Those in favor of spraying maintain that the increasing spread of West Nile disease and the increasing number of deaths argues for intervention and control programs, including spraying.

See Also *Arthropod-Borne Disease; Climate Change and Infectious Disease; Emerging Infectious Diseases; Encephalitis; Meningitis, Viral; Mosquito-Borne Diseases; Vector-Borne Disease*

BIBLIOGRAPHY

Books

Colpitts, Tonya M. *West Nile Virus: Methods and Protocols.* New York: Humana, 2016.

Periodicals

DeFelice, Nicholas B., et al. "Ensemble Forecast of Human West Nile Virus Cases and Mosquito Infection Rates." *Nature Communication* 8 (February 2017).

Simon, Bryan R. "West Nile Virus." *Nursing 2017* 47 (August 2017): 58–60.

Websites

"West Nile Virus." Centers for Disease Control and Prevention. https://www.cdc.gov/westnile/faq/genQuestions.html (accessed November 22, 2017).

"West Nile Virus." World Health Organization. http://www.who.int/mediacentre/factsheets/fs354/en/ (accessed November 22, 2017).

Brian Hoyle

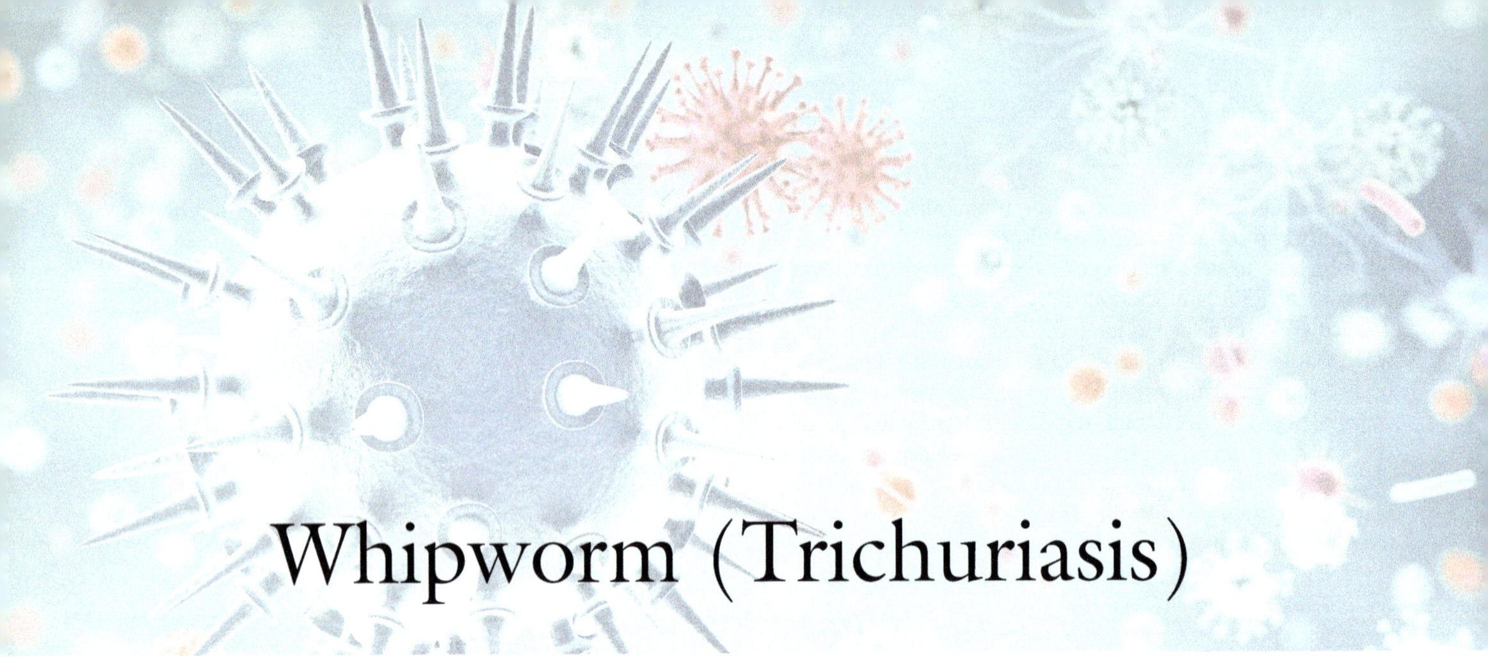

Whipworm (Trichuriasis)

Introduction

Whipworm, or trichuriasis, is caused by an infestation of the helminth (parasitic worm) *Trichuris trichiura*. This roundworm infects human hosts and reproduces within the large intestine. Transmission of the parasite occurs when infective eggs are passed through the feces and contaminate food and soil. Humans ingest contaminated food or soil to become infected. Light infestations often cause no symptoms, or mild symptoms, whereas heavy infestations can cause more serious complications including anemia, rectal prolapse, appendicitis, and colitis.

Treatment for whipworm involves antiparasitic medication containing either mebendazole or albendazole. In addition, treatment may be necessary for accompanying symptoms. Whipworm is a worldwide infection that is prevalent in densely populated tropical countries, especially in regions with poor sanitation methods. Both adults and children can become infected, although children tend to have a higher infection rate. Whipworm can be prevented by avoiding consumption of contaminated foods, maintaining high sanitation practices, and washing hands after working or playing in soil.

WORDS TO KNOW

EMBRYONATED When an embryo has been implanted in a female animal.

HELMINTH A representative of various phyla of wormlike animals.

HOST An organism that serves as the habitat for a parasite or possibly for a symbiont. A host may provide nutrition to the parasite or symbiont, or it may simply provide a place in which to live.

OVA Mature female sex cells produced in the ovaries. (Singular: ovum.)

Disease History, Characteristics, and Transmission

Whipworm infection is a parasitic infection caused by ingestion of the whipworm, or roundworm, *Trichuris trichiura*. The life cycle of *T. trichiura* involves a human host for the maturation of worms and production of eggs. Humans become infested after ingesting food or soil contaminated with embryonated whipworm eggs. The eggs hatch and mature in the small intestine before migrating to the large intestine. Here, the worms attach to the intestine walls, reach about 4 inches (10 centimeters) in length, and become sexually mature. The worms mate, and two to three months after entering the body, the females begin to produce up to 20,000 eggs a day. These eggs pass out of the body with the feces and remain in moist, dark conditions until they are ingested by a new host. Without extremes in temperatures, the eggs can remain viable in soil for years.

In cases where infestation is low—that is, fewer than 100 worms—people usually suffer no symptoms, but some may experience flatulence, abdominal pain, constipation, or diarrhea. If heavily infested, symptoms include weight loss, abdominal pain, nausea, bloody stools, and diarrhea. In severe cases there may be gastrointestinal problems, anemia, and even rectal prolapse, in which the rectum protrudes outside of the body. Children with severe infection may have stunted growth. The disease is diagnosed when a stool ova and parasite exam reveals the presence of *T. trichiura* or their eggs.

Scope and Distribution

Whipworm occurs worldwide. According to the US Centers for Disease Control and Prevention (CDC), this parasitic worm is the third-most common roundworm to infect humans. In 2015 the Global Infectious Diseases and Epidemiology Network (GIDEON) estimated that the prevalence of whipworm was 464.7 million people worldwide. Most whipworm infections occur in regions with dense populations and a tropical climate. Poor sanitation levels also increase the likelihood of the disease. Whipworm is most common in areas of Southeast Asia, Africa, the Caribbean, and Central and South America. Although whipworm infestations can occur in the United States, Japan, Western Europe, or Australasia, they are not common. In the United States infection, though rare, is most common in rural areas in the Southeast.

Children are at the greatest risk of infection. This is generally thought to be a result of infrequent handwashing and their penchant for playing in soil. As soil may be contaminated with whipworm, failure to wash hands thoroughly before contact with the mouth or food increases the chance of infection.

Treatment and Prevention

Whipworm is diagnosed through the identification of whipworm eggs in a patient's stool. Most cases of whipworm tend to be asymptomatic. Treatment usually involves removing the worms through administration of medication containing either mebendazole, which is recommended by the CDC, or albendazole. For symptomatic cases, supportive treatment, in addition to the antiparasitic medication, may be necessary. In cases in which significant blood loss occurs, there is risk of anemia developing. Therefore, iron supplements may be necessary to prevent iron deficiency. Health care providers may repeat a stool analysis following treatment to ensure the patient is free from parasites.

Whipworm infection is prevented by avoiding contact with contaminated soil and food. This may involve wearing protective clothing while working in potentially contaminated soil or washing hands thoroughly after touching soil. Food should be washed and cooked to remove parasites. In addition, crude sanitation, such as the collection of human feces for disposal or for use as fertilizer, is a common way for the infection to spread. Therefore, improved sanitation methods will decrease the likelihood of the infection spreading.

Impacts and Issues

Whipworm infections are most likely to occur in developing countries, or countries with dense populations, tropical weather, or poor sanitation methods. In such countries medical infrastructure is often limited and seldom able to deliver the repeated anthelmintic medication that successful treatment of whipworm infection requires.

Another issue related to whipworm infections involves the complications that can arise following heavy whipworm

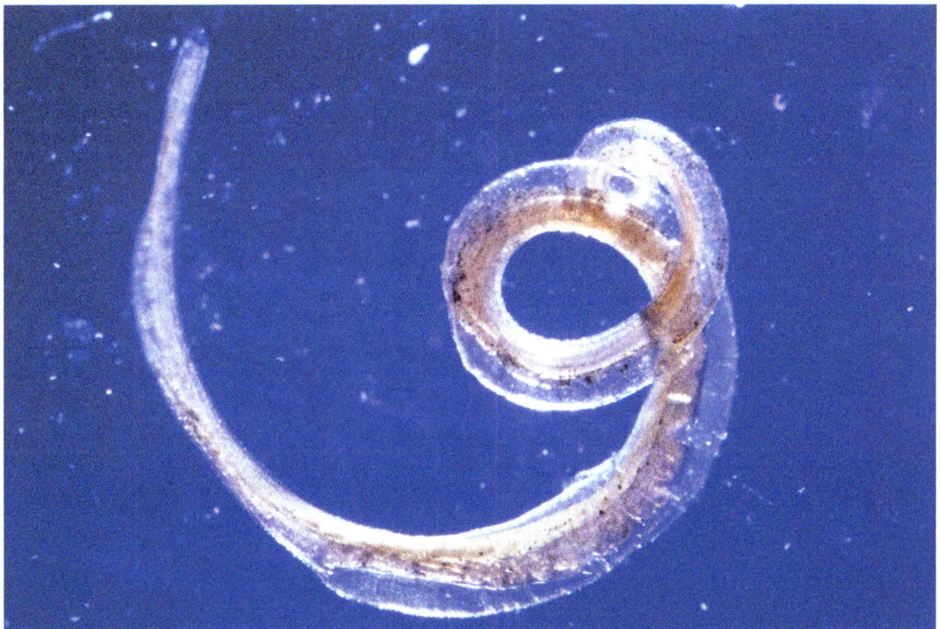

Trichuris trichuria, commonly called the whipworm, is a parasitic roundworm that can grow up to 4 inches (10 centimeters) in length. Whipworms hatch and mature in the small intestine before migrating to the large intestine to reproduce. *© CNRI/Science Source*

infestations. Anemia, a complication that results from a low transfer of oxygen to body tissues, directly affects tissue development. As children are commonly infected, this complication could affect their growth and overall health. Girls with whipworm infection are particularly vulnerable to anemia caused by whipworm infestation, as they experience additional blood loss with menstruation and often begin childbearing at a relatively young age in countries where whipworm is endemic.

The World Health Organization (WHO) has identified several key strategies in reducing whipworm infestation in people living in developing countries. Rather than reduce the number of whipworm infections in people, which was the traditional strategy, health authorities work to reduce the number of worms residing in each person. This strategy recognizes the fact that reinfection will probably occur and thus focuses on lessening the severity of the disease. Drugs are delivered to schools and other long-standing facilities, where minimally trained local citizens can administer them. This strategy has shown more success than relying on mobile medical teams when delivering repeated treatments. In 2017 WHO announced its goal of eliminating soil-transmitted helminthiases in children by 2020. The goal coincides with a plan to regularly treat at least 75 percent of children in endemic areas with albendazole and mebendazole.

PRIMARY SOURCE

WHO Recommends Large-Scale Deworming to Improve Children's Health and Nutrition

SOURCE: *World Health Organization. "WHO Recommends Large-Scale Deworming to Improve Children's Health and Nutrition," World Health Organization, September 29, 2017. http://www.who.int/mediacentre/news/releases/2017/large-scale-deworming/en/ (accessed January 10, 2017).*

INTRODUCTION: *In 2017 the World Health Organization (WHO) launched a new initiative to improve children's health in areas where soil-transmitted helminths such as whipworm are endemic. The following press release announces the initiative.*

Periodic deworming programmes with a single-tablet treatment can drastically reduce the suffering of those infected with parasitic intestinal worms and protect the 1.5 billion people currently estimated to be at risk.

Four main species of intestinal worms (also known as soil-transmitted helminths) affect almost a quarter of the world's poorest and mostly marginalized people. They are a major public health problem because the worms disrupt people's ability to absorb nutrients, impeding the growth and physical development of millions of children.

WHO has long promoted large-scale treatment for intestinal worms, but this is the first guideline approved by WHO's Guidelines Review Committee confirming that deworming improves the health and nutrient uptake of heavily infected children.

"There is now global evidence-based consensus that periodic, large-scale deworming is the best way to reduce the suffering caused by intestinal worms," says Dr Dirk Engels, Director of WHO's Neglected Tropical Diseases Department.

"These new guidelines have been issued at a time when countries where intestinal worms are endemic are accelerating control programmes with the help of partners – to both treat people who are infected and those at risk of infection."

Large-scale deworming programmes are facilitated by WHO, using medicines donated by pharmaceutical companies. WHO coordinates shipment of these medicines to countries requesting them. They are then distributed freely by national disease control programmes during mass treatment campaigns.

"Providing medicines to populations at risk reduces the intensity of intestinal helminth infections," said Dr Francesco Branca, Director of WHO's Department of Nutrition for Health and Development.

Deworming is not the only solution, however.

"Improving basic hygiene, sanitation, health education and providing access to safe drinking-water are also keys to resolving the health and nutritional problems caused by intestinal worms," says Dr Francesco Branca, Director of WHO's Department of Nutrition for Health and Development.

In 2015, just 39% of the global population had access to safe sanitation, while 71% could access safe water.

Treating school-age children for intestinal worms occurs in schools during "deworming days". Teachers supervise the process, freeing up health workers to focus on other demands.

Many countries combine deworming activities for preschool children with other health campaigns, such as vaccination, child health and vitamin supplementation days.

"WHO aims to eliminate the harm caused by worm infections in children by 2020 by regularly treating at least 75% of the estimated 873 million children in areas where prevalence is high," says Dr Antonio Montresor, who heads WHO's global deworming programme. "In 2016, WHO Member States treated 63% of children requiring treatment. Now that the world has agreed standards for deworming at-risk populations, we are in a better position to reach this target."

SEE ALSO *Ascariasis; Handwashing; Helminth Disease; Hookworm (Ancylostoma) Infection; Parasitic Diseases; Pinworm (*Enterobius vermicularis*) Infection; Sanitation*

BIBLIOGRAPHY

Books

Drisdelle, Rosemary. *Parasites: Tales of Humanity's Most Unwelcome Guests.* Berkeley: University of California Press, 2010.

Morand, Serge, Boris R. Krasnov, and D. Timothy J. Littlewood, eds. *Parasite Diversity and Diversification: Evolutionary Ecology Meets Phylogenetics.* Cambridge, UK: Cambridge University Press, 2015.

Periodicals

Kaminsky, Rina G., Renato Valenzuela Castillo, and Coralia Abrego Flores. "Growth Retardation and Severe Anemia in Children with *Trichuris* Dysenteric Syndrome." *Asian Pacific Journal of Tropical Biomedicine* 5, no. 7 (July 2015): 591–597.

Websites

"Soil-Transmitted Helminth Infections: Fact Sheet." World Health Organization, September 2017. http://www.who.int/mediacentre/factsheets/fs366/en/ (accessed January 9, 2018).

"Trichuriasis." Centers for Disease Control and Prevention, January 10, 2013 https://www.cdc.gov/parasites/whipworm/ (accessed January 8, 2018).

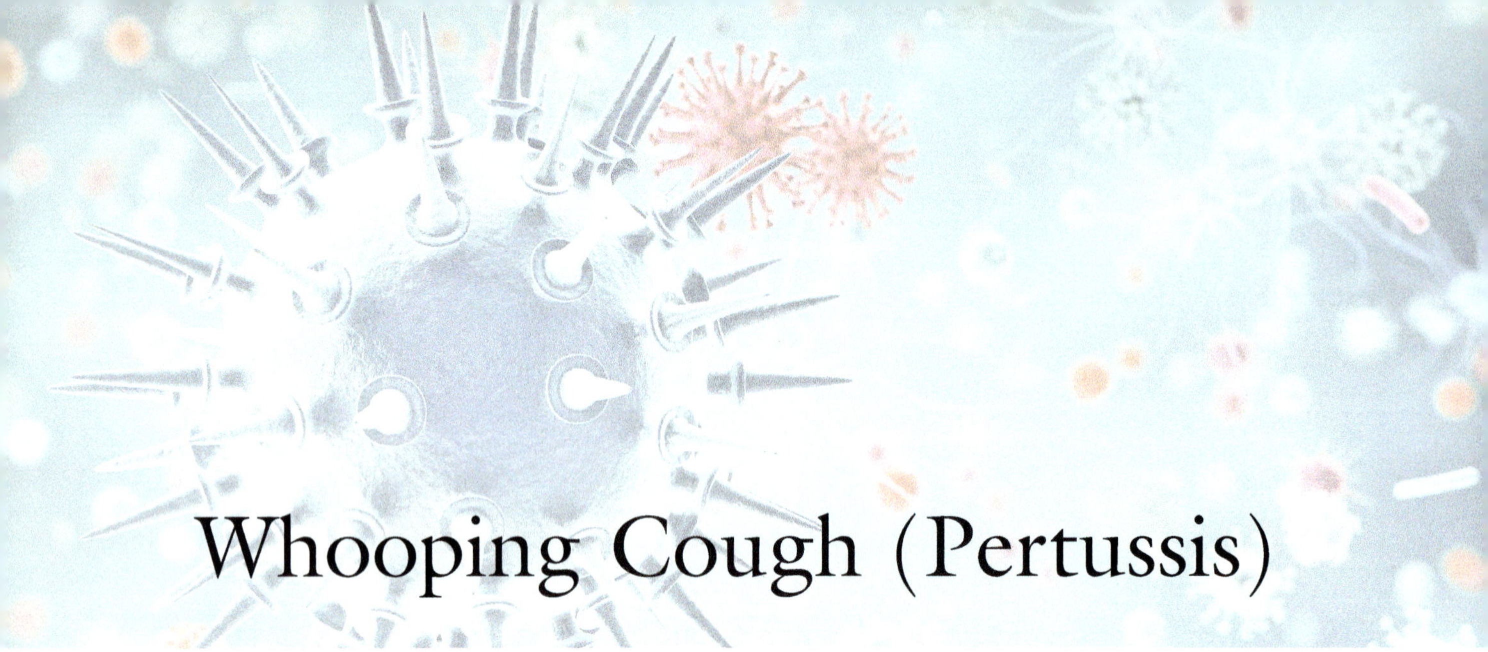

Whooping Cough (Pertussis)

■ Introduction

Whooping cough is also known as pertussis, a word that means "intense cough." It is caused by the bacterium *Bordetella pertussis*, which is a pathogen with a propensity for lung tissue.

Whooping cough was once the leading cause of death in children under age five in the United States. In 1945 it caused more deaths than diphtheria, scarlet fever, measles, and polio combined. Since the introduction of an effective vaccine in the late 1940s, the number of cases of whooping cough has decreased sharply, although there have been increases in recent years. Whooping cough is now one of the leading causes of death from a preventable disease.

Whooping cough is no ordinary cough. The disease is marked by bouts of severe spasmodic coughing that end with a characteristic "whooping" sound and vomiting. Complications from secondary bacterial infection include pneumonia and ear infection. Mortality is greatest among infants, especially those who are born prematurely. Whooping cough is a highly contagious disease, so it is important that children be vaccinated against it.

WORDS TO KNOW

ANTIBIOTIC RESISTANCE The ability of bacteria to resist the actions of antibiotic drugs.

GRAM-NEGATIVE BACTERIA All types of bacteria identified and classified as a group that does not retain crystal-violet dye during the Gram method of staining.

PAROXYSM In medicine, a fit, convulsion, or seizure. It may also be a sudden worsening or recurrence of disease symptoms.

PATHOGEN A disease-causing agent, such as a bacterium, a virus, a fungus, or another microorganism.

PNEUMONIA Inflammation of the lung accompanied by filling of some air sacs with fluid (consolidation). It can be caused by a number of infectious agents, including bacteria, viruses, and fungi.

RESERVOIR The animal or organism in which a virus or parasite normally resides.

VACCINE A substance that is introduced to stimulate antibody production and thus provide immunity to a particular disease.

■ Disease History, Characteristics, and Transmission

The causative agent of whooping cough is *B. pertussis*, which is a Gram-negative coccus (a short, rod-shaped bacterium). The term *Gram-negative* refers to the way the microbe reacts with Gram stain, which is used to prepare samples for microscopy. *B. pertussis* specifically infects the tissue of the lung, and its incubation period is 6 to 20 days.

Whooping cough may last for several weeks and is divided into three distinct stages. The catarrhal stage involves nonspecific symptoms, such as a runny nose, a mild cough, and a mild fever, which may easily be mistaken for a cold. This stage may continue for a week or so, before the second, paroxysmal stage sets in. This is marked by paroxysms (attacks) of severe, repetitive coughing ending in a "whooping" sound and vomiting, usually accompanied by exhaustion. The coughing has a choking quality, and the patient's face may look congested. There may be between 2 and 50 attacks a day, occurring more frequently at night. Between attacks the patient does not usually cough at all.

The whooping sound comes from the voice box (larynx) as the patient finally takes in a proper breath after an attack. Complications of this stage of whooping cough include convulsions and seizures arising from a reduced supply of oxygen to the brain. This is thought to occur either because of the coughing itself or a toxin released by *B. pertussis*. This stage lasts for one to four weeks, during which time secondary bacterial infections such as otitis media (an infection of the middle ear) and pneumonia may set in. The latter is the most common and deadly complication of whooping cough.

The final stage of whooping cough is convalescence and is characterized by a fading away of the cough in both frequency and intensity. The US Centers for Disease Control and Prevention states that the clinical course of whooping cough in adults is complicated by pneumonia in about 2 percent of cases. The pneumonia complication rate is about 23 percent for babies in the hospital with whooping cough (which constitutes about 50 percent of all babies with whooping cough). Mortality rates are highest among infants. In 2016, the last year data was available, there were seven deaths in the United States from whooping cough. Of these, six were infants, and one was older than one year. A case of whooping cough usually gives a patient lifelong immunity to further attacks.

Whooping cough is a highly contagious disease, particularly in the catarrhal stage and up to three weeks after the start of the paroxysmal stage. Adults and adolescents, who may have a milder form of the disease, act as a reservoir of infection. The disease is transmitted through coughing and sneezing, which exposes people to infected respiratory secretions.

■ Scope and Distribution

Whooping cough has been known as a childhood disease for several hundred years. According to a 2017 article in *Lancet Infectious Diseases*, in 2014 there were an estimated 24.1 million cases of whooping cough in children five years old and younger worldwide and 160,700 total deaths. Africa accounted for 33 percent of the cases and 58 percent of the deaths. In many countries regular epidemics occur every three to five years. Those who have not been fully immunized, either because they are too young or for some other reason, are most at risk of dying from whooping cough.

Before the introduction of the whooping cough vaccine, the disease was the leading cause of death from infectious disease in children under age five in the United States. Outbreaks tend to occur in the United States between July and October. Premature babies are particularly at risk of whooping cough and are more likely to develop complications than older children.

The whooping cough vaccine reduced the number of whooping cough cases hundredfold by 1970, compared to figures for 1945. But there has been an increase since then. The increases have been highest among children 7 to 10 years old and in adolescents. A confluence of factors has caused these outbreaks, including the choice of parents not to vaccinate their children against whooping cough for nonmedical reasons, as well as the decreased efficacy of the new whooping cough vaccine DTaP.

Since 2003 the number of whooping cough cases has increased in the United States. Whooping cough outbreaks are associated in part with children who are unvaccinated due to parental objection to vaccinations for personal, nonmedical reasons. In 2016 the CDC reported nearly 15,737

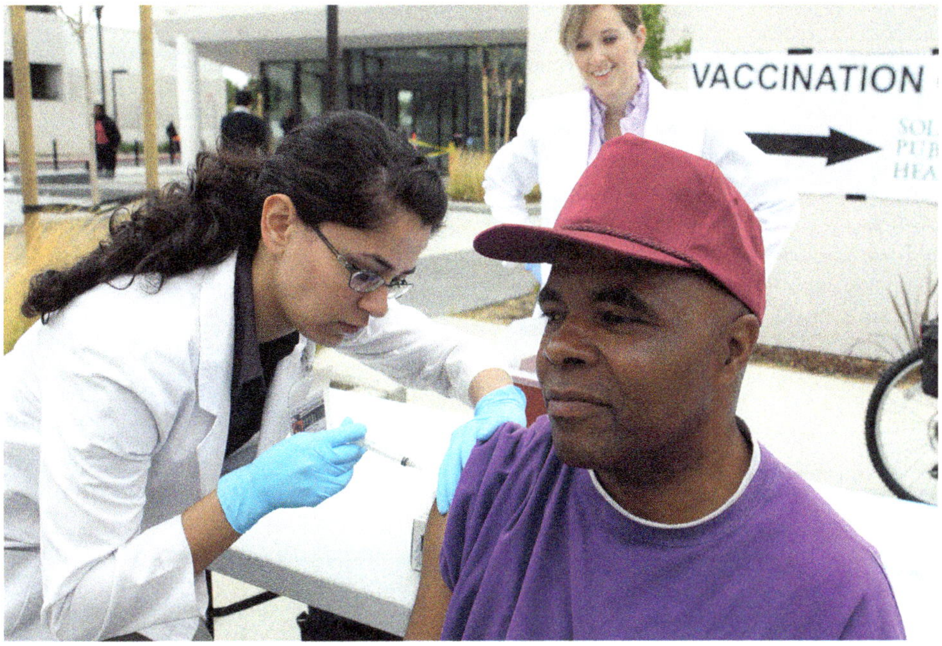

A medical student administers the Tdap (tetanus, diphtheria, and pertussis) vaccine to a resident of Vallejo, California, during a 2010 outbreak of whooping cough (pertussis) responsible for several deaths among infants. Whooping cough, a bacterial infection of the respiratory system, is highly contagious and is particularly dangerous to children. *© Justin Sullivan/Getty Images*

cases in the United States, down from 20,762 cases in 2015. In 2016 there were seven deaths from whooping cough in the United States. As of 2017 the most recent peak year in the United States was 2012, when there were 48,227 cases. The CDC also notes that many instances of whooping cough may not be diagnosed and therefore not reported.

Treatment and Prevention

Antibiotics will shorten the course of whooping cough if given in the early stages of the disease, but they do not tend to shorten the paroxysmal stage. However, antibiotic treatment does help prevent the transmission of the disease. Azithromycin, clarithromycin, and erythromycin are the antibiotics usually recommended for the treatment of whooping cough, but azithromycin should only be taken by those with no previous cardiovascular issues. A major concern is the emergence of strains of *B. pertussis* that are resistant to antibiotics. Patients with whooping cough readily become dehydrated and should be given plenty of fluids.

There are vaccines for pertussis. The pertussis vaccine is generally given in combination with vaccines against diphtheria and tetanus. The World Health Organization (WHO) recommends one injection of a DTP (diphtheria, tetanus, and pertussis) vaccine be given at 6 weeks old, another at 10 to 18 weeks, and the last one at 22 to 30 weeks. Three booster injections should be given between 12 and 23 months, 4 and 7 years, and 9 and 15 years. About a quarter of children receiving the vaccine will become feverish immediately afterward for up to 24 hours and may have soreness and redness at the site of the injection.

There are different types of DTP vaccines. In 1997 the United States stopped using the original whooping cough vaccine known as DTwP (the whole-cell pertussis vaccine) and started using a newer vaccine called DTaP (the acellular pertussis vaccine). The DTaP vaccines had fewer side effects (although the side effects from the DTwP vaccine were generally only mild to moderate). Other countries, including Australia, Norway, and the United Kingdom, also adopted use of the DTaP vaccine. As of August 2017, WHO recommended inactivated DTwP or DTaP vaccines in at least three primary doses combined with diphtheria and tetanus toxoid.

In the United States, the most commonly used whooping cough vaccines are DTaP, which is given to children under seven years old, and Tdap, which is given to adolescents and adults. The CDC recommends that 11- or 12-year-olds should be given a Tdap vaccine. It is also recommended that women who are pregnant should be given a Tdap vaccine at 27 to 36 weeks into their pregnancy.

Impacts and Issues

Whooping cough remains a serious health threat for children around the world, which is why joint efforts of WHO and other agencies are aimed toward universal vaccination for children. As with other diseases, such as diphtheria and polio, the lives of many children around the world are at risk because they have not been vaccinated—either because they do not have access to vaccination or because their parents do not believe vaccinations are safe or effective.

In countries where the health infrastructure is weak or lacking because of socioeconomic and political problems or geographical factors, access to vaccination may be patchy or nonexistent. For example, several children died during two outbreaks of whooping cough in 2003 in Badakhshan, a northeastern province of Afghanistan. An emergency team from the Afghan Ministry of Public Health and WHO mounted a mass distribution of erythromycin. Badakhshan is mountainous, isolated, and has few health workers. Many children who live there are malnourished. These factors put them at risk of whooping cough and many other infections.

An increasing body of evidence shows that the DTaP and Tdap vaccines (both acellular pertussis vaccines) are less effective over time than the whole-cellular pertussis DTwP vaccine. This accounts for one of the reasons why the number of pertussis cases has increased in the United States among older children and adolescents in the 21st century.

PRIMARY SOURCE

"Whooping Cough Vaccine's Protection Fades Quickly"

SOURCE: *Aliferis, Lisa. "Whooping Cough Vaccine's Protection Fades Quickly." NPR, May 5, 2015. https://www.npr.org/sections/health-shots/2015/05/05/404407258/whooping-cough-vaccines-protection-fades-quickly (accessed January 29, 2018).*

INTRODUCTION: *The following article summarizes research published in the journal* Pediatrics *in 2015 that found that the efficacy of a whooping cough vaccine known as TDaP decreases each year after the shot. Nevertheless, the TDaP vaccine should still be administered because it lessens the severity of the disease among people who have had the vaccine. Unlike the measles vaccine, the TDaP vaccine does not prevent people from spreading the disease to others, including infants who are not old enough to receive the vaccine.*

Lately, Californians have been focused on a measles outbreak that got its start at Disneyland. But in the past five years, state health officials have declared epidemics of whooping cough twice—in 2010 and in 2014, when 11,000 people were sickened and three infants died.

Now an analysis of a recent whooping cough epidemic in Washington state shows that the effectiveness of the Tdap vaccine used to fight the illness (also known as pertussis) waned significantly. For adolescents who received all their shots, effectiveness within one year of the final booster was 73 percent. The effectiveness rate plummeted to 34 percent within two to four years.

"This waning is likely contributing to the increase in pertussis among adolescents," the authors wrote.

Tdap protects against three diseases: tetanus, diphtheria and pertussis. The pertussis protection is from the acellular pertussis vaccine. It was introduced in 1997 to replace the whole-cell vaccine, which caused more side effects. Monday's report confirms earlier analysis that the acellular pertussis vaccine may be safer but less effective than the old one.

The study was published Monday in the journal *Pediatrics.*

"The take-home message is that the waning is there," said Dr. Art Reingold, a University of California, Berkeley professor of public health. "You're protected initially but it wanes over time."

It doesn't mean people should skip the vaccine. Someone who is vaccinated, but becomes sick with whooping cough, should have a less severe course of illness.

The authors said that new vaccines are "likely needed to reduce the burden of pertussis disease." But Reingold, who leads the CDC's Advisory Committee on Immunization Practices group on pertussis, said he doesn't know of any pertussis vaccine development in the pipeline.

He also said that adding another dose of the vaccine at a later age wouldn't help much, based on research that was presented to the ACIP group. "[An additional dose] would have very little impact on pertussis," he said, "in terms of cases prevented."

The most severe cases are in very young infants, Reingold said. Babies can't be vaccinated until they are 2 months old. To protect newborns before they can be vaccinated, the CDC recommends that women be vaccinated during the last trimester of every pregnancy—even if they received a vaccine before they became pregnant.

"Babies will be born with circulating antibodies," Reingold said, "and there's pretty good evidence that that will reduce the risk of hospitalization and death in babies."

In an accompanying commentary, Dr. James Cherry at UCLA said the findings about Tdap effectiveness were "disappointing," but he also pointed to other drivers of recent pertussis outbreaks, including increased awareness and better, more sensitive testing.

Previous reports have shown that vaccine refusal played a role in the 2010 whooping cough epidemic in California.

Reingold also drew an interesting distinction between measles and pertussis having to do with herd immunity. If a large enough percentage of the population is immunized against measles, both individuals and the broader community are protected against outbreak. That's because the measles vaccine protects you against the virus that actually causes the measles illness.

But in pertussis, the disease is caused by toxins that are released by bacteria. The pertussis vaccine protects you against those toxins, but it may not prevent you from spreading the bacteria to others—and causing illness in them.

The outbreak of measles earlier this year was most likely caused by someone who brought the disease back from abroad. Measles was eliminated in the United States in 2000.

"Pertussis is not going to go away with the current vaccine," Reingold said.

SEE ALSO *Childhood-Associated Infectious Diseases, Immunization Impacts*

BIBLIOGRAPHY

Books

Bennett, John E., Raphael Dolin, and Martin J. Blaser. *Mandell, Douglas, and Bennett's Principles and Practice of Infectious Diseases.* 8th ed. Philadelphia: Elsevier/Saunders, 2015

Periodicals

Cherry, James D. "The History of Pertussis (Whooping Cough); 1906–2015: Facts, Myths, and Misconceptions." *Current Epidemiology Reports* 2, no. 2 (June 2015): 120–130. This article can also be found online at https://link.springer.com/article/10.1007/s40471-015-0041-9 (accessed January 29, 2018).

Haelle, Tara. "Shooting the Wheeze: Whooping Cough Vaccine Falls Short of Previous Shot's Protection." *Scientific American* (May 21, 2013). This article can also be found online at https://www.scientificamerican.com/article/whooping-cough-vaccine-falls-short-of-previous-shots-protection/ (accessed January 29, 2018).

Haelle, Tara. "Vaccination Opt-Outs Found to Contribute to Whooping Cough Outbreaks in Kids." *Scientific American* (October 2, 2013). This article can also be found online at https://www.scientificamerican.com/article/vaccination-opt-outs-found-to-contribute-to-whooping-cough-outbreaks-in-kids/ (accessed January 29, 2018).

Skoff, T. H., et al. "Sources of Infant Pertussis Infection in the United States." *Pediatrics* 136, no. 4 (October 2015): 635–641. This article can also be found online at https://www.ncbi.nlm.nih.gov/pubmed/26347437 (accessed January 26, 2018).

Yeung, K. H. T., et al. "An Update of the Global Burden of Pertussis in Children Younger than 5 Years: A Modelling Study." *Lancet Infectious Diseases* 17, no. 9 (September 17, 2017): 974–980. This article can also be found online at https://www.ncbi.nlm.nih.gov/pubmed/28623146 (accessed January 26, 2018).

Websites

"Pertussis." World Health Organization, June 21, 2011. http://www.who.int/immunization/topics/pertussis/en/ (accessed January 26, 2018).

"Table 1: Summary of WHO Position Papers—Recommendations for Routine Immunization." World Health Organization, March 2017. http://www.who.int/immunization/policy/Immunization_routine_table1.pdf?ua=1 (accessed January 26, 2018).

"2016 Provisional Pertussis Surveillance Report." Centers for Disease Control and Prevention, January 6, 2017. https://www.cdc.gov/pertussis/downloads/pertuss-surv-report-2016-provisional.pdf (accessed January 26, 2018).

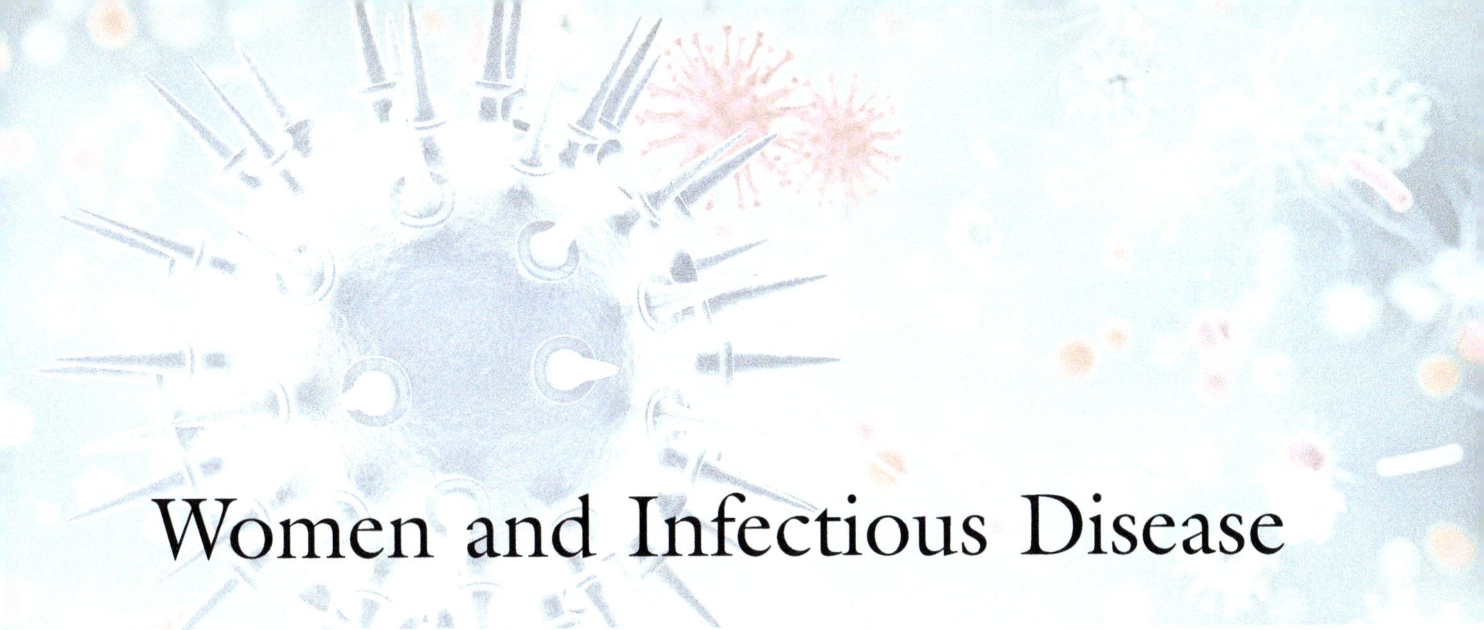

Women and Infectious Disease

Introduction

The medical community did not begin to understand that infectious diseases can affect women differently than men until the late 20th and early 21st centuries. Reasons for the differences between the sexes are still being researched, but it is clear that biology and culture play important roles.

Anatomical differences between the sexes make it easier, for example, for women to contract sexually transmitted infections (STIs) than men. At the same time, however, it has been shown that women have stronger immune systems than men. It seems that both hormones and genetics play a role in women's ability to fight off infection.

Cultural forces, including discrimination against women and power differentials between men and women, can make it difficult for women to access health care, including quality gynecological care. This can leave women more susceptible to infectious diseases than their male counterparts.

History and Scientific Foundations

Medical research historically focused on male participants and applied the results of those studies to women. The assumption that the male body and the female body were similar with the exception of the reproductive system led to lower rates of female research study participants and a one-size-fits-all approach when applying the results from studies that examined men only. Assumptions about infectious disease transmission and progression in women based on such research proved to be incorrect in many instances, especially because studies have shown that women have more robust immune systems than men. The male-only approach is problematic because men and women may react differently to infections and to medication. As the authors of a 2014 study in the *Journal of Infectious Diseases* noted, "Given the inherent men-bias in the enrollment into clinical trials and limited analysis of existing clinical trial data according to sex, focused research in sex-specific differences in infectious diseases is even more critical."

Along with biological differences between men and women, discrimination against women and cultural expectations surrounding women's roles affect women's disease transmission rates (maternal–child transmission, transmission to and from sexual partners, or transmission within the family and community) and the progression of disease in women. Race, nationality, class, age, education level, and other identity issues also play important roles in transmission rates.

According to the World Health Organization (WHO), there are four primary barriers that can prevent women from accessing health care and preventing the spread of

WORDS TO KNOW

IMMUNOCOMPROMISED Having an immune system with reduced ability to recognize and respond to the presence of foreign material.

MICROBICIDE A compound that kills microorganisms such as bacteria, fungi, and protozoa.

MORBIDITY From the Latin *morbus*, "sick," it refers to both the state of being ill and the severity of the illness. A serious disease is said to have a high morbidity.

MORTALITY The condition of being susceptible to death. The term *mortality* comes from the Latin word *mors*, which means death. Mortality can also refer to the rate of deaths caused by an illness or injury (e.g., "Rabies has a high mortality rate.").

infectious disease. They are "unequal power relationships between men and women; social norms that decrease education and paid employment opportunities; an exclusive focus on women's reproductive roles; and potential or actual experience of physical, sexual, and emotional violence."

Pregnancy and childbirth can make women especially vulnerable to infectious diseases because pregnant women experience decreased immunity and increased susceptibility. Malaria, for example, can be more serious for pregnant women than for nonpregnant ones. Pregnancy can also lead to malnutrition and chronic anemia in women of childbearing years. Bacterial infections can occur during or after childbirth.

In areas where birth control is unavailable or constitutes a violation of cultural practices, closely spaced pregnancies weaken women and compromise their overall health, leaving them vulnerable to infectious disease. Repeated pregnancies and breastfeeding can leave women in lower economic conditions chronically malnourished, with weakened immune systems.

Applications and Research

Infectious disease research and programs for women examine a host of factors, including how class, income, religion, geographic location, access to medical care and transportation, and other demographic and environmental issues affect women. Research into infectious disease issues and gender often focuses on mother–child transmission of certain diseases, such as human immunodeficiency virus (HIV)/acquired immunodeficiency syndrome (AIDS).

Tuberculosis (TB), an infectious bacterial disease that is rare in the developed world, is a leading cause of death among women, according to WHO. Historical data on TB rates in developed countries indicate that, from the 1930s through the 1950s, infection rates for women ages 15 to 34 were higher than those of men in the same age range. For women of childbearing years, the time from infection to disease itself is swifter than for similarly aged males, but as prevention and treatment options became more prevalent, infection among women decreased.

In 2004 a study of TB rates among men and women in Bangladesh showed that the female-to-male ratio of TB infections stood at 0.33 to 1, even when women's lower rate of access to health care is factored out. Previous research had questioned whether TB is underreported among women in developing countries. The 2004 findings confirmed a previous study from 2000, but many women's public health researchers questioned the prevailing concept that women consistently underreport or are underrepresented in research studies. In such cases studying women's rates of tuberculosis along with those of men demonstrated that studying only men could lead to erroneous assumptions that affected women's health.

HIV/AIDS and TB have converged in many developing countries. Immunocompromised patients are vulnerable to TB, and the two infectious diseases have posed a

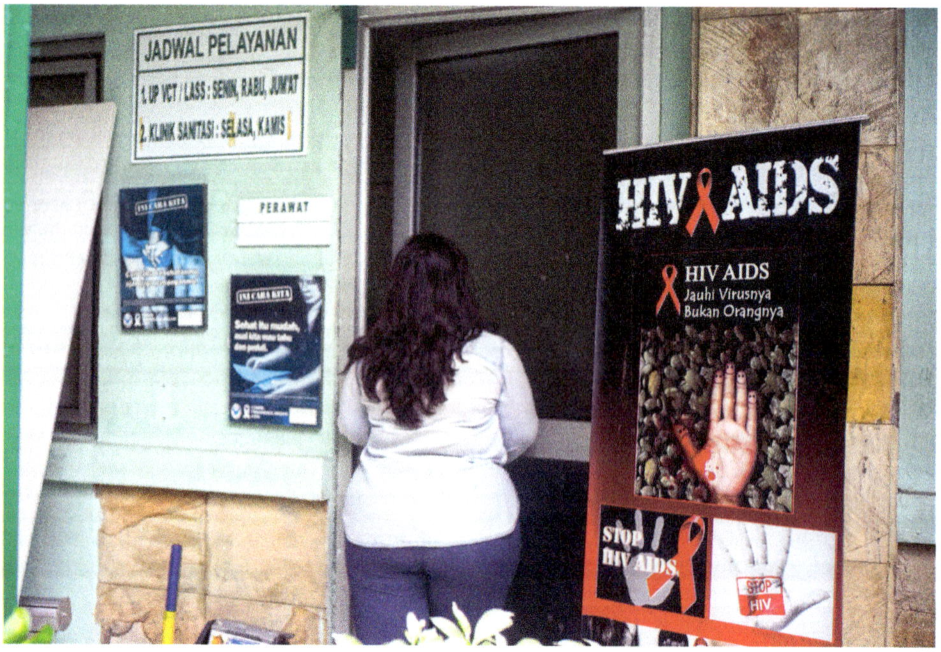

A woman enters a community health center in Jakarta, Indonesia. Globally women and minorities are especially vulnerable to health threats such as HIV, AIDS, and tuberculosis. *© Anton Raharjo/Anadolu Agency/Getty Images*

challenge to public health workers. Pregnant women face even greater obstacles because their lowered immunity makes them more susceptible to infectious disease, and treatment can be limited by concerns about fetal exposure to certain drugs.

HIV/AIDS is the leading cause of death for women between the ages of 15 and 44, according to WHO. HIV/AIDS research and programs for prevention and treatment in developing nations focus a significant amount of resources on sub-Saharan Africa. Fifty-nine percent of all HIV/AIDS cases in sub-Saharan Africa are women, according to United Nations Population Fund data. In eastern and southern Africa, where HIV is more prevalent than any other region on Earth, HIV/AIDS prevalence in women ranges from 14.5 to 39.5 percent.

Women in higher-income countries are affected by HIV/AIDS trends as well. Data from the US Centers for Disease Control and Prevention (CDC) show that diagnoses of HIV/AIDS in women declined in the United States between 2010 and 2014. The disease still disproportionately affects African American women, however. Around 60 percent of all women with HIV/AIDS in the United States are African American.

In general, women can contract STIs more easily than men can. In the case of human papillomavirus (HPV), the STI can cause far more serious repercussions for women if left untreated. HPV is highly treatable in its early stages, but in later stages some strains of the virus can lead to cervical cancer. (HPV can cause cancer in men, but this is less common.) Routine Pap smears can detect precancerous changes in cervical tissue, but women in developing nations and minority women in the United States receive such preventive care at lower rates than white women and those in developed nations. Advanced cervical cancer can be difficult to treat. However, the introduction of a vaccine against cancer-causing strains of HPV has reduced new cases of cervical cancer. From 2003 to 2012, the rate of cervical cancer cases in the United States decreased by 1.3 percent each year, and the mortality rate decreased by 0.9 percent.

Impacts and Issues

Microbicides, rings, gels, or other delivery systems inserted into the vagina prior to sexual intercourse are a promising area of research for women who have partners who do not use condoms during sex. A vaginal microbicide that does not need to be refrigerated, is highly portable, and affords women control over the use of the product could be a powerful tool in public health efforts, according to researchers. Many men in areas of the world where HIV/AIDS is prevalent refuse to use condoms as a cultural matter. Microbicides could be undetected and used by women as a form of protection against infection via sexual violence. Public health officials note that sex workers, who are key transmission points and can often infect hundreds of men, could use the gel to help protect themselves and their clients. While worldwide and US campaigns to promote condom use have had limited success due to cultural bias against condoms, microbicidal gels or creams represent a workaround that takes into account issues unique to women and sexuality.

As of 2017 trials were underway to test microbicides that had shown some effectiveness in preventing the spread of HIV. Two large clinical trials conducted in sub-Saharan Africa showed that a vaginal ring that slowly released an antiretroviral drug (ART) reduced HIV infections by 27 percent. In women older than age 25 who used the vaginal ring most consistently, the reduction rate was much higher, at 61 percent.

PRIMARY SOURCE

Infections Reveal Inequality between the Sexes

SOURCE: *Reardon, Sara. "Infections Reveal Inequality between the Sexes."* Scientific American *(June 22, 2016). This article can also be found online at https://www.scientificamerican.com/article/infections-reveal-inequality-between-the-sexes/ (accessed March 5, 2018).*

INTRODUCTION: *The following article discusses new research that revealed that women's immune systems are stronger at fighting off infection than men's immune systems. Reasons for this immunological difference likely relate to differences in hormones and genes. It is possible that women evolved to have stronger immune systems in order to protect themselves and their fetuses when pregnant.*

The immune systems of men and women respond very differently to infection—and scientists are taking notice. Research presented last week at a microbiology meeting in Boston, Massachusetts, suggests that the split could influence the design of vaccination programmes and lead to more targeted treatment of illness.

Hints that men and women deal with infection differently have been around for some time. In 1992, the World Health Organization hastily withdrew a new measles vaccine after it was linked to a substantial increase in deaths of infant girls in clinical trials in Senegal and Haiti. It is still not clear why boys were unaffected, but the incident was one of the first such examples to catch scientists' attention.

Women might have evolved a particularly fast and strong immune response to protect developing fetuses and newborn babies, says Marcus Altfeld, an immunologist at the Heinrich Pette Institute in Hamburg, Germany. But it comes at a cost: the immune system can overreact and attack the body. This might explain why more women than men tend to develop autoimmune diseases such as multiple sclerosis and lupus.

Yet very few studies assess men and women separately, so any sex-specific effects are masked. And many clinical trials include only men, because menstrual cycles and pregnancies can complicate the results. "It's sort of an inconvenient truth," says Linde Meyaard, an immunologist at University Medical Center Utrecht in the Netherlands. "People really don't want to know that what they study in one sex is different from the other."

Now, scientists are beginning to tease out some precise mechanisms. At the meeting, infectious-disease researcher Katie Flanagan at the University of Tasmania in Australia reported on a tuberculosis vaccine given to Gambian infants. She found that the vaccine suppressed production of an anti-inflammatory protein in girls, but not boys. This boosted the girls' immune responses, and may have made the vaccine more effective.

Hormones also play a part. Estrogen can activate the cells involved in antiviral responses, and testosterone suppresses inflammation.

Treating nasal cells with estrogen-like compounds before exposing them to the influenza virus has revealed further clues, says Sabra Klein, an endocrinologist at Johns Hopkins University in Baltimore, Maryland. Only the cells from females responded to the hormones and fought off the virus (J. Peretz et al. Am. J. Physiol. http://doi.org/bj5w; 2016).

Genetic factors may also guide how the sexes deal with infection. Meyaard studies a protein called TLR7, which detects viruses and activates immune cells. Encoded by a gene on the X chromosome, the protein causes a stronger immune response in women than in men (G. Karnam et al. PLOS Pathogens http://doi.org/bj5x; 2012). Meyaard suspects that this is because it somehow circumvents the process whereby one of the two X chromosomes in women is shut down to avoid overexpression of proteins.

A study set to begin later [in 2016] could help to tease apart the relative influence of genes and hormones on infection. Altfeld and his colleagues will look at 40 adults going through sex-change operations. If female hormones are responsible, the transgender women in the study should begin mounting stronger immune reactions to infections and develop more autoimmune problems than the transgender men.

Whether such results will lead to changes in how drugs are administered is an open question. In 2014, the US National Institutes of Health (NIH) announced that researchers must report the sex of animals used in preclinical research. Similar efforts are under way in Europe. But a 2015 report from the US Government Accountability Office (GAO) found that the NIH does a poor job of enforcing rules requiring that clinical trials include both sexes (see go.nature.com/28ll4nb).

According to the GAO, even if studies include both sexes, the NIH also does not routinely track whether researchers have actually evaluated any differences between them. Klein argues that gathering such data could lead to more-effective programmes—halving vaccine doses for women, for instance.

"People are tending to ignore it for as long as possible," Flanagan says. "People will get a lot of surprises."

SEE ALSO *AIDS (Acquired Immunodeficiency Syndrome); HIV; Sexually Transmitted Infections; United Nations Millennium Goals and Infectious Disease; World Health Organization (WHO)*

BIBLIOGRAPHY

Books

Nelson, Jennifer. *More Than Medicine: A History of the Feminist Women's Health Movement.* New York: New York University Press, 2015.

Periodicals

Hamid Salim, M. A., et al. "Gender Differences in Tuberculosis: A Prevalence Survey Done in Bangladesh." *International Journal of Tuberculosis and Lung Disease* 8, no. 8 (August 2004): 952–957. This article can also be found online at http://www.ingentaconnect.com/content/iuatld/ijtld/2004/00000008/ 00000008/art00005 (accessed March 7, 2018).

Ramjee, Gita, and Brodie Daniels. "Women and HIV in Sub-Saharan Africa." *AIDS Research and Therapy* 10, no. 30 (2013). This article can also be found online at https://aidsrestherapy.biomedcentral.com/articles/10.1186/1742-6405-10-30 (accessed March 5, 2018).

Van Lunzen, Jan, and Marcus Altfeld. "Sex Differences in Infectious Diseases—Common but Neglected." *Journal of Infectious Diseases* 209, suppl. 3 (July 15, 2014): S79–S80. This article can also be found online at https://academic.oup.com/jid/article/209/suppl_3/S79/2192876 (accessed March 5, 2018).

Websites

"Health Equity." Centers for Disease Control and Prevention. https://www.cdc.gov/healthequity/index.html (accessed February 15, 2018).

"Microbicides." HIV.gov. https://www.hiv.gov/hiv-basics/hiv-prevention/potential-future-options/microbicides (accessed March 5, 2018).

"Taking Sex and Gender into Account in Emerging Infectious Disease Programmes: An Analytical Framework." World Health Organization. http://www.wpro.who.int/topics/gender_issues/Takingsexandgenderintoaccount.pdf (accessed March 5, 2018).

"Women's Health." World Health Organization. http://www.who.int/topics/womens_health/en/ (accessed March 5, 2018).

"Women's Health: Fact Sheet." World Health Organization. http://www.who.int/mediacentre/factsheets/fs334/en/ (accessed February 15, 2018).

Melanie Barton Zoltán
Claire Skinner

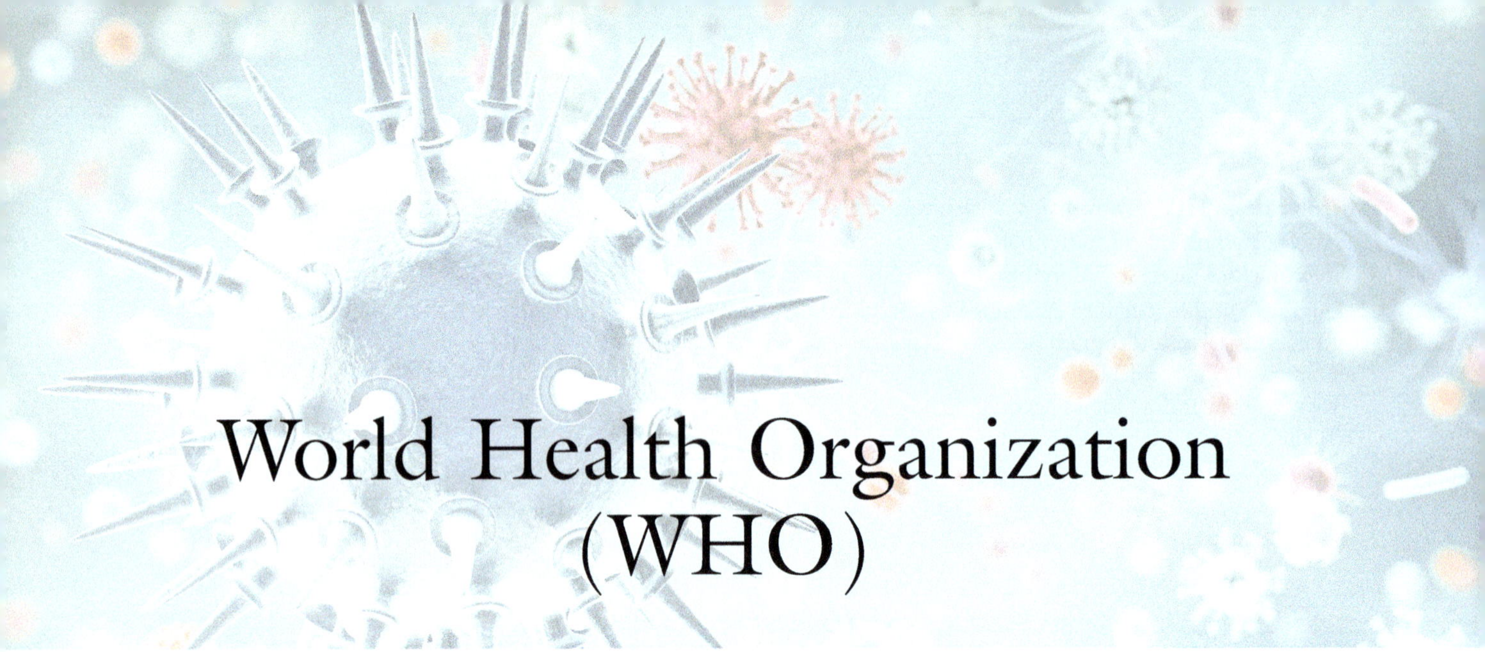

World Health Organization (WHO)

Introduction

The World Health Organization (WHO), as part of the United Nations (UN), has expertise to coordinate international public health matters. Within its constitution, its mission "is the attainment by all peoples of the highest possible level of health." With health as its prime concern, WHO defines health as "a state of complete physical, mental, and social well-being and not merely the absence of disease or infirmity." Its prime concern is to, generally, promote the health of all peoples of the world and to, specifically, combat diseases—especially critical infectious diseases.

The public widely recognizes WHO by much of the work it performs. The organization responds to natural and human-made disasters by providing emergency aid, funds medical research, conducts immunization campaigns against fatal diseases, and improves housing, nutrition, sanitation, and working conditions in developing countries.

WHO is probably best known for its immunization programs and smallpox eradication. In the 21st century it has worked with other health organizations to treat maladies such as tuberculosis, malaria, severe acute respiratory syndrome (SARS), and human immunodeficiency virus/acquired immunodeficiency syndrome (HIV/AIDS).

However, WHO also performs work that is less familiar to the public. It charts statistical health trends and issues warnings about possible health problems. WHO is also responsible for assigning a common international name to each of the drugs used around the world. WHO standards are used for measuring air and water pollution. WHO personnel work with agencies, foundations, governments, nongovernmental organizations, and private-sector groups to address the world's health needs.

Headquartered in Geneva, Switzerland, WHO consists of 194 member states, as of January 2018. It is governed through representatives within its World Health Assembly. A 34-member Executive Board, elected by the World Health Assembly, supports WHO. In addition, six regional committees focus on health concerns within Southeast Asia, the Eastern Mediterranean, the Americas, Africa, the Western Pacific, and Europe. It has offices in over 150 countries around the world.

History and Scientific Foundations

Chinese physician Szeming Sze (1908–1998), Norse physician Karl Evang (1902–1981), and Brazilian physician Geraldo de Paula Souza (1889–1951) proposed the formation of an international health organization in 1945 at the UN Conference on International Organization held in San Francisco, California. The constitution for the international health organization was approved in 1946. The UN approved its charter, and the World Health Organization was established on April 7, 1948, after 61 countries signed its constitution. (This date is celebrated annually as World Health Day.) It became the successor organization of the Health Organization, which was an agency of the League of Nations (an organization founded after World War I, in 1920, to promote peace in the world). The priorities for the fledgling organization were to deal with cholera, malaria, maternal and child health, mental health, nutrition and environmental sanitation, parasitic diseases, plague, smallpox, venereal diseases, yellow fever, and viral diseases. It also expanded immunization programs for diphtheria, measles, poliovirus (commonly called polio), whooping cough, tetanus, and tuberculosis. WHO also worked to improve children and women's health, nutrition, and sanitation around the world. At this time WHO also began to classify diseases according to International Sanitary Regulations, which were renamed International Health Regulations (IHRs) in 1969 to emphasize the importance of combating infectious diseases such as cholera, plague, and yellow fever.

WHO provided health programs for food, food safety, and nutrition; health education; immunizations; prevention and control of endemic diseases; essential drugs; safe water and sanitation; and treatment of diseases and injuries.

After an outbreak of Ebola virus in the Congo went unnoticed by WHO officials for several months in 1995, the organization drastically restructured its surveillance and notification systems and formed the Global Public Health Intelligence Network (GPHIN). The GPHIN enables WHO to search the internet for potential health problems in the world, even when such information is as seemingly inconsequential as a brief note posted on an environmental website. With increasing successes in its operation, the system was expanded in 2000 when it was combined with the Global Outbreak Alert Response Network (GOARN). This allows WHO personnel to analyze data after an outbreak occurred. In all, 120 networks and institutions are linked by this system.

By 2018 WHO had offices in 150 countries of the world, along with six regional offices. It dealt with 194 member countries, while employing more than 7,000 administrators, physicians, epidemiologists, managers, and scientists.

The health priorities for WHO in the 2010s has included communicable diseases (especially Ebola, HIV/AIDS, malaria, and tuberculosis); food security, healthy eating, and nutrition; noncommunicable diseases; occupational health; reproductive and sexual development, health, and aging; and substance abuse. In January 2018 the UN Environment and WHO announced that they would partner to reduce the risks associated with environmental health. The news release stated that approximately 12.6 million deaths per year are caused by such environmental health risks as air and water pollution, climate change, and chemicals and wastes. Of those deaths, the majority occur in the developing countries of Africa, Asia, and Latin America. Other priorities of WHO as of 2018 were acceptance of universal health coverage; authorization of international health regulations; completion of the Sustainable Development Goals (SDGs), which replaced the Millennium Development Goals (MDGs) in 2016; and international access to medical supplies.

WORDS TO KNOW

DIPHTHERIA A potentially fatal, contagious bacterial disease that usually involves the nose, throat, and air passages but may also infect the skin. Its most striking feature is the formation of a grayish membrane covering the tonsils and upper part of the throat.

ENDEMIC Present in a particular area or among a particular group of people.

ERADICATION The process of destroying or eliminating a microorganism or disease.

MULTIBACILLARY The more severe form of leprosy (Hansen's disease). It is defined as the presence of more than five skin lesions on the patient with a positive skin-smear test. The less severe form of leprosy is called paucibacillary leprosy.

PAUCIBACILLARY An infectious condition, such as a certain form of leprosy, characterized by few, rather than many, bacilli, which are a rod-shaped type of bacterium.

SEPSIS A bacterial infection in the bloodstream or body tissues. Sepsis is a very broad term covering the presence of many types of microscopic disease-causing organisms. It is also called bacteremia. Closely related terms include septicemia and septic syndrome.

VENEREAL DISEASE Diseases that are transmitted by sexual contact. They are named after Venus, the Roman goddess of female sexuality.

WATERBORNE DISEASE Diseases that are caused by exposure to contaminated water. The exposure can occur by drinking the water or having the water come in contact with the body. Examples of waterborne diseases are cholera and typhoid fever.

Applications and Research

Three of WHO's largest programs called for the global eradication of smallpox, polio, and leprosy (Hansen's disease). The worldwide campaign to eliminate smallpox, called the Smallpox Eradication Programme, began in 1966 with WHO holding vaccination programs in developing countries. By 1972 only a few countries in Africa and South Asia reported any incidence of smallpox. In 1979 WHO reported that smallpox was eradicated throughout the world. Smallpox was officially declared eradicated a year later, becoming the first disease to be successfully eliminated on a global scale.

In the 1980s WHO led programs to eliminate polio and leprosy worldwide. In 1988 the Global Polio Eradication Initiative (GPEI) was established as a consortium of national governments working to eliminate polio in partnership with five primary organizations: WHO, Rotary International, the US Centers for Disease Control and Prevention (CDC), the United Nations Children's Fund (UNICEF), and the Bill & Melinda Gates Foundation. WHO provides strategic planning, technical direction, and monitoring, evaluation, and certification for the coordinating and planning of GPEI.

As of May 1, 2007, according to the GPEI, the number of polio cases worldwide was 130 (107 in endemic countries and 23 in non-endemic countries). In 2006, 1,997 cases (1,869 in endemic countries and 128 in non-endemic countries) of polio were reported. A decade later, as of January 2018, only three countries (Afghanistan, Nigeria, and Pakistan) continue to have transmission of endemic wild poliovirus. These are called endemic countries. Two countries (Democratic Republic of the Congo and Syrian Arab Republic) are considered outbreak countries. This designation means they have stopped the transmission of domestic wild poliovirus but are encountering external reinfections or vaccine-derived poliovirus. Seventeen other countries are at risk of having polio return.

WHO has been instrumental in reducing the number of leprosy cases around the world. Leprosy, which is caused by the bacterium *Mycobacterium leprae*, primarily affects the skin, along with the eyes, mucous membrane of the upper respiratory tract, and peripheral nerves. The key to this success is a campaign to deliver information, diagnoses, and treatment to endemic countries. The WHO has recommended two types of multidrug therapy (MDT) since 1993: a two-year treatment for multibacillary cases using clofazimine, dapsone, and rifampicin and a six-month treatment for paucibacillary cases using dapsone and rifampicin. Free packs of MDT have been supplied by WHO to all endemic countries since 1995, and this process has been extended into 2020. MDT is provided free of cost to all people with leprosy. It has been funded through the Nippon Foundation (1995–2000) and Novartis (2000–2020).

According to WHO statistics, as of early 2006, approximately 219,826 cases of leprosy were known to exist in 115 countries and territories. In the previous four years, the number of new cases had steadily declined by about 20 percent annually. As of October 2017, 216,108 cases of leprosy have been registered in 145 countries, including Angola, Brazil, Central African Republic, the Congo, India, Madagascar, Mozambique, Nepal, and Tanzania.

In 2016 WHO began its Global Leprosy Strategy 2016–2020, which is dedicated to eliminating leprosy from the planet. The strategy is based on three principles: (1) detecting leprosy before it is visibly discernable; (2) concentrating on high-risk groups through areas and countries most likely to contain leprosy; and (3) improving the accessibility and coverage of health care in populations with the highest risks for leprosy.

Impacts and Issues

In 2000 the United Nations announced the "Water for Life" Decade, a cooperative initiative between several UN agencies and local governments to increase access to clean water and promote sanitation. Contaminated water is a source of infectious disease and parasites. By 2015 their goal was to reduce by half the number of people living without clean water and to aggressively treat or eradicate waterborne diseases and parasites in areas where they have been endemic. As of early 2018 WHO's Water for Life project had provided over 5,800 water wells for people needing clean water. Although billions of people have gained access to safe water and sanitation since 2000, more work needs to be done, with an estimated 2.1 billion people worldwide in 2017 still without safe and readily available drinking water, according to WHO.

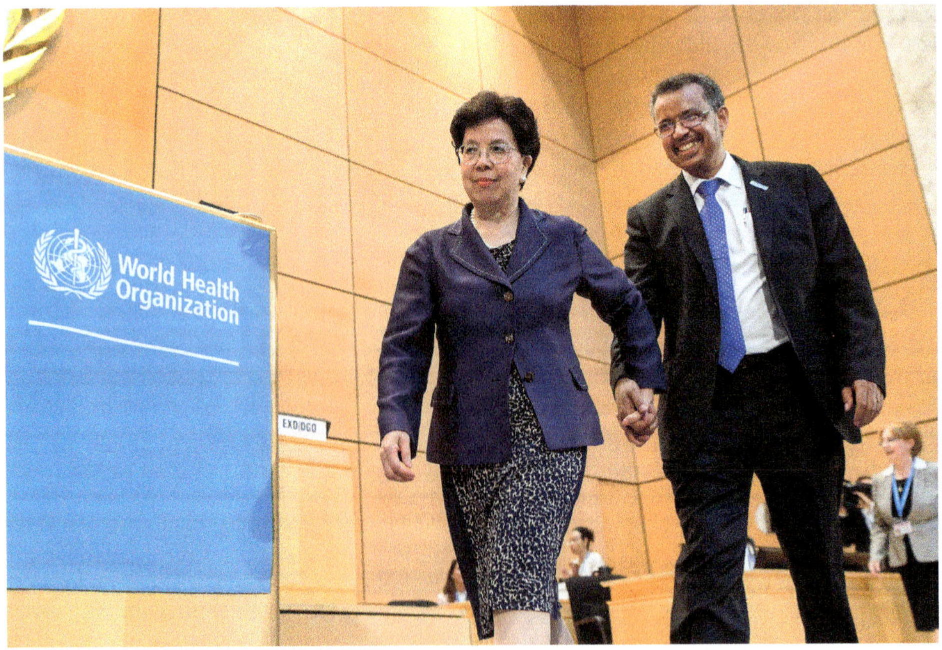

Dr. Tedros Adhanom Ghebreyesus addresses the World Health Assembly in Geneva, Switzerland, on May 23, 2017, after being elected director general of the World Health Organization (WHO), a specialized agency of the United Nations concerned with international public health. Dr. Tedros, an Ethiopian, is the first African to head the WHO. © *FABRICE COFFRINI/AFP/Getty Images*

WHO and UNICEF jointly established the Joint Monitoring Programme for Water Supply, Sanitation and Hygiene (JMP) in 1990. JMP's objectives are threefold: to provide a steady set of reports on drinking water and sanitation with respect to the status of its planning and managing efforts, to support efforts within countries in order to improve their monitoring systems for water and sanitation, and to provide advocacy information.

The JMP's latest status report, *Progress on Drinking Water, Sanitation and Hygiene 2017*, stated that 71 percent (5.2 billion) of the world's population use "safely managed" drinking water services; that is, those readily available and without contamination. In rural areas one out of three people (1.9 billion) have safely managed drinking water services. However, 844 million people remain without basic drinking water services (any improved source within a roundtrip walk of 30 minutes), while another 263 million must walk more than 30 minutes roundtrip to collect water, and still another 159 million people must collect water from surface-water sources.

WHO is also concerned about sepsis because, as of 2018, the bacterial infection was a primary cause of death for infants less than five days old, especially those in the low- and middle-income countries of the world. Antibiotic treatment is recommended in such cases. However, WHO reports in September 2017 that new, more effective antibiotics (those that can control antimicrobial resistance) are not being developed in sufficient quantities. A WHO news release stated that most new antibiotics are only modifications of existing ones. Few treatment options exist for antibiotic-resistant infections. WHO Director-General Tedros Adhanom Ghebreyesus (1965–) stated, "Antimicrobial resistance is a global health emergency that will seriously jeopardize progress in modern medicine."

At the UN Millennium Summit in 2000, 189 governments adopted a set of goals, most aimed at improving the quality of life for people worldwide. The Millennium Development Goals (MDGs) sought to reduce poverty, protect the environment, fight infectious disease, and promote health. WHO was a key organization in the Millennium Goals project. *Millennium Development Goals Report 2015* provided an overview of the accomplishments of the MDGs based on the eight stated goals. (These have since been superseded by 17 Sustainable Development Goals [SDGs] and 169 targets.) The report is summarized with the following: "Although significant achievements have been made on many of the MDG targets worldwide, progress has been uneven across regions and countries, leaving significant gaps." It continued, "Millions of people are being left behind, especially the poorest and those disadvantaged because of their sex, age, disability, ethnicity or geographic location. Targeted efforts will be needed to reach the most vulnerable people."

TEDROS ADHANOM, WHO'S DIRECTOR-GENERAL

As of July 1, 2017, the Director-General of the World Health Organization was Tedros Adhanom Ghebreyesus (1965–). (He goes by the name Tedros Adhanom.) Adhanom is the eighth director-general for the organization, a term that lasts for five years.

Adhanom received a Bachelor of Science degree in biology from the University of Asmara in Eritrea in 1986. Thereafter, he joined the country's Ministry of Health as a junior public health expert. He completed a Master of Science degree in immunology of infectious diseases from the London School of Hygiene & Tropical Medicine and, in 2000, his Doctorate of Philosophy in community health from the University of Nottingham.

In 2001 Adhanom became the head of the Tigray Regional Health Bureau, located in Mekelle, Ethiopia. Two years later, in 2003, he was appointed a Deputy Minister for Health for the country. In 2005 the Ethiopian government named Adhanom its Minister of Health. He held that post into 2012. For the next four years (2012–2016), he was the Minister of Foreign Affairs for Ethiopia.

Through his professional career, Adhanom has authored several professional articles, predominantely on global health issues and especially concerning malaria. In 2003 he received the Young Investigator Award from the Ethiopian Public Health Association. In 2011 he became the first person outside of the United States to receive the Jimmy and Rosalynn Carter Humanitarian Award by the US National Foundation for Infectious Diseases. He was declared one of the 100 most influential Africans of 2015 by *New African* magazine.

In July 2017 WHO reported the perceived benefits and estimated costs of reaching 16 of the 17 SDGs by the year 2030 within 67 low- to middle-income countries of the world. If accomplished, these goals would prevent an estimated 97 million premature deaths between 2017 and 2030. It would also add about 8.4 years of life expectancy to the populations of these countries. However, this accomplishment would come at a cost, what is called the "SDG Health Price Tag." WHO estimated that to reach these targets it would cost $134 billion annually in 2017 and that the price tag would rise steadily to $371 billion by 2030. Furthermore, providing universal health coverage, along with the implementation of the other health targets, would require "not only funding but political will and respect for human rights." Funds would be used to build new health care facilities and improve existing ones, provide currently lacking equipment and medicines, and add over 23 million health care workers worldwide. According to models provided by WHO, approximately 415,000 new health care facilities would need to be built to meet these targets.

SEE ALSO *CDC (Centers for Disease Control and Prevention); Malaria; Polio (Poliomyelitis); Polio Eradication Campaign; Smallpox; Smallpox Eradication and Storage; Tuberculosis*

BIBLIOGRAPHY

Books

Beigbeder, Yves. *The World Health Organization: Achievements and Failures.* New York: Routledge, 2018.

Cooreman, E. A. *Global Leprosy Strategy 2016–2010: Accelerating Towards a Leprosy-Free World.* Geneva: World Health Organization, 2016.

Sze, Szeming. *The Origins of the World Health Organization: A Personal Memoir 1945–1948.* Boca Raton, FL: Lisz, 1982.

The First Ten Years of the World Health Organization (1948–1957). Geneva: World Health Organization, 1958.

The Fourth Ten Years of the World Health Organization (1978–1987). Geneva: World Health Organization, 2011.

The Second Ten Years of the World Health Organization (1958–1967). Geneva: World Health Organization, 1968.

The Third Ten Years of the World Health Organization (1968–1977). Geneva: World Health Organization, 2008.

Websites

"Brief History of WHO." Credible Voice, Columbia University. http://ccnmtl.columbia.edu/projects/caseconsortium/casestudies/112/casestudy/www/layout/case_id_112_id_776.html> (accessed January 18, 2018).

Global Polio Eradication Initiative. http://www.polioeradication.org/ (accessed January 18, 2018).

"The Millennium Development Goals Report 2015." United Nations. http://www.un.org/millenniumgoals/2015_MDG_Report/pdf/MDG%202015%20rev%20(July%201).pdf (accessed January 18, 2018).

"Progress on Drinking Water, Sanitation and Hygiene 2017." World Health Organization and UNICEF. http://apps.who.int/iris/bitstream/10665/258617/1/9789241512893-eng.pdf?ua=1 (accessed January 18, 2018).

"2.1 Billion People Lack Safe Drinking Water at Home, More Than Twice as Many Lack Safe Sanitation." World Health Organization, July 12, 2017. http://www.who.int/mediacentre/news/releases/2017/water-sanitation-hygiene/en/ (accessed January 18, 2018).

"UN Environment and WHO Agree to Major Collaboration on Environmental Health Risks." World Health Organization, January 10. 2018. http://www.who.int/mediacentre/news/releases/2018/environmental-health-collaboration/en/ (accessed January 17, 2018).

"Water for LIFE." LIFE Outreach International. https://lifetoday.org/outreaches/water-for-life/ (accessed January 18, 2018).

"WHO Estimates Cost of Reaching Global Health Targets by 2030." World Health Organization, July 17, 2017. http://www.who.int/mediacentre/news/releases/2017/cost-health-targets/en/ (accessed January 17, 2018).

"WHO/UNICEF Joint Monitoring Program for Water Supply, Sanitation and Hygiene (JMP) —2017 Update and SDG Baselines." UN-WATER, July 12, 2017. http://www.unwater.org/publications/whounicef-joint-monitoring-program-water-supply-sanitation-hygiene-jmp-2017-update-sdg-baselines/ (accessed January 18, 2018).

World Health Organization http://www.who.int/en/ (accessed May 8, 2007).

"World Health Statistics 2017: Monitoring Health for the SDGs." World Health Organization. http://www.who.int/gho/publications/world_health_statistics/2017/en/ (accessed January 17, 2018).

"The World Is Running Out of Antibiotics, WHO Report Confirms." World Health Organization, September 20, 2017. http://www.who.int/mediacentre/news/releases/2017/running-out-antibiotics/en> (accessed January 24, 2018).

William Arthur Atkins

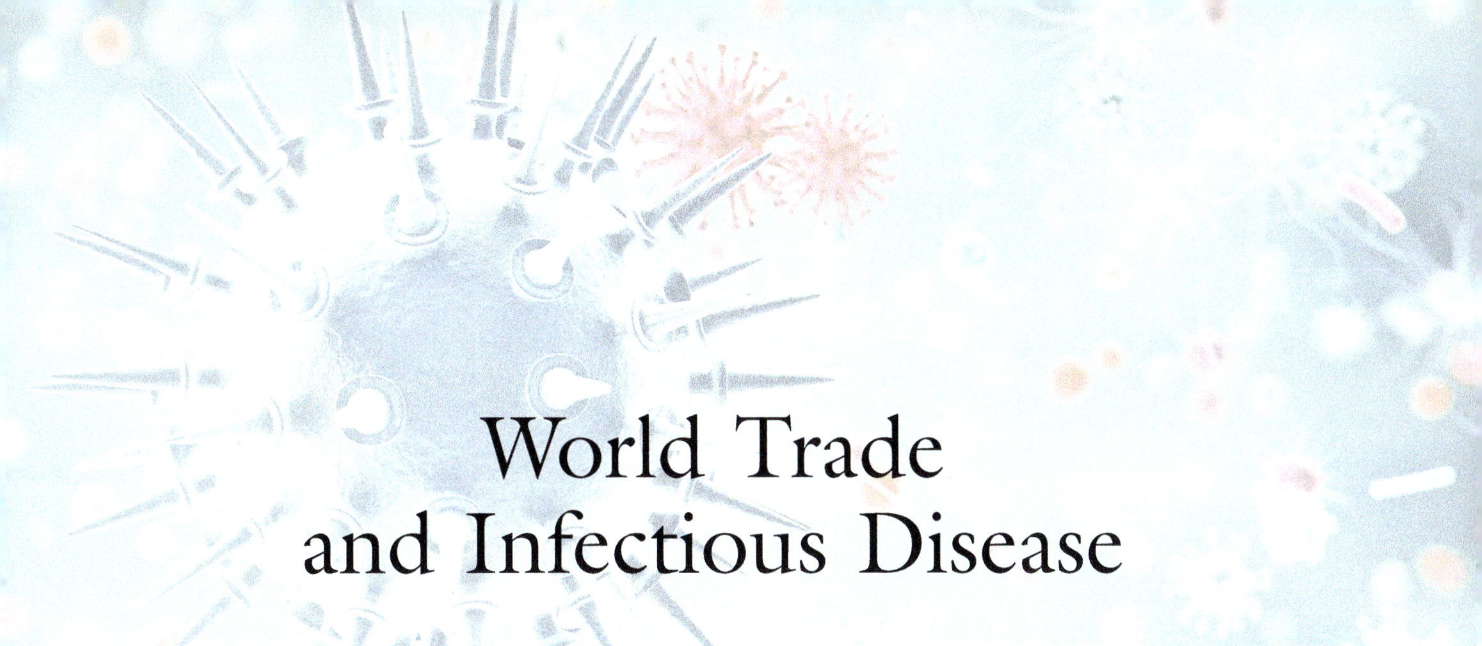

World Trade and Infectious Disease

Introduction

World trade affects the epidemiology of infectious diseases in numerous ways, including commercial travel by air and rail, shipping of contaminated goods, transportation of disease vectors with shipped goods or via commercial transportation, and the consumption of translocated plants and animals that have been infected with nonnative pathogens.

The globalization of world commerce has brought about unprecedented contact between populations and exposure to foreign pathogenic organisms that is radically changing the distribution of communicable diseases worldwide. Consequently, the urgency of international collaboration on public health information and disease control has risen to a point where an outbreak of a serious communicable disease anywhere in the world raises alarms and spawns defensive activity everywhere. The limiting of the severe acute respiratory syndrome (SARS) outbreak in 2004 through quarantine and restriction of wild animal markets and social interaction provides an example of how such collective defense measures can be effective. However, lessons taken from that outbreak and sober reflection on the potential virulence of certain pathogens such as avian influenza, anthrax, and tuberculosis have revealed gaps in international cooperation and preparedness for the consequences of possible pandemics that world trade could facilitate. The future of disease control and local public health will increasingly depend on the processes of globalization and their impact on the distribution of pathogens and on environmental change, which can create new ecological niches for pathogenic organisms.

History and Scientific Foundations

The Impact of Globalization

Human travel and movement have been the main source of epidemics throughout recorded history. Trade caravans, religious pilgrimages, and military maneuvers facilitated the spread of many diseases, including plague and smallpox. Smallpox is presumed to have spread from Egypt or India along historical trade routes, where it was first thought to have become adapted to humans sometime before 1000 BCE. For most of history, human populations were relatively isolated. Only in recent centuries has there been extensive contact between the peoples, flora, and fauna of the Old and New Worlds. Contact between European colonists and Native American populations during trade and exploration led to the transmission of measles, influenza, mumps, smallpox, tuberculosis, and other infections from the crowded urban centers of Europe, which caused the suddenly exposed Native American populations to drop by at least one-third.

Intensifying global trade, which entails deregulated trade and investment, can have a mixed impact on public health. When global trade brings economic growth and disseminates technologies such as antibiotics and other medications that enhance life expectancy, there are broad benefits to public health. However, some aspects of globalization erode public health infrastructure and jeopardize health by causing the deterioration of social and environmental conditions, undermining the livelihoods of certain population groups, and sowing some unhealthful lifestyle patterns. Global environmental changes related to population growth and intensified economic activity include air pollution, deforestation and desertification, depletion of terrestrial aquifers and ocean fisheries, and decreased biodiversity. Some of these processes pose public health risks.

On the positive side, improvements in the public health of industrializing countries have resulted from widespread social, nutritional, and material changes such as rising living standards that make possible improved sanitation and other more deliberate public health interventions, including vaccination and disease vector eradication programs. Health gains have begun more recently in developing nations in the wake of population control efforts, application of knowledge about sanitation and vaccination,

WORDS TO KNOW

BUSHMEAT The meat of terrestrial wild and exotic animals, typically those that live in parts of Africa, Asia, and the Americas; also known as wild meat.

ENDEMIC Present in a particular area or among a particular group of people.

EPIDEMIOLOGY The study of various factors that influence the occurrence, distribution, prevention, and control of disease, injury, and other health-related events in a defined human population. By the application of various analytical techniques, including mathematical analysis of the data, the probable cause of an infectious outbreak can be pinpointed.

GLOBALIZATION The integration of national and local systems into a global economy through increased trade, manufacturing, communications, and migration.

HERD IMMUNITY A resistance to disease that occurs in a population when a proportion of them have been immunized against it. The theory is that it is less likely that an infectious disease will spread in a group where some individuals are less likely to contract it.

PATHOGENIC Causing or capable of causing disease.

VECTOR Any agent that carries and transmits parasites and diseases. Also, an organism or a chemical used to transport a gene into a new host cell.

ZOONOTIC A disease that can be transmitted between animals and humans. Examples of zoonotic diseases are anthrax, plague, and Q fever.

improved nutrition, vector control, and gradually improved treatment of infectious diseases. However, shifts in the ecology of local habitats brought about by environmental change related to globalization can have a profound impact on the distribution of infectious diseases.

Globalization and the Ecology of Infectious Disease

The main reason for the adverse effects of globalization is the disruption of traditional and largely self-contained agricultural societies that produce, consume, and trade on a local basis, using technologies that have a low impact on the environment. The social and environmental determinants of public health for these societies are predominantly local. Over the course of the 20th century, industrialization and modernization have changed the amount of contact, influence, and trade between societies; created new hierarchical business associations; and increased the impact of technology on the environment. The former balance between local populations and the pathogens in their environments is often disturbed, and new pathogens are introduced into local regions, increasing the probability of serious disease outbreaks for which local people either lack herd immunity or the means for effective treatment.

Globalization of commerce and culture has also spurred an increase in human mobility. Much of this travel is voluntary, connected with business, tourism, and movement of labor. Some of this mobility is involuntary, caused by war, which is often connected with trade advantage or resource access issues; social breakdown; and natural disasters. A recent study found that the number of environmental and political refugees has increased about tenfold since 1980. The increased transnational movement of labor generally brings economic benefits to both developed and developing economies but also increases the transmission of ideas, values, and microbiological agents that affect disease patterns.

The globalization of world trade thus fundamentally changes the ecological context of infectious disease epidemiology by opening new opportunities for transmission and environmental niches for pathogens while also increasing the need for transnational public health information sharing and cooperation for disease prevention and treatment. Perhaps more than any other current trend, world trade brings home the importance of viewing epidemiology as more than the analysis of risk factors for disease but rather as the study of ecological systems that mediate disease distribution and causation.

Global Trade and Travel

Global trade necessitates greatly increased travel for transactions, and travel is a major force in disease emergence and spread. According to the US Centers for Disease Control and Prevention (CDC), the current volume, speed, and reach of travel are unprecedented. Travel and trade facilitate the mixing of diverse genetic pools and harbored microorganisms at rates and in combinations unknown. Such massive mobility and other concomitant changes in social, political, climatic, environmental, and technologic factors have converged to favor the emergence of infectious diseases.

Disease emergence or reemergence generally requires several simultaneous events. Travel introduces a potentially pathogenic microbe into a new geographic region. However, to become established and cause disease, a microorganism must survive, proliferate, and find a way to enter a vulnerable host.

Global travel, changing patterns of resistance and susceptibility, and the emergence of infectious diseases also affect plants, animals, and insect vectors. Infectious diseases are dynamic. Most new infections are not caused by genuinely new pathogens. Agents involved in new and reemergent infections include viruses, bacteria, fungi, protozoa, and helminths. Human activities that provide new opportunities for the proliferation of these microbes are the most potent factors driving infectious disease emergence.

Travel is relevant in the emergence of disease if it changes an ecosystem in ways that promote the transmission of disease by introducing new organisms or by altering the ecosystem in ways that facilitate the proliferation of new or endemic pathogens. Travel introduces such organisms by transporting pathogens in or on travelers' bodies, including microbiologic flora or disease vectors, and carrying dormant infections that have been controlled by travelers' immune systems and genetic makeup but to which native populations are not immune. Pathogens are also introduced to new ecosystems by luggage and whatever it contains. Direct change of native ecosystems in ways that favor disease emergence can occur when trade brings about changes in cultural preferences, customs, behavioral patterns, and local technology.

Applications and Research

Worldwide trade in wildlife creates opportunities for infectious disease transmission that cause outbreaks in both humans and livestock. In turn, these outbreaks threaten international trade, agriculture, native wildlife populations, and the integrity of local ecosystems. Disease outbreaks resulting from wildlife trade have caused hundreds of billions of dollars of economic destruction globally.

According to the CDC, estimating the volume of the global wildlife trade is extremely difficult because it encompasses activities ranging from local barter to major international commerce via ships, rail, and aircraft. A significant proportion of this trade is conducted either informally or illegally. It is estimated that 40,000 live primates, 4 million live birds, 640,000 live reptiles, and 350 million live tropical fish are traded globally each year. Guangzhou, China, has live wildlife markets that trade in masked palm civets, ferret badgers, barking deer, wild boars, hedgehogs, foxes, squirrels, bamboo rats, gerbils, snakes, and endangered leopards, as well as domesticated dogs, cats, and rabbits. Lacking precise trade data, the CDC conservatively estimates that, in East and Southeast Asia, tens of millions of wild animals are shipped annually, both within the region and from around the world for food or use in traditional medicine. The estimate for trade and regional consumption of wild animal meat in Central Africa is more than 2.2 billion pounds (1 billion kilograms) per year, and estimates for consumption in the Amazon Basin are in the range of 220 million pounds (100 million kilograms) annually. For mammals this amounts to 6.4 million to 15.8 million individual animals. In Central Africa estimates range over 500 million mammals.

Hunters, brokers/distributors, and consumers have some degree of contact as each animal is traded. Other wildlife in the trade is exposed, as are domesticated animals and wild scavengers in villages and market areas that consume the remnants and wastes from the traded wildlife. The CDC calculates that multiple billions of direct and indirect contacts among wildlife, humans, and domesticated animals result from the wildlife trade annually. The global scope of this trade, together with rapid modern transportation and the role of markets as network hubs rather than as final destinations, dramatically increases the movement and potential cross-species transmission of communicable pathogens that every animal naturally hosts. Because trade in wildlife functions as networks with the markets as major hubs, these markets provide control opportunities to maximize the effects of public health and other regulatory efforts.

Far from being a peripheral public health risk, trade in wild animals presents one of the most severe health threats facing modern society. Perhaps the most significant human disease outbreak in the 21st century directly attributable to wildlife trade, specifically trade in civet cats, was the epidemic of SARS in 2003.

The Guangzhou wildlife markets were visited by experts from the Chinese Ministry of Science and Technology, the Ministry of Health, the World Health Organization (WHO), and the Food and Agriculture Organization (FAO) of the United Nations (UN) to investigate the connection with the SARS epidemic, which spread rapidly to other continents due to travel. Control efforts in Guangzhou involved the confiscation of a reported 838,500 wild animals from the markets. A study of antibody evidence of exposure to the SARS coronavirus demonstrated a dramatic rise from low or zero prevalence of civets at farms to an approximately 80 percent prevalence in civets tested in markets.

Since 1980 more than 35 new infectious diseases have emerged in humans, approximately one every eight months. The origin of HIV is likely linked to human consumption of nonhuman primates. Recent Ebola hemorrhagic fever outbreaks have been traced to index patient contact with infected great apes that are hunted for food.

The collateral transmission of infectious agents due to the wildlife trade is not limited to human pathogens but also involves pathogens of domestic animals and native wildlife. Ominously, H5N1 type A influenza virus was isolated from two mountain hawk eagles illegally imported to Belgium from Thailand in 2005. The virus had been limited to poultry but began infecting migrating birds, as well as mammals and humans. Although human-to-human transmission has not yet been detected, H5N1 presents a clear threat of a pandemic, for which WHO and other organizations are preparing. Monkeypox was transmitted to a native rodent species and then to humans in the United States by imported wild African rodents for the US pet trade. Chytridiomycosis, a fungal disease identified as a major cause of the extinction of 30 percent of amphibian species worldwide, has been spread by the international trade in African clawed frogs.

Many domestic animal diseases are transmitted through the same species of parasites carried by imported animals. Ticks have been removed from nearly 100 shipments of wild animals inspected by the US Department of Agriculture. Ticks carry many diseases that threaten livestock and human health, including heartwater disease, Lyme disease, and babesiosis.

CDC examination of epidemiological data indicates that the possibility of emerging infectious diseases spreading between people and animals is rising due to human activities ranging from the handling of bushmeat and the trade in exotic animals to the destruction or disturbance of wild habitat. The majority (61 percent) of listed human pathogens are known to be zoonotic, and multiple host pathogens are twice as likely to be associated with an emerging human infectious disease. More than three-quarters of pathogens found in livestock are shared with other host species.

The sudden increase of emerging or reemerging livestock disease outbreaks around the world since the mid-1990s, including bovine spongiform encephalopathy (BSE), foot-and-mouth disease, avian influenza, and swine fever, has cost the world economy $80 billion. In early 2003 the UN reported that more than one-third of the global meat trade was embargoed as a result of mad cow disease, avian influenza, and other livestock disease outbreaks. A single reported case of BSE in 2003 brought about an embargo that devastated the beef industry in Canada. Beef prices and exports did not recover until months after the embargo was lifted. Efforts to control the spread of avian influenza in Asian countries since 2003 have required the culling of more than 140 million chickens.

Any attempt to eradicate the trade in wild species is doomed to failure. However, the experience of slowing the spread of SARS by regulating the market in Guangzhou shows that focusing efforts at wildlife markets to regulate, reduce, or in some cases eliminate the trade in particular wildlife species could provide a cost-effective approach to decreasing the risks of disease for humans, domestic animals, wildlife, and ecosystems.

■ Impacts and Issues

The International Health Regulations (IHR) are the only existing global regulations for infectious disease control. These regulations had not been appreciably changed since their original issuance in 1951. WHO is currently attempting to modernize the IHR, in view of the many emerging global public health threats posed by international trade, travel, and other worldwide human activity.

In 2007 revisions to the IHR were adopted obligating member states to "detect, assess, report, and respond to potential public health emergencies of international concern (PHEIC) at all levels of government, and to report such events rapidly to the WHO to determine whether a coordinated, global response is required." Nevertheless, flaws in the international response to public health emergencies were exposed by mistakes made by government and international health agencies in addressing the Ebola outbreak in 2014. In an article published in the *Lancet* in 2017, Rebecca Katz and Scott F. Dowell recommended IHR revisions to improve global health, including the following:

- Metrics that assess national capacity and compliance
- Sample sharing beyond influenza
- International contact tracing to identify and coordinate public health measures for high-risk travelers
- Assigning responsibilities for coordinating the response in a multinational emergency
- Assisting nations with developing the required capacities
- Applying IHR to animal diseases and development of local health systems

Overall, recommendations are for according WHO with sweeping responsibility for enforcing health norms and ensuring state compliance while providing generous economic and technical assistance to developing countries. Enforcement options for WHO remain unclear, but there is an implicit reliance in the recommendations on the power of world public opinion, possibly backed by sanctions imposed by influential countries against those who withhold cooperation. Given the intimacy with which the world is now connected in the struggle against infectious disease, developed and developing nations have an equal stake in ensuring that all countries have the tools to combat emerging and reemerging diseases that result from global trade.

PRIMARY SOURCE

Trafficking Wildlife and Transmitting Disease: Bold Threats in an Era of Ebola

SOURCE: *Bouley, Timothy, and Sara Thompson. "Trafficking Wildlife and Transmitting Disease: Bold Threats in an Era of Ebola." World Bank,*

October 2, 2014. https://blogs.worldbank.org/voices/trafficking-wildlife-and-transmitting-disease-bold-threats-era-ebola (accessed February 26, 2018).

INTRODUCTION: *The illegal trade in wildlife is associated with the spread of infectious diseases. Written during the height of the Ebola outbreak in 2014, this World Bank blog post examines the global threat posed by wildlife trafficking.*

The Ebola epidemic in Guinea, Liberia and Sierra Leone continues to spread despite country and international efforts to stop it in its tracks and make sure it never returns. As of October 1, 3,338 people have died and 7,178 are infected. More people have perished in this latest Ebola outbreak than in all previous outbreaks of the virus on the continent combined. In addition to the large number of people who have died, and the steady march of new infections, the three hardest-hit countries are also suffering heavy economic costs from trade and travel restrictions, food being in short supply, and other impacts. While health workers, international health agencies, and charities work furiously to contain the outbreak, we must also think ahead so that we might avoid similar epidemics in the future. What might the first step be? Better understanding the animal origins of Ebola and other infectious diseases so that we can prevent an epidemic like this from ever happening again.

Ebola is a zoonotic disease, meaning that it is transmitted from animals to humans. In past outbreaks, this has occurred during the handling of wildlife—bats, gorillas, chimpanzees, monkeys, even porcupines. The running hypothesis for this outbreak is that it came from bats, though an early focus of consideration was on primates trafficked through capital cities. Regardless of the precise path of transmission, it is clear that we must examine human relationships with wildlife to ensure we protect against this and other future disease risks.

On one hand, humans embrace our relationship with the wild, advocating for greater protection of natural spaces and species. On another, we exploit it, in sometimes careless and unsustainable ways. As human populations grow, new arcs of deforestation and degradation open, and the climate changes, we enable new wildlife interactions near dense (human) population centers in warm, humid climates, already ripe for disease transmission. Worse yet is that outbreaks are not limited only to those geographies close to wildlife hotspots. International travel and trade mean that these diseases can be exported as easily as any commodity in a shipping crate. In many instances there are measures in place to protect against this, such as regulations of what can be transported abroad coupled with airport and shipyard screenings. Yet, there is much which flies under the radar of these precautions—none of which may pose a more serious threat than wildlife trafficking.

Globally, the illegal wildlife trade market accounts for some $10–20 billion annually, comprising both live and dead species. In Central Africa, the market estimate for wild animal meat is greater than one billion kilograms per year. As wildlife is traded between hunters, middle marketers, and consumers, there are, quite literally, billions of opportunities for disease transmission among wildlife, humans, and domestic animals each year. At the global level, wildlife trafficking is perpetrated by organized criminal networks which illicitly transit wildlife and animal products from country to country. As it is transported, often through densely populated and heavily trafficked cities, countless opportunities for disease transmission occur. In addition to disease risks, wildlife trafficking can also threaten livestock, rural livelihoods, native wildlife populations, and ecosystem health, further imperiling those communities most near the human-animal interface.

The World Bank commits $60 million per year to combat wildlife crime to include projects addressing illegal logging, illegal, unreported, and unregulated (IUU) fishing, elephant poaching, and others. Collectively through our natural resource management, economic, trade facilitation, anti-money laundering, legal, judiciary, and governance expertise, we can play a significant role in combatting wildlife crime. We have also published a roadmap to promote and achieve compliance to mitigate risks from ill-conceived or misdirected enforcement efforts and separately, participate in the International Consortium on Combatting Wildlife Crime (ICCWC)--with UNODC, Interpol, the CITES Secretariat, and WCO. Through these efforts we believe we can better understand and overcome the problems surrounding wildlife crime, which can have rippling effects on the global community.

Though ongoing, the Ebola crisis is helping us better understand our inadequacies in public health and environmental management, and the absolute necessity of better linking the two. Wildlife trafficking is merely but one issue that links environmental sustainability to human health and well-being. If we are to collectively address these issues in the future, we must seize upon the opportunity now to raise the profile of these conversations so that they may be incorporated into general practice and action moving forward.

SEE ALSO *Public Health and Infectious Disease; Travel and Infectious Disease*

BIBLIOGRAPHY

Books

Myers, Norman, and Jennifer Kent. *Environmental Exodus: An Emergent Crisis in the Global Arena.* New York: Climate Institute, 1995.

Periodicals

Gostin, Lawrence O. "International Infectious Disease Law: Revision of the World Health Organization's International Health Regulations." *Journal of the American Medical Association* 291 (2004): 2623–2627. This article can also be found online at http://jama.ama-assn.org/cgi/content/full/291/21/2623 (accessed May 26, 2007).

Karesh, W. B., et al. "Wildlife Trade and Global Disease Emergence." *Emerging Infectious Diseases* 11, no. 7 (July 2005): 1000–1002.

Katz, Rebecca, and Scott F. Dowell. "Revising the International Health Regulations: Call for a 2017 Review Conference." *Lancet Global Health* 3, no. 7 (July 2015): e352–e353. This article can also be found online at http://www.thelancet.com/journals/langlo/article/PIIS2214-109X(15)00025-X/fulltext.

McMichael A. J., and R. Beaglehole. "The Changing Global Context of Public Health." *Lancet* 356, 9228 (August 2000): 495–499.

Kenneth T. LaPensee

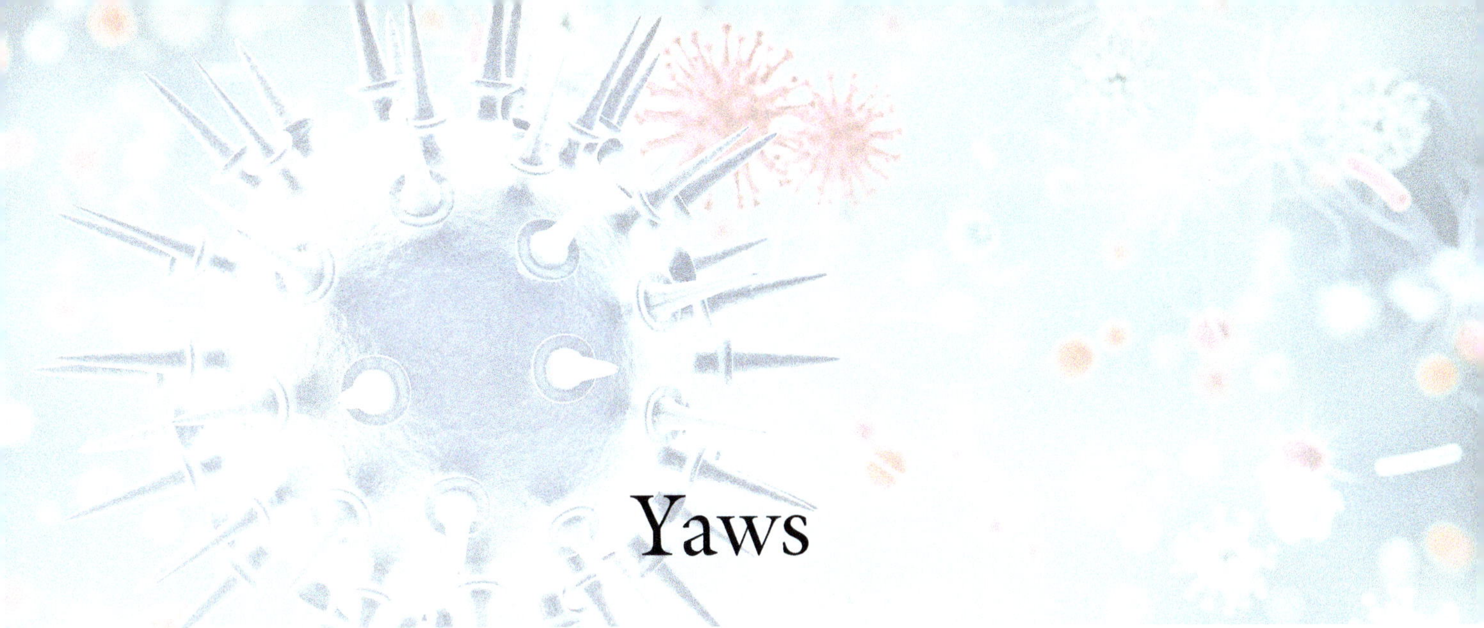

Yaws

Introduction

Yaws is a chronic infection that primarily affects the skin, bones, and cartilage of its victims, who are mostly children. A spiral-shaped bacterium, *Treponema pertenue*, causes yaws. These bacteria, or spirochetes, are closely related to the bacteria that causes syphilis. The spirochetes spread from person to person by direct contact of skin with infectious yaws sores.

Effects of poverty such as overcrowding, poor sanitation, and dirty water all contribute to spreading yaws, and the disease primarily affects the poor in rural tropical areas of Africa, Asia, and Latin America. Yaws is nearly unknown in developed countries.

Disease History, Characteristics, and Transmission

The initial lesion of yaws appears where the bacteria enter the skin, and soon a red bump, or papule, develops. The papule, measuring 0.8 to 2.0 inches (2 to 5 centimeters) in diameter, is painless but often itchy. Scratching results in an open, ulcerated sore. This first sore takes three to six months to heal. Meanwhile, the spirochetes spread to other parts of the body through the lymph system or the bloodstream.

Soon more red papules similar to the initial sore develop. Eventually multiple sores spread over the body of the infected individual. During the wet season in the tropics, these sores may get quite large and resemble fleshy, red, wartlike growths. They eventually heal, but scars often develop at the sites of the sores. The disease is not fatal, but relapses are common up to 10 years after the initial infection.

Other problems caused by the yaws bacteria include enlarged lymph nodes in the armpits, neck, or groin. Sores may develop on the feet (making walking quite difficult) or the palms. The bones, particularly the bones of the fingers and the long bones in the arms and legs, may be affected, as well as the skin. Pain from the affected bones makes sleeping difficult.

The disease may seem to go away after a few years, but the bacteria remain in the skin and bones. The latent (dormant) period may persist, but, in about 10 percent of those afflicted, the sores reappear after five years. When yaws reappears, the individual suffers marked thickening of the skin on the palms and soles, as well as hard nodules under the skin around the joints. Particularly disfiguring are bony growths in the bones of the upper jaw and nose. The skin and membranes of the nose and upper mouth can be in-

WORDS TO KNOW

INCIDENCE The number of new cases of a disease or an injury that occur in a population during a specified period of time.

LATENT INFECTION An infection already established in the body but not yet causing symptoms or having ceased to cause symptoms after an active period.

PAPULE A small, solid bump on the skin.

REEMERGING INFECTIOUS DISEASE Illnesses such as malaria, diphtheria, tuberculosis, and polio that were once nearly absent from the world but are starting to cause greater numbers of infections once again. These illnesses are reappearing for many reasons. Malaria and other mosquito-borne illnesses increase when mosquito-control measures decrease. Other diseases are spreading because people have stopped being vaccinated, as happened with diphtheria after the collapse of the Soviet Union. A few diseases are reemerging because drugs to treat them have become less available or drug-resistant strains have developed.

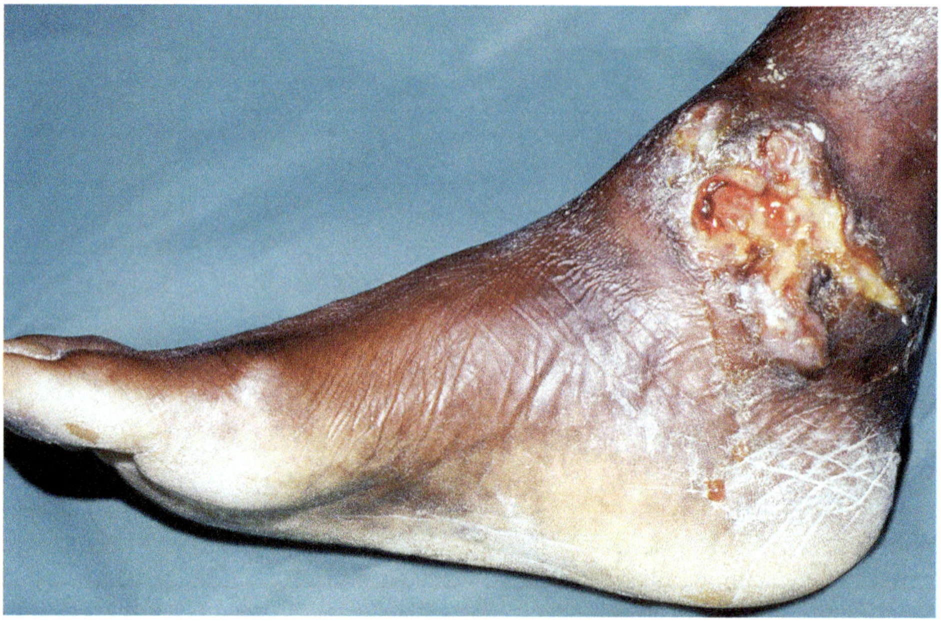

The foot of a patient infected with yaws, a bacterial infection of the skin, bones, and joints common to tropical regions that is caused by the bacterium *Treponema pertenue.* © Clinical Photography, Central Manchester University Hospitals NHS Foundation Trust, UK/Science Source

volved and result in the destruction of the upper mouth and nasal passages. Where the mouth and nose were, a gaping hole develops.

Scope and Distribution

Yaws occurs mostly in children under age 15 and mostly in tropical, forested areas of Africa, Asia, Latin America, and Oceania. The World Health Organization (WHO) reported in 2017 that approximately 89 million people lived in the 13 countries endemic for yaws, although the number of people in those endemic countries infected with yaws remained unknown.

Treatment and Prevention

Yaws is a disease with a cure. WHO has recommended yaws be treated with one dose of the antibiotic azithromycin. If a dose of azithromycin does not cure the disease, or if the patient is allergic to azithromycin, then an injection of the antibiotic penicillin should be given. Patients should be seen by a medical professional one month after antibiotic treatment to confirm they are no longer infected with yaws. Treatment is effective about 95 percent of the time. There is no vaccine for yaws.

Impacts and Issues

In the 1950s WHO mounted a campaign to eliminate yaws. After more than 300 million people received treatment, the global incidence of yaws dropped by more than 95 percent. Unfortunately, interest waned, and with reduced surveillance yaws has made a comeback, reemerging in the 21st century.

In 2007 WHO convened to revive interest in eliminating yaws. The strategy developed at the meeting involves identifying people at risk for yaws, actively treating all infected people and their close contacts, and implementing a renewed surveillance effort. In 2012 WHO established the Yaws Eradication Strategy, which shifted treatment of the disease from penicillin to azithromycin. WHO also announced its goal to eliminate yaws completely by 2020. In 2016 India announced it had eliminated yaws.

Archeologists found evidence of yaws in the bones of human ancient ancestors. Modern medicine has the ability to ensure this disease disappears from the historical record, and no more children (the group most afflicted) suffer the disfigurement of yaws.

PRIMARY SOURCE

Papua New Guinea Struggles to Eradicate Yaws Disease

SOURCE: *Smyth, Jamie. "Papua New Guinea Struggles to Eradicate Yaws Disease."* Financial Times *(April 17, 2017). This article can also be found online at https://www.ft.com/content/9b97ee86-ff65-11e6-8d8e-a5e3738f9ae4 (accessed February 5, 2018).*

INTRODUCTION: *In the following article, the author discusses the treatment of yaws in Papua New Guinea and summarizes the efforts of the World Health Organization (WHO) to eliminate yaws from the globe. The author notes that, although there is an affordable treatment for yaws (namely, the antibiotic drug azithromycin), WHO has not been able to raise enough money to pay for mass treatment.*

At first the lump on Timish Ongula's right leg was barely noticeable, but within six weeks it had developed into a painful, golf ball-sized ulcer that oozed pus and blood, making it difficult for the four-year-old girl to walk. "Timish cried a lot and had a lot of trouble sleeping. The sore grew so fast that we took her to the hospital to get medical treatment," says Noreen Brast, her mother. "Thank God we did."

Timish lives at Landolam migrant settlement, a collection of ramshackle wooden huts on Lihir, a tiny tropical island in the south-west Pacific a two-hour flight from Port Moresby, the capital of Papua New Guinea. Her family is one of many to have moved to Lihir from other parts of the country, lured by work in a local gold mine and its surrounding markets. She was diagnosed with yaws, a disease that affects hundreds of thousands of people living in the world's poorest countries.

Yaws is caused by the bacteria *Treponema pallidum*, another variety of which causes syphilis. Yaws is spread via skin contact rather than sex, however, and typically affects children, who are more prone to cuts and scratches that become infected with the bacteria. It is especially prevalent among those who live in crowded and unsanitary conditions. In its initial stages it causes lesions on the skin, but left untreated, it can lead to disability and deformity.

Yaws is not difficult to treat: just one tablet of an antibiotic, azithromycin, costing about $0.17, is enough. This is what Timish received and "the ulcer improved very fast", according to her doctor, Oriol Mitjà. "After two days the ulcer stopped oozing and bleeding, which indicates that the bacteria have disappeared, and after two weeks there was complete wound healing."

Mitjà has been working at the Lihir medical centre (a facility run jointly by the government and private funding) since 2010 and his research has reignited interest in yaws among global health authorities. It was Mitjà's discovery in 2012 that a single tablet of azithromycin was as effective as the traditional treatment for yaws — an injection of the antibiotic benzathine penicillin — that persuaded the World Health Organisation to design a new strategy the same year to eradicate the disease all over the world by 2020.

"Mitjà's discovery was of great significance, as it makes large-scale treatment of affected populations more practical," says Kingsley Asiedu, the doctor responsible for the WHO eradication campaign. "A dose of azithromycin is cheap and easy to administer. Injections are much more cumbersome as they require administration by healthcare workers and cause a lot of pain for the children."

If it works, this WHO campaign will be only the second ever to result in the successful eradication of a human pathogen. Smallpox, its only success to date, was officially declared eradicated after a global campaign in 1980. But five years after the yaws strategy was launched, the WHO has run into the twin obstacles of a lack of drugs and one of funding. The organisation initiated talks with Pfizer, the pharmaceuticals multinational and manufacturer of azithromycin, over the possible donation of tablets in 2012, but so far these efforts have come to nothing, says Asiedu. "The 2020 timeline is not going to happen now. We have not made the progress we anticipated back in 2012," he says.

This is not the first time the WHO has tried to eradicate yaws. A previous attempt between 1952 and 1964 was unsuccessful. At that time, health workers treated about 50m cases across 46 countries by administering injections of penicillin. By the end of the campaign, the number of cases dropped by 95 per cent to 2.5m, but as the incidence declined, healthcare authorities redirected their attention elsewhere. "Funds dried up, staff moved on to other jobs and surveillance programmes were discontinued, so no one knew how many cases there were," says David Mabey, professor of communicable diseases at the London School of Hygiene and Tropical Medicine. "Yaws was forgotten."

At Lihir medical centre, where Timish is now able to take part in running races with her friends, the consequences of failing to treat the disease quickly are plain to see. Nine-year-old Stanis Malome caught the disease three years ago but did not seek medical attention. The infection has now spread to his shin bone, which is badly misshapen and protrudes out of the skin on his leg, causing a permanent open wound. "I left school because of the sore. It's hard to walk," Stanis says. He will live with the disability for the rest of his life.

Mitjà says such cases demonstrate why the global campaign must be rolled out speedily and effectively. "The treatment is so simple, cheap and effective that there is every reason we can achieve this target," he says. "But it takes a global commitment."

Today, the disease is endemic in 13 countries in west Africa, Asia and the Pacific but it may also be present in other poor countries that do not report cases to the WHO. About 90m people are thought to live in exposed areas. So far, the WHO has funded pilot studies in five endemic countries: Papua New Guinea, Congo, Ghana, the Solomon Islands and Vanuatu. Initial results have been promising, showing that providing a dose of azithromycin to every person in a community whether thought to be infected or not — a strategy known as total community treatment (TCT) — can dramatically cut disease prevalence.

By contrast, in the 1950s, only "active" cases of yaws were targeted. In latent cases, where bacteria were present in the body but did not show noticeable symptoms, the infection was able to recur resulting in a rapid return of the disease. With TCT, health workers believe they can eradicate the bacteria completely.

This new plan is working based on the results of a pilot study in three neighbouring yaws-endemic districts in southern Ghana, says Dr Cynthia Kwakye-Maclean, who co-ordinated the research there. Antibiotics were distributed by volunteers with over 95 per cent coverage across the community. An impact assessment study conducted a year after the trial found a remarkable drop in seroprevalence — the level of a pathogen identified in the population, as measured in blood serum. The main challenges are: the availability of azithromycin; lack of funds to pay the salaries of drug distributors; transportation; supervision; community acceptance, and participation in yaws eradication activities, she adds.

The WHO estimates it will cost about $362m to fund the drugs and outreach programmes needed to eradicate yaws. But it has yet to attract any major donations for its global strategy, despite talks with senior Pfizer executives between 2012 and 2014. In a statement to the FT, Pfizer said it had not studied azithromycin for the treatment of yaws and that the drug was not indicated (authorised by regulators) for this use. "Pfizer does not promote any off-label use of azithromycin or any Pfizer medication. However, we do have a long history of working to address neglected tropical diseases," the company said.

The WHO has begun separate discussions with generic drug manufacturers in the hope that they might donate the millions of tablets that are needed, but so far no agreement has been reached — to the frustration of doctors. "No funds have been raised, no drugs have been donated, there has been no attempt to map the disease globally for over 30 years, so we don't know where it is still a problem or how many cases there are — except in a few countries such as Ghana," says Mabey of the London School of Hygiene and Tropical Medicine.

On Lihir, the Australian mining company Newcrest and International SOS, a medical and travel risk services company, have funded local research efforts. But a major fundraising effort is required if the WHO strategy is to work, says Mitjà. He warns that the unique opportunity to eradicate the disease with azithromycin may not last for ever, as the yaws bacteria could develop resistance — a pattern seen with syphilis. For now, the use of antibiotics in poor countries remains very low, reducing the risk of resistance, but this will increase over time, he says.

Even if enough drugs are provided and funding can be raised, logistical challenges remain. The TCT trial in Lihir in 2012 was initially very successful in reducing the number of cases, but five years on, new cases are being detected. During a spot check by health officials at Kul Destiny primary school, near the Landolam migrant camp, several cases of yaws were identified.

"It really hurts," says Grace Michael, a four-year-old girl, grimacing as Mitjà examines a large ulcer on her ankle. She starts to cry as he pricks her finger to draw some blood to test for yaws. The result is positive.

Later, officials identify more cases at the camp, where families from other areas in Papua New Guinea have recently moved to try and find work in the nearby gold mine and local markets. Many of these children have not been treated and have brought yaws back to the island. Mitjà is seeking funds to extend the Lihir trial to the entire province of New Ireland in Papua New Guinea next year, which would cover 200,000 people and reduce the rate of reinfection.

For Mitjà, the world's failure to deploy a tool that could end their suffering is inexplicable. "If the human race can travel to the moon and back, then it must be able to rid the planet of this debilitating disease," he says. "It now has a powerful tool to do so."

See Also *Reemerging Infectious Diseases*

BIBLIOGRAPHY

Books

Matthews, Philippa C. *Tropical Medicine Notebook.* Oxford, UK: Oxford University Press, 2017.

Periodicals

Ghinai, Rosanna, et al. "A Cross-Sectional Study of 'Yaws' in Districts of Ghana Which Have Previously Undertaken Azithromycin Mass Drug Administration for Trachoma Control." *PLOS Neglected Tropical Diseases* (January 29, 2015). This article can also be found online at http://journals.plos.org/plosntds/article?id=10.1371/journal.pntd.0003496 (accessed February 2, 2018).

Knauf, Sascha, et al. "Isolation of *Treponema* DNA from Necrophagous Flies in a Natural Ecosystem." *EBioMedicine* 11 (September 2016): 85–90. This article can also be found online at http://www.ebiomedicine.com/article/S2352–3964(16)30343–7/fulltext (accessed February 2, 2018).

Mitjà, Oriol, et al. "Global Epidemiology of Yaws: A Systematic Review." *Lancet Global Health* 3, no. 6 (June 2015): e324–331. This article can also be found online at https://www.ncbi.nlm.nih.gov/pubmed/26001576 (accessed February 2, 2018).

Mitjà, Oriol, et al. "Mass Treatment with Single-Dose Azithromycin for Yaws." *New England Journal of Medicine* 372 (February 19, 2015): 703–710. This article can also be found online at http://www.nejm.org/doi/full/10.1056/NEJMoa1408586 (accessed February 2, 2018).

Websites

"Yaws." World Health Organization, March 2017. http://www.who.int/mediacentre/factsheets/fs316/en/ (accessed February 2, 2018).

"Yaws Eradication: Global Experts Meet after Signature of Medicine Donation Agreement." World Health Organization, January 29, 2018. http://www.who.int/neglected_diseases/news/WHO_and_EMS_sign_medicine_donation_agreement/en/ (accessed February 2, 2018).

L. S. Clements
Claire Skinner

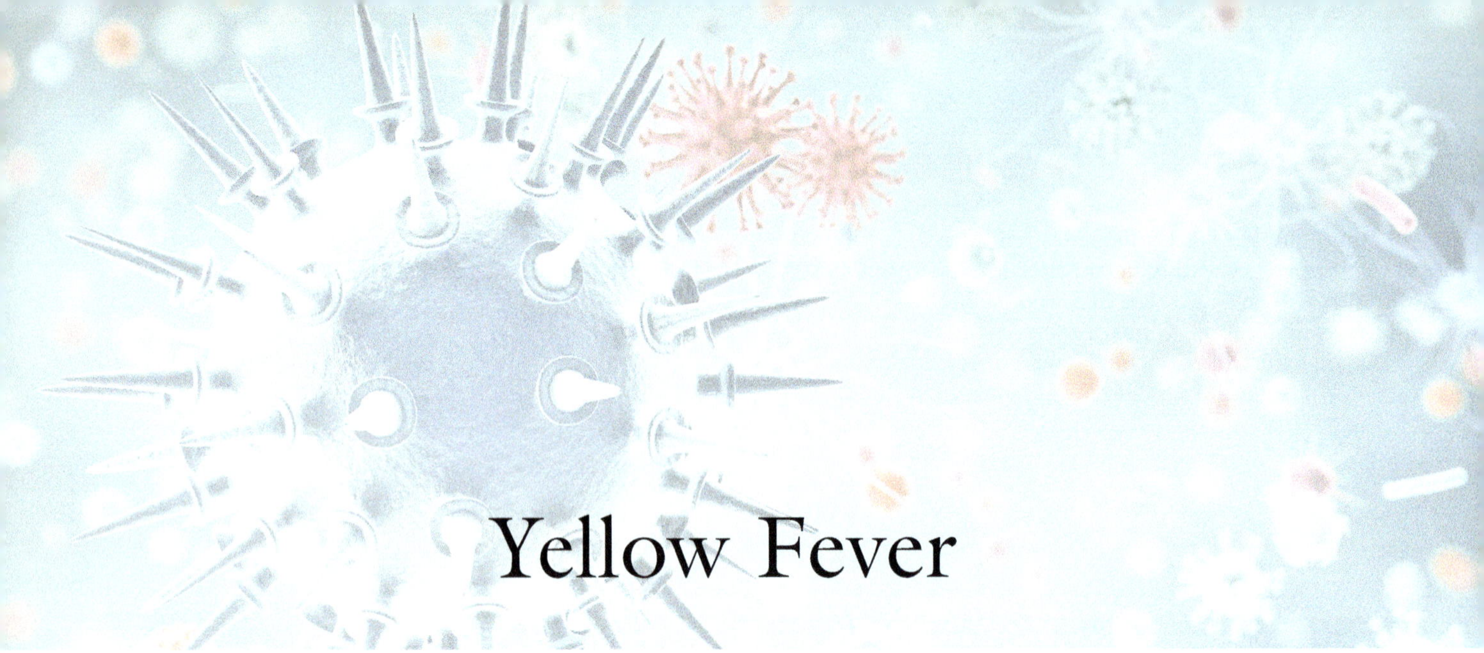

Yellow Fever

Introduction

Yellow fever is an acute viral disease spread by mosquitoes. It occurs in Africa and Central and South America. Although a vaccine is available to prevent the disease, the incidence of yellow fever was growing as of 2017, especially in South America.

Disease History, Characteristics, and Transmission

From the 17th to the early 20th century, the major ports of the United States suffered from periodic epidemics of yellow fever. New York was afflicted in 1668, Boston in 1691, and Philadelphia in 1793, where one in 10 of its inhabitants died. Work on digging the Panama Canal was stalled because of the huge toll of yellow fever and malaria on the workers. In response, the US Army set up a Yellow Fever Commission in Cuba, which was having an epidemic and was at the time under US control.

Yellow fever is transmitted to humans by mosquitoes. It is a classic viral hemorrhagic fever, involving sudden onset of fever, chills, headache, backache, nausea, and vomiting. The infection can cause damage to the liver, kidneys, and heart, as well as hemorrhage. According to the World Health Organization (WHO), the death rate from yellow fever is 20 to 50 percent in severe cases. The liver damage produces the yellow jaundice that gives the disease its name. It is endemic in the jungles of Africa and South America but occasionally breaks out in the cities, especially in West Africa (for example, in Nigeria between 1986 and 1991). WHO estimated in 2017 that yellow fever was capable of causing more than 170,000 cases every year and an estimated 29,000 to 60,000 deaths.

As of 2017, according to WHO, yellow fever was still circulating in the populations of 47 countries in Africa, Central America, and South America.

The best outcomes for people with yellow fever come from prompt recognition of the disease and hospitalization. Laboratory diagnosis is done by isolation of the virus in tissue culture from blood taken within the first five days of illness. The test takes a few days to produce a result.

There was no specific drug for yellow fever as of 2017. However, there was a safe and affordable vaccine. A single injection, administered as a booster injection every 10 years, provides lifetime protection. In rare cases (fewer than one in every 100,000 people vaccinated), there can be serious side effects. The side effects include damage to the liver, kidney, and nervous system. The risks of vaccine-related damage are greater for people over 60 years of age and for anyone whose immune system is not functioning properly, according to WHO.

WORDS TO KNOW

ATTENUATED STRAIN A bacterium or virus that has been weakened. Often used as the basis of a vaccine against the specific disease caused by the bacterium or virus.

ENDEMIC Present in a particular area or among a particular group of people.

HEMORRHAGIC FEVER A high fever caused by viral infection that features a high volume of bleeding. The bleeding is caused by the formation of tiny blood clots throughout the bloodstream. These blood clots, also called microthrombi, deplete platelets and fibrinogen in the bloodstream. When bleeding begins, the factors needed for the clotting of the blood are scarce. Thus, uncontrolled bleeding (hemorrhage) ensues.

VECTOR Any agent that carries and transmits parasites and diseases. Also, an organism or a chemical used to transport a gene into a new host cell.

It was projected that from mid-2017 to mid-2018 the vaccine would be unavailable because of manufacturing delays. Observers warned that, once existing supplies run out, there will be no other vaccination options until manufacture of the vaccine resumes.

Impacts and Issues

An important aspect of control of yellow fever is controlling the spread of the infection. These efforts focus on controlling the spread of *Aedes aegypti*, a type of mosquito. Because these mosquitoes breed in stagnant water, eliminating such water sources can help stop the spread of the virus. Hanging mosquito netting over beds in tropical climates is another way to help reduce the spread of yellow fever. Organizations including WHO and World Vision have conducted campaigns to solicit money for the purchase of mosquito netting and the delivery of the netting to rural villages.

Steps to control mosquito populations, especially during the insect's breeding season, can help lessen the infection. Spraying prime breeding grounds with insecticide is a common strategy. In addition, more high-tech scientific approaches are being used. For example, a program in malaria-prone regions of Africa and in regions of North America such as Florida and California involves the release of sterile male mosquitoes. The males, which are infected with a bacterium called *Wolbachia*, are unable to successfully mate with female mosquitoes. This helps reduce the number of offspring in the next generation.

PRIMARY SOURCE

HAVANA PHYSICIAN WHO SOLVED THE YELLOW FEVER PROBLEM IS EXTOLLED HERE AND ABROAD

SOURCE: *"Dr. Finlay Gets Full Credit Now: Havana Physician Who Solved the Yellow Fever Problem Is Extolled Here and Abroad."* New York Times *(September 3, 1911).*

INTRODUCTION: *Dr. Carlos Finlay began studying yellow fever in the 1870s. In 1881 he became the first to assert that the* Aedes *mosquito was the vector of disease for yellow fever. His research was largely ignored for decades until a team of US researchers posited a substantially similar theory in 1900. The following article from the* New York Times *discusses the scientific community's belated recognition of Finlay's contributions to yellow fever research.*

Dr. Finlay Gets Full Credit Now: Said Mosquitos Carried It

And Allowed a Contaminated Insect to Sting Him to Prove It—Theory Ridiculed at First

Reversing the usual order of things, scientists are determined that the rest of the world shall recognize in his life-

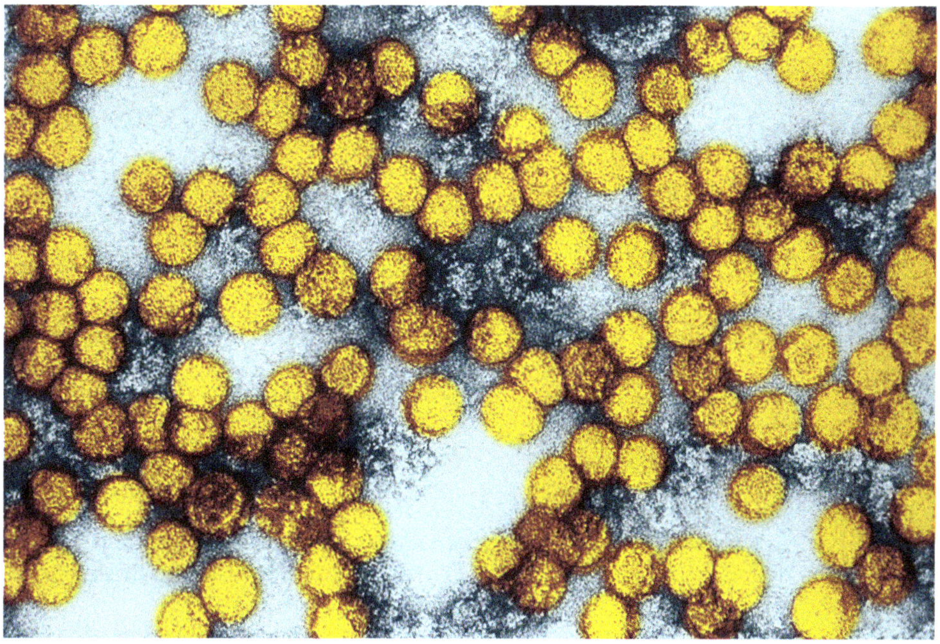

The yellow fever virus under magnification. Most commonly found in Africa and South America, yellow fever is transmitted to humans by infected mosquitoes. *© BSIP/Getty Images*

time the inestimable boon that Dr. Charles (or Carlos) J. Finlay of Havana conferred upon mankind when he formed the correct idea of how yellow fever is transmitted, proved his theory by self-inoculation, and forced it upon enlightened physicians and sanitarians after it had been rejected by contemporaries who regarded him as a nuisance.

Thousands of physicians who are well acquainted with the experiments of Reed, Carroll, and Lazear, who lost their lives in yellow fever investigations, never heard of Finlay. And yet he was their inspiration, and his experiments antedated theirs by a score of years. They succumbed, willing martyrs to the great cause; but he still lives and labors, revered by those working in the higher plains of science, regarded with something akin to awe by those who hear of him casually for the first time, and now, it seems, about to receive full credit, belated though it is, from the wide world.

It is now just thirty years and two weeks since Dr. Finlay read a paper before the Royal Academy of Havana, in which he propounded the novel theory that yellow fever was propagated by through the agency of mosquitos. And it is just six weeks ago that a physician in Edinburgh, commenting on Dr. Finlay and his discovery, in the course of a letter wrote:

"Considering the times, it will eventually be considered one of the most wonderful pieces of constructive work in the history of medicine, but, like every other advance, it was rejected by contemporaries. Unlike nearly all other great medical discoverers, however, he has lived to see the acceptance of his facts and has not had to die of a broken heart; but it has been enough to break any one's heart to see himself so utterly ignored while the world has been singing the praises of the men upon whom he forced his ideas."

Further along the same physician writes:

"No doubt Reed himself, if alive, would blush at the methods used, and would continue to insist upon giving Finlay full credit for the great conception. Too high praise cannot be given also to Lazear and Carroll for their bravery, but Finlay did the self-same inoculation twenty years earlier. Finlay, indeed, used these Americans as one would a tool, and he had to force them, for they, too, laughed at him.

"It seems to me that the credit for initiating the experiments confirming Finlay's discovery is due to Leonard Wood, who, as Governor, forced the matter along in the very city where Spanish generals had positively prohibited such work."

History of the Discovery

The Medical Record, which has all the facts in its possession, has undertaken to establish the brilliant work of Dr. Finlay in such a manner that all may know of it. The editor has written an article embodying the history of the discovery. After relating that Dr. Finlay's theory was received with incredulity and more or less good-natured ridicule, he says:

"Nothing daunted, however, with true grit he continued his observations on the remarkable coincidence between the prevalence of yellow fever and the temporary increase in the number of mosquitos—studied the anatomy, the manner of breeding, and the habits of the mosquitos, and also continued his inoculation experiments. These were begun in July, 1881, at which time he obtained a well-marked attack of yellow fever following a bite by a contaminated mosquito.

"In a paper published in *The American Journal of the Medical Sciences* in October, 1886, Finlay describes the mosquito which he regarded as the agent in the spread of yellow fever. It had a dark-colored body with ventral surface coated thick skin and marked with gray or white rings; on each side of the abdomen was a double row of white spots; its most striking feature was five white rings on the hind legs, present but less marked on the anterior and middle legs; white spots were visible on the side of the thorax and front of the head, while the corselet presented a combination of white lines in the figure of a two-stringed lyre; the wings when closed did not cover the body."

Dr. Finlay made further close observations of this mosquito, which is now known to science as *Stegomyia calopus* (the yellow-fever mosquito,) finding that it did its flying and biting between 9 and 10 o'clock in the morning.

"In the same article," continues the writer, "Finlay argues with much acuteness in support of his theory, and he concludes with the passage, which we quote at length, since it sets forth so clearly the views as to the spread of yellow fever that are universally held to-day.

Dr. Finlay's Argument

"From the evidence adduced in the preceding pages," he writes, "I conclude that while yellow fever is incapable of propagation by its own unaided efforts, it might be artificially communicated by inoculation, and only becomes epidemic when such inoculation can be verified by some external natural agent, such as the mosquito."

"The history and etiology of yellow fever exclude from our consideration as possibly agents of transmission other blood-sucking insects such as fleas &c., the habits and geographical distribution of which in no wise agree with the course of that disease; whereas a careful study of the habits and a natural history of the mosquito shows a remarkable agreement with the circumstances that favor or impede the transmission of yellow fever."

"So far as my information goes this disease appears incapable of propagation wherever tropical do not or are not likely to exist, ceasing to be epidemic at the time limits of temperature and altitude which are incompatible with the functional activity of these insects; while, on the other hand, it spreads readily wherever they abound. From these considerations, taken in connection with my successful attempts in producing experimental yellow fever by means of the mosquito's sting, it is to be inferred that these insects are the habitual agents of transmission."

In an article running through several numbers of *The Edinburgh Medical Journal* in 1894, Dr. Finlay again set forth his mosquito theory, and once more in *The Medical Record*, on May 27, 1899, before the United States Army Commission had proved its correctness in such a manner that there could be no denial. In the latter article he asks:

"Why should not the houses in yellow fever countries be provided with mosquito blinds, such as are used in the United States as a matter of comfort, while here it might be a question of life or death?"

He next went on to tell how the larvae might be destroyed and the mosquitos exterminated, and described ideal sanitary measures and hospital construction. In brief, he foreshadowed conditions which afterward became realities and converted hot-beds of yellow fever into delightful health resorts.

"There can be not doubt that yellow fever might be stamped out from Cuba and Puerto Rico," he said, "and malaria reduced to a minimum. It would then be the business of the port and quarantine officers to prevent the introduction of fresh germs."

His Dreams Realized

"When the United States Army occupied Havana," the writer continues, "Finlay saw his opportunity, and went to the sanitary authorities with his mosquito and his theory, and urged them to investigate the subject and prove the theory which he knew to be a fact. He was received with polite toleration, but without great enthusiasm. He persisted, nevertheless, in season and out of season, and in fact made such a nuisance of himself that an investigation was finally decided upon, his confidence arousing a suspicion that he might, after all, be on the right track.

"The results of this investigation are well known. Major Reed and his associates, Agramonte, Carroll, and Lazear, took Finlay's mosquito and his data and by a series of experiments, the equal of any in the annals of scientific investigation, established beyond cavil the mosquito doctrine of yellow fever transmission.

"Some of his views were found to be erroneous, which is not surprising when one considers the disadvantages under which he labored single-handed, but his basic idea was found to be absolutely correct. Making a practical application of this doctrine and perfecting the measures outlined by Finlay in his *Medical Record* article, the genius of Gorgas converted the two notorious pestholes, Havana and Panama, into health resorts.

"This is all ancient history, but for that very reason it is in danger of being forgotten. Even such a master of medical history as Osler forgot it in an address on the transmission of disease through the agency of blood-sucking insects, which he delivered before the London School of Tropical Medicine last Spring. In this address he omitted all mention of Finlay's work, and only when he was reminded of it by a letter from Guiteras of Havana in *The Lancet* did he apparently recall the great part which this pioneer has taken in the establishment of the mosquito doctrine."

Dr. Finlay was born in Cuba and has devoted his life to the inhabitants of that island, although his work has extended to a wide sphere, but the Scotch really claim and are justly proud of him and his achievements.

SEE ALSO *Arthropod-Borne Disease; Hemorrhagic Fevers; Host and Vector; Tropical Infectious Diseases*

BIBLIOGRAPHY

Books

Dickerson, James L. *Yellow Fever: A Deadly Disease Poised to Kill Again.* New York: Prometheus, 2006.

Periodicals

Woodall, Jack. "Why Mosquitoes Trump Birds." *Scientist* (January 1, 2006). This article can also be found online at https://www.the-scientist.com/?articles.view/articleNo/19704/title/Why-Mosquitoes-Trump-Birds/ (accessed January 15, 2018).

Websites

"Yellow Fever." Centers for Disease Control and Prevention, July 12, 2016. https://www.cdc.gov/yellowfever/ (accessed December 11, 2017).

"Yellow Fever." World Health Organization, May 2016. http://www.who.int/mediacentre/factsheets/fs100/en/ (accessed December 11, 2017).

Jack Woodall
Brian Hoyle

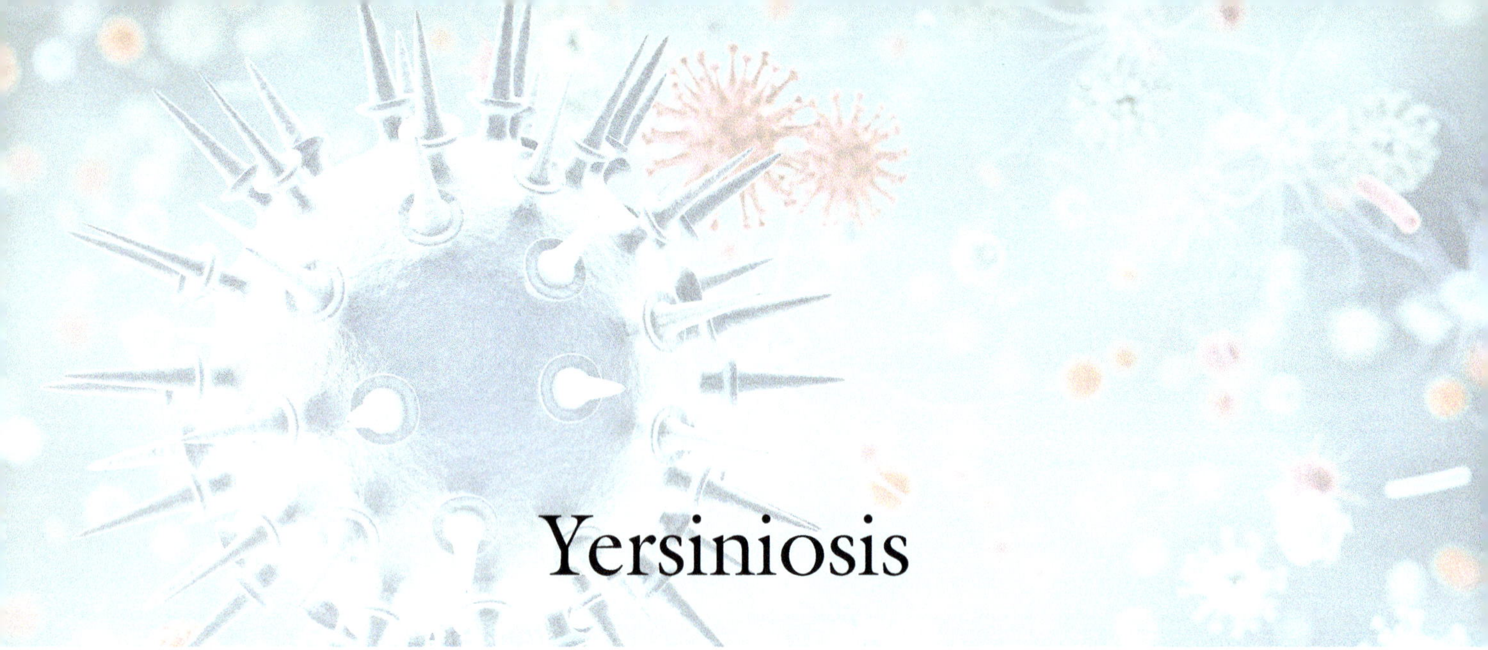

Yersiniosis

■ Introduction

Yersiniosis is an intestinal disease found mostly in children and young adults that is caused by bacteria in the genus *Yersinia*. In the United States, where incidence of the disease is routinely surveilled, the rod-shaped bacterium *Yersinia enterocolitica* causes the most illness from yersiniosis, primarily in young children. This bacterium is found in the feces of infected humans and animals and in some foods. The infectious disease is characterized by intestinal pain and by symptoms that resemble appendicitis.

According to the US Centers for Disease Control and Prevention (CDC), *Y. enterocolitica* causes approximately 117,000 illnesses, 640 hospitalizations, and 35 deaths in the United States annually. Children are infected at higher rates than adults. The infection is more common in the colder months of the year because the bacteria prefer cooler temperatures.

WORDS TO KNOW

BACTEREMIA A condition that occurs when bacteria enter the bloodstream via a wound or infection or via a surgical procedure or injection. Bacteremia may cause no symptoms and resolve without treatment, or it may produce fever and other symptoms of infection. In some cases bacteremia leads to septic shock, a potentially life-threatening condition.

PASTEURIZATION A process where fluids such as wine and milk are heated for a predetermined time at a temperature below the boiling point of the liquid. The treatment kills any microorganisms that are in the fluid but does not alter the taste, appearance, or nutritive value of the fluid.

SURVEILLANCE The systematic analysis, collection, evaluation, interpretation, and dissemination of data. In public health, it assists in the identification of health threats and the planning, implementation, and evaluation of responses to those threats.

■ Disease History, Characteristics, and Transmission

Adults most often acquire yersiniosis when they fail to practice proper hygiene, especially handwashing. Other activities that can lead to transmission of *Y. enterocolitica* include eating contaminated foods, such as undercooked or raw pork (especially chitterlings, which are made from the large intestines of pigs). Sometimes humans contract the disease after coming in contact with the feces or urine of infected animals. Handling contaminated soil or contaminated human feces can also cause the infection.

Children can acquire the infection from drinking contaminated milk that is not pasteurized or untreated water. Babies acquire the infection when adults carelessly handle raw pork or fail to wash their hands before handling the baby or objects in contact with the baby, such as bottles, clothing, and toys.

Infants are especially susceptible to yersiniosis. A medical professional should be consulted as soon as symptoms appear in an infant to ensure that health complications do not result. It is especially important that infants younger than three months of age be immediately treated if yersiniosis is suspected because the blood infection bacteremia can result. An infant with bacteremia is often treated in a hospital or major medical facility due to the seriousness of this condition.

Yersiniosis can cause numerous symptoms, which primarily depend on the age of the patient. Most symptoms appear within three to seven days of being infected. They often last one to three weeks but sometimes longer. In young children common symptoms include abdominal pain, watery diarrhea often containing blood or mucus, and fever. In older children and adults, common symptoms include abdominal pain on the right side of the body (similar to symptoms reported for appendicitis) and fever. Other symptoms include nausea and vomiting. Some people do not have noticeable symptoms, but they still excrete the bacteria in their stool and can infect others. Complications from yersiniosis can include joint pain, skin rashes, and spread of the bacteria into the bloodstream.

■ Scope and Distribution

Yersiniosis is found worldwide, but it is more prevalent in areas where wild or domesticated animals, primarily pigs, are found. The bacterium that causes yersiniosis is also found worldwide; however, the infection itself is more likely to be found in areas with poor sanitary conditions and among people with poor personal hygiene.

Yersiniosis is a relatively uncommon bacterial infection in the United States. According to the Foodborne Diseases Active Surveillance Network (FoodNet), which is monitored by the CDC, about 0.4 *Y. enterocolitica* infections occur for every 100,000 people annually in the United States. The European Centre for Disease Prevention and Control (ECDC) reported that, in 2014, 6,839 cases of yersiniosis were reported by 25 European Union (EU) and European Economic Area (EEA) countries (an overall infection rate of 1.8 cases per 100,000 people). Germany had the highest number of confirmed cases (2,485), followed by Finland (579) and Denmark (434).

■ Treatment and Prevention

Diagnosis of yersiniosis is generally performed through detection of the organism in the feces of infected people. The organism can also be detected through culture samples taken from the bile, blood, joint fluid, lymph nodes, or urine of patients. Stool samples can also distinguish between yersiniosis and appendicitis.

Treatment is usually not necessary when cases are uncomplicated. However, treatment is needed when cases become complicated, such as when severe symptoms occur or when bacteria enter the bloodstream. In these cases antibiotics, such as aminoglycosides, fluoroquinolones, or trimethoprim/sulfamethoxazole, are often prescribed.

Long-term problems caused by lack of treatment can result. Joint pain in the ankles, knees, or wrists sometimes occurs. Such pain often develops about one month after diarrhea occurs. A skin rash sometimes appears on the legs and trunk; women more frequently develop this complication than do men.

Yersiniosis can be prevented by eating only thoroughly cooked meats and, especially, by staying away from raw or undercooked pork. The US Department of Agriculture (USDA) recommends pork, pork products, and organ meats be cooked to an internal temperature of at least

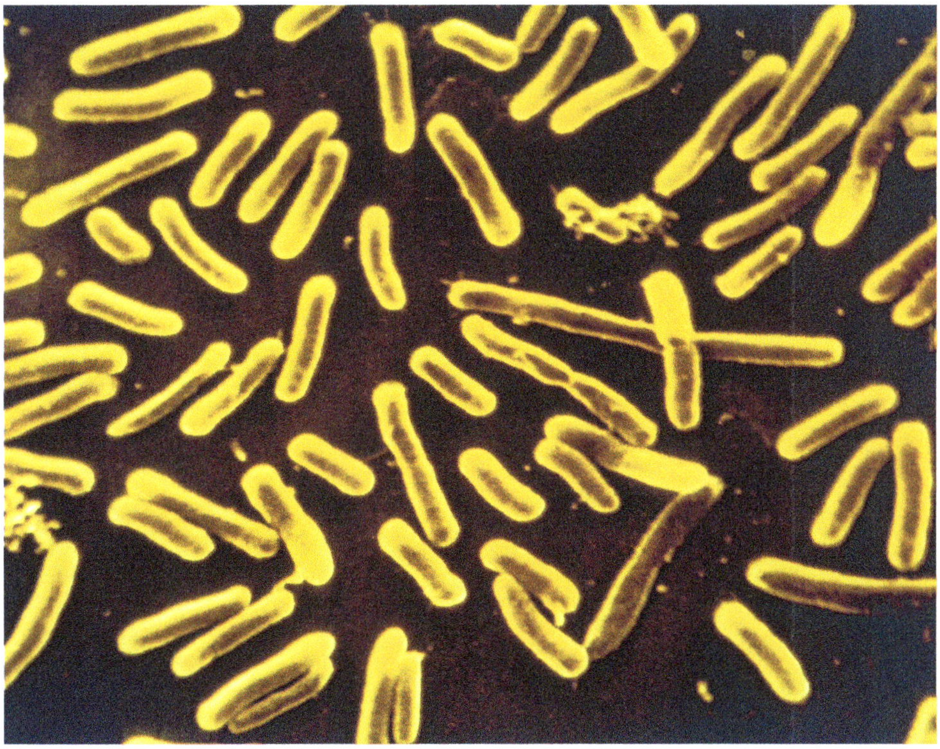

Yersinia enterocolitica bacteria is the most common cause of the intestinal disease yersiniosis in humans.

PERSONAL RESPONSIBILITY AND PREVENTION

In the United States, the primary cause of yersiniosis infections is unsafe preparation of pork products, particularly chitterlings, or pig intestines. Chitlins, as they are commonly known, are a favorite holiday food for many households throughout the southern states. However, because the raw intestines may contain remnants of fecal matter, the risk of contamination by *Y. enterocolitica* is high.

The US Centers for Disease Control and Prevention (CDC) recommends several methods to ensure the safe preparation of chitlins. The safest approach is to purchase them precooked. If chitlins are purchased raw, it is important to store them in a covered container to ensure none of the juices contaminate other foods in the refrigerator or freezer. While preparing raw chitlins, the CDC suggests boiling them for five minutes before cleaning and cooking, which will kill any bacteria without affecting the final flavor of the dish. The US Department of Agriculture (USDA) recommends chitlins be fully cooked to an internal temperature of 160°F (71°C) before tasting or serving.

Cleaning is also an important part of *Y. enterocolitica* prevention. The CDC recommends arranging all necessary cooking utensils and ingredients in the cooking area prior to handling the raw chitlins to avoid cross-contamination. A mixture of 1/4 cup of bleach per gallon of water should be used to clean all surfaces and materials that come into contact with the raw chitlins or their juice. Handwashing with warm water and soap should be performed before and after coming into contact with raw chitlins for a minimum of 20 seconds.

160°F (71°C). In addition, people should only consume milk and milk products that have been pasteurized.

Prevention can be maximized by washing hands after handling raw meat, going to the bathroom, changing diapers (and promptly throwing away soiled diapers), and touching animals. Hands should be washed thoroughly with soap and water before playing with infants or touching their toys, bottles, or other such objects. Kitchen countertops, cutting boards, and other utensils should be cleaned regularly, especially after raw meat is prepared. Animal and human feces should be disposed of in a sanitary manner. Water supplies should be protected from human and animal wastes.

■ Impacts and Issues

Chitterlings (made from pig intestines) are a traditional holiday food in some parts of the world, including parts of the United States. The preparation of chitterlings is a long and messy process that is a primary source of yersiniosis infection. Fecal matter is sometimes contained in the pork intestines, posing a health concern to those in direct contact with the contaminated intestines, and to children and infants who may be exposed to *Y. enterocolitica* by adult caregivers who have handled the contaminated intestines. Public awareness campaigns mounted by the CDC and state and local governments have helped to reduce the risk of such contamination by urging safe food preparation and personal hygiene practices. As a result, the incidence of yersiniosis infections has fallen significantly in the United States since the late 1990s, when it stood at around 1 infection for every 100,000 people, declining to 0.28 per 100,000 in 2015 and 0.42 per 100,000 in 2016, according to FoodNet.

Several US federal agencies are involved in the control and prevention of yersiniosis. The CDC monitors yersiniosis through its FoodNet and also conducts surveillance and investigations whenever outbreaks of the disease occur. This agency also uses public awareness campaigns to publicize the dangers associated with yersiniosis. The US Food and Drug Administration (FDA) inspects food and milk processing plants and restaurants to ensure products are safe for consumption.

The USDA monitors the health of domesticated animals raised for food. It inspects food slaughtering and processing plants to ensure that the human food supply is not contaminated. The US Environmental Protection Agency (EPA) monitors and regulates the safety of drinking water to prevent the transmission of yersiniosis and other infectious diseases through the water supply.

SEE ALSO *Bacterial Disease; Foodborne Disease and Food Safety; Handwashing; Parasitic Diseases*

BIBLIOGRAPHY

Books

Bannister, Barbara, Stephen Gillespie, and Jane Jones. *Infection: Microbiology and Management.* 3rd ed. Malden, MA: Wiley-Blackwell, 2006.

Carniel, Elisabeth, and Bernard J. Hinnebusch, eds. *Yersinia: Systems Biology and Control.* Norfolk, UK: Caister Academic, 2012.

Faruque, Shah M., ed. *Foodborne and Waterborne Bacterial Pathogens: Epidemiology, Evolution and Molecular Biology.* Norfolk, UK: Caister Academic, 2012.

Greenwood, David, et al. *Medical Microbiology: A Guide to Microbial Infections: Pathogenesis, Immunity, Laboratory Diagnosis and Control.* 17th ed. Philadelphia: Churchill Livingstone/Elsevier, 2007.

Periodicals

Bancerz-Kisiel, Agata, and Wojciech Szweda. "Yersiniosis—A Zoonotic Foodborne Disease of Relevance to Public Health." *Annals of Agricultural and Environmental Medicine* 22, no. 3 (2015): 397–402. This article can also be found online at http://www.aaem.pl/Yersiniosis-zoonotic-foodborne-disease-of-relevance-to-public-health,72296,0,2.html (accessed January 9, 2017).

Ong, Kanyin L., et al. "Changing Epidemiology of *Yersinia Enterocolitica* Infections: Markedly Decreased Rates in Young Black Children, Foodborne Diseases Active Surveillance Network (FoodNet), 1996–2009." *Clinical Infectious Diseases* 54, no. S5 (suppl.) (June 2012): S385–S390. This article can also be found online at https://academic.oup.com/cid/article/54/suppl_5/S385/432586 (accessed January 9, 2017).

Websites

"Fresh Pork from Farm to Table." US Department of Agriculture, August 6, 2013. https://www.fsis.usda.gov/wps/portal/fsis/topics/food-safety-education/get-answers/food-safety-fact-sheets/meat-preparation/fresh-pork-from-farm-to-table/CT_Index (accessed January 30, 2018).

"*Yersinia Enterocolitica* (Yersinia)." Centers for Disease Control and Prevention, October 24, 2016. https://www.cdc.gov/yersinia/ (accessed January 9, 2018).

"Yersiniosis—Annual Epidemiological Report 2016 [2014 Data]." European Centre for Disease Prevention and Control, March 13, 2017. https://ecdc.europa.eu/en/publications-data/yersiniosis-annual-epidemiological-report-2016–2014-data (accessed January 30, 2018).

"Yersiniosis and Chitterlings: Tips to Protect You and Those You Care for from Foodborne Illness." Food Safety and Inspection Service, US Department of Agriculture, December 1, 2016. https://www.fsis.usda.gov/wps/portal/fsis/topics/food-safety-education/get-answers/food-safety-fact-sheets/foodborne-illness-and-disease/yersiniosis-and-chitterlings/ct_index (accessed January 11, 2018).

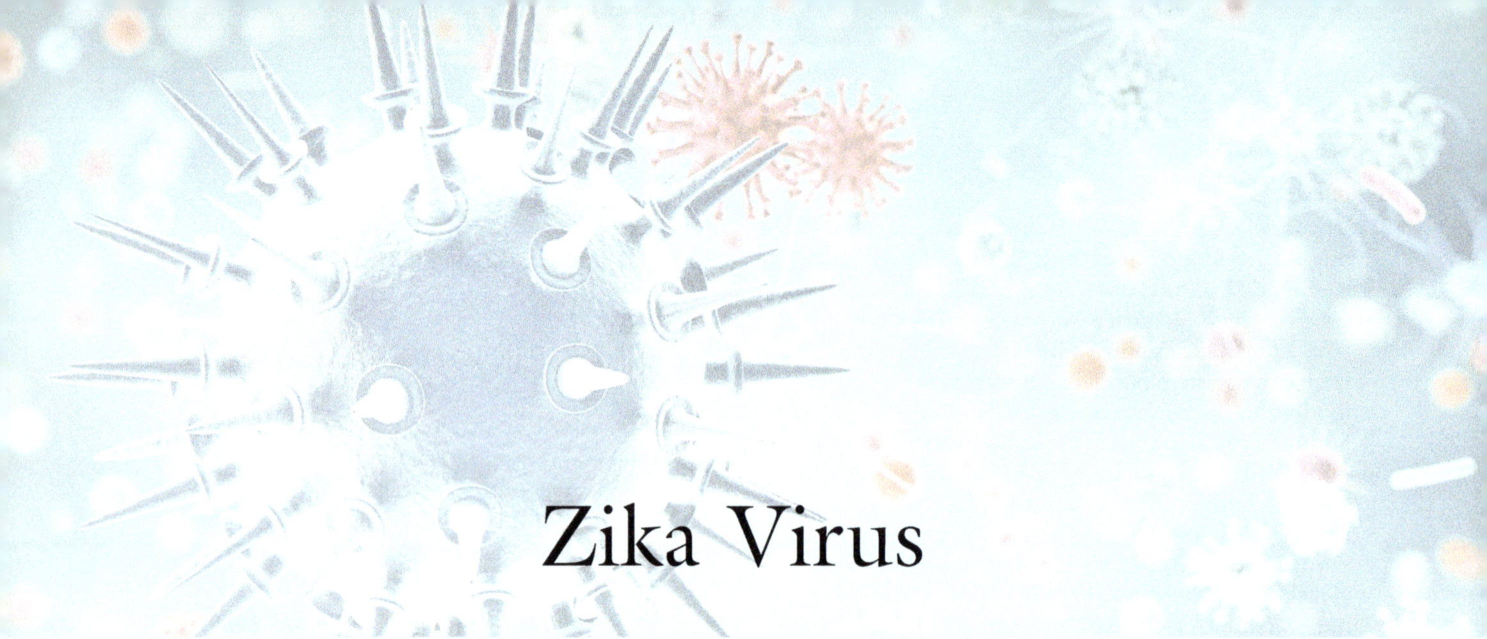

Zika Virus

Introduction

Zika virus (ZIKV) is an arbovirus belonging to the species *Flavivirus* and family Flaviviridae. It is closely related to viruses such as dengue, yellow fever, West Nile, and Japanese encephalitis.

Study of the ZIKV genomes has revealed the presence of two different lineages of the virus: African and Asian. The virus is thought to have originated in Africa, similar to chikungunya and yellow fever. When and how it spread out of Africa is unknown. The virus was isolated in 1966 in Malaysia. However, it was not until genetic analysis was possible that the presence of two separate ZIKV lineages was confirmed. The strain of ZIKV currently found in Africa belongs to the African lineage. Isolates from Asia, the Pacific, and the Americas all belong to the Asian lineage. This is also the viral type responsible for all the known epidemic outbreaks of the disease.

ZIKV infection has symptoms similar to those of dengue virus or chikungunya, as well as mild cases of yellow fever. All of these infections are also transmitted by the same mosquito species. Areas of infection with these viruses

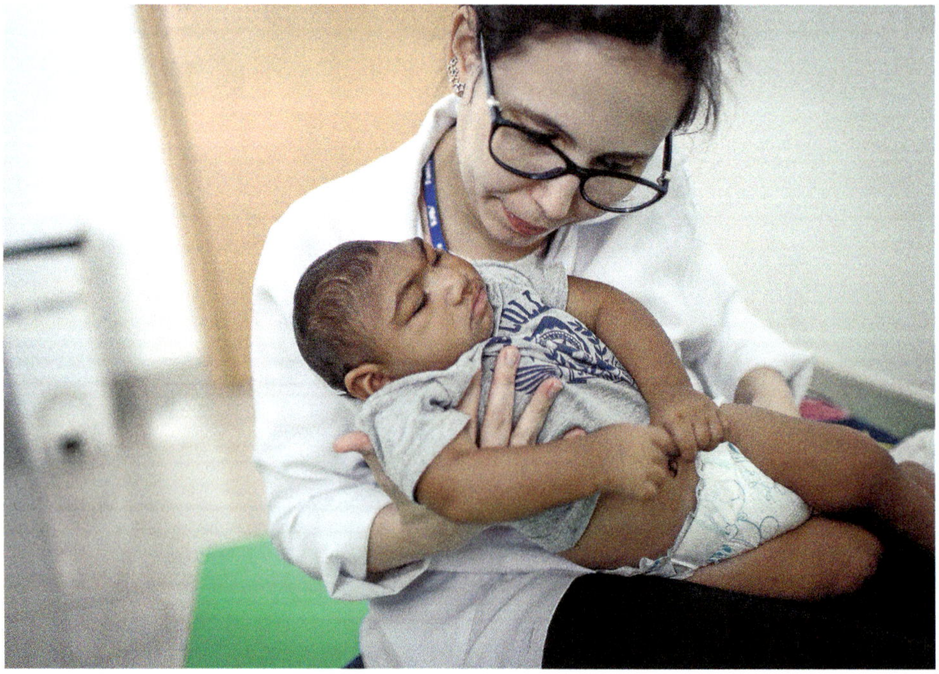

A doctor in Recife, Brazil, examines an infant born to a mother infected with the Zika virus. The baby suffers from microcephaly, or a below-average cranium size, a birth defect common among babies exposed to Zika. *© Mario Tama/Getty Images*

WORDS TO KNOW

ARBOVIRUS A virus that is typically spread by blood-sucking insects, most commonly mosquitoes. Over 100 types of arboviruses cause disease in humans. Yellow fever and dengue fever are two examples.

ASSAY A determination of an amount of a particular compound in a sample (e.g., to make chemical tests to determine the relative amount of a particular substance in a sample). A method used to quantify a biological compound.

CAPSID The protein shell surrounding a virus particle.

ENZOOTIC Affecting animals, naturally present in an environment, and occurring at regular intervals.

FLAVIVIRUS A single genus of ribonucleic acid (RNA) viruses that belong to the family Flaviviridae. Flaviviruses are found in arthropods but can infect humans and animals. Examples are dengue, yellow fever, West Nile, Japanese encephalitis, and Zika.

GUILLAIN-BARRÉ SYNDROME A rare condition in which the body's immune system attacks the nerves. It can cause muscle weakness, nerve tingling, and paralysis and may be triggered by an infection.

MICROCEPHALY A rare neurological condition in which the head of a baby is significantly smaller than that of other children of the same age and sex. This can cause developmental delays, intellectual disability, and movement and coordination difficulties. When detected at birth, it results from abnormal growth in the womb.

VECTOR Any agent that carries and transmits parasites and diseases. Also, an organism or a chemical used to transport a gene into a new host cell.

overlap in the Pacific and the Americas. It is unknown if previous exposure to related viruses can affect the disease progression in humans.

Disease History, Characteristics, and Transmission

ZIKV was discovered in 1947 in monkeys in the Zika forest of Uganda. The first human infections were described in 1952 in Uganda and Tanzania when antibodies were found in patients. ZIKV was first isolated in 1954 in Nigeria. Surveillance of infectious diseases in Africa has uncovered widespread presence of antibodies to ZIKV. However, confirmed human infections in Africa and Asia were relatively sporadic with mild symptoms until the virus emerged in the Pacific and the Americas.

In 2007 a major outbreak of ZIKV occurred on the island of Yap in Micronesia. Six years later, in 2013, the first neurological complications accompanying ZIKV outbreak were reported in French Polynesia. Some of the patients developed Guillain-Barré syndrome. In the 2015 outbreak in Brazil, neonatal microcephaly was reported for the first time. This 2015 epidemic started in the state of Rio Grande do Norte in Brazil and spread rapidly across the Americas, engulfing more than 20 countries. As of November 2017, a total of 85 countries worldwide reported cases of ZIKV.

Most cases outside the Americas were brought back by visitors to the infected regions. Isolated cases of imported virus were reported in Europe, Asia, Australia, and the United States. However, in the United States, limited transmission of the virus occurred in Florida, and no outbreak was reported.

ZIKV appears to follow one of two transmission cycles: enzootic and urban. In an enzootic cycle, the virus circulates between mosquitoes and forest animals. In an urban cycle, the virus circulates between humans and mosquitoes. Enzootic transmission is found primarily in Africa. Viruses spread in this cycle can still infect humans. However, it is the urban cycle that is blamed for the epidemic on Yap and the rapid spread of the virus during the 2015 outbreak.

Mosquitoes remain the main vector of the virus, in particular the genus *Aedes* and its two species, *A. aegypti* and *A. albopictus*. However, there is an alternative transmission mode. During the 2015 outbreak, there was confirmation that ZIKV can be transmitted between humans. There are three routes of non-mosquito transmission: sexual contact, mother-to-child transfer through the placenta, and blood-to-blood contact.

Most human infections are asymptomatic. Those who develop the disease have flu-like symptoms of fever, joint pain, fatigue, muscle pain, headaches, and rash, and these symptoms usually last one to two weeks. In rare cases Guillain-Barré syndrome in adults or microcephaly in neonates can develop. Congenital Zika syndrome (CZS) is a pattern of birth defects that can occur when a fetus is infected with Zika, characterized by microcephaly, damage to the brain and back of the eyes, hypertonia (excessive muscle tension), and congenital contractures (joint abnormalities).

Scope and Distribution

Arboviruses are distributed worldwide but transmitted often by different mosquito species. Their infections have short incubation times, from 3 to 10 days. Most infections are asymptomatic. During the 2015 epidemic, 50 percent of ZIKV cases were asymptomatic. This made tracking the infection difficult.

The spread of ZIKV, dengue, yellow fever, and chikungunya is mediated primarily by *A. aegypti*. The distribution of this mosquito has increased from its traditional tropical and subtropical location. It is primarily present in the Mediterranean, Africa, Southeast Asia, northern Australia, the Pacific, and Central and South America. However, its presence has been shown in northern Europe, southern parts of Australia, and the northeastern United States. The establishment of *A. aegypti* is prevented in those more temperate areas by its inability to survive cold winters, but warmer winters can help establish the mosquito in these regions.

The primary way to determine distribution of ZIKV and confirm infection is serology or an immune assay. This became problematic in Brazil, where antibodies used initially were cross-reacting with other flaviviruses, primarily dengue. The ability to differentiate which virus caused an infection became a priority, and polymerase chain reaction (PCR) tests detecting specific RNA were designed. These assays, together with genome sequencing, allowed researchers to determine relationships between ZIKV involved in all major outbreaks.

Treatment and Prevention

There is no treatment or vaccine for ZIKV. The recommendations in case of infection are to treat symptoms with rest, plenty of fluids, and acetaminophen to reduce fever or pain. Aspirin and nonsteroidal anti-inflammatory drugs (NSAIDs) should be avoided except when dengue virus or yellow fever infection is ruled out. Taking such drugs can lead to bleeding.

The most effective prevention is elimination of viral breeding grounds near human settlements by covering any still water sources and removing any open containers able to collect water. The areas can also be treated with insecticides to kill larvae and adult mosquitoes. Houses should have door and window screens to prevent mosquito entry. Once outside, people should wear protective clothing and use insect repellent.

Because the virus can be transmitted sexually, it is important to either use protection during sex or abstain from sex. Due to the long viability of ZIKV in semen, it is recommended that couples trying to get pregnant refrain from sex for a minimum of six months if a man or both partners traveled to an area with Zika risk. If only the female partner traveled to an area at risk of infection, the minimum abstinence time is eight weeks. Pregnant women should not travel to affected regions.

Impacts and Issues

ZIKV outbreaks in the Pacific, the first large outbreaks of the virus, had affected more than 100,000 people in Polynesia as of 2017. On Yap island the exact numbers were unclear, though there had been at least 900 suspected cases and 185 confirmed cases. Cases in Africa since the discovery of the virus were limited to less than 20 prior to 2015. However, the presence of antibodies to ZIKV was widespread there. In 2015, during the outbreak of the ZIKV epidemic in Brazil, up to 5,000 suspected cases were identified in Cape Verde, an island nation off the northwestern coast of Africa.

The statistics for the Brazilian ZIKV outbreak in 2015–2016 reported 231,725 suspected cases, 137,288 confirmed cases, 2,952 CZS cases, and 11 deaths in Brazil alone. The statistics for the entire Americas at the same time reported 583,451 suspected infections, 223,477 confirmed infections, 3,720 CZS cases, and 20 deaths. The majority of the cases were reported in 2015 and 2016, with the epidemic peaking in 2016.

The 2015 to 2016 outbreak of ZIKV in Brazil led to reduced tourism in the region due to cancelled trips. However, it did not adversely affect the 2016 Olympics in Rio de Janeiro. Accounting of the economic costs of the outbreak is ongoing. In 2016 the World Bank estimated the cost of the epidemic was $3.5 billion. A year later this estimate was increased to between $7 billion and $18 billion.

PRIMARY SOURCE

A Zika Tale in a Favela

SOURCE: *Belluck, Pam, and Tania Franco. "A Zika Tale in a Favela."* New York Times *(March 11, 2017). This article can also be found online at https://www.nytimes.com/2017/03/11/health/zika-virus-favela-360-video.html (accessed March 1, 2018).*

INTRODUCTION: *Brazil was especially devastated by the Zika outbreak, which caused a national health emergency in the country in 2015 and 2016. Although the emergency ended, parents and children continued to struggle in its aftermath. The following article from the* New York Times *describes the experiences of a family caring for a child with disabilities caused by the Zika virus in an impoverished area of Brazil.*

RECIFE, Brazil—At night, rats often scurry on top of the thin gray mattress where Maria de Fátima dos Santos and Paulo Rogério Cavalcanti de Araújo sleep with their two small children in a one-room house with a floor of dirt and concrete, and a green plastic basin for a toilet.

In this achingly poor section of the Brazilian city of Recife, where a water channel has become an acrid open sewer, and clusters of men stand around smoking marijuana while young girls sniff glue from soda bottles, the couple is struggling to raise a baby with disabilities caused by the Zika virus.

Their daughter, Eduarda Vitória, now 17 months old, has a range of problems stemming from brain damage caused by Zika, which her mother contracted when she was bitten by an infected mosquito while pregnant.

When Eduarda was born, her parents had never heard of Zika, and they said doctors at the hospital did not understand it. But they knew something was wrong. In the hospital nursery, Mr. de Araújo said, "I kept looking at her big body and very small head."

The small head, a condition called microcephaly, was the most obvious sign of Zika damage. But Eduarda also suffers from seizures, muscle problems, impaired vision, and problems eating. She cries unless she is held, usually calmed only when her father kisses her belly or her mother plays religious songs on her cellphone and sings along.

Poverty makes it hard for the family to manage Eduarda's needs. Both parents are unemployed and receive a monthly government check of 880 reais (less than $300).

Ms. dos Santos, 21, was abused by a stepmother, ran away to live on the streets at age 8, and became a crack user and prostitute until Mr. de Araújo, 48, met her. She has a stab wound on her left arm from a fight with a client over drugs and has struggled to stay clean since her first child, two-year-old Vitória Maria, was born.

Eduarda, whose eyes cross, waited months for a clinic to have an available pair of glasses. She is supposed to wear braces on her legs and arms, but the leg braces she was given are too loose and the arm braces too tight, her mother says.

Her parents protect Eduarda's seizure medicine from rodents by keeping it in a plastic bag tied to a pipe. Sometimes, their own food is ravaged by giant rats that climb onto the stove the instant Ms. dos Santos turns to help the baby, and grab sausage right out of the pan.

Eduarda has balked at eating much besides formula, and the government quit providing free formula when she turned 1 year old.

"Donations are over, we are not getting anything," Ms. dos Santos said.

The parents, who stow Eduarda's birth certificate and medical records under the mattress of the family's worn bed, don't take her to as many physical therapy sessions as some other Zika families. Getting to a session is a two-and-a-half-hour walk, or a 30-minute walk if they pay to take a bus the rest of the way.

In their one-room house, inside a cabinet door, Ms. dos Santos has taped a strip of paper from a piece of candy. A question printed on the paper reads, "Do que você precisa para ser feliz?" (What do you need to be happy?)

"A better life for my daughters," is Ms. dos Santos answer. "A better future, a future I never had."

See Also *Chikungunya; Dengue and Dengue Hemorrhagic Fever; Japanese Encephalitis; West Nile Virus; Yellow Fever*

BIBLIOGRAPHY

Books

Quereshi, Adnan. *Zika Virus Disease: From Origin to Outbreak*. London: Elsevier, 2018.

Periodicals

Duffy, Mark R., et al. "Zika Virus Outbreak on Yap Island, Federated States of Micronesia." *New England Journal of Medicine* 360, no. 24 (2009): 2536–2543.

Mittal, R., et al. "Zika Virus: An Emerging Global Health Threat." *Frontiers in Cellular and Infection Microbiology* 7 (December 2017): 1–19.

Musso, D., and D. Gubler. "Zika Virus." *Clinical Microbiology Reviews* 29 (2016): 487–524.

Musso, D., E. J. Nilles, and V. M. Cao-Lormeau. "Rapid Spread of Emerging Zika Virus in the Pacific Area." *Clinical Microbiology and Infection* 20, no. 10 (October 2014): O595–O596.

Vorou, Regina. "Zika Virus, Vectors, Reservoirs, Amplifying Hosts, and Their Potential to Spread Worldwide: What We Know and What We Should Investigate Urgently." *International Journal of Infectious Diseases* 48 (July 2016): 85–90.

Weaver, Scott C., et al. "Zika, Chikungunya, and Other Emerging Vector-Borne Viral Diseases." *Annual Review of Medicine* 69 (2018): 395–408.

Websites

"About Zika." Centers for Disease Control and Prevention, September 29, 2016. https://www.cdc.gov/zika/about/index.html (accessed February 26, 2018).

"*Aedes aegypti*—Factsheet for Experts." European Centre for Disease Prevention and Control, December 20, 2016. https://ecdc.europa.eu/en/disease-vectors/facts/mosquito-factsheets/aedes-aegypti (accessed February 26, 2018).

"Oxitec's Eco-Friendly Solution Addresses the Challenges of the *Aedes aegypti* Mosquito." Oxitec, November 4, 2016. http://www.oxitec.com/oxitecs-eco-friendly-solution-addresses-challenges-aedes-aegypti-mosquito/ (accessed February 26, 2018).

Parsons, Tim. "Economic Impact of Zika Outbreak Could Exceed $18B in Latin America, Caribbean." Hub, May 8, 2017. https://hub.jhu.edu/2017/05/08/zika-economic-impact-latin-america-caribbean/ (accessed February 26, 2018).

Ulansky, Elena. "The Economics of Zika." The Hill, June 20, 2016. http://thehill.com/opinion/op-ed/284177-the-economics-of-zika (accessed February 26, 2018).

"Zika Cumulative Cases." Pan American Health Organization, January 4, 2018. http://www.paho.org/hq/index.php?option=com_content&view=article&id=12390&Itemid=42090&lang=en (accessed February 26, 2018).

"Zika Virus." World Health Organization, September 6, 2016. http://www.who.int/mediacentre/factsheets/zika/en/ (accessed February 26, 2018).

"Zika Virus Infection." Pan American Health Organization. http://www.paho.org/hq/index.php?option=com_content&view=article&id=11585&Itemid=41688&lang=en (accessed February 26, 2018).

Agnes Caruso

Zoonoses

Introduction

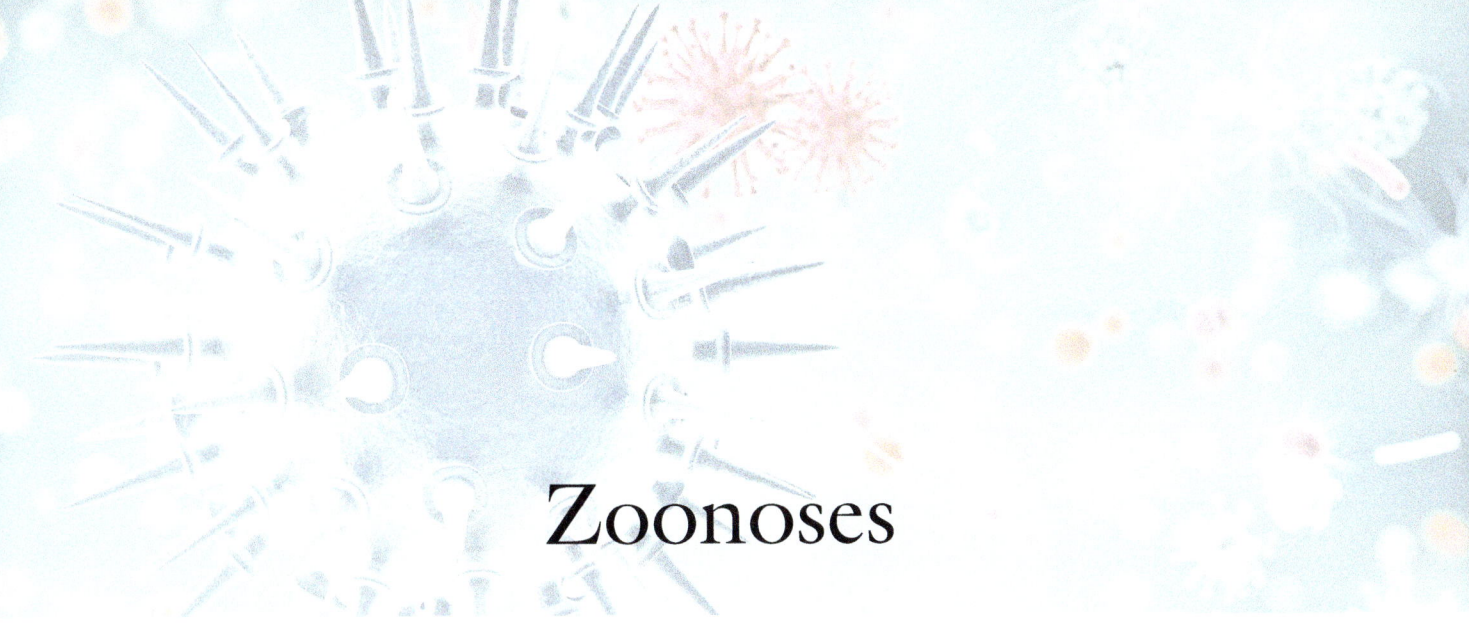

A zoonosis (pronounced ZOO-oh-NO-sis) is a disease that can be transmitted from animals to humans under natural conditions. Zoonoses can be caused by viruses, bacteria, parasites, prions, and fungi. Some zoonoses, after being transmitted from animals to humans, can be transmitted from human to human.

There are hundreds of zoonoses, including some of the most deadly diseases known. For example, avian influenza (flu) pandemics begin as zoonoses transmitted from birds to humans, and malaria is transmitted by mosquitoes to humans and kills about a million people annually. New zoonoses have been emerging in the early 21st century with increased frequency due partly to the incursion of increasing human populations into animal habitats. The World Health Organization (WHO) said in 2014 that 75 percent of new communicable human diseases that have emerged over the last 10 years are zoonoses.

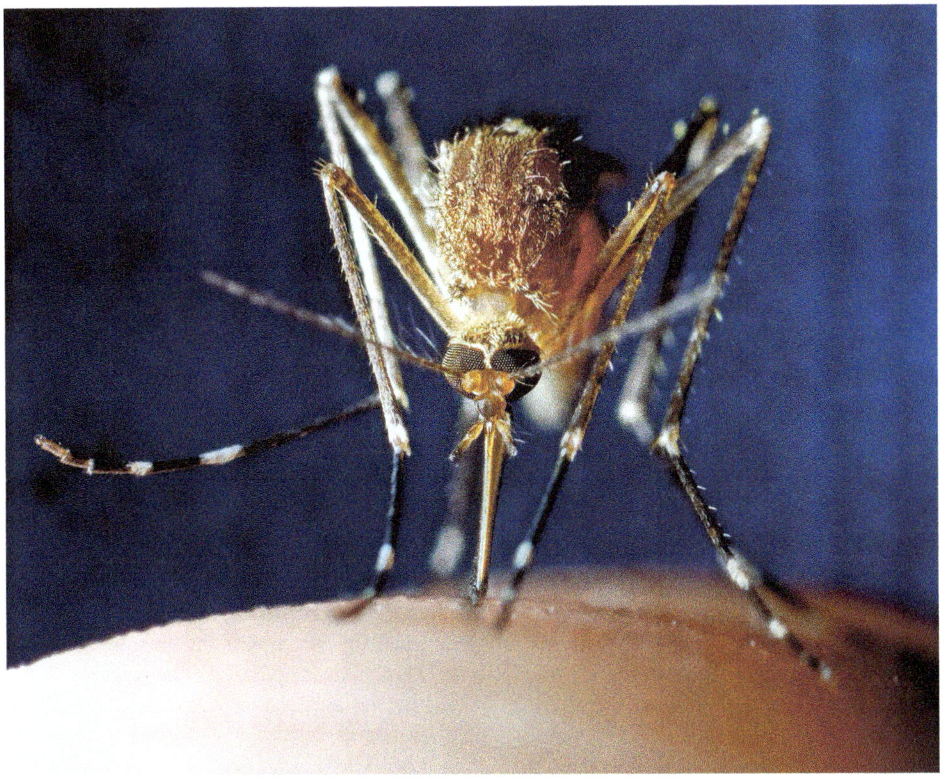

A mosquito feeding on a human finger. Zoonotic diseases are spread through human contact with infected animals and insects. *© CHBD/Getty Images*

WORDS TO KNOW

EMERGING INFECTIOUS DISEASE A new infectious disease such as severe acute respiratory syndrome (SARS) or West Nile virus, as well as a previously known disease such as malaria, tuberculosis, or bacterial pneumonia that is appearing in a new form that is resistant to drug treatments.

HOST An organism that serves as the habitat for a parasite or possibly for a symbiont. A host may provide nutrition to the parasite or symbiont, or it may simply provide a place in which to live.

REEMERGING INFECTIOUS DISEASE Illnesses such as malaria, diphtheria, tuberculosis, and polio that were once nearly absent from the world but are starting to cause greater numbers of infections once again. These illnesses are reappearing for many reasons. Malaria and other mosquito-borne illnesses increase when mosquito-control measures decrease. Other diseases are spreading because people have stopped being vaccinated, as happened with diphtheria after the collapse of the Soviet Union. A few diseases are reemerging because drugs to treat them have become less available or drug-resistant strains have developed.

RESERVOIR The animal or organism in which the virus or parasite normally resides.

VECTOR Any agent that carries and transmits parasites and diseases. Also, an organism or a chemical used to transport a gene into a new host cell.

Zoonoses are found in all societies, but they are most common and most deadly in countries with few resources.

Disease History, Characteristics, and Transmission

Many zoonoses have afflicted human beings throughout their history. Before the development of agriculture in approximately 8,000 BCE, people lived in small nomadic groups. Because their diet included wild game, they were prone to parasitic zoonotic diseases such as hookworm (a disease caused by parasitic nematode worms that attach to the host's intestinal lining). However, members of such groups who survived to adulthood tended to be healthy. Because of the relative mutual isolation of these groups, epidemic disease was rare.

After the domestication of plants and food animals, people began to live in larger groups and in closer contact with a variety of animals, including sheep, pigs, cattle, goats, and chickens. This made the transmission of diseases from animals to humans more likely, as well as the transmission of diseases from person to person. Tuberculosis, measles, smallpox, and influenza first entered human populations through agricultural contact with animals and animal products, and new influenza strains are still transmitted to human populations from domesticated pig and bird populations in Asia.

The development of global trade routes allowed the spread of epidemic diseases that had lost all connection with their original animal hosts, as well as diseases that remained zoonotic, such as bubonic plague. Caused by the bacterium *Yersinia pestis*, bubonic plague first appeared in Europe in 542 CE, but it only devastated the European population after 1346, when flea-infested furs were brought from China over recently opened trade routes. In a few years this zoonosis killed approximately one-third of the population of Europe and about 75 million people worldwide. Bubonic plague is maintained in rodent populations and transmitted to humans by flea and rodent bites.

Since the development of fossil fuel–powered transportation in the 19th century, a whole new set of opportunities has arisen for zoonoses to travel the world. Migrant workers, political and economic refugees, tourists, and military personnel move quickly and in large numbers from one part of the world to another. Animals and animal products are moved globally by airplane and ship, sometimes inadvertently, as when rats and insect eggs are transported along with cargo. The tiger mosquito may have hitchhiked from Asia to the United States in worn tires shipped from the United States to Japan for retreading and then returned to the United States. Some experts warn that these mosquitoes may contribute to increased zoonotic transmission of North American viruses, including La Crosse virus (a virus that causes La Crosse encephalitis), as they spread. West Nile virus, which produced a notorious outbreak in 1999 and is transmitted to humans through mosquito bites, was apparently brought to the United States from Israel on an airplane, either by a stowaway mosquito or an infected human traveler.

Zoonoses can be transmitted to humans by bites, scratches, saliva, dander (skin flakes, similar to dandruff), feces, and blood. Certain zoonoses, such as trichinellosis, are transmitted when humans eat the flesh of certain animals. Dog and bat bites can transmit rabies, cat bites can transmit cat-scratch fever, monkey bites can transmit hepatitis B, and rat bites can transmit leptospirosis, bubonic plague, salmonellosis, and rat-bite fever.

Animals serve as the natural reservoir of some zoonotic diseases and the vector of others. A reservoir is a long-term host organism that maintains an infective agent, usually a virus, bacterium, or parasite. The reservoir is usually not affected by the agent or is without symptoms and can then pass on the infectious agent either by direct contact or through a vector. A vector transfers an infectious agent from an infected host to an uninfected animal or human. Vectors are often arthropods, a group of invertebrate animals including insects. For example, birds are a natural reservoir of West Nile virus, and the disease is transmitted from infected birds to humans by a mosquito vector.

Scope and Distribution

In 2017 the US Centers for Disease Control and Prevention (CDC) reported that "more than 6 out of every 10 known infectious diseases in people are spread from animals." Zoonotic diseases are therefore extremely common.

All parts of the world are affected by zoonotic diseases. The geographical distribution of any given zoonosis depends on the geographical distribution of its host animal or animals. While most zoonoses are most common in developing countries, a few, such as Lyme disease (an acute inflammatory disease transmitted by ticks) and trichinellosis (a disease people can get by eating raw or undercooked meat), are more common in developed countries in North America and Europe.

Treatment and Prevention

Treatment of zoonoses varies by infection type. Bacterial infections can usually be combated with antibiotics. Antifungals, antiparasitics, and antivirals may be used against other infections, but options are generally more limited for fighting nonbacterial infections. For example, there is no available treatment for West Nile virus, which can cause fatal encephalitis in a minority of victims. Treatment of West Nile is supportive—that is, directed at relieving symptoms and helping the patient's own immune system fight off the infection.

Prevention of zoonoses is primarily aimed at reducing the incidence of the zoonosis in the animal population from which it is transmitted to humans. For example, destroying rabid dogs decreases the incidence of rabies in humans. Spraying anti-mosquito pesticide to keep down mosquito populations that can transmit malaria and other diseases has a similar effect. Veterinary medicine and human medicine must cooperate in many of these measures designed to reduce zoonotic disease. This type of coordination can be challenging in low-resource areas.

Humans can also decrease the likelihood of contracting a zoonotic disease by avoiding contact with infected animals and their feces and infected food products. Food products may be rendered safe by excluding infected animals from the food supply, as in the case of anthrax or trichinellosis, or by improved food preparation (e.g., pasteurizing, thorough cooking, and slaughterhouse sanitation).

Impacts and Issues

As noted earlier, 75 percent of recently emerging or reemerging diseases are zoonoses. These include unconventional diseases such as prion diseases (transmissible spongiform encephalopathies), which are caused not by viruses or living organisms but by deformed proteins that, when ingested, cause similar protein deformation in the animal or human who has eaten the meat. These deformed proteins can accumulate in the central nervous system and cause mental degeneration and death.

An emergent pathogen need not be unknown or unusual. A disease is considered emerging if it appears in an area where it has not previously been reported, as, for example, West Nile virus appearing in the United States. As long as an expanding human population continues to encroach on animal habitats, the likelihood that more zoonotic diseases will appear remains high. According to WHO, factors that contribute to the emergence of new zoonoses include "urbanization and destruction of natural habitats, leading to humans and animals living in close proximity; climate change and changing ecosystems; changes in populations of reservoir hosts or intermediate insect vectors; and microbial genetic mutation."

PRIMARY SOURCE

"Poverty Favours the Mosquito": Experts Warn Zika Virus Could Return to Brazil

SOURCE: *Phillips, Dom. "'Poverty Favours the Mosquito': Experts Warn Zika Virus Could Return to Brazil."* Guardian *(July 14, 2017). This article can also be found online at https://www.theguardian.com/global-development/2017/jul/14/poverty-favours-the-mosquito-experts-warn-zika-virus-could-return-to-brazil (accessed January 31, 2018).*

INTRODUCTION: *In the following article, the author reports that ongoing problems in Brazil (such as poor sanitation in impoverished communities) could contribute to another outbreak of Zika virus there. Zika virus is a zoonosis transmitted from mosquitoes to humans. The disease quickly became a global public health concern because it can cause serious birth defects in the children of infected mothers. The first major Zika virus outbreak occurred in Brazil and Colombia in 2014. Between then and January 2018, there were more than two dozen Zika virus outbreaks around the world.*

Weaknesses in the public health system risk another Zika epidemic in Brazil, according to a report published two months after the government declared the mosquito-borne virus was no longer an emergency.

Blamed for the birth defect microcephaly, Zika exposed human rights deficiencies in areas such as sanitation, access to clean water, poverty and sexual health restrictions, the report released on Thursday by Human Rights Watch said.

"The underlying conditions that allowed the outbreak to be so damaging have not been addressed and there is a vulnerability for future outbreaks," said Amanda Klasing, one of the report's authors. She added that millions of people lack proper sanitation or fresh water, and women also need better information and access to contraception and safe abortion – which is illegal in most cases in Brazil.

Zika was first identified in Brazil in 2014 and spread rapidly through the country. There were 191,992 cases in 2016 and by May, 9,351 new cases this year. The ministry of health said Zika was responsible for the majority of the 2,753 cases of the devastating birth defect microcephaly – of which 322 were this year.

Microcephaly, which can also be caused by other infections such as herpes, rubella and syphilis, causes babies to be born with abnormally small heads and leads to cognitive and learning difficulties. Many of the babies come from low-income backgrounds, like Maria Eduarda, born 19 months ago, who is cared for by Cleane Serpa, 19, and Miriam Pereira, 42, who adopted the baby.

They live in a tiny house in a low-income community in Recife, the north-eastern city that was an epicentre for the Zika epidemic, and receive £225 in monthly benefits for the child and two women to live on. They also receive free bus travel to take her to occupational therapy, hearing, physiotherapy and other sessions – spending up to two hours each way on the journey.

"It is not enough. Her milk is expensive, and her medicine is expensive," Serpa said. Caring for a microcephalic baby is intensive, full-time work. Maria Eduarda spent six months feeding through a tube that she has only just been weaned off. "She forgot how to swallow," said Serpa.

Many women interviewed for the report said they lacked information on contraception and were unaware that Zika could be transmitted sexually. Almost half of those with microcephalic babies were single mothers.

Illegal abortions increased in Brazil in the face of the Zika crisis, according to a 2016 study by the *New England Journal of Medicine*. Requests from Brazil to Women on Web, a Dutch organisation that sends abortion medicines to women in countries where it is restricted, increased 108%. Since 2005, more than 900 women have died from unsafe abortion in Brazil.

The HRW report recommended that Brazil's supreme court make abortion legal, a move the country's conservative congress is unlikely to make in this deeply religious country.

"Politically, it is very difficult – but from a public health perspective, criminalising abortion is terrible policy," Klasing said.

The microcephaly outbreak was concentrated last year in the north-east of Brazil – one its poorest and most arid regions – for reasons that scientists and researchers are still trying to understand. The report argues that a lack of proper sanitation and water supply contributed – a view many specialists share.

The *Aedes aegypti* mosquito, which transmits Zika and other arboviruses like Dengue and Chikungunya, lays eggs on damp surfaces near water. Poor sanitation and a lack of water supply, which means people leave their water sitting in buckets or containers, provide ideal conditions for it to spread.

"When you have more conditions for the *Aedes aegypti* mosquito to spread, you have more transmission possibilities," said Jessé Alves, an infectious diseases specialist at the state-run Emilio Ribas hospital in São Paulo.

According to World Health Organisation statistics, 35 million people in Brazil do not have adequate sanitation and 3.8 million do not have access to safe drinking water. In the north-east, just 25% are connected to a wastewater system.

"There is a big deficit in the country," said Alceu Galvão, a sanitation consultant in the north-eastern state of Ceará, following decades of low investment.

In 2013, left President Dilma Rousseff's government launched a 20-year plan to improve sanitation across Brazil. The plan "was overtaken by the economic situation", Galvão said as Brazil has sunk into a debilitating recession. Rousseff was impeached last year for breaking budget rules and her successor, Michel Temer, has introduced a 20-year ceiling on spending to reduce a spiralling £33 billion deficit he blamed on her overspending.

Other specialists agreed that Zika could return.

Danielle Cruz, an infectious diseases specialist in Recife who has treated many microcephalic babies, said Zika could be cyclical, like other arboviruses. While Dengue numbers fell sharply this year, Brazil had to mount an emergency vaccination operation to contain a sylvatic yellow fever outbreak.

"The lack of basic sanitation, the poverty, it all favours the mosquito," Cruz said. "There is a big chance of Zika coming back."

See Also *Animal Importation; Arthropod-Borne Disease; Bovine Spongiform Encephalopathy (Mad Cow Disease); Brucellosis; Cat Scratch Disease; Dengue and Dengue Hemorrhagic Fever; Ebola; Emerging Infectious Diseases; Giardiasis; Hantavirus; Lyme Disease; Malaria; Prion Disease; Rat-Bite Fever; Ringworm; Trichinellosis*

BIBLIOGRAPHY

Books

Bauerfeind, Rolf, et al. *Zoonoses: Infectious Diseases Transmissible from Animals to Humans*. 4th ed. Washington, DC: ASM, 2015.

Torrey, E. Fuller, and Robert H. Yolken. *The Beasts of the Earth: Animals, Humans, and Disease*. New Brunswick, NJ: Rutgers University Press, 2014.

Periodicals

Eisen, Rebecca J. "Tick-Borne Zoonoses in the United States: Persistent and Emerging Threats to Human Health." *ILAR Journal* (March 23, 2017). This article can also be found online at https://academic.oup.com/ilarjournal/advance-article/doi/10.1093/ilar/ilx005/3078806 (accessed January 31, 2018).

Waltner-Toews, David. "Zoonoses, One Health and Complexity: Wicked Problems and Constructive Conflict." *Philosophical Transactions of the Royal Society B* 372, no. 1725 (July 19, 2017).

Welburn, S.C., et al. "The Neglected Zoonoses—The Case for Integrated Control and Advocacy." *Clinical Microbiology and Infection* 21, no. 5 (May 2015): 433–443. This article can also be found online at http://www.clinicalmicrobiologyandinfection.com/article/S1198–743X(15)00419-X/fulltext (accessed January 31, 2018).

Websites

"A Brief Guide to Emerging Infectious Diseases and Zoonoses." World Health Organization, 2014. http://www.searo.who.int/entity/emerging_diseases/ebola/a_brief_guide_emerging_infectious_diseases.pdf?ua=1 (accessed January 31, 2018).

"The Control of Neglected Zoonotic Diseases: Community-Based Interventions for Prevention and Control." World Health Organization, November 2010. http://apps.who.int/iris/bitstream/10665/44746/1/9789241502528_eng.pdf?ua=1 (accessed January 31, 2018).

"Take a Bite out of Rabies!" Centers for Disease Control and Prevention, September 25, 2017. https://www.cdc.gov/features/rabies/index.html (accessed January 31, 2018).

"What Zoonotic Diseases Are Dangerous." Centers for Disease Control and Prevention, December 14, 2016. https://www.cdc.gov/about/facts/cdcfastfacts/zoonotic.html (accessed January 31, 2018).

"Zoonoses." World Health Organization. http://www.who.int/topics/zoonoses/en/ (accessed January 31, 2018).

"Zoonotic Diseases." Centers for Disease Control and Prevention, July 14, 2017. https://www.cdc.gov/onehealth/basics/zoonotic-diseases.html (accessed January 31, 2018).

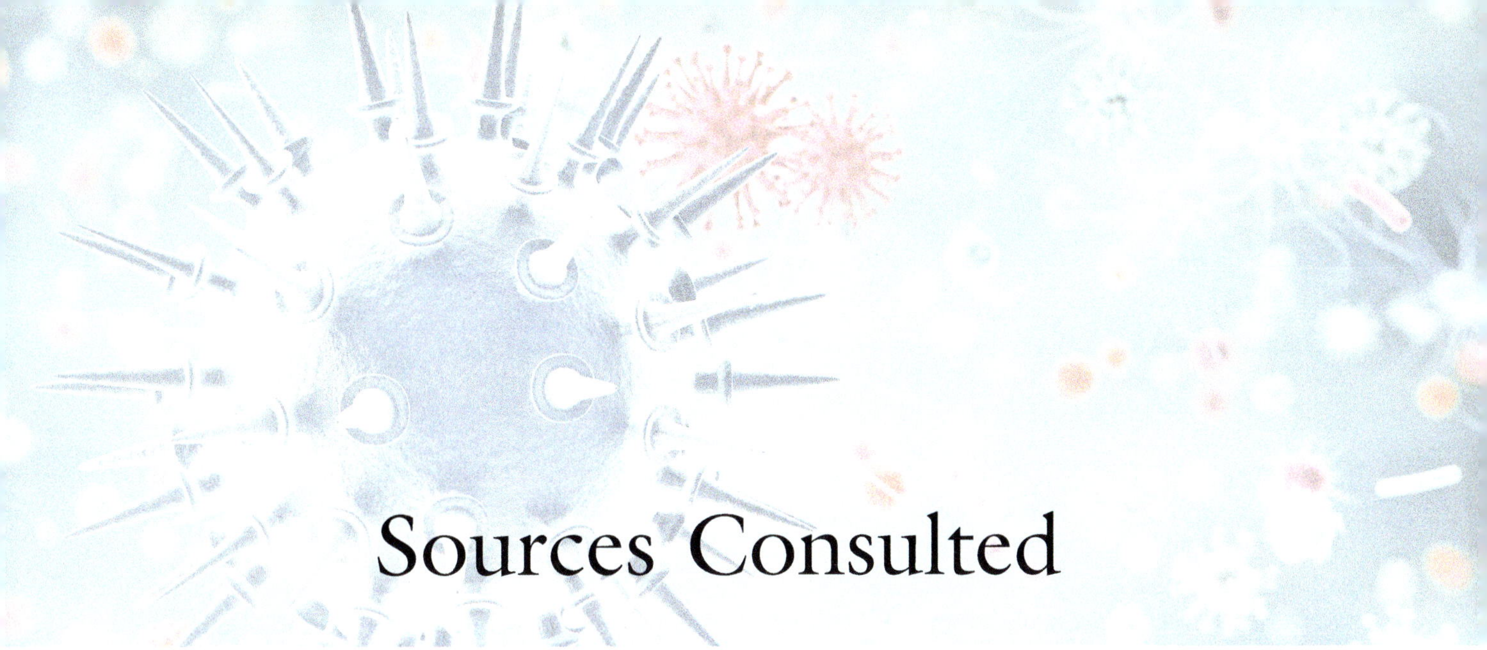

Sources Consulted

BOOKS

Achord, James L. *Understanding Hepatitis.* Oxford: University of Mississippi Press, 2002.

Adams, Vincanne, ed. *Metrics: What Counts in Global Health.* Durham, NC: Duke University Press, 2016.

Adler, Ben, ed. *Leptospira and Leptospirosis.* Berlin: Springer-Verlag, 2016.

Adler, Richard, and Elise Mara. *Typhoid Fever: A History.* Jefferson, NC: McFarland, 2016.

Adley, Catherine C., ed. *Food-Borne Pathogens: Methods and Protocols.* Totowa, NJ: Humana, 2006.

Akyar, Isin, ed. *Toxoplasmosis.* London: InTechOpen, 2017.

Al-Doory, Yousef, and Arthur F. DiSalvo, eds. *Blastomycosis.* New York: Plenum Medical, 1992.

Allman, Toney. *The Importance of Germ Theory.* San Diego, CA: ReferencePoint, 2016.

Alotaibi, Mohammed, and Siraj Amanullah. "*Rickettsia rickettsii* (Rocky Mountain Spotted Fever) Attack." In *Ciottone's Disaster Medicine*, edited by Gregory R. Ciottone et al., 724–725. Philadelphia: Elsevier, 2016.

Amer, Fatma. *Hospital Infection Control, Part 1.* 3rd ed. Saarbrücken, Germany: Noor, 2017.

Angelakis, Andreas N., and Joan B. Rose, eds. *Evolution of Sanitation and Wastewater Technologies through the Centuries.* London: IWA, 2014.

Animal and Plant Health Inspection Service. *Brucellosis: Questions and Answers (Classic Reprint).* London: Forgotten Books, 2017.

Arguin, Paul, ed. *Health Information for International Travel 2005–2006.* Philadelphia: Elsevier, 2005.

Aronson, Susan, and Timothy R. Shope. *Managing Infectious Disease in Child Care and School: A Quick Reference Guide.* Elk Grove Village, IL: American Academy of Pediatrics, 2016.

Artenstein, Andrew W. *In the Blink of an Eye: The Deadly Story of Epidemic Meningitis.* New York: Springer, 2012.

Banerjee, Sudeshna Ghosh, and Elvira Morella. *Africa's Water and Sanitation Infrastructure: Access, Affordability, and Alternatives.* Washington, DC: World Bank, 2011.

Bankston, John. *Joseph Lister and the Story of Antiseptics.* Hockessin, DE: Mitchell Lane, 2005.

Bannister, Barbara A. *Infection: Microbiology and Management.* Malden, MA: Blackwell, 2006.

Bannister, Barbara, Stephen Gillespie, and Jane Jones. *Infection: Microbiology and Management.* 3rd ed. Malden, MA: Wiley-Blackwell, 2006.

Barach, Jeffrey T. *FSMA and Food Safety Systems: Understanding and Implementing the Rules.* Hoboken, NJ: Wiley, 2017.

Barbara, John A. J., Fiona A. M. Regan, and Marcela Contreras, eds. *Transfusion Microbiology.* Cambridge: Cambridge University Press, 2008.

Barbour, Alan G. *Lyme Disease: Why It's Spreading, How It Makes You Sick, and What to Do about It.* 2nd ed. Baltimore: Johns Hopkins University Press, 2015.

Barrett, Ron, and George J. Armelagos. *An Unnatural History of Emerging Infections.* Oxford: Oxford University Press, 2013.

Barry, John M. *The Great Influenza: The Story of the Deadliest Pandemic in History.* New York: Penguin, 2005.

Bartlett, J. G. "Occupational Exposure to Human Immunodeficiency Virus and Other Bloodborne Pathogens." In *Current Surgical Therapy*, edited by John Cameron and Andrew Cameron. Philadelphia: Elsevier Saunders, 2016.

Bartlett, Karen. *The Health of Nations: The Campaign to End Polio and Eradicate Epidemic Diseases.* London: Oneworld, 2017.

Bashford, Alison, ed. *Medicine at the Border: Disease, Globalization, and Security, 1850 to the Present.* New York: Palgrave Macmillan, 2006.

Bastarache, Julie A., and Eric J. Seeley, eds. *Sepsis.* Philadelphia: Elsevier, 2016.

Bauerfeind, Rolf, and Alexander von Graevenitz. *Zoonoses: Infectious Diseases Transmissible from Animals to Humans.* Washington, DC: ASM, 2015.

Bayry, Jagadeesh, ed. *Emerging and Re-emerging Infectious Diseases of Livestock.* New York: Springer, 2017.

Beers, Mark H., ed. *The Merck Manual of Medical Information.* London: Gallery, 2008.

Beers, Mark H., and Robert Berkow. *The Merck Manual of Diagnosis and Therapy.* 18th ed. Whitehouse Station, NJ: Merck Research Laboratories, 2006.

Beigbeder, Yves. *The World Health Organization: Achievements and Failures.* New York: Routledge, 2018.

Beigi, Richard H., ed. *Sexually Transmitted Diseases.* Chichester, UK: John Wiley, 2012.

Bell, Sigall K., Courtney L. McMickens, and Kevin Selby. *AIDS.* Santa Barbara, CA: Greenwood, 2011.

Benedict, Jeff. *Poisoned: The True Story of the Deadly E. coli Outbreak That Changed the Way Americans Eat.* New York: Inspire, 2011.

Bennenson, A. S., ed. *Control of Communicable Diseases Manual.* 20th ed. Washington, DC: American Public Health Association, 2014.

Bennett, John E., Raphael Dolin, and Martin J. Blaser, eds. *Mandell, Douglas, and Bennett's Principles and Practice of Infectious Diseases.* 8th ed. Philadelphia: Elsevier, 2015.

———. *Mandell, Douglas, and Bennett's Infectious Disease Essentials.* Philadelphia: Elsevier, 2017.

Berger, Stephen. *Japanese Encephalitis: Global Status.* Los Angeles: GIDEON Informatics, 2015.

———. *Trichomoniasis: Global Status.* Los Angeles: GIDEON Informatics, 2017.

Biosafety in Microbiological and Biomedical Laboratories. 5th ed. Washington, DC: Government Printing Office, 2009. This book can also be found online at https://www.cdc.gov/biosafety/publications/bmbl5/index.htm> (accessed January 31, 2018).

Birn, Anne-Emanuelle, Yogan Pillay, and Timothy H. Holtz. *Textbook of Global Health.* Oxford; New York: Oxford University Press, 2017.

Blaser, Martin J. *Missing Microbes: How the Overuse of Antibiotics Is Fueling Our Modern Plagues.* New York: Henry Holt, 2014.

Blazina, Christopher, Güler Boyraz, and David Shen-Miller, eds. *The Psychology of the Human-Animal Bond: A Resource for Clinicians and Researchers.* New York: Springer, 2013.

Bloch, Marc. *The Royal Touch: Sacred Monarchy and Scrofula in England and France.* Translated by J. E. Anderson. London: Routledge and Kegan Paul, 1973.

Blume, Stuart. *Immunization: How Vaccines Became Controversial.* London: Reaktion, 2017.

Boccaccio, Giovanni. *The Decameron.* Translated by Mark Musa. New York: Signet, 1992.

Bollet, Alfred J. *Plagues and Poxes: The Impact of Human History on Epidemic Disease.* New York: Demos Medical, 2004.

Boruto, Franco, and Marc de Ridder, eds. *HPV and Cervical Cancer: Achievements in Prevention and Future Prospects.* New York: Springer, 2012.

Botana, Luis M., and Natalia Vilariño, eds. *Climate Change and Marine and Freshwater Toxins.* Berlin: Walter de Gruyter GmbH, 2015.

Bourassa, Erick A. *Infectious Diseases: Pharmacology & Therapeutics.* Seattle: CreateSpace, 2017.

Boutayeb, A. "The Impact of Infectious Diseases on the Development of Africa." In *Handbook of Disease Burdens and Quality of Life Measures*, edited by Victor R. Preedy and Ronald Ross Watson, 1171–1188. New York: Springer-Verlag, 2010.

Bristow, Nancy. *American Pandemic: The Lost Worlds of the 1918 Influenza Pandemic.* Oxford, UK: Oxford University Press, 2017.

Brower, Jennifer, and Peter Chalk. *The Global Threat of New and Reemerging Infectious Diseases: Reconciling U.S. National Security and Public Health Policy.* Santa Monica, CA: RAND, 2003.

Buchanan, Charles M. *Antisepsis and Antiseptics.* 1895. London: Forgotten Books, 2017.

Bustamante, Nirma Dora. "MRSA: A Global Threat." Master's thesis, UT Southwestern Medical School, 2011. This thesis can also be found online at http://www.utsouthwestern.edu/edumedia/edufiles/about_us/admin_offices/global_health/mrsa-bustamante.pdf (accessed February 6, 2018).

Bynum, Helen. *Spitting Blood: The History of Tuberculosis.* Oxford: Oxford University Press, 2012.

Calderone, Richard A. *Candida and Candidiasis.* Washington, DC: ASM, 2012.

Calderone, Richard A., and Ronald Cihlar, eds. *Candida Species: Methods and Protocols.* New York: Humana, 2015.

Carlos, Iracilda Zeppone, ed. *Sporotrichosis: New Developments and Future Prospects.* Cham, Switzerland: Springer, 2015.

Carmichael, Anne G. *Plague and the Poor in Renaissance Florence.* Cambridge: Cambridge University Press, 1986.

Carniel, Elisabeth, and Bernard J. Hinnebusch, eds. *Yersinia: Systems Biology and Control.* Norfolk, UK: Caister Academic, 2012.

Carrell, Jennifer Lee. *The Speckled Monster: A Historical Tale of Battling the Smallpox Epidemic.* New York: Dutton, 2003.

Carter, K. Codell, and Barbara R. Carter. Childbed Fever: *A Scientific Biography* of *Ignaz Semmelweis.* New York: Routledge, 2017.

Carus, W. Seth. *A Short History of Biological Warfare: From Pre-history to the 21st Century.* Washington, DC: National Defense University Press, 2017.

Carvalho, Agostinho. *Immunogenetics of Fungal Diseases.* New York: Springer Berlin Heidelberg, 2017.

Castillo, Victor, and Rodney Harris, eds. *Protozoa: Biology, Classification and Role in Disease.* New York: Nova Biomedical, 2013.

Chander, Jagdish. "Talaromycosis." In *Textbook of Medical Mycology*, 506–523. New Delhi: Jaypee Brothers Medical, 2018.

Cheng, Liang, and David G. Bostwick, eds. *Essentials of Anatomic Pathology.* 3rd ed. New York: Springer, 2010.

Cherry, James, and Gail J. Demmler-Harrison. *Feigen and Cherry's Textbook of Pediatric Infectious Disease.* Philadelphia: Elsevier Saunders, 2014.

Christodoulides, Myron, ed. *Meningitis: Cellular and Molecular Basis.* Wallingford, UK: CAB International, 2013.

Cimaz, Rolando, and Thomas Lehman, eds. *Pediatrics in Systemic Autoimmune Diseases.* 2nd ed. Oxford: Elsevier, 2016.

Closser, Svea. *Chasing Polio in Pakistan: Why the World's Largest Public Health Initiative May Fail.* Nashville: Vanderbilt University Press, 2010.

Coenye, Tom, and Eshwar Mahenthiralingam, eds. *Burkholderia: From Genomes to Function.* Norfolk, UK: Caister Academic Press, 2014.

Cohen J. I. "Herpesviruses." In *Cancer Medicine*, edited by Waun Ki Hong, et al. Shelton, CT: People's Medical, 2010.Mustacchi, Piero. "Parasites." In *Cancer Medicine*, edited by Waun Ki Hong, et al. Shelton, CT: People's Medical, 2010.

Cohen, Jonathan, William G. Powderly, and Steven M. Opal, eds. *Infectious Diseases.* Amsterdam: Elsevier, 2017.

Colbert, Bruce J., and Luis S. Gonzalez III, eds. *Microbiology: Practical Applications and Infection Prevention.* Boston: Cengage Learning, 2016.

Colpitts, Tonya M. *West Nile Virus: Methods and Protocols.* New York: Humana, 2016.

Compans, Richard W., and Michael B.A. Oldstone, eds. *Influenza Pathogenesis and Control—Volume 1.* New York: Springer, 2016.

Connolly, M. A. *Communicable Disease Control in Emergencies: A Field Manual.* Geneva: World Health Organization, 2005.

Conover, Michael R., and Rosanna M. Vail. *Human Diseases from Wildlife.* Boca Raton, FL: CRC, 2015.

Cooreman, E. A. *Global Leprosy Strategy 2016–2010: Accelerating Towards a Leprosy-Free World.* Geneva, Switzerland: World Health Organization, 2016.

Corey, Lawrence, and Anna Wald. "Genital Herpes." In *Sexually Transmitted Diseases,* edited by King K Holmes, et al., 399–437. New York: McGraw-Hill, 2008.

Corsby, Alfred W. *America's Forgotten Pandemic.* New York: Cambridge University Press, 2003.

Cramer, Michael M. *Food Plant Sanitation: Design, Maintenance, and Good Manufacturing Practices.* 2nd ed. Boca Raton, FL: CRC, 2016.

Crawford, Dorothy H., Alan B. Rickinson, and Ingolfur Johannessen. *Cancer Virus: The Discovery of the Epstein-Barr Virus.* Oxford: Oxford University Press, 2014.

Crockett, David, and Nicole Shonka. "Case 1.15: Cough and Dyspnea in a Sarcoma Patient: Appetite for Infection." In *Infections in the Immunosuppressed Patient,* edited by Pranatharthi H. Chandrasekar. New York: Oxford University Press, 2016.

Crompton, D. W. T., and Lorenzo Savioli. *Handbook of Helminthiasis for Public Health.* New York: CRC, 2006.

Crompton, David William Thomasson, et al. *Controlling Disease Due to Helminth Infections.* Geneva: World Health Organization, 2003.

Crosby, Alfred W. *America's Forgotten Pandemic: The Influenza of 1918.* 2nd ed. New York: Cambridge University Press, 2003.

Crosby, Molly Caldwell. *Asleep: The Forgotten Epidemic that Remains One of Medicine's Greatest Mysteries.* Berkley, CA: Berkley Books, 2011.

Dale, Jeremy W., and Simon F. Park. *Molecular Genetics.* 5th ed. Chichester, UK: Wiley-Blackwell, 2010.

David, Michael, and Jean-Luc Benoit, eds. *The Infectious Disease Diagnosis: A Case Approach.* Cham, Switzerland: Springer, 2018.

Davies, Sara E., Adam Kamradt-Scott, and Simon Rushton. *Disease Diplomacy: International Norms and Global Health Security.* Baltimore, MD: Johns Hopkins University Press, 2015.

De Villiers, Ethel-Michele, and Harald zur Hausen, eds. *TT Viruses: The Still Elusive Human Pathogens.* Berlin: Springer, 2009.

Dehner, George. *Influenza: A Century of Science and Public Health Response.* Pittsburgh: University of Pittsburgh Press, 2012.

Delaporte, François. *Chagas Disease: History of a Continent's Scourge.* Translated by Arthur Goldhammer. New York: Fordham University Press, 2012.

Delort, Anne-Marie, and Pierre Amato, eds. *Microbiology of Aerosols.* New York: Wiley-Blackwell, 2017.

Demaitre, Luke. *Leprosy in Premodern Medicine: A Malady of the Whole Body.* Baltimore, MD: Johns Hopkins University Press, 2009.

Despommier, Dickson D. *People, Parasites, and Plowshares: Learning from Our Body's Most Terrifying Invaders.* New York: Columbia University Press, 2013.

Despommier, Dickson D., et al. *Parasitic Diseases,* 6th ed. New York: Parasites without Borders, 2017. This book can also be found online at http://www.parasiteswithoutborders.com/parasitic-diseases-6th-edition/ (accessed January 12, 2018).

Dickerson, James L. *Yellow Fever: A Deadly Disease Poised to Kill Again.* New York: Prometheus, 2006.

Diefenbach, Russell J., and Cornel Fraedel, eds. *Herpes Simplex Virus: Methods and Protocols.* New York: Springer, 2016.

Dingwall, Robert, Lily M. Hoffman, and Karen Staniland, eds. *Pandemics and Emerging Diseases: The Sociological Agenda.* Chichester, UK: Wiley, 2013.

Diniz, Debora. *Zika: From the Brazilian Backlands to Global Threat.* London: Zed, 2017.

Dismukes, William E., Peter G. Pappas, and Jack D. Sobel. *Clinical Mycology.* New York: Oxford University Press, 2003.

Dodd, Christine, and Tim G. Aldsworth. *Foodborne Illnesses.* 3rd ed. New York: Academic Press, 2017.

Dongyou Liu, ed. *Molecular Detection of Human Parasitic Pathogens.* Boca Raton, FL: Taylor & Francis, 2013.

Doudna, Jennifer A., and Samuel H. Sternberg. *A Crack in Creation: Gene Editing and the Unthinkable Power to Control Evolution.* Boston: Houghton Mifflin Harcourt, 2017.

Drisdelle, Rosemary. *Parasites: Tales of Humanity's Most Unwelcome Guests.* Berkeley: University of California Press, 2010.

Dubray, Christine. "Helminths, Soil-Transmitted." In *CDC Yellow Book 2018: Health Information for International Travel.* Oxford: Oxford University Press, 2017.

Dworkin, Mark S., ed. *Cases in Field Epidemiology: A Global Perspective.* Sudbury, MA: Jones & Bartlett Learning, 2011.

Emanuel, Ezekiel J. *The Oxford Textbook of Clinical Research Ethics.* New York: Oxford University Press, 2011.

Enemark, Christian. *Biosecurity Dilemmas: Dreaded Diseases, Ethical Responses, and the Health of Nations.* Washington, DC: Georgetown University Press, 2017.

Engelkirk, Paul G., and Janet Duben-Engelkirk. *Laboratory Diagnosis of Infectious Diseases: Essentials of Diagnostic Microbiology.* Baltimore: Lippincott Williams & Wilkins, 2008.

Ergönül, Önder, and Chris A. Whitehouse, eds. *Crimean-Congo Hemorrhagic Fever: A Global Perspective.* New York: Springer, 2010.

Ergönül, Önder, Füsun Can, Lawrence Madoff, and Murat Akova, eds. *Emerging Infectious Diseases: Clinical Case Studies.* Waltham, MA: Academic Press, 2014.

Ericsson, Charles D., Herbert L. DuPont, and Robert Steffen. *Travelers' Diarrhea.* Hamilton, ON: BC Decker, 2008.

Erlandsen, Stanley L., and Ernest A. Meyer. *Giardia and Giardiasis: Biology Pathogenesis, and Epidemiology.* New York: Springer-Verlag, 2013.

Estenson, Joseph. *Aspergillosis: A Reference Guide.* Washington DC: Capitol Hill Press, 2016.

———. *Chronic Sinusitis.* Washington, DC: Capitol Hill, 2015.

———. *Conjunctivitis: A Reference Guide.* Washington, DC: Capitol Hill Press, 2015.

———. *Epstein-Barr Virus (Mononucleosis): A Reference Guide.* Washington DC: Capitol Hill Press, 2015.

———. *Q Fever: A Reference Guide.* Washington, DC: Capitol Hill Press, 2015.

Fallon, Brian A., and Jennifer Sotsky. *Conquering Lyme Disease: Science Bridges the Great Divide.* New York: Columbia University Press, 2017.

Farb, Daniel. *Bioterrorism Hemorrhagic Viruses.* Los Angeles: University of Health Care, 2004.

Farrar, Jeremy, et al, eds. *Manson's Tropical Diseases.* 23rd ed. New York: Elsevier, 2013.

Faruque, Shah M., ed. *Foodborne and Waterborne Bacterial Pathogens: Epidemiology, Evolution and Molecular Biology.* Norfolk, UK: Caister Academic, 2012.

Ferri, Fred F. *Ferri's Clinical Advisor 2018.* Philadelphia: Elsevier, 2018.

Fidler, David P. *International Law and Infectious Diseases.* Oxford: Clarendon, 1999.

The First Ten Years of the World Health Organization (1948–1957). Geneva, Switzerland: World Health Organization, 1958.

Fitzharris, Lindsey. *The Butchering Art.* New York: Scientific American, 2017.

Flynn, Laura. *All about Infection Control.* Guelph, ON: Mediscript Communications, 2017.

Fong, I. W., and Kenneth Alibek, eds. *Bioterrorism and Infectious Agents: A New Dilemma for the 21st Century.* New York: Springer, 2005.

The Fourth Ten Years of the World Health Organization (1978–1987). Geneva, Switzerland: World Health Organization, 2011.

Fox, Renée C. *Doctors Without Borders: Humanitarian Quests, Impossible Dreams of Médecins Sans Frontières.* Baltimore, MD: Johns Hopkins University Press, 2014.

Freedman, David O., ed. *Immunopathogenetic Aspects of Disease Induced by Helminth Parasites.* New York: Karger, 1997.

Friedman, Ellen M., and James P. Barassi. *My Ear Hurts!: A Complete Guide to Understanding and Treating Your Child's Ear Infections.* New York: Simon & Schuster, 2001.

Gajdusek, D. Carleton. *Journal of Further Explorations in the Kuru Region and in the Kukukuku Country, Eastern Highlands of Eastern New Guinea and of a Return to West New Guinea: December 25, 1963 to May 4, 1964.* Victoria, Australia: Leopold Classic Library, 2016.

Galanda, Claudia D. *AIDS-Related Opportunistic Infections.* New York: Nova Biomedical, 2009.

Gates, Robert H. *Infectious Disease Secrets.* Philadelphia: Hanley & Beltus, 2003.

Gaynes, Robert P. *Germ Theory: Medical Pioneers in Infectious Diseases.* Washington, DC: ASM, 2011.

Gillespie, Stephen H., and Kathleen B. Bamford. *Medical Microbiology and Infection at a Glance.* 4th ed. Hoboken, NJ: Wiley Blackwell, 2012.

Gipe, Abigail. *Keratitis: Essentials in Ophthalmology.* New York: Hayle Medical, 2017.

Goater, Timothy M., Cameron P. Goater, and Gerald W. Esch. *Parasitism: The Diversity and Ecology of Animal Parasites.* 2nd ed. Cambridge: Cambridge University Press, 2014.

Goldsmith, Connie. *Influenza: The Next Pandemic?* Minneapolis: Twenty-First Century Books, 2007.

Gould, Tony. *A Disease Apart: Leprosy in the Modern World.* New York: St. Martin's Press, 2005.

Gratz, Norman. *Vector- and Rodent-Borne Diseases in Europe and North America: Distribution, Public Health Burden, and Control.* Cambridge: Cambridge University Press, 2006.

Graunt, J. *Natural and Political Observations Made upon the Bills of Mortality.* 1662. Reprint, Baltimore: Johns Hopkins Press, 1939.

Greenbaum, Eli. *Emerald Labyrinth: A Scientist's Adventures in the Jungles of the Congo.* Dartmouth, NH: ForeEdge/University Press of New England, 2017.

Greenwood, David, et al. *Medical Microbiology: A Guide to Microbial Infections: Pathogenesis, Immunity, Laboratory Diagnosis and Control.* 17th ed. Philadelphia: Churchill Livingstone/Elsevier, 2007.

Grove, David I. *Tapeworms, Lice, and Prions: A Compendium of Unpleasant Infections.* Oxford: Oxford University Press, 2014.

Gubler, Duane J. "The Global Threat of Emergent/Reemergent Vector-Borne Diseases." In Vector-Borne Diseases: Understanding the Environmental, Human Health, and Ecological Connections: Workshop Summary. Washington, DC: National Academies Press, 2008.

Gubler, Duana J., et al., eds. *Dengue and Dengue Hemorrhagic Fever.* Boston: CABI, 2014.

Guerrant, Richard L., David H. Walker, and Peter F. Weller. *Tropical Infectious Diseases: Principles, Pathogens & Practice.* Philadelphia: Elsevier Health Sciences, 2011.

Guibert, Hervé. *Cytomegalovirus: A Hospitalization Diary.* Translated by Clara Orban. New York: Fordham University Press, 2016.

Gyapong, John, and Boakye Boatin, eds. *Neglected Tropical Diseases—Sub-Saharan Africa.* New York: Springer, 2016.

Hackett, Christopher B. *Salmonella: Prevalence, Risk Factors and Treatment Options.* New York: Nova Science, 2015.

Haddad, S. F. *X-Plain Hand Washing—Preventing Infections.* Coralville, IA: Patient Education Institute, 2016.

Halpin, Kim, and Paul Rota. "A Review of Hendra Virus and Nipah Virus Infections in Man and Other Animals." In *Zoonoses—Infections Affecting Humans and Animals: Focus on Public Health Aspects*, edited by Andreas Sing. Dordrecht, Netherlands: Springer Netherlands, 2015.

Hamborsky, Jennifer, Andrew Kroeger, and Skip Wolfe, eds. *Epidemiology and Prevention of Vaccine-Preventable Diseases.* 13th ed. Atlanta: Centers for Disease Control and Prevention, 2015.

Hamlin, Christopher. *Cholera: The Biography.* Oxford: Oxford University Press, 2009.

Harries, Anthony, Dermot Maher, and Stephen Graham. "Introduction." In *TB/HIV: A Clinical Manual*, 21. Geneva: World Health Organization, 2004. This introduction can also be found online at http://apps.who.int/iris/bitstream/10665/42830/1/9241546344.pdf (accessed November 6, 2017).

Harrison, Mark. *Contagion: How Commerce Has Spread Disease.* New Haven, CT: Yale University Press, 2012.

Hechemy, Karim E., ed. *Rickettsiology and Rickettsial Diseases: Fifth International Conference.* Boston: Blackwell, 2009.

Henderson, Cary G. *Enterococci and Bacterial Diseases: Risk Factors, Molecular Biology, and Antibiotic Resistance.* New York: Nova Science, 2017.

Henderson, Donald A. *Smallpox: The Death of a Disease.* Amherst, NY: Prometheus, 2009.

Hennekens, C. H., and J. E. Buring. *Epidemiology in Medicine.* Boston: Little, Brown, 1987.

Heymann, David L. *Control of Communicable Diseases Manual.* 20th ed. Washington, DC: American Public Health Association, 2014.

Heymann, David L., and Vernon J. M. Lee. "Emerging and Re-emerging Infections." In *Oxford Textbook of Global Public Health*, edited by Roger Detels, Martin Gulliford, Quarraisha Abdool Karim, and Chorh Chuan Tan. 6th ed. Oxford: Oxford University Press, 2015.

Hillery, Anya M., and Kinam Park. *Drug Delivery: Fundamentals and Applications.* 2nd ed. Boca Raton, FL: CRC, 2016.

Holland, Celia V., and Malcolm W. Kennedy, eds. *The Geohelminths: Ascaris, Trichuris, and Hookworm.* Boston: Kluwer Academic, 2002.

Holst, Otto., ed. *Microbial Toxins: Methods and Protocols.* 2nd ed. New York: Humana, 2017.

Homei, Aya, and Michael Worboys. *Fungal Disease in Britain and the United States, 1850–2000: Mycoses and Modernity.* New York: Palgrave Macmillan, 2013.

Hopkins, Donald R., and Alexandra M. Levitt. *Deadly Outbreaks: How Medical Detectives Save Lives Threatened by Killer Pandemics, Exotic Viruses, and Drug-Resistant Parasites.* New York: Skyhorse, 2015.

Hopkins, Donald R., and Ernesto Ruiz-Tiben. "Dracunculiasis (Guinea Worm Disease): Case Study of the Effort to Eradicate Guinea Worm." In *Water and Sanitation-Related Diseases and the Environment: Challenges, Interventions, and Preventive Measures*, edited by Janine M. Selendy, 125–132. Hoboken, NJ: Wiley-Blackwell, 2011.

Horn, Lyle W. *Deadly Diseases and Epidemics: Hepatitis.* Philadelphia: Chelsea House, 2005.

Horn, Lyle W., and Alan Hecht. *Hepatitis.* New York: Chelsea House, 2011.

Hospenthal, Duane R., and Michael G. Rinaldi. *Diagnosis and Treatment of Fungal Infections.* Cham, Switzerland: Springer, 2015.

Hotez, P. J. "The Neglected Tropical Diseases and the Neglected Infections of Poverty." In *The Causes and Impacts of Neglected Tropical and Zoonotic Diseases: Opportunities for Integrated Invention Strategies.* Washington, DC: National Academies Press, 2011.

Howard, Dexter H. *Pathogenic Fungi in Humans and Animals.* New York: Marcel Dekker, 2003.

Ian, Glynn, and Jenifer Glynn. *Life and Death of Smallpox.* New York: Cambridge University Press, 2004.

Inhorn, Marcia C., and Peter J. Brown, eds. *The Anthropology of Disease: International Health Perspectives.* Hoboken, NJ: Taylor and Francis, 2013.

Jackson, Alan C., ed. *Rabies: Scientific Basis of the Disease and its Management.* Amsterdam: Elsevier Academic, 2013.

James, Jenny Lynd. *Microbial Hazard Identification in Fresh Fruits and Vegetables.* New York: Wiley-Interscience, 2006.

Jamieson, Barrie G. M., ed. *Schistosoma: Biology, Pathology, and Control.* Boca Raton, FL: CRC, 2016.

Jamison, Dean T., et al, eds. *Disease and Mortality in Sub-Saharan Africa.* Washington, DC: World Bank, 2006.

Jarvis, William R., ed. *Bennett & Brachman's Hospital Infections.* Philadelphia: Wolters Kluwer Health/Lippincott Williams & Wilkins, 2014.

Johanson, Paula. *HIV and AIDS (Coping in a Changing World).* New York: Rosen, 2007.

Johnson, Kristy Young, and Paul Matthew Nolan. *Biological Weapons: Recognizing, Understanding, and Responding to the Threat.* Hoboken, NJ: Wiley, 2016.

Johnson, Nicholas, ed. *The Role of Animals in Emerging Viral Diseases.* Boston: Elsevier/AP, 2014.

Julius, Henri. *Attachment to Pets: An Integrative View of Human-Animal Relationships with Implications for Therapeutic Practice.* Cambridge, MA: Hogrefe, 2013.

Kahlon, Rachhpal. *Pseudomonas: Molecular and Applied Biology.* New York: Springer, 2016.

Kahn, Laura H. *One Health and the Politics of Antimicrobial Resistance.* Baltimore, MD: Johns Hopkins University Press, 2016.

Kaplan, Justin L., et al. *The Merck Manual of Medical Information.* New York: Pocket Books, 2008.

Kaslow, Richard A., Lawrence R. Stanberry, and James W. Le Duc, eds. *Viral Infections of Humans: Epidemiology and Control.* New York: Springer, 2014.

Kazemi, Samaneth. *Stress Response in Listeria Monocytogenes.* London: Lambert Academic, 2017.

Kek, Peggy, and Penny Whitworth, eds. *Singapore and UNICEF: Working for Children.* Hackensack, NJ: World Scientific, 2016.

Klein, Günter. *Campylobacter: Features, Detection, and Prevention of Foodborne Disease.* New York: Academic Press, 2016.

Kline, Mark W., et al., eds. *Rudolph's Pediatrics.* 23rd ed. New York: McGraw-Hill Education, 2018.

Knodel, Leroy C. "Sexually Transmitted Diseases." In *Pharmacotherapy: A Pathophysiologic Approach*, edited by Joseph T. DiPiro. New York: McGraw-Hill, 2014.

Koata, Gina. *Mercies in Disguise: A Story of Hope, a Family's Genetic Destiny, and the Science Tthat Rescued Them.* New York: St. Martin's, 2017.

Kon, Kateryna. *Antibiotic Resistance: Mechanisms and New Antimicrobial Approaches.* Edited by Mahendra Rai. New York: Academic Press, 2016.

Koplow, David. *Smallpox: The Fight to Eradicate a Global Scourge.* Berkeley: University of California Press, 2004.

Kotar, S. L., and J. E. Gessler. *Smallpox: A History.* Jefferson, NC: McFarland, 2013.

Krauss, Hartmut, et al., eds. *Zoonoses: Infectious Diseases Transmissible from Animals to Humans.* 3rd ed. Washington, DC: ASM, 2003.

Kruel, Donald. *Trypanosomiasis.* New York: Chelsea House, 2007.

Krug, Etienne G., et al., eds. *World Report on Violence and Health.* Geneva: World Health Organization, 2002. This report can also be found online at http://www.who.int/violence_injury_prevention/violence/world_report/chapters/en/ (accessed March 8, 2018).

Kudva, Indira T., et al., eds. *Virulence Mechanisms of Bacterial Pathogens.* 5th ed. Washington DC: American Society for Microbiology, 2016.

Kumar, Awanish. *Leishmania and Leishmaniasis.* New York: Springer, 2013.

Kumar, P. Dileep. *Rabies.* Westport, CT: Greenwood, 2009.

Kumar, Sandeep, Jane C. Benjamin, and Shubhra Shukla. *Pathogenic Bacteria in Bioaerosol of Hospitals: Important of Airborne Pathogen in Hospital.* New York: Lap Lambert Academic, 2013.

Kumar, Vinay, Abul Abbas, and Nelson Fausto. *Robbins and Cotran Pathologic Basis of Disease.* 7th ed. Philadelphia: Saunders, 2004.

Lamb, Tracey J., ed. *Immunity to Parasitic Infections.* Chichester, UK: Wiley-Blackwell, 2012.

Leal, Filho W., Ulisses M. Azeiteiro, and Fátima Alves, eds. Climate Change and Health: Improving Resilience and Reducing Risks. Cham, Switzerland: Springer 2016.

Liaw, Yun-Fan, and Fabien Zoulim, eds. *Hepatitis B Virus in Human Diseases.* New York: Humana, 2015.

Liberski, Pawel P., ed. *Prion Diseases.* New York: Springer, 2017.

Lindler, Luther E., Frank J. Lebeda, and George W. Korch, eds. *Biological Weapons Defense: Infectious Diseases and Counterbioterrorism.* Totowa, NJ: Humana, 2005.

Lindsay, David S., and Louis M. Weiss. *Opportunistic Infections: Toxoplasma, Sarcocystis, and Microsporidia.* New York: Springer, 2011.

Lock, Stephen, Stephen Last, and George M. Dunea, eds. *The Oxford Illustrated Companion to Medicine.* Oxford: Oxford University Press, 2001.

Long, Sarah S., and Charles G. Prober. *Principles and Practice of Pediatric Infectious Disease.* Philadelphia: Elsevier, 2017.

Lopez, Alan D., Colin Mathers, and Majid Ezzati, eds. *Global Burden of Disease and Risk Factors.* New York: World Bank Group, 2006.

Luján, Hugo D., and Staffan Svärd, eds. *Giardia: A Model Organism.* New York: Springer, 2011.

Mackenzie, J. S., A. D. T. Barrett, and V. Deubel, eds. *Japanese Encephalitis and West Nile Viruses.* New York: Springer, 2013.

MacLachlan, N. James, and Edward J. Dubovi. *Fenner's Veterinary Virology.* London: Academic Press, 2016.

Macpherson, Calum N. L., and Philip S. Craig. *Parasitic Helminths and Zoonoses in Africa.* New York: Springer, 1991.

Maddocks, Steven. *UNICEF.* Chicago: Raintree, 2004.

Madkour, M. Monir. *Brucellosis.* Oxford, UK: Butterworth-Heinemann, 2014.

Magez, Stefan, and Magdalena Radwanska, eds. *Trypanosomes and Trypanosomiasis.* Vienna: Springer, 2014.

Markel, Howard. *When Germs Travel: Six Major Epidemics That Have Invaded America since 1900 and the Fears They Have Unleashed.* New York: Pantheon, 2004.

Marr, Lisa. *Sexually Transmitted Diseases: A Physician Tells You What You Need to Know*. 2nd ed. Baltimore, MD: Johns Hopkins University Press, 2007.

Marrin, Albert. *Very, Very, Very Dreadful: The Influenza Pandemic of 1918*. New York: Knopf, 2018.

Matthews, Philippa C. *Tropical Medicine Notebook*. Oxford: Oxford University Press, 2017.

Maule, Aaron G., and Nikki J. Marks, eds. *Parasitic Flatworms: Molecular Biology, Biochemistry, Immunology and Physiology*. Wallingford, UK: CABI, 2006.

Mayer, Kenneth H., and H. F. Pizer, eds. *The AIDS Pandemic: Impact on Science and Society*. San Diego: Academic Press, 2005.

McAuliffe, Kathleen. *This Is Your Brain on Parasites: How Tiny Creatures Manipulate Our Behavior and Shape Society*. New York: Eamon Dolan/Mariner, 2017.

McCormick, Joseph B., and Susan Fisher-Hoch. *Level 4: Virus Hunters of the CDC: Tracking Ebola and the World's Deadliest Viruses*. New York: Sterling, 2016.

McDonnell, Gerald E. *Antisepsis, Disinfection, and Sterilization*. 2nd ed. Washington, DC: ASM, 2017.

McDowell, Mary Ann, and Sima Rafati. *Neglected Tropical Diseases—Middle East and North Africa*. Vienna: Springer, 2014.

McGuire-Wolfe, Christine. *Foundations of Infection Control and Prevention*. Burlington, MA: Jones & Bartlett Learning, 2018.

McKenna, Maryn. *Big Chicken: The Incredible Story of How Antibiotics Created Modern Agriculture and Changed the Way the World Eats*. Washington, DC: National Geographic, 2017.

McNeil, Donald G., Jr. *Zika: The Emerging Epidemic*. New York: Norton, 2017.

McNeill, William Hardy. *Plagues and Peoples*. New York: Doubleday, 1998.

Micheli, Lyle J., ed. *Encyclopedia of Sports Medicine*. Vol. 1. Los Angeles: Sage, 2011.

Miller, Chris H. *Infection Control and Management of Hazardous Materials for the Dental Team*. Toronto: Elsevier Canada, 2017.

Mirete, Salvador, and Marcos López Pérez, eds. *Antibiotic Resistance Genes in Natural Environments and Long-Term Effects*. New York: Nova Biomedical, 2017.

Morand, Serge, Boris R. Krasnov, and D. Timothy J. Littlewood, eds. *Parasite Diversity and Diversification: Evolutionary Ecology Meets Phylogenetics*. Cambridge: Cambridge University Press, 2015.

Morris, Timothy A., Andrew L. Ries, and Richard A. Bordow, eds. *Manual of Clinical Problems in Pulmonary Medicine*. Philadelphia: Wolters Kluwer, 2014.

Mulvey, Matthew A., David J. Klumpp, and Ann E. Stapleton. *Urinary Tract Infections: Molecular Pathogenesis and Clinical Management*. Washington, DC: ASM, 2017.

Muriel, Pablo. *Liver Pathophysiology: Therapies and Antioxidants*. Boston: Elsevier, 2017.

Murphy, Jim, and Alison Blank. *Invincible Microbe: Tuberculosis and the Never-Ending Search for a Cure*. New York: HMH, 2015.

Murray, Patrick, Ken S. Rosenthal, and Michael A. Pfaller. *Medical Microbiology*. Philadelphia: Elsevier, 2016.

Myers, James W., and Jonathan P. Moorman. *Gantz's Manual of Clinical Problems in Infectious Disease*. Philadelphia: Wolters Kluwer, 2015.

Myers, Martin G., and Diego Pineda. *Do Vaccines Cause That?!: A Guide to Evaluating Vaccine Safety Concerns*. Galveston, TX: Immunizations for Public Health, 2008.

Myers, Norman, and Jennifer Kent. *Environmental Exodus: An Emergent Crisis in the Global Arena*. New York: Climate Institute, 1995.

National Academies of Science, Engineering, Medicine. *Human Genome Editing: Science, Ethics, and Governance*. Washington, DC: National Academies Press, 2017.

Nelson, Jennifer. *More Than Medicine: A History of the Feminist Women's Health Movement*. New York: New York University Press, 2015.

Nelson, Kenrad E., and Carolyn F. Masters Williams, eds. *Infectious Disease Epidemiology: Theory and Practice*. 3rd ed. Sudbury, MA: Jones and Bartlett, 2014.

Nester, Eugene W. *Microbiology: A Human Perspective*. 8th ed. New York: McGraw-Hill, 2016.

Nguhiu, Purity, and Dorcas Yole. "Intestinal Protozoa: Human Cyclosporiasis, Emerging Foodborne Zoonosis: The African Green Monkey Model". Saarbrüken, Germany: Noor, 2017.

Nicholson, William L., and Christopher D. Paddock. "Rickettsial (Spotted & Typhus Fevers) & Related Infections, including Anaplasmosis & Ehrlichiosis." In *CDC Health Information for International Travel (Yellow Book)*. New York: Oxford University Press, 2018.

Nuttall, Patricia A., and M. Labuda. "Saliva-Assisted Transmission of Tick-Borne Pathogens." In *Ticks: Biology, Disease and Control*, edited by Alan S. Bowman and Patricia A. Nuttall, 205–219. New York: Cambridge University Press, 2008.

O'Connor, Louise, and Barry Glynn, eds. *Fungal Diagnostics: Methods and Protocols.* New York: Humana, 2013.

O'Neal, Christopher, Raf Rizk, and Marianne Khalil. Clostridium difficile: *A Patient's Guide.* Tustin, CA: Inner Workings, 2011.

Offit, Paul A. *Vaccinated: One Man's Quest to Defeat the World's Deadliest Diseases.* New York: Collins, 2007.

Okeoma, Chioma M., ed. *Chikungunya Virus: Advances in Biology, Pathogenesis, and Treatment.* Cham, Switzerland: Springer, 2016.

Oldstone, Michael B. A. *Viruses, Plagues, and History: Past, Present, and Future.* New York: Oxford University Press, 2010.

Opdycke, Sandra. *The Flu Epidemic of 1918: America's Experience in the Global Health Crisis.* New York, Routledge, 2014.

Ortega-Pierres, Guadalupe. *Giardia and Cryptosporidium: From Molecules to Disease.* Wallingford, UK: CABI, 2009.

Osaro, Erharbor. *Blood Transfusion Services in Sub Saharan Africa: Challenges and Constraints.* Bloomington, IN: AuthorHouse, 2012.

Oshinsky, David M. *Polio: An American Story.* New York: Oxford University Press, 2005.

Osterholm, Michael T., and Mark Olshaker. *Deadliest Enemy: Our War Against Killer Germs.* New York: Little, Brown and Company, 2017.

Oxford, John, Paul Kellam, and Leslie Harold Collier. *Human Virology.* New York: Oxford University Press, 2016.

Palladino, Michael A., and David Wesner. *HIV and AIDS.* Special Topics in Biology Series. San Francisco: Benjamin Cummings, 2005.

Papadakis, Maxine A., and Stephen J. McPhee, eds. *Current Diagnosis & Treatment in Infectious Diseases.* New York: McGraw Hill, 2017.

Parham, Peter. *The Immune System.* 4th ed. New York: Garland Science, 2015.

Payne, Daniel C., and Umesh D. Parashar. "Chapter 13: Rotavirus." In *Manual for the Surveillance of Vaccine-Preventable Diseases.* Atlanta: Centers for Disease Control and Prevention, 1996. This chapter can also be found online at https://www.cdc.gov/vaccines/pubs/surv-manual/chpt13-rotavirus.html (accessed February 13, 2018).

Payne, Susan. *Viruses: From Understanding to Investigation.* New York: Academic Press, 2017.

Pelis, Kim. *Charles Nicolle, Pasteur's Imperial Missionary: Typhus and Tunisia.* Rochester, NY: University of Rochester, 2006.

Persing, David H., et al., eds. *Molecular Microbiology: Diagnostic Principles and Practice.* 3rd ed. Washington, DC: ASM, 2016.

Peters, Wallace, and Geoffrey Pasvol. *Atlas of Tropical Medicine and Parasitology.* 6th ed. London: Elsevier Mosby, 2007.

Petersen, Eskild, Lin H. Chen, and Patricia Schlagenhauf-Lawlor. *Infectious Diseases: A Geographic Guide.* Chichester, UK: Wiley Blackwell, 2017.

Petersen, Lyle R., et al. "Emerging Vector-Borne Diseases in the United States: What Is Next and Are We Prepared?" In Global Health Impacts of Vector-Borne Diseases: Workshop Summary. Washington, DC: National Academies Press, 2016.

Pettit, Dorothy A., and Janice Bailie. *A Cruel Wind: Pandemic Flu in America, 1918–1920.* Murfreesboro, TN: Timberlane, 2008.

Pittet, Didier, John M. Boyce, and Benedetta Allegranzi, eds. *Hand Hygiene: A Handbook for Medical Professionals.* New York: Wiley, 2017.

Plum, Jennifer. *Everything You Need to Know about Chicken Pox and Shingles.* New York: Rosen, 2001.

Prüss-Üstün, Annette, et al. *Preventing Disease through Healthy Environments: Towards an Estimate of the Environmental Burden of Disease.* Geneva, Switzerland: World Health Organization, 2016.

Preciado, Diego, ed. *Otitis Media: State of the Art Concepts and Treatment.* New York: Springer, 2015.

Preston, Richard. *The Hot Zone.* New York: Anchor, 1994.

Preux, Pierre-Marie, and Michel Dumas. *Neuroepidemiology in Tropical Health.* New York: Academic Press, 2017.

Price-Smith, Andrew T. *Contagion and Chaos: Disease, Ecology, and National Security in the Era of Globalization.* Boston: MIT Press, 2008.

Procopius. *History of the Wars.* Translated by H. B. Dewing. Cambridge, MA: Harvard University Press, 1914.

Pulcini, Céline, and Onder Ergonul. *Antimicrobial Stewardship.* Vol. 2 of *Developments in Emerging and Existing Infectious Disease.* New York: Academic Press, 2017.

Quammen, David. *The Chimp and the River: How AIDS Emerged from an African Forest.* New York: Norton, 2015.

Quamann, David. *Ebola: The Natural and Human History of a Deadly Virus.* New York: Norton, 2014.

Quereshi, Adnan. *Zika Virus Disease: From Origin to Outbreak.* London: Elsevier, 2018.

Ramamurthy, T., and S. K. Bhattacharya, eds. *Epidemiological and Molecular Aspects on Cholera.* New York: Springer, 2011.

Redfield, Peter. *Life in Crisis: The Ethical Journey of Doctors Without Borders.* Berkeley: University of California Press, 2013.

Redman, Nina E., and Michele Morrone. *Food Safety: A Reference Handbook.* 3rd ed. Santa Barbara, CA: ABC-CLIO, 2017.

Reinhardt, Bob H. *The End of a Global Pox: America and the Eradication of Smallpox in the Cold War Era.* Chapel Hill: University of North Carolina Press, 2015.

Remington, Jack S., and Christopher B. Wilson. *Infectious Diseases of the Fetus and Newborn Infant.* Philadelphia: Elsevier Saunders, 2016.

Renne, Elisha P. *The Politics of Polio in Northern Nigeria.* Bloomington: Indiana University Press, 2010.

Research and Markets. *Worldwide Facial Injectables Market Drivers, Opportunities, Trends, and Forecasts: 2017–2023.* Dublin: Research and Markets, 2017.

Rezza, Giovanni, and Giuseppe Ippolito, eds. *Emerging and Re-emerging Viral Infections: Advances in Microbiology, Infectious Diseases and Public Health, Volume 6.* Cham, Switzerland: Springer, 2017.

Ribeiro, Janete N. *Human Toxoplasmosis: Clinical Data and Microbiology.* Rio de Janeiro: Luiz Galileu Spoladore, 2016.

Richards, Paul. *Ebola: How a People's Science Helped End an Epidemic.* London: Zed, 2016.

Richardson, Malcolm D., and David W. Warnock. *Fungal Infection: Diagnosis and Management.* New York: Wiley-Blackwell, 2012.

Ridley, Rosalind M., and Harry F. Baker. *Fatal Protein: The Story of CJD, BSE, and Other Prion Diseases.* New York: Oxford University Press, 1998.

Rocco, Fiammetta. *The Miraculous Fever-Tree: Malaria and the Quest for a Cure That Changed the World.* New York: HarperCollins, 2003.

Rodriguez, Ana Maria. *Edward Jenner: Conqueror of Smallpox.* Berkeley Heights, NJ: Enslow, 2006.

Rollinson, D., and J. R. Stothard, eds. *Advances in Parasitology.* New York: Elsevier, 2015.

Rosen, George. *A History of Public Health.* Baltimore, MD: Johns Hopkins University Press, 2015.

Rosen, William. *Miracle Cure: The Creation of Antibiotics and the Birth of Modern Medicine.* New York: Viking, 2017.

Rosner, Lisa. *Vaccination and Its Critics: A Documentary and Reference Guide.* Santa Barbara, CA: Greenwood, 2017.

Ruggeri, Franco Maria, et al. *Hepatitis E Virus: An Emerging Zoonotic and Foodborne Pathogen.* New York: Springer, 2013.

Rupprecht, Charles, and Thirumeni Nagarajan, eds. *Current Laboratory Techniques in Rabies Diagnosis, Research and Prevention.* Amsterdam: Elsevier Academic, 2015.

Rushton, Simon, and Jeremy Youde, ed. *Routledge Handbook of Global Health Security.* London; New York: Routledge, 2014.

Ryan, Jeffrey. *Biosecurity and Bioterrorism: Containing and Preventing Biological Threats.* New York: Butterworth-Heinemann, 2016.

Ryan, Kenneth J., and C. George Ray. *Sherris Medical Microbiology: An Introduction to Infectious Diseases.* 4th ed. New York: McGraw Hill, 2003.

Ryser, Elliot T., and Elmer H. Marth. *Listeria, Listeriosis, and Food Safety.* 3rd ed. Boca Raton, FL: CRC, 2007.

Saint, Sanjay, and Sarah L. Krein. *Preventing Hospital Infections: Real-World Problems, Realistic Solutions.* New York: Oxford University Press, 2014.

Saji, Ben Tsutomu, et al., eds. *Kawasaki Disease: Current Understanding of the Mechanism and Evidence-Based Treatment.* Tokyo: Springer, 2017.

Salman, Mowafak Dauod, Jordi Tarrés-Call, and Agustín Estrada-Pena, eds. *Ticks and Tick-Borne Diseases: Geographical Distribution and Control Strategies in the Euro-Asia Region.* Boston: CAB International, 2013.

Salyers, Abigail A., and Dixie D. Whitt. *Revenge of the Microbes: How Bacterial Resistance Is Undermining the Antibiotic Miracle.* Washington, DC: ASM, 2005.

Sanyahumbi, Amy Sims, et al. "Global Disease Burden of Group A *Streptococcus.*" In Streptococcus Pyogenes: *Basic Biology to Clinical Manifestations,* edited by Joseph J. Ferretti, Dennis L. Stevens, and Vincent A. Fischetti. Oklahoma City: University of Oklahoma Health Sciences Center, 2016.

Sarasin, Philipp. *Anthrax: Bioterror as Fact and Fantasy.* Translated by Giselle Weiss. Cambridge, MA: Harvard University Press, 2006.

Sass, Edmund J. "The History of Polio." In *Polio's Legacy: An Oral History,* edited by Sass. Lanham, MD: University Press of America, 1996.

Satoskar, Abhay R., and Ravi Durvasula, eds. *Pathogenesis of Leishmaniasis: New Developments in Research.* New York: Springer, 2014.

Scheld, W. Michael, et al. *Infections of the Central Nervous System.* 4th ed. Philadelphia: Wolters Kluwer Health, 2014.

Schlossberg, David. *Tuberculosis and Nontuberculosis Mycobacterial Infections.* Washington DC: ASM, 2017.

Schmidt, Robert E., Drury R. Reavill, and David N. Phalen. *Pathology of Pet and Aviary Birds, Vol. 2.* New York: Wiley-Blackwell, 2015.

Schwartz, Eli, ed. *Tropical Diseases in Travelers.* Hoboken, NJ: Wiley-Blackwell, 2009.

Scoones, Ian. *Avian Influenza: Science, Policy and Politics.* London: Earthscan, 2010.

The Second Ten Years of the World Health Organization (1958–1967). Geneva, Switzerland: World Health Organization, 1968.

Secor, W. Evan, and Daniel G. Colley, eds. *Schistosomiasis.* New York: Springer, 2005.

Shah, Sonia. *Pandemic: Tracking Contagions, from Cholera to Ebola and Beyond.* New York: Sarah Crichton Books/Farrar, Straus and Giroux, 2016.

Shenk, Thomas E., and Mark F. Stinski, eds. *Human Cytomegalovirus.* Berlin: Springer Berlin, 2014.

Shephard, David A. E. *John Snow: Anaesthetist to a Queen and Epidemiologist to a Nation.* Cornwall, Canada: York Point, 1995.

Sherman, Irwin W. *Drugs That Changed the World: How Therapeutic Agents Shaped Our Lives.* Boca Raton, FL: CRC, 2017.

Shetty, Kirti, and George Y. Wu. *Chronic Viral Hepatitis.* 2nd ed. New York: Humana, 2012.

Shnayersen, Michael, and Mark J. Plotkin. *The Killers Within: The Deadly Rise of Drug-Resistant Bacteria.* Boston: Little, Brown, 2003.

Shrader, Anthony L., ed. *Meningitis: Symptoms, Management and Potential Complications.* Hauppage, NY: Nova Biomedical, 2014.

Siegel, Mary-Ellen, and Gray Williams. *Shingles: New Hope for an Old Disease.* Lanham, MD: M. Evans 2008.

Simoes, João Carlos Caetano, Sofia Ferreira Anastácio, and Gabriela Jorge Da Silva. *The Principles and Practice of Q Fever: The One Health Paradigm.* Boston: Nova Science, 2017.

Singh G., and S. Prabhakar, eds. *Taenia Solium Cysticercosis: From Basic to Clinical Science.* Chandigarh, India: CABI, 2002.

Singh, Prati Pal, and Vinod P. Sharma. *Water and Health.* New Delhi: Springer, 2014.

Singh, Sunit K., and Daniel Ruzek, eds. *Viral Hemorrhagic Fevers.* Boca Raton, FL: CRC, 2016.

Sipress, Alan. *The Fatal Strain: On the Trail of Avian Flu and the Coming Pandemic.* New York: Penguin, 2014.

Skolnik, Richard. *Global Health 101.* Burlington, MA: Jones & Bartlett, 2016.

Smith, Tara C., and Hilary Babcock. Streptococcus *(Group A).* 2nd ed. New York: Chelsea House, 2010.

Sobel, Jack D. *Contemporary Diagnosis and Management of Fungal Infections.* Longboat Key, FL: Handbooks in Health Care, 2009.

Speilman, Andrew, and Michael D'Antonio. *Mosquito: A Natural History of Our Most Persistent and Deadly Foe.* New York: Hyperion, 2001.

Spinney, Laura. *Pale Rider: The Spanish Flu of 1918 and How It Changed the World.* New York: Public Affairs, 2017.

Sripa, Banchob, and Paul J. Brindley. *Asiatic River Fluke: From Basic Science to Public Health.* New York: Elsevier, 2018.

Staines, Henry M., and Sanjeev Krishna, eds. *Treatment and Prevention of Malaria: Antimalarial Drug Chemistry, Action and Use.* Basel, Switzerland: Springer Basel, 2012.

Stone, C. Keith, and Roger Humphries. *Current Diagnosis and Treatment: Emergency Medicine.* New York: McGraw-Hill Education, 2017.

Stone, Carolyn. *Norovirus: How to Stay Safe.* New York: Eternal Spiral, 2014.

Suárez, Micaela L., and Steffani M. Ortega, eds. *Pneumonia: Symptoms, Diagnosis and Treatment.* New York: Nova Science, 2011.

Sutton, Philip, and Hazel M. Mitchell, eds. *Helicobacter pylori in the 21st Century.* Cambridge, MA: CABI, 2010.

Svensson, Lennart, et al. *Viral Gastroenteritis: Molecular Epidemiology and Pathogenesis.* Amsterdam: Elsevier, 2016.

Sweet, Richard L., and Ronald S. Gibbs. *Infectious Diseases of the Female Genital Tract.* Philadelphia: Wolters Kluwer, 2015.

Swiderski, Richard M. *Anthrax: A History.* Jefferson, NC: McFarland, 2004.

Sze, Szeming. *The Origins of the World Health Organization: A Personal Memoir 1945–1948.* Boca Raton, FL: LISZ, 1982.

Szente, Judit. *Assisting Young Children Caught in Disasters: Multidisciplinary Perspectives and Interventions.* New York: Springer, 2017.

Török, Estée, Ed Moran, and Fiona J. Cooke. *Oxford Handbook of Infectious Diseases and Microbiology.* Oxford: Oxford University Press, 2017.

Tabbara, Khalid, Ahmed M. M. Abu El-Asrar, and Moncef Khairallah. *Ocular Infections.* New York: Springer, 2016.

Tan, Tina Q., John P. Flaherty, and Melvin V. Gerbie. *The Vaccine Handbook: A Practitioner's Guide to Maximizing Use and Efficacy across the Lifespan.* New York: Oxford University Press, 2018.

Tang, John Y. H. *Campylobacter—An Overview.* Saarbrücken, Germany: Lambert Academic Publishing, 2016.

Taylor, Hugh R. *Trachoma: A Blinding Scourge from the Bronze Age to the Twenty-First Century.* East Melbourne, Australia: Centre for Eye Research Australia, 2008.

Telleria, Jenny, and Michel Tibayrenc, eds. *American Trypanosomiasis, Chagas Disease: One Hundred Years of Research.* Amsterdam: Elsevier, 2017.

The Third Ten Years of the World Health Organization (1968–1977). Geneva, Switzerland: World Health Organization, 2008.

Thomas, Howard C., et al., eds. *Viral Hepatitis.* 4th ed. Chichester, UK: Wiley, 2014.

Thompson, Clive, Simon Gillespie, and Emma Goslan, eds. *Disinfection By-products in Drinking Water.* Cambridge: Royal Society of Chemistry, 2016.

Tierno, Philip M. *The Secret Life of Germs: What They Are, Why We Need Them, and How We Can Protect Ourselves against Them.* New York: Atria, 2004.

Torres, Martí Antoni, and Catia Cillóniz. *Clinical Management of Bacterial Pneumonia.* New York: Springer, 2015.

Torrey, E. Fuller, and Robert H. Yolken. *The Beasts of the Earth: Animals, Humans, and Disease.* New Brunswick, NJ: Rutgers University Press, 2014.

Tortora, Gerard J., Berdell R. Funke, and Christine L. Case. *Microbiology: An Introduction.* Boston: Pearson, 2016.

Tripp, Ralph A., and Patricia A. Jorquera. *Human Respiratory Syncytial Virus: Methods and Protocols.* New York: Humana, 2016.

Tselis, Alex C., and John Booss, eds. *Neurovirology.* Amsterdam: Elsevier, 2014.

Tselis, Alexandros Constantine, and Hal B. Jenson. *Epstein-Barr Virus.* New York: Taylor & Francis, 2006.

Tu, Anthony. *Chemical and Biological Weapons and Terrorism.* Boca Raton, FL: CRC, 2018.

Tuberculosis Statistics: States and Cities, 1984. Atlanta: Centers for Disease Control, 1985.

Turksen, Kursad, ed. *Stem Cells: Current Challenges and New Directions.* New York: Humana, 2014.

Turtle, Lance, et al. "Japanese Encephalitis Virus Infection." In *Viral Infections of the Human Nervous System*, edited by Alan C. Jackson, 271–293. Basel, Switzerland: Springer, 2013.

Umar, Constantine S. *New Developments in Epstein-Barr Virus Research.* New York: Nova Science, 2006.

UNICEF. *1946–2006: Sixty Years for Children.* New York: UNICEF, 2006.

USAMRIID's Medical Management of Biological Casualties Handbook. 8th ed. Fort Detrick, MD: US Army Medical Research Institute of Infectious Diseases, 2014. This book can also be found online at http://www.usamriid.army.mil/education/bluebookpdf/USAMRIID%20Blue Book%208th%20Edition%20-%20Sep%202014.pdf (accessed January 31, 2018).

Vargo, Marc E. *The Weaponizing of Biology: Bioterrorism, Biocrime and Biohacking.* Jefferson, NC: McFarland, 2017.

Varlik, Nükhet. *Plague and Empire in the Early Modern Mediterranean World: The Ottoman Experience, 1347–1600.* New York: Cambridge University Press, 2015.

Vercruysse, Jozef. "Schistosomiasis." In *Merck Veterinary Manual.* 11th ed. Whitehouse Station, NJ: Merck, 2016. This article can also be found online at https://www.merckvetmanual.com/circulatory-system/blood-parasites/schistosomiasis (accessed January 12, 2018).

Wadman, Meredith. *The Vaccine Race: Science, Politics, and the Human Costs of Defeating Disease.* New York: Viking, 2017.

Walls, Ron M., Robert S. Hockberger, and Marianne Gausche-Hill, eds. *Rosen's Emergency Medicine: Concepts and Clinical Practice.* 9th ed. Philadelphia: Elsevier, 2018.

Walsh, Christopher, and Timothy Wencewicz. *Antibiotics: Challenges, Mechanisms, Opportunities.* Washington, DC: ASM, 2016.

Wang, Youchun. *Hepatitis E Virus.* New York: Springer, 2016.

Wardlaw, Tessa, Emily White Johansson, and Matthew Hodge. *Pneumonia: The Forgotten Killer of Children.* New York: United Nations Children's Fund/World Health Organization, 2006. This report can also be found online at http://apps.who.int/iris/bitstream/10665/43640/1/9280640489_eng.pdf (accessed January 29, 2017).

Washington, John A. "Principles of Diagnosis." In *Medical Microbiology*, edited by Samuel Baron. 4th ed. Galveston: University of Texas Medical Branch at Galveston, 1996. This article can also be found online at http://www.ncbi.nlm.nih.gov/books/bv.fcgi?rid=mmed.section.5451 (accessed January 26, 2018).

Watson, Ronald. *Health of HIV Infected People: Food, Nutrition and Lifestyle with Antiretroviral Drugs.* Boston: Elsevier, 2015.

Wayne, Marta L., and Benjamin L. Bolker. *Infectious Disease: A Very Short Introduction.* New York: Oxford University Press, 2015.

Webster, Robert G., et al, eds. *Textbook of Influenza.* 2nd ed. Chichester, UK: Wiley-Blackwell, 2013.

Weiss, Louis M., and James J. Becnel, eds. *Microsporidia: Pathogens of Opportunity.* Ames, IA: Wiley Blackwell, 2014.

Weston, Debbie, Alison Burgess, and Sue Roberts. *Infection Prevention and Control at a Glance.* Newark, NJ: Wiley, 2016.

Whitcup, Scott M., ed. *Pharmacologic Therapy of Ocular Disease.* New York: Springer Berlin Heidelberg, 2017.

Whiteside, Alan. *HIV & AIDS: A Very Short Introduction.* 2nd ed. Oxford: Oxford University Press, 2016.

Widmer, Jocelyn. *Investing in Young Children for Peaceful Societies.* Washington, DC: National Academies, 2016.

Wilcox, Mark H., ed. Clostridium difficile *Infection: Infectious Disease Clinics of North America.* London: Elsevier Health Sciences, 2015.

Wilhelm, Klaus-Peter, Hongho Zhai, and Howard I. Maibach. *Dermatotoxicology.* 8th ed. New York: CRC, 2012.

Williams, Gareth. *Angel of Death: The Story of Smallpox.* Basingstoke, UK: Palgrave Macmillan, 2010.

Willrich, Michael. *Pox: An American History.* New York: Penguin, 2011.

Wilson, Daniel J. *Living with Polio: The Epidemic and Its Survivors.* Chicago: University of Chicago Press, 2007.

Wilson, Walter R., and Merle A. Sande. *Current Diagnosis and Treatment in Infectious Diseases.* New York: McGraw-Hill, 2014.

Wiser, Mark F. *Protozoa and Human Disease.* New York: Garland Science, 2011.

Wolf, Jacqueline H. *Don't Kill Your Baby: Public Health and the Decline of Breastfeeding in the 19th and 20th Centuries.* Columbus: Ohio University Press, 2001.

World Health Organization. *Comprehensive Cervical Cancer Control: A Guide to Essential Practice.* Geneva, Switzerland: WHO Press, 2014. This book can also be found online at http://apps.who.int/iris/bitstream/10665/144785/1/9789241548953_eng.pdf?ua=1 (accessed February 20, 2018).

World Health Organization. *Preventing HIV/AIDS in Young People.* Geneva: WHO, 2006.

World Organisation for Animal Health, World Health Organization, and Food and Agriculture Organization of the United Nations. *Anthrax in Humans and Animals.* 4th ed. Geneva, Switzerland: World Health Organization, 2008. This report can also be found online at http://apps.who.int/iris/bitstream/10665/97503/1/9789241547536_eng.pdf (accessed January 11, 2018).

Wrigley, E. A., and R. S. Scofield. *The Population History of England, 1541–1871: A Reconstruction.* Cambridge, MA: Harvard University Press, 1984.

Yamaoka, Yoshio, ed. *Helicobacter Pylori: Molecular Genetics and Cellular Biology.* Norfolk, UK: Caister Academic Press, 2008.

Zhou, Xiao-Nong, et al., eds. *Important Helminth Infections in Southeast Asia: Diversity and Potential for Control and Elimination.* Vol. 72 of *Advances in Parasitology.* New York: Elsevier, 2010.

Zuckerman, Jane N., Gary W. Brunette, and Peter A. Leggat. *Essential Travel Medicine.* New York: Wiley-Blackwell, 2015.

PERIODICALS

Abanyie, F., et al. "2013 Multistate Outbreaks of *Cyclospora cayetanensis* Infections Associated with Fresh Produce: Focus on the Texas Investigations." *Epidemiology & Infection* 143, no. 16 (December 2015): 3451–3458.

Abbasi, Jennifer. "iPhone-Based Device Helps Treat River Blindness." *JAMA* 319, no. 2 (January 9, 2018): 113. This article can also be found online at https://jamanetwork.com/journals/jama/article-abstract/2668328?redirect=true (accessed February 12, 2018).

Abubakar, Ibrahim, Chris Griffiths, and Peter Ormerod. "GUIDELINES: Diagnosis of Active and Latent Tuberculosis: Summary of NICE Guidance." *BMJ: British Medical Journal* 345, no. 7881 (November 2012): 45–47.

Addady, Michal. "FDA Says Processing Plant Linked to Massive Listeria Outbreak Is Impossible to Clean." *Fortune* (May 15, 2016). This article can also be found online at http://fortune.com/2016/05/15/frozen-food-listeria/ (accessed November 20, 2017).

Adler, Nancy E., and Joan M. Ostrove. "Socioeconomic Status and Health: What We Know and What We Don't." *Annals of the New York Academy of Sciences* 896 (1999): 3–15.

Advisory Committee on Immunization Practices, Centers for Disease Control and Prevention. "Preventing Tetanus, Diphtheria, and Pertussis among Adolescents: Use of Tetanus Toxoid, Reduced Diphtheria Toxoid and Acellular Pertussis Vaccines." *Morbidity and Mortality Weekly Report* 55 (February 23, 2006): 1–34. This article can also be found online at http://www.cdc.gov/mmwr/preview/mmwrhtml/rr55e223a1.htm (accessed December 9, 2017).

Aguilar, Patricia V., et al. "Endemic Venezuelan Equine Encephalitis in the Americas: Hidden under the Dengue Umbrella." *Future Virology* 6 (2011): 721–740.

Ahmad, F. A., G. A. Storch, and A. S. Miller. "Impact of an Institutional Guideline on the Care of Neonates at Risk for Herpes Simplex Virus in the Emergency Department." *Pediatric Emergency Care* 33, no. 6 (August 21, 2015): 396–401.

Ahmadiani, Saeed, and Shekoufeh Nikfar. "Challenges of Access to Medicine and the Responsibility of Pharmaceutical Companies: A Legal Perspective." *DARU Journal of Pharmaceutical Sciences* 24 (2016): 13. This article can also be found online at https://www.ncbi.nlm.nih.gov/pmc/articles/PMC4855755/ (accessed March 1, 2018).

Ahmed, Sameer, Nina L. Shapiro, and Neil Bhattacharyya. "Incremental Health Care

Utilization and Costs for Acute Otitis Media in Children." *Laryngoscope* 124, no. 1 (January 2014): 301–305.

Ahn, Joseph, and Robert G. Gish. "Hepatitis D Virus: A Call to Screening." *Journal of Gastroenterology and Hepatology* 10, no. 10 (October 2014): 647–686.

Akpan, A., and R. Morgan. "Oral Candidiasis." *Postgraduate Medical Journal* 78, no. 922 (2002): 455–9. This article can also be found available online at http://pmj.bmj.com/content/78/922/455 (accessed January 25, 2018).

Alawieh, Ali, et al. "Revisiting Leishmaniasis in the Time of War: The Syrian Conflict and the Lebanese Outbreak." *International Journal of Infectious Diseases* 29 (December 2014): 115–119. This article can also be found online at http://www.ijidonline.com/article/S1201-9712(14)01519-7/fulltext (accessed March 8, 2018).

Albariño, Cesar G., et al. "Insights into Reston Virus Spillovers and Adaption from Virus Whole Genome Sequences." *PLOS One* 12, no. 5 (May 25, 2017): e0178224. This article can also be found online at http://journals.plos.org/plosone/article?id=10.1371/journal.pone.0178224 (accessed January 26, 2018).

Allana, Alia. "How War Created the Cholera Epidemic in Yemen." *New York Times* (November 12, 2017). This article can also be found online at https://www.nytimes.com/2017/11/12/opinion/cholera-war-yemen.html (accessed February 12, 2018).

Allegranzi, Benedetta, et al. "Burden of Endemic Health-Care-Associated Infection in Developing Countries: Systematic Review and Meta-Analysis." *Lancet* 377, no. 9761 (January 15, 2011): 228–241. This article can also be found online at http://www.thelancet.com/journals/lancet/article/PIIS0140-6736(10)61458-4/fulltext (accessed February 21, 2018).

AlOtair Hadil A., et al. "Severe Pneumonia Requiring ICU Admission: Revisited." *Journal of Taibah University Medical Sciences* 10, no. 3 (September 2015): 293–299. This article can also be found online at https://www.sciencedirect.com/science/article/pii/S1658361215000682 (accessed January 24, 2018).

Altamimi, Saleh, et al. "Short-Term Late-Generation Antibiotics versus Longer Term Penicillin for Acute Streptococcal Pharyngitis in Children." *Cochrane Database of Systematic Reviews* 8 (2012). This article can also be found online at http://onlinelibrary.wiley.com/wol1/doi/10.1002/14651858.CD004872.pub3/abstract (accessed January 25, 2018).

Alter, M. J. "Epidemiology of Hepatitis C in the West." *Seminars in Liver Disease* 15, no. 1 (1995): 5–14.

Altman, Lawrence K. "After a Phone Tip, Medical Detectives Track Down a Killer." *New York Times* (September 9, 1999). This article can also be found online at http://www.nytimes.com/1999/09/09/nyregion/after-a-phone-tip-medical-detectives-track-down-a-killer.html (accessed November 9, 2017).

Ambrosioni, J., D. Lew, and J. Garbino. "Nocardiosis: Updated Clinical Review and Experience at a Tertiary Center." *Infection* 38, no. 2 (April 2010): 89–97. This article can also be found online at https://link.springer.com/article/10.1007/s15010-009-9193-9#citeas (accessed January 19, 2018).

Amofah, George, et al. "Buruli Ulcer in Ghana: Results of a National Case Search." *Emerging Infectious Diseases* 8, no. 2 (February 2002): 167–170. This article can also be found online at https://www.ncbi.nlm.nih.gov/pmc/articles/PMC2732443/ (accessed January 17, 2018).

Anderson, Dustin, et al. "A Neuropathic Pain Syndrome Associated with Hantavirus Infection." *Journal of Neurovirology* 23 (December 2017): 919–921.

Andraws, R., J. S. Berger, and D. L. Brown. "Effects of Antibiotic Therapy on Outcomes of Patients with Coronary Artery Disease: A Meta-Analysis of Randomized Controlled Trials." *JAMA* 293, no. 21 (2005): 2641–2647.

Anishchenko, M., et al. "From the Cover: Venezuelan Encephalitis Emergence Mediated by a Phylogenetically Predicted Viral Mutation." *Proceedings of the National Academy of Sciences of the United States of America* 103 (2006): 4994–4999.

"Another Lassa Fever Outbreak." *National* (January 23, 2018). http://thenationonlineng.net/another-lassa-fever-outbreak/ (accessed January 24, 2018).

Ansaldi, Filippo, et al. "Real-World Effectiveness and Safety of a Live-Attenuated Herpes Zoster Vaccine: A Comprehensive Review." *Advances in*

Therapy 33 (2016): 1094–1104. This article can also be found online at https://www.ncbi.nlm.nih.gov/pmc/articles/PMC4939147/ (accessed January 24, 2018).

Ansell, Brendan R. E., et al. "Drug Resistance in *Giardia duodenalis*." *Biotechnology Advances* 33, no. 6 (2015): 888–901.

Anselmi, Mariella, et al. "Mass Administration of Ivermectin for the Elimination of Onchocerciasis Significantly Reduced and Maintained Low the Prevalence of *Strongyloides Stercoralis* in Esmeraldas, Ecuador." *PLOS Neglected Tropical Diseases* 9, no. 11 (November 5, 2015). This article can also be found online at https://doi.org/10.1371/journal.pntd.0004150 (accessed January 29, 2018).

Arnold, Carrie. "In the Eye of the Tiger: Global Spread of Asian Tiger Mosquito Could Fuel Outbreaks of Tropical Disease in Temperate Regions." *Science News* 183, no. 13 (June 29, 2013): 26–29.

Aufderheide, Arthur C., et al. "A 9,000-year Record of Chagas' Disease." *Proceedings of the National Academy of Sciences of the United States of America* 101, no. 7 (February 2004): 2034–2039.

Aung, Ar Kar, et al. "Rickettsial Infections in Southeast Asia: Implications for Local Populace and Febrile Returned Travelers." *American Journal of Tropical Medicine and Hygiene* 91, no. 2 (2014): 451–460. This article can also be found online at https://www.ncbi.nlm.nih.gov/pmc/articles/PMC4155544/ (accessed February 15, 2018).

Avasthi R., S. C. Chaudhary, and S. Khanna. "Visceral Leishmaniasis Simulating Chronic Liver Disease: Successful Treatment with Miltefosine." *Indian Journal of Medical Microbiology* 27, no. 1 (January–March 2009): 85–86.

Azevedo, Luiz Sergio, et al. "Cytomegalovirus Infection in Transplant Recipients." *Clinics* 70, no. 7 (2015); 515–523. This article can also be found online at https://www.ncbi.nlm.nih.gov/pmc/articles/PMC4496754/ (accessed February 5, 2018).

Büscher Philippe, Giuliano Cecchi, Vincent Jamonneau, and Gerardo Priotto. "Human African Trypanosomiasis." Lancet (June 30, 2017).

Babigumira, Joseph B., Ian Morgan, and Ann Levin. "Health Economics of Rubella: A Systematic Review to Assess the Value of Rubella Vaccination." *BMC Public Health* 13, no. 406 (2013). This article can also be found online at https://bmcpublichealth.biomedcentral.com/articles/10.1186/1471-2458-13-406 (accessed January 16, 2018).

Babu, Subash, and Thomas B. Nutman. "Immunology of Lymphatic Filariasis." *Parasite Immunology* 36, no. 8 (2014): 338–346. This article can also be found online at https://www.ncbi.nlm.nih.gov/pmc/articles/PMC3990654/ (accessed January 22, 2018).

Badiee, Parisa, and Zahira Hashemizadeh. "Opportunistic Invasive Fungal Infections: Diagnosis & Clinical Management." *Indian Journal of Medical Research* 139, no. 2 (2014): 195–204. This article can also be found online at https://www.ncbi.nlm.nih.gov/pmc/articles/PMC4001330/ (accessed January 25, 2018).

Baggelay, Kate. "Scientists Are Trying to Treat Autoimmune Disease with Intestinal Worms." *Popular Science* (July 28, 2017). This article can also be found online at https://www.popsci.com/can-intestinal-worms-treat-autoimmune-disease

Bahcecioglu, I. H., and A. Sahin. "Treatment of Delta Hepatitis: Today and in the Future." *Infectious Diseases* 49, no. 4 (April 2017): 241–250.

Bakalar, Nicholas. "New Shingles Vaccine Is Cost Effective." *New York Times* (January 4, 2018). This article can also be found online at https://www.nytimes.com/2018/01/04/well/live/new-shingles-vaccine-is-cost-effective.html?mtrref=undefined (accessed January 24, 2018).

Baker, Kate S., et al. "Intercontinental Dissemination of Azithromycin-Resistant Shigellosis through Sexual Transmission: A Cross-Sectional Study." *Lancet* 15, no. 8 (August 2015): 913–921. This article can also be found online at https://www.sciencedirect.com/science/article/pii/S147330991500002X (accessed February 7, 2018).

Balandraud, Nathalie, and Jean Roudier. "Epstein-Barr Virus and Rheumatoid Arthritis." *Joint Bone Spine* (May 9, 2017). This article can also be found online at https://www.sciencedirect.com/science/article/pii/S1297319X17300933 (accessed December 26, 2017).

Ballard, Jimmy D. "Pathogens Boosted by Food Additive." *Nature* (December 21, 2017). This article can also be found online at https://www

.nature.com/articles/d41586-017-08775-4 (accessed February 1, 2018).

Ballard, Mark S, et al. "The Changing Epidemiology of Group B *Streptococcus* Bloodstream Infection: A Multi-National Population-Based Assessment." *Infectious Diseases* 48, no. 5 (2016): 386–391. This article can also be found online at http://www.tandfonline.com/doi/abs/10.3109/23744235.2015.1131330 (accessed January 23, 2018).

Bancerz-Kisiel, Agata, and Wojciech Szweda. "Yersiniosis—A Zoonotic Foodborne Disease of Relevance to Public Health." *Annals of Agricultural and Environmental Medicine* 22, no. 3 (2015): 397–402. This article can also be found online at http://www.aaem.pl/Yersiniosis-zoonotic-foodborne-disease-of-relevance-to-public-health,72296,0,2.html (accessed January 9, 2017).

Banderker, Ebrahim, et al. "Imaging and Management of Childhood Ascariasis." *Journal of Pediatric Infectious Diseases* 12, no. 1 (2017): 20–29.

Barlow, Frank. "The King's Evil." *English Historical Review* 95, no. 374 (January 1980): 3–27.

Barros, Mônica Bastos de Lima, Rodrigo de Almeida Paes, and Armando Oliveira Schubach. "*Sporothrix Schenckii* and Sporotrichosis." *Clinical Microbiology Reviews* 24, no. 4 (2011): 633–654. This article can also be found online at https://www.ncbi.nlm.nih.gov/pmc/articles/PMC3194828/ (accessed January 23, 2018).

Barth Reller, L., et al. "Detection and Identification of Microorganisms by Gene Amplification and Sequencing." *Clinical Infectious Diseases* 44 (2007): 1108–1114.

Bartsch, Sarah M., et al. "The Global Economic and Health Burden of Hookworm Infection." *PLOS Neglected Tropical Diseases* 10, no. 9 (September 8, 2016). This article can also be found online at http://journals.plos.org/plosntds/article?id=10.1371/journal.pntd.0004922 (accessed December 19, 2017).

Baudin, Maria, et al. "Association of Rift Valley Fever Virus Infection with Miscarriage in Sudanese Women: A Cross-Sectional Study." *Lancet: Global Health* 4, no. 11 (November 2016): e864–e871. This article can also be found online at https://www.sciencedirect.com/science/article/pii/S2214109X16301760 (accessed January 18, 2018).

Beachum, Lateshia. "Prisons around the World Are Reservoirs of Infectious Disease." *Washington Post* (July 20, 2016). This article can also be found online at https://www.washingtonpost.com/news/to-your-health/wp/2016/07/20/prisons-around-the-world-are-reservoirs-of-infectious-disease/?utm_term=.5633ed12c8ea (accessed February 9, 2018).

Beer, Karlyn D., et al. "Giardiasis Diagnosis and Treatment Practices among Commercially Insured Persons in the United States." *Clinical Infectious Diseases* 64, no. 9 (May 1, 2017): 1244–1250. This article can also be found online at https://academic.oup.com/cid/article-abstract/64/9/1244/3000619 (accessed January 17, 2018).

Benedict, Kaitlin, et al. "Emerging Issues, Challenges, and Changing Epidemiology of Fungal Disease Outbreaks." *Lancet Infectious Diseases* 17, no. 12 (December 2017): e403–e411.

Benenson, S., et al. "Cluster of Puerperal Fever in an Obstetric Ward: A Reminder of Ignaz Semmelweis." *Infection Control & Hospital Epidemiology* 36, no. 12 (2015): 1488–1490.

Benjak, Andrej, et al. "Phylogenomics and Antimicrobial Resistance of the Leprosy Bacillus *Mycobacterium leprae*." *Nature Communications* 9 (2018): 352. This article can also be found online at https://www.nature.com/articles/s41467-017-02576-z (accessed February 16, 2018).

Berende, Anneleen, et al. "Randomized Trial of Longer-Term Therapy for Symptoms Attributed to Lyme Disease." *New England Journal of Medicine* 374 (2016): 1209–1220. This article can also be found online at http://www.nejm.org/doi/full/10.1056/NEJMoa1505425 (accessed February 6, 2018).

Berlin, Daniel, et al. "A Difficult Case: Eastern Equine Encephalitis."**Practical Neurology** 17 (2017).

Bernardes-Engemann, Andréa Reis, et al. "Validation of a Serodiagnostic Test for Sporotrichosis: A Follow-up Study of Patients Related to the Rio De Janeiro Zoonotic Outbreak." *Medical Mycology* 53, no. 1 (January 1, 2015): 28–33. This article can also be found online at https://academic.oup.com/mmy/article/53/1/28/992696 (accessed January 23, 2018).

Bernardin, F., et al. "Transfusion Transmission of Highly Prevalent Commensal Human Viruses." *Transfusion* 50, no. 11 (November 2010). This article can also be found online at https://www.ncbi.nlm.nih.gov/pubmed/20497515 (accessed February 1, 2018).

Bernstein, D., et al. "Epidemiology, Clinical Presentation, and Antibody Response to Primary Infection with Herpes Simplex Virus Type 1 and Type 2 in Young Women." *Clinical Infectious Diseases* 56 (2013): 344–351.

Bethony J., et al. "Soil-Transmitted Helminth Infections: Ascariasis, Trichuriasis, and Hookworm." *Lancet* 367 (2006): 1521–1532.

Bialek, S. R., et al. "Impact of a Routine Two-Dose Varicella Vaccination Program on Varicella Epidemiology." *Pediatrics* 132, no. 5 (November 2013): e1134–1140. This article can also be found online at https://www.ncbi.nlm.nih.gov/pubmed/24101763 (accessed February 1, 2018).

Bianchi-Jassir, Fiorella, et al. "Preterm Birth Associated with Group B *Streptococcus* Maternal Colonization Worldwide: Systematic Review and Meta-Analyses." *Clinical Infectious Diseases* 65, no. 2 (November 6, 2017): S133–S142. This article can also be found online at https://academic.oup.com/cid/article/65/suppl_2/S133/4589591 (accessed January 23, 2018).

Bick, Joseph A. "Infection Control in Jails and Prisons." *Clinical Infectious Diseases* 45, no. 8 (October 15, 2007): 1047–1055. This article can also be found online at https://academic.oup.com/cid/article/45/8/1047/344842 (accessed February 9, 2018).

Biggs, Holly M., et al. "Diagnosis and Management of Tickborne Rickettsial Diseases: Rocky Mountain Spotted Fever and Other Spotted Fever Group Rickettsioses, Ehrlichioses, and Anaplasmosis—United States." *Morbidity and Mortality Weekly Report* 65, no. 2 (2016): 1–44. This article can also be found online at https://www.cdc.gov/mmwr/volumes/65/rr/rr6502a1.htm (accessed February 15, 2018).

Biji, K. B., et al. "Smart Packaging Systems for Food Applications: A Review." *Journal of Food Science Technology* 52 (October 2015): 6125–6135.

Bird, Brian H., and Anita K. McElroy. "Rift Valley Fever: Unanswered Questions." *Antiviral Research* 132 (August 2016): 274–280. This article can also be found online at https://www.sciencedirect.com/science/article/pii/S0166354216302522 (accessed January 18, 2018).

Blasi, F., P. Tarsia, and S. Aliberti. "*Chlamydophila pneumoniae*." *Clinical Microbiology and Infection* 15, no. 1 (2009): 29–35. This article can also be found online at http://onlinelibrary.wiley.com/doi/10.1111/j.1469-0691.2008.02130.x/full (accessed January 29, 2018).

Boland, Jennifer M., et al. "Pleuropulmonary Infection by *Paragonimus westermani* in the United States: A Rare Cause of Eosinophilic Pneumonia after Ingestion of Live Crabs." *American Journal of Surgical Pathology* 35, no. 5 (May 2011): 707–713.

Boseley, Sarah. "Can You Catch Cancer?" *Guardian* (January 24, 2006). This article can also be found online at https://www.theguardian.com/society/2006/jan/24/cancercare.health (accessed January 26, 2018).

Boussinesq, Michel. "A New Powerful Drug to Combat River Blindness." *Lancet* (January 18, 2018). This article can also be found online at https://www.sciencedirect.com/science/article/pii/S0140673618301016 (accessed February 12, 2018).

Bowerman, Mary. "Mumps Outbreaks Reported across USA." *USA Today* (March 10, 2017). This article can also be found online at https://www.usatoday.com/story/news/nation-now/2017/03/10/mumps-outbreaks-reported-across-country/99002254/ (accessed February 6, 2018).

Bracaglia, Claudia, Giusi Prencipe, and Fabrizio F. Benedetti. "Macrophage Activation Syndrome: Different Mechanisms Leading to a One Clinical Syndrome." *Pediatric Rheumatology* 15 (January 2017): 5–12. This article can also be found online at https://ped-rheum.biomedcentral.com/articles/10.1186/s12969-016-0130-4 (accessed March 12, 2018).

Bradsher, Robert W., Jr. "The Endemic Mimic: Blastomycosis an Illness Often Misdiagnosed." *Transactions of the American Clinical and Climatological Association* 125 (2014): 188–203.

Brady, Oliver J., et al. "Refining the Global Spatial Limits of Dengue Virus Transmission by Evidence-Based Consensus." *PLOS Neglected Tropical Diseases* 6, no. 8 (August 7, 2012): e1760. This article can also be found online at http://journals.plos.org/plosntds/article?id=10.1371/journal.pntd.0001760

Brant, Sara V., et al. "Cercarial Dermatitis Transmitted by Exotic Marine Snail." *Emerging Infectious Diseases* 16, no. 9 (September 2010): 1357–1365.

Brehm, K., and U. Koziol. "*Echinococcus*-Host Interactions at Cellular and Molecular Levels." *Advances in Parasitology* 95 (2017): 147–212.

Brighenti, Susanna, and Jan Andersson. "Local Immune Responses in Human Tuberculosis: Learning from the Site of Infection?" *Journal of Infectious Diseases* 205, no. 2. (May 2012): S316–S324

Broad, William J. "Anthrax Not Weapons-Grade, Official Says." *New York Times* (September 26, 2006). This article can also be found online at http://www.nytimes.com/2006/09/26/us/26anthrax.html (accessed January 12, 2018).

Brody, Jane E. "An Itchy Torment, Often Misdiagnosed." *New York Times* (September 22, 2008): F6. This article is also available online at http://www.nytimes.com/2008/09/23/health/23brod.html (accessed November 13, 2017).

Brody, Jane E. "That Dreaded Nemesis, Head Lice." *New York Times* (June 2, 2015): D5. This article can also be found online at https://well.blogs.nytimes.com/2015/06/01/new-tactics-for-battling-head-lice/ (accessed November 14, 2017).

Brouwer, Willem Pieter, et al. "Adding Pegylated Interferon to Entecavir for Hepatitis B e Antigen-Positive Chronic Hepatitis B: A Multicenter Randomized Trial (ARES Study)." *Hepatology* 61, no. 5 (May 2015): 1512–1522. This article can also be found online at http://onlinelibrary.wiley.com/doi/10.1002/hep.27586/full (accessed February 2, 2018).

Brown, Katrina F., et al. "Factors Underlying Parental Decisions about Combination Childhood Vaccinations Including MMR: A Systematic Review." *Vaccine* 28, no. 26 (June 11, 2010): 4235–4248. This article can also be found online at https://www.sciencedirect.com/science/article/pii/S0264410X10005761 (accessed February 15, 2018).

Brown, Katy, and Peter A. Leggat. "Human Monkeypox: Current State of Knowledge and Implications for the Future." *Tropical Medicine and Infectious Disease* 1, no. 8 (2016). This article can also be found online at http://www.mdpi.com/2414–6366/1/1/8/htm (accessed January 24, 2018).

Bucci, Cristina, et al. "Anisakis, Just Think about It in an Emergency!" *International Journal of Infectious Diseases* 17, no. 11 (2013): e1071–e1072.

Buckee, Caroline O., Andrew J. Tatem, and Jessica E. Metcalf. "Seasonal Population Movements and the Surveillance and Control of Infectious Diseases." *Trends in Parasitology* 33, no. 1 (January 2017): 10–20.

Budke Christine M., Adriano Casulli, Peter Kern, and Dominique A. Vuitton. "Cystic and Alveolar Echinococcosis: Successes and Continuing Challenges." *PLOS Neglected Tropical Diseases* 11, no. 4 (2017).

Buehler, Kelsey, Julie Spencer-Rogers, and Kaiping Peng. "HIV/AIDS, Treatment Adherence, and Lifestyle: A Qualitative Study." *Journal of HIV/AIDS & Social Services* 6, no. 4 (October–December 2017): 367–381.

Bulger, Eileen M., et al. "A Novel Drug for Treatment of Necrotizing Soft-Tissue Infections: A Randomized Clinical Trial." *JAMA Surgery* 149, no. 6 (2014): 528–536. This article can also be found online at https://jamanetwork.com/journals/jamasurgery/fullarticle/1859986 (accessed February 12, 2018).

Burnett, Eleanor, et al. "Global Impact of Rotavirus Vaccination on Childhood Hospitalizations and Mortality from Diarrhea." *Journal of Infectious Diseases* 215, no. 11 (2017): 1666–1672. This article can also be found online at https://academic.oup.com/jid/article/215/11/1666/3738521 (accessed January 23, 2018).

Burnham, Jason P., and Marin H. Kollef. "Understanding Toxic Shock Syndrome." *Intensive Care Medicine* 41, no. 9 (September 2015): 1707–1710.

Buti, Maria, et al. "Seven-Year Efficacy and Safety of Treatment with Tenofovir Disoproxil Fumarate for Chronic Hepatitis B Virus Infection." *Digestive Diseases and Sciences* 60, no. 5 (May 2015): 1457–1464. This article can also be found online at https://link.springer.com/article/10.1007/s10620–014-3486–7 (accessed February 2, 2018).

Butler, T. "Plague History: Yersin' Discovery of the Causative Bacterium in 1894 Enabled, in the Subsequent Century, Scientific Progress in Understanding the Disease and the Development of Treatments and Vaccines." *Clinical Microbiology and Infection* 20, no. 3 (March 2014): 202–209.

Byrd, Allyson L., and Julia A. Segre. "Adapting Koch's Postulates." *Science* 351, no. 6270 (January 15, 2016): 224–226. This article can also be found online at http://science.sciencemag.org/content/351/6270/224 (accessed January 16, 2018).

Cabral, Maria P., et al. "Design of Live Attenuated Bacterial Vaccines Based on D-Glutamate Auxotrophy." *Nature Communications* 8 (May 2017).

Callaway, Ewen. "One in 2,000 UK People Might carry vCJD Proteins." *Nature* (October 15, 2013). This article can also be found online at https://www.nature.com/news/one-in-2–000-uk-people-might-carry-vcjd-proteins-1.13962 (accessed January 29, 2018).

Cardemil, Cristina V., Umesh D. Parashar, and Aron J. Hall. "Norovirus Infection in Older Adults: Epidemiology, Risk Factors, and Opportunities for Prevention and Control." *Infectious Diseases Clinics of North America* 31 (December 2017): 839–870.

Carey Daniel E., and Patrick J. McNamara. "The Impact of Triclosan on the Spread of Antibiotic Resistance in the Environment." *Frontiers in Microbiology* (January 15, 2015). This article can also be found online at https://www.frontiersin.org/articles/10.3389/fmicb.2014.00780/full (accessed November 16, 2017).

Carignan, Sylvia. "Fort Detrick's $10 Million Fire." *Frederick News-Post* (March 17, 2014). This article can also be found online at https://www.fredericknewspost.com/news/disasters_and_accidents/fires/fort-detrick-s-million-fire/article_6b0025de-2989–5e29–8005-edc9297cc984.html (accessed January 31, 2018).

Carlos W. G., et al. Blastomycosis in Indiana: Digging Up More Cases. *Chest* 138, no. 6 (2010): 1377–1382.

Carnaud, Claude. "Is There Still Hope after Prions Have Spread within the Brain." *Journal of Infectious Diseases* 204, no. 7 (October 2011): 978–979.

Carrel, Margaret, Eli N. Perencevich, and Michael Z. David. "USA300 Methicillin-Resistant *Staphylococcus aureus*, United States, 2000–2013." *Emerging Infectious Diseases* 21, no. 11 (November 2015): 1973–1980.

Cashman, Kathleen A., et al. "A DNA Vaccine Delivered by Dermal Electroporation Fully Protects Cynomolgus Macaques against Lassa Fever." *Human Vaccines and Immunotherapies* 13, no. 12 (2017): 2902–2911. This article can also be found online at http://www.tandfonline.com/doi/full/10.1080/21645515.2017.1356500?scroll=top&needAccess=true (accessed January 24, 2018).

Castro, Jose G., and Maya Morrison-Bryant. "Management of *Pneumocystis Jirovecii* Pneumonia in HIV Infected Patients: Current Options, Challenges and Future Directions." *HIV/AIDS—Research and Palliative Care* 2 (2010): 123–134. This article can also be found online at https://www.ncbi.nlm.nih.gov/pmc/articles/PMC3218692/ (accessed February 14, 2018).

Caulfield, Laura E., et al. "Undernutrition as an Underlying Cause of Child Deaths Associated with Diarrhea, Pneumonia, Malaria, and Measles." *American Journal of Clinical Nutrition* 80, no. 1 (July 2004): 193. This article can also be found online at http://ajcn.nutrition.org/content/80/1/193.full (accessed January 30, 2018).

Cetinkaya, Yesim, Pamela Falk, and C. Glen Mayhall. "Vancomycin-Resistant *Enterococci*." *Clinical Microbiology Reviews* 13, no. 4 (2000): 686–707. This article can also be found online at https://www.ncbi.nlm.nih.gov/pmc/articles/PMC88957/ (accessed March 7, 2018).

Chakrabarti, Arunaloke, et al. "Global Epidemiology of Sporotrichosis." *Medical Mycology* 53, no. 1 (January 1, 2015): 3–14. This article can also be found online at https://academic.oup.com/mmy/article/53/1/3/992886 (accessed January 23, 2018).

Chakraborty, A., et al. "Evolving Epidemiology of Nipah Virus Infection in Bangladesh: Evidence from Outbreaks during 2010–2011." *Epidemiology and Infection* 144, no. 2 (January 2016): 371–380. This article can also be found online at https://www.cambridge.org/core/journals/epidemiology-and-infection/article/evolving-epidemiology-of-nipah-virus-infection-in-bangladesh-evidence-from-outbreaks-during-20102011/B613FF64EDFA3F105C7FAC390F32FB4B (accessed January 19, 2018).

Chakravarthy, Kalyana, et al. "Paediatric Brucellosis: A Case Series from a Tertiary Care Center in Karnataka." *Indian Journal of Applied Research* 7, no. 6 (2017): 738–739.

Chalker, V., et al. "Genome Analysis Following a National Increase in Scarlet Fever in England 2014." *BMC Genomics* 18 (2017): 224.

Chamany, S., et al. "A Large Histoplasmosis Outbreak among High School Students in Indiana, 2001." *Pediatric Infectious Disease Journal* 23, no. 10 (2004): 909–914.

Chan, Emily H., et al. "Global Capacity for Emerging Infectious Disease Detection." *Proceedings of the National Academy of Sciences of the United States of America* 107, no. 50 (2010): 21701–21706.

Chan, Jasper F. W., et al. "*Talaromyces* (*Penicillium*) *marneffei* Infection in Non-HIV-Infected Patients." *Emerging Microbes & Infections* 5, no. 3 (2016): e19. This article can also be found online at https://www.nature.com/articles/emi201618 (accessed February 21, 2018).

Chan, K. C. Allen, et al. "Analysis of Plasma Epstein-Barr Virus DNA to Screen for Nasopharyngeal Cancer." *New England Journal of Medicine* (August 10, 2017): 513–522. This article can also be found online at http://www.nejm.org/doi/full/10.1056/NEJMoa1701717 (accessed December 26, 2017).

Chang, Daniel. "Florida Has Reported More Mumps Cases in 2017 Than the Last Five Years Combined." *Miami Herald* (December 19, 2017). This article can also be found online at http://www.miamiherald.com/news/health-care/article190625819.html (accessed February 6, 2018).

Chang, Quizhi, et al. "Antibiotics in Agriculture and the Risk to Human Health: How Worried Should We Be?" *Evolutionary Applications* 8, no. 3 (2015): 240–247. This article can also be found online at https://www.ncbi.nlm.nih.gov/pmc/articles/PMC4380918/ (accessed February 26, 2018).

Charlier, Caroline, et al. "MONOLISA: A Grim Picture of Listeriosis." *Lancet Infectious Diseases* 17 (May 2017): 464–466.

Chauchet, Adrien, et al. "Increased Incidence and Characteristics of Alveolar Echinococcosis in Patients with Immunosuppression-Associated Conditions." *Clinical Infectious Diseases* 59, no. 8 (October 15, 2014): 1095–1104.

Check, Erika. "Heightened Security after Flu Scare Sparks Biosafety Debate." *Nature* 432 (2005): 943.

Cheng, Allen C., and Bart J. Currie. "Melioidosis: Epidemiology, Pathophysiology, and Management." *Clinical Microbiology Reviews* 18 (April 2005): 383–416. This article can also be found online at http://cmr.asm.org/cgi/content/full/18/2/383 (accessed February 7, 2018).

Cherry, James D. "The History of Pertussis (Whooping Cough); 1906–2015: Facts, Myths, and Misconceptions." *Current Epidemiology Reports* 2, no. 2 (June 2015): 120–130. This article can also be found online at https://link.springer.com/article/10.1007/s40471-015-0041-9 (accessed January 29, 2018).

Chitsulo, L., et al. "The Global Status of Schistosomiasis and Its Control." *Acta Tropica* 77, no. 1 (October 2000): 41–51. This article can also be found online at http://www.sciencedirect.com/science/article/pii/S0001706X00001224 (accessed January 12, 2018).

Chiu, C. H. et al. "Leptospirosis and Depression: A Nationwide Cohort Analysis." *Journal of Clinical Psychiatry* 78, no. 4 (April 2017): e398–e403. This article can also be found online at https://www.ncbi.nlm.nih.gov/pubmed/28297597 (accessed January 19, 2018).

"Cholera Vaccines: WHO Position Paper, August 2017." *World Health Organization Weekly Epidemiological Record* 92, no. 34 (August 25, 2017): 477–500. This article can also be found online at http://apps.who.int/iris/bitstream/10665/258763/1/WER9234.pdf?ua=1 (accessed February 12, 2018).

Chowdhary, Anuradha, Cheshta Sharma, and Jacques F. Meis "*Candida auris*: A Rapidly Emerging Cause of Hospital-Acquired Multidrug-Resistant Fungal Infections Globally." *PLOS Pathogens* 13, no. 5 (2017). This article can also be found online at http://journals.plos.org/plospathogens/article?id=10.1371/journal.ppat.1006290 (accessed January 25, 2018).

Clendinen, C., et al. "Manufacturing Costs of HPV Vaccines for Developing Countries." *Vaccine* 34, no. 48 (November 2016): 5984–5989.

Cleveland, Angela Ahlquist, et al. "Declining Incidence of Candidemia and the Shifting Epidemiology of *Candida* Resistance in Two

US Metropolitan Areas, 2008–2013: Results from Population-Based Surveillance." *PLOS ONE* (March 30, 2015). This article can also be found online at http://journals.plos.org/plosone/article?id=10.1371/journal.pone.0120452 (accessed January 25, 2018).

"Climate Change: The Role of the Infectious Disease Community." Lancet Infectious Diseases 17, no. 12 (December 2017): 1219. This article can also be found online at http://www.thelancet.com/journals/laninf/article/PIIS1473–3099(17)30645-X/fulltext (accessed March 2, 2018).

Cohen Hillel W., Robert M. Gould, and Victor W. Sidel. "The Pitfalls of Bioterrorism Preparedness: The Anthrax and Smallpox Experiences." *American Journal of Public Health* 94 (October 2004): 1667–1671.

Cohen, Jeffrey I., et al. "Recommendations for Prevention of and Therapy for Exposure to B Virus (*Cercopithecine Herpesvirus* 1)." **Clinical Infectious Diseases** 35, no. 10 (2002): 1191–1203. This article can also be found online at https://academic.oup.com/cid/article/35/10/1191/296729 (accessed December 15, 2017).

Cohen, Jon. "AIDS Vaccine May Be 'Functional Cure' for Some." *Science* (February 22, 2017). This article can also be found online at http://www.sciencemag.org/news/2017/02/aids-vaccine-may-be-functional-cure-some (accessed December 23, 2017).

———. "Swine Flu Pandemic Reincarnates 1918 Virus." *Science* (March 24, 2010). This article is also available online at http://www.sciencemag.org/news/2010/03/swine-flu-pandemic-reincarnates-1918-virus (accessed January 16, 2018).

———. "Zika Has All but Disappeared in the Americas. Why?" *Science* (August 16, 2017). This article can also be found online at http://www.sciencemag.org/news/2017/08/zika-has-all-disappeared-americas-why (accessed February 9, 2018).

Cole, S. T., et al. "Massive Gene Decay in the Leprosy Bacillus." *Nature* 409 (February 22, 2001): 1007–1011. This article can also be found online at https://www.nature.com/articles/35059006 (accessed February 9, 2018).

Coller, Beth-Ann, et al. "Clinical Development of a Recombinant Ebola Vaccine in the Midst of an Unprecedented Epidemic." *Vaccine* 35 (August 16, 2017): 4465–4469.

Collins, J., et al. "Dietary Trehalose Enhances Virulence of Epidemic *Clostridium difficile*." *Nature* 553 (2018): 291–294. This article can also be found online at https://www.nature.com/articles/nature25178 (accessed February 1, 2018).

Collison, Lauren W., and Dario A. A. Vignali. "In Vitro Treg Suppression Assays." *Methods in Molecular Biology* 707 (2011): 21–37.

Connor, Bradley, and William B. Bunn. "The Changing Epidemiology of Japanese Encephalitis and New Data: The Implications for New Recommendations for Japanese Encephalitis Vaccine." *Tropical Disease, Travel Medicine and Vaccines* 3, no. 14 (August 1, 2017). This article can also be found online at https://tdtmvjournal.biomedcentral.com/articles/10.1186/s40794–017-0057-x (accessed February 15, 2018).

Cooper, Chester R., and Nongnuch Vanittanakom. "Insights into the Pathogenecity of *Penicillium marneffei*." *Future Microbiology* 3, no. 1 (2008): 43–55. This article can also be found online at https://www.futuremedicine.com/doi/abs/10.2217/17460913.3.1.43?rfr_dat=cr_pub%3Dpubmed&url_ver=Z39.88–2003&rfr_id=ori%3Arid%3Acrossref.org&journalCode=fmb (accessed February 21, 2018).

Cope, Jennifer R., et al. "Contact Lens Wearer Demographics and Risk Behaviors for Contact Lens-Related Eye Infections—United States, 2014." *Morbidity and Mortality Weekly* 64, no. 32 (2015): 865–870.

———. "Risk Behaviors for Contact Lens-Related Eye Infections among Adults and Adolescents—United States, 2016." *Morbidity and Mortality Weekly* 66, no. 32 (2017): 841–845.

Corbett, Elizabeth, et al. "The Growing Burden of Tuberculosis: Global Trends and Interactions with the HIV Epidemic." *Archives of Internal Medicine* 163, no. 9 (May 12, 2003): 1009–1021. This article can also be found online at https://www.ncbi.nlm.nih.gov/pubmed/12742798 (accessed March 9, 2018).

Corrado, Minetti, et al. "Giardiasis." *BMJ* 355 (2016): i5369. This article can also be found online at http://www.bmj.com/content/355/bmj.i5369 (accessed January 16, 2018).

Cossaboom, Caitlin M., et al. "Risk Factors and Sources of Foodborne Hepatitis E Virus Infection in the United States." *Journal of Medical Virology* 88, no.9 (September 2016): 1641–1645.

Costa, Federico, et al. "Global Morbidity and Mortality of Leptospirosis: A Systematic Review." *PLOS Neglected Tropical Diseases* (September 17, 2015). This article can also be found online at http://journals.plos.org/plosntds/article?id=10.1371/journal.pntd.0003898 (accessed January 19, 2018).

Costerus, Joost M., et al. "Community-Acquired Bacterial Meningitis." *Current Opinion in Infectious Diseases* 30, no. 1 (February 2017): 135–141.

Cowan, George. "Rickettsial Diseases: The Typhus Group of Fevers—a Review." *Postgraduate Medical Journal* 76 (May 2000): 269–272.

Cowart, Leigh. "Women Are Still Getting Toxic Shock Syndrome, and No One Quite Knows Why." *Washington Post* (March 21, 2016). This article can also be found online at https://www.washingtonpost.com/news/speaking-of-science/wp/2016/03/21/women-are-still-getting-toxic-shock-syndrome-and-no-one-quite-knows-why/?utm_term=.eccd5e2bcc05 (accessed January 17, 2018).

Cunha, Burke A. "Effective Antibiotic-Resistance Control Strategies." *Lancet* 357 (2001): 1307–1308.

Curi, Andre L., and Rim Kahloun. "Cat-Scratch Disease." *Emerging Infectious Uveitis* (June 2017): 57–63.

Dalke, Brian, et al. "Gonorrhea: Treatment and Management Considerations for the Male Patient." *U.S. Pharmacist* 41, no. 8 (2016): 41–44.

Dans, L. F., and E. G. Martinez. "Amoebic Dysentery." *BMJ Clinical Evidence* (2007): 0918.

Davies, Julian, and Dorothy Davies. "Origins and Evolutions of Antibiotic Resistance." *Microbiology and Molecular Biology Reviews* 74, no. 3 (2010): 417–433. This article can also be found online at https://www.ncbi.nlm.nih.gov/pmc/articles/PMC2937522/ (accessed February 25, 2018).

De La Monte, S., et al. "The Systemic Pathology of Venezuelan Equine Encephalitis Virus Infection in Humans." *American Journal of Tropical Medicine and Hygiene* 34 (1985): 194–202.

De Martel C., et al. "Global Burden of Cancers Attributable to Infections in 2008: A Review and Synthetic Analysis." *Lancet Oncology* 13, no. 6 (June 2012): 607–615.

De Vincenzi, I. "A Longitudinal Study of Human Immunodeficiency Virus Transmission by Heterosexual Partners." *New England Journal of Medicine* 331 (August 11, 1994): 341–346.

DeFelice, Nicholas B., et al. "Ensemble Forecast of Human West Nile Virus Cases and Mosquito Infection Rates." *Nature Communication* 8 (February 2017).

Dellinger, R. Phillip, et al. "Surviving Sepsis Campaign: International Guidelines for Management of Severe Sepsis and Septic Shock: 2012." *Critical Care Medicine* 41, no. 2 (February 2013): 580–637. This article can also be found online at https://www.sccm.org/Documents/SSC-Guidelines.pdf (accessed February 28, 2018).

Delzo, Janissa. "Utah Hit by National Hepatitis Outbreak That Has Left 41 Dead in California and Michigan." *Newsweek* (November 30, 2017). This article can also be found online at http://www.newsweek.com/utah-hit-national-hepatitis-outbreak-which-has-left-41-dead-california-and-727616 (accessed January 22, 2018).

DeMuri, Gregory P., and Ellen R. Wald. "The Group A Streptococcal Carrier State Reviewed: Still an Enigma." *Journal of the Pediatric Infectious Diseases Society* 3, no. 4 (December 1, 2014): 336–342. This article can also be found online at https://academic.oup.com/jpids/article/3/4/336/909914 (accessed January 31, 2018).

Denis, Martine, et al. "No Clear Differences between Organic and Conventional Pig Farms in the Genetic Diversity or Virulence of *Campylobacter coli* Isolates." *Frontiers in Microbiology* 6 (2017).

Deresiewicz, Robert L., et al. "Clinical and Neuroradiographic Manifestations of Eastern Equine Encephalitis."**New England Journal of Medicine** 336 (June 26, 1997): 1867–1874. This article can also be found online at http://www.nejm.org/doi/full/10.1056/NEJM199706263362604#t=abstract (accessed December 17, 2017).

Desjardins, Christopher A., et al. "Population Genetics and the Evolution of Virulence in the Fungal Pathogen *Cryptococcus neoformans.*" *Genome Research* 27 (2015): 1207–1219.

Devleesschauwer, Brecht, et al. "The Low Global Burden of Trichinellosis: Evidence and Implications." *International Journal for*

Parasitology 45 (2015): 95–99. This article can also be found online at http://www.cbra.be/publications/Devleesschauwer2015.pdf (accessed January 11, 2018).

———. "Taenia Solium in Europe: Still Endemic?" *Acta Tropica* 165 (2017): 96–99.

Dewey-Mattia, Daniel, et al. "Foodborne and Waterborne Disease Outbreaks—United States, 1971–2012." *Morbidity and Mortality Weekly Report* 62, no. 54 (October 23, 2015): 86–89.

DeWitte, Sharon. "Mortality Risk and Survival in the Aftermath of the Medieval Black Death." *PLOS ONE* 9, no. 5 (2015): e96513.

Diaz, James H. "Paragonimiasis Acquired in the United States: Native and Nonnative Species." *Clinical Microbiology Reviews* 26, no. 3 (July 2013): 493–504.

Didier E. S., and L. M. Weiss. "Microsporidiosis: Current Status." *Current Opinion in Infectious Diseases* 19, no. 5 (2006): 485.

Didier, E. S., et al. "Epidemiology of Microsporidiosis: Sources and Modes of Transmission." *Veterinary Parasitology* 126, no. 1–2 (December 2004):145–166.

Doherty, Mark, et al. "Vaccine Impact: Benefits for Human Health." *Vaccine* 34, no. 52 (December 20, 2016): 6707–6714. This article can also be found online at https://www.sciencedirect.com/science/article/pii/S0264410X16309434 (accessed February 13, 2018).

Dolan, Kate, et al. "Global Burden of HIV, Viral Hepatitis, and Tuberculosis in Prisoners and Detainees." *Lancet* 388, no. 10049 (September 10, 2016):1089–1102. This article can also be found online at http://www.thelancet.com/journals/lancet/article/PIIS0140–6736(16)30466–4/fulltext (accessed February 9, 2018).

Dollard, Sheila C., et al. "National Prevalence Estimates for Cytomegalovirus IgM and IgG Avidity and Association between High IgM Antibody Titer and Low IgG Avidity." *Clinical and Vaccine Immunology* 18, no. 11 (2011): 1895–1899.

Dominguez, Antonia A., Wendell A. Lim, and Lei S. Qi. "Beyond Editing: Repurposing CRISPR-Cas9 for Precision Genome Regulation and Interrogation." *Nature Reviews Molecular Cell Biology* 17, no. 1 (January 2016): 5–15.

Doolan, Denise L., Carlota Dobaño, and J. Kevin Baird. "Acquired Immunity to Malaria." *Clinical Microbiology Reviews* 22, no. 1 (2009): 13–36. This article can also be found online at https://www.ncbi.nlm.nih.gov/pmc/articles/PMC2620631/ (accessed February 23, 2018).

Downham, Christina, et al. "Season of Infectious Mononucleosis as a Risk Factor for Multiple Sclerosis: A UK Primary Care Case-Control Study." *Multiple Sclerosis and Related Disorders* 17 (2017): 103–106.

Drancourt, M., and D. Raoult. "Molecular Insights into the History of Plague." *Microbes and Infection* 4, no. 1 (January 2002): 105–109.

Drexler, Naomi. A., et al. "Fatal Rocky Mountain Spotted Fever along the United States–Mexico Border, 2013–2016." *Emerging Infectious Diseases* 10 (October 23, 2017): 1621–1626.

Du, Rebecca, et al. "Old World Cutaneous Leishmaniasis and Refugee Crises in the Middle East and North Africa." *PLOS Neglected Tropical Diseases* 10, no. 5 (May 26, 2016). This article can also be found online at http://journals.plos.org/plosntds/article?id=10.1371/journal.pntd.0004545 (accessed February 3, 2018).

Ducrot, Christian, et al. "Modelling BSE Trend over Time in Europe, a Risk Assessment Perspective." *European Journal of Epidemiology* 25, no. 6 (2010): 411–419.

Duffy, Mark R., et al. "Zika Virus Outbreak on Yap Island, Federated States of Micronesia." *New England Journal of Medicine* 360, no. 24 (2009): 2536–2543.

Duggan, Ana T., et al. "17th Century Variola Virus Reveals the Recent History of Smallpox." *Current Biology* 26, no. 24 (December 2016): 3407–3412. This article can also be found online at https://www.sciencedirect.com/science/article/pii/S0960982216313240 (accessed January 30, 2018).

Dunne, Eileen F., et al. "CDC Grand Rounds: Reducing the Burden of HPV-Associated Cancer and Disease." *Morbidity and Mortality Weekly* 63, no. 4 (January 31, 2014): 68–72. This article can also be found online at https://www.cdc.gov/mmwr/preview/mmwrhtml/mm6304a1.htm?s_cid=mm6304a1_e (accessed February 20, 2018).

DuPont, Herbert L. "The Growing Threat of Foodborne Bacterial Enteropathogens of Animal Origin." *Clinical Infectious Diseases* 45, no. 10 (2007): 1353–1361.

Dworkin, Mark S., et al. "Tick-Borne Relapsing Fever." *Infectious Disease Clinics of North America* 22, no. 3 (September 2008): 449–468.

Eamsobhana, Praphathip. "Angiostrongyliasis in Thailand: Epidemiology and Laboratory Investigations." *Hawaii Journal of Medicine and Public Health* 72, no. 6 (June 2013): 28–32.

Ebel, G. D. "Update on Powassan Virus: Emergence of a North American Tick-Borne Flavivirus." *Annual Review of Entomology* 55 (2010): 95–110.

Ebel, G. D., A. Spielman, and S. R. Telford. "Phylogeny of North American Powassan Virus." *Journal of General Virology* 82 (2001): 1657–1665.

Ebel, G. D., and L. D. Kramer. "Short Report: Duration of Tick Attachment Required for Transmission of Powassan Virus by Deer Ticks." *American Journal of Tropical Medicine and Hygiene* 71 (2004): 268–271.

Einarsson, Elin, Showgy Ma'ayeh, and Staffan G. Svärd. "An Update on *Giardia* and Giardiasis." *Current Opinion in Microbiology* 34 (December 2016): 47–52.

Eisen, Rebecca J. "Tick-Borne Zoonoses in the United States: Persistent and Emerging Threats to Human Health." *ILAR Journal* (March 23, 2017). This article can also be found online at https://academic.oup.com/ilarjournal/advance-article/doi/10.1093/ilar/ilx005/3078806 (accessed January 31, 2018).

Eldin, Carole, et al. "From Q Fever to *Coxiella burnetii* Infection: A Paradigm Change." *Clinical Microbiology Reviews* 30, no. 1 (January 2017): 115–190.

Eliopoulus, George M., and H. S. Gold. "Vancomycin-Resistant *Enterococci*: Mechanisms and Clinical Observations." *Clinical Infectious Diseases* 33, no. 2 (July 2001): 210–219. This article can also be found online at https://doi.org/10.1086/321815 (accessed March 7, 2018).

Elliott, Sean P. "Rat Bite Fever and *Streptobacillus moniliformis*." *Clinical Microbiology Reviews* 20, no. 1 (January 2007): 13–22. This article can also be found online at http://cmr.asm.org/content/20/1/13.full (accessed January 19, 2018).

Elschner, Mandy C., Heinrich Neubauer, and Lisa D. Sprague. "The Resurrection of Glanders in a New Epidemiological Scenario: A Beneficiary of 'Global Change.'" *Current Clinical Microbiology Reports* 4, no. 1 (2017): 54–60.

Elsenberg, Tobias, et al. "Approved and Novel Strategies in Diagnostics of Rat Bite Fever and Other *Streptobacillus* Infections in Humans and Animals." *Virulence* 7, no. 6 (August 2016): 630–648.

Elston, Dirk M. "Drugs Used in the Treatment of Pediculosis." *Journal of Drugs in Dermatology* 4, no. 2 (March–April 2005): 207–211.

Eltagouri, Marwa, and Cleve R. Wootson Jr. "Rats Used to Spread the Black Death. Now, Poverty Plays a Role." *Washington Post* (October 7, 2017). This article can also be found online at https://www.washingtonpost.com/news/to-your-health/wp/2017/10/05/black-death-outbreak-strikes-madagascar-killing-30-and-triggering-panic/?utm_term=.a3517d7c2c49 (accessed November 6, 2017).

Emanuel, Ezekiel J. "How to Develop New Antibiotics." *New York Times* (February 24, 2015). This article can also be found online at https://www.nytimes.com/2015/02/24/opinion/how-to-develop-new-antibiotics.html (accessed November 14, 2017).

Engelman, Daniel, et al. "Toward the Global Control of Human Scabies: Introducing the International Alliance for the Control of Scabies." *PLOS Neglected Tropical Diseases* 7, no. 8 (August 2013): e2167. This article is also available online at https://www.ncbi.nlm.nih.gov/pmc/articles/PMC3738445/ (accessed November 13, 2017).

Enserink, Martin, and Jocelyn Kaiser. "Accidental Anthrax Shipment Spurs Debate over Safety." *Nature* 304 (June 2004): 1726–1727.

Erbelding, Emily J., et al. "A Universal Influenza Vaccine: The Strategic Plan for the National Institute of Allergy and Infectious Diseases." *Journal of Infectious Diseases* (February 28, 2018). This article can also be found online at https://academic.oup.com/jid/advance-article/doi/10.1093/infdis/jiy103/4904047 (accessed February 28, 2018).

"Estimates of Deaths Associated with Seasonal Influenza—United States, 1976–2007." *Morbidity and Mortality Weekly Report* 59, no. 33 (August 27, 2010): 1057–1062.

Evans, Sam Weiss. "Biosecurity Governance for the Real World." *Issues in Science and Technology* 33, no. 1 (2016): 84–88.

Factor, Stephanie H., et al. "Invasive Group A Streptococcal Disease: Risk Factors for Adults." *Emerging Infectious Diseases* 9, no. 8 (2003): 970–977. The article can also be found online at https://www.ncbi.nlm.nih.gov/pmc/articles/PMC3020599/ (accessed February 12, 2018).

———. "Risk Factors for Pediatric Invasive Group A Streptococcal Disease." *Emerging Infectious Diseases* 11, no. 7 (2005): 1062–1066. This article can also be found online at https://wwwnc.cdc.gov/eid/article/11/7/pdfs/04-0900.pdf (accessed February 21, 2018).

Fallah, Mosoka P., et al. "Quantifying Poverty as a Driver of Ebola Transmission." *PLOS Neglected Tropical Disease* 9, no. 12 (2015): e0004260. This article can also be found online at https://doi.org/10.1371/journal.pntd.0004260 (accessed March 5, 2018).

Farmer, P. "Social Inequalities and Emerging Infectious Diseases." *Emerging Infectious Diseases* 2, no. 4 (October–December 1996): 259–269. This article can also be found online at https://wwwnc.cdc.gov/eid/article/2/4/pdfs/96-0402.pdf (accessed February 26, 2018).

Fast, Shannon M., Marta C. González, and Natasha Markuzon. "Cost-Effective Control of Infectious Disease Outbreaks Accounting for Societal Reaction." *PLOS One* 8 (2015): 211–223.

Feasey, Nicholas A., et al. "Rapid Emergence of Multidrug Resistant, H58-Lineage *Salmonella* Typhi in Blantyre, Malawi." *PLOS Neglected Tropical Diseases* 9, no. 4 (2015): e0003748. This article can also be found online at http://journals.plos.org/plosntds/article?id=10.1371/journal.pntd.0003748 (accessed January 29, 2018).

Feinberg, Mark B., and Rafi Ahmed. "Advancing Dengue Vaccine Development." *Science* 358, no. 6365 (November 17, 2017): 865–866.

Feldstein, Leora R., et al. "Global Routine Vaccination Coverage, 2016." *Morbidity and Mortality Weekly Report* 66, no. 45 (November 17, 2017): 1252–1255. This article can also be found online at https://www.cdc.gov/mmwr/volumes/66/wr/mm6645a3.htm (accessed February 13, 2018).

Felitti, Vincent J. "GIDEON: Global Infectious Diseases and Epidemiology Online Network." *JAMA* 293 (2005): 1674–1675.

Fernandez, Sonia. "Undetected Infection: Raccoon Roundworm—a Hidden Human Parasite?" *Current* (July 24, 2017). This article can also be found online at http://www.news.ucsb.edu/2017/018138/undetected-infection (accessed December 17, 2017).

Fetters, Ashley. "The Tampon: A History." *Atlantic* (June 1, 2015). This article can also be found online at https://www.theatlantic.com/health/archive/2015/06/history-of-the-tampon/394334/ (accessed January 17, 2018).

Fine, D. L., et al. "Venezuelan Equine Encephalitis Virus Vaccine Candidate (V3526) Safety, Immunogenicity and Efficacy in Horses." *Vaccine* 25 (2007): 1868–1876.

Fitzpatrick, Christopher, et al. "The Cost-Effectiveness of an Eradication Programme in the End Game: Evidence from Guinea Worm Disease." *PLOS Neglected Tropical Diseases* 11, no. 10 (October 2017): 1–21.

Fleischmann, C., et al. "Assessment of Global Incidence and Mortality of Hospital-Treated Sepsis: Current Estimates and Limitations ."**American Journal of Respiratory and Critical Care Medicine** 193, no. 3 (February 2016): 259–272.

Fletcher SM, et al. "Enteric Protozoa in the Developed World: A Public Health Perspective." *Clinical Microbiology Reviews* 25, no. 3 (July 2012): 420–449

Forrester, Joseph D., et al. "Assessment of Ebola Virus Disease, Health Care Infrastructure, and Preparedness—Four Counties, Southeastern Liberia, August 2014." *Morbidity and Mortality Weekly Report* 63, no. 40 (2014): 891–893.

Forrester, N. L., et al. "Evolution and Spread of Venezuelan Equine Encephalitis Complex Alphavirus in the Americas" *PLOS Neglected Tropical Diseases* 11 (2017): e0005693.

Foster, Scott A., Scott Parker, and Randall Lanier. "The Role of Brincidofovir in Preparation for a Potential Smallpox Outbreak." *Viruses* 9, no. 11 (2017). This article can also be found online at http://www.mdpi.com/1999-4915/9/11/320 (accessed January 30, 2018).

Fox, Cherie, et al. "Use of a Patient Hand Hygiene Protocol to Reduce Hospital-Acquired Infections and Improve Nurses' Hand Washing." *American Journal of Critical Care* 24 (2015): 216–224.

Franco Jose R., Pere P. Simarro, Abdoulaye Diarra, and Jean G. Jannin. "Epidemiology of Human African Trypanosomiasis." *Clin Epidemiol* 6 (2014): 257–275.

Frank, C., et al. "The Role of Parenteral Antischistosomal Therapy in the Spread of Hepatitis C Virus in Egypt." *Lancet* 355 (2000): 887–891.

Frazer, Jennifer. "Bed Bugs, Kissing Bugs Linked to Deadly Chagas Disease in U.S." *Scientific American* (December 10, 2014). This article can also be found online at https://www.scientificamerican.com/article/bed-bugs-kissing-bugs-linked-to-deadly-chagas-disease-in-u-s/ (accessed January 18, 2017).

Frederick, Adzitey, Nurul Huda, and Gulam Rusul Rahmat Ali. "Molecular Techniques for Detecting and Typing of Bacteria, Advantages and Application to Foodborne Pathogens Isolated from Ducks." *3 Biotech* 3, no. 2 (2013): 97–107.

Freeman, E. E., et al. "Herpes Simplex Virus 2 Infection Increases HIV Acquisition in Men and Women: Systematic Review and Meta-Analysis of Longitudinal Studies." *AIDS* 20 (2006): 73–83.

Fried, Susana T. "Telling Women to Avoid Pregnancy Is Not a Solution for HIV and the Zika Virus." *Guardian* (May 28, 2016). This article can also be found online at https://www.theguardian.com/global-development/2016/may/28/women-avoid-pregnancy-not-solution-hiv-zika-virus-internation-day-action-womens-health-conservative-religious-ideologies (accessed January 24, 2018).

Gagnon, Alain, et al. "Pandemic Paradox: Early Life H2N2 Pandemic Influenza Infection Enhanced Susceptibility to Death during the 2009 H1N1 Pandemic." *MBio* 9, no. 1 (January 16, 2018): 1–15. This article can also be found online at http://mbio.asm.org/content/9/1/e02091-17.full.pdf (accessed January 22, 2018).

Galgiani, John N., et al. "Coccidioidomycosis." *Clinical Infectious Diseases*, 41, 9 (2005): 1217–1223. This article can also be found online at https://doi.org/10.1086/496991 (accessed February 6, 2018).

Gally, David L., and Mark P. Stevens. "Microbe Profile: *Escherichia coli* O157:H7—Notorious Relative of the Microbiologist's Workhorse." *Microbiology Society* 163 (2017): 1–3.

Ghinai, Rosanna, et al. "A Cross-Sectional Study of 'Yaws' in Districts of Ghana Which Have Previously Undertaken Azithromycin Mass Drug Administration for Trachoma Control." *PLOS Neglected Tropical Diseases* (January 29, 2015). This article can also be found online at http://journals.plos.org/plosntds/article?id=10.1371/journal.pntd.0003496 (accessed February 2, 2018).

Ghooi, Ravindra B. "The Nuremberg Code—A Critique." *Perspectives in Clinical Research* 2, no. 2 (April–June 2011): 72–76. This article can also be found online at https://www.ncbi.nlm.nih.gov/pmc/articles/PMC3121268/ (accessed February 12, 2018).

Gillespie, Portia M., et al. "Status of Vaccine Research and Development of Vaccines for Leishmaniasis." *Vaccine* 34, no. 26 (June 2016): 2992–2995. This article can also be found online at https://www.sciencedirect.com/science/article/pii/S0264410X16002899 (accessed February 3, 2018).

Giuliano, Anna R., et al. "Efficacy of Quadrivalent HPV Vaccine against HPV Infection and Disease in Males." *New England Journal of Medicine* 364 (2011): 401–411. This article can also be found online at http://www.nejm.org/doi/full/10.1056/nejmoa0909537 (accessed February 20, 2018).

Goldmann, Donald. "System Failure versus Personal Accountability—The Case for Clean Hands" *New England Journal of Medicine* 355 (July 13, 2006): 121–123.

Gomez, Gabriela B., et al. "Untreated Maternal Syphilis and Adverse Outcomes of Pregnancy: A Systematic Review and Meta-Analysis." *Bulletin of the World Health Organization* 91 (2013): 217–226. This article can also be found online at https://www.scielosp.org/pdf/bwho/v91n3/a13v94n3.pdf (accessed February 16, 2018).

Gompper, Matthew E., and Amber N. Wright. "Altered Prevalence of Raccoon Roundworm (*Baylisascaris procyonis*) Owing to Manipulated Contact Rates of Hosts." *Journal of Zoology* 266, no. 2 (June 2005): 215–219.

Gonzales, Maria Liza M., Leonila F. Dans, and Elizabeth G. Martinez. "Antiamoebic Drugs for Treating Amoebic Colitis." *Cochrane Database of Systematic Reviews* (April 15, 2009). This article can also be found online at http://onlinelibrary.wiley.com/doi/10.1002/14651858.CD006085.pub2/abstract;jsessionid=F46287E3F4291C657AAA1B8E09315CD4.f02t02 (accessed March 15, 2018).

Goodyear, Dana. "Death Dust." *New Yorker* (January 20, 2014). This article can also be found online at https://www.newyorker.com/magazine/2014/01/20/death-dust (accessed February 6, 2018).

Gostin, Lawrence O. "International Infectious Disease Law: Revision of the World Health Organization's International Health Regulations." *Journal of the American Medical Association* 291 (2004): 2623–2627. This article can also be found online at http://jama.ama-assn.org/cgi/content/full/291/21/2623 (accessed May 26, 2007).

Gottlieb, M. S., et al. "*Pneumocystis* Pneumonia—Los Angeles." *Morbidity and Mortality Weekly Report* 30, no. 21 (June 5, 1981): 1–3.

Graham, Judith. "In Flu Season, Use a Mask. but Which One?" *New York Times* (January 16, 2013). This article can also be found online at https://newoldage.blogs.nytimes.com/2013/01/16/in-flu-seasonuse-a-mask-but-which-one/ (accessed November 6, 2017).

Graham, W. J., et al. "Childbed Fever: History Repeats Itself?" *BJOG* 122, no. 2 (2015): 156–159.

Gray, Penelope, et al. "Evaluation of HPV Type-Replacement in Unvaccinated and Vaccinated Adolescent Females—Post-Hoc Analysis of A Community-Randomized Clinical Trial (II)." *International Journal of Cancer* (February 12, 2018). This article can also be found online at https://www.ncbi.nlm.nih.gov/pubmed/29377141 (accessed February 20, 2018).

Gross, C. P., and K. A. Sepkowitz. "The Myth of the Medical Breakthrough: Smallpox, Vaccination, and Jenner Reconsidered." *International Journal of Infectious Disease* 3 (1998): 54–60.

Grossman, Nina T., and Arturo Casadevall. "Physiological Differences in *Cryptococcus neoformans* Strains *in vitro* versus *in vivo* and Their Effects on Antifungal Susceptibility." *Antimicrobial Agents and Chemotherapy* 61 (2017): e02108–e02116.

Grote, Alexandra, et al. "Defining Brugia Malayi and Wolbachia Symbiosis by Stage-Specific Dual RNA-Seq." *PLOS Neglected Tropical Diseases* 11, no. 3 (2017). This article can also be found online at https://doi.org/10.1371/journal.pntd.0005357 (accessed January 22, 2018).

Guerra, Marta A. "Leptospirosis: Public Health Perspectives." *Biologicals* 41, no. 5 (September 2013): 295–297. This article can also be found online at http://www.sciencedirect.com/science/article/pii/S1045105613000687 (accessed January 19, 2018).

"Guidelines for Prevention of Herpesvirus Simiae (B Virus) Infection in Monkey Handlers." *Morbidity and Mortality Weekly Report* 36, no. 41 (October 23, 1987): 680+. This article can also be found online at http://www.cdc.gov/mmwr/preview/mmwrhtml/00015936.htm (accessed December 15, 2017).

Gupta, Neil, and Paul Farmer. "We Can Cure Hepatitis C. But We're Now Making the Same Mistake We Did with AIDS." *Washington Post* (July 28, 2017). This article can also be found online at https://www.washingtonpost.com/opinions/we-can-cure-hepatitis-c-but-were-now-making-the-same-mistake-we-did-with-aids/2017/07/28/503a4b02-72f9-11e7-9eac-d56bd5568db8_story.html (accessed February 20, 2018).

Gupta, P., et al. "Potentiation of Antibiotic against Pseudomonas Aeruginosa Biofilm: A Study with Plumbagin and Gentamicin." *Journal of Applied Microbiology* 123 (July 2017): 246–261.

Guris, Dalya, et al. "Changing Varicella Epidemiology in Active Surveillance Sites—United States, 1995–2005." *Journal of Infectious Diseases* 197, supplement no. 2 (March 1, 2008): S71–S75. This article can also be found online at https://academic.oup.com/jid/article/197/Supplement_2/S71/848964 (accessed January 31, 2018).

Gurley, Emily S., et al. "Convergence of Humans, Bats, Trees, and Culture in Nipah Virus Transmission, Bangladesh." *Emerging Infectious Diseases* 23, no. 9 (September 2017): 1446–1453. This article can also be found online at https://www.ncbi.nlm.nih.gov/pmc/articles/PMC5572889/ (January 19, 2018).

Guy, W., et al. "Increase in Scarlet Fever Notifications in the United Kingdom, 2013/2014." *Eurosurveillance* 19, no. 12 (2014): 1–2.

Hadchouel, Michelle, Anne-Marie Prieur, and Claude Griscelli. "Acute Hemorrhagic, Hepatic and Neurologic Manifestations in Juvenile Rheumatoid Arthritis: Possible Relationship to Drugs or Infection." *Journal of Pediatrics* 106 (1985): 561–566.

Haelle, Tara. "Shooting the Wheeze: Whooping Cough Vaccine Falls Short of Previous Shot's Protection." *Scientific American* (May 21, 2013). This article can also be found online at https://www.scientificamerican.com/article/whooping-cough-vaccine-falls-short-of-previous-shots-protection/ (accessed January 29, 2018).

———. "Vaccination Opt-Outs Found to Contribute to Whooping Cough Outbreaks in Kids." *Scientific American* (October 2, 2013). This article can also be found online at https://www.scientificamerican.com/article/vaccination-opt-outs-found-to-contribute-to-whooping-cough-outbreaks-in-kids/ (accessed January 29, 2018).

Hahn, James Duaine. "8-Year-Old Dies from Rare Flesh-Eating Bacteria: Doctors 'Kept Cutting and Hoping,' Mother Says." *People* (January 25, 2018). This article can also be found online at http://people.com/human-interest/flesh-eating-bacteria-kills-boy/ (accessed February 13, 2018).

Halden, Rol U. "On the Need and Speed of Regulating Triclosan and Tricarban in the United States." *Environmental Science and Technology* 48, no. 7 (April 2014): 3603–3611. This article can also be found online at https://www.ncbi.nlm.nih.gov/pmc/articles/PMC3974611/ (accessed November 27, 2017).

Hale, Malika, et al. "Engineering HIV-Resistant, Anti-HIV Chimeric Antigen Receptor T Cells." *Molecular Therapy* 25, no. 3 (2017): 570–579. This article can also be found online at http://www.cell.com/molecular-therapy-family/molecular-therapy/fulltext/S1525–0016(17)30004–7 (accessed March 12, 2018).

Hamid Salim, M. A., et al. "Gender Differences in Tuberculosis: A Prevalence Survey Done in Bangladesh." *International Journal of Tuberculosis and Lung Disease* 8, no. 8 (August 2004): 952–957. This article can also be found online at http://www.ingentaconnect.com/content/iuatld/ijtld/2004/00000008/00000008/art00005 (accessed March 7, 2018).

Hans, Rekha, and Neelam Marwhara. "Nucleic Acid Testing—Benefits and Constraints." *Asian Journal of Transfusion Science* 8, no. 1 (January–June 2014): 2–3. This article can also be found online at https://www.ncbi.nlm.nih.gov/pmc/articles/PMC3943139/ (accessed February 12, 2018).

Harmon, Katherine. "Why Is Cholera Spreading in Haiti Now?" *Scientific American* October 25, 2010. This article can also be found online at https://www.scientificamerican.com/article/cholera-outbreak-haiti/ (accessed February 12, 2018).

Harris, Aaron, M., et al. "Increases in Acute Hepatitis B Virus Infections—Kentucky, Tennessee, and West Virginia, 2006–2013." *Morbidity and Mortality Weekly Report* 65, no. 3 (2016): 47–50. This article can also be found online at https://www.cdc.gov/mmwr/volumes/65/wr/mm6503a2.htm (accessed February 2, 2018).

Harris, Patrick N. A., et al. "An Outbreak of Scrub Typhus in Military Personnel Despite Protocols for Antibiotic Prophylaxis: Doxycycline Resistance Excluded by a Quantitative PCR-based Susceptibility Assay." *Microbes and Infection* 18, no. 6 (June 2016): 406–411.

Hartman, Amy. "Rift Valley Fever." *Clinics in Laboratory Medicine* 37, no. 2 (June 2017): 285–301. This article can also be found online at https://www.sciencedirect.com/science/article/pii/S0272271217300069 (accessed January 18, 2018).

Hauri, A. M., G. L. Armstrong, and Y. J. Hutin. "The Global Burden of Disease Attributable to Contaminated Injections Given in Health Care Settings." *International Journal of STD and AIDS* 15 (2004): 7–16.

Hecht, Robert, et al. "Putting It Together: AIDS and the Millennium Development Goals." *PLOS Medicine* 3, no. 11 (2006): e455. This article can also be found online at http://journals.plos.org/plosmedicine/article?id=10.1371/journal.pmed.0030455 (accessed March 9, 2018).

Hector, Richard F., and Rafael Laniado-Laborin. "Coccidioidomycosis—A Fungal Disease of the Americas." *PLOS Medicine* (January 25, 2005). This article can also be found online at https://doi.org/10.1371/journal.pmed.0020002 (accessed February 6, 2018).

Heijne, J. C., et al. "Uptake of Regular Chlamydia Testing by U.S. Women: A Longitudinal Study." *American Journal of Preventive Medicine* 39 (2010): 243–250.

Hemilä, Harri, et al. "Zinc Acetate Lozenges May Improve the Recovery Rate of Common Cold Patients: An Individual Patient Data Meta-Analysis." *Open Forum Infectious Diseases* 4 (2017): 59.

Henry, Ronnie, and Frederick A. Murphy. "Etymologia: Marburg Virus." *Emerging Infectious Diseases* 23, no. 10 (October 2017): 1689. This article can also be found online at https://wwwnc.cdc.gov/eid/article/23/10/et-2310_article (accessed January 18, 2018).

Herfst, Sander, et al. "Airborne Transmission of Influenza A/H5N1 Virus between Ferrets." *Science* 336, no. 6088 (June 22, 2012): 1534–1541. This article can also be found online at http://science.sciencemag.org/content/336/6088/1534.full (accessed February 22, 2018).

Hernandez, Nelson, and Philip Rucker. "Anthrax Case Raises Doubt on Security." *Washington Post* (August 8, 2008): A01. This article can also be found online at http://www.washingtonpost.com/wp-dyn/content/story/2008/08/07/ST2008080703559.html (accessed January 31, 2018).

Herwaldt, B. L., et al. "Endemic Babesiosis in Another Eastern State: New Jersey." *Emerging Infectious Diseases* 9 (February 2003): 184–188.

Hicar, Mark D., Kathryn Edwards, and Karen Bloch. "Powassan Virus Infection Presenting as Acute Disseminated Encephalomyelitis in Tennessee." *Pediatric Infectious Disease Journal* 30, no. 1 (2011): 86–88.

Hill, C. A., et al. "Arthropod-Borne Diseases: Vector Control in the Genomics Era." *Nature Reviews Microbiology* 3 (March 2005): 262–268.

Hilts, Philip J. "79 Anthrax Traced to Soviet Military." *New York Times* (November 18, 1994).

Hobson, C., et al. "Detection of Bartonella in Cat Scratch Disease Using a Single-Step PCR Assay Kit." *Journal of Medical Microbiology* 66 (2017).

Hodal, Kate. "Rohingya Children Close to Starvation Amid 'Health Crisis on an Unimaginable Scale.'" *Guardian* (November 10, 2017). This article can also be found online at https://www.theguardian.com/global-development/2017/nov/10/rohingya-kids-starvation-health-crisis-unimaginable-scale-malnutrition-myanmar-bangladesh (accessed February 5, 2018).

Hoerauf, Achim. "Filariasis: New Drugs and New Opportunities for Lymphatic Filariasis and Onchocerciasis." *Current Opinion in Infectious Disease* 21, no. 6 (2008): 673–681. This article can also be found online at https://insights.ovid.com/pubmed?pmid=18978537 (accessed January 22, 2018).

Hoffmann, Constanze, et al. "Persistent Anthrax as a Major Driver of Wildlife Mortality in a Tropical Rainforest." *Nature* 548 (2017): 82–86.

Hogerwerf, L., et al. "Chlamydia Psittaci (Psittacosis) as a Cause of Community-Acquired Pneumonia: A Systematic Review and Meta-Analysis." *Epidemiology & Infection* 145, no. 15 (2017): 3096–3105.

Hopkins, Donald R., et al. "Progress toward Global Eradication of Dracunculiasis, January 2016–June 2017." *Morbidity and Mortality Weekly Report* 66, no. 48 (December 8, 2017): 1327–1331. This article can also be found online at https://www.cdc.gov/mmwr/volumes/66/wr/mm6648a3.htm (accessed January 9, 2018).

Hotez, Peter J. "Helminth Infections: The Great Neglected Tropical Diseases." *Journal of Clinical Investigation* 118, no. 4 (April 2008): 1311–1321. This article can also be found online at https://www.ncbi.nlm.nih.gov/pmc/articles/PMC2276811/

———. "Tropical Diseases: The New Plague of Poverty." *New York Times* (August 19, 2012): SR4. This article can also be found online at http://www.nytimes.com/2012/08/19/opinion/sunday/tropical-diseases-the-new-plague-of-poverty.html (accessed January 30, 2018).

Hotez, Peter J., et al. "Hookworm Infection." *New England Journal of Medicine* 351, no. 8 (August 19, 2004): 799–807.

Huang, Ying, et al. "Parainfluenza Virus 5 Expressing the G protein of Rabies Virus Protected Mice after Rabies Virus Infection." *Journal of Virology* (December 31, 2014). This article can also be found online at http://jvi.asm.org/content/early/2014/12/26/JVI.03656–14.full.pdf+html (accessed February 26, 2018).

Huff, Jennifer L., and Peter A. Barry. "B-Virus (*Cercopithecine Herpesvirus* 1) Infection in Humans and Macaques: Potential for Zoonotic Disease." *Emerging Infectious Diseases* 9 (February 2003): 246–250. This article can also be found online at https://wwwnc.cdc.gov/eid/article/9/2/02–0272_article (accessed December 15, 2017).

Hugh-Jones, Martin. "Global Awareness of Disease Outbreaks: The Experience of ProMED-Mail." *Public Health Reports* 116, no. 2 (2001): 27–31.

Hyland, Ryan. "Polio's Last Stand: Frantic Effort to Eradicate Pakistan's 'Badge of Shame.'" *Guardian* (March 15, 2017). This article can also be found online at https://www.theguardian.com/global-development-professionals-network/2017/mar/15/polio-in-pakistan-the-frantic-effort-to-eradicate-the-countrys-badge-of-shame (accessed February 2, 2018).

Hymes, K. B., et al. "Kaposi's Sarcoma in Homosexual Men: A Report of Eight Cases." *Lancet* 2 (September 19, 1981): 598–600.

Iacono, Giovanni Lo, et al. "Using Modelling to Disentangle the Relative Contributions of Zoonotic and Anthroponotic Transmission: The Case of Lassa Fever." *PLOS Neglected Tropical Diseases* (January 8, 2015). This article can also be found online at http://journals.plos.org/plosntds/article?id=10.1371/journal.pntd.0003398 (accessed January 24, 2018).

"Illegal Giant Snails Threatening America." *New York Post* (August 29, 2014). This article can also be found online at https://nypost.com/2014/08/29/illegal-giant-snails-threatening-america/ (accessed January 12, 2018).

Ishak, Kamal, et al. "Histological Grading and Staging of Chronic Hepatitis." *Journal of Hepatology* 22, no. 6 (1995): 696–699.

Ishaq, Sauid, and Lois Nunn. "*Helicobacter pylori* and Gastric Cancer: A State of the Art Review." *Gastroenterology and Hepatology from Bed to Bench* 8, sup. 1 (2015): S6–S14. This article can also be found online at https://www.ncbi.nlm.nih.gov/pmc/articles/PMC4495426/ (accessed March 6, 2018).

Jain, Seema, et al. "Community-Acquired Pneumonia Requiring Hospitalization among U.S. Adults." *New England Journal of Medicine* 373 (July 30, 2015): 415–427. This article can also be found online at http://www.nejm.org/doi/full/10.1056/NEJMoa1500245 (accessed February 15, 2018).

Jason, Leonard A., et al. "A Prospective Study of Infectious Mononucleosis in College Students." *International Journal of Psychiatry* 2, 1 (2017): 1–8. This article can also be found online at https://www.ncbi.nlm.nih.gov/pmc/articles/PMC5510613/ (accessed January 24, 2018).

Jensen, Ramon Gordon, et al. "Recurrent Otorrhea in Chronic Suppurative Otitis Media: Is Biofilm the Missing Link?" *European Archives of Oto-Rhino-Laryngology* 274, no. 7 (July 2017): 2741–2747.

Jernigan, D. B., et al. "Investigation of Bioterrorism-Related Anthrax, United States, 2001: Epidemiologic Findings." *Emerging Infectious Diseases* 8, no. 10 (October 2002): 1019–1028.

Jiggins, Francis M. "The Spread of *Wolbachia* through Mosquito Populations." *PLOS Biology* 15 (June 2017): e2002780.

Johnson, D. K., et al. "Tickborne Powassan Virus Infections among Wisconsin Residents." *Wisconsin Medical Journal* 109, no. 2 (2010): 91–97.

Johnson, Niall P. A. S., and Jeurgen Mueller. "Updating the Accounts: Global Mortality of the 1918–1920 'spanish' Influenza Pandemic." *Bulletin of the History of Medicine* 76, no. 1 (2002): 105–115.

Jordan, Vanessa. "Cochrane Corner: Preventing Cold Sores: Do Antivirals Work?" *Journal of Primary Health Care* 7, no. 4 (2015): 348.

Jouan, Y., et al. "Long-Term Outcome of Severe Herpes Simplex Encephalitis: A Population-Based Observational Study." *Critical Care* 19 (September 21, 2015): 345.

June, Carl H., and Bruce L. Levine. "T Cell Engineering as Therapy for Cancer and HIV: Our Synthetic Future." *Philosophical Transactions of the Royal Society B* 370, no. 1680 (2015): 20140374. This article can also be found online at http://rstb.royalsocietypublishing.org/content/370/1680/20140374 (accessed March 12, 2018).

Kabwama, Steven Ndugwa, et al. "A Large and Persistent Outbreak of Typhoid Fever Caused by Consuming Contaminated Water and Street-Vended Beverages: Kampala, Uganda, January–June 2015." *BMC Public Health* 17, no. 23 (October 2017). This article can also be found online at https://bmcpublichealth.biomedcentral.com/articles/10.1186/s12889-016-4002-0 (accessed January 29, 2018).

Kaiser, Jocelyn. "Quick Save for Infectious-Disease Grants at NIAID." *Science* 303 (2004): 941.

Kaiser, Pete. "Advances in Avian Immunology—Prospects for Disease Control: A Review." *Avian Pathology* 39, no. 5 (2010): 309–324.

Kaminsky, Rina G., Renato Valenzuela Castillo, and Coralia Abrego Flores. "Growth Retardation and Severe Anemia in Children with *Trichuris* Dysenteric Syndrome." *Asian Pacific Journal of Tropical Biomedicine* 5, no. 7 (July 2015): 591–597.

Kamradt-Scott, Adam. "WHO's to Blame? The World Health Organization and the 2014 Ebola Outbreak in West Africa." *Third World Quarterly* 37, no. 3 (2016): 401–418. This article can also be found online at https://www.tandfonline.com/doi/abs/10.1080/01436597.2015.1112232 (accessed February 28, 2018).

Kandi, Venkataramana, et al. "Chronic Pulmonary Histoplasmosis and Its Clinical Significance: An Under-Reported Systemic Fungal Disease." *Cureus* 8, no. 8 (2016): e751. This article can also be found online at https://www.ncbi.nlm.nih.gov/pmc/articles/PMC5037059/ (accessed January 23, 2018).

Kane, A., et al. "Transmission of Hepatitis B, Hepatitis C and Human Immunodeficiency Viruses through Unsafe Injections in the Developing World: Model-Based Regional Estimates." *Bulletin of the World Health Organization* 77, no. 10 (1999): 801–807.

Karesh, W. B., et al. "Wildlife Trade and Global Disease Emergence." *Emerging Infectious Diseases* 11, no. 7 (July 2005): 1000–1002.

Karlamangla, Soumya. "California Hospitals Face a 'War Zone' of Flu Patients—And Are Setting Up Tents to Treat Them." *Los Angeles Times* (January 16, 2018). This article can also be found online at http://www.latimes.com/local/lanow/la-me-ln-flu-demand-20180116-htmlstory.html (accessed January 17, 2018).

Kashangura, Rufaro, et al. "Effects of MVA85A Vaccine on Tuberculosis Challenge in Animals: Systematic Review." International Journal of Epidemiology 44, no. 6 (December 2015): 1970–1981. This article can also be found online at https://academic.oup.com/ije/article/44/6/1970/2572503 (accessed March 16, 2018).

Kato, Hirofumi, et al. "Epidemiological and Clinical Features of Severe Fever with Thrombocytopenia Syndrome in Japan, 2013–2014." *PLOS ONE* 11, 10 (2016). This article can also be found online at https://doi.org/10.1371/journal.pone.0165207 (accessed March 1, 2018).

Katz, Rebecca, and Scott F. Dowell. "Revising the International Health Regulations: Call for a 2017 Review Conference." *Lancet Global Health* 3, no. 7 (July 2015): e352–e353. This article can also be found online at http://www.thelancet.com/journals/langlo/article/PIIS2214-109X(15)00025-X/fulltext.

Kauffman, Carol A. "Histoplasmosis: A Clinical and Laboratory Update." *Clinical Microbiology Reviews* 20, no. 1 (2007): 115–132. This article can also be found online at https://www.ncbi.nlm.nih.gov/pmc/articles/PMC1797635/ (accessed January 23, 2018).

Kaufmann, Arnold F., Martin I. Meltzer, and George P. Schmid. "The Economic Impact of a Bioterrorist Attack: Are Prevention and Postattack Intervention Programs Justifiable?" *Emerging Infectious Diseases* 3, no. 2 (June 1997): 83–94. This article can also be found online at https://wwwnc.cdc.gov/eid/article/3/2/97-0201_article (accessed January 12, 2018).

Kavanagh, Kevin T., Said Abusalem, and Lindsey E. Calderon. "The Incidence of MRSA Infections in the United States: Is a More Comprehensive Tracking System Needed?" *Antimicrobial Resistance & Infection Control* 6, no. 34 (April 2017). This article can also be found online at https://aricjournal.biomedcentral.com/articles/10.1186/s13756-017-0193-0 (accessed December 7, 2017).

Kelley, Shana O. "New Technologies for Rapid Bacterial Identification and Antibiotic Resistance." *SLAS Technology* 22 (April 2017): 113–121.

Kelly, Michelle N., and Judd E. Shellito. "Current Understanding of *Pneumocystis* Immunology." *Future Microbiology* 5, no. 1 (2010): 43–65. This article can also be found online at https://www.ncbi.nlm.nih.gov/pmc/articles/PMC3702169/ (accessed February 15, 2018).

Kennedy, Peter G. E., et al. "A Comparison of Herpes Simplex Virus Type 1 and Varicella-Zoster Virus Latency and Reactivation." *Journal of General Virology* 96 (2015): 1581–1602.

Kennedy, Peter G. E., Phenix-Lan Quan, and W. Ian Lipkin. "Viral Encephalitis of Unknown Cause: Current Perspective and Recent Advances." *Viruses* 9, no. 6 (2017): 138.

Kenyon, C., et al. "Incident *Trichomonas vaginalis* Is Associated with Partnership Concurrency: A Longitudinal Cohort Study." *Sexually Transmitted Infections* 93, no. 2 (2017). This article can also be found online at http://sti.bmj.com/content/93/Suppl_2/A109.1 (accessed January 22, 2018).

Khalifa, Mohammed Mahdy, Radwa Raed Sharaf, and Ramy Karim Aziz. "*Helicobacter pylori*: A Poor Man's Gut Pathogen?" **Gut Pathogens** 2, no. 2 (2010).

Khamnuan, Patcharin, et al. "Necrotizing Fasciitis: Risk Factors of Mortality." *Risk Management Healthcare Policy* 8 (2015): 1–7. This article can also be found online at https://www.ncbi.nlm.nih.gov/pmc/articles/PMC4337692/ (accessed January 31, 2018).

Khan, K., et al. "WHO Analysis of Causes of Maternal Death: A Systematic Review." *Lancet* 367, no. 9516 (2006):1066–1074.

Kharsany, Ayesha B.M., and Quarraisha A. Karim. "HIV Infection and AIDS in Sub-Saharan Africa: Current Status, Challenges and Opportunities." *Open AIDS Journal* 10 (2016): 34–48.

Khorsandi, Danial, and Ghasemi Mahtab. "Childhood Skin Disorders: Genetic Study of the Erythema Infectiosum (Fifth Disease)." *Journal of Pregnancy and Child Health* 4 (2017): 1–4.

Khuu, Diana, et al. "Blastomycosis Mortality Rates, United States, 1990–2010." *Emerging Infectious Diseases* 20, no. 11 (2014): 1789–1794. This article can also be found online at https://wwwnc.cdc.gov/eid/article/20/11/13-1175_article (accessed January 26, 2018).

———. "Malaria-Related Hospitalizations in the United States, 2000–2014." *American Journal of Tropical Medicine and Hygiene* 97, no. 1 (July 2017): 213–221. This article can also be found online at https://www.ajtmh.org/content/journals/10.4269/ajtmh.17-0101 (accessed February 23, 2018).

Kiatsimkul, Porntip. "Increasing Incidence of Blastomycosis Infection in Vermont." Supplement, *Open Forum Infectious Diseases* 4 (2017): S84–S85. This article can also be found online at https://www.ncbi.nlm.nih.gov/pmc/articles/PMC5631645/ (accessed January 25, 2018).

"Kids' Tonsillectomies Make More Sense for Sleep Apnea Than for Strep Throat." *Washington Post* (January 20, 2017). This article can also be found online at https://www.washingtonpost.com/national/health-science/tonsillectomies-may-not-be-wise-for-stopping-throat-infections/2017/01/20/6655bbf6-ddb7-11e6-ad42-f3375f271c9c_story.html?utm_term=.40825a7e9193 (accessed January 25, 2018).

Kim, W. Ray. "Epidemiology of Hepatitis B in the United States." *Hepatology* 49, no. 5 Suppl. (2009): S28–S34. This article can also be found online at https://www.ncbi.nlm.nih.gov/pmc/articles/PMC3290915/ (accessed December 15, 2017).

Kim, Young Eun, Elisa Sicuri, and Fabrizio Tediosi. "Financial and Economic Costs of the Elimination and Eradication of Onchocerciasis (River Blindness) in Africa." *PLOS Neglected Tropical Diseases* (September 11, 2015). This article can also be found online at http://journals.plos.org/plosntds/article?id=10.1371/journal.pntd.0004056 (accessed February 12, 2018).

Kimberlin, David W., and Richard J. Whitley. "Varicella-Zoster Vaccine for the Prevention of Herpes Zoster." *New England Journal of Medicine* 356 (March 29, 2007): 1338–1343.

King, Charles H. "The Evolving Schistosomiasis Agenda 2007–2017: Why We Are Moving beyond Morbidity Control toward Elimination of Transmission." *PLOS Neglected Tropical Diseases* 11, no. 4 (2017): e0005517. This article can also be found online at https://doi.org/10.1371/journal.pntd.0005517 (accessed January 12, 2018).

Kirkland, Theo N., and Joshua Fierer. "Coccidioidomycosis: A Reemerging Infectious Disease." *Emerging Infectious Diseases* 2, no. 3 (July 1996). This article can also be found online at https://wwwnc.cdc.gov/eid/article/2/3/96-0305_article (accessed March 9, 2018).

Kissinger, Patricia. "*Trichomonas vaginalis*: A Review of Epidemiologic, Clinical and Treatment Issues." BMC Infectious Diseases 15, no. 307 (August 5, 2015). This article can also be found online at https://bmcinfectdis.biomedcentral.com/articles/10.1186/s12879-015-1055-0 (accessed January 22, 2018).

Klass, Perri. "Mumps Makes a Comeback, Even among the Vaccinated." *New York Times* (November 6, 2017). This article can also be found online at https://www.nytimes.com/2017/11/06/well/family/mumps-makes-a-comeback-even-among-the-vaccinated.html (accessed January 24, 2018).

———. "When Athletes Share Infections." *New York Times* (October 3, 2017): D4. This article is also available online at https://www.nytimes.com/2017/09/25/well/family/when-athletes-share-infections.html (accessed November 13, 2017).

Klein, Eili Y., et al. "Trends in Methicillin-Resistant *Staphylococcus Aureus* Hospitalizations in the United States, 2010–2014." *Clinical Infectious Diseases* 65 (November 2017): 1921–1923.

Klimek, Ludger, et al. "Factors Associated with Efficacy of an Ibuprofen/Pseudoephedrine Combination Drug in Pharmacy Customers with

Common Cold Symptoms." *International Journal of Clinical Practice* 71 (2017): e12907.

Kluger, Jeffrey. "Is 2018 the Year for Polio's Extinction?" *Time* (December 18, 2017). This article can also be found online at http://time.com/5068516/is-2018-the-year-for-polios-extinction/ (accessed February 2, 2018).

Knauf, Sascha, et al. "Isolation of *Treponema* DNA from Necrophagous Flies in a Natural Ecosystem." *EBioMedicine* 11 (September 2016): 85–90. This article can also be found online at http://www.ebiomedicine.com/article/S2352-3964(16)30343-7/fulltext (accessed February 2, 2018).

Koelle, Katia, et al. "Epochal Evolution Shapes the Phylodynamics of Interpandemic Influenza A (H3N2) in Humans." *Science* 314 (2006): 1898–1903.

Koepke, Ruth., et al. "Estimating the Effectiveness of Tetanus-Diphtheria-Acellular Pertussis Vaccine (Tdap) for Preventing Pertussis: Evidence of Rapidly Waning Immunity and Difference in Effectiveness by Tdap Brand." *Journal of Infectious Diseases* 210, no. 6 (September 15, 2014): 942–953.

Kolata, Gina. "A Dangerous Form of Strep Stirs Concern in Resurgence." *New York Times* (June 8, 1994). This article can also be found online at http://www.nytimes.com/1994/06/08/us/a-dangerous-form-of-strep-stirs-concern-in-resurgence.html?pagewanted=all (accessed February 12, 2018).

Kotloff, Karen L., et al. "Shigellosis." *Lancet* (forthcoming). This article can also be found online at https://www.sciencedirect.com/science/article/pii/S0140673617332968 (accessed February 7, 2018).

Krain, Lisa J., Kenrad E. Nelson, and Alain B. Labrique. "Host Immune Status and Response to Hepatitis E Virus Infection." *Clinical Microbiology Reviews* 27, no. 1 (January 2014): 139–165. This article can also be found online at http://cmr.asm.org/content/27/1/139.full (accessed February 7, 2018).

Kralievits, Katherine E., et al. "The Global Blood Supply: A Literature Review." *Lancet* 385 (April 27, 2015). This article can also be found online at http://www.thelancet.com/journals/lancet/article/PIIS0140-6736(15)60823-6/fulltext (accessed February 12, 2018).

Kreston, Rebecca. "Baylisascariasis! The Tragic Parasitic Implications of Raccoons in Your Backyard." Discover (March 29, 2012). This article can also be found online at http://blogs.discovermagazine.com/bodyhorrors/2012/03/29/baylisascariasis/#.WjgSkFQ-dN1 (accessed December 17, 2017).

Kubiak, K., E. Dzika, and Ł. Paukszto. "Enterobiasis Epidemiology and Molecular Characterization of *Enterobius vermicularis* in Healthy Children in North-Eastern Poland." **Helminthologia** 54, no. 4 (2017): 284–291. This article can also be found online at https://www.degruyter.com/downloadpdf/j/helm.2017.54.issue-4/helm-2017-0042/helm-2017-0042.pdf (accessed January 10, 2018).

Kuchinsky, Sarah Catherine, et al. "Assessing the Infection Rates and Pathogenesis of *Borrelia burgdorferi* in Wild Rodents and Ticks in Western Maryland." *Journal of Immunology* 198, no. 1 (May 1, 2017): S7–S13.

Kugelman, Jeffrey R., et al. "Informing the Historical Record of Experimental Nonhuman Primate Infections with Ebola Virus: Genomic Characterization of USAMRIID Ebola Virus/H.sapiens-tc/COD/1995/Kikwit-9510621 Challenge Stock 'R4368' and Its Replacement 'R4415.'" *PLOS One* (March 22, 2016). This article can also be found online at http://journals.plos.org/plosone/article?id=10.1371/journal.pone.0150919 (accessed January 31, 2018).

Kulkarni, D. D., et al. "Nipah Virus Infection: Current Scenario." *Indian Journal of Virology* 24, no. 3 (December 2013): 398–408. This article can also be found online at https://www.ncbi.nlm.nih.gov/pmc/articles/PMC3832692/ (accessed January 22, 2018).

Kullberg, Bart Jan, and Maiken C. Arendrup. "Invasive Candidiasis." *New England Journal of Medicine* 373 (2015): 1445–1456.

Kunze, Ursula. "Tick-Borne Encephalitis—Still on the Map." *Ticks and Tick-Borne Diseases* 7, no. 5 (July 2016): 911–914.

Kuo, Cho-Chou, et al. "*Chlamydia pneumoniae* (TWAR)." *Clinical Microbiology Reviews* 8, no. 4 (1995): 451–461. This article can also be found online at http://cmr.asm.org/content/8/4/451.long (accessed January 26, 2018).

Kwok, Roberta. "Vaccines: The Real Issues in Vaccine Safety." *Nature* 473 (May 26, 2011): 436–438. This article can also be found online at https://www.nature.com/news/2011/110525/full/473436a.html (accessed February 14, 2018).

Lagunas-Rangel, Francisco. A., et al. "Current Trends in Zika Vaccine Development." *Journal of Virus Eradication* 3 (2017): 124–127.

Lahariya, Chandrakant. Global Eradication of Polio: The Case for "Finishing the Job." *Bulletin of the World Health Organization* 85 (2007): 421. This article can also be found online at http://www.who.int/bulletin/volumes/85/6/06–037457/en/ (accessed February 6, 2018).

Lamoth, Frederic, et al. "Changes in the Epidemiological Landscape of Invasive Candidiasis." *Journal of Antimicrobial Chemotherapy* 73 (January 2018): i4–i13.

Land, Stephanie. "Kids Shouldn't Be Sent Home for Lice, but Schools Can't Ignore the Issue Either." *Washington Post* (October 24, 2017). This article can also be found online at https://www.washingtonpost.com/news/parenting/wp/2017/10/24/easing-up-on-the-no-nit-policy-at-schools-hurts-low-income-families/?utm_term=.8e360f99b675 (accessed November 14, 2017).

Landro, Laura. "The Rising Risk of a Contaminated Blood Supply." *Wall Street Journal* (September 27, 2015). This article can also be found online at https://www.wsj.com/articles/the-rising-risk-of-a-contaminated-blood-supply-1443407428 (accessed February 12, 2018).

Lane, J. Michael, and Gregory A. Poland. "Why Not Destroy the Remaining Smallpox Virus Stocks?" *Vaccine* 29, no. 16 (April 5, 2011): 2823–2824. This article can also be found online at https://www.sciencedirect.com/science/article/pii/S0264410X1100329X?via%3Dihub (accessed January 29, 2018).

Larsson, Mattias, et al. "Clinical Characteristics and Outcome of *Penicillium marneffei* Infection among HIV-Infected Patients in Northern Vietnam." *AIDS Research and Therapy* 9, no. 1 (2012): 24. This article can also be found online at https://aidsrestherapy.biomedcentral.com/articles/10.1186/1742–6405-9–24 (accessed February 21, 2018).

Lee, Kyung Yeon. "Enterovirus 71 Infection and Neurological Complications." *Korean Journal of Pediatrics* 59, no. 10 (October 2016): 395–401. This article can also be found online at https://www.ncbi.nlm.nih.gov/pmc/articles/PMC5099286/ (accessed February 5, 2018).

Lee, Szu-Chia, et al. "Comparative Effectiveness of Azithromycin for Treating Scrub Typhus: A PRISMA-Compliant Systematic Review and Meta-Analysis." *Medicine* 96, no. 36 (September 2017). This article can also be found online at https://journals.lww.com/md-journal/Fulltext/2017/09080/Comparative_effectiveness_of_azithromycin_for.37.aspx (accessed January 23, 2018).

Leroy, E. M., et al. "Fruits Bats as Reservoirs of Ebola Virus." *Nature* (December 1, 2005): 575–576.

Leshem, Eyal, et al. "National Estimates of Reductions in Acute Gastroenteritis–Related Hospitalizations and Associated Costs in US Children After Implementation of Rotavirus Vaccines."**Journal of the American Pediatric Infectious Diseases Society** 91 (2017): 6.

Lesho, Emil, et al. "Mitigating *Candida auris* at a Busy Community Hospital: A Quasi-Experimental Near Real-Time Approach." *Open Forum Infectious Diseases* 4, suppl. 1 (2017): S72. This article can also be found online at https://doi.org/10.1093/ofid/ofx163.001 (accessed January 25, 2018).

Lessler, Justin, and C. Jessica E. Metcalf. "Balancing Evidence and Uncertainty When Considering Rubella Vaccine Introduction." *PLOS One* 8, no. 7 (July 2013). This article can also be found at http://journals.plos.org/plosone/article?id=10.1371/journal.pone.0067639 (accessed January 16, 2018).

Lester, Robert S., et al. "Novel Cases of Blastomycosis Acquired in Toronto, Ontario." *Canadian Medical Association Journal* 163 (November 14, 2000): 1309–1312.

Leventhal, Gabriel E., et al. "Evolution and Emergence of Infectious Diseases in Theoretical and Real-World Networks." *Nature Communications* 6, no. 6101 (2015). This article can also be found online at https://www.nature.com/articles/ncomms7101 (accessed February 9, 2018).

Lewis, Katharine Kranz. "The Pandemic Threat: Is Massachusetts Prepared?" *Massachusetts Health Policy Forum* (June 2006): 1–8. This article can also be found online at https://masshealthpolicyforum.brandeis.edu/publications/pdfs/29-Jun06/PolicyBrief29.pdf (accessed March 6, 2018).

Li, De-Kun, et al. "Genital Herpes and Its Treatment in Relation to Preterm Delivery." *American Journal of Epidemiology* 180, no. 11 (2014): 1109–1117. This article can also be found online at https://academic.oup.com/aje/article/180/11/1109/147904 (accessed February 28, 2018).

Lim, Jae Hoo. "Liver Flukes: The Malady Neglected." *Korean Journal of Radiology* 12, no. 3 (May–June 2011): 269–279. This article can also be found online at https://www.ncbi.nlm.nih.gov/pmc/articles/PMC3088844/ (accessed January 4, 2018).

Limbago, Brandi M., et al. "Report of the 13th Vancomycine-Resistant *Staphylococcus aureus* Isolate from the United States." *Journal of Clinical Microbiology* 52, no. 3 (March 2014): 998–1002.

Limmathurotsakul, Direk, and Sharon J. Peacock. "Melioidosis: A Clinical Overview." *British Medical Bulletin* 99, no. 1 (2011): 125–139. This article can also be found online at https://doi.org/10.1093/bmb/ldr007 (accessed February 7, 2018).

Limmathurotsakul, Direk, et al. "Predicted Global Distribution of *Burkholderia pseudomallei* and Burden of Melioidosis." *Nature Microbiology* 1, no. 1 (2016): 15008.

Lin, Derek M., Britt Koskella, and Henry C. Lin. "Phage Therapy: An Alternative to Antibiotics in the Age of Multi-drug Resistance." *World Journal of Gastrointestinal and Pharmacology and Therapeutics* 8, no. 3 (August 2017): 162–173.

Lindoso, José Angelo Lauletta, et al. "Leishmaniasis–HIV Coinfection: Current Challenges." *HIV/AIDS* 8 (2016): 147–156. This article can also be found online at https://www.ncbi.nlm.nih.gov/pmc/articles/PMC5063600/ (accessed February 3, 2018).

Lindstrom, Lauren. "More Than 300 People Now Affected by Norovirus Outbreak." *Toledo Blade* (August 11, 2017). This article can also be found online at http://www.toledoblade.com/Medical/2017/08/11/Officials-to-keep-an-eye-on-outbreak-of-novovirus.html (accessed November 20, 2017).

Lipsitch, Marc, and Matthew H. Samore. "Antimicrobial Use and Antimicrobial Resistance: A Population Perspective." *Emerging Infectious Diseases* 8 (2002): 347–354. This article can also be found online at https://www.ncbi.nlm.nih.gov/pmc/articles/PMC2730242/ (accessed February 26, 2018).

Lipton, Eric. "Bid to Stockpile Bioterror Drugs Stymied by Setbacks." *New York Times* (September 18, 2006). This article can also be found online at http://www.nytimes.com/2006/09/18/washington/18anthrax.html (accessed January 12, 2018).

Lite, Jordan. "Medical Mystery: Only One Person Has Survived Rabies without Vaccine—But How?" *Scientific American* (October 8, 2008). This article can also be found online at https://www.scientificamerican.com/article/jeanna-giese-rabies-survivor/ (accessed February 19, 2018).

Littman, R. J., and M. L. Littman. "Galen and the Antonine Plague." *American Journal of Philology* 94, no. 3 (Autumn 1973): 243–255.

Liu, Yan, et al. "The Pathogenesis of Severe Fever with Thrombocytopenia Syndrome Virus Infection in Alpha/Beta Interferon Knockout Mice: Insights into the Pathologic Mechanisms of a New Viral Hemorrhagic Fever." *Journal of Virology* 88, no. 3 (2014): 1781–1786. This article can also be found online at https://www.ncbi.nlm.nih.gov/pmc/articles/PMC3911604/ (accessed March 1, 2018).

Lo, Nathan C., et al. "A Call to Strengthen the Global Strategy against Schistosomiasis and Soil-Transmitted Helminthiasis: The Time Is Now." *Lancet Infectious Diseases* 17, no. 2 (2017): e64–e69.

Lomax, Elisabeth. "Hereditary of Acquired Disease? Early Nineteenth Century Debates on the Cause of Infantile Scrofula and Tuberculosis." *Journal of the History of Medicine and Allied Sciences* (October 1977): 356–374.

Low, Nicola, Nathalie Broutet, and Richard Turner. "A Collection on the Prevention, Diagnosis, and Treatment of Sexually Transmitted Infections," *PLOS Medicine* 14, no. 6 (2017): e1002333.

Lu Han, Kang Li, et al. "Human Enterovirus 71 Protein Interaction Network Prompts Antiviral Drug Repositioning." *Scientific Reports* 7, no. 43143 (2017). This article can also be found online at https://www.nature.com/articles/srep43143 (accessed February 5, 2018).

Lu Lu, Andrew J. Leigh Brown, and Samantha J. Lycett. "Quantifying Predictors for the Spatial Diffusion of Avian Influenza Virus in China."

BMC Evolutionary Biology 17 (January 13, 2017): 1–14. This article can also be found online at https://bmcevolbiol.biomedcentral.com/articles/10.1186/s12862-016-0845-3 (accessed January 22, 2018).

Lv, Shan, et al. "Human Angiostrongyliasis Outbreak in Dali, China." *PLOS Neglected Tropical Diseases* (September 22, 2009). This article can also be found online at http://journals.plos.org/plosntds/article?id=10.1371/journal.pntd.0000520 (accessed January 12, 2018).

Lyons, Kate. "Yemen's Cholera Outbreak Now the Worst in History as Millionth Case Looms." *Guardian* (October 12, 2017). This article can also be found online at https://www.theguardian.com/global-development/2017/oct/12/yemen-cholera-outbreak-worst-in-history-1-million-cases-by-end-of-year (accessed March 8, 2018).

MacKenzie, Debora. "Many More People Could Still Die from Mad Cow Disease in the UK." *New Scientist* (January 18, 2017). This article can also be found online at https://www.newscientist.com/article/2118418-many-more-people-could-still-die-from-mad-cow-disease-in-the-uk/ (accessed January 29, 2018).

MacMillan, Amanda. "A New Mom Became a Quadruple Amputee from Flesh-Eating Bacteria. Here's What You Need to Know." *Time* (October 16, 2017). This article can also be found online at http://time.com/4984752/flesh-eating-bacteria-necrotizing-fasciitis/ (accessed February 12, 2018).

Madoff, Lawrence C. "ProMED-Mail: An Early Warning System for Emerging Diseases." *Clinical Infectious Diseases* 39, no. 2 (July 2004): 227–232.

Maggi, F., and M. Bendinelli. "Human Anelloviruses and the Central Nervous System." *Reviews in Medical Virology* 20, no. 6 (November 2010): 392–407. This article can also be found online at https://www.ncbi.nlm.nih.gov/pubmed/20925048 (accessed February 2, 2018).

Mahajan, Vikram K. "Sporotrichosis: An Overview and Therapeutic Options." *Dermatology Research and Practice* 2014 (2014). This article can also be found online at https://www.hindawi.com/journals/drp/2014/272376/ (accessed January 23, 2018).

Majumder, Maimuna S., et al. "Substandard Vaccination Compliance and the 2015 Measles Outbreak." *JAMA Pediatrics* 169, no. 5 (May 2015): 494–495. This article can also be found online at https://jamanetwork.com/journals/jamapediatrics/fullarticle/2203906 (accessed February 15, 2018).

Mandell, L. A., et al. "Infectious Diseases Society of America/American Thoracic Society Consensus Guidelines on the Management of Community-Acquired Pneumonia in Adults." *Clinical Infectious Diseases* 44, suppl. 2 (2007): S27–S72.

Mani, Satchin, Thomas Wierzba, and Richard I. Walker. "Status of Vaccine Research and Development for *Shigella*." *Vaccine* 34, no. 26 (June 3, 2016): 2887–2894. This article can also be found online at https://www.sciencedirect.com/science/article/pii/S0264410X16002863 (accessed February 8, 2018).

Manicklal, Sheetal, et al. "The 'silent' Global Burden of Congenital Cytomegalovirus." *Clinical Microbiology Reviews* 26, no. 1 (2013): 86–102. This article can also be found online at https://www.ncbi.nlm.nih.gov/pmc/articles/PMC3553672/ (accessed February 5, 2018).

Mansfield, K. L., et al. "Tick-Borne Encephalitis Virus: A Review of an Emerging Zoonosis." *Journal of General Virology* 90 (2009): 1781–1794.

Mansfield, Karen, et al. "Rift Valley Fever Virus: A Review of Diagnosis and Vaccination, and Implications for Emergence in Europe." *Vaccine* 33, no. 42 (October 13, 2015): 5520–5531. This article can also be found online at https://www.sciencedirect.com/science/article/pii/S0264410X15011342 (accessed January 18, 2018).

Marin, Mona, et al. "Global Varicella Vaccine Effectiveness: A Meta-Analysis." *Pediatrics* (February 2016). This article can also be found online at http://pediatrics.aappublications.org/content/early/2016/02/14/peds.2015-3741 (accessed January 31, 2018).

Marineli, Filio, et al. "Mary Mallon (1869–1938) and the History of Typhoid Fever." *Annals of Gastroenterology* 26, no. 2 (2013): 132–134. This article can also be found online at https://www.ncbi.nlm.nih.gov/pmc/articles/PMC3959940/ (accessed January 29, 2018).

Markowitz, Lauri E., et al. "Reduction in Human Papillomavirus (HPV) Prevalence among Young Women Following HPV Vaccine Introduction in the United States, National Health and Nutrition Examination Surveys, 2003–2010." *Journal of Infectious Diseases* 208, 3 (August 1, 2013): 385–393. This article can also be found online at https://academic.oup.com/jid/article/208/3/385/2192839 (accessed February 20, 2018).

Marlow, Jeffrey. "The Virus Hunters." *Scientific American* (May 26, 2017). This article can also be found online at https://www.scientificamerican.com/article/the-virus-hunters/ (accessed January 31, 2018).

Maron, Dina Fine. "How to Get More Parents to Vaccinate Their Kids." *Scientific American* (February 19, 2015). This article can also be found online at https://www.scientificamerican.com/article/how-to-get-more-parents-to-vaccinate-their-kids/ (accessed February 13, 2018).

Marston, Barbara J., et al. "Ebola Response Impact on Public Health Programs, West Africa, 2014–2017." *Emerging Infectious Diseases* 23, no. 13 (December 2017): S25–S32. This article can also be found online at https://wwwnc.cdc.gov/eid/article/23/13/17–0727_article (accessed March 6, 2018).

Martin, Steven J., and Raymond J. Yost. "Infectious Diseases in the Critically Ill Patients." *Journal of Pharmacy Practice* 24 (March 2011): 35.

Marzec, Natalie S., et al. "Serious Bacterial Infections Acquired during Treatment of Patients Given a Diagnosis of Chronic Lyme Disease—United States." *Morbidity and Mortality Weekly Report* 66, no. 23 (June 16, 2017): 607–609. This article can also be found online at https://www.cdc.gov/mmwr/volumes/66/wr/mm6623a3.htm (accessed February 6, 2018).

Massolo, Alessandro, Stefano Liccioli, Christine Budke, and Claudia Klein. "*Echinococcus multilocularis* in North America: The Great Unknown. *Parasite* 21 (2014): 73–86.

Mathis, Alexander, Rainer Weber, and Peter Deplazes. "Zoonotic Potential of the Microsporidia." *Clinical Microbiological Reviews* 18, no. 3 (July 2005): 423–445.

Matthews, Melissa. "Buruli Ulcer: Will the Flesh-Eating Bacteria Spreading through Australia Come to the U.S.?" *Newsweek* (September 22, 2017). This article can also be found online at http://www.newsweek.com/buruli-ulcer-australia-flesh-eating-bacteria-come-us-669684 (accessed January 17, 2018).

Mazer, Dale M., et al. "*In vitro* Activity of Ceftolozane-Tazobactam and Other Antimicrobial Agents against *Burkholderia cepacia* Complex and *Burkholderia gladioli*." *Antimicrobial Agents and Chemotherapy* 61, no. 9 (2017).

McAllister, Rebecca, and Janice Allwood. "Recurrent Multidrug Resistant Urinary Tract Infections in Geriatric Patients." *Federal Practitioner* 31, no. 7 (July 2014): 32–35.

McAuley, James B. "Congenital Toxoplasmosis." *Journal of the Pediatric Infectious Diseases Society* 3, no. S1 (September 2014): S30–S35.

McCollum, Eric D., et al. "Reduction of Childhood Pneumonia Mortality in the Sustainable Development Era." *Lancet Respiratory Medicine* 4, no. 12 (December 2016): 932–933. This article can also be found online at http://www.thelancet.com/journals/lanres/article/PIIS2213–2600(16)30371-X/fulltext (accessed January 24, 2018).

McCrindle, Brian W., et al. "Diagnosis, Treatment, and Long-Term Management of Kawasaki Disease: A Scientific Statement for Health Professionals from the American Heart Association." *Circulation* 135, no. 17 (2017): e927–e999. This article can also be found online at http://circ.ahajournals.org/content/135/17/e927.short (accessed February 5, 2018).

McGill F., M. J. Griffiths, and T. Solomon. "Viral Meningitis: Current Issues in Diagnosis and Treatment." *Current Opinion in Infectious Diseases* 30, no. 2 (April 2017): 248–256. This article can also be found online at https://www.ncbi.nlm.nih.gov/pubmed/28118219 (accessed February 22, 2018).

McKenna, Maryn. "After Years of Debate, the FDA Finally Curtails Antibiotic Use in Livestock." *Newsweek* (January 13, 2017). This article can also be found online at http://www.newsweek.com/after-years-debate-fda-curtails-antibiotic-use-livestock-542428 (accessed February 24, 2018).

———. "Fatal Fungus Linked to 4 New Deaths—What You Need to Know." *National Geographic* (November 7, 2016). This article can also be found online at https://news.nationalgeographic.com/2016/11/deadly-fungus-drug-resistance-candida-auris-health-science/ (accessed January 25, 2018).

McMichael A. J., and R. Beaglehole. "The Changing Global Context of Public Health." *Lancet* 356, 9228 (August 2000): 495–499.

McNeil, Donald G., Jr. "A Step Closer to the Defeat of Polio." *New York Times* (November 23, 2015). This article can also be found online at https://www.nytimes.com/2015/11/24/health/a-move-closer-to-total-disappearance-of-polio.html (accessed February 2, 2018).

———. "Fearsome Plague Epidemic Strikes Madagascar." *New York Times* (October 7, 2017): A12. This article can also be found online at https://www.nytimes.com/2017/10/06/health/madagascar-plague.html (accessed November 6, 2017).

———. "Fight against Tropical Diseases Is Framed as Efficient." *New York Times* (July 28, 2015): D5. This article can also be found online at https://www.nytimes.com/2015/07/28/health/fight-against-tropical-diseases-is-framed-as-efficient.html (accessed January 30, 2018).

———. "For Polio Vaccines, a Worldwide Switch to a New Version." *New York Times* (April 11, 2016). This article can also be found online at https://www.nytimes.com/2016/04/12/health/for-polio-vaccines-a-worldwide-switch-to-new-version.html (accessed February 2, 2018).

———. "How the Response to Zika Failed Millions." *New York Times* (January 16, 2017). This article can also be found online at https://www.nytimes.com/2017/01/16/health/zika-virus-response.html (accessed February 28, 2018).

———. "The Next Flu Pandemic Will Appear When You Least Expect It." *New York Times* (December 8, 2017). This article can also be found online at https://www.nytimes.com/2017/12/08/health/next-flu-pandemic.html (accessed January 22, 2018).

———. "Progress Against AIDS, but Not Enough." *New York Times* (November 8, 2017): D3. This article can also be found online at https://www.nytimes.com/2017/11/20/health/aids-drugs-united-nations.html (accessed December 6, 2017).

———. "Wary of Attack with Smallpox, U.S. Buys Up a Costly Drug." *New York Times* (March 12, 2013). This article can also be found online at http://www.nytimes.com/2013/03/13/health/us-stockpiles-smallpox-drug-in-case-of-bioterror-attack.html (accessed January 30, 2018).

———. "Worrisome New Link: AIDS Drugs and Leprosy." *New York Times* (October 24, 2006). This article can also be found online at http://www.nytimes.com/2006/10/24/health/24lepr.html (accessed February 9, 2018).

McNeil, Michael M., et al. "Trends in Mortality Due to Invasive Mycotic Diseases in the United States, 1980–1997." *Clinical Infectious Diseases* 33, no. 5 (2001): 641–647. This article can also be found online at https://doi.org/10.1086/322606 (accessed January 25, 2018).

McPartlin, Daniel A., et al. "Biosensors for the Monitoring of Harmful Algal Blooms." *Current Opinion in Biotechnology* 45 (June 2017): 164–169.

Meites, Elissa, et al. "A Review of Evidence-Based Care of Symptomatic Trichomoniasis and Asymptomatic *Trichomonas vaginalis* Infections." *Clinical Infectious Diseases* 61, no. 8 (December 15, 2015). This article can also be found online at https://academic.oup.com/cid/article/61/suppl_8/S837/344844 (accessed January 22, 2018).

Mell, H. K. "Management of Oral and Genital Herpes in the Emergency Department." *Emergency Medicine Clinics of North America* 26, no. 2 (May 26, 2008): 457–473.

Merritt, Richard W., et al. "Ecology and Transmission of Buruli Ulcer Disease: A Systematic Review." *PLOS Neglected Tropical Diseases* (December 4, 2010). This article can also be found online at http://journals.plos.org/plosntds/article?id=10.1371/journal.pntd.0000911 (accessed January 17, 2018).

Metsky, Harold C., et al. "Zika Virus Evolution and Spread in the Americas." *Nature* 546 (June 2017): 411–415.

Metsky, Hayden C., et al. "Zika Virus Evolution and Spread into the Americas." *Nature* 546 (June 2017): 411–415.

Miller, Taylor, Patrick Olivieri, and Elizabeth Singer. "The Utility of Tdap in the Emergency Department." *American Journal of Emergency Medicine* 35, no. 9 (September 2017): 1348–1349.

Mills, Christina E., James M. Robins, and Marc Lipsitch. "Transmissibility of 1918 Pandemic Influenza." *Science* 432 (December 16, 2004): 904–906.

Min, Sea C., et al. "In-Package Inhibition of *E. coli* O157:H7 on Bulk Romaine Lettuce Using Cold Plasma." *Food Microbiology* 65 (2017): 1–6.

Minoia, Francesca, et al. "Clinical Features, Treatment, and Outcome of Macrophage Activation Syndrome Complicating Systemic Juvenile Idiopathic Arthritis." *Arthritis & Rheumatology* 66 (2014): 3160–3169. This article can also be found online at http://onlinelibrary.wiley.com/doi/10.1002/art.38802/full (accessed March 12, 2018).

Mira, Marcelo T., et al. "Susceptibility to Leprosy is Associated with PARK2 and PACRG." *Nature* 427 (2004): 636–640.

Mitjà, Oriol, et al. "Global Epidemiology of Yaws: A Systematic Review." *Lancet Global Health* 3, no. 6 (June 2015): e324–331. This article can also be found online at https://www.ncbi.nlm.nih.gov/pubmed/26001576 (accessed February 2, 2018).

———. "Mass Treatment with Single-Dose Azithromycin for Yaws." *New England Journal of Medicine* 372 (February 19, 2015): 703–710. This article can also be found online at http://www.nejm.org/doi/full/10.1056/NEJMoa1408586 (accessed February 2, 2018).

Mittal, R., et al. "Zika Virus: An Emerging Global Health Threat." *Frontiers in Cellular and Infection Microbiology* 7 (December 2017): 1–19.

Miyamoto, Yukiko, and Lars Eckmann. "Drug Development against the Major Diarrhea-Causing Parasites of the Small Intestine, *Cryptosporidium* and *Giardia*." *Frontiers in Microbiology* 6 (2015): 1208. This article can also be found online at https://www.frontiersin.org/articles/10.3389/fmicb.2015.01208/full (accessed January 16, 2018).

Mogasale, Vittal, et al. "Burden of Typhoid Fever in Low-Income and Middle-Income Countries: A Systematic, Literature-Based Update with Risk-Factor Adjustment." *Lancet Global Health* 2, no. 10 (October 2014): 570–580. This article can also be found online at http://www.thelancet.com/journals/langlo/article/PIIS2214–109X(14)70301–8/fulltext (accessed January 29, 2018).

Monot, Marc, et al. "On the Origin of Leprosy." *Science* 308 (June 2005): 1040–1042.

Moore, S. Jason, et al. "Clinical Characteristics and Antibiotic Utilization in Pediatric Patients Hospitalized with Acute Bacterial Skin and Skin Structure Infection." *Pediatric Infectious Disease Journal* 33, no. 8 (2014): 825–828.

Morgan, Thomas E. "Plague or Poetry? Thucydides on the Epidemic at Athens." *Transactions of the American Philological Association* 124 (1994: 197–209.

Morillo C. A., et al. "Randomized Trial of Benznidazole for Chronic Chagas' Cardiomyopathy." *New England Journal of Medicine* 373 (October 2015): 1295–1306. This article can be found online at http://www.nejm.org/doi/full/10.1056/NEJMoa1507574.

Morris, Alison, et al. "Epidemiology and Clinical Significance of *Pneumocystis* Colonization." *Journal of Infectious Diseases* 197, no. 1 (2008): 10–17. This article can also be found online at https://academic.oup.com/jid/article/197/1/10/795412 (accessed February 15, 2018).

Morris, Shaun K. et al. "Rotavirus Mortality in India: Estimates Based on a Nationally Representative Survey of Diarrhoeal Deaths." *Bulletin of the World Health Organization* 90 (2012):720–727. This article can also be found online at http://www.who.int/bulletin/volumes/90/10/12–101873/en/ (accessed February 13, 2018).

Morrison, Jim. "Can Virus Hunters Stop the Next Pandemic Before It Happens?" *Smithsonian Magazine* (January 25, 2018). This article can also be found online at https://www.smithsonianmag.com/science-nature/how-to-stop-next-animal-borne-pandemic-180967908/#FW1WmlrbGHJa2jjj.99 (accessed January 31, 2018).

Mubarak, Mohammad Yousuf, et al. "Hygienic Behaviors and Risks for Ascariasis among College Students in Kabul, Afghanistan." *American Journal of Tropical Medicine and Hygiene* 97, no. 2 (August 2017): 563–566.

Murray, Kristy O., et al. "Typhus Group Rickettsiosis, Texas, USA, 2003–2013." *Emerging Infectious Diseases* 23, no. 4 (April 2017): 645–648. This article can also be found online at https://wwwnc.cdc.gov/eid/article/23/4/16–0958_article (accessed January 23, 2018).

Musher, Daniel M., et al. "Trends in Bacteremic Infection Due to *Streptococcus pyogenes* (Group A Streptococcus), 1986–1995." *Emerging Infectious Diseases* 2 (1996): 54–56. This article can also be found online at https://wwwnc.cdc.gov/eid/article/2/1/96–0107_article (accessed February 12, 2018).

Musso, D., and D. Gubler. "Zika Virus." *Clinical Microbiology Reviews* 29 (2016): 487–524.

Musso, D., E. J. Nilles, and V. M. Cao-Lormeau. "Rapid Spread of Emerging Zika Virus in the Pacific Area." *Clinical Microbiology and Infection* 20, no. 10 (October 2014): O595–O596.

Mylne, Adrian Q. N., et al. "Mapping the Zoonotic Niche of Lassa Fever in Africa." *Transactions of the Royal Society of Tropical Medicine and Hygiene* 109.8 (August 1, 2015): 483v492. This article can also be found online at https://academic.oup.com/trstmh/article/109/8/483/1910156 (accessed January 24, 2018).

Nagata, N., et al. "Predictive Value of Endoscopic Findings in the Diagnosis of Active Intestinal Amebiasis." *Endoscopy* 44, no. 4 (2012): 425–428.

Naidoo, Levashni, et al. "HAART in Hand: The Change in Kaposi's Sarcoma Presentation in KwaZulu-Natal, South Africa." *South African Medical Journal* 106, no. 6 (2016): 611–616.

Nakashima, Allyn K., et al. "Epidemic Bullous Impetigo in a Nursery Due to a Nasal Carrier of *Staphylococcus aureus*: Role of Epidemiology and Control Measures." *Infection Control* 5, no. 7 (1984): 326–331.

Navarro, J., et al. "Postepizootic Persistence of Venezuelan Equine Encephalitis Virus, Venezuela." *Emerging Infectious Diseases* 11 (2005): 1907–1915.

Neal, David J. **"It's** a Mysterious Infection. It**'s** on the Rise. Here**'s** How to Recognize It.**" Miami Herald** (October 2, 2017). This article can also be found online at http://www.miamiherald.com/news/health-care/article176512621.html (accessed December 18, 2017).

Nelson, Andrew, et al. "Polymicrobial Challenges to Koch's Postulates: Ecological Lessons from the Bacterial Vaginosis and Cystic Fibrosis Microbiomes." *Innate Immunity* 18, no. 5 (2012): 774–783. This article can also be found online at http://journals.sagepub.com/doi/pdf/10.1177/1753425912439910 (accessed January 16, 2018).

Nelson, Christina A., et al. "Incidence of Clinician-Diagnosed Lyme Disease, United States, 2005–2010." *Emerging Infectious Diseases* 21, no. 9 (September 2015): 1625–1631. This article can also be found online at https://www.ncbi.nlm.nih.gov/pmc/articles/PMC4550147/ (accessed February 6, 2018).

Nelson, Christina A., Shubhayu Saha, and Paul S. Mead. "Cat-Scratch Disease in the United States, 2005–2013." *Emerging Infectious Diseases* 22, no. 10 (2016): 1741–1746.

Nelson, Christina, et al. "Tularemia—United States, 2001–2010." *Morbidity and Mortality Weekly Report* 62, no. 47 (November 29, 2013): 963–966. This article can also be found online at https://www.ncbi.nlm.nih.gov/pmc/articles/PMC4585636/ (accessed February 9, 2018).

Newman, Lori, et al. "Global Estimates of Syphilis in Pregnancy and Associated Adverse Outcomes: Analysis of Multinational Antenatal Surveillance Data." *PLOS Medicine* (February 26, 2013). This article can also be found online at http://journals.plos.org/plosmedicine/article?id=10.1371/journal.pmed.1001396 (accessed February 16, 2018).

———. "Global Estimates of the Prevalence and Incidence of Four Curable Sexually Transmitted Infections in 2012 Based on Systematic Review and Global Reporting." *PLOS One* 10, no. 12 (2015): e0143304. This article can also be found online at https://www.ncbi.nlm.nih.gov/pmc/articles/PMC4672879/ (accessed February 16, 2018).

Ng-Nguyen, Dinh, Mark A. Stevenson, and Rebecca J. Traub. "A Systematic Review of Taeniasis, Cysticercosis and Trichinellosis in Vietnam." *Parasites & Vectors* 10 (March 2017): 150.

Ngonghala, Calistus N., et al. "General Ecological Models for Human Subsistence, Health and Poverty." *Nature Ecology & Evolution* 1 (2017): 1153–1159.

Nicolle, Lindsay E. "Catheter Associated Urinary Tract Infections." *Antimicrobial Resistance and Infection Control* 3 (2014): 23.

Nikaido, Hiroshi. "Multidrug Resistance in Bacteria." *Annual Review of Biochemistry* 78 (2009): 119–146. This article can also be found online at https://www.ncbi.nlm.nih.gov/pmc/articles/PMC2839888/ (accessed February 26, 2018).

Ninomiya M., et al. "Development of PCR Assays with Nested Primers Specific for Differential Detection of Three Human Anelloviruses and Early Acquisition of Dual or Triple Infection During Infancy." *Journal of Clinical Microbiology* 46 (2008): 507–514. This article can also be found online at http://jcm.asm.org/content/46/2/507 (accessed February 1, 2018).

Nishiyama, Shoko, et al. "Identification of Novel Anelloviruses with Broad Diversity in UK Rodents." *Journal of General Virology* 95 (July 2014): 1544–1553. This article can also be found online at https://www.ncbi.nlm.nih.gov/pmc/articles/PMC4059270 (accessed February 1, 2018).

Nixon, Lance. "At Rocky Mountain Labs, 'Virus Ecology' Helps Scientists Understand Threats Such as Zika." *Missoulian* (August 29, 2016). This article can also be found online at http://missoulian.com/lifestyles/health-med-fit/at-rocky-mountain-labs-virus-ecology-helps-scientists-understand-threats/article_8f13f9c8–1d99–53fe-a51d-c90d63bfa13d.html (accessed February 28, 2018).

Noble, Ronald K. "Keeping Science in the Right Hands: Policing the New Biological Frontier." *Foreign Affairs* 92, no. 6 (November/December 2013): 47–53.

Nolen, Leisha Diane, et al. "Introduction of Monkeypox into a Community and Household: Risk Factors and Zoonotic Reservoirs in the Democratic Republic of the Congo." *American Journal of Tropical Medicine and Hygiene* 93, 2 (August 2015): 410–415. This article can also be found online at http://www.ajtmh.org/content/journals/10.4269/ajtmh.15–0168 (accessed January 24, 2018).

Nordmann, Patrice, Aurélie Jayol, and Laurent Poirel. "Rapid Detection of Polymyxin Resistance in *Enterobacteriaceae*." *Emerging Infectious Diseases* 22 (June 2016): 1038–1043.

Nordmann, Patrice, Laurent Poirel, and Laurent Dortet. "Rapid Detection of Carbapenemase-Producing *Enterobacteriaceae*." *Emerging Infectious Diseases* 18 (September 2012): 1503–1507.

Nunez, Christina. "Mad Cow Disease Still Menaces U.K. Blood Supply." *National Geographic* (February 16, 2015). This article can also be found online at https://news.nationalgeographic.com/news/2015/02/150215-mad-cow-disease-vcjd-blood-supply-health/ (accessed February 12, 2018).

O'Carroll, Lisa. "Ebola Crisis Brutally Exposed Failures of the Aid System, Says MSF." *Guardian* (March 23, 2014). This article can also be found online at https://www.theguardian.com/global-development/2015/mar/23/ebola-crisis-response-aid-who-msf-report-sierra-leone-guinea (accessed February 27, 2018).

O'Driscoll, Tristan, and Christopher W. Crank. "Vancomycin-Resistant Enterococcal Infections: Epidemiology, Clinical Manifestations, and Optimal Management." *Infection and Drug Resistance* 8 (2015): 217–230. This article can also be found online at https://www.ncbi.nlm.nih.gov/pmc/articles/PMC4521680/ (accessed March 8, 2018).

Okamoto, H. "History of Discoveries and Pathogenicity of TT Viruses." *Current Topics in Microbiology and Immunology* 331 (2009): 1–20. This article can also be found online at https://www.ncbi.nlm.nih.gov/pubmed/19230554 (accessed February 1, 2018).

Okello, Anna L., and Lian Francesca Thomas. "Human Taeniasis: Current Insights into Prevention and Management Strategies in Endemic Countries." *Risk Management and Healthcare Policy* 10 (April 2017): 107–116.

Oliver, Sara E, et al. "Ocular Syphilis—Eight Jurisdictions, United States, 2014–2015." *Morbidity and Mortality Weekly* 65, no. 43 (November 4, 2016): 1185–1188. This article can also be found online at https://www.cdc.gov/mmwr/volumes/65/wr/mm6543a2.htm (accessed February 16, 2018).

Ong, Kanyin L., et al. "Changing Epidemiology of *Yersinia Enterocolitica* Infections: Markedly Decreased Rates in Young Black Children, Foodborne Diseases Active Surveillance Network (FoodNet), 1996–2009." Supplement, *Clinical Infectious Diseases* 54, no. S5 (June 2012): S385–S390. This article can also be found online at https://academic.oup.com/cid/article/54/suppl_5/S385/432586 (accessed January 9, 2017).

Ordóñez-Mena, José M., Noel D. McCarthy, and Thomas R. Fanshawe. "Comparative Efficacy of Drugs for Treating Giardiasis: A Systematic Update of the Literature and Network Meta-Analysis of Randomized Clinical Trials." *Journal of Antimicrobial Chemotherapy* (November 27, 2017). This article can also be found online at https://academic.oup.com/jac/advance-article-abstract/doi/10.1093/jac/dkx430/4662983?redirectedFrom=fulltext (accessed January 17, 2018).

Osumi, Magdalena. "Anisakis Infections from Raw Fish on Rise, Health Ministry Warns." *Japan Times* (May 12, 2016). This article can also be found online at https://www.japantimes.co.jp/news/2017/05/12/national/science-health/

anisakis-infections-raw-fish-rise-health-ministry-warns/#.WjQ64baZNN0 (accessed January 18, 2018).

Ozawa, Sachiko, et al. "Return on Investment from Childhood Immunization in Low- and Middle-Income Countries, 2011–20." *Health Affairs* 35, no. 2 (February 2016).

Pöhlmann, Stefan, et al. "Herpes B Virus Replication and Viral Lesions in the Liver of a Cynomolgus Macaque Which Died from Severe Disease with Rapid Onset." **Journal Medical Primatology** 46, no. 5 (October 2017): 256–259.

Paessler, S., and S. C. Weaver. "Vaccines for Venezuelan Equine Encephalitis." *Vaccine* 27, no. S4 (2009): D80–D85

Pal, Mahendra. "Chlamydophila Psittaci as an Emerging Zoonotic Pathogen of Global Significance." *International Journal of Vaccines and Vaccination* 4, no. 3 (2017): 80.

Pal, Mahendra, et al. "An Overview on Biological Weapons and Bioterrorism." *American Journal of Biomedical Research* 5, no. 2 (2017): 24–34. The article can also be found online at https://www.researchgate.net/profile/Mahendra_Pal2/publication/316189350_An_Overview_on_Biological_Weapons_and_Bioterrorism/links/58f8f149a6fdcc770be54143/An-Overview-on-Biological-Weapons-and-Bioterrorism.pdf (accessed January 29, 2018).

Papa, Anna, et al. "Crimean-Congo Hemorrhagic Fever: Tick-Host-Virus Interactions." *Frontiers in Cellular and Infection Microbiology* (May 26, 2017). This article can also be found online at https://www.frontiersin.org/articles/10.3389/fcimb.2017.00213/full (accessed January 19, 2018).

Pappas, P. G., et al. "Clinical Practice Guideline for the Management of Candidiasis: 2016 Update by the Infectious Diseases Society of America." *Clinical Infectious Diseases* 62, no. 4 (2016): e1–e50.

Park, Sun-Whan, et al. "Severe Fever with Thrombocytopenia Syndrome Virus, South Korea, 2013." *Emerging Infectious Diseases* 20, no. 11 (2014). This article can also be found online at https://wwwnc.cdc.gov/eid/article/20/11/14-0888_article (accessed March 1, 2018).

Parodi, Allesandro, et al. "Macrophage Activation Syndrome in Juvenile Systemic Lupus Erythematosus: A Multinational Multicenter Study of Thirty-Eight Patients." *Arthritis & Rheumatism* 60, no. 11 (2009): 3388–3399. This article can also be found online at http://onlinelibrary.wiley.com/doi/10.1002/art.24883/pdf (accessed March 12, 2018).

Patton, Monica E., et al. "Primary and Secondary Syphilis—United States, 2005–2013." *Morbidity and Mortality Weekly* 63, no. 18 (May 9, 2014): 402–406. This article can also be found online at https://www.cdc.gov/mmwr/preview/mmwrhtml/mm6318a4.htm (accessed February 16, 2018).

Paules, Catharine I., and Anthony S. Fauci. "Emerging and Reemerging Infectious Diseases: The Dichotomy between Acute Outbreaks and Chronic Endemicity." *JAMA* 317, no. 7 (February 2017): 691–692. This article can also be found online at https://jamanetwork.com/journals/jama/article-abstract/2598516?redirect=true (accessed February 9, 2018).

Paulson, Michael. "'Brilliant,' 41 and Lost to AIDS: The Theater World Asks Why." *New York Times* (October 15, 2017): AR1. This article can also be found online at https://www.nytimes.com/2017/10/11/theater/michael-friedman-aids-death-theater.html (accessed December 6, 2017).

Peeters, Ben, et al. "Genetic versus Antigenic Differences among Highly Pathogenic H5N1 Avian Influenza A Viruses: Consequences for Vaccine Strain Selection." *Virology* 503 (2017): 83–93.

Peletz, Rachel, et al. "Preventing Cryptosporidiosis: The Need for Safe Drinking Water." *Bulletin of the World Health Organization* 91, no. 4 (2013): 237–312. This article can also be found online at http://www.who.int/bulletin/volumes/91/4/13-119990/en/ (accessed January 16, 2018).

Peplies, Jorg, Frank Oliver Glockner, and Rudolf Amann. "Optimization Strategies for DNA Microarray-Based Detection of Bacteria with 16S rRNA-Targeting Oligonucleotide Probes." *Applied and Environmental Microbiology* 69 (2003): 1397–1407.

Petousis-Harris, Helen, et al. "Effectiveness of a Group B Outer Membrane Vesicle Meningococcal Vaccine against Gonorrhoea in New Zealand: A Retrospective Case-Control Study. *Lancet* 39, no. 10102 (September 20, 2017): 1603–1610. This article can also be found online at http://www.thelancet.com/journals/lancet/article/

PIIS0140–6736(17)31449–6/fulltext?elscal =tlpr (accessed January 31, 2018).

Pfeffer, Martin, and Gerhard Dobler. "Emergence of Zoonotic Arboviruses by Animal Trade and Migration." *Parasites and Vectors* 3 (2010): 35–49. This article can also be found online at https://parasitesandvectors.biomedcentral.com/articles/10.1186/1756–3305-3–35 (accessed February 25, 2018)

Phadke, Varun K., Robert A. Bednarczyk, and Daniel A. Salmon. "Association between Vaccine Refusal and Vaccine-Preventable Diseases in the United States: A Review of Measles and Pertussis." *JAMA* 315, no. 11 (2016): 1149–1158. This article can also be found online at https://jamanetwork.com/journals/jama/article-abstract/2503179?tab=cme&redirect =true (accessed February 13, 2018).

Phillips, Richard Odame. "Effectiveness of Routine BCG Vaccination on Buruli Ulcer Disease: A Case-Control Study in the Democratic Republic of Congo, Ghana and Togo." *PLOS Neglected Tropical Diseases* (January 8, 2015). This article can also be found online at http://journals.plos .org/plosntds/article?id=10.1371/journal.pntd .0003457 (accessed January 26, 2018).

Phutthichayanon, Thanyada, and Surapol Naowarat. "Effects of Hand Washing Campaign on Dynamical Model of Hand Foot Mouth Disease." *International Journal of Modeling and Optimization* 5, no. 2 (2015): 104–108.

Piantadosi, A., et al. "Emerging Cases of Powassan Virus Encephalitis in New England: Clinical Presentation, Imaging, and Review of the Literature." *Clinical Infectious Diseases* 62 (2016): 707–713.

Piarroux, Martine, et al. "Populations at Risk for Alveolar Echinococcosis, France." *Emerging Infectious Diseases* 19, no. 5 (May 2013): 721–728.

Picardeau, Mathieu. "Leptospirosis: Updating the Global Picture of an Emerging Neglected Disease." *PLOS Neglected Tropical Diseases* (September 24, 2015). This article can also be found online at http://journals.plos.org/plosntds/article?id=10.1371/journal.pntd .0004039 (accessed January 19, 2018).

Piedrahita, Christina T., et al. "Environmental Surfaces in Healthcare Facilities are a Potential Source for Transmission of *Candida auris* and Other *Candida* Species." *Infection Control & Hospital Epidemiology* 38, no. 9 (September 2017): 1107–1109. This article can also be found online at https://www.cambridge.org/core/journals/infection-control-and-hospital-epidemiology/article/environmental-surfaces-in-healthcare-facilities-are-a-potential-source-for-transmission-of-candida-auris-and-other-candida-species/AC2A27472832F4304BD55D2 4D3B4638F (accessed February 21, 2018).

Pierce, Harold. "Unprecedented Six Bills Introduced within Days of Each Other to Address Valley Fever." *Bakersfield Californian* (January 16, 2018). This article can also be found online at http://www.bakersfield.com/news/unprecedented-six-bills-introduced-within-days-of-each-other-to/article_fe783238-fb2f-11e7-a3ce-03cfff6cb9ff.html (accessed February 6, 2018).

Pinches, Helene, et al. "Asymptomatic Kawasaki Disease in a 3-Month Old Infant." *Pediatrics* 138, no. 2 (2016): e1–4. This article can also be found online at http://pediatrics .aappublications.org/content/pediatrics/138/2/e20153936.full.pdf (accessed February 5, 2018).

Plevin, Rebecca, and Rachael Callcut. "Update in Sepsis Guidelines: What Is Really New?" *Trauma Surgery & Acute Care Open* 2, no. 1 (2017): e000088. This article can also be found online at http://tsaco.bmj.com/content/2/1/e000088 (accessed February 28, 2018).

Polgreen, Philip M., et al. "Using Internet Searches for Influenza Surveillance." *Clinical Infectious Diseases* 47, no. 11 (December 1, 2008): 1442–1448. This article can also be found online at https://academic.oup.com/cid/article/47/11/1443/282247 (accessed January 26, 2018).

"Polio Vaccines: WHO Position Paper, March 2016." *Vaccine* 35, no. 9 (March 2017): 1197–1199.

Porter, Tom. "Sushi Fans Warned of Raw Fish Infection Risk." *Newsweek* (May 12, 2017). This article can also be found online at http://www .newsweek.com/sushi-rise-parasitic-infection-608240 (accessed January 18, 2018).

Potera, Carol. "Obama's Battle Plan for Antibiotic-Resistant Bacteria." *BioScience* 65, no. 7 (2015): 740. This article can also be found online at https://academic.oup.com/bioscience/article/65/7/740/258364 (accessed February 25, 2018).

Pramodh, Nathaniel. "Limiting the Spread of Communicable Diseases Caused by Human Population Movement." *Journal of Rural and Remote Environmental Health.* (2003): 2,no. 1: 23–32. This article can also be found online at http://jrtph.jcu.edu.au/vol/v02nathaniel.pdf (accessed February 5, 2018).

Principi, Nicola, Donato Rigante, and Susanna Esposito. "The Role of Infection in Kawasaki Syndrome." *Journal of Infection* 67, no. 1 (July 2013): 1–10. This article can also be found online at http://www.journalofinfection.com/article/S0163-4453(13)00077-7/abstract (accessed February 5, 2018).

Prusinski, Melissa A. et al. "Sylvatic Typhus associated with Flying Squirrels (*Glaucomys volans*) in New York State, United States. *Vector-Borne and Zoonotic Diseases* 14.4 (2014): 1–5. This article can also be found online at https://www.researchgate.net/publication/261290069_Sylvatic_Typhus_Associated_with_Flying_Squirrels_Glaucomys_volans_in_New_York_State_United_States.

Puvanendran, Rukshini, Jason Chan Meng Huey, and Shanker Pasupathy. "Necrotizing Fasciitis." *Canadian Family Physician* 55, no. 10 (2009): 981–987. This article can also be found online at https://www.ncbi.nlm.nih.gov/pmc/articles/PMC2762295/ (accessed February 12, 2018).

Quach, Jeanie, Joëlle St-Pierre, and Kris Chadee. "The Future for Vaccine Development against *Entamoeba histolytica*." *Human Vaccines & Immunotherapies* 10, no. 6 (2014): 1514–1521.

Quiner, Claire A., et al. "Presumptive Risk Factors for Monkeypox in Rural Communities in the Democratic Republic of the Congo." *PLOS ONE* 12, 2 (February 13, 2017). This article can also be found online at http://journals.plos.org/plosone/article?id=10.1371/journal.pone.0168664 (accessed January 24, 2018).

Rac, Hana, et al. "Successful Treatment of Necrotizing Fasciitis and Streptococcal Toxic Shock Syndrome with the Addition of Linezolid." *Case Reports in Infectious Diseases* (2017). This article can also be found online at https://www.hindawi.com/journals/criid/2017/5720708/ (accessed January 31, 2018).

Radford, Anthony, and Roy Scragg. "Discovery of Kuru Revisited: How Anthropology Hindered Then Enhanced Kuru Research." *Health and History* 15, no. 2 (2013): 29–52.

Raja, N. S., M. Z. Ahmed, and N. N. Singh. "Melioidosis: An Emerging Infectious Disease." *Journal of Postgraduate Medicine* 51, no. 2 (2005): 140–145. This article can also be found online at http://www.jpgmonline.com/article.asp?issn=0022-3859;year=2005;volume=51;issue=2;spage=140;epage=145;aulast=Raja (accessed February 7, 2018).

Ramachandran, Prashanth, et al. "Adult Food Borne Botulism in Australia: The Only 2 Cases from the Last 15 Years." *Journal of Clinical Neuroscience* 41 (2017): 86–87.

Ramjee, Gita, and Brodie Daniels. "Women and HIV in Sub-Saharan Africa." *AIDS Research and Therapy* 10, no. 30 (2013). This article can also be found online at https://aidsrestherapy.biomedcentral.com/articles/10.1186/1742-6405-10-30 (accessed March 5, 2018).

Ramsey, C. "A Sore Throat, Fever and Rash." *Prescriber* 25, no. 12 (2014): 22.

Rasmussen, Sonja A., et al. "Zika Virus and Birth Defects—Reviewing the Evidence for Causality." *New England Journal of Medicine* 374, no. 20 (May 19, 2016): 1981–1987. This article can also be found online at http://www.nejm.org/doi/full/10.1056/NEJMsr1604338#t=article (accessed January 16, 2018).

Rassi, A., Jr., A. Rassi, and J. A. Marin-Neto. "Chagas Disease." *Lancet* 375, no. 9723 (April 17, 2010): 1388–1402.

Ravelli, Angello, et al. "2016 Classification Criteria for Macrophage Activation Syndrome Complicating Systemic Juvenile Idiopathic Arthritis." *Annals of the Rheumatic Diseases* 75, no. 3 (2016): 481–489. This article can also be found online at http://ard.bmj.com/content/75/3/481.info (accessed March 12, 2018).

"Raw Water: The Unsterilised Health Craze That Could Give You Diarrhea." *Guardian* (January 3, 2018). This article can also be found online at https://www.theguardian.com/lifeandstyle/shortcuts/2018/jan/03/raw-water-the-unsterilised-health-craze-that-could-give-you-diarrhoea (accessed January 16, 2018).

Read, Timothy D., et al. "Comparative Genome Sequencing for Discovery of Novel Polymorphisms in *Bacillus anthracis*." *Science* 296 (June 14, 2002): 2028–2033.

Rebman, Alison W., et al. "The Clinical, Symptom, and Quality-of-Life Characterization of a Well-Defined Group of Patients with Posttreatment

Lyme Disease Syndrome." *Frontiers in Medicine* 4 (December 14, 2017). This article can also be found online at https://www.frontiersin.org/articles/10.3389/fmed.2017.00224/full?&u (accessed February 6, 2018).

Rebmann, Terri. "Pandemic Preparedness: Implementation of Infection Prevention Emergency Plans." *Infection Control and Hospital Epidemiology* 31, no. S1 (November 2010): S63–S65.

Regules, Jason A., et al. "A Recombinant Vesicular Stomatitis Virus Ebola Vaccine." *New England Journal of Medicine* 376 (2017): 330–341.

Reinhart, Konrad, et al. "Recognizing Sepsis as a Global Health Priority: A WHO Resolution." *New England Journal of Medicine* 377 (August 3, 2017): 414–417. This article can also be found online at http://www.nejm.org/doi/full/10.1056/NEJMp1707170 (accessed February 28, 2018).

Restrepo, Marcos I., Paola Faverio, and Antonio Anzuetoa. "Long-Term Prognosis in Community-Acquired Pneumonia." *Current Opinion in Infectious Diseases* 26, no. 2 (April 2013): 151–158. This article can also be found online at https://www.ncbi.nlm.nih.gov/pmc/articles/PMC4066634/ (accessed January 24, 2018).

Reynolds, Pierce, and Andrea Marzi. "Ebola and Marburg Virus Vaccines." *Virus Genes* 53, no. 4 (August 2017): 501–515.

Rhodes, Katherine A., and Herbert P. Schweizer. "Antibiotic Resistance of *Burkholderia* Species." *Drug Resistance Update* 28, no. 8 (2017): 82–90.

Rice, Louis B. "Emergence of Vancomycin-Resistant *Enterococci*." *Emerging Infectious Diseases* 7, no. 2 (March–April 2001): 183–187. This article can also be found online at https://wwwnc.cdc.gov/eid/article/7/2/70-0183_article (accessed March 8, 2018).

Rice, Philip. "Viral Meningitis and Encephalitis." *Medicine* 45, no. 11 (November 2017): 664–669.

Rico-Torres C. P., et al. "Molecular Diagnosis and Genotyping of Cases of Perinatal Toxoplasmosis in Mexico." *Pediatric Infectious Disease Journal* 31, no. 4 (December 14, 2011).

Robert-Gangneux, Florence, et al. "Diagnosis of *Pneumocystis jirovecii* Pneumonia in Immunocompromised Patients by Real-Time PCR: A 4-Year Prospective Study." *Journal of Clinical Microbiology* 52, no. 9 (2014): 3370–3376. This article can also be found online at https://www.ncbi.nlm.nih.gov/pmc/articles/PMC4313164/ (accessed February 14, 2018).

Robine, J. M., et al. "Death Toll Exceeded 70,000 in Europe during the Summer of 2003." Comptes rendus Biologies 331, no. 2 (February 2008): 171–178. This article can also be found online at https://www.ncbi.nlm.nih.gov/pubmed/18241810 (accessed March 2, 2018).

Rock Kat S., Steve J. Torr, Crispin Lumbala, and Matt J. Keeling. "Quantitative Evaluation of the Strategy to Eliminate Human African Trypanosomiasis in the Democratic Republic of Congo." *Parasit Vectors* 8, no. 1 (2015): 532.

Roett, M. A., M. T. Mayor, and K. A. Uduhiri. "Diagnosis and Management of Genital Ulcers." *American Family Physician* 85 (2012): 254–262.

Rogers, Adam. "Ebola Returns, and Central Africa's Virus Hunters Are Ready." *Wired* (May 12, 2017). This article can also be found online at https://www.wired.com/2017/05/ebola-returns-central-africas-virus-hunters-ready/ (accessed January 31, 2018).

Rosovitz, M. J., and Stephen H. Leppla. "Virus Deals Anthrax a Killer Blow." *Nature* 418 (August 2002): 825–826. This article can also be found online at https://www.nature.com/articles/418825a (accessed January 12, 2018).

Ross, John J., and Daniel S. Shapiro. "Evaluation of the Computer Program GIDEON for the Diagnosis of Fever in Patients Admitted to a Medical Service." *Clinical Infectious Diseases* 26, no. 3: (March 1998): 766–767.

Ross, John J., and Douglas N. Keeling. "Cutaneous Blastomycosis in New Brunswick: Case Report." *Canadian Medical Association Journal* 163 (November 14, 2000): 1303–1305.

Rostami, Ali, et al. "Meat Sources of Infection for Outbreaks of Human Trichinellosis." *Food Microbiology* 64 (June 2017): 65–71.

Rothman, Tiran. "The Cost of Influenza Disease Burden in U.S Population." *International Journal of Economics & Management Sciences* 6, no. 4 (2017). This article can also be found online at https://www.omicsonline.org/open-access/the-cost-of-influenza-disease-burden-in-us-population-2162-6359-1000443.pdf (accessed January 17, 2018).

Russell, Clark D., et al. "The Human Immune Response to Respiratory Syncytial Virus Infection." *Clinical Microbiology Reviews* 30, no. 2 (April 2017): 481–502.

Russell, Colin A., et al. "The Potential for Respiratory Droplet–Transmissible A/H5N1 Influenza Virus to Evolve in a Mammalian Host." *Science* 336, no. 6088 (June 22, 2012): 1541–1547. This article can also be found online at http://science.sciencemag.org/content/336/6088/1541 (accessed February 22, 2018).

Russell, Josiah C. "That Earlier Plague." *Demography* 5, no. 1 (1968): 174–184.

Rychman, Brent J., et al. "Human Cytomegalovirus Entry into Epithelial and Endothelial Cells Depends on Genes UL128 to UL150 and Occurs by Endocytosis and Low-pH Fusion." *Journal of Virology* 80, no. 2 (2006): 710–722. This article can also be found online at http://jvi.asm.org/content/80/2/710.full (accessed February 5, 2018).

Saguil, Aaron, and Matthew Fargo. "Diagnosis and Management of Kawasaki Disease." *American Family Physician* 91, no. 6 (March 15, 2015): 365–371. This article can also be found online at https://www.aafp.org/afp/2015/0315/p365.html (accessed February 5, 2018).

Sahadeo, N. S. D., et al. "Understanding the Evolution and Spread of Chikungunya Virus in the Americas Using Complete Genome Sequences." *Virus Evolution* 3, no. 1 (January 2017). This article can also be found online at https://academic.oup.com/ve/article/3/1/vex010/3792090 (accessed January 31, 2018).

Samiphak, Sara, and S. Leonard Syme. "The Battle of Worldviews: A Case Study of Liver Fluke Infection in Khon Kaen, Thailand." *Journal of Evidence-Based Integrative Medicine* 22, no. 4 (2017): 902–908. This article can also be found online at http://journals.sagepub.com/doi/full/10.1177/2156587217723497 (accessed January 4, 2018).

Sands, Peter, Carmen Mundaca-Shah, and Victor J. Dzau. "The Neglected Dimension of Global Security—A Framework for Countering Infectious-Disease Crises." *New England Journal of Medicine* 374 (2016): 1281–1287. This article can also be found online at http://www.nejm.org/doi/full/10.1056/NEJMsr1600236 (accessed March 6, 2018).

Sanglard, Dominique. "Emerging Threats in Antifungal-Resistant Fungal Pathogens." *Frontiers in Medicine* (March 15, 2016). This article can also be found online at https://www.frontiersin.org/articles/10.3389/fmed.2016.00011/full (accessed February 21, 2018).

Santín, M., and R. Fayer. "*Enterocytozoon bieneusi* Genotype Nomenclature Based on the Internal Transcribed Spacer Sequence: A Consensus." *Journal of Eukaryotic Microbiology* 56 (2009): 34.

Santer, Melvin. "Joseph Lister: First Use of a Bacterium as a 'Model Organism' to Illustrate the Cause of Infectious Disease of Humans." *Notes and Records of the Royal Society of London* 64, no. 1 (March 2010): 59–65.

Santosham, Mathuram, and Duncan Steele. "Rotavirus Vaccines—A New Hope." *New England Journal of Medicine* 376 (2017): 1170–1172.

Savaris, R. F., et al. "Antibiotic Therapy for Pelvic Inflammatory Disease." *Cochrane Database of Systematic Reviews* 4 (April 2017): CD010285.

Sawhney, S., P. Woo, and K. J. Murray. "Macrophage Activation Syndrome: A Potentially Fatal Complication of Rheumatic Disorders." *Archives of Disease in Childhood* 85 (June 2001): 421–426. This article can also be found online at http://adc.bmj.com/content/archdischild/85/5/421.full.pdf (accessed March 12, 2018).

Saxena, Astha. "Delhi Hit by Dengue and Malaria Outbreaks as Monsoon Rains Boost Mosquito Numbers." Daily Mail India (July 18, 2017). This article can also be found online at http://www.dailymail.co.uk/indiahome/indianews/article-3696319/Delhi-hit-dengue-malaria-outbreaks-monsoon-rains-boost-mosquito-numbers.html (accessed March 2, 2018).

Say, Lale, et al. "Global Causes of Maternal Death: A WHO Systematic Analysis." *Lancet Global Health* 2, no. 6 (June 2014): e323–e333. This article can also be found online at http://www.thelancet.com/journals/langlo/article/PIIS2214–109X(14)70227-X/fulltext (accessed January 31, 2018).

Sayre, Carolyn. "Students Still Getting Mono After All These Years." *New York Times* (January 21, 2009). This article can also be found online at http://www.nytimes.com/ref/health/healthguide/esn-mono-ess.html (accessed January 24, 2018).

Schleiss, Mark R. "Cytomegalovirus Vaccines under Clinical Development." *Journal of Virus Eradication* 2, no. 4 (2016): 198–207. This article can also be found online at https://www.ncbi.nlm.nih.gov/pmc/articles/PMC5075346/ (accessed February 13, 2018).

Schuster, F.L., and L. Ramirez-Avila. "Current World Status of *Balantidium coli*." *Clinical Microbiology Reviews* 21, no. 4 (October 2008): 626–638. http://cmr.asm.org/content/21/4/626.full (accessed November 10, 2017).

Scollard, David M. "Infection with *Mycobacterium lepromatosis*." *American Journal of Tropical Medicine and Hygiene* 95, no. 3 (September 2016): 500–501. This article can also be found online at https://www.ncbi.nlm.nih.gov/pmc/articles/PMC5014247/ (accessed February 12, 2018).

"Scrofula and Pork." *Scientific American* 8, no. 7 (October 1852): 54.

Seale, Anna C, et al. "Stillbirth with Group B *Streptococcus* Disease Worldwide: Systematic Review and Meta-Analyses." *Clinical Infectious Diseases* 65, no. 2 (November 6, 2017): S125–S132. This article can also be found online at https://academic.oup.com/cid/article/65/suppl_2/S125/4589583 (accessed January 23, 2018).

Seibert, Grace, et al. "What Do Visitors Know and How Do They Feel about Contact Precautions?" *American Journal of Infection Control* 45 (2017).

Sempere, J. M., V. Soriano, and J. M. Benito. "T Regulatory Cells and HIV Infection." *AIDS Reviews* 9, no. 1 (January–March 2007): 54–60.

Senkomago, Virginia. "CDC Activities for Improving Implementation of Human Papillomavirus Vaccination, Cervical Cancer Screening, and Surveillance Worldwide." Global Health Security Supplement 23 (December 2017). This article can also be found online at https://wwwnc.cdc.gov/eid/article/23/13/17–0603_article (accessed January 26, 2018).

Serradell, Marianela C., et al. "Vaccination of Domestic Animals with a Novel Oral Vaccine Prevents *Giardia* Infections, Alleviates Signs of Giardiasis and Reduces Transmission to Humans." *Nature* (September 15, 2016). This article can also be found online at https://www.nature.com/articles/npjvaccines201618?utm_source=feedburner&utm_medium=feed&utm_campaign=Feed%3A+npjvaccines%2Frss%2Fcurrent+(npj+Vaccines) (accessed January 17, 2018).

Shapiro, E. D. "Clinical Practice: Lyme Disease." *New England Journal of Medicine* 370, no. 18 (May 2014): 1724–1731.

Sharapov, Umid M., et al. "Multistate Outbreak of *Escherichia coli* O157:H7 Infections Associated with Consumption of Fresh Spinach: United States, 2006." *Journal of Food Protection* 79 (2016): 2024–2030.

Sharara, Sima L., and Souha S. Kanj. "War and Infectious Diseases: Challenges of the Syrian Civil War." *PLOS Pathogens* 10, no. 11 (November 13, 2014): e1004438. This article can also be found online at http://journals.plos.org/plospathogens/article?id=10.1371/journal.ppat.1004438 (accessed March 8, 2018).

Sharma Monica, Shashank Singh, and Sidharth Sharma. "New Generation Antibiotics/Antibacterials: Deadly Arsenal for Disposal of Antibiotic Resistant Bacteria." *Journal of Microbial & Biochemical Technology* 7, no. 6 (January 2015): 374–379. This article can also be found online at https://www.researchgate.net/publication/288859488_New_Generation_AntibioticsAntibacterials_Deadly_Arsenal_for_Disposal_of_Antibiotic_Resistant_Bacteria (accessed November 8, 2017).

Sharp, Paul M., and Beatrice H. Hahn. "Origins of HIV and the AIDS Pandemic." *Cold Springs Harbor Perspectives in Medicine* 1 (2011): a006841.

Shayan, Sara, et al. "Crimean-Congo Hemorrhagic Fever." *Laboratory Medicine* 46, no. 3 (2015): 180–189. This article can also be found online at https://academic.oup.com/labmed/article/46/3/180/2657762 (accessed January 19, 2018).

Shea, Katherine M. "Antibiotic Resistance: What Is the Impact of Agricultural Uses of Antibiotics on Children's Health?" *Pediatrics* 112 (2003): 253–258. This article can also be found online at http://pediatrics.aappublications.org/content/112/Supplement_1/253 (accessed February 26, 2018).

Shechter, Sharon, et al. "Novel Inhibitors Targeting Venezuelan Equine Encephalitis Virus Capsid Protein Identified Using *In Silico* Structure-Based-Drug-Design." *Scientific Reports* 7, no. 1 (December 2017): 17705.

Shin, H., and A. Iwasaki. "Generating Protective Immunity against Genital Herpes." *Trends in Immunology* 34 (2013): 487–494.

Shives, Katherine D., Kenneth L. Tyler, and J. David Beckham. "Molecular Mechanisms of Neuroinflammation and Injury during Acute Viral Encephalitis." *Journal of Neuroimmunology* 308 (July 2017): 102–111.

Short, Erica E., Cyril Caminade, and Bolaji N. Thomas. "Climate Change Contribution to the Emergence or Re-emergence of Parasitic Diseases." *Infectious Diseases: Research and Treatment* 10 (2017): 1–7. This article can also be found online at http://journals.sagepub.com/doi/pdf/10.1177/1178633617732296 (accessed March 12, 2018).

Shragai, Talya, et al. "Zika and Chikungunya: Mosquito-Borne Viruses in a Changing World." *Annals of the New York Academy of Sciences* 1399 (July 2017): 61–77. This article can also be found online at http://onlinelibrary.wiley.com/doi/10.1111/nyas.13306/full (accessed January 31, 2018).

Shrivastava, Arpit Kumar, et al. "Revisiting the Global Problem of Cryptosporidiosis and Recommendations." *Tropical Parasitology* 7, no. 1 (2017): 8–17. This article can also be found online at https://www.ncbi.nlm.nih.gov/pmc/articles/PMC5369280/ (accessed January 16, 2018).

Shulman, Stanford T., et al. "Clinical Practice Guideline for the Diagnosis and Management of Group A Streptococcal Pharyngitis: 2012 Update by the Infectious Diseases Society of America." *Clinical Infectious Diseases* 55, no. 10 (November 15, 2012): e86–e102. This article can also be found online at https://academic.oup.com/cid/article/55/10/e86/321183 (accessed January 25, 2018).

Shuster, Evelyn. "Fifty Years Later: The Significance of the Nuremberg Code." *New England Journal of Medicine* 337 (November 13, 1997): 1436–1440. This article can also be found online at http://www.nejm.org/doi/full/10.1056/NEJM199711133372006 (accessed February 12, 2018).

Siedner, Mark J., et al. "Strengthening the Detection of and Early Response to Public Health Emergencies: Lessons from the West African Ebola Epidemic." *PLOS Medicine* 12, no. 3 (March 24, 2015): e1001804. This article can also be found online at http://journals.plos.org/plosmedicine/article?id=10.1371/journal.pmed.1001804 (accessed February 28, 2018).

Siegel-Itzkovich, Judy. "First-Ever Case of 'Cave Disease' Diagnosed in the Middle East." *Jerusalem Post* (December 11, 2017). This article can also be found online at http://www.jpost.com/HEALTH-SCIENCE/First-ever-case-of-cave-disease-diagnosed-in-the-Middle-East-517728 (accessed January 23, 2018).

Silva-Costa, C. "Scarlet Fever Is Caused by a Limited Number of *Streptococcus pyogenes* Lineages and Is Associated with the Exotoxin Genes ssa, speA and speC." *Pediatric Infectious Disease Journal* 33, no. 3 (2014): 306–310.

Silver, Bronywn J., et al. "*Trichomonas vaginalis* as a Cause of Perinatal Morbidity: A Systematic Review and Meta-Analysis." *Sexually Transmitted Diseases* 41, no. 6 (June 2014): 369–376. This article can also be found online at https://journals.lww.com/stdjournal/Abstract/2014/06000/Trichomonas_vaginalis_as_a_Cause_of_Perinatal.5.aspx (accessed January 22, 2018).

Simmons, Bryan P., and Elaine L. Larson. "Multiple Drug Resistant Organisms in Healthcare: The Failure of Contact Precautions." *Journal of Infection Prevention* 16, no. 4: 178–181. This article can also be found online at https://www.ncbi.nlm.nih.gov/pmc/articles/PMC5074191/ (accessed February 26, 2018).

Simms, I., et al. "Intensified Shigellosis Epidemic Associated with Sexual Transmission in Men Who Have Sex with Men—*Shigella flexneri and S. sonnei* in England, 2004 to End of February 2015." *Eurossurveillance* 20, no. 15 (April 16, 2015). This article can also be found online at http://www.eurosurveillance.org/content/10.2807/1560-7917.ES2015.20.15.21097 (accessed February 7, 2018).

Simon, Bryan R. "West Nile Virus." *Nursing 2017* 47 (August 2017): 58–60.

Simonsen, L., et al. "Unsafe Injections in the Developing World and Transmission of Bloodborne Pathogens." *Bulletin of the World Health Organization* 77, no. 10 (1999): 789–800.

Simor, Andrew E., et al. "Prevalence of Colonization and Infection with Methicillin-Resistant *Staphylococcus aureus* and Vancomycin-Resistant *Enterococcus* and of *Clostridium difficile* Infection in Canadian Hospitals." *Infection Control and Hospital Epidemiology* 34, no. 7 (July 2013): 687–693. This article can also be found online at http://www.jstor.org/stable/10.1086/670998 (accessed March 9, 2018).

Singer, Mervyn, et al. "The Third International Consensus Definitions for Sepsis and Septic Shock (Sepsis-3)." *JAMA* 315 (2016): 801–810. This article can also be found online at https://www.ncbi.nlm.nih.gov/pmc/articles/PMC4968574/ (accessed February 28, 2018).

Singh, Preeti, Bijay Mirdha, Vineet Ahuja, and Sundeep Singh. "Loop-Mediated Isothermal Amplification (LAMP) Assay for Rapid Detection of *Entamoeba histolytica* in Amoebic Liver Abscess. *World Journal of Microbiology and Biotechnology* 29, no. 1 (2013): 27–32.

Sircar, Anita D., et al. "Raccoon Roundworm Infection Associated with Central Nervous System Disease and Ocular Disease." *Morbidity and Mortality Weekly Report* 65, no. 35 (September 9, 2016): 930–933. This article can also be found online at https://www.cdc.gov/mmwr/volumes/65/wr/mm6535a2.htm (accessed December 17, 2017).

Skarp, C. P. Astrid, et al. "Campylobacteriosis: The Role of Poultry Meat." *Clinical Microbiology and Infection* 22 (2016): 103–109.

Skinner, Ginger. "Pinworm Treatments Are an Expensive Drug Mistake You Don't Need to Make." **Consumer Reports** (January 27, 2017). This article can also be found online at https://www.consumerreports.org/drugs/pinworm-treatments-expensive-drug-mistake-you-dont-need-to-make/ (accessed January 9, 2018).

Skoff, T.H., et al. "Sources of Infant Pertussis Infection in the United States." *Pediatrics* 136, no. 4 (October 2015): 635–641. This article can also be found online at https://www.ncbi.nlm.nih.gov/pubmed/26347437 (accessed January 26, 2018).

Slomski, Anita. "Vaccines for Enterovirus 71." *JAMA* 311, no. 16 (2014): 1602.

Smalley, Claire, et al. "Status of Research and Development of Vaccines for Chikungunya." *Vaccine* 34, no. 26, (June 2016): 2976–2981. This article can also be found online at https://www.sciencedirect.com/science/article/pii/S0264410X16300731 (accessed January 31, 2018).

Smith, David L., et al. "Agricultural Antibiotics and Human Health" *PLOS Medicine* 2 (2005): 731–735. This article can also be found online at http://journals.plos.org/plosmedicine/article?id=10.1371/journal.pmed.0020232 (accessed February 26, 2018).

Smith, J. P. "Healthy Bodies and Thick Wallets: The Dual Relationship between Health and Economic Status." *Journal of Economic Perspectives* 13, no. 2 (1999): 145–166.

Smith, Jennie Erin. "America's War on the Kissing Bug." *New Yorker* (November 20, 2015). This article can also be found online at https://www.newyorker.com/tech/elements/americas-war-on-the-kissing-bug-and-chagas-disease (accessed January 18, 2017).

Soto, S. M. "Human Migration and Infectious Diseases." *Clinical Microbiology and Infection* 15, no. 1 (January 2009): 26–28. This article can also be found online at http://onlinelibrary.wiley.com/doi/10.1111/j.1469–0691.2008.02694.x/full (accessed February 6, 2018.)

Spandole, S., et al. "Human Anelloviruses: An Update of Molecular, Epidemiological and Clinical Aspects." *Archives of Virology* 160, no. 4 (April 2015): 893–908. This article can also be found online at https://www.ncbi.nlm.nih.gov/pubmed/25680568 (accessed February 1, 2018).

Squire, Sylvia Afriyie, and Una Ryan. "*Cryptosporidium* and *Giardia* in Africa: Current and Future Challenges." *Parasites & Vectors* 10, no. 1 (2017): 195. This article can also be found online at https://parasitesandvectors.biomedcentral.com/articles/10.1186/s13071-017-2111-y#Sec8 (accessed January 16, 2018).

Stahlman, Shauna. "Incident Diagnoses of Leishmaniasis, Active and Reserve Components, U.S. Armed Forces, 2001–2016." *Medical Surveillance Monthly Report* 24, no. 2 (February 2017): 2–7. This article can also be found online at https://health.mil/MSMRArchives (accessed February 3, 2018).

Staples J. Erin, Robert F. Breiman, and Ann M. Powers. "Chikungunya Fever: An Epidemiological Review of a Re-emerging Infectious Disease." *Clinical Infectious Diseases* 49, no. 6 (2009): 942–948.

Starling, Shimona. "Viral Infection: Competing Membrane Proteins Regulate Picornavirus Genome Delivery." *Nature Reviews Microbiology* 15 (2017): 132–133.

Stein, Richard A. "Hopes and Challenges for the Common Cold." *International Journal of Clinical Practice* 71 (2017): e12921.

Stevens, Dennis L. "Streptococcal Toxic-Shock Syndrome: Spectrum of Disease, Pathogenesis, and New Concepts in Treatment." *Emerging*

Infectious Diseases 1 (1995): 69–76. This article can also be found online at https://www.ncbi.nlm.nih.gov/pmc/articles/PMC2626872/pdf/8903167.pdf (accessed February 12, 2018).

Stevens, Hilde, and Isabelle Huys. "Innovative Approaches to Increase Access to Medicines in Developing Countries." *Frontiers in Medicine* 4 (2017): 218. This article can also be found online at https://www.ncbi.nlm.nih.gov/pmc/articles/PMC5725781/ (accessed March 1, 2018).

Steverding, Dietmar. "The History of Leishmaniasis." *Parasites & Vectors* 10, no. 82 (2017). This article can also be found online at https://parasitesandvectors.biomedcentral.com/articles/10.1186/s13071-017-2028-5 (accessed February 2, 2018).

Stocks, Meredith E., et al. "Effect of Water, Sanitation, and Hygiene on the Prevention of Trachoma: A Systematic Review and Meta-Analysis." *PLOS Medicine* (February 25, 2014). This article can also be found online at http://journals.plos.org/plosmedicine/article?id=10.1371/journal.pmed.1001605 (accessed January 18, 2018).

Stone, B., et al. "Brave New Worlds: The Expanding Universe of Lyme Disease." *Vector Borne and Zoonotic Diseases* 17, no. 9 (2017): 619–629.

Stone, Lewi, Ronen Olinky, and Amit Huppert. "Seasonal Dynamics of Recurrent Epidemics." *Nature* (April 2007): 533–536. This article can also be found online at https://www.researchgate.net/publication/6416975_Seasonal_dynamics_of_recurrent_epidemics (accessed February 5, 2018).

Sullivan, Con, et al. "Using Zebrafish Models of Human Influenza A Virus Infections to Screen Antiviral Drugs and Characterize Host Immune Cell Responses." *Journal of Visualized Experiments* 119 (2017): e55235.

Sun, Jimin, et al. "Factors Associated with Severe Fever with Thrombocytopenia Syndrome Infection and Fatal Outcome." *Scientific Reports* 6 (2016). This article can also be found online at https://www.nature.com/articles/srep33175 (accessed March 1, 2018).

Sun, Lena H. "Chasing a Killer." *Washington Post* (November 3, 2017). This article can also be found online at https://www.washingtonpost.com/graphics/2017/national/health-science/monkeypox/?utm_term=.fb1ed3443a41 (accessed January 24, 2018).

———. "Rise in Mumps Outbreaks Prompts U.S. Officials to Weigh Third Vaccine Dose." *Washington Post* (February 23, 2017). This article can also be found online at https://www.washingtonpost.com/news/to-your-health/wp/2017/02/23/rise-in-mumps-outbreaks-prompts-u-s-officials-to-weigh-third-vaccine-dose (accessed January 26, 2018).

Tabrah, Frank L. "Koch's Postulates, Carnivorous Cows, and Tuberculosis Today." *Hawaii Medical Journal* 70, no. 7 (2011): 144–148. This article can also be found online at https://www.ncbi.nlm.nih.gov/pmc/articles/PMC3158372/ (accessed January 16, 2018).

Tate, Jacqueline E., et al. "Global, Regional, and National Estimates of Rotavirus Mortality in Children <5 Years of Age, 2000–2013." Supplement 2. *Clinical Infectious Diseases* 62 (2016): S96–S105. This article can also be found online at https://academic.oup.com/cid/article/62/suppl_2/S96/2478843 (accessed January 23, 2018).

Taubenberger, Jeffery K., et al. "Reconstruction of the 1918 Influenza Virus: Unexpected Rewards from the Past" *mBio* 3, no. 5 (2012). This article can also be found online at http://mbio.asm.org/content/3/5/e00201-12.full (accessed January 16, 2018).

Tee, Kok Keng, et al. "Evolutionary Genetics of Human Enterovirus 71: Origin, Population Dynamics, Natural Selection, and Seasonal Periodicity of the VP1 Gene." *Journal of Virology* 84, no. 7 (2010): 3339–3350. This article can also be found online at http://jvi.asm.org/content/84/7/3339.full (accessed February 5, 2018).

TeKippe, Erin McElvania, et al. "Increased Prevalence of Anellovirus in Pediatric Patients with Fever." *PLOS One* (November 30, 2012). This article can also be found online at http://journals.plos.org/plosone/article?id=10.1371/journal.pone.0050937 (accessed February 1, 2018).

Terrault, Norah A., et al. "AASLD Guidelines for Treatment of Chronic Hepatitis B." *Hepatology* 63, no. 1 (2016): 261–283. This article can also be found online at https://www.aasld.org/sites/default/files/Terrault_et_al-2016-Hepatology.pdf (accessed February 2, 2018).

Thornton, S. A., et al. "Gastroenteritis in US Marines during Operation Iraqi Freedom." *Clinical Infectious Diseases* 40, no. 4 (February 15, 2005): 519–525. This article can also be found online at https://www.ncbi.nlm.nih.gov/pubmed/15712073 (accessed March 8, 2018).

Toich, Laurie. "Will Hepatitis C Virus Medication Costs Drop in the Years Ahead?" *Pharmacy Times* (February 8, 2017). This article can also be found online at http://www.pharmacytimes.com/resource-centers/hepatitisc/will-hepatitis-c-virus-medicaton-costs-drop-in-the-years-ahead (accessed February 20, 2018).

Tong, Michael Xiaoliang, et al. "Infectious Diseases, Urbanization and Climate Change: Challenges in Future China." *International Journal of Environmental Research and Public Health* 12, no. 9 (September 2015): 11025–11036. This article can also be found online at https://www.ncbi.nlm.nih.gov/pmc/articles/PMC4586659/ (accessed March 12, 2018).

Torgerson, Paul R., and Pierpaolo Mastroiacovo. "The Global Burden of Toxoplasmosis: A Systematic Review." *Bulletin of the World Health Organization* 91 (May 2013): 501–508.

Torgerson, Paul R., et al. "Global Burden of Leptospirosis: Estimated in Terms of Disability Adjusted Life Years." *PLOS Neglected Tropical Diseases* (October 2, 2015). This article can also be found online at http://journals.plos.org/plosntds/article?id=10.1371/journal.pntd.0004122 (accessed January 19, 2018).

Torjesen, Ingrid. "World Leaders Are Ignoring Worldwide Threat of Ebola, Says MSF." *BMJ* 349 (September 5, 2014). This article can also be found online at http://www.bmj.com/content/349/bmj.g5496 (accessed February 27, 2018).

Torres, Rolando, et al. "Enzootic Mosquito Vector Species at Equine Encephalitis Transmission Foci in the República de Panamá" *PLOS ONE* 12 (2017): e0185491. This article can also be found online at https://doi.org/10.1371/journal.pone.0185491 (accessed February 25, 2018).

Townsend-Payne, Kelly, et al. "Children with *Haemophilus Influenzae* Type B (Hib) Vaccine Failure Have Long-Term Bactericidal Antibodies against Virulent Hib Strains with Multiple Capsular Loci."**Vaccine** 34 (July 2016): 3931–3934

Tran, D. Q. "In vitro Suppression Assay for Functional Assessment of Human Regulatory T Cells." *Methods in Molecular Biology* 979 (2013): 199–212.

"Treatment of Aspergillosis: Clinical Practice Guidelines of the Infectious Disease Society of America." *Clinical Infectious Diseases* 46, no. 3 (2008): 327–360.

Tronstein, Elizabeth, et al. "Genital Shedding of Herpes Simplex Virus among Symptomatic and Asymptomatic Persons with HSV-2 Infection." *JAMA* 14 (April 13, 2011): 1441–1449.

Tumpey, Terrence M., et al. "Characterization of the Reconstructed 1918 Spanish Influenza Pandemic Virus." *Science* 310 (October 7, 2005): 77–80.

Turelli, Michael, and Nicholas H. Barton. "Deploying Dengue-Suppressing *Wolbachia*: Robust Models Predict Slow but Effective Spatial Spread in *Aedes aegypti*." *Theoretical Population Biology* 115 (June 2017): 45–60.

Turkan, Togal, et al. "Intensive Care of a Weil's Disease with Multiorgan Failure." *Journal of Clinical Medicine Research* 2, no. 3 (June 2010): 145–149. This article can also be found online at https://www.ncbi.nlm.nih.gov/pmc/articles/PMC3104646/ (accessed January 19, 2018).

Tutolo, Jessica W., et al. "Notes from the Field: Powassan Virus Disease in Infant—Connecticut, 2016." *Morbidity and Mortality Weekly Report* 66 (April 2017): 408–409. This article can also be found online at https://www.cdc.gov/mmwr/volumes/66/wr/mm6615a3.htm (accessed February 12, 2018).

Tutty, Jacinda. "Country Faces Largest Mumps Outbreak in 20 Years." *Sunshine Coast Daily* (March 16, 2017). This article can also be found online at https://www.sunshinecoastdaily.com.au/news/country-faces-largest-mumps-outbreak-in-20-years/3155104/ (accessed February 6, 2018).

Uehara, Ritei, and Ermias D. Belay. "Epidemiology of Kawasaki Disease in Asia, Europe, and the United States." *Journal of Epidemiology* 22, no. 2 (2012): 79–85. This article can also be found online at https://www.jstage.jst.go.jp/article/jea/22/2/22_JE20110131/_article/-char/ja/ (accessed February 5, 2018).

Unuabonah, Emmanuel I., et al. "Clays for Efficient Disinfection of Bacteria in Waters." *Applied Clay Science* 151 (January 2018): 211–223.

Vacca, Irene. "Bacterial Pathogenesis: *Campylobacter* Follows the Clues." *Nature Reviews Microbiology* 15 (May 2017): 381.

Vaidya, Sunil R., et al. "Measles & Rubella Outbreaks in Maharashtra State, India." *Indian Journal of Medical Research* 143, no. 2 (February 2016): 227–231. This article can also be found online at https://www.ncbi.nlm.nih.gov/pmc/articles/PMC4859132/ (accessed February 12, 2018).

Van den Berg, Henk. "Global Status of DDT and Its Alternatives for Use in Vector Control to Prevent Disease." *Environmental Health Perspectives* 117, no. 11 (November 2009): 1656–1663.

Van Dillen, J., et al. "Maternal Sepsis: Epidemiology, Etiology and Outcome." *Current Opinion in Infectious Diseases* 23, no. 3 (2010): 249–254.

Van Duin, David, and David Paterson. "Multidrug Resistant Bacteria in the Community: Trends and Lessons Learned." *Infectious Disease Clinics of North America* 30, no. 2 (2016): 377–390. This article can also be found online at https://www.ncbi.nlm.nih.gov/pmc/articles/PMC5314345/ (accessed February 26, 2018).

Van Dyke, Melissa K., et al. "Etiology of Acute Otitis Media in Children Less Than 5 Years of Age: A Pooled Analysis of 10 Similarly Designed Observational Studies?" *Pediatric Infectious Diseases* 36, no. 3 (March 2017): 274–281.

Van Lunzen, Jan, and Marcus Altfeld. "Sex Differences in Infectious Diseases—Common but Neglected." *Journal of Infectious Diseases* 209, suppl. 3 (July 15, 2014): S79–S80. This article can also be found online at https://academic.oup.com/jid/article/209/suppl_3/S79/2192876 (accessed March 5, 2018).

Van Nunen, S., et al. "The Association between *Ixodes holocyclus* Tick Bite Reactions and Red Meat Allergy." *Internal Medicine Journal* 39, no. S5 (2007): A132.

Van Weyenbeg, S. J. B., and N. K. De Boer. "*Enterobiasis vermicularis*." *Video Journal and Encyclopedia of GI Endoscopy* 1, no. 2 (October 2013): 359–360.

Van Zandt, Kristopher E., Marek T. Greer, and H. Carl Gelhaus. "Glanders: An Overview of Infection in Humans." *Orphanet Journal of Rare Diseases* 8 (2013): 131. This article can also be found online at https://doi.org/10.1186/1750-1172-8-131 (accessed February 7, 2018).

Vannier, Edouard, and Peter J. Krause. "Human Babesiosis." *New England Journal of Medicine* 366 (June 21, 2012): 2397–2407.

Vasilyev, Evgeny V, et al. "Torque Teno Virus (TTV) Distribution in Healthy Russian Population." *Virology Journal* 6 (September 7, 2009). This article can also be found online at https://www.ncbi.nlm.nih.gov/pmc/articles/PMC2745379 (accessed February 1, 2018).

Ventola, C. L. "The Antibiotic Resistance Crisis. Part 1: Causes and Threats." *Pharmacy & Therapeutics* 40, no. 4 (2015): 277–283.

Vergano, Dan. "Mystery of 1918 Flu That Killed 50 Million Solved?" *National Geographic* (April 29, 2014). This article can also be found online at https://news.nationalgeographic.com/news/2014/04/140428-1918-flu-avian-swine-science-health-science/ (accessed January 16, 2018).

Verma, Dinesh, Jacob Thompson, and Sankar Swaminathan. "Spironolactone Blocks Epstein-Barr Virus Production by Inhibiting EBV SM Protein Function." *Proceedings of the National Academy of Sciences* 113 (2016): 3609–3614. This article can also be found online at http://www.pnas.org/content/113/13/3609.full.pdf (accessed November 16, 2017).

Viboud, Cécile, et al. "Global Mortality Impact of the 1957–1959 Influenza Pandemic." *Journal of Infectious Diseases* 213, no. 5 (March 1, 2016): 738–745. This article can also be found online at https://academic.oup.com/jid/article/213/5/738/2459470 (accessed January 22, 2018).

Vitek, Charles R., and Melinda Wharton. "Diphtheria in the Former Soviet Union: Reemergence of a Pandemic Disease." *Emerging Infectious Diseases* 4 (October–December 1998). This article can also be found online at https://wwwnc.cdc.gov/eid/article/4/4/98-0404_article (accessed February 14, 2018).

Vorou, Regina. "Zika Virus, Vectors, Reservoirs, Amplifying Hosts, and Their Potential to Spread Worldwide: What We Know and What We Should Investigate Urgently." *International Journal of Infectious Diseases* 48 (July 2016): 85–90.

Wójcik, Oktawia P., et al. "Public Health for the People: Participatory Infectious Disease Surveillance in the Digital Age." *Emerging Themes in*

Epidemiology 11, no. 7 (June 20, 2014). This article can also be found online at https://ete-online.biomedcentral.com/articles/10.1186/1742-7622-11-7 (accessed March 6, 2018).

Walker, Mark J., et al. "Disease Manifestations and Pathogenic Mechanisms of Group A *Streptococcus*." *Clinical Microbiology Reviews* 27, no. 2 (April 1, 2014): 264–301. This article can also be found online at http://cmr.asm.org/content/27/2/264.full (accessed January 25, 2018).

Waltner-Toews, David. "Zoonoses, One Health and Complexity: Wicked Problems and Constructive Conflict." *Philosophical Transactions of the Royal Society B* 372, no. 1725 (July 19, 2017).

Wang, Mengmei, Jinjing Zuo, and Ke Hu. "Identification of Severe Fever with Thrombocytopenia Syndrome Virus in Ticks Collected from Patients." *International Journal of Infectious Diseases* 29 (2014): 82–83. This article can also be found online at https://www.sciencedirect.com/science/article/pii/S1201971214016464 (accessed March 1, 2018).

Waterman, Stephen H., et al. "A New Paradigm for Quarantine and Public Health Activities at Land Borders: Opportunities and Challenges." *Public Health Reports* 124, no. 2 (2009): 203–211.

Waters, Andrew E., et al. "Multidrug-Resistant Staphylococcus aureus in US Meat and Poultry." *Clinical Infectious Diseases* 52, no. 10 (2011): 1227–1230.

Watkins, Richard R., and Lars Eckmann. "Treatment of Giardiasis: Current Status and Future Directions." *Current Infectious Disease Report* 16, no. 2 (2014): 396. This article can also be found online at https://link.springer.com/article/10.1007/s11908-014-0396-y (accessed January 17, 2018).

Weaver, Scott C., et al. "Venezuelan Equine Encephalitis." *Annual Review of Entomology* 49 (2004): 141–174.

———. "Zika, Chikungunya, and Other Emerging Vector-Borne Viral Diseases" *Annual Review of Medicine* 69 (2018): 395–408.

Webber Mark A., et al. "Quinolone-Resistant Gyrase Mutants Demonstrate Decreased Susceptibility to Triclosan." *Journal of Antimicrobial Chemotherapy* 72, no. 10 (October 2017): 2755–2763.

Weber, Ingrid B., et al. "Clinical Recognition and Management of Tularemia in Missouri: A Retrospective Records Review of 121 Cases." *Clinical Infectious Diseases* 55, no. 10 (November 15, 2012): 1283–1290. This article can also be found online at https://academic.oup.com/cid/article/55/10/1283/323868 (accessed February 9, 2018).

Wee, Ian, Adeline Lo, and Chaturaka Rodrigo. "Drug Treatment of Scrub Typhus: A Systematic Review and Meta-Analysis of Controlled Clinical Trials." *Transactions of the Royal Society of Tropical Medicine and Hygiene* 111, no. 8 (December 2017): 336–344.

Weinberg, Geoffrey A. "Respiratory Syncytial Mortality among Young Children." *Lancet Global Health* 5 (October 2017): e951–e952.

Weinstein, A. "Topical Treatment of Common Superficial Tinea Infections." *American Family Physician* 65, no. 10 (May 15, 2002): 2095–2102.

Weintraub, Pamela. "The Dr. Who Drank Infectious Broth, Gave Himself an Ulcer, and Solved a Medical Mystery." *Discover* (April 8, 2010). This article can also be found online at http://discovermagazine.com/2010/mar/07-dr-drank-broth-gave-ulcer-solved-medical-mystery (accessed March 6, 2018).

Welburn, S.C., et al. "The Neglected Zoonoses—The Case for Integrated Control and Advocacy." *Clinical Microbiology and Infection* 21, no. 5 (May 2015): 433–443. This article can also be found online at http://www.clinicalmicrobiologyandinfection.com/article/S1198-743X(15)00419-X/fulltext (accessed January 31, 2018).

West, Sheila K., et al. "The 'F' in SAFE: Reliability of Assessing Clean Faces for Trachoma Control in the Field." *PLOS Neglected Tropical Diseases* (November 30, 2017). This article can also be found online at http://journals.plos.org/plosntds/article?id=10.1371/journal.pntd.0006019 (accessed January 18, 2018).

Wheeler, Susan. "Henry IV of France Touching for Scrofula by Pierre Firens." *Journal of the History of Medicine and Allied Sciences* 58 (2003): 79–81.

White, Gregory S., et al. "Reemergence of St. Louis Encephalitis Virus, California, 2015." *Emerging Infectious Diseases* 22, no. 1 (December 2016): 2185–2188. This article can also be found online at https://wwwnc.cdc.gov/eid/article/22/12/pdfs/16-0805.pdf (accessed November 10, 2017).

Whitney, Laura C., and Tihana Bicanic. "Treatment Principles for *Candida* and *Cryptococcus*." *Cold Spring Harbor Perspectives in Medicine* 5, no. 6 (2014):1–12.

Whittaker, Robert, et al. "Epidemiology of Invasive *Haemophilus influenza* Disease, Europe, 2007–2014." *Emerging and Infectious Disease* 23 (March 2017): 396–404.

Whitty, Christopher J. M., Peter L. Chiodini, and David G. Lalloo. "Investigation and Treatment of Imported Malaria in Non-Endemic Countries." *BMJ* 346, no. 7909 (May 25, 2013): 31–34.

Wilkinson, Lise. "Glanders: Medicine and Veterinary Medicine in Common Pursuit of a Contagious Disease." *Medical History* 25 (1981): 363–384. This article can also be found online at https://www.ncbi.nlm.nih.gov/pmc/articles/PMC1139069/pdf/medhist00089–0026.pdf (accessed February 18, 2018).

Willyard, Cassandra. "The Drug-Resistant Bacteria That Pose the Greatest Health Threats." *Nature* (February 28, 2017). This article can also be found online at https://www.nature.com/news/the-drug-resistant-bacteria-that-pose-the-greatest-health-threats-1.21550 (accessed February 26, 2018).

Wilson, John W. "Nocardiosis: Updates and Clinical Overview." *Mayo Clinic Proceedings* 87, no. 4 (April 2012): 403–407. This article can also be found online at http://www.sciencedirect.com/science/article/pii/S0025619612002042 (accessed January 19, 2018).

Witte, L., D. Droemann, K. Dalhoff, and J. Rupp. "*Chlamydia pneumoniae* Is Frequently Detected in the Blood after Acute Lung Infection." *European Respiratory Journal* 37 (2011): 712–714. This article can also be found online at http://erj.ersjournals.com/content/37/3/712 (accessed January 26, 2018).

Wong, Alia. "When the Last Patient Dies." *Atlantic* (May 27, 2015). This article can also be found online at https://www.theatlantic.com/health/archive/2015/05/when-the-last-patient-dies/394163/ (accessed February 9, 2018).

Wong, K. T. "Enterovirus Encephalitis Including Enterovirus 71 and D68." *International Journal of Infectious Diseases* 45 (2016): 25.

Wong, Vanessa K., et al. "Phylogeographical Analysis of the Dominant Multidrug-Resistant H58 Clade of *Salmonella* Typhi Identifies Inter- and Intracontinental Transmission Events." *Nature Genetics* 47, no. 6 (June 2015): 632–639. This article can also be found online at https://www.nature.com/articles/ng.3281 (accessed January 29, 2018).

Woodall, Jack. "Why Mosquitoes Trump Birds." *Scientist* (January 1, 2006). This article can also be found online at https://www.the-scientist.com/?articles.view/articleNo/19704/title/Why-Mosquitoes-Trump-Birds/ (accessed January 15, 2018).

Woodworth, M. H., et al. "Increasing *Nocardia* Incidence Associated with Bronchiectasis at a Tertiary Care Center." *Annals of the American Thoracic Society* 14, no. 3 (March 2017): 347–354. This article can also be found online at https://www.ncbi.nlm.nih.gov/pubmed/28231023 (accessed January 19, 2018).

Workowski, Kimberly A., and Gail A. Bolan. "Sexually Transmitted Diseases Treatment Guidelines, 2015." *Morbidity and Mortality Weekly Report* 64, no. 3 (June 15, 2015): 1–137. This article can also be found online at https://www.cdc.gov/mmwr/preview/mmwrhtml/rr6403a1.htm (accessed March 15, 2018).

Worobey, Michael, Andrew Rambaut, and Guan-Zhu Han. "Genesis and Pathogenesis of the 1918 Pandemic H1N1 Influenza A Virus." *Proceedings of the National Academy of Sciences of the United States of America* 111, no. 22 (June 2014): 8107–8112. This article can also be found online at http://www.pnas.org/content/111/22/8107.full (accessed January 16, 2018).

Wroblewski, Lydia E., Richard M. Peek Jr., and Keith T. Wilson. "*Helicobacter pylori* and Gastric Cancer: Factors That Modulate Disease Risk." *Clinical Microbiology Reviews* 23, no 4 (2010): 713–739. This article can also be found online at https://www.ncbi.nlm.nih.gov/pmc/articles/PMC2952980/ (accessed March 6, 2018).

Xu, Y., et al. "Monitoring of the Bacterial and Fungal Biodiversity and Dynamics during Massa Medicata Fermentata Fermentation." *Applied Microbiology and Biotechnology* 97, no. 22 (2013): 9647–9655.

Yan, Yongyong, et al. "A Combinatory Mucosal Vaccine against Influenza and Botulism." *Journal of Immunology* 196, no. 1 Supplement (May 1, 2016): 145–158.

Yanagida, Tetsuya, et al. "Taeniasis and Cysticercosis Due to *Taenia solium* in Japan." *Parasites & Vectors* 5 (January 2012): 18.

Yates, Tom A., et al. "The Transmission of *Mycobacterium tuberculosis* in High Burden Settings." *Lancet* 16, no. 2 (February 2016): 227–238.

Yeung, K. H. T., et al. "An Update of the Global Burden of Pertussis in Children Younger than 5 Years: A Modelling Study." *Lancet Infectious Diseases* 17, no. 9 (September 17, 2017): 974–980. This article can also be found online at https://www.ncbi.nlm.nih.gov/pubmed/28623146 (accessed January 26, 2018).

Yong, Ed. "A Strange Type of Anthrax Is Killing Chimpanzees." *Atlantic* (August 2, 2017). This article can also be found online at https://www.theatlantic.com/science/archive/2017/08/a-strange-type-of-anthrax-is-killing-chimpanzees/535521/ (accessed January 11, 2018).

Young, Andrew T. Y., et al. "From SARS to Avian Influenza Preparedness in Hong Kong." *Clinical Infectious Diseases* 64 (May 2017): S98–S104.

Young, Bob. "King County Toddler May Have Rare Disease Linked to Roundworms Found in Raccoon Droppings." *Seattle Times* (May 8, 2017). This article can also be found online at https://www.seattletimes.com/seattle-news/health/king-county-toddler-may-have-rare-disease-linked-to-roundworms-found-in-raccoon-droppings/ (accessed December 17, 2017).

Young, Lawrence S., Lee Fah Yap, and Paul G Murray. "Epstein-Barr Virus: More Than 50 Years Old and Still Providing Surprises." *Nature Reviews Cancer* 16, no. 12 (2016): 789–802.

Yu, Xue-Jie, et al. "Fever with Thrombocytopenia Associated with a Novel Bunyavirus in China." *New England Journal of Medicine* 364, 16 (2011): 1523–1532. This article can also be found online at http://www.nejm.org/doi/full/10.1056/NEJMoa1010095 (accessed March 2, 2018).

Zühlke, Liesl J., and Andrew C. Steer. "Estimates of the Global Burden of Rheumatic Heart Disease." *Global Heart* 8, no. 3 (September 2013): 189–195. This article can also be found online at https://www.sciencedirect.com/science/article/pii/S2211816013001142 (accessed January 30, 2018).

Zacharioudaki, Maria E., and Emmanouil Galanakis. "Management of Children with Persistent Group A Streptococcal Carriage." *Expert Review of Anti-infective Therapy* 15, no. 8 (2017): 787–795. This article can also be found online at http://www.tandfonline.com/doi/abs/10.1080/14787210.2017.1358612 (accessed January 31, 2018).

Zagari, Rocco Maurizio, Stefano Rabitti, Leonardo Henry Eusebi, and Franco Bazzoli. "Treatment of Helicobacter pylori infection: A Clinical Practice Update." *European Journal of Clinical Investigation* 48, no. 1 (2018). This article can also be found online at http://onlinelibrary.wiley.com/doi/10.1111/eci.12857/full (accessed March 6, 2018).

Zezima, Katie. "Another Outbreak Related to the Nation's Opioid Crisis: Hepatitis C." *Washington Post* (October 17, 2017). This article can also be found online at https://www.washingtonpost.com/national/another-outbreak-related-to-the-nations-opioid-crisis-hepatitis-c/2017/10/17/eb24e7b6-a063–11e7–9083-fbfddf6804c2_story.html (accessed February 20, 2018).

Zhang, Jun, et al. "Long-Term Efficacy of a Hepatitis E Vaccine." *New England Journal of Medicine* 372 (2015): 914–922. This article can also be found online at http://www.nejm.org/doi/full/10.1056/nejmoa1406011 (accessed February 7, 2018).

Zhou, Min, et al. "Effects of Chlamydia Pneumonia Infection on Progression of Coronary Heart Disease in Elderly Patients." *Biomedical Research* 28, no. 7 (2017). This article can also be found online at http://www.alliedacademies.org/articles/effects-of-chlamydia-pneumonia-infection-on-progression-of-coronary-heart-disease-in-elderly-patients.html (accessed January 26, 2018).

Zhu, Shimao, and Caiping Guo. "Rabies Control and Treatment: From Prophylaxis to Strategies with Curative Potential." *Viruses* 8, no. 11 (November 2016): 279. This article can also be found online at https://www.ncbi.nlm.nih.gov/pmc/articles/PMC5127009/ (accessed February 26, 2018).

Zipprich, Jennifer, et al. "Measles Outbreak—California, December 2014–February 2015." *Morbidity and Mortality Weekly Report* 64, no. 6 (February 15, 2018): 153–154. This article can also be found online at https://www.cdc.gov/mmwr/preview/mmwrhtml/mm6406a5.htm?s_cid=mm6406a5_w (accessed February 15, 2018).

Zumla, Alimuddin, et al. "Rapid Point of Care Diagnostic Tests for Viral and Bacterial Respiratory Tract Infections—Needs, Advances, and Future Prospects." *Lancet* 14 (2014): 1123–1135.

WEBSITES

"$8.9 Million Collaborative Grant to Understand How Dangerous Virus 'Hides' to Attack Another Day." EurekAlert, January 23, 2018. https://www.eurekalert.org/pub_releases/2018–01/uoah-cg012318.php (accessed February 2, 2018).

"10 Facts on Malaria." World Health Organization, December 2016. http://www.who.int/features/factfiles/malaria/en/ (accessed March 14, 2018).

"10 Facts on Polio Eradication." World Health Organization, April 2017. http://www.who.int/features/factfiles/polio/en/ (accessed February 2, 2018).

"The 10 Hottest Global Years on Record." Climate Central, January 18, 2018. http://www.climatecentral.org/gallery/graphics/the-10-hottest-global-years-on-record (accessed March 2, 2018).

"17 Million People with Access to Antiretroviral Therapy." World Health Organization, May 31, 2016. http://www.who.int/hiv/mediacentre/news/global-aids-update-2016-news/en/ (accessed March 1, 2018).

"2.1 Billion People Lack Safe Drinking Water at Home, More Than Twice as Many Lack Safe Sanitation." World Health Organization, July 12, 2017. http://www.who.int/mediacentre/news/releases/2017/water-sanitation-hygiene/en/ (accessed January 18, 2018).

"2015 Sexually Transmitted Diseases Treatment Guidelines: Trichomoniasis." Centers of Disease Control and Prevention, August 12, 2016. https://www.cdc.gov/std/tg2015/trichomoniasis.htm (accessed January 22, 2018).

"2016 Provisional Pertussis Surveillance Report." Centers for Disease Control and Prevention, January 6, 2017. https://www.cdc.gov/pertussis/downloads/pertuss-surv-report-2016-provisional.pdf (accessed January 26, 2018).

"2016 Sexually Transmitted Diseases Surveillance." Centers for Disease Control and Prevention, January 2018. https://www.cdc.gov/std/stats16/default.htm (accessed March 7, 2018).

"2017 National Notifiable Infectious Diseases." Centers for Disease Control and Prevention. https://wwwn.cdc.gov/nndss/conditions/notifiable/2017/infectious-diseases/ (accessed November 20, 2017).

"45 CFR 46." US Department of Health & Human Services, January 15, 2009. https://www.hhs.gov/ohrp/regulations-and-policy/regulations/45-cfr-46/index.html (accessed February 12, 2018).

"5 Opportunistic Infections and Coinfections." HIV i-BASE, January 1, 2016. http://i-base.info/ttfa/5-opportunistic-infections-ois-and-coinfections/ (accessed January 28, 2018).

"5 Things to Know About Triclosan." Food and Drug Administration (FDA). https://www.fda.gov/ForConsumers/ConsumerUpdates/ucm205999.htm (accessed November 17, 2017).

"85 Million People Treated for Trachoma through Expanded Access to Medicine." World Health Organization. July 13, 2017. http://www.who.int/neglected_diseases/news/85_million_people_treated_for_trachoma/en/ (accessed January 18, 2018).

"About Antibiotic Resistance." Centers for Disease Control and Prevention, September 19, 2017. https://www.cdc.gov/drugresistance/about.html (accessed February 26, 2018).

"About Blastomycosis." Minnesota Department of Health. http://www.health.state.mn.us/divs/idepc/diseases/blastomycosis/basics.html (accessed January 25, 2018).

"About Trachoma." International Trachoma Initiative. 2017. http://www.trachoma.org/about-trachoma (accessed January 18, 2018).

"About USAMRIID." US Army Medical Research Institute of Infectious Diseases. http://www.usamriid.army.mil/aboutpage.htm (accessed January 31, 2018).

"About Zika." Centers for Disease Control and Prevention, September 29, 2016. https://www.cdc.gov/zika/about/index.html (accessed February 26, 2018).

"Access to Antiretroviral Therapy in Africa: Status Report on Progress to the 2015 Targets." UNAIDS, 2013. http://www.unaids.org/sites/default/files/media_asset/20131219_AccessARTAfricaStatusReportProgresstowards2015Targets_en_0.pdf (accessed March 1, 2018).

"Administration of Rabies Immunoglobulin." World Health Organization. http://www.who.int/rabies/human/adminimmuno/en/ (accessed February 19, 2018).

"Advantages and Disadvantages of FDA-Approved HIV Assays Used for Screening, by Test Category." Centers for Disease Control and Prevention. https://www.cdc.gov/hiv/pdf/testing/hiv-tests-advantages-disadvantages.pdf (accessed December 5, 2017).

"Advisory Group of Independent Experts to Review the Smallpox Research Programme (AGIES): Comments on the Scientific Review of Variola Virus Research 1999–2010." World Health Organization, December 2010. http://apps.who.int/iris/bitstream/10665/70509/1/WHO_HSE_GAR_BDP_2010.4_eng.pdf (accessed January 29, 2018).

"*Aedes aegypti*—Factsheet for Experts." European Centre for Disease Prevention and Control, December 20, 2016. https://ecdc.europa.eu/en/disease-vectors/facts/mosquito-factsheets/aedes-aegypti (accessed February 26, 2018).

"African Programme for Onchocerciasis Control (APOC)." World Health Organization. http://www.who.int/apoc/about/en/ (accessed March 1, 2018).

"AIDS 2000, a Laboratory Simulation." University of Arizona. http://www.biology.arizona.edu/immunology/tutorials/AIDS (accessed March 6, 2018).

"All about BSE (Mad Cow Disease)." US Food and Drug Administration. https://www.fda.gov/animalveterinary/resourcesforyou/animalhealthliteracy/ucm136222.htm (accessed January 29, 2017).

"Alveolar Echinococcosis AE) FAQs." Centers for Disease Control and Prevention. https://www.cdc.gov/parasites/echinococcosis/gen_info/ae-faqs.html (accessed November 6, 2017).

Alwan, Ala. "The Cost of War." World Health Organization, November 6, 2015. http://www.who.int/mediacentre/commentaries/war-cost/en/ (accessed March 8, 2018).

"Amebiasis." Centers for Disease Control and Prevention. https://www.cdc.gov/parasites/amebiasis/(accessed January 16, 2018).

"Americas Region Is Declared the World's First to Eliminate Rubella." Pan American Health Organization, April 29, 2015. http://www.paho.org/hq/index.php?option=com_content&view=article&id=10798&Itemid=1926 (accessed January 16, 2018).

Andrews, Michelle. "FDA's Approval of a Cheaper Drug for Hepatitis C Will Likely Expand Treatment." NPR. https://www.npr.org/sections/health-shots/2017/10/04/555156577/fdas-approval-of-a-cheaper-drug-for-hepatitis-c-will-likely-expand-treatment (accessed February 20, 2018).

"Anellovirus." ScienceDirect. https://www.sciencedirect.com/topics/immunology-and-microbiology/anellovirus (accessed February 2, 2018).

"Angiostrongyliasis." Centers for Disease Control and Prevention, December 28, 2015. https://www.cdc.gov/parasites/angiostrongylus/index.html (accessed January 12, 2018).

"Angiostrongyliasis." World Health Organization. http://www.who.int/ith/diseases/angiostrongyliasis/en/ (accessed January 12, 2018).

"Anisakiasis." Centers for Disease Control and Prevention. 2016. https://www.cdc.gov/parasites/anisakiasis/ (accessed December 15, 2017).

"Anisakiasis." Merck Manuals. 2017. https://www.merckmanuals.com/professional/infectious-diseases/nematodes-roundworms/anisakiasis (accessed December 15, 2017).

"Anthrax." Centers for Disease Control and Prevention, January 31, 2017. https://www.cdc.gov/anthrax/index.html (accessed January 11, 2018).

"Antibiotic Resistance." World Health Organization. http://www.who.int/mediacentre/factsheets/antibiotic-resistance/en (accessed November 15, 2017).

"Antibiotic Resistance Threats in the United States, 2013." Centers for Disease Control and Prevention, April 10, 2017. https://www.cdc.gov/drugresistance/threat-report-2013/index.html (accessed January 23, 2018).

"Antibiotic Use in the United States, 2017: Progress and Opportunities." Centers for Disease Control and Prevention, October 6, 2017. https://www.cdc.gov/antibiotic-use/stewardship-report/outpatient.html (accessed March 14, 2018).

"Antibiotic/Antimicrobial Resistance." Centers for Disease Control and Prevention. https://www.cdc.gov/drugresistance/index.html (accessed November 8, 2017).

"Antimicrobial Resistance." World Health Organization, January 2018. http://www.who.int/mediacentre/factsheets/fs194/en/ (accessed February 26, 2018).

"Antimicrobial Resistance Fact Sheet." World Health Organization, November 2017. http://www.who.int/mediacentre/factsheets/fs194/en/ (accessed November 8, 2017).

"Antimicrobial Resistance: Global Report on Surveillance 2014." World Health Organization. http://www.who.int/drugresistance/documents/surveillancereport/en/ (accessed February 25, 2018).

"Antiviral Drugs." Centers for Disease Control and Prevention, January 24, 2018. http://www.cdc.gov/flu/professionals/treatment (accessed March 11, 2018).

"Are You Prepared?" Centers for Disease Control and Prevention, 2017. https://www.cdc.gov/phpr/areyouprepared/ (accessed January 15, 2018).

"Ascariasis." Centers for Disease Control and Prevention, May 24, 2016. https://www.cdc.gov/parasites/ascariasis/ (accessed January 10, 2018).

"Ascariasis." Mayo Clinic. https://www.mayoclinic.org/diseases-conditions/ascariasis/symptoms-causes/syc-20369593 (accessed January 10, 2018).

"Aspergillosis." Centers for Disease Control and Prevention. https://www.cdc.gov/fungal/diseases/aspergillosis/index.html (accessed November 14, 2017).

"Avian and Other Zoonotic Influenza." World Health Organization. http://www.who.int/influenza/human_animal_interface/en (accessed December 6, 2017).

"Avian Influenza." Centers for Disease Control and Prevention, April 13, 2017.http://www.cdc.gov/flu/avian/gen-info/pdf/avian_facts.pdf (accessed February 9, 2018).

"B Virus (Herpes B, Monkey B Virus, Herpesvirus Simiae, and Herpesvirus B)." Centers for Disease Control and Prevention, July 18, 2014. https://www.cdc.gov/herpesbvirus/index.html (accessed December 15, 2017).

"Babesiosis." Centers for Disease Control and Prevention. https://www.cdc.gov/parasites/babesiosis/ (accessed January 8, 2018).

"Babesiosis." Columbia University Medical Center Lyme and Tick-Borne Diseases Research Center. http://columbia-lyme.org/patients/tbd_babesia.html (accessed January 8, 2018).

"Babesiosis." New York State Department of Health. https://www.health.ny.gov/diseases/communicable/babesiosis/fact_sheet.htm (accessed January 8, 2018).

"Back to the Future: Asilomar and the Upcoming *NIH Guidelines* Workshop." National Institutes of Health. https://osp.od.nih.gov/2017/07/05/back-to-the-future-asilomar-and-the-upcoming-nih-guidelines-workshop/ (accessed November 14, 2017).

"Balantidiasis." National Organization for Rare Disorders (NORD). https://rarediseases.org/rare-diseases/balantidiasis/ (accessed November 10, 2017).

Balasegaram, Manica. "Drugs for the Poor, Drugs for the Rich: Why the Current R&D Model Doesn't Deliver." *PLOS* Speaking of Medicine Community Blog, February 14, 2014. http://blogs.plos.org/speakingofmedicine/2014/02/14/drugs-poor-drugs-rich-current-rd-model-doesnt-deliver/ (accessed March 1, 2018).

"Bartonella Infection (Cat Scratch Disease, Trench Fever, and Carrión's Disease)." Centers for Disease Control and Prevention. https://www.cdc.gov/bartonella/index.html (accessed November 14, 2017).

"Basic Concepts in Microscopy." Zeiss. http://zeiss-campus.magnet.fsu.edu/articles/basics/index.html (accessed January 29, 2018).

"Basics of Fungal Keratitis." Centers for Disease Control and Prevention. https://www.cdc.gov/contactlenses/fungal-keratitis.html (accessed November 14, 2017).

"Baylisascaris Infection." Centers for Disease Control and Prevention. https://www.cdc.gov/parasites/baylisascaris/ (accessed December 17, 2017).

"Behind Bars II: Substance Abuse and America's Prison Population." National Center on Addiction and Substance Abuse at Columbia University, February 2010. https://www.centeronaddiction.org/addiction-research/reports/behind-bars-ii-substance-abuse-and-america%E2%80%99s-prison-population (accessed February 9, 2018).

Bell, Melissa, Michael M. McNeil, and June M. Brown. "*Nocardia* species (Nocardiosis)." Antimicrobe, 2014. http://www.antimicrobe.org/b117.asp (accessed January 19, 2018).

Bennett, Nicholas John. "*Pneumocystis jiroveci* Pneumonia (PJP) Overview of *Pneumocystis jiroveci* Pneumonia." Medscape, August 8, 2017. https://emedicine.medscape.com/article/225976-overview (accessed February 14, 2018).

Berkley, Seth. "A New Vaccine against Typhoid Fever Will Also Help Fight Antimicrobial Resistance." STAT, November 30, 2017. https://www.statnews.com/2017/11/30/typhoid-fever-antimicrobial-resistance/ (accessed January 29, 2018).

"Biological Weapons." United Nations Office for Disarmament Affairs. https://www.un.org/disarmament/wmd/bio/ (accessed January 29, 2018).

"Biological Weapons Convention Signatories and States-Parties." Arms Control Association, September 27, 2017. https://www.armscontrol.org/factsheets/bwcsig (accessed January 29, 2018).

"Biomedical Advanced Research and Development Authority (BARDA)." US Department of Health and Human Services. https://www.medicalcountermeasures.gov/barda/ (accessed January 7, 2018).

"Bioterrorism." Centers for Disease Control and Prevention. https://www.cdc.gov/anthrax/bioterrorism/index.html (accessed January 7, 2018).

"Bioterrorism Agents/Diseases." Centers for Disease Control and Prevention, January 4, 2018. https://emergency.cdc.gov/agent/agentlist.asp (accessed March 8, 2018).

"Blastomycosis." Centers for Disease Control and Prevention, January 26, 2017. https://www.cdc.gov/fungal/diseases/blastomycosis/index.html (accessed January 25, 2018).

"Blood Safety and Availability." World Health Organization, June 2017. http://www.who.int/mediacentre/factsheets/fs279/en/ (accessed February 12, 2018).

"Blood Safety Basics." Centers for Disease Control and Prevention, January 31, 2013. https://www.cdc.gov/bloodsafety/basics.html (accessed February 12, 2018).

"Bloodborne Infectious Diseases: HIV/AIDS, Hepatitis B, Hepatitis C." Centers for Disease Control and Prevention. https://www.cdc.gov/niosh/topics/bbp/genres.html (accessed November 20, 2017).

Bolan, Gail. "Syphilis and HIV: A Dangerous Duo Affecting Gay and Bisexual Men." HIV.gov, December 13, 2012. https://www.hiv.gov/blog/syphilis-and-hiv-a-dangerous-duo-affecting-gay-and-bisexual-men (accessed February 16, 2018).

"Botulism." Centers for Disease Control and Prevention. https://www.cdc.gov/botulism/resources.html (accessed December 3, 2017).

"Botulism." US Food and Drug Administration. https://www.foodsafety.gov/poisoning/causes/bacteriaviruses/botulism/index.html (accessed November 14, 2017).

"Bovine Spongiform Encephalopathy (BSE), or Mad Cow Disease." Centers for Disease Control and Prevention, August 9, 2017. https://www.cdc.gov/prions/bse/index.html (accessed January 29, 2017).

Brady, Virginia A., Chad R. Marion, and Charles S. Dela Cruz. "Hospital Acquired Pneumonia." Clinical Advisor, 2017. https://www.clinicaladvisor.com/pulmonary-medicine/hospital-acquired-pneumonia/article/625521/ (accessed January 24, 2018).

Branswell, Helen. "A 'Perfect Storm' Superbug: How an Invasive Fungus Got Health Officials' Attention." STAT, July 31, 2017. https://www.statnews.com/2017/07/31/superbug-fungus-candida-auris/ (accessed January 25, 2018).

Branswell, Helen. "History Credits This Man with Discovering Ebola on His Own. History Is Wrong." STAT, July 14, 2017. https://www.statnews.com/2016/07/14/history-ebola-peter-piot/ (accessed January 31, 2018).

Breene, Keith. "7 Deadly Diseases the World Has (Almost) Eliminated." World Economic Forum, May 26, 2017. https://www.weforum.org/agenda/2017/05/7-deadly-diseases-the-world-has-almost-eradicated/ (accessed February 13, 2018).

Bresnahan, Samantha. "Virus Hunters Search for the Next Deadly Disease Outbreak." CNN, August 23, 2016. http://www.cnn.com/2016/08/23/health/virus-hunters-bat-cave-south-africa/index.html (accessed December 11, 2017).

"A Brief Guide to Emerging Infectious Diseases and Zoonoses." World Health Organization, 2014. http://www.searo.who.int/entity/emerging

_diseases/ebola/a_brief_guide_emerging_infectious_diseases.pdf?ua=1 (accessed January 31, 2018).

"Brief History of WHO." Credible Voice, Columbia University. http://ccnmtl.columbia.edu/projects/caseconsortium/casestudies/112/casestudy/www/layout/case_id_112_id_776.html> (accessed January 18, 2018).

"Bringing an Animal into the United States." Centers for Disease Control and Prevention, September 1, 2016. https://www.cdc.gov/importation/bringing-an-animal-into-the-united-states/index.html (accessed January 26, 2018).

"Britain's 'Anthrax Island.'" British Broadcasting Corporation, July 25, 2001. http://news.bbc.co.uk/2/low/uk_news/scotland/1457035.stm (accessed January 11, 2018).

"Brucellosis." Centers for Disease Control and Prevention. https://www.cdc.gov/brucellosis/index.html (accessed November 14, 2017).

Brundtland, Gro Harlem. "Bioterrorism and Military Health Risks." World Health Organization. http://www.who.int/dg/brundtland/speeches/2003/DAVOS/en/ (accessed January 15, 2018).

"BSE and Other Transmissible Spongiform Encephalopathies." Food Standards Agency, September 28, 2015. https://www.food.gov.uk/science/bse-and-other-transmissible-spongiform-encephalopathies (accessed January 29, 2017).

"BSE: Frequently Asked Questions." Department for Environment, Food and Rural Affairs, October 3, 2006. http://webarchive.nationalarchives.gov.uk/20080908074619/http://www.defra.gov.uk/animalh/bse/faq.html (accessed January 29, 2017).

"The BSE Inquiry." The National Archives. http://webarchive.nationalarchives.gov.uk/20060802142310/http://www.bseinquiry.gov.uk/ (accessed January 29, 2018).

"BSE Situation in the World and Annual Incidence Rate (1989–31/12/2016)." World Organisation for Animal Health, December 31, 2016. http://www.oie.int/en/animal-health-in-the-world/bse-specific-data (accessed January 29, 2017).

Buensalido, Joseph Adrian L. "Haemophilus Influenzae Infections Treatment & Management." Medscape. Last modified November 29, 2017. https://emedicine.medscape.com/article/218271-treatment.

Bugl, Paul. "Immune System." University of Hartford, March 2001. http://uhaweb.hartford.edu/BUGL/immune.htm (accessed March 8, 2018).

"Burkholderia Mallei and Pseudomallei (Glanders and Melioidosis)." Center for Health Security, December 1, 2013. http://www.centerforhealthsecurity.org/our-work/publications/glanders-and-melioidosis-fact-sheet (accessed February 7, 2018).

"Buruli Ulcer." Centers for Disease Control and Prevention, January 26, 2015. https://www.cdc.gov/buruli-ulcer/index.html (accessed January 17, 2018).

"Buruli Ulcer." World Health Organization, February 2017. http://www.who.int/mediacentre/factsheets/fs199/en/ (accessed January 30, 2018).

"*C. difficile* Control: Handwashing Practices Lax at Quebec Hospitals." CBC News, November 12, 2015. http://www.cbc.ca/news/canada/montreal/c-difficile-handwashing-quebec-hospitals-study-investigation-chart-1.3314788 (accessed December 6, 2017).

"*C. Difficile* Infection." American College of Gastroenterology, July 2016. http://patients.gi.org/topics/c-difficile-infection/ (accessed January 31, 2018).

"C. neoformans Infection." Centers for Disease Control and Prevention. https://www.cdc.gov/fungal/diseases/cryptococcosis-neoformans/index.html (accessed November 15, 2017).

"*Campylobacter* (Campylobacteriosis)." Centers for Disease Control and Prevention. https://www.cdc.gov/campylobacter/index.html (accessed November 14, 2017).

"Cancer Vaccines." National Cancer Institute, December 18, 2015. https://www.cancer.gov/about-cancer/causes-prevention/vaccines-fact-sheet (accessed January 26, 2018).

"CAR T Cells: Engineering Patients' Immune Cells to Treat Their Cancers." National Cancer Institute. https://www.cancer.gov/about-cancer/treatment/research/car-t-cells (accessed March 8, 2018).

"CDC Media Statement on Newly Discovered Smallpox Specimens." Centers for Disease Control and Prevention, July 8, 2014. https://

www.cdc.gov/media/releases/2014/s0708-NIH.html (accessed January 29, 2018).

"CDC Report: CDC Arboviral Disease Case Definition." Centers for Disease Control and Prevention. https://wwwn.cdc.gov/nndss/conditions/arboviral-diseases-neuroinvasive-and-non-neuroinvasive/case-definition/2015/ (accessed February 12, 2018).

"CDC Updates Guidance Related to Local Zika Transmission in Miami-Dade County, Florida." Centers for Disease Control and Prevention. https://www.cdc.gov/media/releases/2016/p1019-zika-florida-update.html (accessed January 25, 2018).

"CDC Urges Early Recognition, Prompt Treatment of Sepsis." Centers for Disease Control and Prevention. https://www.cdc.gov/media/releases/2017/p0831-sepsis-recognition-treatment.html (accessed January 25, 2018).

"CDC Warns of Common Parasites Plaguing Millions in U.S." CBS News, May 8, 2014. https://www.cbsnews.com/news/parasites-causing-infections-in-the-us-cdc-says/ (accessed March 2, 2018).

"Cercarial Dermatitis (Also Known as Swimmer's Itch)." Centers for Disease Control and Prevention, January 10, 2012. https://www.cdc.gov/parasites/swimmersitch/index.html (accessed November 14, 2017).

"Chagas Disease (American trypanosomiasis)." World Health Organization, March 2017. http://www.who.int/mediacentre/factsheets/fs340/en/ (accessed January 18, 2017).

Cheng, Allen. "Explainer: What Is the Flesh-eating Bacterium that Causes Buruli Ulcer and How Can I Avoid It?" Conversation, September 21, 2017. http://theconversation.com/explainer-what-is-the-flesh-eating-bacterium-that-causes-buruli-ulcer-and-how-can-i-avoid-it-84432 (accessed January 17, 2018).

Cheng, Lily, and Scott Smith. "Parasites and Pestilence: Infectious Public Health Challenges." Stanford University, 2006. https://web.stanford.edu/class/humbio103/ParaSites2006/Microsporidiosis/microsporidia1.html (accessed February 5, 2018).

"Chengdu Declaration on Cestode Infections Calls for Global Collaboration into Research and Control." World Health Organization, December 13, 2017. http://www.who.int/neglected_diseases/news/Chengdu_Declaration_on_cestode_infections_calls/en/ (accessed January 10, 2018).

Christian, N. "Everything You Should Know about Dysentery." Medical News Today. https://www.medicalnewstoday.com/articles/171193.php (accessed January 16, 2018).

"Chicken Pox (Varicella)." Centers for Disease Control and Prevention, July 1, 2016. https://www.cdc.gov/chickenpox/index.html (accessed January 24, 2018).

"Chickenpox Vaccine FAQs." National Health Service, March 31, 2016. https://www.nhs.uk/conditions/vaccinations/chickenpox-vaccine-questions-answers/ (accessed February 1, 2018).

"Chikungunya." Pan American Health Organization. http://www.paho.org/hq/index.php?Itemid=40931 (accessed January 31, 2018).

"Chikungunya." World Health Organization, April 2017. http://www.who.int/mediacentre/factsheets/fs327/en/ (accessed January 31, 2018).

"Chikungunya Virus." Centers for Disease Control and Prevention, August 29, 2017. https://www.cdc.gov/chikungunya/index.html (accessed January 31, 2018).

"Child Protection." UNICEF. https://www.unicef.org/protection/ (accessed January 16, 2018).

"Chlamydia." Centers for Disease Control and Prevention, September 26, 2017. https://www.cdc.gov/std/stats16/chlamydia.htm (accessed January 24, 2018).

"Chlamydia—CDC Fact Sheet (Detailed)." Centers for Disease Control and Prevention, September 26, 2017. https://www.cdc.gov/std/chlamydia/stdfact-chlamydia-detailed.htm (accessed January 25, 2018).

"*Chlamydia pneumoniae* Infection." Centers for Disease Control and Prevention, September 26, 2016. https://www.cdc.gov/pneumonia/atypical/cpneumoniae/index.html (accessed January 26, 2018).

"Cholera." World Health Organization. http://www.who.int/gho/epidemic_diseases/cholera/en/ (accessed February 12, 2018).

"Cholera—Mozambique." World Health Organization, February 19, 2018. http://www.who.int/csr/don/19-february-2018-cholera-mozambique/en/ (accessed February 28, 2018).

"Cholera—Vibrio Holerae Infection." Centers for Disease Control and Prevention, October 27, 2014. https://www.cdc.gov/cholera/index.html (accessed February 12, 2018).

"Climate Change and Health." World Health Organization, July 2017. http://www.who.int/mediacentre/factsheets/fs266/en/ (accessed March 2, 2018).

"Climate Effects on Health." Centers for Disease Control and Prevention, July 26, 2016. https://www.cdc.gov/climateandhealth/effects/default.htm (accessed March 2, 2018).

"Clinical Advisory: Ocular Syphilis in the United States." Centers for Disease Control and Prevention, March 24, 2016. https://www.cdc.gov/std/syphilis/clinicaladvisoryos2015.htm (accessed February 16, 2018).

"Clonorchiasis." World Health Organization. http://www.who.int/foodborne_trematode_infections/clonorchiasis/en/> (accessed January 5, 2018).

"*Clostridium difficile* Colitis—Overview." WebMD. https://www.webmd.com/digestive-disorders/tc/clostridium-difficile-colitis-overview#1 (accessed November 17, 2017).

"*Clostridium difficile* Infection Information for Patients." Centers for Disease Control and Prevention, February 24, 2015. https://www.cdc.gov/hai/organisms/cdiff/cdiff-patient.html (accessed January 31, 2018).

"*Clostridium difficile* Infections." MedlinePlus, October 20, 2017. https://medlineplus.gov/clostridiumdifficileinfections.htmlhttps://medlineplus.gov/clostridiumdifficileinfections.html (accessed January 31, 2018).

Cobra, Claudine, and David A. Sack. *The Control of Epidemic Dysentery in Africa: Overview, Recommendations, and Checklists.* Technical Paper No. 37. US Agency for International Development, 1996. http://pdf.usaid.gov/pdf_docs/pnaby890.pdf (accessed January 25, 2018).

"Coccidioidomycosis." American Lung Association. http://www.lung.org/lung-health-and-diseases/lung-disease-lookup/coccidioidomycosis/ (accessed February 6, 2018).

"Coccidioidomycosis." Center for Food Security and Public Health. http://www.cfsph.iastate.edu/Factsheets/pdfs/coccidioidomycosis.pdf (accessed February 6, 2018).

"Cold Sore." Mayo Clinic, May 15, 2015. https://www.mayoclinic.org/diseases-conditions/cold-sore/symptoms-causes/syc-20371017 (accessed December 6, 2017).

"Cold Sores: Overview." American Academy of Dermatology Association. https://www.aad.org/public/diseases/contagious-skin-diseases/cold-sores> (accessed December 6, 2017).

Collins, Francis. "Resurgence of Measles, Pertussis Fueled by Vaccine Refusals." Directors Blog, National Institutes of Health, March 22, 2016. https://directorsblog.nih.gov/2016/03/22/resurgence-of-measles-pertussis-fueled-by-vaccine-refusals/ (accessed February 13, 2018).

Columbus, Courtney. "Drug for 'Neglected' Chagas Disease Gains FDA Approval Amid Price Worries." NPR, September 10, 2017. https://www.npr.org/sections/health-shots/2017/09/10/547351794/drug-for-neglected-chagas-disease-gains-fda-approval-amid-price-worries (accessed January 18, 2017).

"Common Cold." Mayo Clinic, 2017. https://www.mayoclinic.org/diseases-conditions/common-cold/symptoms-causes/syc-20351605 (accessed December 6, 2017).

"Common Cold." MedlinePlus, 2017. https://medlineplus.gov/commoncold.html (accessed January 5, 2018).

"Common Cold." PubMed Health, 2017. https://www.ncbi.nlm.nih.gov/pubmedhealth/PMHT0024671/ (accessed December 6, 2017).

"Conjunctivitis (Pink Eye)." Centers for Disease Control and Prevention, October 2, 2017. https://www.cdc.gov/conjunctivitis/index.html (accessed November 20, 2017).

"Conjunctivitis (Pinkeye)." WebMD. https://www.webmd.com/eye-health/eye-health-conjunctivitis#1 (accessed November 20, 2017).

"The Control of Neglected Zoonotic Diseases: Community-Based Interventions for Prevention and Control." World Health Organization, November 2010. http://apps.who.int/iris/bitstream/10665/44746/1/9789241502528_eng.pdf?ua=1 (accessed January 31, 2018).

"Co-Receptors: CCR5—Understanding HIV." The Body Pro, January 2003. http://www.thebodypro.com/content/art4978.html (accessed March 6, 2018).

Corey, Lawrence. “Designing CAR T Cells for HIV: A Link between Cancer and Infectious Disease Therapy.” International AIDS Society, 2017. http://www.iasociety.org/Web/WebContent/File/HIV_Cure_Forum_2017/Session%206_RT/2%20IS5-2_Corey.pdf (accessed March 8, 2018).

“Correctional Health.” Centers for Disease Control and Prevention, May 13, 2016. https://www.cdc.gov/correctionalhealth/ (accessed February 9, 2018).

“Cost to Develop New Pharmaceutical Drug Now Exceeds $2.5B.” Scientific American, 2014. https://www.scientificamerican.com/article/cost−to−develop−new−pharmaceutical−drug−now−exceeds−2−5b/ (accessed November 8, 2017).

“Countries with the Most Dogs Worldwide.” WorldAtlas.com, April 25, 2017. https://www.worldatlas.com/articles/countries-with-the-most-dogs-worldwide.html (accessed January 26, 2018).

“Creutzfeldt-Jakob Disease, Classic (CJD).” Centers for Disease Control and Prevention, February 6, 2015. https://www.cdc.gov/prions/cjd/index.html (accessed January 29, 2018).

“Creutzfeldt-Jakob Disease Fact Sheet. National Institute of Neurological Disorders and Stroke, May 10, 2017. https://www.ninds.nih.gov/Disorders/Patient-Caregiver-Education/Fact-Sheets/Creutzfeldt-Jakob-Disease-Fact-Sheet (accessed January 29, 2018).

“Creutzfeldt-Jakob Disease Surveillance in the UK.” National CJD Research and Surveillance Unit, University of Edinburgh, 2016. https://www.cjd.ed.ac.uk/sites/default/files/report25.pdf (accessed January 29, 2018).

“Crimean-Congo Hemorrhagic Fever.” Centers for Disease Control and Prevention, May 9, 2015. https://www.cdc.gov/vhf/crimean-congo/index.html (accessed January 19, 2018).

“Crimean-Congo Haemorrhagic Fever.” European Center for Disease Prevention and Control. https://ecdc.europa.eu/en/crimean-congo-haemorrhagic-fever (accessed January 19, 2018).

“Crimean-Congo Haemorrhagic Fever.” World Health Organization. http://www.who.int/csr/disease/crimean_congoHF/en/ (accessed January 19, 2018).

“Crypto Outbreaks Linked to Swimming Have Doubled Since 2014.” CDC Newsroom, May 18, 2017. https://www.cdc.gov/media/releases/2017/p0518-cryptosporidium-outbreaks.html (accessed January 16, 2018).

“Cryptosporidiosis.” European Centre for Disease Prevention and Control. https://ecdc.europa.eu/en/cryptosporidiosis (accessed January 16, 2018).

“Cumulative Number of Confirmed Human Cases for Avian Influenza A(H5n1) Reported to WHO, 2003–2018.” World Health Organization, January 25, 2018. http://www.who.int/influenza/human_animal_interface/2018_01_25_tableH5N1.pdf?ua=1 (accessed February 22, 2018).

“The Current Evidence for the Burden of Group A Streptococcal Diseases.” Department of Child and Adolescent Health and Development, World Health Organization. http://apps.who.int/iris/bitstream/10665/69063/1/WHO_FCH_CAH_05.07.pdf?ua=1&ua=1 (accessed January 30, 2018).

“Cyclosporiasis (Cyclospora Infection).” Centers for Disease Control and Prevention, July 28, 2016. https://www.cdc.gov/parasites/cyclosporiasis/index.html (accessed December 18, 2017).“Increase in Reported Cases of *Cyclospora cayetanensis* Infection, United States, Summer 2017.” Centers for Disease Control and Prevention Health Alert Network, August 7, 2017. https://emergency.cdc.gov/han/han00405.asp (accessed December 18, 2017).

“Cytomegalovirus (CMV) and Congenital CMV Infection.” Centers for Disease Control and Prevention, June 5, 2017. https://www.cdc.gov/cmv/index.html (accessed February 2, 2018).

“Declaration of the Rights of the Child.” UNICEF. https://www.unicef.org/malaysia/1959-Declaration-of-the-Rights-of-the-Child.pdf (accessed January 16, 2018).

De Lima Corvino, Daniela F., and Steve S. Bhimji. “Ascariasis.” National Center for Biotechnology Information, May 25, 2017. https://www.ncbi.nlm.nih.gov/books/NBK430796/ (accessed January 10, 2018).

“Dengue.” Centers for Disease Control and Prevention. https://www.cdc.gov/dengue/epidemiology/index.html (accessed January 14, 2018).

“Dengue and Severe Dengue.” World Health Organization, April 2017. http://www.who.int/mediacentre/factsheets/fs117/en/ (accessed December 11, 2017).

"Dengue: Epidemiology." Centers for Disease Control and Prevention, June 9, 2014. http://www.cdc.gov/dengue/epidemiology/index.html (accessed December 11, 2017).

Dewan, Angela, and Henrik Pettersson. "Cholera Outbreak Hits Record 1 Million." CNN, December 21, 2017. https://www.cnn.com/2017/12/21/health/yemen-cholera-intl/index.html (accessed February 12, 2018).

"Diagnosis and Management of Gonococcemia: Differential Diagnoses." Medscape, 2010. https://www.medscape.org/viewarticle/724973 (accessed January 21, 2017).

"Diarrhoea." World Health Organization. http://www.who.int/topics/diarrhoea/en (accessed November 16, 2017).

Díaz, Herminio R. Hernández. "The Common Cold." Pan American Health Organization. http://www.paho.org/English/AD/DPC/CD/AIEPI-1–3.9.pdf (accessed December 6, 2017).

Di Bisceglie, Adrian M. "TT Virus and Other Anelloviruses." UpToDate, September 5, 2017. https://www.uptodate.com/contents/tt-virus-and-other-anelloviruses (accessed February 1, 2018).

"Diphtheria." Mayo Clinic, December 8, 2016. https://www.mayoclinic.org/diseases-conditions/diphtheria/symptoms-causes/syc-20351897 (accessed February 14, 2018).

"Diphtheria." Todar's Online Textbook of Bacteriology. http://textbookofbacteriology.net/diphtheria.html (accessed February 14, 2018).

"Diphtheria." World Health Organization. http://www.who.int/topics/diphtheria/en/ (accessed February 14, 2018).

"Diphtheria: Clinicians." Centers for Disease Control and Prevention, January 15, 2016. https://www.cdc.gov/diphtheria/clinicians.html (accessed February 14, 2018).

"Diphtheria, Tetanus, and Whooping Cough Vaccination: What Everyone Should Know." Centers for Disease Control and Prevention, November 22, 2016. https://www.cdc.gov/vaccines/vpd/dtap-tdap-td/public/index.html (accessed February 14, 2018).

"Diphtheria Vaccination." Centers for Disease Control and Prevention, November 22, 2016. https://www.cdc.gov/vaccines/vpd/diphtheria/index.html (accessed February 14, 2018).

"Disease Outbreak Alerts." Equine Disease Communication Center. http://www.equinediseasecc.org/alerts/outbreaks (accessed December 17, 2017)."Eastern Equine Encephalitis." Centers for Disease Control and Prevention, April 5, 2016. https://www.cdc.gov/easternequineencephalitis/index.html (accessed December 17, 2017).

"Disease Outbreak News." World Health Organization. http://www.who.int/csr/don/en (accessed December 11, 2017).

"Division of Vector-Borne Diseases." Centers for Disease Control and Prevention. https://www.cdc.gov/ncezid/dvbd/index.html (accessed December 6, 2017).

Doucleff, Michaeleen. "Why Mumps and Measles Can Spread Even When We're Vaccinated." NPR, April 18, 2014. https://www.npr.org/sections/health-shots/2014/04/18/304155213/why-mumps-and-measles-can-spread-even-when-were-vaccinated (accessed February 15, 2018).

"Dracunculiasis Eradication." World Health Organization. http://www.who.int/dracunculiasis/en/ (accessed November 15, 2017).

"Drinking-Water." World Health Organization, July 2017. http://www.who.int/mediacentre/factsheets/fs391/en/ (accessed March 2, 2018).

"Drinking Water Requirements for States and Public Water Systems: Stage 1 and Stage 2 Disinfectants and Disinfection Byproducts Rule." United States Environmental Protection Agency. https://www.epa.gov/dwreginfo/stage-1-and-stage-2-disinfectants-and-disinfection-byproducts-rules (accessed November 15, 2017).

"Drug-Resistant TB: XDR-TB FAQ." World Health Organization. http://www.who.int/tb/areas-of-work/drug-resistant-tb/xdr-tb-faq/en/ (accessed March 7, 2018).

"Drug Treatments." Medical Research Council Prion Unit, 2018. http://www.prion.ucl.ac.uk/clinic-services/research/drug-treatments (accessed January 29, 2018).

"Drugs Used in HIV-Related Infections." World Health Organization, 1999. http://apps.who.int/medicinedocs/en/d/Js2215e/7.3.html#Js2215e.7.3 (accessed February 5, 2018).

"*E. coli (Escherichia coli)*." Centers for Disease Control and Prevention. http://www.cdc.gov/ecoli/index.html (accessed January 12, 2018).

"Ear Infections in Children." National Institute on Deafness and Other Communication Disorders. https://www.nidcd.nih.gov/health/ear-infections-children (accessed November 15, 2017).

"Eastern, Western and Venezuelan Equine Encephalomyelitis." Iowa State University Center for Food Security and Public Health, January 2015. http://lib.dr.iastate.edu/cfsph_factsheets/49 (accessed February 25, 2018).

"Ebola Virus Disease." World Health Organization, June 2017. http://www.who.int/mediacentre/factsheets/fs103/en/ (accessed November 15, 2017).

"Echinococcosis Fact Sheet." World Health Organization, March 2017. http://www.who.int/mediacentre/factsheets/fs377/en/ (accessed November 6, 2017).

"ECOSOC." United Nations Economic and Social Council. https://www.un.org/ecosoc/ (accessed January 16, 2018).

"Eliminating Malaria." World Health Organization, 2016. http://apps.who.int/iris/bitstream/10665/205565/1/WHO_HTM_GMP_2016.3_eng.pdf (accessed February 23, 2018).

Ellerington, Alina. "Japanese Encephalitis." Encephalitis Society, December 2017. https://www.encephalitis.info/japaneseencephalitis?gclid=Cj0KCQiA_JTUBRD4ARIsAL7_VeU9jpuLE074M7r78ZxAUvongEtvtrzzHLkH19KNR9SHV-6MDT2Ps5IaAqaDEALw_wcB (accessed February 15, 2018).

"Emergency Preparedness and Response." Centers for Disease Control and Prevention. https://emergency.cdc.gov/planning/index.asp (accessed January 31, 2018).

"Emergency Preparedness and Response: Tularemia." Centers for Disease Control and Prevention, November 18, 2015. https://emergency.cdc.gov/agent/tularemia/index.asp (accessed February 9, 2018).

"Emerging Infectious Diseases/Pathogens." National Institute of Allergy and Infectious Diseases. https://www.niaid.nih.gov/research/emerging-infectious-diseases-pathogens (accessed November 15, 2017).

"Emerging Pandemic Threats." USAID, May 24, 2016. https://www.usaid.gov/news-information/fact-sheets/emerging-pandemic-threats-program (accessed January 31, 2018).

"Ending AIDS: Progress Towards the 90–90–90 Targets." UNAIDS, July 20, 2017. http://www.unaids.org/en/resources/documents/2017/20170720_Global_AIDS_update_2017 (accessed December 17, 2017).

Engelberg, Stephen. "New Evidence Adds Doubt to FBI's Case against Anthrax Suspect." ProPublica, October 10, 2011. https://www.propublica.org/article/new-evidence-disputes-case-against-bruce-e-ivins (accessed January 11, 2018).

"Enterobiasis (Also Known as Pinworm Infection): Epidemiology & Risk Factors." Centers for Disease Control and Prevention, January 10, 2013. https://www.cdc.gov/parasites/pinworm/epi.html (accessed March 10, 2018).

"Enterovirus 71 (EV71) Infection—Including Symptoms, Treatment and Prevention." SA Health, Government of South Australia. http://www.sahealth.sa.gov.au/wps/wcm/connect/public+content/sa+health+internet/health+topics/health+conditions+prevention+and+treatment/infectious+diseases/enterovirus+71+ev71+infection/enterovirus+71+%28ev71%29+infection+-+inlcuding+symptoms+treatment+and+prevention (accessed February 5, 2018).

"Enterovirus 71 (EV71) Neurological Disease." Queensland Government, December 10, 2017. http://conditions.health.qld.gov.au/HealthCondition/condition/14/217/45/Enterovirus-71-EV71-Neurological-Disease (accessed February 5, 2018).

"Enterovirus 71 Infection." Centre for Health Protection, Department of Health, Government of the Hong Kong Special Administrative Region, April 5, 2017. https://www.chp.gov.hk/en/healthtopics/content/24/12431.html (accessed February 5, 2018).

"Epidemiological Notes: Influenza." World Health Organization, 1957. http://www.who.int/iris/handle/10665/211117 (accessed January 20, 2018).

"Epidemiology and Ecology of Eastern Equine Encephalomyelitis." US Department of Agriculture, April 2004. https://www.aphis.usda.gov/animal_health/emergingissues/downloads/EEE042004.pdf (accessed December 17, 2017).

"Epidemiology and Statistics." Centers for Disease Control and Prevention, December 26, 2017. https://www.cdc.gov/qfever/stats/index.html (accessed February 25, 2018).

"Epidemiology of HIV Infection through 2016." Centers for Disease Control and Prevention. https://www.cdc.gov/hiv/pdf/library/slidesets/cdc-hiv-surveillance-genepi-2016.pdf (accessed December 5, 2017).

"Epstein-Barr Virus and Infectious Mononucleosis." Centers for Disease Control and Prevention, September 14, 2016. https://www.cdc.gov/epstein-barr/index.html (accessed January 24, 2018).

"Essential Medicines." World Health Organization. http://www.who.int/topics/essential_medicines/en/ (accessed March 1, 2018).

"Estimates of Foodborne Illness in the United States." Centers for Disease Control and Prevention. http://www.cdc.gov/foodborneburden/burden/index.html (accessed November 16, 2017).

"Estimating Seasonal Influenza-Associated Deaths in the United States." Centers for Disease Control and Prevention, December 9, 2016. https://www.cdc.gov/flu/about/disease/us_flu-related_deaths.htm (accessed January 22, 2018).

"EU/3/16/1777." European Medicines Agency, December 14, 2016. http://www.ema.europa.eu/ema/index.jsp?curl=pages/medicines/human/orphans/2016/12/human_orphan_001896.jsp&mid=WC0b01ac058001d12b (accessed January 24, 2018).

"European Creutzfeldt-Jakob Disease Surveillance Network (EuroCJD)." European Centre for Disease Prevention and Control. https://ecdc.europa.eu/en/about-us/partnerships-and-networks/disease-and-laboratory-networks/european-creutzfeldt-jakob (accessed February 1, 2018).

Executive Order 13676 of September 18, 2014, Combating Antibiotic-Resistant Bacteria. Obama White House. https://obamawhitehouse.archives.gov/the-press-office/2014/09/18/executive-order-combating-antibiotic-resistant-bacteria (accessed February 25, 2018).

"Exposure to Blood: What Healthcare Personnel Need to Know." Centers for Disease Control and Prevention, July 2003. https://www.cdc.gov/hai/pdfs/bbp/exp_to_blood.pdf (accessed February 23, 2018).

"Extraordinary Progress against AIDS." NBC News, July 14, 2015. https://www.nbcnews.com/health/health-news/extraordinary-progress-against-aids-report-n391861 (accessed March 6, 2018.)

"Fact Sheet: Gonorrhea." Centers for Disease Control and Prevention (CDC), June 2017. https://www.cdc.gov/std/gonorrhea/Gonorrhea-FS-June-2017.pdf (accessed January 21, 2017).

"Fact Sheet: World Malaria Report 2016." World Health Organization, December 13, 2016. http://www.who.int/malaria/media/world-malaria-report-2016/en/ (accessed December 6, 2017).

"Fact Sheets: Neglected Tropical Diseases." World Health Organization. http://www.who.int/topics/tropical_diseases/factsheets/neglected/en/ (accessed January 20, 2018).

"Fact Sheets: Tropical Diseases." World Health Organization. http://www.who.int/topics/tropical_diseases/factsheets/en/ (accessed January 19, 2018).

"Factors Increasing the Risk of Acquiring or Transmitting HIV." Centers for Disease Control and Prevention. https://www.cdc.gov/hiv/risk/estimates/riskfactors.html (accessed December 3, 2017).

"Facts about Louse-Borne Relapsing Fever." European Centre for Disease Prevention and Control. https://ecdc.europa.eu/en/louse-borne-relapsing-fever/facts (accessed November 16, 2017).

"Fascioliasis (Fasciola Infection)." Centers for Disease Control and Prevention, January 10, 2013. https://www.cdc.gov/parasites/fasciola/index.html (accessed January 5, 2018).

"FDA Review of the 2014 Discovery of Vials Labeled '*Variola*' and Other Vials Discovered in and FDA-Occupied Building on the NIH Campus." US Food and Drug Administration, December 13, 2016. https://www.fda.gov/downloads/AboutFDA/ReportsManualsForms/Reports/UCM532877.pdf (accessed January 29, 2018).

"Federal Engagement in Antimicrobial Resistance." Centers for Disease Control and Prevention. https://www.cdc.gov/drugresistance/federal-engagement-in-ar/index.html (accessed February 26, 2018).

"Filariasis." National Organization for Rare Disorders. https://rarediseases.org/rare-diseases/filariasis/ (accessed January 22, 2018).

"Final Results Confirm Ebola Vaccine Provides High Protection against Disease." World Health Organization, December 23, 2016. http://www

.who.int/mediacentre/news/releases/2016/ebola-vaccine-results/en/ (accessed November 15, 2017).

"Final Trial Results Confirm Ebola Vaccine Provides High Protection against Disease." World Health Organization. http://www.who.int/mediacentre/news/releases/2016/ebola-vaccine-results/en/ (accessed November 15, 2017).

"Founding of MSF." Doctors Without Borders/Médecins Sans Frontières. http://www.doctorswithoutborders.org/founding-msf (accessed February 27, 2018).

"Fresh Pork from Farm to Table." US Department of Agriculture, August 6, 2013. https://www.fsis.usda.gov/wps/portal/fsis/topics/food-safety-education/get-answers/food-safety-fact-sheets/meat-preparation/fresh-pork-from-farm-to-table/CT_Index (accessed January 30, 2018).

Fried, Susana T., and Debra J. Lebowitz. "What the Solution Isn't: The Parallel of the Zika and HIV Viruses for Women. Lancet Global Health Blog, February 16, 2016. http://globalhealth.thelancet.com/2016/02/16/what-solution-isnt-parallel-zika-and-hiv-viruses-women (accessed January 24, 2018).

"Funding for HIV and AIDS." Avert. https://www.avert.org/professionals/hiv-around-world/global-response/funding (accessed December 30, 2017).

"Fungal Diseases." Centers for Disease Control and Prevention, September 6, 2017. https://www.cdc.gov/fungal/index.html (accessed January 25, 2018).

"Fungal Diseases: People Living with HIV/AIDS." Centers for Disease Control and Prevention. https://www.cdc.gov/fungal/infections/hiv-aids.html (accessed January 25, 2018).

Gamache, Justina. "Bacterial Pneumonia Medication." Medscape, June 20, 2017. https://emedicine.medscape.com/article/300157-medication (accessed January 24, 2018).

"Gastrointestinal Amebiasis." Harvard Health Publishing. https://www.health.harvard.edu/digestive-health/gastrointestinal-amebiasis (accessed November 7, 2017).

"GenBank Overview." National Center for Biotechnology Information (NCBI). https://www.ncbi.nlm.nih.gov/genbank/ (accessed February 28, 2018).

"General Background: About Antibiotic Resistance." Alliance for the Prudent Use of Antibiotics. http://emerald.tufts.edu/med/apua/about_issue/about_antibioticres.shtml (accessed November 15, 2017).

"Genital Herpes." Centers for Disease Control and Prevention, September 1, 2017. https://www.cdc.gov/std/herpes/stdfact-herpes.htm (accessed January 29, 2018).

"Genital Herpes: CDC Fact Sheet." Centers for Disease Control and Prevention, September 1, 2017. https://www.cdc.gov/std/herpes/stdfact-herpes.htm (accessed February 27, 2018).

"Genital HSV Infections." Centers for Disease Control and Prevention, June 8, 2015. http://www.cdc.gov/std/tg2015/herpes.htm (accessed February 17, 2018).

"Genotypes of Hepatitis C." Hepatitis C Trust. http://www.hepctrust.org.uk/information/about-hepatitis-c-virus/genotypes-hepatitis-c (accessed February 19, 2018).

Georges, Helen. "Alliance for Cervical Cancer Prevention Receives $50 Million Gift from Bill and Melinda Gates." Bill & Melinda Gates Foundation. https://www.gatesfoundation.org/Media-Center/Press-Releases/1999/09/Alliance-for-Cervical-Cancer-Prevention (accessed January 26, 2018).

"Germ Theory." *Contagion: Historical Views of Diseases and Epidemics.* Harvard University Library. http://ocp.hul.harvard.edu/contagion/germtheory.html (accessed December 1, 2017).

"GIDEON Content-Outbreaks." GIDEON, 2018. https://www.gideononline.com (accessed December 11, 2017).

Gilbert, Charles E. "Concern with Communicable (Infectious) Diseases of Raccoons." Epidemiology and Toxicology Institute. http://www.epidemiologyandtoxicology.org/raccoons.html (accessed December 17, 2017).

"Glanders." Centers for Disease Control and Prevention, October 31, 2017. https://www.cdc.gov/glanders/index.html (accessed February 7, 2018).

"Global Enteric Multicenter Study (GEMS)." University of Maryland School of Medicine. http://www.medschool.umaryland.edu/GEMS/ (accessed January 16, 2018).

"Global Foodborne Infections Network (GFN)." World Health Organization. http://www.who.int/gfn/en/ (accessed November 21, 2017).

"Global Health Observatory (GHO) Data: Vaccination Coverage." World Health Organization. http://www.who.int/gho/immunization/en/ (accessed February 13, 2018).

"Global Health Sector Strategy on Sexually Transmitted Infections 2016–2021: Towards Ending STIs." World Health Organization, June 2016. http://apps.who.int/iris/bitstream/10665/246296/1/WHO-RHR-16.09-eng.pdf?ua=1 (accessed March 6, 2018).

"Global Hepatitis Report, 2017." World Health Organization. http://apps.who.int/iris/bitstream/10665/255016/1/9789241565455-eng.pdf?ua=1 (accessed February 19, 2018).

"Global HIV/AIDS Timeline." Henry J. Kaiser Family Foundation, November 29, 2016. https://www.kff.org/global-health-policy/timeline/global-hivaids-timeline/ (Accessed December 23, 2017).

"Global Incidence and Prevalence of Selected Curable Sexually Transmitted Infections—2008." World Health Organization, 2012. http://apps.who.int/iris/bitstream/10665/75181/1/9789241503839_eng.pdf (accessed January 25, 2018).

"Global Outbreak Alert and Response Network (GOARN)." World Health Organization. http://www.who.int/csr/outbreaknetwork/en (accessed February 27, 2018).

Global Polio Eradication Initiative. http://www.polioeradication.org/ (accessed January 18, 2018).

"Global WASH Fact Facts." Centers for Disease Control and Prevention, April 11, 2016. https://www.cdc.gov/healthywater/global/wash_statistics.html (accessed January 31, 2018).

"Gonococcal Isolate Surveillance Project (GISP) Supplement & Profiles." Centers for Disease Control and Prevention (CDC), Division of STD Prevention, February 2016. https://www.cdc.gov/std/gisp2014/gisp-2014-text-fig-tables.pdf (accessed January 21, 2017).

"GPEI: Wild Poliovirus List. Global Polio Eradication Initiative, 2018. http://polioeradication.org/polio-today/polio-now/wild-poliovirus-list/ (accessed February 1, 2018).

"Group A Streptococcal (GAS) Disease." Centers for Disease Control and Prevention, September 16, 2016. https://www.cdc.gov/groupAstrep/index.html> (accessed December 9, 2017).

"Group B Strep (GBS)." Centers for Disease Control and Prevention (CDC), May 23, 2016. https://www.cdc.gov/groupbstrep/about/index.html (accessed January 23, 2018).

"Group B Strep Infection: GBS." American Pregnancy Association, March 2, 2017. http://americanpregnancy.org/pregnancy-complications/group-b-strep-infection/ (accessed January 23, 2018).

Guerina, Nicholas, and Lucila Marquez. "Congenital Toxoplasmosis: Clinical Features and Diagnosis." UpToDate. http://www.uptodate.com/contents/congenital-toxoplasmosis-clinical-features-and-diagnosis (accessed on November 22, 2017).

"Guidance for Managing Ethical Issues in Infectious Disease Outbreaks." World Health Organization, 2016. http://apps.who.int/iris/bitstream/10665/250580/1/9789241549837-eng.pdf (accessed February 28, 2018).

"Guidelines for Prevention and Treatment of Opportunistic Infections in HIV-Infected Adults and Adolescents: Recommendations from CDC, the National Institutes of Health, and the HIV Medicine Association of the Infectious Diseases Society of America." Centers for Disease Control and Prevention. https://www.cdc.gov/mmwr/preview/mmwrhtml/rr58e324a1.htm (accessed December 5, 2017.

"Guidelines for the Prevention, Care and Treatment of Persons with Chronic Hepatitis B Infection." World Health Organization (WHO), March 2015. http://apps.who.int/iris/bitstream/10665/154590/1/9789241549059_eng.pdf?ua=1&ua=1 (accessed February 2, 2018)

"Guidelines for the Screening, Care and Treatment of Persons with Chronic Hepatitis C Infection." World Health Organization. http://apps.who.int/iris/bitstream/10665/205035/1/9789241549615_eng.pdf?ua=1 (accessed February 19, 2018).

"Guidelines for the Surveillance and Control of Anthrax in Humans and Animals." World Health Organization. http://www.who.int/csr/resources/publications/anthrax/WHO_EMC_ZDI_98_6/en (accessed January 11, 2018).

"Guidelines for the Treatment of Malaria, 3rd ed." World Health Organization, 2015. http://apps.who.int/iris/bitstream/10665/162441/1/9789241549127_eng.pdf?ua=1&ua=1 (accessed February 26, 2018).

"Guinea Worm Case Totals." The Carter Center, November 13, 2017. https://www.cartercenter.org/health/guinea_worm/case-totals.html (accessed November 15, 2017).

Haelle, Tara. "CDC Endorses a More Effective HPV Vaccine to Prevent Cancer." NPR, February 1, 2016. https://www.npr.org/sections/health-shots/2016/02/01/465160937/cdc-endorses-a-more-effective-hpv-vaccine-to-prevent-cancer (accessed February 20, 2018).

"Haemophilus Influenza Type B (Hib)." World Health Organization. http://www.who.int/immunization/diseases/hib/en/ (accessed November 17, 2017).

"*Haemophilus influenzae* Disease (Including Hib)." Centers for Disease Control and Prevention. https://www.cdc.gov/hi-disease/index.html (accessed November 17, 2017).

"Haemorrhagic Fevers, Viral." World Health Organization. http://www.who.int/topics/haemorrhagic_fevers_viral/en (accessed November 17, 2017).

"Hand Hygiene in Healthcare Settings." Centers for Disease Control and Prevention, March 24, 2017. https://www.cdc.gov/handhygiene/index.html (accessed January 16, 2017).

"Hand, Foot & Mouth Disease." Centers for Disease Control and Prevention, June 26, 2017. https://www.cdc.gov/features/handfootmouthdisease/index.html (accessed February 5, 2018).

"Handwashing: Clean Hands Save Lives." Centers for Disease Control and Prevention, December 8, 2017. https://www.cdc.gov/handwashing/index.html (accessed December 4, 2017).

"Hand-washing: Do's and Don't's." Mayo Clinic. https://www.mayoclinic.org/healthy-lifestyle/adult-health/in-depth/hand-washing/art-20046253 (accessed December 11, 2017).

"Hansen's Disease (Leprosy)." Centers for Disease Control and Prevention, February 10, 2017. https://www.cdc.gov/leprosy/ (accessed February 9, 2018).

"Hantavirus." Centers for Disease Control and Prevention. http://www.cdc.gov/hantavirus/hps/index.html (accessed December 11, 2017).

"Hantavirus Pulmonary Syndrome." Mayo Clinic. https://www.mayoclinic.org/diseases-conditions/hantavirus-pulmonary-syndrome/symptoms-causes/syc-20351838 (accessed December 11, 2017).

Hartmann, Erica. "Banned Antimicrobial Chemicals Found in Many Household Products." CNN. January 25, 2017. http://www.cnn.com/2017/01/25/health/triclosan-household-items-partner/index.html (accessed November 17, 2017).

Hataway, James. "Beating the Clock: UGA Researchers Develop New Treatment for Rabies." UGAToday, January 26, 2015. https://news.uga.edu/beating-the-clock-researchers-develop-new-rabies-treatment-0115/ (accessed February 19, 2018).

Hays, Brooks. "Scientists Develop Potential Late-Stage Rabies Treatment." UPI, January 29, 2015. https://www.upi.com/Science_News/2015/01/29/Scientists-develop-potential-late-stage-rabies-treatment/9691422485373/ (accessed February 20, 2018).

"Health Alert: Increased Flea-Borne (Murine) Typhus Activity in Texas." Texas Department of State Health Services, November 30, 2017. http://www.dshs.texas.gov/news/releases/2017/HealthAlert-11302017.aspx (accessed January 22, 2018).

"Health Care-Associated Infections: Fact Sheet." World Health Organization. http://www.who.int/gpsc/country_work/gpsc_ccisc_fact_sheet_en.pdf?ua=1 (accessed February 21, 2018).

"Health Equity." Centers for Disease Control and Prevention. https://www.cdc.gov/healthequity/index.html (accessed February 15, 2018).

"Health in 2015: From MDGs to SDGs." World Health Organization, 2015. http://apps.who.int/iris/bitstream/10665/200009/1/9789241565110_eng.pdf?ua=1 (accessed March 9, 2018).

"Health Systems Dangerously Inadequate for Dealing with Emergencies Like Ebola." UK Parliament, Commons Select Committee, December 18, 2014. http://www.parliament.uk/business/committees/committees-a-z/commons-select/international-development-committee/news/report-responses-to-ebola-crisis/ (accessed February 10, 2018).

"Health Workers Urged to Work with Communities to Stop Marburg." World Health Organization, November 4, 2017. http://www.afro.who.int/news/health-workers-urged-work-communities-stop-marburg (accessed November 29, 2017).

"Healthcare-Associated Infections." Centers for Disease Control and Prevention, July 14, 2017. https://www.cdc.gov/hai/index.html (accessed November 17, 2017).

"Healthy Swimming." Centers for Disease Control and Prevention. https://www.cdc.gov/healthywater/swimming/swimmers/rwi/rashes.html (accessed November 17, 2017).

"Heartland Virus." Centers for Disease Control and Prevention. https://www.cdc.gov/heartland-virus/index.html (accessed March 2, 2018).

Helicobacter Foundation. http://www.helico.com/ (accessed March 6, 2018).

"*Helicobacter pylori* (*H. pylori*) infection." Mayo Clinic, May 17, 2017. https://www.mayoclinic.org/diseases-conditions/h-pylori/symptoms-causes/syc-20356171 (accessed March 6, 2018).

"Helminth Parasites." Australian Society of Parasitology. http://parasite.org.au/para-site/contents/helminth-intoduction.html (accessed January 29, 2017).

"Hepatitis A." World Health Organization, July 2017. http://www.who.int/mediacentre/factsheets/fs328/en/ (accessed January 22, 2018).

"Hepatitis B VIS." Center for Disease Control and Prevention, October 18, 2016 https://www.cdc.gov/vaccines/hcp/vis/vis-statements/hep-b.html (accessed January 26, 2018).

"Hepatitis B." World Health Organization (WHO), July 2017. http://www.who.int/mediacentre/factsheets/fs204/en/ (accessed February 2, 2018).

"Hepatitis C." World Health Organization. http://www.who.int/mediacentre/factsheets/fs164/en/ (accessed February 19, 2018).

"Hepatitis D." Centers for Disease Control and Prevention, December 8, 2015. https://www.cdc.gov/hepatitis/hdv/index.htm (accessed January 9, 2018).

"Hepatitis D." World Health Organization, July 2017. http://www.who.int/mediacentre/factsheets/hepatitis-d/en/ (accessed January 9, 2017).

Hepatitis Delta. http://hepatitis-delta.org/ (accessed January 10, 2017).

"Hepatitis E." World Health Organization, July 2017. http://www.who.int/mediacentre/factsheets/fs280/en/ (accessed February 7, 2018).

"Herpes Simplex Virus." World Health Organization, January 2017. http://www.who.int/mediacentre/factsheets/fs400/en/ (accessed March 15, 2018).

Hewings-Martin, Yella. "Food Additive to Blame for *C. difficile* epidemic." Medical News Today, January 4, 2018. https://www.medicalnewstoday.com/articles/320520.php (accessed January 31, 2018).

"Hib Initiative: A GAVI Success Story." Global Alliance for Vaccines and Immunization. http://www.gavi.org/library/news/roi/2010/hib-initiative--a-gavi-success-story/ (accessed November 17, 2017).

Highleyman, Liz. "Hepatitis C Vaccine Shows Progress but Scientific Barriers Remain." World Hepatitis Alliance, September 12, 2016. http://www.worldhepatitisalliance.org/latest-news/infohep/3084554/hepatitis-c-vaccine-development-shows-progress-scientific-barriers-remain (accessed February 26, 2018).

"Highly Pathogenic Asian Avian Influenza A (H5N1) Virus." Centers for Disease Control and Prevention, October 14, 2015. https://www.cdc.gov/flu/avianflu/h5n1-virus.htm (accessed February 22, 2018).

"Histoplasmosis." Centers for Disease Control and Prevention, November 21, 2015. https://www.cdc.gov/fungal/diseases/histoplasmosis/index.html (accessed January 23, 2018).

"Histoplasmosis." Mayo Clinic. https://www.mayoclinic.org/diseases-conditions/histoplasmosis/symptoms-causes/syc-20373495 (accessed January 23, 2018).

"HIV and AIDS in Asia and the Pacific Regional Overview." Avert. https://www.avert.org/professionals/hiv-around-world/sub-saharan-africa/overview (accessed January 1, 2018).

"HIV and AIDS in East and Southern Africa Regional Overview." Avert. https://www.avert.org/professionals/hiv-around-world/sub-saharan-africa/overview> (accessed January 1, 2018).

"HIV and AIDS in Western Europe and North America Regional Overview." Avert. https://www.avert.org/professionals/hiv-around-world/western europe and north america/overview (accessed January 1, 2018).

"HIV and Viral Hepatitis." Centers for Disease Control and Prevention. https://www.cdc.gov/hiv/pdf/library/factsheets/hiv-viral-hepatitis.pdf (accessed February 20, 2018).

"HIV Vaccine Development." World Health Organization. http://www.who.int/immunization/research/development/hiv_vaccdev/en/ (accessed February 26, 2018).

Hooker, Edmond, "Biological Warfare." eMedicineHealth, November 20, 2017. https://www.emedicinehealth.com/biological_warfare/article_em.htm (accessed January 29, 2018).

"Hookworm." Centers for Disease Control and Prevention. https://www.cdc.gov/parasites/hookworm/ (accessed December 19, 2017).

"Horn of Africa: Emergency-Affected Countries, 2007." World Health Organization, 2007 http://www.who.int/diseasecontrol_emergencies/toolkits/Hoa2.pdf (accessed January 28, 2018).

Hotez, Peter, and Jennifer Herricks. "One Million Deaths by Parasites." *PLOS* Speaking of Medicine Community Blog, January 16, 2015. http://blogs.plos.org/speakingofmedicine/2015/01/16/one-million-deaths-parasites/ (accessed February 23, 2018).

Hotez, Peter, and Serap Aksoy. "Eliminating Lymphatic Filariasis in Cameroon." Speaking of Medicine Community Blog, June 29, 2017. http://blogs.plos.org/speakingofmedicine/2017/06/29/eliminating-lymphatic-filariasis-in-cameroon/ (accessed January 22, 2018).

"How CRISPR Could Snip Away Some of Humanity's Worst Diseases." Wired, May 5, 2017. https://www.wired.com/2017/05/crispr-snip-away-humanitys-worst-diseases (accessed November 21, 2017).

"Human Papillomavirus (HPV)." Centers for Disease Control and Prevention, January 4, 2017. https://www.cdc.gov/std/hpv/default.htm (accessed February 20, 2018).

"Human Papillomavirus (HPV) and Cervical Cancer." World Health Organization, June 2016. http://www.who.int/mediacentre/factsheets/fs380/en/ (accessed February 20, 2018).

"Immunization Coverage." World Health Organization, January 2018. http://www.who.int/mediacentre/factsheets/fs378/en/ (accessed February 13, 2018).

"Immunization, Vaccines and Biologicals: Diphtheria." World Health Organization, August 8, 2017. http://www.who.int/immunization/monitoring_surveillance/burden/diphtheria/en/ (accessed February 14, 2018).

"Impact of an Innovative Approach to Prevent Mother-to-Child Transmission of HIV—Malawi, July 2011–September 2012." Centers for Disease Control and Prevention. https://www.cdc.gov/mmwr/preview/mmwrhtml/mm6208a3.htm (accessed December 2, 2017).

"Impetigo." Medline Plus, December 5, 2017. http://www.nlm.nih.gov/medlineplus/ency/article/000860.htm (accessed December 8, 2017).

"Impetigo: Guidance, Data and Analysis." Public Health England, July 1, 2014. https://www.gov.uk/government/collections/impetigo-guidance-data-and-analysis (accessed December 8, 2017).

"Import Live Animals." United States Department of Agriculture, January 29, 2018. https://www.aphis.usda.gov/aphis/ourfocus/animalhealth/animal-and-animal-product-import-information/import-live-animals (accessed January 26, 2018).

"Increase in Scarlet Fever across England." Public Health England, March 11, 2016. https://www.gov.uk/government/news/increase-in-scarlet-fever-across-england (accessed December 9, 2017).

"Increased Antiviral Medication Sales before the 2005–06 Influenza Season—New York City." Centers for Disease Control and Prevention, March 16, 2006. http://www.cdc.gov/mmwr/preview/mmwrhtml/mm5510a3.htm (accessed March 11, 2018).

"Infection Control." Centers for Disease Control and Prevention. https://www.cdc.gov/infectioncontrol/index.html (accessed November 15, 2017).

"Infection Prevention and Control." World Health Organization. http://who.int/infection-prevention/en/ (accessed November 21, 2017).

"Influenza." World Health Organization. http://www.who.int/influenza/en/ (accessed January 19, 2018).

"Influenza (Avian and Other Zoonotic)." World Health Organization, January 2018. http://www.who.int/mediacentre/factsheets/avian_influenza/en/ (accessed February 22, 2018).

"Influenza (Flu)." Centers for Disease Control and Prevention (January 19, 2018). https://www.cdc.gov/flu/ (accessed January 19, 2018).

"Influenza Pandemics." The History of Vaccines, 2018. https://www.historyofvaccines.org/content/articles/influenza-pandemics (accessed March 11, 2018).

"Influenza Surveillance and Monitoring." World Health Organization. http://www.who.int/influenza/surveillance_monitoring/en/ (accessed March 11, 2018).

"Infographic: Progress Toward an HIV Vaccine." National Institute of Allergy and Infectious Diseases, May 18, 2016. https://www.niaid.nih.gov/news-events/progress-toward-hiv-vaccine (accessed March 14, 2018).

"Information on Avian Influenza." Centers for Disease Control and Prevention. http://www.cdc.gov/flu/avianflu/index.htm (accessed December 6, 2017).

International Alliance for the Control of Scabies. http://www.controlscabies.org/ (accessed November 13, 2017).

"International Health Regulations (IHR)." World Health Organization. http://www.who.int/topics/international_health_regulations/en/ (accessed February 25, 2018).

"Intestinal Worms." World Health Organization. http://www.who.int/intestinal_worms/en/ (accessed December 19, 2017).

"Introduction to Superresolution Microscopy." Zeiss. http://zeiss-campus.magnet.fsu.edu/articles/superresolution/introduction.html (accessed January 29, 2018).

"Japanese Encephalitis." World Health Organization. 2015. http://www.who.int/mediacentre/factsheets/fs386/en/ (accessed November 16, 2017).

"John Snow." UCLA Department of Epidemiology, Fielding School of Public Health. http://www.ph.ucla.edu/epi/snow.html (accessed March 30, 2007).

"Kawasaki Disease." US National Library of Medicine—Genetics Home Reference, January 30, 2018. https://ghr.nlm.nih.gov/condition/kawasaki-disease#statistics (accessed February 5, 2018).

"Kawasaki Syndrome." Centers for Disease Control and Prevention, December 13, 2013. https://www.cdc.gov/kawasaki/ (accessed February 5, 2008).

"Kawasaki Syndrome." US Department of Health & Human Services—National Heart, Lung, and Blood Institute. https://www.nhlbi.nih.gov/health-topics/kawasaki-disease (accessed February 5, 2018).

"Keeping You Safe 24–7." Centers for Disease Control and Prevention. https://www.cdc.gov/about/24–7/index.html (accessed January 25, 2018).

"Key Facts about the World's Refugees." Pew Charitable Trust. http://www.pewresearch.org/fact-tank/2016/10/05/key-facts-about-the-worlds-refugees/ (accessed February 6, 2018).

"Key Facts from JMP 2015 Report." World Health Organization. http://www.who.int/water_sanitation_health/monitoring/jmp-2015-key-facts/en/ (accessed February 12, 2018).

Khan, Zartash Zafar. "Kuru." Medscape, February 17, 2016. http://www.emedicine.com/med/topic1248.htm (accessed December 8, 2017).

Kodjak, Alison. "Hepatitis Drug among the Most Costly for Medicaid." NPR. https://www.npr.org/sections/health-shots/2015/12/15/459873815/hepatitis-drug-among-the-most-costly-for-medicaid (accessed February 20, 2018).

Koerth-Baker, Maggie. "To Keep the Blood Supply Safe, Screening Blood Is More Important Than Banning Donors." FiveThirtyEight, June 16, 2016. https://fivethirtyeight.com/features/to-keep-the-blood-supply-safe-screening-blood-is-more-important-than-banning-donors/ (accessed February 12, 2018).

Kohn, Melissa. "Herpes Simplex in Emergency Medicine." Medscape, June 26, 2017

Konkel, Lindsey. "Fungal Diseases Are on the Rise. Is Environmental Change to Blame?" Ensia, April 26, 2017. https://ensia.com/features/19036/ (accessed January 25, 2018).

"Kuru Information Page." National Institute of Neurological Disorders and Stroke, February 14, 2007. https://www.ninds.nih.gov/Disorders/All-Disorders/Kuru-Information-Page (accessed December 8, 2017).

LaMotte, Sandee. "During a Hepatitis A Emergency, There's a Nationwide Shortage of Vaccine." CNN, January 12, 2018. http://www.cnn.com/2017/11/15/health/hepatitis-a-outbreak-vaccine-shortage/index.html (accessed January 22, 2018).

"Lassa Fever." Centers for Disease Control and Prevention. https://www.cdc.gov/vhf/lassa/pdf/factsheet.pdf (accessed February 27, 2018).

"Lassa Fever." World Health Organization (WHO), July 2017. http://www.who.int/mediacentre/factsheets/fs179/en/ (accessed January 24, 2018).

"Latest Information." United Nations Office at Geneva. https://www.unog.ch/bwc/news (accessed January 29, 2018).

Legionella.org. http://www.legionella.org/ (accessed December 7, 2017).

"Legionella (Legionnaires' Disease and Pontiac Fever)." Centers for Disease Control and Prevention, June 1, 2017. https://www.cdc.gov/legionella/fastfacts.html (accessed November 15, 2017).

"Leishmaniasis." Centers for Disease Control and Prevention. https://www.cdc.gov/parasites/leishmaniasis/index.html (accessed February 3, 2018).

"Leishmaniasis." European Centre for Disease Prevention and Control. https://ecdc.europa.eu/en/leishmaniasis (accessed February 3, 2018).

"Leishmaniasis." World Health Organization. http://www.who.int/leishmaniasis/en/// (accessed February 2, 2018).

"Leishmaniasis Fact Sheet." World Health Organization, April 2017. http://www.who.int/mediacentre/factsheets/fs375/en/ (accessed March 1, 2018).

"Leprosy." World Health Organization, January 2018. http://www.who.int/mediacentre/factsheets/fs101/en/ (accessed February 9, 2018).

"Leptospirosis." Centers for Disease Control and Prevention, October 13, 2017. https://www.cdc.gov/leptospirosis/index.html (accessed January 19, 2018).

"Leptospirosis." World Health Organization, August 13, 2012. http://www.wpro.who.int/mediacentre/factsheets/fs_13082012_leptospirosis/en/ (accessed January 19, 2018).

Lessnau, Klaus-Dieter. "Psittacosis (Parrot Fever)." eMedicine, September 8, 2017. https://emedicine.medscape.com/article/227025-overview (accessed December 8, 2017).

Lewis, Michael R. "Scrofula." Medscape. https://emedicine.medscape.com/article/858234-overview (accessed November 6, 2017).

"Life Cycle of Hard Ticks That Spread Disease." Centers for Disease Control and Prevention, April 20, 2017. https://www.cdc.gov/ticks/life_cycle_and_hosts.html (accessed February 25, 2018).

Lindsey, Rebecca. "Climate Change: Global Sea Level." Climate.gov, September 11, 2017. https://www.climate.gov/news-features/understanding-climate/climate-change-global-sea-level (accessed March 2, 2018).

"Listeria (Listeriosis)." Centers for Disease Control and Prevention. https://www.cdc.gov/listeria/index.html (accessed November 20, 2017).

"Listeria Monocytogenes: Policy, Procedures, Guidance." United States Department of Agriculture, June 11, 2015. https://www.fsis.usda.gov/wps/portal/fsis/topics/regulatory-compliance/listeria (accessed November 20, 2017).

Liu, Angus. "Vical's Astellas-Partnered CMV Vaccine Falls Short Again, This Time in Stem Cell Transplant Recipients." FiercePharma, January 22, 2018. https://www.fiercepharma.com/vaccines/vical-s-astellas-partnered-cmv-vaccine-failed-phase-3 (accessed February 2, 2018).

Lo, Bruce M. "Emergent Management of Gonorrhea." Medscape, March 24, 2016. https://emedicine.medscape.com/article/782913-overview#a1 (accessed January 21, 2017).

Locke, Susannah. "The Painful, Mosquito-Borne Chikungunya Virus Has Reached the US." Vox, July 19, 2014. https://www.vox.com/2014/7/19/5916249/chikungunya-fever-virus-caribbean-florida-disease-symptoms-explained (accessed January 31, 2018).

"Lyme Borreliosis (Lyme Disease)." World Health Organization. http://www.who.int/ith/diseases/lyme/en/ (accessed February 6, 2018).

"Lyme Disease." Centers for Disease Control and Convention, January 19, 2018. https://www.cdc.gov/lyme/index.html (accessed February 6, 2018).

"Lyme Disease." National Institute of Allergy and Infectious Diseases, April 6, 2016. https://www.niaid.nih.gov/diseases-conditions/lyme-disease (accessed February 6, 2018).

"Lymphatic Filariasis." Centers for Disease Control and Prevention, June 14, 2013. https://www.cdc.gov/parasites/lymphaticfilariasis/ (accessed January 22, 2018).

"Lymphatic Filariasis." World Health Organization. http://www.who.int/lymphatic_filariasis/en/ (January 22, 2018).

"Lymphatic Filariasis: Scabies." World Health Organization. http://www.who.int/lymphatic_filariasis/epidemiology/scabies/en/ (accessed November 13, 2017).

MacKay, Robert. "Eastern Equine Encephalitis (EEE)." University of Florida Large Animal Hospital. http://largeanimal.vethospitals.ufl.edu/eastern-equine-encephalitis-eee/ (accessed December 17, 2017).

Maginnis, Robert. "Al Qaeda and the Plague." Human Events, January 23, 2009. http://humanevents.com/2009/01/23/alqaeda-and-the-plague/ (accessed January 15, 2018).

"Malaria." Centers for Disease Control and Prevention, January 26, 2018. https://www.cdc.gov/malaria/ (accessed February 9, 2018).

"Malaria." World Health Organization. http://www.who.int/topics/malaria/en (accessed February 21, 2018).

"Malaria Control: The Power of Integrated Action." World Health Organization. http://www.who.int/heli/risks/vectors/malariacontrol/en/ (accessed December 6, 2017).

"Malaria—Strategy Overview." Bill & Melinda Gates Foundation. https://www.gatesfoundation.org/What-We-Do/Global-Health/Malaria (accessed January 14, 2018).

"Malaria Vaccine Development." World Health Organization, May 27, 2016. http://www.who.int/malaria/areas/vaccine/en/ (accessed March 7, 2018).

"Man 'Lucky' to Be Alive after Getting Powassan Virus from Tick Bite." CBS News, June 12, 2017. https://www.cbsnews.com/news/tick-bite-coma-powassan-virus-cape-cod-man/ (accessed February 12, 2018).

Mandt, Rebecca. "The Road to Guinea Worm Eradication: Running the Final Mile." *Science in the News* (blog), December 14, 2015. http://sitn.hms.harvard.edu/flash/2015/the-road-to-guinea-worm-eradication-running-the-final-mile/ (accessed November 15, 2017).

"Marburg Hemorrhagic Fever." Centers for Disease Control and Prevention, December 1, 2014. https://www.cdc.gov/vhf/marburg/index.html (accessed November 20, 2017).

"Marburg Virus Disease." World Health Organization, October 2017. http://www.who.int/mediacentre/factsheets/fs_marburg/en/ (accessed November 20, 2017).

"Marine Environments." Centers for Disease Control and Prevention. https://www.cdc.gov/habs/illness-symptoms-marine.html (accessed November 20, 2017).

Markel, Howard. "The Day We Discovered the Cause of the 'White Death.'" PBS NewsHour, March 24, 2015. https://www.pbs.org/newshour/health/march-24–1882-robert-koch-announces-his-discovery-of-the-cause-of-tuberculosis (accessed January 16, 2018).

Mastny, Lisa. "Eradicating Polio: A Model for International Cooperation." Worldwatch Institute, January 25, 1999. https://web.archive.org/web/20060608165205/http://www.worldwatch.org/node/1644 (accessed February 2, 2018).

"Maternal Deaths Disproportionately High in Developing Countries." World Health Organization, October 20, 2003. http://www.who.int/mediacentre/news/releases/2003/pr77/en/index.html (accessed December 9, 2017).

Mauroni, Al. "We Don't Need Another National Biodefense Strategy." Modern War Institute, August 1, 2017. https://mwi.usma.edu/dont-need-another-national-biodefense-strategy/ (accessed January 7, 2018).

McColl, Karen. "High Levels of Paralytic Shellfish Poisoning Found off Haines, Alaska." CBC News, December 23, 2015. http://www.cbc.ca/news/canada/north/psp-levels-high-along-haines-coast-says-report-1.3371953 (accessed November 20, 2017).

"Measles." World Health Organization, January 2018. http://www.who.int/mediacentre/factsheets/fs286/en/ (accessed February 13, 2018).

"Measles (Rubeola)." Centers for Disease Control and Prevention, February 5, 2018. https://www.cdc.gov/measles/index.html (accessed February 13, 2018).

Médecins Sans Frontières Access Campaign. https://www.msfaccess.org/ (accessed March 1, 2018).

"Melioidosis." Centers for Disease Control and Prevention. https://www.cdc.gov/melioidosis/index.html (accessed November 14, 2017).

"Meningitis." Centers for Disease Control and Prevention, April 10, 2017. https://www.cdc.gov/meningitis/index.html (accessed February 9, 2018).

"Meningitis and You—the Facts." Meningitis Now. https://www.meningitisnow.org/fight-for-now/wtf-meningitis/identifying-disease/meningitis-and-you-facts/ (accessed February 16, 2018).

"Meningococcal Meningitis." World Health Organization, December 2017. http://www.who.int/mediacentre/factsheets/fs141/en/ (accessed November 29, 2017).

"Meningococcal Vaccination: What Everyone Should Know." Centers for Disease Control and Prevention, May 19, 2017. https://www.cdc.gov/vaccines/vpd/mening/public/index.html (accessed November 20, 2017).

"Methicillin-Resistant *Staphylococcus aureus* (MRSA)." Centers for Disease Control and Prevention, July 6, 2017. https://www.cdc.gov/mrsa/tracking/index.html (accessed November 17, 2017).

"Michigan Hepatitis A Outbreak." Michigan Department of Health and Human Services, January 17, 2018. http://www.michigan.gov/mdhhs/0,5885,7-339-71550_2955_2976_82305_82310-447907--,00.html (accessed January 22, 2018).

"Microbial Identification and Strain Typing Using Molecular Techniques." Rapidmicrobiology. http://www.rapidmicrobiology.com/test-method/molecular-techniques-for-microbial-identification-and-typing/ (accessed February 1, 2018).

"Microbicides." HIV.gov. https://www.hiv.gov/hiv-basics/hiv-prevention/potential-future-options/microbicides (accessed March 5, 2018).

"Microsporidiosis." Centers for Disease Control and Prevention, 2017. https://www.cdc.gov/dpdx/microsporidiosis/index.html (accessed February 5, 2018).

"Milestones in the U.S. HIV Epidemic." Centers for Disease Control and Prevention, 2002. https://stacks.cdc.gov/view/cdc/40914 (accessed December 23, 2017).

"Millennium Development Goals Report." United Nations. http://www.un.org/millenniumgoals/reports.shtml (accessed January 7, 2018).

Minghui, Ren. "Endemic Infectious Diseases: The Next 15 Years." World Health Organization, August 17, 2016. http://www.who.int/mediacentre/commentaries/2016/Endemic-infectious-diseases-next-15-years/en/ (accessed February 9, 2018).

"Modern History Sourcebook: Oliver Wendell Holmes (1809–1894): Contagiousness of Puerperal Fever, 1843." Fordham University, August 1998. http://www.fordham.edu/halsall/mod/1843holmes-fever.html (accessed December 9, 2017).

"Monkeypox." Centers for Disease Control and Prevention, May 11, 2015. https://www.cdc.gov/poxvirus/monkeypox/ (accessed January 24, 2018).

"Monkeypox." World Health Organization, November 2016. http://www.who.int/mediacentre/factsheets/fs161/en/ (accessed January 24, 2018).

"Mononucleosis." Mayo Clinic. https://www.mayoclinic.org/diseases-conditions/mononucleosis/symptoms-causes/syc-20350328 (accessed January 24, 2018).

Morgan, Kate. "Use Tampons? Don't Panic about Toxic Shock Syndrome." CNN, December 22, 2017. http://www.cnn.com/2017/12/22/health/toxic-shock-syndrome-partner/index.html (accessed January 17, 2018).

"Mosquitoes Found with Eastern Equine Encephalitis Virus." Associated Press, July 14, 2017. https://www.usnews.com/news/best-states/rhode-island/articles/2017-07-14/mosquitoes-found-with-eastern-equine-encephalitis-virus (accessed December 17, 2017).

Moyer, Melinda Wenner. "What to Do If You Get Invited to a Chickenpox Party." Slate, November 15, 2013. http://www.slate.com/articles/double_x/the_kids/2013/11/chickenpox_vaccine_is_it_really_necessary.html (accessed February 1, 2018).

"Multiple Cause of Death Data." Centers for Disease Control and Prevention, December 20, 2017. https://wonder.cdc.gov/mcd.html (accessed January 7, 2108).

"Mumps." Centers for Disease Control and Prevention, November 20, 2017. https://www.cdc.gov/mumps/index.html (accessed January 24, 2018).

"Mumps—Annual Epidemiological Report for 2015." European Centre for Disease Control and Prevention, November 28, 2017. https://

ecdc.europa.eu/en/publications-data/mumps-annual-epidemiological-report-2015 (accessed February 6, 2018).

"Mumps—Number of Reported Cases (Vaccine-Preventable Communicable Diseases)." World Health Organization. http://apps.who.int/gho/data/node.imr.WHS3_53?lang=en (accessed January 21, 2018)

"Mycotic Diseases Branch." Centers for Disease Control and Prevention, Division of Foodborne, Waterborne, and Environmental Diseases, January 27, 2017. https://www.cdc.gov/ncezid/dfwed/mycotics/index.html (accessed January 25, 2018).

"National Action Plan for Combating Antibiotic-Resistance Bacteria." Obama White House, March 27, 2015. https://obamawhitehouse.archives.gov/sites/default/files/docs/national_action_plan_for_combating_antibotic-resistant_bacteria.pdf (accessed February 24, 2018).

"National Action Plan for Combating Antibiotic-Resistance Bacteria Progress Report for Years 1 and 2. " Office of the Assistant Secretary for Planning and Evaluation. https://aspe.hhs.gov/pdf-report/national-action-plan-combating-antibiotic-resistant-bacteria-progress-report-years-1-and-2 (accessed February 24, 2018).

"National B Virus Resource Center." Georgia State University. http://www2.gsu.edu/~wwwvir/ (accessed December 15, 2017).

"National Center for Emerging and Zoonotic Infectious Diseases (NCEZID)." Centers for Disease Control and Prevention, March 8, 2018. https://www.cdc.gov/ncezid/index.html (accessed March 7, 2018).

National Institute of Allergy and Infectious Diseases, 2018. https://www.niaid.nih.gov/ (accessed February 27, 2018).

National Necrotizing Fasciitis Foundation, January 28, 2007. http://www.nnff.org/ (accessed February 14, 2007).

"National Notifiable Diseases Surveillance System (NNDSS)." Centers for Disease Control and Prevention, February 16, 2018. https://wwwn.cdc.gov/nndss/ (accessed March 6, 2018).

"National Strategy for Pandemic Flu." US Department of Homeland Security, July 6, 2009. https://www.dhs.gov/national-strategy-pandemic-flu (accessed January 22, 2007).

"National Vital Statistics Reports." Centers for Disease Control and Prevention, November 27, 2017. https://www.cdc.gov/nchs/products/nvsr.htm (accessed January 22, 2018).

Nature"Creutzfeldt-Jakob Disease: Diagnosis." National Health Service (NHS), January 21, 2015. https://www.nhs.uk/conditions/creutzfeldt-jakob-disease-cjd/diagnosis/ (accessed January 29, 2018).

"Nearly Half a Million Americans Suffered from *Clostridium difficile* Infections in a Single Year." Centers for Disease Control and Prevention, February 25, 2015. https://www.cdc.gov/media/releases/2015/p0225-clostridium-difficile.html

"Necrotizing Fasciitis." Centers for Disease Control and Prevention, October 26, 2017. https://www.cdc.gov/features/necrotizingfasciitis/index.html (accessed February 12, 2018).

"New Export Market Opens for UK Beef." Agricultural and Horticultural Development Board, August 9, 2017. http://beefandlamb.ahdb.org.uk/wp-content/uploads/2017/08/090817-Export-release.pdf (accessed January 20, 2017).

"New Hepatitis C Infections Nearly Tripled over Five Years." Centers for Disease Control and Prevention. https://www.cdc.gov/nchhstp/newsroom/2017/Hepatitis-Surveillance-Press-Release.html (accessed February 20, 2018).

New Scientist<https://www.newscientist.com/article/2118418-many-more-people-could-still-die-from-mad-cow-disease-in-the-uk/"Variant Creutzfeldt-Jakob Disease (vCJD)." Centers for Disease Control and Prevention, February 6, 2015. https://www.cdc.gov/prions/vcjd/index.html (accessed January 29, 2018).

"NIAID Emerging Infectious Diseases/Pathogens." National Institute of Allergy and Infectious Diseases. https://www.niaid.nih.gov/research/emerging-infectious-diseases-pathogens (accessed November 15, 2017).

"NIAID's Antibacterial Research Program: Current Status and Future Directions." National Institute of Allergy and Infectious Diseases, 2014. https://www.niaid.nih.gov/sites/default/files/arstrategicplan2014.pdf (accessed February 28, 2018).

"Nipah Virus (NiV)." Centers for Disease Control and Prevention, March 20, 2014. https://www.cdc.gov/vhf/nipah/index.html (accessed January 19, 2018).

"Nipah Virus (NiV) Infection." World Health Organization. http://www.who.int/csr/disease/nipah/en/ (accessed January 19, 2018).

"The Nobel Peace Prize 1965." Nobelprize.org. http://nobelprize.org/nobel_prizes/peace/laureates/1965/ (accessed January 16, 2018).

"The Nobel Peace Prize 1999: Médecins Sans Frontières." Nobelprize.org. http://nobelprize.org/peace/laureates/1999/index.html (accessed February 26, 2018).

"The Nobel Prize in Chemistry 2014." Nobelprize.org. http://www.nobelprize.org/nobel_prizes/chemistry/laureates/2014/ (accessed January 29, 2018).

"The Nobel Prize in Physiology or Medicine 2005." Nobelprize.org, October 3, 2005. https://www.nobelprize.org/nobel_prizes/medicine/laureates/2005/press.html (accessed March 6, 2018).

"Nocardiosis." Centers for Disease Control and Prevention, October 13, 2005. https://www.cdc.gov/nocardiosis/ (accessed January 19, 2018).

Nordqvist, Christian. "Everything You Need to Know about Cytomegalovirus." Medical News Today, January 11, 2018. https://www.medicalnewstoday.com/articles/173811.php (accessed February 2, 2018).

"Norovirus Worldwide." Centers for Disease Control and Prevention. https://www.cdc.gov/norovirus/worldwide.html (accessed November 20, 2017).

"Norovirus: U.S. Trends and Outbreaks." Centers for Disease Control and Prevention. https://www.cdc.gov/norovirus/trends-outbreaks.html (accessed November 20, 2017).

"The Nuremberg Code." National Institutes of Health, 1949. https://history.nih.gov/research/downloads/nuremberg.pdf (accessed February 12, 2018).

"Nursing Homes and Assisted Living (Long-Term Care Facilities [LTCFs])." Centers for Disease Control and Prevention, February 28, 2018. https://www.cdc.gov/longtermcare/ (accessed February 9, 2018).

"Onchocerciasis." World Health Organization, September 2017. http://www.who.int/mediacentre/factsheets/fs374/en/ (accessed February 12, 2018).

"Onchocerciasis (River Blindness)—Disease Information." World Health Organization. http://www.who.int/blindness/partnerships/onchocerciasis_disease_information/en/ (accessed February 12, 2018).

"One Million Deaths by Parasites." *PLOS* Speaking of Medicine Community Blog, January 16, 2015. http://blogs.plos.org/speakingofmedicine/2015/01/16/one-million-deaths-parasites/ (accessed March 2, 2018).

"Opisthorchiasis." Centers for Disease Control and Prevention, December 14, 2017 https://www.cdc.gov/dpdx/opisthorchiasis/index.html (accessed January 5, 2018).

"Opportunistic Infections." Centers for Disease Control and Prevention, May 30, 2017. https://www.cdc.gov/hiv/basics/livingwithhiv/opportunisticinfections.html (accessed January 28, 2018).

"Origin of HIV & AIDS." Avert, December 5, 2017. https://www.avert.org/professionals/history-hiv-aids/origin (accessed December 17, 2017).

"OSHA Fact Sheet: OSHA's Bloodborne Pathogens Standard." United States Department of Labor, Occupational Safety and Health Administration, January 2011. https://www.osha.gov/OshDoc/data_BloodborneFacts/bbfact01.pdf (accessed February 25, 2018).

"Outbreaks Chronology: Ebola Virus Disease." Centers for Disease Control and Prevention, July 28, 2017. https://www.cdc.gov/vhf/ebola/outbreaks/history/chronology.html (accessed January 26, 2018).

"Oxitec's Eco-Friendly Solution Addresses the Challenges of the *Aedes aegypti* Mosquito." Oxitec, November 4, 2016. http://www.oxitec.com/oxitecs-eco-friendly-solution-addresses-challenges-aedes-aegypti-mosquito/ (accessed February 26, 2018).

Padmanabha, Disha. "Gene Therapy Using CAR-T Could Interfere with the Ability of HIV to Infect Cells." BioTecNika, December 30, 2017. https://www.biotecnika.org/2017/12/gene-therapy-using-car-t-interfere-ability-hiv-infect-cells/ (accessed March 6, 2018).

"Pandemic Influenza." Centers for Disease Control and Prevention, January 2, 2018. https://www.cdc.gov/flu/pandemic-resources/index.htm (accessed January 22, 2018).

"Pandemic Influenza." US Department of Health and Human Services. https://www.hhs.gov/about/agencies/oga/global-health-security/pandemic-influenza/index.html (accessed January 22, 2018).

"Pandemic Influenza." US Department of Health and Human Services, January 2, 2018. http://www.pandemicflu.gov/index.html (accessed April 28, 2007).

"Pandemic Influenza Plan: 2017 Update." US Department of Health and Human Services. https://www.cdc.gov/flu/pandemic-resources/pdf/pan-flu-report-2017v2.pdf (accessed January 19, 2018).

"Pandemic Intervals Framework (PIF)." Centers for Disease Control and Prevention, November 30, 2016. https://www.cdc.gov/flu/pandemic-resources/national-strategy/intervals-framework.html (accessed March 7, 2018).

"Pandemic Preparedness." World Health Organization. http://www.who.int/influenza/preparedness/pandemic/en/ (accessed February 27, 2018).

"Paragonimiasis." World Health Organization. http://www.who.int/foodborne_trematode_infections/paragonimiasis/en/ (accessed November 14, 2017).

"Paragonimus Westermani–Lung Fluke." Parasites in Humans. http://www.parasitesinhumans.org/paragonimus-westermani-lung-fluke.html (accessed November 14, 2017).

"Parasites." Centers for Disease Control and Prevention, September 27, 2017. https://www.cdc.gov/parasites/ (accessed February 25, 2018).

"Parasites—African Trypanosomiasis (also known as Sleeping Sickness)." Centers for Disease Control and Prevention. https://www.cdc.gov/parasites/sleepingsickness/index.html (accessed November 6, 2017).

"Parasites—Amebiasis—*Entamoea histolytica* Infection." Centers for Disease Control and Prevention. https://www.cdc.gov/parasites/amebiasis/index.html (accessed November 7, 2017).

"Parasites—American Trypanosomiasis (also known as Chagas Disease)." Centers for Disease Control and Prevention, May 24, 2016. https://www.cdc.gov/parasites/chagas/ (accessed January 18, 2017).

"Parasites—Babesiosis." Centers for Disease Control and Prevention, May 24, 2016. https://www.cdc.gov/parasites/babesiosis/index.html (accessed March 1, 2018).

"Parasites—Balantidiasis (also known as Balantidium coli infection)." Centers for Disease Control and Prevention. https://www.cdc.gov/parasites/balantidium/ (accessed November 10, 2017).

"Parasites—Cryptosporidium (Also Known as 'Crypto')." Centers for Disease Control and Prevention, April 1, 2015. https://www.cdc.gov/parasites/crypto/index.html (accessed January 16, 2018).

"Parasites: Giardia." US Centers for Disease Control and Prevention, July 22, 2015. https://www.cdc.gov/parasites/giardia/index.html (accessed January 16, 2018).

"Parasites—Hymenolepis." Centers for Disease Control and Prevention, January 10, 2012. https://www.cdc.gov/parasites/hymenolepis/ (accessed January 23, 2018).

"Parasites—Leishmaniasis. Epidemiology & Risk Factors." Centers for Disease Control and Prevention, January 10, 2013. http://www.cdc.gov/parasites/leishmaniasis/epi.html (accessed March 1, 2018).

"Parasites—Lice—Body Lice." Centers for Disease Control and Prevention. https://www.cdc.gov/parasites/lice/body/index.html (accessed November 14, 2017).

"Parasites—Onchocerciasis (Also Known as River Blindness)." Centers for Disease Control and Prevention, August 10, 2015. https://www.cdc.gov/parasites/onchocerciasis/index.html (accessed February 12, 2018).

"Parasites—Paragonimiasis (also known as Paragonimus Infection)." Centers for Disease Control and Prevention. https://www.cdc.gov/parasites/paragonimus/index.html (accessed November 14, 2017).

"Parasites: Scabies." Centers for Disease Control and Prevention. https://www.cdc.gov/parasites/scabies/index.html (accessed November 17, 2017).

"Parasites: Toxoplasmosis (Toxoplasma Infection)." Centers for Disease Control and Prevention. https://www.cdc.gov/parasites/toxoplasmosis/index.html (accessed on November 22, 2017).

"Parasites—Trichinellosis (also known as Trichinosis)." Centers for Disease Control and Prevention, August 8, 2012. http://www.cdc

.gov/ncidod/dpd/parasites/trichinosis/factsht_trichinosis.htm (accessed January 12, 2018).

Parsonnet, Julie. "Infectious Disease: A Surprising Cause of Cancer." Stanford Medicine Newsletter, Spring 2008. http://stanfordmedicine.org/communitynews/2008spring/infectiousdisease.html (accessed January 26, 2018).

Parsons, Tim. "Economic Impact of Zika Outbreak Could Exceed $18B in Latin America, Caribbean." Hub, May 8, 2017. https://hub.jhu.edu/2017/05/08/zika-economic-impact-latin-america-caribbean/ (accessed February 26, 2018).

"Parvovirus B19 and Fifth Disease." Centers for Disease Control and Prevention. http://www.cdc.gov/parvovirusb19/fifth-disease.html (accessed November 16, 2017).

PATH. "Accelerating Access to Rotavirus Vaccine." http://www.path.org/projects/rvp.php (accessed January 23, 2018).

"Patient Education: Methicillin-resistant *Staphylococcus aureus* (MRSA) (Beyond the Basics)." UpToDate, August 15, 2017. https://www.uptodate.com/contents/methicillin-resistant-staphylococcus-aureus-mrsa-beyond-the-basics (accessed November 20, 2017).

"Penicilliosis and HIV." HIV InSite. http://hivinsite.ucsf.edu/InSite?page=kb-00&doc=kb-05–02-07 (accessed February 21, 2018).

"People with Natural Immunity to HIV May Serve as Basis for New Vaccine." Medical Xpress. https://medicalxpress.com/news/2012–11-people-natural-immunity-hiv-basis.html (accessed December 28, 2017).

"Pertussis." World Health Organization, June 21, 2011. http://www.who.int/immunization/topics/pertussis/en/ (accessed January 26, 2018).

Petri, William A. "Overview of Rickettsial Infections." Merck Manual: Consumer Version. https://www.merckmanuals.com/home/infections/rickettsial-and-related-infections/overview-of-rickettsial-infections (accessed February 15, 2018).

"Pinworm Infection." Mayo Clinic, April 8, 2015. https://www.mayoclinic.org/diseases-conditions/pinworm/symptoms-causes/syc-20376382 (accessed January 9, 2018).

"Plague." Centers for Disease Control and Prevention. https://www.cdc.gov/plague/index.html (accessed January 29, 2018).

"Plague: Fact Sheet." World Health Organization, October 2017. http://www.who.int/mediacentre/factsheets/fs267/en (accessed January 29, 2018).

"Plague Outbreak Highlighted Ongoing Problem in Africa." Center for Infectious Disease Research and Policy, May 27, 2005. http://www.cidrap.umn.edu/cidrap/content/bt/plague/news/may2705plag.html (accessed January 29, 2018).

"*Pneumocystis* pneumonia." Centers for Disease Control and Prevention, April 26, 2017. https://www.cdc.gov/fungal/diseases/pneumocystis-pneumonia/index.html (accessed February 14, 2018).

"*Pneumocystis jirovecii* Pneumonia." AIDS Info, National Institutes of Health, November 6, 2013. https://aidsinfo.nih.gov/guidelines/html/5/pediatric-opportunistic-infection/415/pneumocystis-jirovecii-pneumonia (accessed March 13, 2018).

"Pneumonia." Mayo Clinic, August 11, 2017. https://www.mayoclinic.org/diseases-conditions/pneumonia/symptoms-causes/syc-20354204 (accessed January 22, 2018).

"Pneumonia." World Health Organization, September 2016. http://www.who.int/mediacentre/factsheets/fs331/en/ (accessed January 24, 2018).

Pockros, Paul J. "Direct-Acting Antivirals for the Treatment of Hepatitis C Virus Infection." UpToDate. https://www.uptodate.com/contents/direct-acting-antivirals-for-the-treatment-of-hepatitis-c-virus-infection (accessed November 16, 2017).

"Poliomyelitis." World Health Organization, April 2017. http://www.who.int/mediacentre/factsheets/fs114/en/ (accessed February 1, 2018).

"Poliomyelitis. Immunization, Vaccines and Biologicals." World Health Organization, February 2017. http://www.who.int/immunization/diseases/poliomyelitis/en/ (accessed February 4, 2018).

Pollard, Andrew, et al. "Using New Genomic Techniques to Identify the Causes of Meningitis in UK Children." Meningitis Research Foundation, May 14, 2015. https://www.meningitis.org/research-projects/genomic-techniques-identify-causes-of-meningitis (accessed February 16, 2018).

"Powassan Virus." Centers for Disease Control and Prevention, November 2, 2017. https://www.cdc.gov/powassan/index.html (accessed February 13, 2018).

"Preventing the Spread of Bloodborne Pathogens." American National Red Cross, 2011. http://www.in.gov/isdh/files/BBP_American_Red_Cross_Fact_Sheet_xps(1).pdf (accessed February 23, 2018).

"Progress on Drinking Water, Sanitation and Hygiene 2017." World Health Organization and UNICEF. http://apps.who.int/iris/bitstream/10665/258617/1/9789241512893-eng.pdf?ua=1 (accessed January 18, 2018).

"Progress towards the Millennium Development Goals, 1990–2005." United Nations, 2005. http://mdgs.un.org/unsd/mdg/Host.aspx?Content=Products/Progress2005.htm (accessed March 6, 2018).

"Project BioShield Annual Report to Congress." US Department of Health and Human Services, 2016. https://www.medicalcountermeasures.gov/barda/cbrn/project-bioshield-overview/project-bioshield-annual-report.aspx (accessed January 7, 2018).

ProMED-Mail. http://www.promedmail.org (accessed December 11, 2017).

"A Promise to Children." UNICEF. http://www.unicef.org/wsc/ (accessed January 16, 2018).

"Protozoan Parasites." Parasites in Humans. http://www.parasitesinhumans.org/protozoa.html (accessed March 1, 2018).

"Psittacosis." Centers for Disease Control and Prevention, June 29, 2017. https://www.cdc.gov/pneumonia/atypical/psittacosis.html (accessed December 8, 2017).

"Psittacosis." Medline Plus, December 5, 2017. https://medlineplus.gov/ency/article/000088.htm (accessed December 8, 2017).

"Psittacosis Fact Sheet." NSW Government Health, July 1, 2012. http://www.health.nsw.gov.au/Infectious/factsheets/Pages/psittacosis.aspx (accessed December 8, 2017).

"A Public Health Action Plan to Combat Antibiotic Resistance." Centers for Disease Control and Prevention, February 9, 2005. http://www.cdc.gov/drugresistance/actionplan/aractionplan.pdf (accessed February 26, 2007).

"Pulse Polio Programme." National Health Portal (NHP), April 6, 2015. https://www.nhp.gov.in/pulse-polio-programme_pg (accessed February 2, 2018).

"Pushed to the Limit and Beyond: A Year into the Largest Ever Ebola Outbreak." Doctors Without Borders/Médecins Sans Frontières, March 19, 2015. https://www.msf.org.uk/sites/uk/files/ebola_-_pushed_to_the_limit_and_beyond.pdf (accessed February 27, 2018).

"Q Fever." *CDC Health Information for International Travel.* Centers for Disease Control and Prevention, May 31, 2017. https://wwwnc.cdc.gov/travel/yellowbook/2018/infectious-diseases-related-to-travel/q-fever (accessed November 20, 2017).

"Q Fever Fact Sheet." New South Wales Government. http://www.health.nsw.gov.au/Infectious/factsheets/Pages/q-fever.aspx (accessed November 20, 2017).

"Quick Reference Guide to the Bloodborne Pathogens Standard." United States Department of Labor, Occupational Safety and Health Administration. https://www.osha.gov/SLTC/bloodbornepathogens/bloodborne_quickref.html (accessed November 20, 2017).

"Rabies." Centers for Diseases Control and Prevention, National Center for Infectious Diseases, September 28, 2017. https://www.cdc.gov/rabies/ (accessed February 19, 2018).

"Rabies." World Health Organization, September 2017. http://www.who.int/mediacentre/factsheets/fs099/en (accessed February 19, 2018).

"Rapid Detection of Methicillin-Resistant *Staphylococcus aureus.*" UpToDate. https://www.uptodate.com/contents/rapid-detection-of-methicillin-resistant-staphylococcus-aureus (accessed November 21, 2017).

"Rat-Bite Fever." Centers for Disease Control and Prevention, April 24, 2015. https://www.cdc.gov/rat-bite-fever/index.html (accessed January 19, 2018).

Rathore, Mobeen H. "Rickettsial Infection." Medscape, June 14, 2016. https://reference.medscape.com/article/968385-overview (accessed February 15, 2018).

"Recognizing the Biosafety Levels." Centers for Disease Control and Prevention. https://www.cdc.gov/training/quicklearns/biosafety/ (accessed January 31, 2018).

"Report of the Secretary-General on the Work of the Organization." United Nations, 2006. http://mdgs.un.org/unsd/mdg/Resources/Static/Products/SGReports/61_1/a_61_1_e.pdf (accessed March 6, 2018).

"Report on Global Sexually Transmitted Infection Surveillance 2013." World Health Organization, June 2014. http://apps.who.int/iris/bitstream/10665/112922/1/9789241507400_eng.pdf?ua=1 (accessed March 6, 2018).

"Report on the Burden of Endemic Health Care-Associated Infection Worldwide: A Systematic Review of the Literature." World Health Organization, 2011. http://apps.who.int/iris/bitstream/10665/80135/1/9789241501507_eng.pdf?ua=1 (accessed February 21, 2018).

Resnick, Brian. "The Entire World Has 2 Weeks to Switch Over to a New Oral Polio Vaccine. Here's Why." Vox, April 18, 2016. https://www.vox.com/2016/4/18/11450362/polio-opv-eradication (accessed February 2, 2018).

"Respiratory Syncytial Virus." Centers for Disease Control and Prevention. January 1, 2005. http://www.cdc.gov/rsv/index.html (accessed November 21, 2017).

"Respiratory Syncytial Virus (RSV)." Mayo Clinic. https://www.mayoclinic.org/diseases-conditions/respiratory-syncytial-virus/symptoms-causes/syc-20353098 (accessed November 21, 2017).

"Revision to OSHA's Bloodborne Pathogens Standard." United States Department of Labor, Occupational Safety and Health Administration, April 2001. https://www.osha.gov/needlesticks/needlefact.html (accessed February 23, 2018).

"Rickettsial Infections—including Symptoms, Treatment and Prevention." South Australia Health. http://www.sahealth.sa.gov.au/wps/wcm/connect/public+content/sa+health+internet/health+topics/health+conditions+prevention+and+treatment/infectious+diseases/rickettsial+infections/rickettsial+infections+-+including+symptoms+treatment+and+prevention (accessed February 15, 2018).

"Rift Valley Fever in China." World Health Organization, August 2, 2016. http://www.who.int/csr/don/02-august-2016-rift-valley-fever-china/en/ (accessed January 18, 2018)/

"Rift Valley Fever (RVS)." Centers for Disease Control and Prevention, October 19, 2016. https://www.cdc.gov/vhf/rvf/ (accessed January 18, 2018).

"Ringworm." American Academy of Dermatology. https://www.aad.org/public/diseases/contagious-skin-diseases/ringworm (accessed January 10, 2017).

"Ringworm." Centers for Disease Control and Prevention. https://www.cdc.gov/fungal/diseases/ringworm/index.html (accessed January 10, 2017).

"Risks and Complications." American Red Cross. https://www.redcrossblood.org/learn-about-blood/blood-transfusions/risks-complications (accessed February 12, 2018).

"River Blindness Elimination Program." The Carter Center. https://www.cartercenter.org/health/river_blindness/index.html (accessed February 12, 2018).

"Rocky Mountain Spotted Fever." Centers for Disease Control and Prevention, June 26, 2017. http://www.cdc.gov/ncidod/dvrd/rmsf/index.htm (accessed December 9, 2017).

"Rocky Mountain Spotted Fever." Illinois Department of Public Health. http://www.idph.state.il.us/public/hb/hbrmsf.htm (accessed December 9, 2017).

Ross, Adam, and Hugh W. Shoff. "Toxic Shock Syndrome." National Center for Biotechnology Information, US National Library of Medicine, October 6, 2017. https://www.ncbi.nlm.nih.gov/books/NBK459345/ (accessed January 17, 2018).

"Rotavirus." Centers for Disease Control and Prevention. https://www.cdc.gov/rotavirus/index.html (accessed November 16, 2017).

"Rotavirus." Mayo Clinic. https://www.mayoclinic.org/diseases-conditions/rotavirus/symptoms-causes/syc-20351300 (accessed January 23, 2018).

"Rotavirus." World Health Organization, June 3, 2016. http://www.who.int/immunization/diseases/rotavirus/en/ (accessed January 23, 2018).

"Rotavirus Vaccine Support." Global Alliance for Vaccines and Immunization. http://www.gavi.org/support/nvs/rotavirus (accessed November 16, 2017).

"Rubella." World Health Organization, January 2018. http://www.who.int/mediacentre/factsheets/fs367/en/ (accessed January 16, 2018).

"Rubella (German Measles, Three-Day Measles)." Centers for Disease Control and Prevention, September 15, 2017. https://www.cdc.gov/rubella/index.html (accessed January 16, 2018).

Sachdev, Chhavi. "Why Does India Lead the World in Deaths from TB?" NPR, November 9, 2017. https://www.npr.org/sections/goatsandsoda/2017/11/09/561834263/why-does-india-lead-the-world-in-deaths-from-tb (accessed March 5, 2018).

"Saint Louis Encephalitis." Centers for Disease Control and Prevention. https://www.cdc.gov/sle/ (accessed November 9, 2017).

Saldana, José Ignacio. "Macrophages." British Society for Immunology. https://www.immunology.org/public-information/bitesized-immunology/cells/macrophages (accessed March 12, 2018).

"Salmonella." Centers for Disease Control and Prevention. https://www.cdc.gov/salmonella/ (accessed November 21, 2017).

Santacroce, Luigi. "*Helicobacter pylori* Infection." Medscape, October 12, 2017. https://emedicine.medscape.com/article/176938-overview (accessed March 6, 2018).

Santosham, Mathuram. "5 Reasons the Global Gap in Rotavirus Vaccine Access Is Shrinking. *Impatient Optimists*, January 9, 2018. https://www.impatientoptimists.org/Posts/2018/01/5-reasons-the-global-gap-in-rotavirus-vaccine-access-is-shrinking#.WmexOSOZPGK (accessed January 23, 2018).

"Scabies." American Academy of Dermatology. https://www.aad.org/public/diseases/contagious-skin-diseases/scabies (accessed November 13, 2017).

"Schistosomiasis (Bilharzia)." National Health Service, June 1, 2016. https://www.nhs.uk/conditions/schistosomiasis/ (accessed January 12, 2018).

"Schistosomiasis." Centers for Disease Control and Prevention, November 7, 2012. https://www.cdc.gov/parasites/schistosomiasis/index.html (accessed January 12, 2018).

"Schistosomiasis." Sabin Vaccine Institute. http://www.sabin.org/programs/schistosomiasis (accessed January 12, 2018).

"Schistosomiasis." World Health Organization, October 2017. http://www.who.int/mediacentre/factsheets/fs115/en/ (accessed January 12, 2018).

"Schistosomiasis Control Initiative." Imperial College London. http://www.imperial.ac.uk/schistosomiasis-control-initiative/ (accessed January 12, 2018).

"Seasonal Flu Death Estimate Increases Worldwide." Centers for Disease Control and Prevention, December 13, 2017. https://www.cdc.gov/media/releases/2017/p1213-flu-death-estimate.html (accessed January 17, 2018).

"Secretary-General Warns of Glaring Gaps in Ability to Prevent, Respond to Catastrophic Biological Attack, at Review Conference Opening." United Nations, November 7, 2016. https://www.un.org/press/en/2016/sgsm18256.doc.htm (accessed January 29, 2018).

"Selective Vaccinations: Japanese Encephalitis." International Association for Medical Assistance to Travelers, September 20, 2016. https://www.iamat.org/country/thailand/risk/japanese-encephalitis (accessed February 15, 2018).

"Sepsis." World Health Organization. http://www.who.int/sepsis/en/ (accessed February 28, 2018).

"Sepsis: Basic Information." Centers for Disease Control and Prevention, January 23, 2018.

"Severe Acute Respiratory Syndrome (SARS)." Centers for Disease Control and Prevention. http://www.cdc.gov/sars/index.html (accessed December 11, 2017).

"Severe Acute Respiratory Syndrome (SARS)." World Health Organization. http://www.who.int/csr/sars/en (accessed December 11, 2017).

"Sexually Transmitted Infections (STIs)." World Health Organization, August 2016. http://www.who.int/mediacentre/factsheets/fs110/en/ (accessed January 31, 2018).

Sharp, Andy. "North Korea Begins Tests to Load Anthrax onto ICBMs, Report Says." Bloomberg, December 19, 2017. https://www.bloomberg.com/news/articles/2017–12-20/north-korea-begins-tests-to-load-anthrax-onto-icbms-asahi-says (accessed January 11, 2018).

Sheridan, Jackie. "Diphtheria Outbreak among Rohingya Refugees Enters Third Month." The Disease Daily, January 25, 2018. http://www.healthmap.org/site/diseasedaily/article/

diphtheria-outbreak-among-rohingya-refugees-enters-third-month-12518. (accessed January 27, 2018).

"Shigella." World Health Organization. http://www.who.int/immunization/topics/shigella/en/ (accessed February 7, 2018).

"Shigella—Shigellosis." Centers for Disease Control and Prevention. https://www.cdc.gov/shigella/ (accessed January 16, 2018).

"Shingles." American Academy of Dermatology Association. https://www.aad.org/public/diseases/contagious-skin-diseases/shingles (accessed January 24, 2018).

"Shingles." Centers for Disease Control and Prevention, January 30, 2018. https://www.cdc.gov/shingles/ (accessed February 1, 2018).

"Shingles (Herpes Zoster)." Centers for Disease Control and Prevention, October 17, 2017. https://www.cdc.gov/shingles/index.html (accessed January 24, 2018).

Singh, Maanvi. "Why College Campuses Get Hit by Meningitis Outbreaks." NPR, November 19, 2013. https://www.npr.org/sections/health-shots/2013/11/19/246178160/why-college-campuses-get-hit-by-meningitis-outbreaks (accessed February 9, 2018).

"Six Common Misconceptions about Immunization." World Health Organization. http://www.who.int/vaccine_safety/initiative/detection/immunization_misconceptions/en/index1.html (accessed February 14, 2018).

"Smallpox." Centers for Disease Control and Prevention, July 12, 2017. https://www.cdc.gov/smallpox/index.html (accessed January 29, 2018).

"Smallpox." World Health Organization. http://www.who.int/csr/disease/smallpox/en/ (accessed January 29, 2018).

"Smallpox: Preparedness." Centers for Disease Control and Prevention, December 19, 2016. https://www.cdc.gov/smallpox/bioterrorism/public/preparedness.html (accessed January 29, 2018).

"Soil-Transmitted Helminth Infections Fact Sheet." World Health Organization, September 2017. http://www.who.int/mediacentre/factsheets/fs366/en/ (accessed December 19, 2017).

"Sporotrichosis." Centers for Disease Control and Prevention, January 30, 2017. https://www.cdc.gov/fungal/diseases/sporotrichosis/index.html (accessed January 23, 2018).

Springer, Yuri P., et al. "Two Outbreaks of Trichinellosis Linked to Consumption of Walrus Meat—Alaska, 2016–2017." Centers for Disease Control and Prevention, July 7, 2017. https://www.cdc.gov/mmwr/volumes/66/wr/mm6626a3.htm (accessed January 25, 2018).

"St. Louis encephalitis." Vector Disease Control International. http://www.vdci.net/vector-borne-diseases/st-louis-encephalitis-education-and-mosquito-management-to-protect-public-health (accessed November 9, 2017).

"The State of the World's Children 2016." UNICEF. https://www.unicef.org/sowc2016/ (accessed January 16, 2018).

Stop Pneumonia. https://stoppneumonia.org/ (accessed January 24, 2018).

"Streptococcal Toxic Shock Syndrome (STSS) (*Streptococcus pyogenes*) 2010 Case Definition." Centers for Disease Control and Prevention, 2010. https://wwwn.cdc.gov/nndss/conditions/streptococcal-toxic-shock-syndrome/case-definition/2010/ (accessed January 31, 2018).

"Strongyloidiasis." World Health Organization. http://www.who.int/intestinal_worms/epidemiology/strongyloidiasis/en/ (accessed January 12, 2018).

"Strongyloidiasis Infection FAQs." Centers for Disease Control and Prevention, July 10, 2014. https://www.cdc.gov/parasites/strongyloides/gen_info/faqs.html (accessed January 12, 2018).

"A Study on Public Health and Socioeconomic Impact of Substandard and Falsified Medical Products: Executive Summary." World Health Organization, 2017. http://www.who.int/medicines/regulation/ssffc/publications/SummarySESTUDY-WEB.pdf?ua=1 (accessed March 1, 2018).

"Summary of the Global HIV Epidemic 2016." World Health Organization. http://www.who.int/hiv/data/epi_core_2016.png?ua=1 (accessed December 2, 2017).

"Swimmer's Ear." American Academy of Otolaryngology. http://www.entnet.org/content/swimmers-ear (accessed November 15, 2017).

"Syphilis." Centers for Disease Control and Prevention, November 30, 2017. https://www.cdc.gov/std/syphilis/default.htm (accessed February 15, 2018).

"Table 1: Summary of WHO Position Papers —Recommendations for Routine Immunization." World Health Organization, March 2017. http://www.who.int/immunization/policy/Immunization_routine_table1.pdf?ua=1 (accessed January 26, 2018).

"Taeniasis." Centers for Disease Control and Prevention, January 10, 2013. https://www.cdc.gov/parasites/taeniasis/index.html (accessed January 10, 2018).

"Take a Bite out of Rabies!" Centers for Disease Control and Prevention, September 25, 2017. https://www.cdc.gov/features/rabies/index.html (accessed January 31, 2018).

"Taking Sex and Gender into Account in Emerging Infectious Disease Programmes: An Analytical Framework." World Health Organization. http://www.wpro.who.int/topics/gender_issues/Takingsexandgenderintoaccount.pdf (accessed March 5, 2018).

"Talaromycosis (Formerly Penicilliosis)." Centers for Disease Control and Prevention, September 26, 2017. https://www.cdc.gov/fungal/diseases/other/talaromycosis.html#four (accessed February 21, 2018).

"Tapeworm Infestation." Medscape, September 11, 2017. https://emedicine.medscape.com/article/786292-overview (accessed January 23, 2018).

"TB Statistics India—National, Treatment Outcome & State Statistics." TBFacts.org. https://www.tbfacts.org/tb-statistics-india/ (accessed March 5, 2018).

"Tetanus." Centers for Disease Control and Prevention, April 14, 2017. https://www.cdc.gov/tetanus/index.html (accessed December 9, 2017).

"Tetanus." Mayo Clinic, August 8, 2017. https://www.mayoclinic.org/diseases-conditions/tetanus/symptoms-causes/syc-20351625 (accessed December 9, 2017).

"Tetanus Vaccination." Centers for Disease Control and Prevention, November 28, 2017. https://www.cdc.gov/vaccines/vpd/tetanus/index.html (accessed December 9, 2017).

Tetro, Jason. "This Natural Chemical May Replace Triclosan and Improve Oral Health. Huffington Post, May 25, 2015. http://www.huffingtonpost.ca/jason-tetro/triclosan-oral-health_b_7421152.html (accessed November 27, 2017).

"Tick Allergy." Australasian Society of Clinical Immunology and Allergy, 2016. https://allergy.org.au/images/pcc/ASCIA_PCC_Tick_allergy_2016.pdf (accessed February 25, 2018).

"Tickborne Diseases of the United States: A Reference Manual for Health Care Providers." Centers for Disease Control and Prevention, 2017. https://www.cdc.gov/lyme/resources/TickborneDiseases.pdf (accessed February 25, 2018).

"Tick-Borne Diseases." European Centre for Disease Prevention and Control, 2018. https://ecdc.europa.eu/en/tick-borne-diseases (accessed February 25, 2018).

"Tick-Borne Relapsing Fever (TBRF)." Center for Disease Control and Prevention, October 15, 2015. https://www.cdc.gov/relapsing-fever/index.html (accessed November 15, 2017).

"Ticks." Centers for Disease Control and Prevention, May 22, 2017. https://www.cdc.gov/ticks/index.html (accessed February 25, 2018).

"Ticks and Tick-Borne Diseases Protecting Yourself." Australian Association of Bush Regenerators, May 2, 2014. http://aabr.org.au/site/wp-content/uploads/2013/12/AABR-Ticks-and-tick-borne-diseases-protecting-yourself1.pdf (accessed February 25, 2018).

"Trachoma." National Library of Medicine, National Institutes of Health. December 21, 2017. http://www.nlm.nih.gov/medlineplus/ency/article/001486.htm (accessed January 18, 2018).

"Trachoma." World Health Organization. July 2017. http://www.who.int/mediacentre/factsheets/fs382/en/ (accessed January 18, 2018).

"Trachoma: Epidemiological Situation." World Health Organization. http://www.who.int/trachoma/epidemiology/en/ (accessed February 10, 2018).

"Transmission-Based Precautions" Centers for Disease Control and Prevention, February 28, 2017. https://www.cdc.gov/infectioncontrol/basics/transmission-based-precautions.html (accessed December 4, 2017).

"Travelers' Health: Japanese Encephalitis." Centers for Disease Control and Prevention, November 24, 2015. https://wwwnc.cdc.gov/travel/diseases/japanese-encephalitis (accessed February 15, 2018).

"Trichinellosis." European Center for Disease Prevention and Control. https://ecdc.europa.eu/en/trichinellosis (accessed January 11, 2018).

"Trichomoniasis—CDC Fact Sheet." Centers of Disease Control and Prevention, July 14, 2017. https://www.cdc.gov/std/trichomonas/stdfact-trichomoniasis.htm (accessed January 22, 2018).

"Trichomoniasis." Office on Women's Health, US Department of Health and Human Services, June 12, 2017. https://www.womenshealth.gov/a-z-topics/trichomoniasis (accessed January 22, 2018).

"Trichuriasis." Centers for Disease Control and Prevention, January 10, 2013 https://www.cdc.gov/parasites/whipworm/ (accessed January 8, 2018).

"Trypanosomiasis, Human African (Sleeping Sickness)." World Health Organization. http://www.who.int/mediacentre/factsheets/fs259/en/ (accessed November 6, 2017).

"Tuberculosis." World Health Organization, January 2018. http://www.who.int/mediacentre/factsheets/fs104/en/ (accessed March 7, 2018).

"Tuberculosis (TB)." Centers for Disease Control and Prevention. https://www.cdc.gov/tb/default.htm (accessed November 22, 2017).

"Tuberculosis and Air Travel: Guidelines for Prevention and Control." World Health Organization, 2006. http://www.who.int/tb/publications/2006/who_htm_tb_2006_363.pdf (accessed May 17, 2007).

"Tuberculosis Data and Statistics." Centers for Disease Control and Prevention, February 1, 2018. https://www.cdc.gov/tb/statistics/default.htm (accessed March 7, 2018).

"Tularemia." Centers for Disease Control and Prevention, September 27, 2016. https://www.cdc.gov/tularemia/ (accessed February 9, 2018).

Turbert, David. "Histoplasmosis." American Academy of Ophthalmology, September 1, 2017. https://www.aao.org/eye-health/diseases/what-is-histoplasmosis (accessed January 23, 2018).

"Types of Healthcare-Associated Infections." Centers for Disease Control and Prevention. https://www.cdc.gov/hai/infectiontypes.html (accessed January 21, 2018).

"Types of Influenza Viruses." Centers for Disease Control and Prevention. https://www.cdc.gov/flu/about/viruses/types.htm (accessed January 25, 2018).

"Typhoid Fever." Centers for Disease Control and Prevention, July 18, 2016. https://www.cdc.gov/typhoid-fever/index.html (accessed January 29, 2018)

"Typhoid." World Health Organization, April 13, 2015. http://www.who.int/immunization/diseases/typhoid/en/ (accessed January 29, 2018).

"Typhus Fevers." Centers for Disease Control and Prevention, March 7, 2017. https://www.cdc.gov/typhus/ (accessed January 22, 2018).

"Typhus." National Library of Medicine. https://medlineplus.gov/ency/article/001363.htm (accessed January 21, 2018)

Ulansky, Elena. "The Economics of Zika." The Hill, June 20, 2016. http://thehill.com/opinion/op-ed/284177-the-economics-of-zika (accessed February 26, 2018).

"UN Environment and WHO Agree to Major Collaboration on Environmental Health Risks." World Health Organization, January 10. 2018. http://www.who.int/mediacentre/news/releases/2018/environmental-health-collaboration/en/ (accessed January 17, 2018).

"UN Millennium Development Goals." United Nations. http://www.un.org/millenniumgoals/ (accessed June 8, 2007).

"UNICEF Eastern and Southern Africa Overview." UNICEF. https://www.unicef.org/esaro/5482_HIV_AIDS.html (accessed January 1, 2018).

"UNICEF's Engagement in the Global Polio Eradication Initiative." UNICEF. https://www.unicef.org/partners/files/Partnership_profile_2012_Polio_revised.pdf (accessed February 2, 2018).

United Nations–Water. "World Toilet Day." http://www.worldtoiletday.info/ (accessed February 12, 2018).

"Update: Investigations of Patients Who Have Been Treated by HIV-Infected Health-Care Workers." Centers for Disease Control and Prevention. https://www.cdc.gov/mmwr/preview/mmwrhtml/mm5753a3.htm (accessed December 2, 2017).

"Urinary Tract Infection (UTI)." Mayo Clinic. https://www.mayoclinic.org/diseases-conditions/urinary-tract-infection/symptoms-causes/syc-20353447 (accessed November 22, 2017).

"US BSL Laboratories." Federation of American Scientists, 2013. https://fas.org/programs/bio/research.html (accessed January 29, 2018).

"USDA Begins 2017 Field Trials to Evaluate New Oral Rabies Vaccine in Raccoons, Other Wildlife." United States Department of Agriculture, August 7, 2017. https://www.aphis.usda.gov/aphis/newsroom/news/sa_by_date/sa-2017/new-rabies-vaccine (accessed February 19, 2018).

"USDA Detects a Case of Atypical Bovine Spongiform Encephalopathy in Alabama." US Food and Drug Administration, July 18, 2017 https://www.aphis.usda.gov/aphis/newsroom/stakeholder-info/sa_by_date/sa-2017/sa-07/bse-alabama (accessed January 29, 2017).

"USDA Expands Field Trials of New Oral Rabies Vaccine for Use in Raccoons and Other Wildlife in 5 States." United States Department of Agriculture, August 31, 2016. https://www.aphis.usda.gov/aphis/newsroom/news/sa_by_date/sa_2012/sa_08/ct_rabies_vaccine_expanded (accessed February 20, 2018).

"Vaccine Evidence." ROTA Council. http://rota-council.org/vaccine-evidence/ (accessed February 15, 2018).

"Vaccine-Preventable Diseases, Immunizations, and MMWR --- 1961—2011" https://www.cdc.gov/mmwr/preview/mmwrhtml/su6004a9.htm

"Vaccines and Immunizations." *Centers for Disease Control and Prevention*, February 8, 2017. https://www.cdc.gov/vaccines/index.html (accessed February 13, 2018).

"Valley Fever (Coccidioidomycosis)." Centers for Disease Control and Prevention. https://www.cdc.gov/fungal/diseases/coccidioidomycosis/index.html (accessed February 6, 2018).

"Vancomycin-Resistant *Enterococci* (VRE) Overview." National Institute of Allergy and Infectious Disease, March 9, 2009. https://www.niaid.nih.gov/research/vre-overview (accessed March 7, 2018).

"Vancomycin-Resistant *Enterococcus* (VRE)." New York State Department of Health. http://www.health.state.ny.us/diseases/communicable/vancomycin_resistant_enterococcus/fact_sheet.htm (accessed March 7, 2018).

Vanderlinden, Caree. "USAMRIID Supports Ebola Virus Disease Outbreak Response in West Africa." US Army, October 22, 2014. https://www.army.mil/article/136531/usamriid_supports_ebola_virus_disease_outbreak_response_in_west_africa> (accessed January 31, 2018).

"Variant CJD Cases Worldwide." University of Edinburgh, December 4, 2017. https://www.cjd.ed.ac.uk/sites/default/files/worldfigs.pdf (accessed January 29, 2018).

"Variant Creutzfeldt-Jakob Disease (vCJD)." Centers for Disease Control and Prevention, February 10, 2015. https://www.cdc.gov/prions/vcjd/index.html (accessed January 26, 2018).

"Varicella." World Health Organization, April 4, 2015. http://www.who.int/immunization/diseases/varicella/en/ (accessed February 1, 2018).

"Varicella and Herpes Zoster Vaccination Position Paper." World Health Organization, June 2014. http://www.who.int/immunization/position_papers/WHO_pp_varicella_herpes_zoster_june2014_summary.pdf?ua=1 (accessed February 1, 2018).

"Vector-Borne Diseases." World Health Organization. http://www.who.int/mediacentre/factsheets/fs387/en/ (accessed January 14, 2018).

"Venezuelan Equine Encephalitis." World Organisation for Animal Health, April 2013. http://www.oie.int/fileadmin/Home/eng/Animal_Health_in_the_World/docs/pdf/Disease_cards/VEE.pdf (accessed February 25, 2018)

"Viral Hepatitis." Centers for Disease Control and Prevention, September 29, 2017. https://www.cdc.gov/hepatitis/hav/index.htm (accessed January 22, 2018).

"Viral Hepatitis and Young Persons Who Inject Drugs." Centers for Disease Control and Prevention (CDC), April 17, 2017. https://www.cdc.gov/hepatitis/featuredtopics/youngpwid.htm (accessed February 2, 2018).

"Viral Hepatitis: Hepatitis B Information." Centers for Disease Control and Prevention (CDC), May 31, 2015. https://www.cdc.gov/hepatitis/hbv/index.htm (accessed February 2, 2018).

"Viral Hepatitis: Hepatitis C Information." Centers for Disease Control and Prevention. https://www.cdc.gov/hepatitis/hcv/index.htm (accessed February 19, 2018).

"Viral Hepatitis: Hepatitis E." Centers for Disease Control and Prevention, April 28, 2015. https://www.cdc.gov/hepatitis/hev/index.htm (accessed February 7, 2018).

"Viral Meningitis." Centers for Disease Control and Prevention, April 15, 2016 https://www.cdc.gov/meningitis/viral.html (accessed February 16, 2018).

"Viral Meningitis." Meningitis Research Foundation. https://www.meningitis.org/meningitis/what-is-meningitis/viral-meningitis (accessed February 16, 2018).

"VRE in Healthcare Settings." Centers for Disease Control and Prevention, May 10, 2011. https://www.cdc.gov/hai/organisms/vre/vre.html (accessed March 7, 2018).

"Vulvovaginal Candidiasis." Centers for Disease Control and Prevention, June 4, 2015. https://www.cdc.gov/std/tg2015/candidiasis.htm (accessed January 23, 2018).

Walker, Cameron. "Bubonic Plague Traced to Ancient Egypt." National Geographic News, March 10, 2004. http://news.nationalgeographic.com/news/2004/03/0310_040310_blackdeath.html (accessed May 17, 2007).

Wan, Cordia. "Viral Meningitis." Medscape, August 22, 2017. https://emedicine.medscape.com/article/1168529-overview (accessed February 16, 2018).

Waseem, Muhammad. "Otitis Media Treatment & Management." Medscape. https://emedicine.medscape.com/article/994656-treatment (accessed November 15, 2017).

"Water." United Nations. http://www.un.org/en/sections/issues-depth/water/ (accessed November 22, 2017).

"Water for LIFE." LIFE Outreach International. https://lifetoday.org/outreaches/water-for-life/ (accessed January 18, 2018).

"Water Related Diseases." World Health Organization. http://www.who.int/water_sanitation_health/diseases-risks/diseases/ascariasis/en/ (accessed January 10, 2018).

"Weekly Epidemiological Record." World Health Organization, June 10, 2014. http://www.who.int/wer/2014/wer8925.pdf?ua=1 (accessed February 1, 2018).

"Welcome to Headlice.org." National Pediculosis Association. 2007. http://www.headlice.org/ (accessed November 14, 2017).

Wellcome Trust Sanger Institute. "Out of Europe: Researchers Look at the Spread of Dysentery from Europe to Industrializing Countries." ScienceDaily. https://www.sciencedaily.com/releases/2012/08/120805144818.htm (accessed January 16, 2018).

"West Nile Virus." Centers for Disease Control and Prevention. https://www.cdc.gov/westnile/index.html (accessed January 15, 2018).

"West Nile Virus." World Health Organization. http://www.who.int/mediacentre/factsheets/fs354/en/ (accessed November 22, 2017).

"WHA Adopts Resolution on Sepsis." Global Sepsis Alliance, May 26, 2017. https://www.global-sepsis-alliance.org/news/2017/5/26/wha-adopts-resolution-on-sepsis (accessed February 28, 2018).

"What Are Genome Editing and CRISPR-Cas9?" National Institutes of Health. https://ghr.nlm.nih.gov/primer/genomicresearch/genomeediting (accessed November 14, 2017).

"What Are Opportunistic Infections?" HIV.gov, May 15, 2017. https://www.hiv.gov/hiv-basics/staying-in-hiv-care/other-related-health-issues/opportunistic-infections (accessed January 28, 2018).

"What Is Hepatitis D?" Hepatitis B Foundation. http://www.hepb.org/research-and-programs/hepdeltaconnect/whatishepatitisd/ (accessed January 9, 2017).

"What Is Herpes Keratitis?" American Academy of Ophthalmology, March 1, 2017. https://www.aao.org/eye-health/diseases/herpes-keratitis (accessed January 27, 2018).

"What We Do: Prepare Countries to Prevent, Detect, and Respond to Global Health Threats." Centers for Disease Control and Prevention. https://www.cdc.gov/globalhealth/healthprotection/ghs/about.html (accessed January 25, 2018).

"What Zoonotic Diseases Are Dangerous." Centers for Disease Control and Prevention, December 14, 2016. https://www.cdc.gov/about/facts/cdcfastfacts/zoonotic.html (accessed January 31, 2018).

"WHO Estimates Cost of Reaching Global Health Targets by 2030." World Health Organization, July 17, 2017. http://www.who.int/mediacentre/news/releases/2017/cost-health-targets/en/ (accessed January 17, 2018).

"WHO Guide to Identifying the Economic Consequences of Disease and Injury." World Health Organization, 2009. http://www.who.int/choice/publications/d_economic_impact_guide.pdf?ua=1 (accessed February 8, 2018).

"WHO Guidelines for the Treatment of *Neisseria gonorrhoeae*, 2016." World Health Organization. http://apps.who.int/iris/bitstream/10665/246114/1/9789241549691-eng.pdf?ua=1 (accessed January 21, 2017).

"WHO Guidelines for the Treatment of *Treponema pallidum* (Syphilis)." World Health Organization, 2016. http://apps.who.int/iris/bitstream/10665/249572/1/9789241549806-eng.pdf?ua=1 (accessed February 15, 2018).

"WHO Guidelines on Tularaemia." World Health Organization, 2007. http://www.who.int/csr/resources/publications/WHO_CDS_EPR_2007_7.pdf?ua=1 (accessed February 9, 2018).

"WHO/UNICEF Joint Monitoring Program for Water Supply, Sanitation and Hygiene (JMP)—2017 Update and SDG Baselines." UN-WATER, July 12, 2017. http://www.unwater.org/publications/whounicef-joint-monitoring-program-water-supply-sanitation-hygiene-jmp-2017-update-sdg-baselines/ (accessed January 18, 2018).

"Why Is CDC Concerned about Lyme Disease?" Centers for Disease Control and Prevention, December 1, 2017. https://www.cdc.gov/lyme/why-is-cdc-concerned-about-lyme-disease.html (accessed February 25, 2018).

Wild Poliovirus List. Global Polio Eradication Initiative, 2018. http://polioeradication.org/polio-today/polio-now/wild-poliovirus-list/ (accessed February 1, 2018).

"WMA Declaration of Helsinki—Ethical Principles for Medical Research Involving Human Subjects." World Medical Association, March 29, 2017. https://www.wma.net/policies-post/wma-declaration-of-helsinki-ethical-principles-for-medical-research-involving-human-subjects/ (accessed February 12, 2018)

"Women's Health." World Health Organization. http://www.who.int/topics/womens_health/en/ (accessed March 5, 2018).

"Women's Health: Fact Sheet." World Health Organization. http://www.who.int/mediacentre/factsheets/fs334/en/ (accessed February 15, 2018).

"World Health Statistics 2017: Monitoring Health for the SDGs." World Health Organization. http://www.who.int/gho/publications/world_health_statistics/2017/en/ (accessed January 17, 2018).

"The World Is Running Out of Antibiotics, WHO Report Confirms." World Health Organization, September 20, 2017. http://www.who.int/mediacentre/news/releases/2017/running-out-antibiotics/en> (accessed January 24, 2018).

"World Malaria Report 2017." World Health Organization, 2017. http://apps.who.int/iris/bitstream/10665/259492/1/9789241565523-eng.pdf?ua=1 (accessed February 23, 2018).

"Yaws." World Health Organization, March 2017. http://www.who.int/mediacentre/factsheets/fs316/en/ (accessed February 2, 2018).

"Yaws Eradication: Global Experts Meet after Signature of Medicine Donation Agreement." World Health Organization, January 29, 2018. http://www.who.int/neglected_diseases/news/WHO_and_EMS_sign_medicine_donation_agreement/en/ (accessed February 2, 2018).

"Year in Review: Measles Linked to Disneyland." Centers for Disease Control and Prevention, December 2, 2015. https://blogs.cdc.gov/publichealthmatters/2015/12/year-in-review-measles-linked-to-disneyland/ (accessed February 15, 2018).

"Yellow Fever." Centers for Disease Control and Prevention, July 12, 2016. https://www.cdc.gov/yellowfever/ (accessed December 11, 2017).

"Yellow Fever." World Health Organization, May 2016. http://www.who.int/mediacentre/factsheets/fs100/en/ (accessed December 11, 2017).

"Yellow Fever. Fact Sheet." World Health Organization, May 2016. http://www.who.int/mediacentre/factsheets/fs100/en (accessed January 19, 2018).

"*Yersinia Enterocolitica* (Yersinia)." Centers for Disease Control and Prevention, October 24, 2016. https://www.cdc.gov/yersinia/ (accessed January 9, 2018).

"Yersiniosis and Chitterlings: Tips to Protect You and Those You Care for from Foodborne Illness." Food Safety and Inspection Service, US Department of Agriculture, December 1, 2016. https://www.fsis.usda.gov/wps/portal/fsis/topics/food-safety-education/get-answers/food-safety-fact-sheets/foodborne-illness-and-disease/yersiniosis-and-chitterlings/ct_index (accessed January 11, 2018).

"Yersiniosis—Annual Epidemiological Report 2016 [2014 Data]." European Centre for Disease Prevention and Control, March 13, 2017. https://ecdc.europa.eu/en/publications-data/yersiniosis-annual-epidemiological-report-2016–2014-data (accessed January 30, 2018).

"Your Guide to Urinary Tract Infections (UTIs)." WebMD. https://www.webmd.com/women/guide/your-guide-urinary-tract-infections#1 (accessed November 22, 2017).

"Zika Cumulative Cases." Pan American Health Organization, January 4, 2018. http://www.paho.org/hq/index.php?option=com_content&view=article&id=12390&Itemid=42090&lang=en (accessed February 26, 2018).

"Zika Situation Report." World Health Organization. Last modified April 7, 2016. http://www.who.int/emergencies/zika-virus/situation-report/7-april-2016/en/ (accessed December 10, 2017).

"Zika Virus." Centers for Disease Control and Prevention. https://www.cdc.gov/zika/index.html (accessed January 14, 2018).

"Zika Virus." World Health Organization, September 6, 2016. http://www.who.int/mediacentre/factsheets/zika/en/ (accessed February 26, 2018).

"Zika Virus Disease." World Health Organization. http://www.who.int/csr/disease/zika/en/ (accessed February 27, 2018).

"Zika Virus Infection." Pan American Health Organization. http://www.paho.org/hq/index.php?option=com_content&view=article&id=11585&Itemid=41688&lang=en (accessed February 26, 2018).

"Zoonoses." World Health Organization. http://www.who.int/topics/zoonoses/en/ (accessed January 31, 2018).

"Zoonotic Diseases." Centers for Disease Control and Prevention, July 14, 2017. https://www.cdc.gov/onehealth/basics/zoonotic-diseases.html (accessed January 31, 2018).

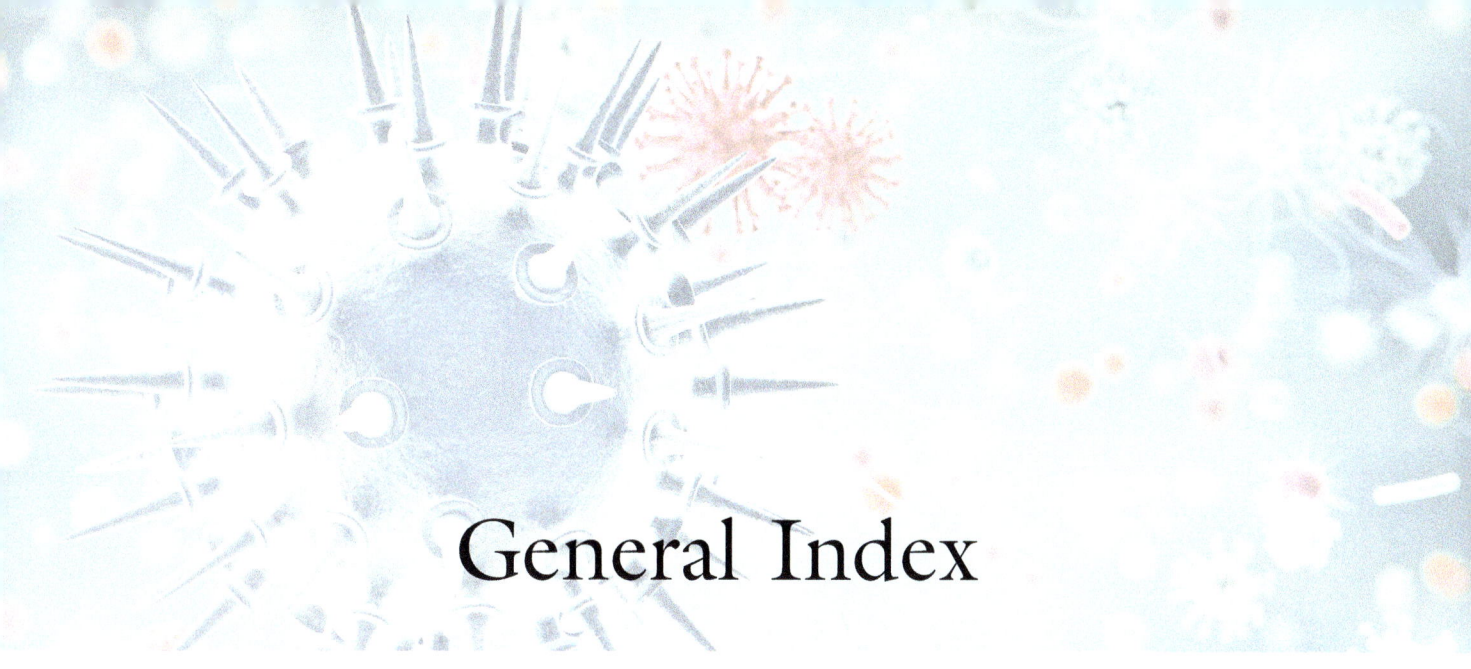

General Index

Page numbers in **boldface** indicate the main essay for a topic. An *italicized* page number indicates a photo, illustration, chart, or other graphic. An *s* following a page number indicates the use of a term in a sidebar and a *t* indicates a table appears within an entry.

A

AB103, 2:963
Abbott Laboratories, 1:64
Abdominal bleeding and balantidiasis, 1:103
Abdominal cramps
- AIDS, 1:12
- balantidiasis, 1:103
- *Campylobacter* infection, 1:151
- cholera, 1:201
- cryptosporidiosis, 1:251
- cyclosporiasis, 1:259
- giardiasis, 1:371
- hand, foot, and mouth disease, 1:397
- hookworm infection, 1:458
- listeriosis, 1:556
- marine toxins, 2:591
- protozoan diseases, 2:754
- rotavirus infection, 2:828
- *Salmonella* infection, 2:841
- shigellosis, 2:880, 881
- water-borne disease, 2:1054

Abdominal pain
- alveolar echinococcosis, 1:24
- amebiasis, 1:27
- angiostrongyliasis, 1:35
- anisakiasis, 1:45
- *Clostridium difficile* infection, 1:209, 210
- Crimean-Congo hemorrhagic fever, 1:244
- Ebola, 1:302
- glanders, 1:379
- gonorrhea, 1:389
- helminth disease, 1:415
- hemorrhagic fevers, 1:420*s*
- hepatitis B, 1:426
- hepatitis C, 1:430
- hepatitis D, 1:434
- hookworm infection, 1:458
- influenza, 1:488
- Legionnaires' disease, 1:530
- liver fluke infections, 1:560
- lung flukes, 1:566
- Marburg hemorrhagic fever, 2:586
- marine toxins, 2:590
- microsporidiosis, 2:623
- mononucleosis, 2:631
- puerperal fever, 2:767
- Q fever, 2:772
- Rocky Mountain spotted fever, 2:824
- schistosomiasis, 2:861
- severe fever with thrombocytopenia syndrome, 2:871
- sexually transmitted infections, 2:877
- shigellosis, 2:883
- tapeworm infections, 2:948
- trichinellosis, 2:972
- typhoid fever, 2:993, 995
- typhus, 2:997
- whipworm, 2:1062
- yersiniosis, 2:1096–1097

Abelcet. *See* Amphotericin B
Abortion, 1:76*s*, 2:1108
Abrams, Rachel, 2:671
Abscesses
- blastomycosis, 1:122
- *Chlamydia* infection, 1:191
- dysentery, 1:290
- glanders, 1:379, 380
- gonorrhea, 1:389
- nocardiosis, 2:666
- pneumonia, 2:726
- protozoan diseases, 2:755
- rat-bite fever, 2:786
- ringworm, 2:817
- tsunami lung, 2:730

Abstinence, sexual
- AIDS prevention, 1:14
- *Chlamydia* infection prevention, 1:191
- Ebola prevention, 1:303*s*
- gonorrhea, 1:389
- herpes simplex virus 2, 1:446*s*

ACAM2000, 2:893
Acanthamoeba, 2:643
Acaricides, 2:826
Accelerate Action to End Child Marriage, 2:1005–1006
Accelerate to Zero strategy, 1:77
Access to clean water and sanitation. *See* Sanitation
Access to health care resources
- African sleeping sickness, 1:5
- AIDS, 1:15
- arthropod-borne disease, 1:76
- Brazil, 2:1108
- CDC, 1:169
- diphtheria, 1:277
- economic development, 1:307, 308–309
- glanders, 1:381
- globalization, 1:385
- group B streptococcal infections, 2:925
- hepatitis B, 1:428
- hepatitis C, 1:432, 435
- HIV/AIDS, 2:1008, 1009, 1010
- immigration, 1:472
- Japanese encephalitis, 1:512, 513*s*
- liver fluke infections, 1:563
- malaria, 2:582, 583

measles, 2:595
microsporidiosis, 2:623
monkeypox, 2:628, 628*s*
puerperal fever, 2:769
rotavirus infection, 2:828, 829, 830–831
sepsis, 2:869
sexually transmitted infections, 2:879
syphilis, 2:936
Syrians, 1:264
tropical infectious diseases, 2:981
tuberculosis, 2:987
typhoid fever, 2:995
vaccines, 2:1023
viral disease, 2:1041
wars and conflicts, 1:314
whooping cough, 2:1068
women, 2:1072
See also Developing nations and drug delivery
Acetaminophen
chikungunya, 1:182
mononucleosis, 2:634
RSV infection, 2:834
strep throat, 2:918
Zika virus, 2:1102
Acetylcholine, 1:133
Aches. *See* Body aches
Acid-fast staining tests, 1:260, 545
Acinetobacter baumannii, 1:59
Aciphex. *See* Rabeprazole
Acquired immunity. *See* Adaptive immunity
Acquired immunodeficiency syndrome. *See* AIDS
Acquired Immunodeficiency Syndrome Program, 2:654
Active case findings, 2:763
Active immunization, 1:185, 2:893
Active tuberculosis, 2:983
Acupuncture and AIDS transmission, 1:11
Acute forms of diseases. *See* specific diseases
Acute respiratory distress syndrome, 1:405
Acyclovir
antiviral drugs, 1:72
encephalitis, 1:318
genital herpes, 1:365
herpes simplex 1 virus, 1:442
herpes simplex virus 2, 1:445, 446
shingles, 2:886
Adam, Jessica K, 2:787
Adamantanes, 1:490
Adams Waldorf, Kristina, 2:926, 927
Adaptive immunity, 1:455, 478, 2:792
Adenoviruses, 1:228, 2:1039
Adhanom Ghebreyesus, Tedros, 2:*1078,* 1079, 1079*s*
Adhesins, 2:841
Adolescents
ADHD medications and sexually transmitted infections, 2:977
child marriage, 2:1005
Chlamydia infection, 1:191
cohorted communities, 1:224*s*
Creutzfeldt-Jakob disease, 1:240
diphtheria vaccine, 1:276, 277
encephalitis, 1:317
Epstein-Barr virus, 1:335, 337
gonorrhea, 1:389
hepatitis B vaccine, 1:428*s*
herpes simplex virus 2, 1:445
HPV vaccine, 1:470–471
Kawasaki disease, 1:517
mononucleosis, 2:630, 631, 632, 633–635
mumps, 2:647
pneumonia, 2:726
tetanus, 2:954
tuberculosis, 2:985
viral meningitis, 2:609
whooping cough, 2:1067, 1068, 1069
Adoption, international, 1:474–475
Adoptive cell transfer, 1:479
Adult T-cell leukemia, 1:155
Adults
chickenpox, 1:177
diphtheria, 1:275, 276, 277
encephalitis, 1:317
fifth disease, 1:347, 348
influenza epidemiology, 1:505
mononucleosis, 2:632
mumps, 2:645, 646
pinworm infection, 2:706
pneumonia, 2:728
polio, 2:737
re-emerging infectious diseases, 2:791
rotavirus infection, 2:829
rubella, 2:837
scabies, 2:852
war, 2:1050
whooping cough, 2:1067
yersiniosis, 2:1097
Advanced Diagnostics Program, 2:783*s*
Adverse effects
AIDS drugs, 1:13
measles vaccine clinical trials, 2:1073
MMR vaccine, 2:838
public health, 2:763
typhus drugs, 2:1000
vaccines, 2:1022, 1023
yellow fever vaccine, 2:1092
See also Side effects
Advisory Committee on Immunization Practices, 2:646, 887
Advisory Committee on Variola Virus Research, 2:898
Advisory Group of Independent Experts, WHO, 2:898
Aedes mosquitoes, 2:*815*
chikungunya, 1:181
congenital Zika syndrome, 2:1102
dengue and dengue hemorrhagic fever, 1:266, 268
Eastern equine encephalitis, 1:296
globalization, 1:385
mosquito-borne diseases, 2:637
Rift Valley fever, 2:813
tropical infectious diseases, 2:980
vector-borne disease, 2:1029
Venezuelan equine encephalitis virus, 2:1033
yellow fever, 2:1093
Zika virus, 2:1101, 1108
Aerosols
Ebola, 1:303
hemorrhagic fevers, 1:419, 420*s*
histoplasmosis, 1:451
hot tub rash, 1:466–467
measles, 2:594
plague, 2:719
rabies, 2:776
Rift Valley fever, 2:816
tularemia, 2:990, 991, 991*s*
war, 2:1050, 1051, 1052
Afghan Ministry of Public Health, 2:1068
Afghanistan
avian influenza, 1:89
bioterrorism, 1:116
diphtheria, 1:278
dysentery, 1:*291*
glanders, 1:381
leishmaniasis, 1:539, *539,* 541
outbreaks, field-level response to, 2:686
polio, 1:184, 2:733, 734, 734*s,* 738, 740
rotavirus, 2:831
whooping cough, 2:1068
Afghanistan, war in, 1:59
Africa
African sleeping sickness, 1:1
AIDS, 1:14, 15, 18, 19, 20
amebiasis, 1:28
anellovirus, 1:30
angiostrongyliasis, 1:36
animal importation, 2:1084
anthrax, 1:48–49
antiviral drug types, 1:72–73
arthropod-borne diseases, 1:77
ascariasis, 1:79
avian influenza, 1:88
babesiosis, 1:96
bacterial meningitis, 2:605, *605,* 606
blastomycosis, 1:122
brucellosis, 1:141
burkholderia, 1:142, 145
Buruli ulcer, 1:147–150
candidiasis, 1:160
chikungunya, 1:180, 181, 2:614
cholera, 1:198, 201

climate change, 1:206, 207
contact precautions, 1:237–238
cryptosporidiosis, 1:251
demographics, 1:262, 263
dengue and dengue hemorrhagic fever, 1:266
dracunculiasis, 1:283, 285
drug delivery, 1:270, 271, 272*s*
Ebola, 1:41, 301–302
economic development, 1:308
emerging infectious diseases, 1:313–314
encephalitis, 1:317
environmental health risks, 2:1077
epidemiology, 1:332–333
Epstein-Barr virus, 1:335
filariasis, 1:351
gastroenteritis, 1:358–361
glanders, 1:380
Haemophilus influenzae, 1:395, 396
helminth disease, 1:415
hemorrhagic fevers, 1:420
hepatitis D, 1:434, 435
hepatitis E, 1:438
herpes simplex 1 virus, 1:442
H5N1, 1:496
hookworm infection, 1:58
hosts and vectors, 1:463
immigration, 1:474
leishmaniasis, 1:539
leprosy, 1:544
leptospirosis, 1:549
liver fluke infections, 1:561
Lyme disease, 1:571
malaria, 1:462, 2:581, 582–583
Marburg hemorrhagic fever, 2:585, 586
maternal mortality, 2:768
microsporidiosis, 2:623
monkeypox, 2:626, 627, 628
mosquito-borne diseases, 2:637
necrotizing fasciitis, 2:659
opportunistic infections, 2:684
pinworm infection, 2:705
plague, 2:715, 716, 717, 719
Pneumocystis jirovecii pneumonia, 2:723
polio eradication campaign, 2:734
protozoan diseases, 2:755
rabies, 2:775, 777
rat-bite fever, 2:786
re-emerging infectious diseases, 2:791*s,* 792
relapsing fever, 2:796, 797, 798
Rift Valley fever, 2:813, 814, 815, 816
river blindness, 2:820, 821
rotavirus, 1:361, 2:831
rubella, 2:838
SARS, 2:849
schistosomiasis, 2:861, 863
smallpox, 2:1077
syphilis, 2:936
taeniasis, 2:942, 943
tapeworm infections, 2:949
tick-borne diseases, 2:957
trachoma, 2:967
travel, 2:970, 971
tropical infectious diseases, 2:981
typhoid fever, 2:993, 994, 996
typhus, 2:997, 999
United Nations Millennium Goals, 2:1008, 1009
vector-borne disease, 2:1030
virus hunters, 2:1043
water-borne disease, 2:1055, 1056
West Nile virus, 2:1057, 1060
whipworm, 2:1063
whooping cough, 2:1067
yaws, 2:1087, 1088, 1089
yellow fever, 2:1092, 1093
Zika virus, 1:169, 2:1100, 1102
Africa, ancient, 2:890
African Americans
AIDS, 1:13
blastomycosis, 1:122
syphilis, 2:936
trichomoniasis, 2:976
Tuskegee syphilis study, 2:937–938
women, 2:1073
African clawed frogs, 2:1084
African green monkeys, 2:585
African Program for Onchocerciasis, 1:270, 2:822
African sleeping sickness, 1:**1–6,** *2*
Médecins Sans Frontières, 2:600
protozoan diseases, 2:753, 755, 756
travel, 2:971
tropical infectious diseases, 2:980, 981
Agency for Healthcare Research and Quality, 1:256*s*
Agitation, 2:776, 997
Agramonte, Aristides, 1:342–343, 2:1043, 1095
Agriculture
climate change and protozoan diseases, 2:757
encephalitis, 1:317
keratitis, 1:232
See also Livestock
Ahmedabad, India, 1:*99*
AIDS, 1:**7–16**
antiviral drugs, 1:72–73
aspergillosis risk factors, 1:85
candidiasis risk factors, 1:158, 159
climate change, 1:206
CMV infection risk factors, 1:214, 215
Cryptococcus neoformans infection, 1:248, 249
cryptosporidiosis, 1:251, 253
demographics, 1:262
developing nations and drug delivery, 1:271, 272*s*
diagnosis, 1:12–13
diseases that weaken the immune system, 2:667*s*
economic development, 1:309
emerging infectious diseases, 1:312
epidemiology, 1:331–332
fifth disease, 1:349
first reports of, 1:19*s*
gastroenteritis, 1:358
helminth disease, 1:416
history, 1:13, 17–20
HIV, 1:453–456
impacts and issues, 1:14–15
Koch's postulates, 1:521
Legionnaires' disease, 1:530
leishmaniasis, 1:541
measles, 2:595
Médecins Sans Frontières, 2:600–601
microsporidiosis, 2:622, 623–624
mosquito-borne diseases, 2:638
mycotic disease, 2:650
National Institute of Allergy and Infectious Diseases, 2:654
opportunistic infections, 2:682, 683, 684
Pneumocystis jirovecii pneumonia, 2:721–724, *723*
pneumonia, 2:725–726
prevalence, 1:13
protozoan diseases, 2:755
re-emerging infectious diseases, 2:792
retroviruses, 2:805, 806
ringworm, 2:819
scrofula, 2:867
sexually transmitted infections, 2:876–877, 878
signs and symptoms, 1:11
talaromycosis, 2:944, 945
toxoplasmosis, 2:964, 966
transmission, 1:7–11
travel, 2:970, 971
treatment and prevention, 1:13–14
tuberculosis, 2:983
UNICEF, 2:1006
United Nations Millennium Goals, 2:1007, 1008–1009, 1010
vancomycin-resistant *Enterococci,* 2:1026
viral disease, 2:1038, 1039, 1041
water-borne disease, 2:1055
West Nile virus, 2:1060
women, 2:1072–1073
See also HIV
AIDS: origin of the modern pandemic, 1:7–8, 13, *17,* **17–20**
AIDS drugs and leprosy, 1:547
AIDS test kit, 1:*454*
AIDS vaccine, 1:*9*

Air filtration, 1:22, 23
Air pressure and airborne precautions, 1:22
Air quality and pneumonia, 2:729
Air travel
  emerging infectious diseases, 1:313
  epidemiology, 1:332
  globalization, 1:383
  immigration, 1:472, 474
  SARS, 2:850
  travel, 2:970
  vaccinations, 1:186
Airborne precautions, 1:**21–23,** 21*t,* *22,* 484–485
Airborne transmission
  anthrax, 1:47
  botulinum toxin, 1:134
  Burkholderia bacteria, 1:381
  chickenpox, 1:175, 176
  Chlamydia infection, 1:190, 193
  colds, 1:229
  diphtheria, 1:275
  droplet precautions, 1:286–288
  Ebola, 1:237, 303
  encephalitis, 1:316, 317
  endemicity, 1:322
  fifth disease, 1:348
  glanders, 1:378
  group A streptococcal infections, 2:921
  Haemophilus influenzae, 1:395
  hemorrhagic fevers, 1:419, 420*s*
  herpes simplex 1 virus, 1:440–441
  histoplasmosis, 1:451
  H5N1 virus, 1:393
  hot tub rash, 1:466–467
  influenza, 1:488–489
  influenza pandemic of 1918, 1:495
  influenza pandemic of 1957, 1:500
  Legionnaires' disease, 1:530, 531
  measles, 2:593, 594
  monkeypox, 2:626
  MRSA, 2:643
  mumps, 2:645, 646
  mycotic disease, 2:650, 651
  necrotizing fasciitis, 2:659
  nocardiosis, 2:666
  personal protective equipment, 2:700
  plague, 2:712
  Pneumocystis jirovecii pneumonia, 2:722
  psittacosis, 2:759
  Q fever, 2:771
  Rift Valley fever, 2:816
  RSV infection, 2:833
  rubella, 2:837
  scarlet fever, 2:857
  shingles, 2:885
  smallpox, 1:115, 2:890, 891, 892, 893
  strep throat, 2:917
  tropical infectious diseases, 2:980
  tuberculosis, 2:983
  tularemia, 2:991, 991*s*
  viral disease, 2:1041
  viral meningitis, 2:609
Airway obstruction, 2:857
Alabama, 1:139
Alaska, 2:591, 973
Albania, 1:89
Albendazole
  anisakiasis, 1:45
  ascariasis, 1:80
  costs, 2:707, 708
  filariasis, 1:351
  hookworm infection, 1:58
  liver fluke infections, 1:562
  microsporidiosis, 2:624
  pinworm infection, 2:706
  taeniasis, 2:942
  tapeworm infections, 2:950
  toxocariasis, 1:80*s*
  tropical infectious diseases, 2:981
  whipworm, 2:1062, 1063, 1064
Albenza. *See* Albendazole
Alberta, Quebec, 1:142, 406
Albuminuria, 1:404
Alcohol and disinfection, 1:56, 69, 281, 485
Alcohol-based hand sanitizers
  CDC recommendations, 1:69
  contact precautions, 1:237
  hospital settings, 1:400, 402
  infection control and asepsis, 1:486*s*
  MRSA prevention, 2:642
  standard precautions, 1:486*s,* 2:*909,* 910
  strep throat prevention, 2:918
  vancomycin-resistant *Enterococci* prevention, 2:1027
Alcoholism, 2:667*s*
Aldehyde, 1:281
Alexander the Great, 1:544, 2:579
Algae and algal blooms, 2:592, 1054
Algeria, 1:116, 539
Aliferis, Lisa, 2:1068
"All That Glitters: Gold Nanoparticles Yield Possible Vaccine for Common Childhood Virus," 2:*834–835*
Allen, Arthur, 1:186
Allergies
  after giardiasis, 1:373
  aspergillosis, 1:85, 86
  colds, 1:230*s*
  disinfection as contributing to, 1:370
  pink eye, 2:702–703
  ringworm, 2:817
  swimmer's ear and swimmer's itch, 2:931
  tick bites, 2:958
  tick-borne diseases, 2:957, 958
Alliance for Cervical Cancer Prevention, 1:156
Alliance for the Global Elimination of Trachoma, 2:968*s*
Allworth, Anthony, 2:730
Alpers, Michael, 1:524–525
Alphaviruses, 2:1033
al-Qaeda, 1:116
Altered mental state. *See* Mental status changes
Altfeld, Marcus, 2:1074
Alveolar echinococcosis, 1:**24–26**
Alves, Jessé, 2:1108
Alzheimer's disease, 1:195, 524, 525
Amantadine
  H5N1 virus, 1:393
  influenza, 1:490, 505
  rabies, 2:778
Amazonian snails, 1:36
Amebiasis, 1:**27–29**
  climate change and protozoan diseases, 2:757
  dysentery, 1:289, 290
  protozoan diseases, 2:754–755, 756
  water-borne diseases, 2:1054
Amebicides, 1:28
Amedra Pharmaceuticals, 2:708
American Academy of Pediatrics, 1:135, 470
American Association of Pediatrics, 2:606
American Civil War, 1:290
American dog ticks, 2:824
American Foundation for AIDS Research, 1:19*s*
American Journal of Obstetrics & Gynecology, 2:926
The American Journal of the Medical Sciences, 2:1094
American Mosquito Control Association, 2:638–639
American Optometric Association, 1:233
American Osteopathic College of Dermatology, 2:933
American Public Health Association, 1:332
American Red Cross
  blood supply, 1:126, 127
  Measles and Rubella Initiative, 2:595
  parasitic disease screening, 2:695
American Samoa, 1:182
American Thoracic Society, 2:728
American trypanosomiasis. *See* Chagas disease
Americaninhas, Brazil, 2:863
Americas
  chikungunya, 1:*180,* 181, 182
  helminth disease, 1:415, 417
  herpes simplex 1 virus, 1:442
  herpes simplex virus 2, 1:445
  hookworm infection, 1:58, 457
  microsporidiosis, 2:623

polio, 2:733, 734, 738, 740
rubella, 2:838
tick-borne diseases, 2:957
tropical infectious diseases, 2:981
Zika virus, 2:1100, 1102
Amgen, 1:114
Amikacin, 2:668
Aminoglycoside antibiotics, 1:58, 2:1097
Amish communities, 1:487, 2:837
Amnesic shellfish poisoning, 2:591
Amoxicillin
antibiotic resistance, 1:59
dysentery, 1:290
group A streptococcal infections, 2:922
Helicobacter pylori, 1:411
leptospirosis, 1:549
Lyme disease, 1:571
pneumonia, 2:718
Q fever, 2:773
strep throat, 2:918
Amphibians, importation of, 2:1084
Amphotericin B
blastomycosis, 1:122
candidiasis, 1:159
coccidioidomycosis, 1:221
Cryptococcus neoformans infection, 1:248
Fusarium keratitis, 1:232
sporotrichosis, 2:903
talaromycosis, 2:945
Ampicillin
antibiotic resistance, 1:59
cholera, 1:198
dysentery, 1:290
leptospirosis, 1:549
nocardiosis, 2:668
typhoid fever, 2:994
Amplification, 1:287–288, 304
Amprenivir, 1:13
Amputation
necrotizing fasciitis, 2:659
toxic shock, 2:963
war, 2:1050
Amur River, 2:*609*
Amyotrophic lateral sclerosis, 1:573
Anal cancer
cancer, 1:155
HPV, 1:468, 470
opportunistic infections, 2:683
Analamanga region, Madagascar, 2:717
Analgesics
chikungunya, 1:182
colds, 1:230
dracunculiasis, 1:284
emergency preparedness kits, 2:766
mononucleosis, 2:632
mumps, 2:646
shingles, 2:886–887
strep throat, 2:918–919
viral meningitis, 2:610
Zika virus, 2:1102
Anaphylaxis, 2:957, 958
Anaplasmosis, 2:810, 811, 957
Anatomical issues, 2:1013, 1071
Ancient cultures
animal importation, 1:39
anthrax, 1:47
brucellosis, 1:140
cholera, 1:199
colds, 1:228
diphtheria, 1:277
glanders, 1:378–379
gonorrhea, 1:387
helminth disease, 1:414
influenza, 1:488
leprosy, 1:543, 544
lice infestation, 1:552–553
malaria, 2:579
mumps, 2:644
plague, 2:710, 713–714
rabies, 2:775
scrofula, 2:865
smallpox, 2:890, 1081
tetanus, 2:952
trachoma, 2:967
tuberculosis, 2:983, *984*
zoonoses, 2:1106
Ancylostoma. See Hookworm infection
Anders, Kelto, 2:601
Andes virus, 1:405, 406
Andrews, Travis M., 2:882
Anellovirus, 1:**30–34**
Anemia
arthropod-borne diseases, 1:75
ascariasis, 1:80
babesiosis, 1:96
fifth disease, 1:347, 349
hookworm infection, 1:58, 458, 459
protozoan diseases, 2:753
puerperal fever, 2:767
rubella, 2:837
talaromycosis, 2:944
whipworm, 2:1062, 1063, 1064
women, 2:1072
Aneurysms and Kawasaki disease, 1:515, 516, 517
Angiostrongyliasis, 1:**35–38,** *37*
Angiostrongylus infection. *See* Angiostrongyliasis
Angola
African sleeping sickness, 1:3
cholera, 1:201
leprosy, 2:1078
Marburg hemorrhagic fever, 2:585, 587
Rift Valley fever, 2:814
yellow fever, 1:169
Anhui Province, China, 2:849
Animal experimentation
anellovirus, 1:31
B virus infection, 1:91–92
coccidioidomycosis, 1:221
Creutzfeldt-Jakob disease, 1:241
disinfection byproducts, 1:282
DNA technology, 1:81
Ebola vaccine, 2:1022
group B streptococcal infection, 2:926–927
H5N1 virus, 1:393
importation of animals for, 1:40, 41
influenza, 1:495, 496
kuru, 1:524
leprosy, 1:545
Marburg hemorrhagic fever, 2:585
nosocomial infections, 2:675–676
pigmentation research, 1:478*s*
rabies vaccine research, 2:779
retroviruses, 2:808
Rift Valley fever, 2:815
SARS, 2:850
sex of animals used in, 2:1074
smallpox drugs, 1:115
toxic shock, 2:963
typhus, 2:1001
virus hunters, 2:1045
Animal feed
antibiotics in, 2:1027–1028
bovine spongiform encephalopathy, 1:137, 138–139, 241
Animal handlers
animal importation, 1:41
B virus infection, 1:91–92, 93
Baylisascaris infection, 1:107
brucellosis, 1:141
cat scratch disease, 1:163
cryptosporidiosis, 1:251
protozoan diseases, 2:754
rabies, 2:777
Animal importation, 1:**39–42,** *40*
angiostrongyliasis, 1:38
Ebola, 1:303
giant African land snail ban, 1:38
globalization, 1:384
hemorrhagic fevers, 1:420*s*
Marburg hemorrhagic fever, 2:585
mosquito-borne diseases, 2:637
psittacosis, 2:759–760
Q fever, 2:773
rabies, 2:778
world trade, 2:1083–1085
zoonoses, 2:1106
Animals
anthrax, 1:51
DDT effects, 1:77
deticking, 1:245
leishmaniasis, 1:541
leptospirosis, 1:549*s,* 550
tetanus, 2:953
See also Livestock; Zoonoses; specific animals

Anisakiasis, 1:*43,* **43–46,** *44*
Anisakis simplex. See Anisakiasis
Annals of the Rheumatic Diseases, 2:576
Annual Review of Biochemistry, 2:801
Annual Review of Immunology, 1:53
Anopheles mosquitoes
- climate change and re-emerging infectious diseases, 2:791*s*
- immigration, 1:472
- malaria, 2:578–582
- mosquito-borne diseases, 2:638
- treated bed nets and the life span of, 2:1031–1032

Antelopes, 1:1
Anthelmintic drugs
- ascariasis, 1:80
- costs, 2:707–708
- helminth disease, 1:416
- hookworm infection, 1:58, 459–460
- liver fluke infections, 1:562
- lung flukes, 1:567
- pinworm infection, 2:706
- schistosomiasis, 2:860, 862
- strongyloidiasis, 2:929, 930
- taeniasis, 2:942
- tapeworm infections, 2:948, 950
- toxocariasis, 1:80*s*
- trichinellosis, 2:974
- whipworm, 2:1062, 1063, 1064

Anthrasil, 1:116
Anthrax, 1:**47–52,** *48,* 2:*696*
- bacterial diseases, 1:99, 100
- biodefense research and development, 1:119
- bioterrorism, 1:113–114, 115–116, 2:*751,* 894, 1051*s*
- disinfection, ineffectiveness of, 1:282
- genetic identification of microorganisms, 1:364
- germ theory of disease, 1:367
- microorganisms, 2:615
- personal protective equipment, 2:701
- re-emerging infectious diseases, 2:790, 792
- USAMRIID, 2:1017, 1018
- war, 2:1050–1051
- zoonoses, 2:1107

Antibacterial drugs, 1:*56,* **56–59,** *57. See also* Antibiotic resistance; Antibiotics
Antibacterial soaps. *See* Antimicrobial soaps
Antibiotic ointment. *See* Topical medications
Antibiotic resistance, 1:*61,* **61–65**
- antibacterial drug issues, 1:59
- antimicrobial soaps, 1:66, 67–68
- bacterial diseases, 1:100, 101
- biodefense research and development, 1:119
- burkholderia, 1:145–146
- candidiasis risk factors, 1:160
- *Chlamydia* infection, 1:191
- cholera, 1:198
- *Clostridium difficile* infection, 1:209, 211
- cohorted communities, 1:224
- contact precautions, 1:237
- demographics, 1:263
- drug development research, 2:675–676
- emerging infectious diseases, 1:313–314
- gonorrhea, 1:389, 389*s*
- group A streptococcal infections, 2:920, 922
- *Haemophilus influenzae,* 1:396
- *Helicobacter pylori,* 1:412
- infection control and asepsis, 1:487
- isolation and quarantine, 1:509
- leprosy, 1:545, 547
- microbial evolution, 2:611, 612, *613*
- MRSA, 2:640–643
- National Institute of Allergy and Infectious Diseases, 2:654–655
- nosocomial infections, 2:674–675
- and overreliance on fluoroquinolones, 1:257
- plague, 2:716–717, 718
- pneumonia, 2:728, 729
- President's Initiative on Combating Antibiotic Resistance, 2:744–746
- rapid diagnostic tests, 2:783
- re-emerging infectious diseases, 2:791
- resistant organisms, 2:799–803
- *Salmonella* infection, 2:842
- scarlet fever, 2:858
- sexually transmitted infections, 2:878–879
- shigellosis, 2:882
- *Staphylococcus aureus* infections, 2:912–913
- sterilization, 2:916*s*
- strep throat, 2:919
- superbugs, 2:1027*s*
- topical antibiotics, 2:704
- tuberculosis, 2:984, 985, 986
- typhoid fever, 2:994, 996
- typhus, 2:1000
- urinary tract infection, 2:1013, 1014
- vancomycin-resistant *Enterococci,* 2:1025–1028
- war, 2:1050
- whooping cough, 2:1068
- *See also* Antimicrobial resistance; Drug resistance

Antibiotic Resistance Solutions Initiative, 2:803
Antibiotics
- anthrax, 1:51, 115
- antiviral drugs compared to, 1:70
- babesiosis, 1:95
- bacterial diseases, 1:101
- bacterial infections with chickenpox, 1:177
- bacterial meningitis, 2:606, 610
- balantidiasis, 1:102, 103
- bioterrorism, 1:116
- brucellosis, 1:142
- burkholderia, 1:142, 145–146
- Buruli ulcer, 1:149
- *Campylobacter* infection, 1:152
- cancer, 1:155
- candidiasis risk factors, 1:157, 158, 159
- cat scratch disease, 1:162
- CDC, 1:169
- *Chlamydia* infection, 1:189–191
- *Chlamydia pneumoniae,* 1:193, 195
- cholera, 1:198
- *Clostridium difficile* infection, 1:209, 210, 211
- colds, 1:229
- cryptosporidiosis, 1:252
- culture and sensitivity, 1:254–257
- cyclosporiasis, 1:260
- diphtheria, 1:276
- drug development research, 2:675–676
- dysentery, 1:290
- ear infections, 1:293
- gastroenteritis, 1:360
- genetic identification of microorganisms, 1:363
- glanders, 1:380
- gonorrhea, 1:388, 389
- group A streptococcal infections, 2:920, 922
- group B streptococcal infections, 2:925, 926, 927
- *Helicobacter pylori,* 1:409, 411, 412
- hot tub rash, 1:466
- impetigo, 1:481
- Legionnaires' disease, 1:531
- leprosy, 1:546
- leptospirosis, 1:548, 549, 550
- Lyme disease, 1:569, 571, 573, 574
- measles and secondary infections, 2:595
- microorganisms, 2:617
- microsporidiosis, 2:624
- mononucleosis, secondary infections with, 2:632
- MRSA, 2:642
- mycotic disease as a side effect of, 2:650
- necrotizing fasciitis, 2:657, 659, 660

nocardiosis, 2:668
nosocomial infections, 2:674–675
opportunistic infections, 2:682, 683
plague, 2:718
Pneumocystis jirovecii pneumonia, 2:721
pneumonia, 2:728
post-treatment Lyme disease syndrome, 1:572
prescriptions, by state, 1:*57*
psittacosis, 2:759, 760
Q fever, 2:773
rat-bite fever, 2:786
relapsing fever, 2:796–797
resistant organisms, 2:799–803
rickettsial disease, 2:809, 811
Rocky Mountain spotted fever, 2:824, 825–826
Salmonella infection, 2:842
scarlet fever, 2:857, 858
scrofula, 2:866
secondary infections, 1:490, 501, 507
severe fever with thrombocytopenia syndrome, 2:871, 872
sexually transmitted infections, 2:878–879
shigellosis, 2:880, 882, 883
Staphylococcus aureus infections, 2:912–913
stockpiling, 2:700*s*
strep throat, 2:917, 918
substandard and falsified medical products, 1:272
swimmer's ear and swimmer's itch, 2:933
syphilis, 2:934, 936
tetanus, 2:954
tick-borne diseases, 2:958
toxic shock, 2:962
trachoma, 2:968–969
trichomoniasis, 2:976, 977
tropical infectious diseases, 2:981
tsunami lung, 2:730
tuberculosis, 2:984, 985, 986
tularemia, 2:989, 991, 991*s*
Tuskegee syphilis study, 2:937
typhoid fever, 2:994
typhus, 2:998, 999–1000
urinary tract infection, 2:1013, 1014
vancomycin-resistant *Enterococci*, 2:1026–1027
war, 2:1049–1050
whooping cough, 2:1068
World Health Organization, 2:1078, 1079
yaws, 2:1003, 1088, 1089, 1090
yersiniosis, 2:1097
zoonoses, 2:1107
See also Antibacterial drugs

Antibodies
AIDS, 1:12
anti-cytokine antibody syndrome, 1:53–54
dysentery, 1:290
HIV, 1:12
mononucleosis, 2:634
Zika virus, 2:1101, 1102

Antibody tests
AIDS, 1:12
botulism, 1:135
brucellosis, 1:142
Crimean-Congo hemorrhagic fever, 1:244, 245
dengue and dengue hemorrhagic fever, 1:267–268
dysentery, 1:290
encephalitis, 1:318
Epstein-Barr virus, 1:337
glanders, 1:380
hantavirus, 1:407
herpes simplex 1 virus, 1:442
influenza, 1:490
Legionnaires' disease, 1:531
mononucleosis, 2:632
Powassan virus, 2:743
rapid diagnostic tests, 2:781–782, 782–783
RSV infection, 2:833–834
St. Louis encephalitis, 2:906
strep throat, 2:919

Antibody treatment for Creutzfeldt-Jakob disease, 1:241
Anticancer drugs from marine microorganisms, 2:591*s*
Anticonvulsants, 1:513
Anti-cytokine antibody syndrome, 1:**53–55**
Antidepressants, 2:887
Antidiarrheal drugs, 1:252
Antifungal drugs
alveolar echinococcosis, 1:25
aspergillosis, 1:85
blastomycosis, 1:122, 123
candidiasis, 1:159
coccidioidomycosis, 1:221
Cryptococcus neoformans infection, 1:248
Fusarium keratitis, 1:232
histoplasmosis, 1:451
mycotic disease, 2:649
for opportunistic infections, 2:683
parasitic diseases, 2:695
ringworm, 2:818
sporotrichosis, 2:901, 902, 903
talaromycosis, 2:945–946
zoonoses, 2:1107

Antigen-antibody tests. *See* Antibody tests
Antigenic drift and shift, 1:489–490, 503
Antigenic variation, 1:2
Antigens
aspergillosis, 1:85
colds, 1:229
immune response, 1:478

Anti-GM-CSF antibodies, 1:53, 54
Antihistamines
colds, 1:230
ear infections, 1:294
scabies, 2:854
swimmer's itch, 2:933

Anti-infective drugs, 1:375
Anti-inflammatory drugs, 1:182
Antimalarial drugs
malaria, 2:578–579, 581
resistant organisms, 2:800–801
UNICEF, 2:1005

Antimicrobial resistance
disinfection, 1:281, 282
germ theory of disease, 1:369–370
hot tub rash, 1:465
re-emerging infectious diseases, 2:790
sterilization, 2:915–916
Task Force on Antimicrobial Resistance, 1:256*s*

"Antimicrobial Resistance: Global Report on Surveillance," 2:802
Antimicrobial soaps, 1:*66*, **66–69**
contact precautions, 1:236
disinfection, 1:281
resistant organisms, 2:803
sterilization, 2:915–916
tularemia prevention, 2:991

Antiminth. *See* Pyrantel pamoate
Antimonials, 1:540
Antimony and parasitic diseases, 2:695
Antiox. *See* Anthelmintic drugs
Antiparasitic drugs
babesiosis, 1:95, 97
Chagas disease, 1:173
costs, 2:707–708
filariasis, 1:350, 351–352
giardiasis, 1:373
helminth disease, 1:416
hookworm infection, 1:458
leishmaniasis, 1:540
lung flukes, 1:567
microsporidiosis, 2:624
pinworm infection, 2:706
river blindness, 2:820, 821
taeniasis, 2:942
tapeworm infections, 2:948, 950
toxoplasmosis, 2:966
tropical infectious diseases, 2:981
whipworm, 2:1062, 1063, 1064
zoonoses, 2:1107

Antiprotozoal drugs, 2:695
Antipyretics
mononucleosis, 2:632
RSV infection, 2:834
shigellosis, 2:882
viral meningitis, 2:610

Antiretroviral therapy
AIDS, 1:8, 13, 15
antiviral drug types, 1:72

cryptosporidiosis, 1:252
developing nations and drug delivery, 1:272*s*
HIV prevention, 2:1010
microsporidiosis, 2:623
Pneumocystis jirovecii pneumonia, 2:721, 722
sexually transmitted infections, 2:878
talaromycosis, 2:945, 946
United Nations Millennium Goals, 2:1008, 1009
women, 2:1073
Antiseptic soaps. *See* Antimicrobial soaps
Antismoking campaigns, 1:167
Antitoxins
bioterrorism, 1:114, 116
botulism, 1:135
diphtheria, 1:276
tetanus, 2:952
"Anti-Vaccine Activists Spark a State's Worst Measles Outbreak in Decades," 2:*596–598*
Anti-VD campaigns, 2:936
Antiviral drugs, 1:**70–73**
avian influenza, 1:89, 90
B virus infection, 1:93
bioterrorism, 1:114, 115
chickenpox, 1:175, 177
CMV infection, 1:215, 216–217
cold sores, 1:226
colds, 1:230
Crimean-Congo hemorrhagic fever, 1:245
encephalitis, 1:318
genital herpes, 1:365
hantavirus, 1:407
hepatitis B, 1:427
hepatitis C, 1:431–432
hepatitis E, 1:438
herpes simplex 1 virus, 1:442
herpes simplex virus 2, 1:444, 445, 446, 446*s*
H5N1 virus, 1:393
influenza, 1:490, 496, 505, 507
Lassa fever, 1:526, 528
measles, 2:595
microorganisms, 2:617
monkeypox, 2:628
Nipah virus infection, 2:663
opportunistic infections, 2:683
rabies, 2:778
Rift Valley fever, 2:815
RSV infection, 2:834
severe fever with thrombocytopenia syndrome, 2:872
sexually transmitted infections, 2:878
shingles, 2:885, 886
smallpox, 2:892–893
zoonoses, 2:1107
Antivomiting drugs, 1:252
Anxiety and Creutzfeldt-Jakob disease, 1:240
Apes, 1:304, 2:1083
Appalachia, 2:929
Appalachian Mountain disease. *See* Histoplasmosis
Appendicitis, 2:1062, 1097
Appendix obstruction, 2:942
Appetite loss
cat scratch disease, 1:161–163
Chagas disease, 1:172
Clostridium difficile infection, 1:210
cyclosporiasis, 1:259
enterovirus 71 infection, 1:325
glanders, 1:379
hand, foot, and mouth disease, 1:397
hepatitis A, 1:422–425
hepatitis B, 1:426
hookworm infection, 1:458
mononucleosis, 2:634
mumps, 2:645
Rocky Mountain spotted fever, 2:824
Salmonella infection, 2:841
scarlet fever, 2:856
schistosomiasis, 2:861
sexually transmitted infections, 2:877
syphilis, 2:935
talaromycosis, 2:944
typhoid fever, 2:993
viral meningitis, 2:608
West Nile virus, 2:1058
Aquaculture, 2:591*s*
Araraquara virus, 1:406
Arboviruses. *See* Arthropod-borne diseases
Archives of Virology, 1:31
Arenaviruses
hemorrhagic fevers, 1:418, 419
Lassa fever, 1:526–528
viral disease, 2:1041
Argasid ticks, 1:243
Argentina
Chagas disease, 1:173
coccidioidomycosis, 1:218, 220
hantavirus, 1:406
Rocky Mountain spotted fever, 2:825
trichinellosis, 2:974
Argentine hemorrhagic fever, 1:418, 420
Aristotle, 2:775
Arizona
coccidioidomycosis, 1:218, 220, 221
hantavirus, 1:407
hemorrhagic fevers, 1:420
hepatitis A vaccine, 1:425
plague, 2:717
relapsing fever, 2:795
St. Louis encephalitis, 2:906
Arkansas, 1:449, 2:873*s*
Armadillos, 1:107, 545
Armenia, 1:277
Arrhenius, Svante, 1:205
ART. *See* Antiretroviral therapy
Artemether and lumefantrine, 2:581
Artemisinin, 2:581, 802
Arthralgia. *See* Joints and joint pain
Arthritis
Campylobacter infection as risk factor for, 1:152
chikungunya, 1:181, 182
Cryptococcus neoformans infection, 1:248
gonorrhea, 1:388
Haemophilus influenzae, 1:395
Kawasaki disease, 1:517
Lyme disease, 1:569, 570, 571
macrophage activation syndrome, 2:575–576
microsporidiosis, 2:624*s*
mumps, 2:645
rat-bite fever, 2:786
retroviruses, 2:808
Salmonella infection, 2:841
shigellosis, 2:881
viral disease, 2:1041
Arthritis & Rheumatism, 2:576
Arthritis & Rheumatology, 2:575
Arthropod-borne diseases, 1:*74,* **74–77**
African sleeping sickness, 1:1–5
Brazil, 2:1108–1109
Buruli ulcer, 1:148
Chagas disease, 1:171–174
chikungunya, 1:180–182
climate change, 1:204
Crimean-Congo hemorrhagic fever, 1:243–246
dysentery, 1:289
Eastern equine encephalitis, 1:296–298
emerging infectious diseases, 1:312
encephalitis, 1:316, 317, 318
endemicity, 1:321, 322
filariasis, 1:350–352
hemorrhagic fevers, 1:419, 420
hosts and vectors, 1:461
infection control and asepsis, 1:486
Japanese encephalitis, 1:511–514
leishmaniasis, 1:538–541
Lyme disease, 1:569–574
malaria, 2:578–583
mosquito-borne diseases, 2:636–639
parasitic diseases, 2:694
Powassan virus, 2:741–743
protozoan diseases, 2:753–754
re-emerging infectious diseases, 2:790–791, 792
rickettsial disease, 2:809–812
river blindness, 2:820–822

Rocky Mountain spotted fever, 2:824–826
severe fever with thrombocytopenia syndrome, 2:871–873
St. Louis encephalitis, 2:905–907
tapeworm infections, 2:948
tick-borne diseases, 2:956–959
tropical infectious diseases, 2:979–980, 981
typhus, 2:997–1001
vector-borne disease, 2:1029, 1030–1031
Venezuelan equine encephalitis virus, 2:1033–1035
viral disease, 2:1041, 1042
viral meningitis, 2:609
virus hunters, 2:1046
West Nile virus, 2:1057–1061
yellow fever, 2:1092–1095
Zika virus, 2:1100–1103
zoonoses, 2:1105, 1106–1107
ARV therapy. *See* Antiretroviral therapy
Ascariasis, 1:**78–80**
Ascaris lumbricoides infection. *See* Ascariasis
Asepsis. *See* Infection control and asepsis
Aseptic meningitis, 2:606*s*, 607–610, 736
Asia
AIDS, 1:14, 15
alveolar echinococcosis, 1:24
anellovirus, 1:30
arthropod-borne diseases, 1:75
avian influenza, 1:88, 89–90
B virus infection, 1:93
babesiosis, 1:96
bloodborne infections transmitted through barber shops, 1:131*s*
bovine spongiform encephalopathy, 1:242
brucellosis, 1:141
burkholderia, 1:142
carbapenem-resistant Enterobacteriaceae, 1:59
chikungunya, 1:181, 2:614
cholera, 1:198
cryptosporidiosis, 1:251
dengue and dengue hemorrhagic fever, 1:266
developing nations and drug delivery, 1:271
dracunculiasis, 1:285
dysentery, 1:290
encephalitis, 1:318
environmental health risks, 2:1077
extremely drug-resistant tuberculosis, 1:23
gastroenteritis, 1:358–361
glanders, 1:380
Haemophilus influenzae, 1:396
hantavirus, 1:404
hepatitis E, 1:438
H5N1, 1:391–393, 496
hookworm infection, 1:58
hosts and vectors, 1:463
influenza pandemics, 1:496
Japanese encephalitis, 1:513–514
leishmaniasis, 1:539
liver fluke infections, 1:561, 562
lung flukes, 1:565
Lyme disease, 1:571
malaria, 2:581
maternal mortality, 2:769
microsporidiosis, 2:623
mosquito-borne diseases, 2:637
necrotizing fasciitis, 2:659
Nipah virus infection, 2:664
pinworm infection, 2:705
plague, 2:716–717
protozoan diseases, 2:755
rabies, 2:775, 777
rat-bite fever, 2:786
relapsing fever, 2:796
Rift Valley fever, 2:814
rotavirus, 2:831
sanitation, 2:844, 845
SARS, 2:678
scrofula, 2:867
taeniasis, 2:943
tapeworm infections, 2:949
tick-borne diseases, 2:957
tularemia, 2:990
typhoid fever, 2:993, 994, 996
typhus, 2:999
vector-borne disease, 2:1031
West Nile virus, 2:1060
yaws, 2:1087, 1088, 1089
Zika virus, 1:169, 2:1100, 1101
Asian Americans, 1:122
Asia-Pacific region, 1:325, 326
Asiatic cholera. *See* Cholera
Asiedu, Kingsley, 2:1089
Asilomar Conference, 1:**81–83**
Aspergillosis, 1:53, *84,* **84–86**
Aspiration
Legionnaires' disease, 1:530
pneumonia, 2:727
tsunami lung, 2:730–731
Aspirin
chikungunya precautions, 1:182
Kawasaki disease, 1:515
Reye's syndrome, 2:632, 634, 918–919
Zika virus cautions, 2:1102
Association for Professionals in Infection Control and Epidemiology, 1:483
Asthma
aspergillosis, 1:84–85
Chlamydia pneumoniae, 1:194, 195
RSV infection, 2:834
Astrodome, 2:670
Astrology, 2:712
Asymptomatic carriers
candidiasis, 1:159
diphtheria, 1:276*s*
group A streptococcal infections, 2:921
polio, 2:734
SARS, 2:850
scarlet fever, 2:856
typhoid fever, 2:993, 994, 995, 995*s*
"At Rocky Mountain Labs, 'Virus Ecology' Helps Scientists Understand Threats Such as Zika," *2:655–656*
Ataxia, 1:240, 2:749
Atazanavir, 1:13
Athens, ancient, 2:710
Atherosclerotic plaques, 1:195
Athlete's foot, 2:650, *650,* 651, 817–818
Athletic facilities
MRSA, 2:641, 642–643
mycotic disease, 2:650
scabies prevention, 2:854*s*
See also Sports and athletes
Atlanta, GA, 1:165, 166, 2:894, 1051
Atlantic Ocean, 1:43
Atlantic states, 1:297, 2:591
Atopy, 2:853
Atovaquone, 1:97, 2:581
Attention deficit hyperactivity disorder, 2:977
Attention deficits and hookworm infection, 1:459
Attenuated vaccines
anthrax, 1:50
polio, 2:734, 739
rabies, 2:779
rubella, 2:838
smallpox, 2:897
typhoid fever, 2:994
vaccines and vaccine development, 2:1022*s*
Atypical measles, 2:594
Aum Shinrikyo, 1:304, 2:1050
Australasia, 2:1063
Australia
AIDS history, 1:18
angiostrongyliasis, 1:36
antimicrobial soaps, 1:67
burkholderia, 1:144, 145
Buruli ulcer, 1:147
candidiasis, 1:160
chickenpox vaccine, 1:177
cryptosporidiosis, 1:251
enterovirus 71 infection, 1:326
fruit bats, 2:663
glanders, 1:378, 380, 381
globalization, 1:384
group B streptococcal infection, 2:926
hepatitis A, 1:424
influenza epidemiology, 1:506
Japanese encephalitis, 1:514
kuru, 1:523
microsporidiosis, 2:623
MRSA, 2:640

mumps, 2:647
necrotizing fasciitis, 2:659
psittacosis, 2:760
Q fever, 2:771, 772
re-emerging infectious diseases, 2:791*s*
talaromycosis, 2:945
tapeworm infections, 2:949
tick-borne diseases, 2:957, 958
triclosan, 2:916
typhus, 2:997, 999, 1000
whooping cough vaccine, 2:1068
Zika virus, 2:1101, 1102
Australian Department of Health, 2:760
Austria, 1:89
Autism and MMR vaccines, 2:597, 598, 837, 838*s*, 1021
Autoantibodies, 1:53, 54
Autoclaving, 2:910, 914–915, *915*
Autoimmune disorders
anti-cytokine antibody syndrome, 1:53
group A streptococcal infections, 2:920
histoplasmosis risk factors, 1:449, 451
immune response, 1:478–479
retroviruses, 2:808
women, 2:1074
Autoimmune polyendocrinopathy, candidiasis, ectodermal dystrophy syndrome, 1:53
Autolysins, 1:58
Aventis Pasteur Smallpox Vaccine, 2:893
Avert, 1:262, 272*s*
Avian influenza, 1:*87*, **87–90,** *489*
CDC, 1:169
dangers of, 1:491, 496
endemicity, 1:322
globalization, 1:385
H5N1, 1:391–393
human encroachment into wildlife areas, 1:304
microbial evolution, 2:614
personal protective equipment, 2:700
public health, 2:764, 765–766
viral disease, 2:1041
world trade, 2:1083–1084
zoonoses, 2:1105
"Avian Influenza--Necessary Precautions to Prevent Human Infection of H5N1, Need for Virus Sharing," 1:*89–90*
Awareness, public. *See* Public awareness and education
Axid. *See* Nizatidine
Azerbaijan, 1:88, 89, 277
Azidothymidine. *See* AZT
Azithromycin
babesiosis, 1:97
Chlamydia infection, 1:191
cholera, 1:198
gonorrhea, 1:389, 389*s*
Legionnaires' disease, 1:531
pneumonia, 2:718
shigellosis, 2:882
trachoma, 2:968, 969
tropical infectious diseases, 2:981
typhus, 2:999–1000
yaws, 2:1088, 1089, 1090
Azoles, 2:945–946
AZT, 1:13, 72
Aztecs, 2:890
Aztreonam, 2:728
Azvedo, Luiz Sergio, 1:216

B

B cells
anti-cytokine antibody syndrome, 1:54
Epstein-Barr virus, 1:335
HIV, 1:455
immune response, 1:478
re-emerging infectious diseases, 2:792
RSV infection, 2:835
B virus infection, 1:**91–94**
Baba Raghav Das Hospital, 1:*315*
Babes, Victor, 1:95
Babesia infection. *See* Babesiosis
Babesiosis, 1:*95*, **95–98,** *96*, 571, 2:957, 958
Babies. *See* Infants
Baboons and histoplasmosis, 1:449
Baby boomers and hepatitis C, 1:431
Bacillus anthracis. See Anthrax
Bacillus Calmette-Guérin vaccine, 1:149, 2:791, 985
Bacillus stearothermophilus, 2:915
Bacillus subtilus, 2:915
Back pain
Crimean-Congo hemorrhagic fever, 1:244
hantavirus, 1:404
hemorrhagic fevers, 1:419
monkeypox, 2:626, 628*s*
rat-bite fever, 2:785
West Nile virus, 2:1058
yellow fever, 2:1092
Bacteremia, 2:926, 1096, 1097
Bacteria
antimicrobial soaps, 1:66–69
Asilomar Conference guidelines, 1:82
filariasis, 1:352
food-borne disease, 1:354
infection control and asepsis, 1:484, 485, 486, 487
marine microorganisms, 2:591*s*
microbial evolution, 2:611–614
microorganisms, 2:616
microscopes and microscopy, 2:619
positive role of, 1:412*s*
Bacterial diseases, 1:*99*, **99–101**
with AIDS, 1:12
anthrax, 1:47–51
antibacterial drugs, 1:56–59
antibiotic drug development, 2:675–676
antibiotic resistance, 1:61–64
anti-cytokine antibody syndrome, 1:53
avian influenza, 1:156
biodefense research and development, 1:119
blood supply, 1:126
botulism, 1:133–135
brucellosis, 1:140–142
Campylobacter infection, 1:151–153
cancer, 1:155
cat scratch disease, 1:161–163
with chickenpox, 1:175, 177
Chlamydia infection, 1:189–191
Chlamydia pneumoniae, 1:193–195
cholera, 1:197–201
climate change, 1:205
Clostridium difficile infection, 1:209–213
cohorted communities, 1:223–224
colds, 1:229
contact precautions, 1:236
culture and sensitivity, 1:254–257
diphtheria, 1:274–278
disinfection, 1:280–282
droplet precautions, 1:286
dysentery, 1:289, 292
ear infections, 1:293, 294, 295
Escherichia coli O157:H7, 1:338–341
food-borne disease, 1:355, 356
gastroenteritis, 1:359, 360
glanders, 1:378–381
gonorrhea, 1:387–390
group B streptococcal infections, 2:924–927
Haemophilus influenzae, 1:394–396
Helicobacter pylori, 1:409–412
hemorrhagic fevers, 1:418
hot tub rash, 1:465–467
impetigo, 1:480–482
with influenza, 1:488, 490
influenza and secondary infections, 1:501
Japanese encephalitis secondary infections, 1:512
Legionnaires' disease, 1:529–531
leprosy, 1:543–547
leptospirosis, 1:548–550
listeriosis, 1:556–558
louse-borne disease, 1:554
Lyme disease, 1:569–574
marine toxins, 2:590
meningitis, 2:604–606
with mononucleosis, 2:632

MRSA, 2:640–643
necrotizing fasciitis, 2:657–660
nosocomial infections, 2:673–675
opportunistic infections, 2:682, 683
pink eye, 2:702, 703
plague, 2:715–719
pneumonia, 2:726, 727–728, 729
President's Initiative on Combating Antibiotic Resistance, 2:744–746
psittacosis, 2:759–760
puerperal fever, 2:767–769
Q fever, 2:771–773
rat-bite fever, 2:785–788
re-emerging infectious diseases, 2:791–792
relapsing fever, 2:795–798
resistant organisms, 2:799–803
rickettsial disease, 2:809–812
with ringworm, 2:818, 819
Rocky Mountain spotted fever, 2:824–826
Salmonella infection, 2:840–842
sanitation, 2:844–845
scarlet fever, 2:856–858
scrofula, 2:865–867
secondary infections and influenza, 1:507
sexually transmitted infections, 2:877, 878–879
shigellosis, 2:880–883
Staphylococcus aureus infections, 2:911–913
sterilization, 2:915–916, 916*s*
strep throat, 2:917–919
streptococcal infections, group A, 2:920–922
syphilis, 2:934–939
tetanus, 2:952–955
tick-borne diseases, 2:957, 958
toxic shock, 2:961–963
trachoma, 2:967–969
trichomoniasis, 2:975–977
tropical infectious diseases, 2:980
tuberculosis, 2:983–988
tularemia, 2:989–991
typhoid fever, 2:993–996
typhus, 2:997–1001
urinary tract infection, 2:1012, 1013, 1014
vaccine-preventable bacterial diseases, 1:100*t*
vancomycin-resistant *Enterococci,* 2:1025–1028
vector-borne disease, 2:1029
war, 2:1051–1052
water-borne diseases, 2:1053–1054, 1054–1055
whooping cough, 2:1066–1069
World Health Organization, 2:1078–1079
yaws, 2:1087–1090
yersiniosis, 2:1096–1099

Bacterial meningitis. *See* Meningitis, bacterial
Bacterial pneumonia, 1:101
Bacteriology, 1:369*s,* 519
Bacteriophage therapy. *See* Phage therapy
Bacteriophages, 2:612, 642
Badgers, 1:31
Baggelay, Kate, 1:417
Baghdad boil. *See* Leishmaniasis
Bahta, Lyn, 2:597
Bairnsdale ulcer. *See* Buruli ulcer
Baja California, 1:406
Bakersfield Californian, 1:221
Balance issues and ear infections, 1:293
Balantidiasis, 1:*102,* **102–104,** 2:754
Ballard, Jimmy D., 1:211, 212
Bamboo rats, 2:944, 945, *945,* 1083
Ban Ki-moon, 1:111
Bananas, edible vaccines in, 1:82*s*
Bandicoot rats and hantavirus, 1:405
Bang, Oluf, 1:154
Bangkok, Thailand, 1:514
Bangladesh
child marriage, 2:1005
cholera, 1:197, 199, 201
demographics, 1:261
leishmaniasis, 1:539, 540, 541
leprosy, 1:546
Nipah virus infection, 2:663, 664
outbreaks, field-level response to, 2:686
rotavirus, 1:361, 2:831
smallpox, 2:*892,* 897
women, 2:1072
Bans
antimicrobial soap substances, 1:66
beef imports, 2:750
enrofloxacin, 2:803
giant African land snail importation, 1:38
nontherapeutic antibiotics, 1:64
triclosan, 2:916
UK beef, 1:241–242
Baranska, Anna, 1:478*s*
Barbare, Shannon, 1:425
Barber shops, 1:131*s*
Barking deer, 2:1083
Barr, Yvonne, 1:335, 2:631
Bartonella henselae. See Cat scratch disease
Bas, 2:*587*
Basidiospores, 1:247–248
Basil and cyclosporiasis outbreaks, 1:258
Basse-Guinée, Guinea, 2:1022
Bassi, Agostino, 1:367
Bats
Ebola, 1:301, 303, 304
hemorrhagic fevers, 1:419, 420*s*
Marburg hemorrhagic fever, 2:586
Nipah virus infection, 2:662–663, 664
rabies, 2:776, 777, 778
virus hunters, 2:1045, 1046
zoonoses, 2:1106
Battlefield medicine, 2:1018
Bausch & Lomb, 1:232
Bayer, 1:64
Bayesian formulas, 1:377
Baylisascaris infection, 1:**105–108,** *106*
Baylor College of Medicine, 1:212
Bayou virus, 1:405
Beach, Doug, 2:671
Bear meat, 2:973, 974
Beaver fever. *See* Giardiasis
Beavers, 1:372, 2:931, 973
Bed netting. *See* Netting, bed
Bed rest
encephalitis, 1:318
mononucleosis, 2:635
nocardiosis, 2:668
pneumonia, 2:729
viral meningitis, 2:610
Bedding
chlamydia, 1:190
lice infestation, 1:552, 553
monkeypox, 2:628
mosquito-borne diseases, 2:639
scabies, 2:854, 854*s*
standard precautions, 2:910
yellow fever transmission theories, 1:342–343, 345
Beef. *See* Cattle; Meat
Behavior changes
AIDS prevention, 1:15
Baylisascaris infection, 1:107
encephalitis, 1:316
Japanese encephalitis, 1:512
Beijing, China
food-borne disease, 1:*355*
public health, 2:764
SARS, 2:849
Beira, Mozambique, 1:200
Belarus, 1:277
Belém, Brazil, 2:1046
Belgium, 2:778, 1083
Bell, Erin, 2:887
Belluck, Pam, 2:1102
Benin, 1:149
Benjak, Andrej, 1:545
Benzalkonium chloride, 1:68
Benzathine penicillin G, 2:936
Benzethonium chloride, 1:68
Benznidazole
alveolar echinococcosis, 1:25
Chagas disease, 1:171, 173–174
protozoan diseases, 2:756
tropical infectious diseases, 2:981
Benzole. *See* Anthelmintic drugs
Berg, Paul, 1:81
Bergantino, Michelle, 2:*1015*
Bergen-Belsen concentration camp, 2:999
Bermejo virus, 1:405

Berries, 1:258, *259*
Beta-hemolytic *Streptococci,* 2:921
Beta-lactam antibiotics
antibacterial drugs, 1:57–58
antibiotic resistance, 1:63
dysentery, 1:290
nosocomial infections, 2:674
resistant organisms, 2:801
Betatorquevirus, 1:30
Bethesda, MD, 2:894, 898
Betzig, Eric, 2:620
Beurmann, Charles Lucien de, 2:901
Bhutan, 1:540
Bias, gender, 2:1071
Biblical texts
bacterial disease, 1:99
leprosy, 1:543
marine toxins, 2:589
plague, 2:710
vector-borne disease, 2:1029
Bihar, India, 1:513*s*
Bile ducts and microsporidiosis, 2:623
Bilharz, Theodor, 2:860
Bilharzia. *See* Schistosomiasis
Biliary duct obstruction, 2:942
Bill & Melinda Gates Foundation
African sleeping sickness, 1:4
arthropod-borne diseases, 1:77
cervical cancer prevention, 1:156
emerging infectious diseases, 1:312
Global Alliance for Vaccines and Immunization, 2:1005
Global Polio Eradication Initiative, 2:740, 1077
helminth disease, 1:417
mosquito-borne disease research and prevention, 2:638
parasitic diseases, 2:696
rabies, 2:779
rotavirus vaccine, 1:361
Schistosomiasis Control Initiative, 2:863
tropical infectious diseases, 2:981*s*
UNICEF, 2:1004
United Nations Millennium Goals, 2:1009
Billroth, Christian Theodor, 2:658, 920, 925
Biltricide. *See* Praziquantel
bin Laden, Osama, 1:116, 2:734*s*
Biocontainment laboratories, 2:792
Biodefense
Project Bioshield, 1:51, 114, 2:654
re-emerging infectious diseases, 2:792
USAMRIID, 2:1015–1016
"Biodefense R&D: Anticipating Future Threats, Establishing a Strategic Environment," 1:*118–119*
Biodiversity and climate change, 2:697–698
Bioengineering
bioweapons, 1:118, 119
edible vaccines, 1:82*s*
HIV prevention, 1:455
pathogens, 2:783*s*
See also Genetic engineering
Bioethics. *See* Ethical issues
Biofilms
disinfection, 1:282
ear infections, 1:293
hot tub rash, 1:465
infection control and asepsis, 1:485, 487
Legionnaires' disease, 1:530
resistant organisms, 2:802*s*
urinary tract infection, 2:1014
Biohazardous waste, 1:485
Bioindicators, 2:915
Bioinformatics, 1:363, 375–377
Biological magnification, 2:590
Biological mosquito control methods, 2:638
Biological weapons
Advanced Diagnostics Program, 2:783*s*
anthrax, 1:47–48, 49, 50, 51
bacterial diseases, 1:101
Baylisascaris procyonis, 1:108
Biological Weapons Convention, 1:109–111
bioterrorism preparedness, 2:1051*s*
botulism, 1:134*s*
brucellosis, 1:142
burkholderia, 1:144, 146, 146*s*
Ebola, 1:304
genetic identification of microorganisms, 1:363*s*
glanders, 1:378, 381
monkeypox, 2:628
Operation Sea Spray, 2:1014*s*
plague, 2:719
preparedness, 2:700*s*
Rift Valley fever, 2:816
shigellosis, 2:880, 882
smallpox, 2:890, 893–894, 896
tularemia, 2:991, 991*s*
war, 2:1050–1052
Biological Weapons Convention, 1:47, **109–112,** *110,* 2:893–894
Biologics Control Laboratory, 2:654
Biomedical Advanced Research and Development Authority, 1:114, 115, 117
Biopsy
blastomycosis, 1:122
Buruli ulcer, 1:149
coccidioidomycosis, 1:220
nocardiosis, 2:667
Biosafety and the hantavirus, 1:407
Biosafety in Microbiological and Biomedical Laboratories, 2:1016
Biosafety level 1 laboratories, 2:1017*s*
Biosafety level 3 laboratories, 1:142
Biosafety level 4 laboratories
at CDC, 1:168
Crimean-Congo hemorrhagic fever, 1:246
hemorrhagic fevers, 1:420*s,* 421
Marburg hemorrhagic fever, 2:587
personal protective equipment, 2:700
Rocky Mountain Laboratory, 2:656
safety requirements, 2:1017*s*
smallpox eradication and storage, 2:897–898
USAMRIID, 2:1016
viral disease, 2:1041
Biosensor Technologies Program, 1:363*s*
Biosensors and the Advanced Diagnostics Program, 2:783*s*
Biosynthetic vaccines, 2:1022*s,* 1023
Biotechnology and microbial evolution, 2:613–614
Bioterrorism, 1:*113,* **113–120**
Advanced Diagnostics Program, 2:783*s*
anthrax, 1:47, 48, 51
anthrax-by-mail scare, 2:*751*
biological warfare, 1:111*s*
Ebola, 1:304
food-borne disease, 1:357
genetic identification of microorganisms, 1:363*s*
GIDEON, 1:375, 377
glanders, 1:381
Lassa fever, 1:528
Marburg hemorrhagic fever, 2:587
microbial evolution, 2:614
National Institute of Allergy and Infectious Diseases, 2:654
plague, 2:715, 719
preparedness, 2:700*s,* 1051*s*
re-emerging infectious diseases, 2:790, 792
shigellosis, 2:882
smallpox, 2:894, 896, 899, 1022
tularemia, 2:989, 991*s*
war, 2:1050
Bird flu. *See* Avian influenza
Birds, 2:*760*
aspergillosis, 1:86
avian influenza, 1:87–90
Baylisascaris infection, 1:107
Chlamydia infection, 1:189
Cryptococcus neoformans infection, 1:248
cryptosporidiosis, 1:251
DDT effects, 1:77
Eastern equine encephalitis, 1:296, 297, 298
encephalitis, 1:317
endemic disease, 1:322
histoplasmosis, 1:449
H5N1 virus, 1:391–393

influenza, 1:488, 491, 505
Japanese encephalitis, 1:512
mosquito-borne diseases, 2:637
psittacosis, 2:759–760
Salmonella infection, 2:841
schistosomes, 2:931
St. Louis encephalitis, 2:905
vector-borne diseases, 2:1029, 1030
West Nile virus, 2:1057, 1058, 1060
world trade, 2:1083
zoonoses, 2:1106, 1107
Birmingham, England, 1:397
Birth control pills, 1:517
Birth defects
maternal chickenpox, 1:177
parasitic diseases, 2:695
sexually transmitted infections, 2:877
vector-borne disease, 2:1030
Venezuelan equine encephalitis virus, 2:1035
viral disease, 2:1042
Zika virus, 2:687, 1101, 1107–1108
Birth rates, 1:261–262
Bismuth subsalicylates, 1:411, 2:882
Bison and brucellosis, 1:140, 142, 143
Bites and scratches
B virus infection, 1:92, 93
cat scratch disease, 1:161, 162, 162*s*, 163
human bites and AIDS transmission, 1:9
rabies, 2:775–779
rat-bite fever, 2:785–788
sporotrichosis, 2:902
zoonoses, 2:1106
See also Arthropod-borne diseases
Bithionol, 1:562
Biting midges, 1:244
Black Bane, 1:47
Black Creek Canal virus, 1:405
Black Death
arthropod-borne diseases, 1:75
bioterrorism, 1:116
immigration, 1:472
plague, early history of, 2:711–712
policies regarding, 1:533
theories, 2:713–714
Black flies and river blindness, 2:820, 821, 822
Black market in animals, 1:384
Black people and coccidioidomycosis, 1:219
Black stools, 1:244
Blackburn, Christine Crudo, 1:264
Blacklegged ticks
babesiosis, 1:95
Lyme disease, 1:569, 570
tick-borne diseases, 2:959
Bladder cancer, 1:155, 2:863
Bladder disease or symptoms
blastomycosis, 1:122
schistosomiasis, 2:861
urinary tract infection, 2:1012, 1013
viral disease, 2:1039
Blaser, Martin J., 1:412*s*
Blastomycosis, 1:*121*, **121–124**
Bleach, 2:915
Bleeding
chikungunya, 1:181, 182
dengue and dengue hemorrhagic fever, 1:267
Ebola, 1:300, 302, 303
hantavirus, 1:404
hemorrhagic fevers, 1:418, 420
macrophage activation syndrome, 2:575
Marburg hemorrhagic fever, 2:586
plague, 2:715
puerperal fever, 2:767
relapsing fever, 2:795, 796
river blindness, 2:820
typhoid fever, 2:995*s*
yellow fever, 2:1092
Blepharitis, 1:442*s*
Blindness. *See* Eye and vision disorders
Blinking, 2:703*s*
Blisters
chickenpox, 1:176, 177
cold sores, 1:226
dracunculiasis, 1:283
enterovirus 71 infection, 1:325, 326, 327
genital herpes, 1:365
hand, foot, and mouth disease, 1:397
herpes simplex 1 virus, 1:440, 441–442
impetigo, 1:480
ringworm, 2:817
scabies, 2:852
sexually transmitted infections, 2:877
shingles, 2:885, 886, 887
swimmer's itch, 2:932
trachoma, 2:967
Bloating
cyclosporiasis, 1:259
hookworm infection, 1:458
strongyloidiasis, 2:929
Blood agar, 2:921
Blood clotting, 1:289, 2:997
Blood count abnormalities and protozoan diseases, 2:754
Blood flukes. *See* Schistosomes
Blood infection
blastomycosis, 1:122
burkholderia, 1:145
cat scratch disease, 1:161–163
Chagas disease, 1:172, 173
Clostridium difficile infection, 1:210
glanders, 1:379–380
Haemophilus influenzae, 1:395
plague, 2:716
pneumonia, 2:726
relapsing fever, 2:795
Salmonella infection, 2:841
severe fever with thrombocytopenia syndrome, 2:872
strongyloidiasis, 2:929
tsunami lung, 2:730
See also Bacteremia; Sepsis; Septicemia
Blood replacement and *Escherichia coli* O157:H7, 1:340
Blood supply, 1:*125*, **125–128**
AIDS, 1:8, 19–20
babesiosis, 1:96
bloodborne pathogens, 1:129–131
BSE inquiry, 1:138*s*
Chagas disease, 1:171, 173
Creutzfeldt-Jakob disease, 1:241, 242
hepatitis B, 1:426, 428
hepatitis C, 1:430, 431, 432*s*
hepatitis D, 1:434
leishmaniasis, 1:539
malaria, 2:580
Marburg hemorrhagic fever, 2:585
mosquito-borne diseases, 2:637
parasitic diseases, 2:695
rickettsial disease, 2:810
St. Louis encephalitis, 2:906
West Nile virus, 1:317, 2:1060
Blood tests
amebiasis, 1:29
ascariasis, 1:79
blastomycosis, 1:122
botulism, 1:135
brucellosis, 1:142
burkholderia, 1:145–146
coccidioidomycosis, 1:220, 221
Crimean-Congo hemorrhagic fever, 1:244
glanders, 1:380
herpes simplex virus 2, 1:446*s*
histoplasmosis, 1:451
Japanese encephalitis, 1:512, 513
lung flukes, 1:567
macrophage activation syndrome, 2:576
malaria, 2:582
mononucleosis, 2:632, 634
parasitic diseases, 2:695
Powassan virus, 2:743
protozoan diseases, 2:756
relapsing fever, 2:797
St. Louis encephalitis, 2:906
strongyloidiasis, 2:930
typhoid fever, 2:993
yellow fever, 2:1092

Blood vessels
  Buruli ulcer, 1:147
  Chlamydia pneumoniae, 1:195
  rickettsial disease, 2:810
Bloodborne pathogens, 1:**129–132**
  cohorted communities, 1:224
  personal protective equipment, 2:701
  universal precautions, 2:908
Bloodborne Pathogens Standard, 1:131, 2:701
Bloody diarrhea
  Campylobacter infection, 1:151
  dysentery, 1:289
  Ebola, 1:302
  Salmonella infection, 2:841
  shigellosis, 2:883
  water-borne disease, 2:1054
  yersiniosis, 2:1097
Bloody mucus and dysentery, 1:289
Bloody sputum
  lung flukes, 1:566
  tuberculosis, 2:983
  tularemia, 2:990
Bloody stools and whipworm, 2:1062
Bloody urine
  aspergillosis, 1:85
  Crimean-Congo hemorrhagic fever, 1:244
  helminth disease, 1:415
  schistosomiasis, 2:861
  urinary tract infection, 2:1012
Bloody vomit and Ebola, 1:302
Bloom, Marshall, 2:655, 656
Blue Cross Blue Shield Association, 1:470
BMC Infectious Diseases, 2:976
BMJ, 1:372
Boars, 1:31, 2:973, 1083
Boccaccio, Giovanni, 2:712
Boceprevir, 1:432
Body aches
  Chagas disease, 1:172
  chikungunya, 1:*180,* 182
  Epstein-Barr virus, 1:337
  herpes simplex virus 2, 1:444
  Lassa fever, 1:526
  leptospirosis, 1:548
  liver fluke infections, 1:560
  Lyme disease, 1:569
  psittacosis, 2:759
  shingles, 1:176
  tick-borne diseases, 2:957
Body fluids
  AIDS, 1:9, 10
  CMV infection, 1:215
  Ebola, 1:303
  fifth disease, 1:348
  hepatitis B, 1:426
  hepatitis C, 1:430
  hepatitis D, 1:434
  Lassa fever, 1:526
  Marburg hemorrhagic fever, 2:585
  personal protective equipment, 2:700
  standard precautions, 2:908
Body lice
  lice infestation, 1:552, 553, *553*
  relapsing fever, 2:795
  typhus, 2:998, 999
Body piercing, 1:11, 432, 2:952
Boko Haram, 1:200, 473, 2:734
Bolivia
  balantidiasis, 1:103
  hantavirus, 1:405
  leishmaniasis, 1:539
  sanitation, 2:846
  Venezuelan equine encephalitis virus, 2:1034
  virus hunters, 2:1045
Bolivian hemorrhagic fever, 1:418, 2:1045
Bone lesions and blastomycosis, 1:122
Bone marrow
  brucellosis, 1:141
  immune response, 1:*476,* 477
Bone marrow tests
  brucellosis, 1:142
  protozoan diseases, 2:756
Bone marrow transplantation and mononucleosis, 2:633
Bone pain
  aspergillosis, 1:85
  burkholderia, 1:145
  cat scratch disease, 1:161–163
  yaws, 2:1087
Bones
  blastomycosis, 1:122
  Buruli ulcer, 1:147, 148
  coccidioidomycosis, 1:218, 219
  Cryptococcus neoformans infection, 1:248
  group B streptococcal infections, 2:925
  nocardiosis, 2:666
Booster vaccinations
  diphtheria, 1:276*s,* 277
  tetanus, 2:954
  typhoid fever, 2:993
Bordeaux, France, 2:778
Borderline leprosy, 1:545
Bordetalla pertussis. See Whooping cough
Borrelia burgdorferi. See Lyme disease
Borreliosis, 2:958
Bosley, Sarah, 2:664
Bosnia and Herzegovina, 1:89, 2:1050
Boston, MA, 2:671
Boston College, 2:671, 672
Botox, 1:135
Botswana, 1:3, 15
Botulinum toxin and bioterrorism, 1:114–115, 116
Botulism, 1:**133–135,** *134*
  disinfection, ineffectiveness of, 1:282
  food-borne disease, 1:356, 357
  USAMRIID, 2:1018
  war, 2:1051–1052
Boulder, CO, 1:186–187
Bouley, Timothy, 2:1084
Bourbon virus, 2:957
Bovine pleuropneumonia, 1:39
Bovine spongiform encephalopathy, 1:*39,* **136–139,** *137*
  animal importation, 1:40
  Creutzfeldt-Jakob disease, 1:240
  prion disease, 2:748, 749, 750
  variant Creutzfeldt-Jakob disease, 1:239
  world trade, 2:1084
Bowel incontinence. *See* Incontinence
Bowel obstruction and taeniasis, 2:942
Boyer, Herbert, 1:81
Brady, Oliver J., 1:266
Brady, Sean, 2:676
Brain development and maternal chickenpox, 1:177
Brain disease or symptoms
  amebiasis, 1:27
  bacterial meningitis, 2:604
  Baylisascaris infection, 1:105
  blastomycosis, 1:122
  congenital Zika syndrome, 2:1101
  encephalitis, 1:316, 317
  enterovirus 71 infection, 1:325
  Escherichia coli O157:H7, 1:340
  glanders, 1:379
  helminth disease, 1:415
  Japanese encephalitis, 1:511–514
  kuru, 1:522–525
  lung flukes, 1:566, 567
  malaria, 2:580
  marine toxins, 2:591, 592
  measles, 2:593, 594
  microsporidiosis, 2:623
  nocardiosis, 2:666
  Powassan virus, 2:741, 742
  protozoan diseases, 2:753
  rabies, 2:775–779
  rubella, 2:837
  syphilis, 2:935
  taeniasis, 2:942–943
  tapeworm infections, 2:948, 949
  tsunami lung, 2:730
  typhus, 2:998
  viral disease, 2:1041
  viral meningitis, 2:608
  water-borne disease, 2:1054
  See also Neurological disease or symptoms

Brain imaging, 1:240, 318
Brain inflammation. *See* Encephalitis
Branca, Francesco, 2:1064
Brazil
AIDS, 1:15
animal importation, 1:40
balantidiasis, 1:103
burkholderia, 1:145
CMV infection, 1:215
coccidioidomycosis, 1:220
hantavirus, 1:406
leishmaniasis, 1:539
leprosy, 1:546, 2:1078
outbreaks, field-level response to, 2:687
plague, 2:717
re-emerging infectious diseases, 2:*791s*
river blindness, 2:821
Rocky Mountain spotted fever, 2:825
sanitation, 2:*845*
schistosomiasis, 2:863
smallpox, 2:897
sporotrichosis, 2:902, 903
typhus, 2:999
vector-borne disease, 2:1029, 1030
viral disease, 2:1042
virus hunters, 2:1043, 1046
Zika virus, 1:169, 462, 2:655, 1022, 1101, 1102–1103
zoonoses, 2:1107
Brazilian hemorrhagic fever, 1:418
Breastfeeding
AIDS, 1:8
brucellosis, 1:141, 142*s*
Chagas disease, 1:173
CMV infection, 1:215
Ebola, 1:303*s*
immune system, 1:478
scrofula transmission, 2:866
UNICEF, 2:1003
West Nile virus, 2:1060
women and infectious disease, 2:1072
Breathing issues
AIDS, 1:12
aspergillosis, 1:85
avian influenza, 1:89
blastomycosis, 1:122
botulism, 1:135
burkholderia, 1:142
diphtheria, 1:276
enterovirus 71 infection, 1:326
hantavirus, 1:405
hookworm infection, 1:458
Legionnaires' disease, 1:531
lung flukes, 1:566
marine toxins, 2:591
opportunistic infections, 2:682
Pneumocystis jirovecii pneumonia, 2:722
pneumonia, 2:726
SARS, 2:847, 850
strongyloidiasis, 2:929
tularemia, 2:990
typhus, 2:997
West Nile virus, 2:1059
Breeding season for hosts and vectors, 1:463
Brest, France, 2:1048
Brill-Zinsser disease, 2:998
Brincidofovir, 1:115
British Columbia, 1:142
British Columbia Cancer Agency, 2:850
British Medical Bulletin, 1:381
Britton, Robert A., 1:212, 213
Broad-spectrum antibiotics
antibacterial drug types, 1:57
candidiasis risk factors, 1:159
Chlamydia infection, 1:189–191
Clostridium difficile infection, 1:211
scrofula, 2:866
without culturing, 1:257
Broad-spectrum disinfectants, 1:282
Bronchiolitis and RSV infection, 2:832, 834
Bronchitis
Chlamydia infection, 1:190
Chlamydia pneumoniae, 1:194
glanders, 1:379
Haemophilus influenzae, 1:394
infections for which cultures are not possible, 1:256
Brouwer, Stephan, 2:859
Browne Sarah K., 1:53
Bruce, David, 1:1, 140
Brucellosis, 1:**140–143,** *141,* 536*s*, 2:1051
Brugia infection. *See* Filariasis
Bruising
Crimean-Congo hemorrhagic fever, 1:244
dengue and dengue hemorrhagic fever, 1:267
Brundtland, Gro Harlem, 1:114–115
BSE. *See* Bovine spongiform encephalopathy
BSE Inquiry, 1:137, 138*s*
Buboes, 2:710, 711, 715
Bubonic plague. *See* Black Death; *Yersinia pestis*
"Bucking the Herd: Parents Who Refuse Vaccination for Their Children May Be Putting Entire Communities at Risk," 1:*186–187*
Budget, CDC, 1:164
Budgets. *See* Economic and financial issues; Funding and budgets
Bulbar polio, 2:736–737
Bulgaria, 1:325, 2:973
Bulletin of the World Health Organization, 1:130
Bull's eye rash, Erythema migrans rash
Bunyaviruses
hemorrhagic fevers, 1:418–419
Rift Valley fever, 2:813–816
severe fever with thrombocytopenia syndrome, 2:871–873
Burack, Victoria, 2:708
Burgdorfer, Willy, 1:570
Burholderia pseudomallei, 2:730
Burial and mourning customs
Ebola, 1:287–288, 303*s*, 304
hemorrhagic fevers, 1:421
kuru, 1:522, 523–525
Marburg hemorrhagic fever, 2:586, 587
personal protective equipment, 2:701
prion disease, 2:749
Burkholder, Walter, 1:144
Burkholderia, 1:**144–146,** *145. See also* Glanders
Burkina Faso, 1:89, 2:1005
Burkitt's lymphoma
cancer, 1:154, 155
Epstein-Barr virus, 1:335, 337
viral disease, 2:1039
Burma. *See* Myanmar
Burning sensation
candidiasis, 1:159
Chlamydia infection, 1:189
dracunculiasis, 1:283
protozoan diseases, 2:754
sexually transmitted infections, 2:877
swimmer's itch, 2:932
trichomoniasis, 2:976
urinary tract infection, 2:1012
Burns
bacterial diseases, 1:100
candidiasis risk factors, 1:159
opportunistic infections, 2:682, 683
Burton, Dennis, 1:12
Buruli ulcer, 1:**147–150,** *148, 149,* 2:980, 981
Burundi, 1:554, 2:999, 1000
Bush, George W.
Hurricane Katrina aftermath, 1:201
SARS, 2:850–851
USA PATRIOT Act, 1:111*s*
Bushmeat
AIDS, origins of, 1:17, 18
Ebola, 1:304
world trade, 2:1083–1084
Business settings and AIDS transmission, 1:11
Businesses and pandemic preparedness, 2:692, 693

C

Cabo Verde, 2:1042
Calambra, Philippines, 2:*994*
Calciviruses, 2:1039

Calcutta, India, 1:181
California
AIDS pandemic history, 1:18, 19
Asilomar Conference, 1:81–83
babesiosis, 1:96
chickenpox, 1:179
coccidioidomycosis, 1:218, 220, 221
encephalitis, 1:317
globalization, 1:384, 385
hantavirus, 1:406
hepatitis A, 1:424–425
Legionnaires' disease, 1:531
lung flukes, 1:567
measles, 1:487, 2:597
norovirus infection, 2:670, 671
plague, 2:717
rat-bite fever, 2:787–788
relapsing fever, 2:795
rubella, 2:837
shigellosis, 2:882
St. Louis encephalitis, 2:906
tularemia, 2:989–990
typhus, 2:999
West Nile virus, 2:*1058,* 1060
whooping cough, 2:1069
yellow fever, 2:1093
Calmette, Albert, 2:985
Cambodia
angiostrongyliasis, 1:36
avian influenza, 1:88
burkholderia, 1:145
glanders, 1:380
trachoma, 2:968*s*
Camels, 1:31, 386
Cameroon, 1:169
Caminade, Cyril, 2:756
"Camp Devens Letter," 1:*497–498*
Camp fever. *See* Typhus
Camp Forrest, GA, 2:1048
Camp Funston, KS, 2:1047–1048
Camp Greenleaf, GA, 2:1048
Campaign for Access to Essential Medicines, 1:271, 2:601
Campylobacter infection, 1:**151–153,** *152*
bacterial diseases, 1:100
food-borne disease, 1:355, 356
handwashing, 1:401
infection control and asepsis, 1:485
Canada
alveolar echinococcosis, 1:24, 25
animal importation, 1:40
antimicrobial soaps, 1:67
Biosafety level 4 facilities, 1:246
blastomycosis, 1:122, 123
bovine spongiform encephalopathy, 1:137, 139
brucellosis, 1:141
Clostridium difficile infection, 1:211, 212, 486
Cryptococcus neoformans infection, 1:248
cyclosporiasis, 1:258
diphtheria, 1:275
Ebola virus research, 1:304
encephalitis, 1:317
Escherichia coli O157:H7, 1:339, *339,* 341
food-borne disease, 1:355
group B streptococcal infection, 2:926
Haemophilus influenzae, 1:396
hand, foot, and mouth disease, 1:397
hantavirus, 1:406
hosts and vectors, 1:463
immigration, 1:474
influenza pandemic of 1957, 1:500
listeriosis, 1:558
marine microorganisms, 2:591*s*
marine toxins, 2:592
measles, 2:595, 597
notifiable diseases, 2:678, 681
polio, 2:737
Powassan virus, 2:741–743
public health, 2:764–765
relapsing fever, 2:796
SARS, 2:848, 849, 850
shingles, 2:888
travel, 2:970–971
triclosan, 2:916
UNICEF, 2:1004
vector-borne disease, 2:1030
West Nile virus, 2:1059, 1060
world trade, 2:1084
Canadian Food Inspection Agency, 1:558
Cancer, 1:**154–156**
AIDS, 1:8, 12, 14
candidiasis risk factors, 1:159
chickenpox, 1:177, 178
disinfection byproducts, 1:282
Epstein-Barr virus, 1:337
Helicobacter pylori, 1:409, 411, 412
hepatitis B, 1:428
hepatitis C, 1:432
hepatitis D, 1:434
HPV, 1:468–469, 470–471
immune response, 1:479
immune system, diseases that weaken the, 2:667*s*
liver fluke infections, 1:561, 562–564
marine microorganisms as treatment for, 2:591*s*
microscopy, 2:620
mycotic disease, 2:650, 651
opportunistic infections, 2:683
paraneoplastic limbic encephalitis, 1:316
Pneumocystis jirovecii pneumonia, 2:722
retroviruses, 2:806
schistosomiasis, 2:863
sexually transmitted infections, 2:878
tuberculosis risk factors, 2:984
viral disease, 2:1039, 1041
Cancer treatment
aspergillosis risk factors, 1:85
candidiasis risk factors, 1:159
marine microorganisms, 2:591*s*
Candidiasis, 1:**157–160,** *158*
anti-cytokine antibody syndrome, 1:53–54
mycotic disease, 2:650, 651–652
nosocomial infections, 2:675
opportunistic infections, 2:682
sexually transmitted infections, 2:878
Canned foods and canning, 1:133, 135, 356, 357
Caño Delgadito virus, 1:405
Cape York Peninsula, Australia, 1:514
Capsids, 1:30, 493, 494, 500, 2:1033
Capsules
Brucella's lack of, 1:140
conjugate Hib vaccines, 1:396
Cryptococcus neoformans, 1:247
Haemophilus influenzae, 1:394, 395
retroviruses, 2:806
Trichinella spiralis, 2:972
vaccines, 2:606
Carbapenemase-producing organisms, 2:1027*s*
Carbapenem-resistant *Enterobacteriaceae*
antibiacterial drugs, 1:59
bacterial diseases, 1:100
contact precautions, 1:237
isolation and quarantine, 1:509
nosocomial infections, 2:675
Carbapenems and antibacterial resistance, 2:676
Carbolic acid, 1:56, 367
CARB-X, 2:803
Cardiac arrest and Chagas disease, 1:173
Cardiac pacemakers. *See* Implanted devices
Cardiff University, 1:229
Cardiovascular syphilis, 2:935
Carditis and Lyme disease, 1:571
Cargo. *See* World trade
Caribbean
angiostrongyliasis, 1:36
anthrax, 1:49
arthropod-borne diseases, 1:75
avian influenza, 1:156
brucellosis, 1:141
chikungunya, 1:180, 181, 182, 2:614
cholera, 1:199
dengue and dengue hemorrhagic fever, 1:266
Eastern equine encephalitis, 1:296, 297
glanders, 1:380

immigration, 1:472
leprosy, 1:544
maternal mortality, 2:769
retroviruses, 2:806
sanitation, 2:844
schistosomiasis, 2:861
St. Louis encephalitis, 2:906
United Nations Millennium Goals, 2:1009
whipworm, 2:1063
Caribou and brucellosis, 1:140
Carlson, Colin J., 2:697, 698
Carriers. *See* Asymptomatic carriers
Carriers, 2:1017
Carroll, James, 1:342–343, 344, 345, 2:1043, 1094, 1095
Carroll, Patti, 2:597
Carson, Rachel Louise, 2:638*s*
Carter, Jimmy, 1:285, 417
Carter Center, 1:284–285, 417
Carville, LA, 1:545
Case reports and epidemiology, 1:332
Cash, Sydney, 2:730–731
Castelos dos Sonhos virus, 1:406
Casual contact transmission, 1:9
Cat scratch disease, 1:**161–163,** *162,* 2:1106
Catalonian Rebellion, 2:712
Cataracts and rubella, 2:837
Catheters
biofilms, 2:802*s*
candidiasis risk factors, 1:158–159
nosocomial infections, 1:257, 2:674, 675
opportunistic infections, 2:683
sterilization, 2:914
urinary tract infection, 2:1013, 1014
Catholic Church, 2:712
Cation dyes, 1:255
Cats
alveolar echinococcosis, 1:25, 25*f*
anellovirus, 1:31
animal importation, 1:40
burkholderia, 1:145
cat scratch disease, 1:161–163
cryptosporidiosis, 1:251
DDT susceptibility, 2:1045
giardiasis vaccine, 1:373
glanders, 1:378
histoplasmosis, 1:449
leptospirosis, 1:*549*
lung flukes, 1:567
parasitic diseases, 2:695
plague, 2:716, 719
protozoan diseases, 2:754, 755
rabies, 2:775
rat-bite fever, 2:785
ringworm, 2:817
sporotrichosis, 2:903
taeniasis, 2:940, 941
tapeworm infections, 2:948
tetanus, 2:953
toxocariasis, 1:80*s*
toxoplasmosis, 2:964, 965*s*
trade, 2:1083
typhus, 2:998, 999
West Nile virus, 2:1060
zoonoses, 2:1106
Cattle
African sleeping sickness, 1:1
animal importation, 1:39, *40*
anthrax, 1:47, 50
antibiotic resistance, 1:63
bovine spongiform encephalopathy, 1:136–139, 239, 241–242
brucellosis, 1:140, 141
burkholderia, 1:145
Campylobacter infection, 1:152
Crimean-Congo hemorrhagic fever, 1:244
cryptosporidiosis, 1:251
Escherichia coli O157:H7, 1:338, 339, 340–341
food-borne disease, 1:356
hemorrhagic fevers, 1:419
leptospirosis, 1:548
listeriosis, 1:556
liver fluke infections, 1:561, 562
prion disease, 2:748, 750
Q fever, 2:771–773, *772,* 773
rabies, 2:*777*
Rift Valley fever, 2:814
ringworm, 2:817
Staphylococcus aureus infections, 2:912
taeniasis, 2:940, 941
tapeworm infections, 2:948, 949, 950
tetanus, 2:953
toxoplasmosis, 2:964
transmissible spongiform encephalopathies, 1:523
Venezuelan equine encephalitis virus, 2:1033
world trade, 2:1084
zoonoses, 2:1106
Cattle feed. *See* Animal feed
Cattle ranchers, 1:141
Caucasus, 2:769
Causation, disease. *See* Germ theory; Koch's postulates
Cavalcanti de Araújo, Paulo Rogério, 2:1103
Cave disease. *See* Histoplasmosis
Caves and histoplasmosis, 1:448, 449
CCR5 gene, 2:1060
CD4+ T cells
AIDS, 1:8, 12
HIV, 1:454, 2:790
Pneumocystis jirovecii pneumonia, 2:723–724
CDC, 1:**164–170,** *166*
African sleeping sickness, 1:3
AIDS, 1:8, 9, 10, 11, 18–19, 19*s*
airborne precautions, 1:21–22, 23
animal importation, 1:39, 40, 41
anthrax, 1:49, 50, 51, 116
antibiotic resistance, 1:62, 2:676, 746
aspergillosis, 1:85
avian influenza, 1:88, 89
B virus, 1:91–92, 93
babesiosis, 1:97
bacteria identification, 1:340*s*
bacterial disease-related deaths, 2:744
Baylisascaris infection, 1:105
biodefense research and development, 1:118–119
biological weapons, 1:111*s*
Biomedical Advanced Research and Development Authority, 1:114
bioterrorism, 1:115, 117–118, 2:1051*s*
blastomycosis, 1:122, 123
blood supply, 1:125, 126
bloodborne pathogens, 1:130
botulism, 1:134*s,* 135
bovine spongiform encephalopathy, 1:137
brucellosis, 1:142*s*
Campylobacter infection, 1:151, 152*s*
candidiasis, 1:157, 160
cat scratch disease, 1:162*s*
Chagas disease, 1:171, 173
chickenpox, 1:178, 178*s*
chikungunya, 1:182
childhood-associated infectious diseases vaccines, 1:184
Chlamydia infection, 1:190, 191
Chlamydia pneumoniae, 1:193
cholera, 1:201
Clostridium difficile infection, 1:209–210, 211, 212
CMV infection, 1:215
coccidioidomycosis, 1:220, 221
cohorted communities, 1:225
contact precautions, 1:235–238, 236, 237–238
Crimean-Congo hemorrhagic fever, 1:243, 246
Cryptococcus neoformans infection, 1:248
cryptosporidiosis, 1:251, 252
cyclosporiasis, 1:258, 260
diphtheria, 1:276*s,* 277, 278
diseases that weaken the immune system, 2:667*s*
disinfection recommendations for Ebola control, 1:281
dracunculiasis, 1:285
droplet precautions, 1:286–288
dysentery, 1:291
Eastern equine encephalitis, 1:296, 297
Ebola, 1:301, 303

elbow bump greeting, 1:402
emerging infectious diseases, 1:313
encephalitis, 1:316, 317, 319
epidemiology, 1:332
Epstein-Barr virus, 1:335
Escherichia coli infection, 2:672
Escherichia coli O157:H7, 1:338, 339
fifth disease, 1:348
filariasis, 1:351
food-borne disease, 1:354
gastroenteritis, 1:358, 359, 361
genital herpes, 1:365
germ theory of disease, 1:369
giardiasis, 1:371*s*, 372
Global Polio Eradication Initiative, 2:732, 740, 1077
globalization, 1:385
gonorrhea, 1:389–390
group A streptococcal infections, 1:481*s*, 2:922, 922*s*
group B streptococcal infections, 2:925
Haemophilus influenzae, 1:394, 395
handwashing, 1:402
hantavirus, 1:405, 407
Helicobacter pylori, 1:411
helminth disease, 1:417
hepatitis A, 1:423, 424–425
hepatitis B, 1:426, 427
hepatitis C, 1:431, 432*s*
hepatitis E, 1:438
herpes simplex virus 2, 1:444, 445, 446*s*
histoplasmosis, 1:451
HIV Risk Reduction Tool, 1:455*s*
HIV testing of pregnant women, 1:13
HIV/AIDS treatment, 1:13
H5N1 vaccine research, 2:614
hosts and vectors, 1:463
hot tub rash, 1:466
HPV, 1:469, 470
immigration, 1:472
infection control and asepsis, 1:485, 486, 487
influenza epidemiology, 1:491, 503, 505, 506, 507
influenza pandemic of 1918, 1:496
influenza pandemic of 1957, 1:499
isolation and quarantine, 1:508
keratitis, 1:232
Lassa fever, 1:383, 527
legislation and international law, 1:536
leprosy, 1:546
listeriosis, 1:556, 558
liver fluke infections, 1:562
Lyme disease, 1:571, 573
malaria, 2:581
measles, 2:594, 595, 595*s*
MERS in the Arabian Peninsula, 1:386
MMR vaccine, 2:646, 647, 838*s*
monkeypox, 2:627–628, 628*s*
mononucleosis, 2:630
MRSA, 2:640
mycotic disease, 2:651, 652
necrotizing fasciitis, 2:659
Nipah virus infection, 2:663
nocardiosis, 2:666, 667, 668
norovirus infection, 2:669, 670
nosocomial infections, 1:257, 483, 2:675
notifiable diseases, 2:678–679, 680*s*
otitis media *vs.* swimmer's ear, 1:294*s*
outbreaks, field-level response to, 2:685, 686, 687
parasitic diseases, 2:696
pinworm infection, 2:706
plague, 2:718, 719
Pneumocystis jirovecii pneumonia, 2:721
pneumonia, 2:726
post-treatment Lyme disease syndrome, 1:572
protozoan diseases, 2:756
public health, 2:764*s*, 765, 766
Q fever, 2:773
rabies, 2:777
rapid diagnostic tests, 2:783
rat-bite fever, 2:786
re-emerging infectious diseases, 2:790, 791, 792–793
relapsing fever, 2:796–797
research laboratory worker contamination, 2:1016
resistant organisms, 2:801, 803
Rocky Mountain spotted fever, 2:825
rotavirus, 2:830
rubella, 2:838
Salmonella infection, 2:841, 842
sanitation, 2:845–846
SARS, 2:849, 849*s*, 850–851
scabies prevention, 2:854*s*
sepsis, 2:868
sexually transmitted infections, 2:877–878, 878–879
shigellosis, 2:881
shingles, 1:177, 2:885, 886, 887
smallpox, 2:893, 894, 897
sporotrichosis, 2:903
sports and infection control, 1:442*s*
standard precautions, 2:908
strep throat prevention, 2:918*s*
Streptococcus pneumoniae vaccine, 2:606
superbugs, 2:1027*s*
swimmer's ear and swimmer's itch, 2:932
syphilis, 2:936
taeniasis, 2:942
Task Force on Antimicrobial Resistance, 1:256*s*
tetanus, 2:952, 954
tick-borne diseases, 2:958
timeline, 1:*164*
toxocariasis, 1:80*s*
toxoplasmosis, 2:964–966, 965*s*, 966
trichinellosis, 2:973, 973*s*, 974
trichomoniasis, 2:975
tuberculosis, 1:101, 2:986
tularemia, 2:990, 991
vaccines and vaccine development, 2:1021–1022
vancomycin-resistant *Enterococci,* 2:1027, 1028
Venezuelan equine encephalitis virus, 2:1035*s*
virus hunters, 2:1045
war, 2:1051
water-borne diseases, 1:466*s*, 2:1053, 1055–1056
West Nile virus, 2:1060, 1061
whipworm, 2:1063
whooping cough, 2:1067–1068, 1069
wildlife trade, 2:1083
women, 2:1073
world trade and travel, 2:1082
yersiniosis, 2:1096–1099, 1097, 1098, 1098*s*
zoonoses, 2:1107
"CDC Media Statement on Newly Discovered Smallpox Specimens," 2:*894*
CDC Travel Notice: MERS in the Arabian Peninsula, 1:*386*
CDC Yellow Book 2018, 1:416
Cefalexin, 2:674
Cefepime, 2:728
Cefixime, 1:389
Cefotaxime, 2:728
Ceftazidime, 1:380, 2:730
Ceftriaxone
gonorrhea, 1:389, 389*s*
nocardiosis, 2:668
relapsing fever, 2:797
Cefuroxime, 2:728
Cefuroxime axetil, 1:571
Cell death, 2:809, 824
Cell-free filtrate anthrax vaccine, 1:50
Center for Drug Evaluation and Research, FDA, 1:68
Center for Food Safety and Applied Nutrition, 1:43
Center for Global Health, 1:167
Center for Infectious Disease Dynamics, 2:1032
Center for Law and the Public's Health, 1:117
Centers for Disease Control and Prevention. *See* CDC
Centers for Medicare and Medicaid Services, 1:256*s*

Centers of Excellence for Biodefense and Emerging Infectious Disease Research, 2:792
Central Africa
monkeypox, 2:627, 628, 628*s*
river blindness, 2:821
typhus, 2:999
wildlife trade, 2:1083, 1085
Central African Republic
African sleeping sickness, 1:3
Biological Weapons Convention, 1:111
leprosy, 2:1078
monkeypox, 2:628
Central America
blastomycosis, 1:122
brucellosis, 1:141
burkholderia, 1:142
Buruli ulcer, 1:147–150
Chagas disease, 1:171, 173, 174
coccidioidomycosis, 1:220
dysentery, 1:290
Eastern equine encephalitis, 1:296, 297
encephalitis, 1:317
filariasis, 1:351
glanders, 1:380
hantavirus, 1:404, 405
histoplasmosis, 1:449
immigration, 1:474
influenza, 1:490
lung flukes, 1:566
malaria, 2:581
mosquito-borne diseases, 2:637
outbreaks, field-level response to, 2:687
parasitic diseases, 2:695
protozoan diseases, 2:755
re-emerging infectious diseases, 2:791*s*
river blindness, 2:821
St. Louis encephalitis, 2:906
tropical infectious diseases, 2:981
typhoid fever, 2:994
typhus, 2:999
Venezuelan equine encephalitis virus, 2:1033, 1034, 1035
water-borne disease, 2:1055
whipworm, 2:1063
yellow fever, 2:1092
Zika virus, 2:1102
Central Asia
anthrax, 1:50
hemorrhagic fevers, 1:418
maternal mortality, 2:769
taeniasis, 2:942
tropical infectious diseases, 2:981
Central Europe, 2:721, 942
Central line-associated bloodstream infection, 1:257
Central nervous system. *See* Neurological disease or symptoms
Central Plata virus, 1:405
Central United States
blastomycosis, 1:122
encephalitis, 1:317
hantavirus, 1:406
histoplasmosis, 1:449
Lyme disease, 1:572
Central venous catheters and nosocomial infections, 2:674
Cephalexin, 2:918
Cephalosporins
antibacterial resistance, 2:676
antibiotic types, 1:58
gonorrhea, 1:388
pneumonia, 2:728
Cercariae, 1:566
Cercarial dermatitis. *See* Swimmer's ear and swimmer's itch
Cercomonas intestinalis. See Giardiasis
Cercopithecine herpesvirus 1. *See* B virus infection
Cerebral malaria, 2:580
Cerebral palsy, 1:135
Cerebral toxoplasmosis, 1:53
Cerebrospinal fluid tests
enterovirus 71 infection, 1:326
Japanese encephalitis, 1:512, 513
mumps, 2:646
Powassan virus, 2:743
St. Louis encephalitis, 2:906
viral meningitis, 2:607, 609
Cervarix, 1:155*s*, 156, 469, 2:878
Cervical cancer
AIDS, 1:12
avian influenza, 1:156
cancer, 1:154, 155
HPV, 1:468–469, 470
opportunistic infections, 2:683
sexually transmitted infections, 2:877–878
women, 2:1073
Cervical intraepithelial dysplasia, 1:469
Cervicitis, 1:387, 2:976
Cesarean delivery for AIDS prevention, 1:8
Cestoda. *See* Tapeworm infections
Cetaceous anthrax, 1:*48*
Cetus Corporation, 2:616*s*
Ceviche and anisakiasis, 1:45
Chad, 1:283, 285
Chagas, Carlos, 1:*171,* 171–172
Chagas disease, 1:**171–174,** *172*
parasitic diseases, 2:695
protozoan diseases, 2:753–754, 755, 756
trypanosomiasis, 1:3
Chagas Disease: History of a Continent's Scourge (Delaporte), 1:171–172
Chancres
African seeping sickness, 1:2
sexually transmitted infections, 2:877
syphilis, 2:934, 936
Chancroid and AIDS susceptibility, 1:11
Charity Navigator, 2:1004
Cheeses, 1:141, 556, 557
Chemical sterilization of water, 2:915
Chemotherapy
Buruli ulcer, 1:149
candidiasis risk factors, 1:158
Chagas disease, 1:173
histoplasmosis risk factors, 1:449, 451
opportunistic infections, 2:682, 683
scrofula, 2:866
taeniasis, 2:943
vancomycin-resistant *Enterococci,* 2:1026
Chen, Johnny, 2:847–848
Chen, Mu-Hong, 2:977
Chengdu Declaration for Action, 2:943
Chennai, India, 1:197
Cherry, James, 2:1069
Chesapeake Bay, 1:567
Chest pain
aspergillosis, 1:85
histoplasmosis, 1:448
Marburg hemorrhagic fever, 2:586
nocardiosis, 2:666
pneumonia, 2:726
tularemia, 2:990
Chest x-rays
avian influenza, 1:89
coccidioidomycosis, 1:220, 221
Legionnaires' disease, 1:531
nocardiosis, 2:667
pneumonia, 2:726
Chiang Mai Valley, Thailand, 1:514
Chicago, IL, 1:195, 258
Chicago disease. *See* Blastomycosis
Chickenpox, 1:**175–179**
antiviral drugs, 1:72
immigration, 1:474
vaccine, 1:*176*
vaccine refusal, 1:186
viral disease, 2:1039
Chickens
avian influenza, 1:88
Campylobacter infection, 1:152–153
hosts and vectors, 1:*462*
tetanus, 2:953
Venezuelan equine encephalitis virus, 2:1033
world trade, 2:1084
zoonoses, 2:1106
Chikungunya, 1:*180,* **180–183,** *181,* 2:614, *1030*
Child care settings
bacterial meningitis, 2:606
giardiasis, 1:371*s*, 372
infection control and asepsis, 1:485

norovirus infection, 2:670
pneumonia, 2:727
RSV infection, 2:833, 834
shigellosis, 2:882
strongyloidiasis, 2:930
Child marriage, 1:15, 2:1005–1006
Child mortality, 2:1007, 1008, 1050
Child Survival and Development Revolution, 2:1003
Childbed fever. *See* Puerperal fever
Childbirth
group A streptococcal infections, 2:921–922
nosocomial infections, 2:673–674
puerperal fever, 2:767–769
skilled health personnel, attended by, 2:768*t*
women, 2:1072
See also Maternal-to-fetal/child transmission
Childhood-associated infectious diseases, immunization impacts, 1:**184–188,** *185*
Children
African sleeping sickness, 1:4
AIDS, 1:12–13, 15, 20
anellovirus, 1:30, 31, 32–33
angiostrongyliasis, 1:38
antiviral drugs, 1:73
ascariasis, 1:78, 80
avian influenza, 1:89
babesiosis, 1:96
bacterial meningitis, 2:606
Baylisascaris infection, 1:107
Buruli ulcer, 1:148
cancer, 1:154
CDC vaccination programs, 1:167
Chagas disease drugs, 1:171
chickenpox, 1:176
Chlamydia pneumoniae, 1:195
cholera, 1:198
Clostridium difficile infection, 1:211
cryptosporidiosis, 1:251, 252
cyclosporiasis, 1:259
demographics, 1:263
deworming, 2:1064
diphtheria, 1:275, 277
dracunculiasis, 1:283, 285
dysentery, 1:289, 290
ear infections, 1:293–294
emerging infectious diseases, 1:312, 314
encephalitis, 1:316, 317
enterovirus 71 infection, 1:324, 325, 327
Epstein-Barr virus, 1:335, 336
Escherichia coli O157:H7, 1:340
fifth disease, 1:347, 348*s,* 349
filariasis, 1:350
food-borne disease, 1:357
gastroenteritis, 1:358–361, 359–360
giardiasis, 1:373
group A streptococcal infections, 2:921
Haemophilus influenzae, 1:394, 395, 396
hand, foot, and mouth disease, 1:397, 398
handwashing, 1:402
Helicobacter pylori, 1:411
helminth disease, 1:415, 417
hepatitis A, 1:422, 423
hepatitis B, 1:426, 428, 428*s*
hepatitis C, 1:432*s*
hepatitis E, 1:437
histoplasmosis, 1:449
hookworm infection, 1:457, 459
immunization impacts on childhood-associated infectious diseases, 1:184–187
impetigo, 1:480, 482
influenza, 1:488–489, 490, 505
international adoption, 1:475
Japanese encephalitis, 1:513, 513*s*
Kawasaki disease, 1:517
kuru, 1:522, 523
Lassa fever, 1:527
Legionnaires' disease, 1:530
lice infestation, 1:554
liver fluke infections, 1:563
Lyme disease, 1:570
macrophage activation syndrome, 2:575, 576
malaria, 2:578, *578,* 580, 581–582
of maternally fatal deliveries, 2:769
measles, 2:593, 595
Médecins Sans Frontières, 2:600–601
monkeypox, 2:627
mononucleosis, 2:631, 632
mosquito-borne diseases, 2:637, 639
mumps, 2:645, 646
norovirus infection, 2:669
opportunistic infections, 2:684
parasitic diseases, 2:695, 696
pink eye, 2:703, 704
pinworm infection, 2:705, 706, 707
pneumococcal vaccines, 2:729
Pneumocystis jirovecii pneumonia, 2:721, 723
pneumonia, 2:725–730
polio, 2:732, 736–739
psittacosis, 2:760
rabies, 2:775, 777
rat-bite fever, 2:785, 787–788
Reye's syndrome, 2:919
ringworm, 2:818, 819
Rocky Mountain spotted fever, 2:825
rotavirus infection, 1:361, 2:828, 829
RSV infection, 2:832, 834
rubella, 2:837, 838, 839
sanitation-related diseases, 2:845
scabies, 2:852, 853
scarlet fever, 2:856, 857, 858
shigellosis, 2:880, 882
strep throat, 2:918
strongyloidiasis, 2:930
tapeworm infections, 2:949
tetanus, 2:954
trachoma, 2:967, 968
trichomoniasis, 2:977
tropical infectious diseases, 2:981
tuberculosis, 2:984, 985
tularemia, 2:991
typhoid fever, 2:994–995
UNICEF, 2:1003–1006
United Nations Millennium Goals, 2:1007, 1008–1009
vaccines, 2:1021
vector-borne disease, 2:1029, 1031
viral disease, 2:1039, 1041
viral meningitis, 2:607, 609, 610
war, 2:1049, 1050
water-borne disease, 2:1055
whipworm, 2:1062, 1063, 1064
whooping cough, 2:1068
yaws, 2:1088
yersiniosis, 2:1096–1097, 1098
Children's Hospitals and Clinics of Minnesota, 2:596
Chile, 1:406
Chills
aspergillosis, 1:85
B virus infection, 1:92
babesiosis, 1:95, 96
blastomycosis, 1:122
brucellosis, 1:141
chikungunya, 1:*180,* 181
colds, 1:228
hantavirus, 1:404, 405
helminth disease, 1:415
hemorrhagic fevers, 1:420*s*
histoplasmosis, 1:448
Legionnaires' disease, 1:530
malaria, 2:579, 581
Marburg hemorrhagic fever, 2:586
necrotizing fasciitis, 2:660
nocardiosis, 2:666
plague, 1:116, 2:715
pneumonia, 2:726
protozoan diseases, 2:753
rat-bite fever, 2:785
relapsing fever, 2:795
Salmonella infection, 2:841
scrofula, 2:866
shingles, 2:885, 886
tick-borne diseases, 2:956
trichinellosis, 2:973
tuberculosis, 2:983
typhoid fever, 2:993, 995*s*
typhus, 2:997
yellow fever, 2:1092

Chimeric antigen receptor T cell therapy, 1:479
Chimpanzees
AIDS, origins of, 1:17–18
anthrax, 1:48–49
colds, 1:228
Ebola, 1:304, 2:1085
lice infestation, 1:552
typhus research, 2:1001
China
AIDS deaths, 1:15, 20
angiostrongyliasis, 1:36
avian influenza, 1:88
bacterial meningitis, 2:606
carbapenem-resistant Enterobacteriaceae, 1:59
chickenpox vaccine, 1:177
cholera, 1:533
dysentery, 1:290
encephalitis, 1:318
enterovirus 71 infection, 1:325, 326, *326*
filariasis eradication, 1:350, 352
food-borne disease, 1:*355*
glanders, 1:380, 381
Haemophilus influenzae, 1:396
helminth disease, 1:415
hepatitis E, 1:437, 438
hookworm infection, 1:58, 457
immigration, 1:474
infection control, 1:*384*
influenza, 1:*489,* 499, 500, 501, 506
international adoption, 1:475
Japanese encephalitis, 1:514
liver fluke infections, 1:561, 562
lung flukes, 1:566
mitten crabs, 1:567
pandemic preparedness, 2:692
plague, 2:712–713, 716
polio eradication campaign, 2:733
ProMED, 2:752
protozoan diseases, 2:755
public health, 2:764
rabies, 2:*775,* 778
Rift Valley fever, 2:814
sanitation, 2:846
SARS, 2:847, 848, *848,* 849
schistosomiasis, 2:863
severe fever with thrombocytopenia syndrome, 2:871–872
smallpox, 2:890, 899, 1020
taeniasis, 2:942
talaromycosis, 2:944, 945, 946
tick-borne diseases, 2:957
trachoma, 2:968*s*
travel, 2:970
typhus research, 2:1000
United Nations Millennium Goals, 2:1009
wildlife trade, 2:1083, 1084
zoonoses, 2:1106
China, ancient, 2:710
China Information System for Disease Control and Prevention, 2:872
Chinese prisoners of war, 1:50
Chipmunks
Baylisascaris infection, 1:107
encephalitis, 1:317
hantavirus, 1:406
plague, 2:715
"Chipotle Is Subpoenaed in Criminal Inquiry over Norovirus outbreak," 2:*671–672*
Chipotle Mexican Grill restaurants, 2:671–672
Chitterlings, 2:1098, 1098*s*
Chlamydia infection, 1:**189–192,** *190*
AIDS susceptibility, 1:14
cancer, 1:155
sexually transmitted infections, 2:877, 879
urinary tract infection, 2:1013
Chlamydia pneumoniae, 1:**193–196,** *194*
Chlamydia psittaci. See Psittacosis
Chloramphenicol
plague, 2:718
relapsing fever, 2:796
rickettsial disease, 2:811
Rocky Mountain spotted fever, 2:825
typhoid fever, 2:994
typhus, 2:999
Chlorhexidine, 1:281
Chlorination for water-borne disease prevention, 2:1054, 1055
Chlorine
antimicrobial soaps, 1:67
disinfection, 1:281
puerperal fever prevention, 2:768, 769
sterilization, 2:915
Chloroquine
developing nations and drug delivery, 1:271
malaria, 2:581
mosquito-borne diseases, 2:638
re-emerging infectious diseases, 2:790
resistant organisms, 2:800, 802
Chloroxylenol, 1:68
Choclo virus, 1:405
Choice, patients' right to, 2:987
Cholangitis, 2:623
Cholera, 1:**197–202,** *199*
bacterial diseases, 1:100, 101
demographics, 1:261
epidemiology, 1:329, 333–334
immigration, 1:473, 474
legislation and international law, 1:533–534
outbreaks, field-level response to, 2:686–687
quarantine, 1:508
sanitation, 2:844
war, 2:1049
water-borne disease, 2:1054–1055
WHO childhood vaccination recommendations, 1:185
Choriomeningitis, 2:1041
Chromogenicity, 1:255
Chromosomes and antibiotic resistance, 1:62
Chronic diseases
CDC, 1:168
coccidioidomycosis, 1:219, 221
ear infections, 1:293, 294, 295
giardiasis, 1:372
glanders, 1:379
hepatitis B, 1:426, 427, 428*s*
hepatitis C, 1:430–432, 431
hepatitis D, 1:435
histoplasmosis, 1:448, 451
hookworm, 1:458
with influenza, 1:489
liver fluke infections, 1:560–561
Lyme disease, 1:572–574
mononucleosis, 2:631
nocardiosis, 2:667, 668
Q fever, 2:771–773, 772
schistosomiasis, 2:860, 861
sepsis, 2:868
strongyloidiasis with, 2:929
tick-borne diseases, 2:958
toxoplasmosis, 2:964
yaws, 2:1087
Chronic fatigue syndrome, 1:373, 2:633
Chronic obstructive pulmonary disease (COPD), 1:195, 330
Chronic suppressive therapy, 2:668
Chronic wasting disease, 1:136
The Chronicles of Gilles de Muisit, 2:*709*
Chuuk Islands, 2:757
Chytridiomycosis, 2:1084
Cidofovir, 1:115, 215, 2:893
Ciero, Alessandra, 2:797
Ciguatera poisoning, 2:*589,* 590–591
Cilantro and cyclosporiasis outbreaks, 1:258
Cimetidine, 1:411
Cincinnati, OH, 1:166
Ciprofloxacin
anthrax, 1:115
cholera, 1:198
gonorrhea, 1:389
hot tub rash, 1:466
nosocomial infections, 2:674
plague, 2:718
pneumonia, 2:728
shigellosis, 2:882
typhoid fever, 2:994
typhus, 2:1000
war, 2:1049
"What If Cipro Stopped Working?", 1:64

Circumcision, 2:977
Cirrhosis. *See* Liver disease or symptoms
Civets, 2:1083
Civil liberties, 1:509, 535–536
Civilian biodefense strategy, 1:118–119
CJD. *See* Creutzfeldt-Jakob disease
Clam digger's itch. *See* Swimmer's ear and swimmer's itch
Clams, 2:591
Clarithromycin, 1:149, 411
Classification of diseases, World Health Organization, 2:1076
Clayton, Dale, 1:554
Clemens, John, 2:664
Clement VI, Pope, 2:712
Climate and impetigo, 1:482
Climate change, 1:**203–208**
  African sleeping sickness, 1:4
  algal blooms, 2:592
  Cryptococcus neoformans infection, 1:248–249
  emerging infectious diseases, 1:313
  endemicity, 1:322
  helminth disease, 1:416
  hosts and vectors, 1:463
  Japanese encephalitis, 1:514
  leptospirosis, 1:550
  Lyme disease, 1:571
  malaria, 2:582
  marine toxins, 2:591
  mycotic disease, 2:649, 652
  parasitic diseases, 2:696
  plague, 2:719
  protozoan diseases, 2:757
  re-emerging infectious diseases, 2:791*s*, 793
  Rocky Mountain Laboratory research, 2:655
  St. Louis encephalitis, 2:905, 907
  swimmer's ear and swimmer's itch, 2:933
  tropical infectious diseases, 2:982
"Climate Change Contribution to the Emergence or Re-emergence of Parasitic Diseases," 2:*756–757*
"Climate change May Accelerate Infectious Disease Outbreaks, Say Researchers," 1:*206–207*
"Climate Change Threatens the World's Parasites (That's Not Good)", 2:*697–698*
Clindamycin
  babesiosis, 1:97
  MRSA, 2:642
  necrotizing fasciitis, 2:659
  nosocomial infections, 2:674
  protozoan diseases, 2:755
  scarlet fever, 2:857
  Staphylococcus aureus infections, 2:913
  toxic shock, 2:962
Clinical and Vaccine Immunology, 1:215
Clinical Infectious Diseases, 1:373, 2:828
Clinical Microbiology and Infection, 1:195
Clinical Microbiology Reviews, 1:215, 216, 2:579, 1025
Clinical Practice Guidelines, 2:728
Clinical trials
  African sleeping sickness drugs, 1:4
  antibiotic resistance, 1:59, 63
  Buruli ulcer, 1:149
  chikungunya vaccine, 1:182
  Chlamydia infection vaccine, 1:191
  Chlamydia pneumoniae, 1:195
  CMV infection vaccine, 1:216
  coccidioidomycosis drugs, 1:221
  ear infection vaccine, 1:295
  Ebola vaccine, 1:303–304, 419
  enterovirus 71 infection vaccine, 1:326
  epidemiology, 1:331
  herpes simplex virus 2 vaccine, 1:445
  HIV vaccine, 2:654
  Japanese encephalitis vaccine, 1:514
  leishmaniasis vaccine, 1:540
  malaria vaccine, 1:205, 2:791
  polio vaccine, 2:739
  rabies vaccine, 2:779
  retroviral gene therapy, 2:806
  schistosomiasis vaccine, 2:863
  shingles vaccine, 2:888
  smallpox drugs, 2:893
  typhus drugs, 2:1000
  vaccines and vaccine development, 2:1023
  women, 2:1073
  worm therapy, 1:417
  Zika virus vaccine, 2:1022–1023
Clinics, 1:216–217
Clinton, William Jefferson, 2:937–938
Clofazimine, 1:545, 546, 2:981, 1078
Clonazepam, 1:241, 2:750
Clonorchiasis. *See* Liver fluke infections
Clostridium botulinum. See Botulism
Clostridium difficile infection, 1:**209–213**
  cohorted communities, 1:224
  infection control and asepsis, 1:485–486
  nosocomial infections, 2:675
  President's Initiative on Combating Antibiotic Resistance, 2:746
Clostridium tetani. See Tetanus
Clothing, protective, 1:*236*
  African sleeping sickness, 1:4
  AIDS, 1:10
  alveolar echinococcosis, 1:25
  angiostrongyliasis, 1:37
  avian influenza, 1:90
  B virus infection, 1:92
  babesiosis, 1:97
  Baylisascaris infection, 1:107
  bloodborne pathogens, 1:131
  brucellosis, 1:143
  chikungunya, 1:180, 182
  colds, 1:230
  contact precautions, 1:237–238
  Crimean-Congo hemorrhagic fever, 1:245
  droplet precautions, 1:287
  Eastern equine encephalitis, 1:296, 298
  Ebola, 1:304
  encephalitis, 1:318
  filariasis, 1:352
  hemorrhagic fevers, 1:420–421
  histoplasmosis, 1:451
  infection control and asepsis, 1:484, 485, 486
  Lassa fever, 1:528
  leishmaniasis, 1:540
  leptospirosis, 1:549*s*, 550
  Lyme disease, 1:572
  malaria, 2:581
  Marburg hemorrhagic fever, 2:586
  Médecins Sans Frontières, 2:602
  mosquito-borne disease, 2:639
  mycotic disease, 2:651
  Nipah virus infection, 2:663
  nosocomial infection, 2:*674*, 675
  Powassan virus, 2:742
  psittacosis, 2:759, 760
  Q fever, 2:773
  rat-bite fever, 2:786, 788
  relapsing fever, 2:797
  rickettsial disease, 2:809, 811
  Rift Valley fever, 2:815
  river blindness, 2:821
  Rocky Mountain spotted fever, 2:826
  smallpox, 2:893
  sporotrichosis, 2:903
  St. Louis encephalitis, 2:907
  standard precautions, 2:909
  tick-borne diseases, 2:958
  typhus, 2:1000
  vector control, 1:462
  vector-borne diseases, 2:1031
  Venezuelan equine encephalitis virus, 2:1035, 1035*s*
  viral diseases, 2:1041
  West Nile virus, 2:1061
  whipworm, 2:1063
  Zika virus, 2:1102
  See also Personal protective equipment

Clotrimazole, 2:818
Clovis I, 2:865, *866*
CMV infection, 1:**214–217,** *215, 216*
anti-cytokine antibody syndrome, 1:53
antiviral drugs, 1:72
mononucleosis, 2:634
viral disease, 2:1039
CNN, 2:963
Coagulation and rickettsial disease, 2:811
Coartem. *See* Artemether and lumefantrine
Cocci meningitis, 1:218, 219, 221
Coccicium parasites. *See* Cyclosporiasis
Coccidioidomycosis, 1:121, **218–222,** *219, 220*
Cochlea, 2:606
Cod and anisakiasis, 1:45
Cod worm, 1:43
Codeine, 2:886
Cognitive issues, 1:230, 2:845
Cohen, Jeffrey I., 1:91, 93
Cohen, Stanley, 1:81
Cohorted communities, 1:**223–225,** *224*
airborne precautions, 1:22
Chlamydia pneumoniae, 1:195
cyclosporiasis, 1:258
droplet precautions, 1:286
dysentery, 1:289, 290, 292
gastroenteritis, 1:358
hand, foot, and mouth disease, 1:398
helminth disease, 1:415
hepatitis A, 1:423
impetigo, 1:482
infection control, 1:484
influenza epidemiology, 1:504, 507
mumps, 2:647
norovirus infection, 2:670
pandemic preparedness, 2:692
pinworm infection, 2:706
pneumonia, 2:727
RSV infection, 2:833, 834
viral disease, 2:1039
viral meningitis, 2:610
Coinfection
AIDS, 2:1010
avian and human influenza, 1:90
chickenpox, 1:175, 177
chronic diseases, 1:489, 2:929
glanders, 1:379
hepatitis infections, 1:423, 435, 436
HIV and hepatitis C, 1:432
leishmaniasis and HIV, 1:541
Lyme disease, 1:571
MRSA, 2:641–642, 1026
protozoan diseases, 2:755
ringworm, 2:818, 819
strongyloidiasis, 2:929
tuberculosis, 2:987
Cold sores, 1:*226,* **226–227**
herpes simplex 1 virus, 1:440
herpes simplex virus 2, 1:444
viral disease, 2:1039
Cold weather, 1:229–230, 230*s,* 2:833
Cold-like symptoms
Chlamydia pneumoniae, 1:194
fifth disease, 1:347
measles, 2:593
mononucleosis, 2:631
RSV infection, 2:832
Colds, 1:**228–231,** *229*
influenza *vs.,* 1:489*t*
pneumonia, 2:726
viral disease, 2:1039
Colitis
balantidiasis, 1:102
Clostridium difficile infection, 1:210, 212
protozoan diseases, 2:754
whipworm, 2:1062
Collaborating Center for Reference and Research on Plague Control, WHO, 2:718
Collaborating Centre for Orthopoxvirus Diagnosis and Repository for Variola Virus Strains and DNA, 2:897
Collaborating Centre for Research and Control of Opisthorchiasis, 1:562, 563
Collaborating Centres for Reference and Research on Influenza, 1:506
Collective case reports and epidemiology, 1:332
Colleges as cohorted communities, 1:223–224, 225
Collinge, John, 1:524, 525
Colombia
coccidioidomycosis, 1:220
encephalitis, 1:317
leishmaniasis, 1:539
river blindness, 2:821
Rocky Mountain spotted fever, 2:825
Venezuelan equine encephalitis virus, 2:1034, 1035
viral disease, 2:1042
Colon inflammation, 1:173, 209
Colon perforation and *Clostridium difficile* infection, 1:210
Colonialism and leprosy, 1:544
Colonization
opportunistic infections, 2:683
Staphylococcus aureus, 2:641
strep throat, 2:917
vancomycin-resistant *Enterococci,* 2:1026
Colorado
encephalitis, 1:317
hantavirus, 1:407
hepatitis A vaccine, 1:425
plague, 2:717
relapsing fever, 2:795
tuberculosis, 2:986
vaccination, 1:186–187
Colorado tick fever, 2:957
Colorectal cancer, 1:155
Colostridium infection, 2:658
Columbus, Christopher, 2:983
Coma
B virus infection, 1:92
bacterial meningitis, 2:604
Baylisascaris infection, 1:105, 107
Eastern equine encephalitis, 1:296
encephalitis, 1:316, 317
hemorrhagic fevers, 1:420
Japanese encephalitis, 1:512
Lassa fever, 1:527
macrophage activation syndrome, 2:575
malaria, 2:580
St. Louis encephalitis, 2:905
typhus, 2:997, 998
West Nile virus, 2:1059
Combantrin-A. *See* Anthelmintic drugs
Combination therapy
AIDS, 1:13
Cryptococcus neoformans infection, 1:248
hepatitis C, 1:431
leishmaniasis, 1:540
leprosy, 1:545, 546, 2:1078
malaria, 2:581
MRSA, 2:642
nocardiosis, 2:668
pneumonia, 2:728
resistant organisms, 2:802
Staphylococcus aureus infections, 2:913
tropical infectious diseases, 2:981
vancomycin-resistant *Enterococci,* 2:1027
Comfort care
Creutzfeldt-Jakob disease, 1:241
Ebola, 1:303
prion disease, 2:750
Committee on the Rights of the Child, 2:1004
Common colds. *See* Colds
Communicable Disease Center, 1:165–166
Communicable Disease Surveillance and Response Unit, WHO, 1:4–5
Communication, 2:766, 849*s*
"Community Strategy for Pandemic Influenza Mitigation in the United States," 2:*692–693*
Community-acquired infections
antibiotic resistance, 1:62
Chlamydia infection, 1:190
Chlamydia pneumoniae, 1:195
mycotic disease, 2:651, 652
necrotizing fasciitis, 2:659

overreliance on fluoroquinolones, 1:257
pneumonia, 2:726–727, 727–728, 729
RSV infection, 2:833
sepsis, 2:869
Community-associated MRSA
antibiotic resistance, 1:63–64
demographics, 1:263
MRSA types, 2:640, 641, 642–643
Staphylococcus aureus infections, 2:912
Compliance
handwashing by health care workers, 2:642, 910
tuberculosis patients' responsibilities, 2:988
Computed tomography (CT) scans
aspergillosis, 1:85
coccidioidomycosis, 1:220
lung flukes, 1:567
nocardiosis, 2:667
pneumonia, 2:726
Computer modeling
bioterrorism, 1:116
climate change, 1:205
emergency department use, 2:763
Concentration problems and protozoan diseases, 2:753
Condominial sewer systems, 2:846
Condoms
AIDS prevention, 1:11, 14, 15
Ebola prevention, 1:303*s*
gonorrhea prevention, 1:389–390
hepatitis C prevention, 1:431
herpes simplex virus 2 prevention, 1:446*s*
HIV prevention, 2:1010
trichomoniasis prevention, 2:977
viral disease prevention, 2:1041
women and infectious disease, 2:1073
Confidentiality, patients' right to, 2:987
Conflicts. *See* War
Confusion
AIDS, 1:12
bacterial meningitis, 2:608
Crimean-Congo hemorrhagic fever, 1:244
glanders, 1:379
Japanese encephalitis, 1:512
necrotizing fasciitis, 2:659
nocardiosis, 2:666
pneumonia, 2:726
Powassan virus, 2:741
protozoan diseases, 2:753
rat-bite fever, 2:787
taeniasis, 2:943
toxic shock, 2:961
typhus, 2:997
Congenital rubella syndrome, 2:595, 836, 837–838
Congenital syphilis, 2:936
Congenital Zika syndrome, 2:1101
Congestive heart failure and Kawasaki disease, 1:515
Congo hemorrhagic fever. *See* Crimean-Congo hemorrhagic fever
Conjunctivitis
avian influenza, 1:89
Chlamydia infection, 1:190
Cryptococcus neoformans infection, 1:248
gonorrhea, 1:388, 389
herpes gladiatorum, 1:442*s*
Lassa fever, 1:526
pink eye, 2:702–704
trachoma, 2:967–969
Connecticut, 1:96, 570, 571
Connective tissue disorders, 2:667*s*
Conservationism, 1:304
Constipation
typhoid fever, 2:993, 995*s*
whipworm, 2:1062
Construction and coccidioidomycosis, 1:218, 221
Construction workers, 1:531
Consumer Reports, 2:707, 708
Consumers Union, 2:708
Consumption. *See* Tuberculosis
Contact dermatitis, 2:819
Contact lenses and *Fusarium* keratitis, 1:**232–234**
Contact precautions, 1:**235–238,** *236*
cryptosporidiosis, 1:251
infection control and asepsis, 1:485, 486
MRSA, 2:642
Contact tracing
gonorrhea, 1:389
plague, 2:717, 718
public health, 2:762
travelers, 1:510
See also Sexual contact notification
Contagion (film), 2:664
Contraception, 1:76*s,* 158, 2:1108
Contractures and congenital Zika syndrome, 2:1101
Convention on the Prohibition of the Development, Production, and Stockpiling of Bacteriological and Toxin Weapons. *See* Biological Weapons Convention
Convention on the Rights of the Child, 2:1003
Convict Creek virus, 1:406
Convulsions. *See* Seizures
Cook, Albert, 1:147
Cooking temperatures
anisakiasis, 1:45
campylobacteriosis, 1:152*s*
Escherichia coli, 1:341
listeriosis, 1:557
liver flukes, 1:562, 563
lung flukes, 1:567
tapeworm, 2:950
trichinellosis, 2:974
Yersiniosis, 2:1098
Cooks, Graham, 1:117
Coordinating Center for Infectious Diseases, 1:481*s*
Coordination problems
AIDS, 1:12
marine toxins, 2:591
Powassan virus, 2:741
Venezuelan equine encephalitis virus, 2:1035
West Nile virus, 2:1059
Copegus. *See* Ribavirin
Copepods, 1:283, 284, 463
Copper sulfate, 2:933
Coquillettidia mosquitoes, 1:296
Corbett, Elizabeth L., 2:791
Cornea
contact lenses and *Fusarium* keratitis, 1:232–233
pink eye, 2:703*s,* 704
trachoma, 2:967, 968, 969
Corneal transplantation and rabies, 2:777
Coronary artery dilatation, 1:515, 516
Coronary heart disease. *See* Heart disease or symptoms
Coronaviruses, 1:228, 2:1039, 1041
Cortes, Hernando, 1:289
Corticosteroids
ascariasis, 1:80
aspergillosis, 1:85
blastomycosis, 1:123
encephalitis, 1:318
lung flukes, 1:567
macrophage activation syndrome, 2:576
mycotic disease as a side effect of, 2:650
swimmer's ear and swimmer's itch, 2:933
Corynebacterium diphtheriae. See Diphtheria
Cosmetic procedures, 1:135
Costa, Federico, 1:550
Costa Rica, 1:550, 2:825
Costs. *See* Economic and financial issues
Cote d'Ivoire
anthrax, 1:49
avian influenza, 1:89
Buruli ulcer, 1:148, *148*
Ebola, 1:41
hemorrhagic fevers, 1:420, 420*s*
Co-trimoxazole drugs, 2:668
Cough
AIDS, 1:12
ascariasis, 1:79
aspergillosis, 1:85
avian influenza, 1:89
blastomycosis, 1:122, 123

chickenpox, 1:176
Chlamydia infection, 1:190
Chlamydia pneumoniae, 1:193, 194
colds, 1:228, 229
diphtheria, 1:275
encephalitis, 1:317
enterovirus 71 infection, 1:325, 327
glanders, 1:379
group A streptococcal infections, 2:921
helminth disease, 1:415
histoplasmosis, 1:448
influenza, 1:488, 504
Legionnaires' disease, 1:530
leprosy, 1:546
lung flukes, 1:566
measles, 2:593, 594
mumps, 2:645
necrotizing fasciitis, 2:659
nocardiosis, 2:666
opportunistic infections, 2:682
pneumonia, 2:726
psittacosis, 2:759
RSV infection, 2:833
rubella, 2:837
SARS, 2:847, 850
scarlet fever, 2:857
schistosomiasis, 2:861
smallpox, 2:890, 891
strep throat, 2:917, 918*s*
strongyloidiasis, 2:929
talaromycosis, 2:944
tuberculosis, 2:983
tularemia, 2:990
typhoid fever, 2:993
typhus, 2:997
viral meningitis, 2:608, 609
whooping cough, 2:1066
Cough suppressants, 1:230
Coughing up blood, 2:726, 929
Cowpox, 2:891, 1020, 1039
Coxiella burnetii, 2:773
Coxsackievirus A16, 1:397
Coyotes
alveolar echinococcosis, 1:24, 25, 25*f*
lung flukes, 1:567
rabies, 2:776
Crab lice. *See* Pubic lice
Crabs
anisakiasis, 1:45
lung flukes, 1:566, 567–568
marine toxins, 2:591
Craigie, David, 1:333
Cramps, abdominal. *See* Abdominal cramps
Cranberry juice, 2:1013
Crank, Christopher W., 2:1026, 1027
Crayfish and lung flukes, 1:566, 567
Crepitus and necrotizing fasciitis, 2:659
Creutzfeldt-Jakob disease, 1:**239–242,** *240*
animal importation, 1:40
blood supply, 1:126
bovine spongiform encephalopathy, 1:136
kuru, 1:522–523, 524
prion disease, 2:748–750
Crimea, 2:711, 1050
Crimean-Congo hemorrhagic fever, 1:**243–246,** *244, 245*
hemorrhagic fevers, 1:418
tick-borne diseases, 2:957
Crispr-Cas9 technology, 1:82, 2:808
Croatia
avian influenza, 1:89
babesiosis, 1:96
trichinellosis, 2:974
Crockett, David, 2:722
Cross-resistance, 2:1026, 1028
Crowded conditions
Chlamydia infection, 1:190
cohorted communities, 1:224
demographics, 1:261
diphtheria, 1:275, 277
hepatitis A, 1:422, 423
re-emerging infectious diseases, 2:793
scabies, 2:853
shigellosis, 2:880, 882
St. Louis encephalitis, 2:906
trachoma, 2:967, 968
typhus, 2:998
yaws, 2:1087
Crowe, James, 2:835
Cruise ships
gastroenteritis, 1:358
norovirus infection, 2:670
viral disease, 2:1039
Crustaceans. *See* Seafood
Cryptococcal meningitis, 1:53, 247–248, 2:651
Cryptococcus neoformans infection, 1:**247–249,** *248, 249*
CryptoNet, 1:252
Cryptosporidiosis, 1:**250–253,** *251*
anti-cytokine antibody syndrome, 1:53
gastroenteritis, 1:359–360
opportunistic infections, 2:683
protozoan diseases, 2:756
water-borne disease, 2:1054, 1055
CT scans. *See* Computed tomography (CT) scans
Cuba
angiostrongyliasis, 1:36
cholera, 1:198
dengue and dengue hemorrhagic fever, 1:266
virus hunters, 2:1043
yellow fever research, 2:1092, 1093–1095
Culex mosquitoes, 2:*906*
Japanese encephalitis, 1:511, 512, 513
St. Louis encephalitis, 2:905, 907
Venezuelan equine encephalitis virus, 2:1033
West Nile virus, 2:1058
Culicoides, 1:244
Culiseta melanura, 1:296, 297, 298, 298*s*
Culling, animal
avian influenza, 1:90, 2:1084
bovine spongiform encephalopathy, 1:40, 138–139, 241
brucellosis, 1:141, 142, 2:1051
glanders, 1:381
H5N1 virus, 1:393
Nipah virus infection, 2:664
Q fever, 2:773
Rift Valley fever, 2:815
Slaughter and slaughterhouses, 1:393
world trade, 2:1084
Cultural issues
burial and mourning customs, 1:287–288
Ebola, 1:303*s,* 304
hemorrhagic fevers, 1:420–421
kuru, 1:522, 523–525
Marburg hemorrhagic fever, 2:587
personal protective equipment, 2:701
prion disease, 2:749
women, 2:1071–1072, 1073
Culture and sensitivity (tests), 1:**254–257,** 331
Cultures (tests)
bacterial meningitis, 2:605
blastomycosis, 1:122
brucellosis, 1:142
Buruli ulcer, 1:149
coccidioidomycosis, 1:220
dysentery, 1:290
enterovirus 71 infection, 1:326
Fusarium keratitis, 1:233
glanders, 1:380
gonorrhea, 1:389
hantavirus, 1:407
herpes simplex virus 2, 1:445
histoplasmosis, 1:451
microbial identification, traditional, 1:363
mononucleosis, 2:634
ringworm, 2:818
sporotrichosis, 2:902
talaromycosis, 2:945
tuberculosis, 2:984
viral meningitis, 2:609
yellow fever, 2:1092
yersiniosis, 2:1097
Cutaneous forms
anthrax, 1:49, *49,* 50, 115
diphtheria, 1:275

leishmaniasis, 1:538, 539–540, 541
mycotic disease, 2:649, 650
protozoan diseases, 2:756
Cuts and tetanus, 2:953
Cuttlefish and anisakiasis, 1:45
Cyclones and cholera, 1:200
Cyclophosphamide, 1:54, 2:576
Cyclosporiasis, 1:*258*, **258–260**, 2:1054
Cyclosporine A, 2:576
Cyprus, 1:89, 2:998
Cystic fibrosis
bacterial diseases, 1:100
burkholderia, 1:144, 145–146
hot tub rash, 1:467
with MRSA, 2:642
opportunistic infections, 2:683
pneumonia, 2:728
pneumonia risk factors, 2:727
Cysticercosis
parasitic diseases, 2:695
taeniasis, 2:943
tapeworm infections, 2:949
Cystitis, 2:1012, 1039
Cysts
amebiasis, 1:27
balantidiasis, 1:103
climate change and protozoan diseases, 2:757
dysentery, 1:289
giardiasis, 1:371, 372
helminth disease, 1:415
liver fluke infections, 1:560, 561
parasitic diseases, 2:695
protozoan diseases, 2:754
sanitation, 2:845
taeniasis, 2:941
tapeworm infections, 2:948
trichinellosis, 2:972
Cytokine storm, 1:495
Cytokines, 1:53–54
Cytomegalovirus infection. *See* CMV infection
Czech Republic, 1:89, 474

D

Daclatasvir, 1:432
Dairy products
brucellosis, 1:140, 141, 142*s*
listeriosis, 1:556, 557
pasteurization, 1:356
Q fever, 2:773
rat-bite fever, 2:786
Salmonella infection, 2:841
scrofula, 2:866
tuberculosis, 2:983
yersiniosis, 2:1096, 1098
Dalbavancin, 2:1027
Damon, Matt, 2:664
"Dangerous Unproven Treatments for 'Chronic Lyme Disease' Are on the Rise," 1:*572–574*
Dapsone, 1:545, 546, 2:981, 1078
Daptomycin, 2:676, 1027
Darfur region, 1:200, 201, 261
Darling, Samuel, 1:448
Darling's disease. *See* Histoplasmosis
DARPA. *See* Defense Advanced Research Projects Agency
Darwinian evolution, 2:611, 612
Dasabuvir, 1:432
Daschle, Tom, 1:48
Data collection, 1:328–329, 2:763
Databases
DNA databases, 1:363, 364
notifiable diseases, 2:679, 681
PREDICT, 2:1046
Date palm sap, 2:662, 663, 664
Day care settings. *See* Child care settings
ddC, 1:13
ddI, 1:13
DDT
arthropod-borne disease, 1:77
CDC, 1:165
malaria, 1:321, 2:579
mosquito-borne diseases, 2:638, 638*s*
parasitic disease prevention, 2:696
vector control, 1:462, 2:1030
virus hunters, 2:1045
Dead virus vaccines. *See* Inactivated vaccines
Deafness and hearing loss
bacterial meningitis, 2:604, 606, 608
CMV infection, 1:215, 216
ear infections, 1:295
Lassa fever, 1:527
measles, 2:593, 1009
mumps, 2:644
Rocky Mountain spotted fever, 2:825
rubella, 2:836, 837
shingles, 2:886, 888
Dean, William, 1:343
Deaths
African sleeping sickness, 1:4
AIDS, 1:14, 15, 19, 20, 453
alveolar echinococcosis prevention, 1:25–26
amebiasis, 1:28
anthrax, 1:47, 48, 49, 115
antibiotic resistant infections, 1:62
antimicrobial resistant infections, 2:799, 801
ascariasis, 1:78, 80
aspergillosis, 1:86
avian influenza, 1:87, 89, 156
B virus infection, 1:91
bacterial diseases, 1:101, 2:744
bacterial meningitis, 2:604
Baylisascaris infection, 1:105, 107
blastomycosis, 1:122, 123
botulism, 1:135
bovine spongiform encephalopathy, 1:136
brucellosis, 1:141
cervical cancer, 1:469
chickenpox, 1:176, 177, 178, 178*s*
chikungunya, 1:182
childhood-associated infectious diseases, 1:184
Chlamydia pneumoniae, 1:195
cholera, 1:198, 201, 2:686
Clostridium difficile infection, 1:210, 212
coccidioidomycosis, 1:218
Creutzfeldt-Jakob disease, 1:240
Crimean-Congo hemorrhagic fever, 1:245
cryptosporidiosis, 1:251, 252, 253
demographics, 1:261–262
dengue and dengue hemorrhagic fever, 1:267
diphtheria, 1:275, 276, 277
dysentery, 1:289
Eastern equine encephalitis, 1:296, 297, 298
Ebola, 1:41, 300–301, 302
economic development, 1:306, 308, 309
emerging infectious diseases, 1:313
encephalitis, 1:316, 317, 318
enterovirus 71 infection, 1:325
environmental health risks, 2:1077
epidemiology, 1:329, 330
Escherichia coli O157:H7, 1:338, 340, 341
extreme weather, 1:204
food-borne disease, 1:354, 355, 356, 357
gastroenteritis, 1:358–361, 359–360, 361
glanders, 1:379–380, 380–381
gonorrhea, 1:388
group A streptococcal infections, 2:920, 922
group B streptococcal infection, 2:925–926
Haemophilus influenzae, 1:394, 395, 396
hand, foot, and mouth disease, 1:398–399
hantavirus, 1:404
hemorrhagic fevers, 1:419, 420
hepatitis A, 1:423, 424–425
hepatitis B, 1:426
hepatitis C, 1:431
hepatitis D, 1:434
herpes simplex 1 virus, 1:443
histoplasmosis, 1:448, 449
HIV/AIDS, 2:1006
H5N1 infection, 1:391
influenza, 1:49, 490, 496, 504

influenza pandemic of 1918, 1:493, 495, 497
influenza pandemic of 1957, 1:499, 500
invasive candidiasis, 1:159
Japanese encephalitis, 1:511, 512, 513*s*
Kawasaki disease, 1:517
kuru, 1:522, 523
Lassa fever, 1:526, 527
leading causes of, 1:166
Legionnaires' disease, 1:530, 531
leishmaniasis, 1:538, 541
leptospirosis, 1:550
listeriosis, 1:556, 558
macrophage activation syndrome, 2:576
malaria, 1:462, 2:580, 582
Marburg hemorrhagic fever, 2:585, 586, 587
marine toxins, 2:591, 592
measles, 1:186, 2:593, 594, 595
Médecins Sans Frontières, 2:601
meningitis, 1:223–224, 2:607
monkeypox, 2:627, 628
mononucleosis, 2:633
mosquito-borne diseases, 2:636
MRSA, 1:485, 2:640, 643
mumps, 2:645
mycotic disease, 2:649, 650, 651, 652
necrotizing fasciitis, 2:657, 659
Nipah virus infection, 2:662, 663, 664
nocardiosis, 2:666
norovirus infection, 2:669
nosocomial infections, 1:487, 2:673–674, 675
opportunistic infections, 2:683, 684
pandemic preparedness, 2:691
parasitic diseases, 2:695, 696
plague, 1:116, 2:710, 712–713, 715, 717, 718
Pneumocystis jirovecii pneumonia, 2:722, 723
pneumonia, 2:725, 726, 727, 729–730
polio, 2:737, 739
Powassan virus, 2:742
protozoan diseases, 2:753, 755, 756
psittacosis, 2:759
public health, 2:764
puerperal fever, 2:767–769, 768
Q fever, 2:772
rabies, 2:775, 777, 779
rat-bite fever, 2:786, 787
re-emerging infectious diseases, 2:790, 791, 792
relapsing fever, 2:796
retroviruses, 2:808
rickettsial disease, 2:810, 811
Rift Valley fever, 2:813–816, 815, 816
Rocky Mountain spotted fever, 2:826
rotavirus, 2:818, 828, 829
rotavirus vaccine, 2:830
RSV infection, 2:832
rubella, 2:837
Salmonella infection, 2:842
sanitation-related diseases, 2:844, 845
SARS, 2:847, 848, 849, 850
scarlet fever, 2:856, 857
schistosomiasis, 2:863
sepsis, 1:168, 257, 2:868, 869, 1079
severe fever with thrombocytopenia syndrome, 2:871, 872
shigellosis, 2:882
smallpox, 2:891, 892, 1020
smallpox vaccine, 2:628*s*
sporotrichosis, 2:901, 902
St. Louis encephalitis, 2:905, 906
Staphylococcus aureus infections, 2:913
superbugs, 2:1027*s*
taeniasis, 2:942
talaromycosis, 2:945, 946
tapeworm infections, 2:949, 950
tetanus, 2:953, 954
tick-borne diseases, 2:957, 958
toxic shock, 2:961, 962
travel, 2:970–971
trichinellosis, 2:974
tropical infectious diseases, 2:980, 981
tuberculosis, 2:983, 984, 986
tularemia, 2:989, 990, 991
typhoid fever, 2:993, 994, 995, 995*s*
typhus, 2:997–1001, 998, 999, 1001
United Nations Millennium Goals, 2:769, 1007, 1008, 1009, 1010
unsafe abortion, 2:1108
vaccine reactions, 2:1022
vaccine-preventable diseases, 2:1005
vancomycin-resistant *Enterococci,* 2:1025, 1027
vector-borne disease, 2:1029, 1031
Venezuelan equine encephalitis virus, 2:1035
viral disease, 2:1039, 1041
virus hunters, 2:1043
war, 2:1047, 1048, 1050
water-borne diseases, 2:1053, 1054, 1055
West Nile virus, 2:1058, 1059, 1060
whooping cough, 2:1066, 1067, 1068
women, 2:1073
yellow fever, 2:1092–1095
yersiniosis, 2:1096–1099
Zika virus, 2:1102
Debridement, 2:659, 1050
Decameron, 2:712
DEC-fortified salt, 1:351
Declaration of Commitment on HIV/AIDS, 2:1009
Declaration of Helsinki, 1:344, 2:937
Declaration of the Rights of the Child, 2:1003
Decongestants, 1:294
Deer
babesiosis, 1:97
Lyme disease, 1:571, 572
rabies, 2:777
transmissible spongiform encephalopathies, 1:136
Deer flies, 2:990
Deer mice, 1:406, 407, *407*
Deer ticks, 2:*742*
babesiosis, 1:95
climate change, 2:698
Lyme disease, 1:569, 570, 572
Deerfly fever. *See* Tularemia
DEET insect repellents
Crimean-Congo hemorrhagic fever, 1:245
Japanese encephalitis, 1:513
Lyme disease, 1:572
malaria, 2:581
St. Louis encephalitis, 2:907
swimmer's ear and swimmer's itch, 2:933
typhus, 2:1000
Venezuelan equine encephalitis virus, 2:1035*s*
West Nile virus, 2:1061
Defense Advanced Research Projects Agency, 1:363*s*, 2:783*s*
Deforestation
alveolar echinococcosis, 1:26
antibacterial drugs, 1:57
Chagas disease, 1:174
Ebola, 1:304
leismaniasis, 1:541
malaria, 1:205
wildlife, 2:1085
world trade, 2:1084, 1085
Deformities
Buruli ulcer, 1:149
leprosy, 1:543
sexually transmitted infections, 2:877
syphilis, 2:936
Degenerative brain disease research, 1:524–525
Dehydration
amebiasis, 1:27
balantidiasis, 1:103
Campylobacter infection, 1:151
cholera, 1:197–198, 197–201
Clostridium difficile infection, 1:211

cryptosporidiosis, 1:250, 251, 252
dysentery, 1:290
Escherichia coli O157:H7, 1:340
food-borne disease, 1:354–355
gastroenteritis, 1:359–360
hand, foot, and mouth disease, 1:398
norovirus infection, 2:669, 670
protozoan diseases, 2:754
rotavirus infection, 2:829, 830
Salmonella infection, 2:841
sanitation-related diseases, 2:844
shigellosis, 2:882
typhoid fever, 2:995*s*
viral disease, 2:1041
water-borne disease, 2:1054
Delaporte, François, 1:172
Delavridine, 1:13
Delaware, 1:571
Delhi, India, 1:267
Delicatessen-style meat, 1:557
Delirium and scarlet fever, 2:857
Dellinger, R. Phillip, 2:868
Delousing, 1:553, 554
Delusions, 1:316, 2:935
Dementia
Creutzfeldt-Jakob disease, 1:240
kuru research, 1:525
prion disease, 2:749
sexually transmitted infections, 2:877
syphilis, 2:934
Democratic Republic of the Congo
African sleeping sickness, 1:3, 5
AIDS, origin of, 1:17–18
Buruli ulcer, 1:149
cholera, 1:201
Crimean-Congo hemorrhagic fever, 1:243
disinfection recommendations for Ebola control, 1:281
Ebola, 1:300, 301, 302, 2:1022
leprosy, 1:546, 2:1078
malaria, 2:*578*
monkeypox, 2:627, *627*
plague, 2:715, 716, 717
rotavirus, 2:829, 831
typhoid fever, 2:995
United Nations Millennium Goals, 2:1009
virus hunters, 2:1045
yaws, 2:1089
Demographics, 1:**261–265**
Dendritic cells, 1:455, 2:835
Dengue and dengue hemorrhagic fever, 1:*204*, **266–269,** *267, 268*
arthropod-borne diseases, 1:75, 77
chikungunya *vs.,* 1:181, 182
climate change, 1:205, 207
globalization, 1:385
hemorrhagic fevers, 1:419
mosquito-borne diseases, 2:637
tropical infectious diseases, 2:979–980
vector-borne disease, 2:1029, *1030*
Dengue shock syndrome, 1:267, 268
Dengvaxia, 1:269
Denmark
avian influenza, 1:89
group B streptococcal infection, 2:926
vancomycin-resistant *Enterococci,* 2:1027
yersiniosis, 2:1097
Dental problems, 2:876
Denver, CO, 2:986
Department of Health, Australia, 2:647
Depression
Creutzfeldt-Jakob disease, 1:240
dengue and dengue hemorrhagic fever, 1:267
economic development, 1:307
mononucleosis, 2:631
rickettsial disease, 2:809
Dermatitis
hot tub rash, 1:465–467
ringworm, 2:819
river blindness, 2:820, 821
strongyloidiasis, 2:929
swimmer's itch, 2:931–933
Dermatology Research and Practice, 2:902
Dermatophytosis. *See* Ringworm
Derrick, Edward H., 2:771
Desorption electrospray ionization, 1:117
De-ticking of animals, 1:245
Detroit Free Press, 2:883
Developed nations
bacterial meningitis, 2:605
blood supply screening, 1:126
botulism, 1:135
childhood vaccinations, 1:186
dysentery, 1:290, 291
economic development, 1:306–307
gastroenteritis, 1:360
giardiasis, 1:372
hepatitis A, 1:422
hepatitis E, 1:438
Legionnaires' disease, 1:531
lice infestation, 1:553, 554
measles, 2:595
mononucleosis, 2:632
mumps, 2:647
protozoan diseases, 2:756
puerperal fever, 2:768
resistant organisms, 2:802
scarlet fever, 2:856
sepsis, 2:869
trachoma, 2:968
water-borne diseases, 2:1053, 1055
zoonoses, 2:1107
Developing nations
AIDS, 1:8
anthrax, 1:50
ascariasis, 1:78–79
bacterial meningitis, 2:604, 606
balantidiasis, 1:103
blood supply, 1:127
bloodborne pathogens, 1:130
botulism, 1:135
brucellosis, 1:141–142
cat scratch disease, 1:163
Chagas disease, 1:173
chickenpox, 1:178
Chlamydia infection, 1:189, 190
cholera, 1:197
cryptosporidiosis, 1:251
cyclosporiasis, 1:259
dengue and dengue hemorrhagic fever, 1:268
diphtheria, 1:277
dysentery, 1:290, 291–292
economic development, 1:306–309
emerging infectious diseases, 1:312
endemicity, 1:321
environmental health risks, 2:1077
Epstein-Barr virus, 1:336, 337
filariasis, 1:350, 352
food-borne disease, 1:357
gastroenteritis, 1:358–361, 359–360
globalization and infectious disease, 1:385
group A streptococcal infections, 2:922
group B streptococcal infections, 2:925
Haemophilus influenzae, 1:395, 396
helminth disease, 1:414, 415, 416, 417
hepatitis A, 1:423
hepatitis E, 1:438, 439
hookworm infection, 1:458
impetigo, 1:482
Japanese encephalitis, 1:513*s*
lice infestation, 1:553
liver fluke infections, 1:562
measles, 2:595
Médecins Sans Frontières, 2:601
microsporidiosis, 2:623–624
mononucleosis, 2:632
norovirus infection, 2:669
nosocomial infections, 2:675
opportunistic infections, 2:684
outbreaks, field-level response to, 2:687
pneumonia, 2:727, 729
polio, 2:738
protozoan diseases, 2:754–755, 756
puerperal fever, 2:768
rabies, 2:777

rapid diagnostic tests, 2:783
retroviruses, 2:808
river blindness, 2:822
rotavirus, 1:361, 2:829, 830
sanitation, 2:846, 846*s*
scarlet fever, 2:856, 857
schistosomiasis, 2:860, 862, 863
scrofula, 2:866
sepsis, 2:868, 869
shigellosis, 2:880, 881, 882
smallpox research, opposition to, 2:899
syphilis, 2:936
tapeworm infections, 2:950
tetanus, 2:954
toxic shock, 2:962*s*
trachoma, 2:967
tropical infectious diseases, 2:982
tuberculosis, 1:101, 2:984
typhoid fever, 2:995
UNICEF, 2:1003
vaccines and vaccine development, 2:1023
virus hunters, 2:1045
water-borne diseases, 2:1053, *1053*, 1054–1055, 1055*s*
whipworm, 2:1063
women, 2:1072
World Health Organization, 2:1077
yaws, 2:1089
zoonoses, 2:1107

Developing nations and drug delivery, 1:**270–273**, *271*
antibiotics, 1:58
emerging infectious diseases, 1:313
globalization, 1:385
leishmaniasis, 1:541
leprosy, 1:547
Médecins Sans Frontières, 2:600–601
river blindness, 2:822
rotavirus vaccine, 2:831
schistosomiasis, 2:863
trachoma, 2:969
tropical infectious diseases, 2:981*s*, 982
World Health Organization, 2:1078
yaws, 2:1089, 1090

Devon, Frye, 2:977
DeWitte, Sharon, 2:712
Deworming
children, 2:1064
helminth disease prevention, 1:416
liver fluke infection, 1:562
tapeworm infection prevention, 2:950

Dexilant. *See* Dexlansoprazole
Dexlansoprazole, 1:411
d4T, 1:13
Diabetes
candidiasis risk factors, 1:158, 159
coccidioidomycosis risk factors, 1:219
diseases that weaken the immune system, 2:667*s*
with glanders, 1:379
group A streptococcal infections, 2:921
mycotic disease, 2:650
opportunistic infections, 2:683
rubella, 2:837
swimmer's ear, 2:933
tuberculosis risk factors, 2:984
urinary tract infection, 2:1013

Diagnosis
Advanced Diagnostics Program, 2:783*s*
GIDEON, 1:375, 376–377
rapid diagnostic tests, 2:781–783
See also Misdiagnosis; specific diseases

Dialysis, 1:340, 341, 432*s*, 531
Diaper rash, 1:159
Diarrhea
AIDS, 1:12
amebiasis, 1:27
anisakiasis, 1:45
ascariasis, 1:79
avian influenza, 1:89
bacterial diseases, 1:99, 100
balantidiasis, 1:103
Campylobacter infection, 1:151, 152*s*
Chagas disease, 1:172
cholera, 1:197, 198, 201
climate change, 1:205
Clostridium difficile infection, 1:209, 210, 211, 212
cohorted communities, 1:224
Crimean-Congo hemorrhagic fever, 1:244
cryptosporidiosis, 1:250–253
cyclosporiasis, 1:258, 259, 260
dysentery, 1:289
Ebola, 1:302
Escherichia coli O157:H7, 1:338–339, 340
fifth disease, 1:347
food-borne disease, 1:354–355, 357
gastroenteritis, 1:358–361, 359–360
giardiasis, 1:371
glanders, 1:379
heartland virus, 2:873*s*
helminth disease, 1:415
hemorrhagic fevers, 1:419, 420*s*
hepatitis A, 1:422–425
hepatitis B, 1:426
hepatitis D, 1:434
hepatitis E, 1:437
hookworm infection, 1:458
influenza, 1:488
Lassa fever, 1:526
Legionnaires' disease, 1:530
leptospirosis, 1:548
listeriosis, 1:556
liver fluke infections, 1:560
lung flukes, 1:566
malaria, 2:580
Marburg hemorrhagic fever, 2:586
marine toxins, 2:590, 591
measles, 2:593
microsporidiosis, 2:623
norovirus infection, 2:669, 670
opportunistic infections, 2:683, 684
protozoan diseases, 2:754
Rocky Mountain spotted fever, 2:824
rotavirus, 2:828–829, 831
Salmonella infection, 2:841
sanitation, 2:844, 845
schistosomiasis, 2:861
severe fever with thrombocytopenia syndrome, 2:871
sexually transmitted infections, 2:877
shigellosis, 2:883
strongyloidiasis, 2:929
tapeworm infections, 2:948
toxic shock, 2:961
travel, 2:971
trichinellosis, 2:972, 973
tularemia, 2:989, 990
typhoid fever, 2:995*s*
viral disease, 2:1041
viral meningitis, 2:608
water-borne disease, 2:1054, 1055
West Nile virus, 2:1059
whipworm, 2:1062
yersiniosis, 2:1097

Diatoms, 2:591
Dichloro-diphenyl-trichloroethane. *See* DDT
Dick, George Frederick, 2:858
Dick, Gladys Henry, 2:858
Dideoxyinosine, 1:13
Die-offs and West Nile virus, 2:1058
Diet and *Clostridium difficile* infection, 1:210, 211
Diethylcarbamazine citrate (DEC), 1:351
Differential diagnoses, 1:377
Diflucan. *See* Fluconazole
Digenetic trematodes, 1:415
Dignity, patients' right to, 2:987
Dinoflagellates, 2:591
Diphtheria, 1:**274–279**
bacterial disease vaccines, 1:101
childhood vaccination, 1:186, 187
demographics, 1:261
vaccines, 1:184, 185, *275*, 2:1022*s*

WHO childhood vaccination recommendations, 1:185
Diptera. *See* Mosquito-borne diseases
Direct immunofluorescence assays, 1:191*s*
Direct-acting antiviral drugs, 1:431–432
Directly Observed Therapy, 2:985–986
Directors of Health Promotion and Education, 2:826
Disability
bacterial meningitis, 2:604
Buruli ulcer, 1:148
Chlamydia infection, 1:191
filariasis, 1:350, 351, 352
helminth disease, 1:416
Japanese encephalitis, 1:511, 512
leprosy, 1:543
polio, 2:736, 737
viral meningitis, 2:607
yaws, 2:1089
Discharge
Chlamydia infection, 1:189
gonorrhea, 1:387–388
influenza, 1:504
protozoan diseases, 2:754
puerperal fever, 2:767
sexually transmitted infections, 2:877, 878
swimmer's ear, 2:933
trachoma, 2:967
trichomoniasis, 2:976
Discoloration and necrotizing fasciitis, 2:659
Discrimination, gender, 2:1071
Disease causation. *See* Germ theory; Koch's postulates
Disfigurement
Buruli ulcer, 1:148
filariasis, 1:350
leishmaniasis, 1:540, 541
river blindness, 2:820
smallpox, 2:890
yaws, 2:1087
Disinfection, 1:**280–282**, *281*
antibacterial agents, 1:56
Baylisascaris infection prevention, 1:107
enterovirus 71 infection, 1:327
germ theory of disease, 1:367, 370
glanders, 1:380
handwashing, 1:400–402
hot tub rash, 1:465, 466
infection control and asepsis, 1:484–485
leptospirosis, 1:549*s*
MRSA prevention, 2:642
mycotic disease, 2:651
pinworm infection, 2:706
plague, 2:*717*
protozoan diseases, 2:757
See also Sterilization
Disneyland, 1:384, 531, 2:595
Disorientation
bacterial meningitis, 2:605, 608
encephalitis, 1:316, 317
Japanese encephalitis, 1:512
Nipah virus infection, 2:663
nocardiosis, 2:666
St. Louis encephalitis, 2:905
West Nile virus, 2:1059
Disparities in AIDS deaths, 1:14
Displaced persons
demographics, 1:261, 263
diphtheria, 1:278
emerging infectious diseases, 1:314
immigration, 1:472
measles, 2:595
Médicins Sans Frontières, 2:600
Syria, 2:*1049*
Disseminated forms
coccidioidomycosis, 1:219, 221
gonococcal infection, 1:388
histoplasmosis, 1:448–449
intravascular coagulation, 2:716
nocardiosis, 2:666
sporotrichosis, 2:901, 902
strongyloidiasis, 2:929
Divine right of kings, 2:865
Division of Bacterial and Mycotic Diseases, CDC, 1:122, 2:668
Division of Global HIV & TB, CDC, 1:8
Division of Global Migration and Quarantine, CDC, 1:508, 2:850
Division of HIV/AIDS Prevention, 2:965*s*
Division of Select Agents and Toxins, CDC, 2:898
Division of Vector-Borne Diseases, CDC, 2:991*s*
Dizziness
Crimean-Congo hemorrhagic fever, 1:244
hemorrhagic fevers, 1:419
hookworm infection, 1:458
marine toxins, 2:591
nocardiosis, 2:666
Rift Valley fever, 2:813
toxic shock, 2:961
Djibouti, 1:88, 2:*979*
DNA
Advanced Diagnostics Program, 2:783*s*
antibiotic resistance, 1:62
Asilomar Conference and genetic research, 1:81–82
edible vaccines, 1:82*s*
Epstein-Barr virus, 1:335
genetic identification of microorganisms, 1:362
rapid diagnostic tests, 2:782
viral disease, 2:1039
DNA Data Bank of Japan, 1:363
DNA databases, 1:363, 364
DNA fingerprinting, 1:340*s*
DNA viruses
hepatitis B, 1:426
herpes simplex 1 virus, 1:440–443
herpes simplex virus 2, 1:444–446
HPV, 1:468–470
Dobrava-Belgrade virus, 1:404–405
Doctors Without Borders. *See* Médecins Sans Frontières
"Doctors Without Borders Has Mixed Feelings about Award for Ebola Work," 2:*601–602*
Dog ticks, 2:824
Dogs
alveolar echinococcosis, 1:25, 25*f*
anellovirus, 1:31
animal importation, 1:40
Baylisascaris infection, 1:107
brucellosis, 1:140
burkholderia, 1:145
Campylobacter infection, 1:152
cat scratch disease, 1:163
cryptosporidiosis, 1:251
giardiasis vaccine, 1:373
glanders, 1:378
histoplasmosis, 1:449
hosts and vectors, 1:461
leishmaniasis, 1:539, 540
leptospirosis, 1:548
lung flukes, 1:567
parasitic diseases, 2:695
plague, 2:716, 719
rabies, 2:775, 777, 778
rat-bite fever, 2:785
ringworm, 2:817
taeniasis, 2:940, 941
tapeworm infections, 2:948
tetanus, 2:953
toxocariasis, 1:80*s*
trade, 2:1083
typhus, 2:998
Venezuelan equine encephalitis virus, 2:1033
West Nile virus, 2:1060
zoonoses, 2:1106, 1107
"Dole under U.S. Probe after Deadly Listeria Outbreak," 1:*558*
Doll, Richard, 1:328
Domesticated animals. *See* Livestock; Pets
Dominican Republic, 1:198
Doner, Sam, 2:937
Donkeys
burkholderia, 1:144
glanders, 1:378
Venezuelan equine encephalitis virus, 2:1033, 1035
Donohue, Mark, 2:708
Dormancy
CMV infection, 1:214
herpes simplex virus 2, 1:444

shingles, 2:885
See also Latency
Dos Santos, Maria de Fátima, 2:1102–1103
Dowell, Scott F., 2:1084
Dox, Gwendolyn, 2:937
Doxycycline
anthrax, 1:115
brucellosis, 1:142
Chlamydia infection, 1:191
cholera, 1:198
glanders, 1:380
leptospirosis, 1:549
Lyme disease, 1:571
malaria, 2:581
MRSA, 2:642
nosocomial infections, 2:674
plague, 2:718
pneumonia, 2:728
psittacosis, 2:760
Q fever, 2:772
relapsing fever, 2:796, 797
rickettsial disease, 2:811
river blindness, 2:821
Rocky Mountain spotted fever, 2:825
Staphylococcus aureus infections, 2:913
syphilis, 2:936
trachoma, 2:968
typhus, 2:999, 1000
war, 2:1049
"Dr. Finlay Gets Full Credit Now," *2:1093–1095*
Dracunculiasis, 1:**283–285,** *284*
helminth disease, 1:417
hosts and vectors, 1:463
tropical infectious diseases, 2:981*s*
water-borne disease, 2:1055–1056
Drancourt, M, 2:713
Drinking water. *See* Water-borne diseases
Droplet precautions, 1:**286–288,** *287*
contact precautions, 1:237
Ebola prevention, 1:237
infection control, 1:484–485
Droplet transmission
airborne precautions, 1:21–23
Chlamydia infection, 1:190
diphtheria, 1:275
disinfection, 1:281
encephalitis, 1:316, 317
fifth disease, 1:348
group A streptococcal infections, 2:921
Haemophilus influenzae, 1:395
herpes simplex 1 virus, 1:440–441
influenza, 1:488–489
influenza pandemic of 1918, 1:495
influenza pandemic of 1957, 1:499, 500
Legionnaires' disease, 1:529, 530, 531*s*
leprosy, 1:546
measles, 2:593, 594
monkeypox, 2:626
mumps, 2:645
necrotizing fasciitis, 2:659
personal protective equipment, 2:700
psittacosis, 2:759
rickettsial disease, 2:809
RSV infection, 2:833
SARS, 2:847
shingles, 2:885
smallpox, 2:890, 891
tropical infectious diseases, 2:980
tuberculosis, 1:473, 2:983
viral disease, 2:1041
viral meningitis, 2:610
Drought, 2:664, 757
Drowsiness. *See* Sleepiness
Drug abuse
gonorrhea risk factors, 1:389
hepatitis A, 1:424–425
See also Injection drug users
Drug companies. *See* Pharmaceutical companies
Drug delivery and developing nations. *See* Developing nations and drug delivery
Drug development
antibiotic resistance, 1:59, 63
antibiotics, 2:803
epidemiology, 1:331–332
marine microorganisms, 2:591*s*
See also Pharmaceutical companies; Vaccines and vaccine development
Drug donation programs. *See* Developing nations and drug delivery
Drug interactions, 1:13
Drug resistance
candidiasis, 1:158
CDC, 1:169
helminth disease, 1:416
HIV, 1:13
H5N1 virus, 1:393
influenza epidemiology, 1:507
leishmaniasis, 1:540
lice, 1:553, 554
malaria, 2:581
microorganisms, 2:617
mosquito-borne diseases, 2:638
mycotic disease, 2:649, 651–652
sepsis, 2:869
tropical infectious diseases, 2:981
world trade, 2:1083
See also Antibiotic resistance
Drug stockpiling. *See* Stockpiling, drug
Drugs. *See* Pharmaceutical companies; specific drugs and drug classes
Drugs for Neglected Diseases Initiative, 1:174
Dry mouth and cryptosporidiosis, 1:252
DT vaccine, 1:276
DTaP vaccine, 1:276, 2:954, 1067, 1068
DTP vaccine, 1:276–277, 2:*952,* 1068
DTwP vaccine, 2:1068
Dual use aspect of bioscience, 1:119
Dubray, Christine, 1:416
Duck itch. *See* Swimmer's ear and swimmer's itch
Ducks and schistosomes, 2:931
Duesberg, Peter, 1:521
Dumb rabies, 2:776
Duodenal fluid tests, 2:929
Duration of disease and epidemiology, 1:330
Dust, 2:666, 771
Dutch National Institute for Public Health and the Environment, 2:*957*
Dwarf tapeworm infection, 2:949
Dysentery, 1:**289–292,** *291*
balantidiasis, 1:103
protozoan diseases, 2:754
sanitation, 2:844–845
shigellosis, 2:880, 881
water-borne disease, 2:1054
Dysphagia. *See* Swallowing problems
Dysplasia and HPV, 1:469
Dystonia and botulinum toxin, 1:135
Dysuria. *See* Urination issues

E

Ear discharge and swimmer's ear, 2:933
Ear infections, 1:**293–295,** *294*
AIDS, 1:12
bacterial meningitis, 2:604–605
Cryptococcus neoformans infection, 1:248
Epstein-Barr virus, 1:337
Haemophilus influenzae, 1:394
infections for which cultures are not possible, 1:256
measles, 2:593
scarlet fever, 2:857
strep throat, 2:917
swimmer's ear, 2:931–933
Earthquakes
cholera, 1:198
climate change, 1:207
typhoid fever, 2:995
East Africa
developing nations and drug delivery, 1:272*s*
leishmaniasis, 1:541
leprosy, 1:544
plague, 2:716

resistant organisms, 2:800
river blindness, 2:821
United Nations Millennium Goals, 2:1009
East African trypanosomiasis, 1:1, 2, 3
East Asia
AIDS deaths, 1:15
helminth disease, 1:415
hepatitis B, 1:427
hepatitis E, 1:437
Kawasaki disease, 1:515
maternal mortality, 2:769
tropical infectious diseases, 2:981
wildlife trade, 2:1083
East Asian descent and Kawasaki disease, 1:515, 517
East Indies, 2:637
Eastern Africa, 2:791*s*, 814
Eastern equine encephalitis, 1:**296–299,** 317
Eastern Europe
anthrax, 1:50
brucellosis, 1:141
climate change, 1:206
Crimean-Congo hemorrhagic fever, 1:245
developing nations and drug delivery, 1:271
hemorrhagic fevers, 1:418
international adoption, 1:475
Jewish immigration, 2:712
liver fluke infections, 1:561
malaria, 2:579
Pneumocystis jirovecii pneumonia, 2:721
rabies, 2:777
relapsing fever, 2:797
trichinellosis, 2:972, 973
typhus, 2:999, 1001
West Nile virus, 2:1057
Eastern Mediterranean region, 1:431, 2:734
Eastern Russia, 2:957
Eastern United States
botulism, 1:134
Eastern equine encephalitis, 1:296, 297
encephalitis, 1:317
hantavirus, 1:406
mitten crabs, 1:567
typhus, 2:999
Eating problems and Zika virus, 2:1103
Ebers Papyrus, 2:710
Ebola, 1:**300–305,** *301, 419,* 2:*1044*
airborne transmission and droplet precautions, 1:287–288
animal importation, 1:41
bioterrorism, 1:114
CDC, 1:169
economic development, 1:308
emerging infectious diseases, 1:312
epidemiology, 1:332–333
field-level response to Ebola outbreak, 2:*685*
fruit bats, 2:664
globalization and infectious disease, 1:385
hemorrhagic fevers, 1:419, 420–421, 420*s*
isolation and quarantine, 1:510
Médecins Sans Frontières, 2:599, 601–602
National Institute of Allergy and Infectious Diseases, 2:655
outbreaks, field-level response to, 2:687, 688
personal protective equipment, 2:701
public health, 2:765
Rocky Mountain Laboratory, 2:655–656
standard precautions, 2:909
travel, 2:970, 971
USAMRIID, 2:1017, 1018
vaccines and vaccine development, 2:1022
viral disease, 2:1041
virus hunters, 2:1045
wildlife trade, 2:1083, 1085
World Health Organization, 2:1077
"Ebola Diaries: Hitting the Ground Running," 2:*688*
EBV. *See* Epstein-Barr virus
Ecchymoses, 1:267
Echinococcosis, 2:943
Echinococcus multicocularis infection. See Alveolar echinococcosis
Ecological issues, 2:656, 1082, 1107
Econazole, 2:818
Economic and financial issues
African sleeping sickness, 1:4
alveolar echinococcosis treatment, 1:26
anthrax, 1:50, 51
antiviral drugs, 1:72–73, 496
bovine spongiform encephalopathy, 1:139
Brazil, 2:1108
cancer-related infection vaccines, 1:156
candidiasis, 1:160
childhood vaccinations, 1:185
Chipotle Mexico Grill stock prices, 2:672
Clostridium difficile infection, 1:209, 212
cryptosporidiosis, 1:252
demographics, 1:263
developing nations and drug delivery, 1:271–272
dracunculiasis, 1:284–285
ear infections, 1:295
Ebola, 2:1085
effective antibiotics, 2:802*s*
filariasis, 1:350
food-borne disease, 1:166
handwashing, 1:402
hepatitis C drugs, 1:432
influenza, 1:491
leprosy, 1:547
leptospirosis, 1:550
Lyme disease vaccine, 1:572
malaria prevention, 2:583
marine toxins, 2:592
microsporidiosis, 2:623
Nipah virus infection, 2:663–664
pesticides, 2:638
pinworm treatments, 2:707–708
plague, 2:712
pneumonia, 2:729
polio eradication, 2:740
rapid diagnostic tests, 2:783
Rift Valley fever, 2:815
river blindness, 2:821, 822
rotavirus vaccine, 2:831
rubella, 2:839
Salmonella infection, 2:842
schistosomiasis, 2:863
sexually transmitted infections, 2:877*s*
shingles vaccines, 2:887, 888
trachoma, 2:969
trichinellosis, 2:974
tropical infectious disease drugs, 2:982
vaccines, 1:167, 2:1022
vancomycin-resistant *Enterococci,* 2:1027
vector-borne disease, 2:1031
viral disease, 2:1041
viral meningitis, 2:610
water-borne disease, 2:1055
women, 2:1072
world trade, 2:1082, 1084
Zika virus, 2:1102
See also Funding and budgets
Economic development, 1:**306–310**
Economic status. *See* Socioeconomic status
Ecosystems
climate change and parasites, 2:697–698
ecosystems health approach, 1:562–564
lung fluke eradication issues, 1:568
mosquito-borne diseases, 2:638*s*
protozoan diseases, 2:756
Rocky Mountain Laboratory research, 2:655
world trade, 2:1082, 1085
zoonoses, 2:1107
Ectoparasites, 2:694
Ectopic pregnancy, 1:389
Ecuador
burkholderia, 1:145
climate change, 1:207
river blindness, 2:821
strongyloidiasis, 2:930
Venezuelan equine encephalitis virus, 2:1034

Eczema herpeticum, 1:442
Edible vaccines, 1:82*s*
The Edinburgh Medical Journal, 2:1095
Education, public. *See* Public awareness and education
Edward the Confessor, 2:865
EEE. *See* Eastern equine encephalitis
"Effectiveness of Routine BCG Vaccination On Buruli Ulcer Disease," 1:149
Eflornithine, 1:4
Efravirenz, 1:13
Eggs, 1:357, 392*s,* 2:841, 842
Egypt
  angiostrongyliasis, 1:36
  Biological Weapons Convention, 1:111
  bloodborne pathogens, 1:130
  cholera, 1:200
  demographics, 1:263
  hepatitis C, 1:*431*
  plague, 2:713
  Rift Valley fever, 2:815
  schistosomiasis, 2:861, 863
  smallpox and trade, 2:1081
Egypt, ancient
  anthrax, 1:47
  colds, 1:228
  diphtheria, 1:277
  helminth disease, 1:414
  leprosy, 1:544
  lice infestation, 1:552
  plague, 2:710
  trachoma, 2:967
  tuberculosis, 2:983, *984*
Egyptian ophthalmia. *See* Trachoma
Ehrenberg, Christian Gottfried, 1:255
Ehrlich, Paul, 1:57, 254
Ehrlichiosis, 1:571, 2:810, 811, 957
"8-Year-Old Dies from Rare Flesh-Eating Bacteria: Doctors 'Kept Cutting and Hoping,' Mother Says," 2:*659–660*
El Niño, 1:207
El Tor serotype, 1:197, 199
Elbow bump greeting, 1:402
Elderly. *See* Older adults and the elderly
Electrical nerve stimulation, 2:887
Electrocardiograms, 2:695, 796
Electroencephalograms, 1:240
Electrolyte balance
  cholera, 1:198, 201
  Crimean-Congo hemorrhagic fever, 1:245
  cryptosporidiosis, 1:252
  Lassa fever, 1:528
Electron microscopy, 2:619, 620*s,* 1045
Elephantiasis
  filariasis, 1:350, 351*s,* 352
  tropical infectious diseases, 2:980
Elephants and the wildlife trade, 2:1085
Elk, 1:136, 140, 141, 143
Ellerman, Wilhelm, 1:154
Emergency Operations Center, CDC, 1:166, 169, 2:1051*s*
Emergency Preparedness and Response Department, CDC, 2:687
Emergency response
  anthrax emergency response training, 1:116
  bioterrorism, 1:114, 117, 2:1051*s*
  field-level response to outbreaks, 2:685–688
  legislation and international law, 1:535–536
  Médecins Sans Frontières, 2:600
  outbreaks, field-level response to, 2:685–688
  pandemic preparedness, 2:690–693
  SARS, 2:849*s*
  USAMRIID, 2:1017, 1018
Emergency risk management for health plan, 2:690–691
Emergency room visits, 2:763, 828
Emergency situations and shigellosis outbreaks, 2:880, 882
Emergency Use Authorization, 2:1018
Emerging infectious diseases, 1:*311,* **311–314,** *312*
  avian influenza, 1:88, 89
  demographics, 1:263
  Eastern equine encephalitis, 1:297
  encephalitis, 1:319
  enterovirus 71 infection, 1:327
  epidemiology, 1:332
  infection control and asepsis, 1:486
  leptospirosis, 1:548
  microorganisms, 2:617
  Nipah virus infection, 2:662, 663
  notifiable diseases, 2:678
  parasitic diseases, 2:756–757
  ProMED, 2:751–752
  relapsing fever, 2:798
  Rocky Mountain Laboratory, 2:656
  severe fever with thrombocytopenia syndrome, 2:871–873
  tick-borne diseases, 2:957
  vector-borne disease, 2:1030
  viral disease, 2:1041
  world trade, 2:1083, 1084
  zoonoses, 2:1105, 1107
  See also Re-emerging infectious diseases
Emerging Infectious Diseases
  blastomycosis, 1:122
  CDC journals, 1:168
  plague, 2:713
  typhus, 2:999
Emory University, 1:91–92, 166
Emotional instability and toxic shock, 2:961
Emphysema, 2:667
Employment. *See* Labor and employment issues; Occupational risk
Emverm. *See* Mebendazole
Encephalitis, 1:*315,* **315–319**
  arthropod-borne diseases, 1:75, 77
  chickenpox, 1:176
  Eastern equine encephalitis, 1:296–298
  enterovirus 71 infection, 1:326
  hand, foot, and mouth disease, 1:397, 398–399
  hemorrhagic fevers, 1:419
  herpes simplex 1 virus, 1:441, 442, 443
  Japanese encephalitis, 1:511–514
  measles, 2:593, 594
  mumps, 2:645
  Nipah virus infection, 2:662, 664
  Powassan virus, 2:741–743, 742
  protozoan diseases, 2:755
  rubella, 2:837
  shingles, 2:886
  St. Louis encephalitis, 1:418, 2:905–907
  tick-borne diseases, 2:957, 958
  toxoplasmosis, 2:964
  vaccine reactions, 2:1022
  vector-borne disease, 2:1029, 1030, 1031
  Venezuelan equine encephalitis virus, 2:1033–1035
  viral disease, 2:1039, 1041, 1042
  viral meningitis, 2:608
  West Nile virus, 2:1057, 1059, 1060, 1061
  zoonoses, 2:1107
Encephalitizoon species. *See* Microsporidiosis
Encephalomyelitis, 1:91, 92
Encroachment, human. *See* Human encroachment into wildlife areas
End TB Strategy, WHO, 2:986
Endangered and threatened species, 2:697–698
Endemic typhus, 2:997, 998, 999
Endemicity, 1:**320–323**
  Buruli ulcer, 1:147, 149–150
  Chagas disease, 1:171, 172, *172,* 173
  chikungunya, 1:180, 181, 182
  cholera, 1:198, 199, 200
  climate change and parasitic diseases, 2:756
  coccidioidomycosis, 1:218, 220, 221
  Crimean-Congo hemorrhagic fever, 1:244, 245
  cyclosporiasis, 1:259

demographics, 1:262
dengue and dengue hemorrhagic fever, 1:267, 268
diphtheria, 1:276, 277
dracunculiasis, 1:285
dysentery, 1:292
Eastern equine encephalitis, 1:297
epidemiology, 1:332
filariasis, 1:350, 351
glanders, 1:*379*
globalization, 1:384
histoplasmosis, 1:449, *449*
immigration, 1:474
Japanese encephalitis, 1:512, 513
leishmaniasis, 1:538, 541
leprosy, 1:546
Lyme disease, 1:572
malaria, 2:579, 580, 581
Marburg hemorrhagic fever, 2:586
monkeypox, 2:627
mycotic disease, 2:651, 652
Nipah virus infection, 2:662, 664
plague, 2:715, 718, 719
polio, 2:732, 733, 737–738, 740, 1078
Powassan virus, 2:743
protozoan diseases, 2:755
puerperal fever, 2:768
re-emerging infectious diseases, 2:790, 792
rickettsial disease, 2:810, 811
Rift Valley fever, 2:813, 814
river blindness, 2:821
schistosomiasis, 2:860, 861, 862
severe fever with thrombocytopenia syndrome, 2:873
strongyloidiasis, 2:929, *930*
taeniasis, 2:*942*
talaromycosis, 2:945
tapeworm infections, 2:950
trachoma, 2:967
trichinellosis, 2:974
tropical infectious diseases, 2:982
tularemia, 2:989, 990, 991
typhoid fever, 2:993, 994
whipworm, 2:1064
WHO childhood vaccination recommendations, 1:185
yaws, 2:1088, 1089
yellow fever, 2:1092
Enders, John F., 2:736, 739
Endocarditis
bacterial meningitis, 2:604–605
brucellosis, 1:142
gonorrhea, 1:388
hand, foot, and mouth disease, 1:398–399
psittacosis, 2:759
Q fever, 2:772
rat-bite fever, 2:786
Staphylococcus aureus infections, 2:912
vancomycin-resistant *Enterococci*, 2:1025
Endocytosis, 2:1039
Endoscopy, 1:45
End-stage renal disease, 1:428*s*
Energix-B, 1:155*s*
Enfuvirtide, 1:13
Engels, Dirk, 2:1064
England. *See* United Kingdom
Ennals, David, 1:*110*
Enrofloxacin ban, 2:803
Entacyl. *See* Piperazine
Entamoeba histolytica infection. *See* Amebiasis
Enteric fever. *See* Typhoid fever
Enterobius vermicularis. See Pinworm infection
Enterococcus infections. *See* Vancomycin-resistant *Enterococci*
Enterotoxin type B, 2:1018
Enterovirus 71 infection, 1:**324–327,** *325, 326*
hand, foot, and mouth disease, 1:397, 398–399
meningitis, 2:607
Enteroviruses
hand, foot, and mouth disease, 1:397–399
meningitis, 2:607, 609
polio, 2:736–740
viral meningitis, 2:610
Environmental concerns
antibiotics, 1:64
antimicrobial soaps, 1:68
burkholderia, benefits of, 1:146
Chagas disease, 1:174
climate change and parasites, 2:697–698
DDT, 1:165
Eastern equine encephalitis prevention, 1:298
insecticide use, 1:76
integrated mosquito management practices, 2:639
lung fluke eradication, 1:568
mosquito-borne diseases, 2:638*s*
parasitic disease prevention, 2:696
plague, 2:711
sanitation, 2:846
West Nile virus prevention, 2:1061
wildlife, 2:1085
world trade, 2:1081–1082, 1083
zoonoses, 2:1107
Environmental health risks, 2:1077
Environmental infection control measures, 1:237, 2:909–910
Environmental Protection Agency (EPA)
antimicrobial resistance, 1:256*s*
cryptosporidiosis prevention, 1:252–253
disinfection byproducts, 1:282
microsporidiosis, 2:624
mosquito-borne disease prevention, 2:639
yersiniosis, 2:1098
Environmental Science and Technology, 1:68
Environmental transmission of AIDS, 1:9
Enzootic transmission, 2:1034, 1035, 1101
Enzyme-linked immunosorbent assay (ELISA), 1:244–245
Enzymes and antiviral drugs, 1:70, 72
Eosinophilia and ascariasis, 1:79
Eosinophilic meningitis, 1:35, 36
Eosinophils and lung flukes, 1:567
EPA. *See* Environmental Protection Agency (EPA)
Epic of Gilgamesh, 2:710
Epidemic and Pandemic Alert and Response Initiative, WHO, 1:314
Epidemic arthritic erythema. *See* Rat-bite fever
Epidemic cholera. *See* Cholera
Epidemic typhus
rickettsial disease, 2:809, 810, 811
typhus types, 2:997, 999, 1000, 1001
Epidemics
African sleeping sickness, 1:1, 3
AIDS, 1:14
among livestock, 1:39
arthropod-borne diseases, 1:75
bovine spongiform encephalopathy, 1:137, 138–139
cholera, 1:199, 200, 201
Clostridium difficile infection, 1:211–213
cohorted communities, 1:225
demographics, 1:261, 263–264
diphtheria, 1:277–278
endemicity, 1:320, 322
enterovirus 71 infection, 1:325
epidemiology, 1:331
group A streptococcal infections, 2:922
Haemophilus influenzae, 1:394
hand, foot, and mouth disease, 1:398
hepatitis A, 1:422, 423
immigration, 1:473
influenza, 1:488, 489, 504
kuru, 1:522, 523
legislation and international law, 1:535
Médecins Sans Frontières, 2:601
mosquito-borne diseases, 2:637
plague, 2:709–714, 717
polio, 2:732, 736
prion disease, 2:750
public health, 2:765
puerperal fever, 2:767
Q fever, 2:773

Rift Valley fever, 2:814–815, 816
rubella, 2:836, 837
typhus, 2:998–999, 1000, 1001
vaccines and vaccine development, 2:1022
viral disease, 2:1041
virus hunters, 2:1045
war, 2:1047
weather's relationship to, 1:203–204
whooping cough, 2:1067, 1069
Zika virus, 2:1102, 1108
zoonoses, 2:1106
Epidemiologic Surveillance Project, 2:679
Epidemiology, 1:**328–334,** *329*
germ theory of disease, 1:369
GIDEON, 1:375
influenza, 1:503–507
influenza pandemic of 1918, 2:1047
liver fluke infections, 1:563–564
Médecins Sans Frontières, 2:600, 602
notifiable diseases, 2:678–681
outbreaks, field-level response to, 2:685–688
SARS, 2:847–849, 849*s*
trachoma, 2:968*s*
Epidemiology and Disease Control Program, 1:260
Epidemiology and Toxicology Institute, 1:107
Epididymitis, 1:388, 2:877, 976
Epiglottitis, 1:394
Epilepsy and tapeworm infections, 2:950
Epinephrine, 2:590, 958
Epizootic transmission, 1:39, 2:1034, 1035
Epstein, Anthony, 1:154
Epstein, Michael, 1:335, 2:631
Epstein-Barr virus, 1:**335–337,** *336, 336t*
antiviral drugs, 1:72
cancer, 1:154–156, 155
mononucleosis, 2:630–633, 634
Equine encephalitis viruses
Eastern equine encephalitis, 1:296–298
encephalitis, 1:317
Venezuelan equine encephalitis virus, 1:317, 2:1033–1036
Western equine encephalitis, 1:317, 2:1029, 1033
Equine rabies immunoglobulin, 2:777
Equipment, protective. *See* Personal protective equipment
Eradication
childhood-associated infectious diseases, 1:184–185, 187
dracunculiasis, 1:284*s*
endemic diseases, 1:320, 321
filariasis, 1:350, 352
leprosy, 1:543, 546
measles, 2:597
microorganisms, 2:617
mosquito-borne diseases, 2:637
polio, 2:732–734, 736, 737
rabies eradication, 2:777–778
re-emerging infectious diseases, 2:789
river blindness, 2:822
smallpox, 2:738, 890, 896–899, *898*
taeniasis, 2:943
trachoma, 2:968*s*
vaccines, 2:1021, 1023
World Health Organization, 2:1077–1078
yaws, 2:1088–1090
Eriocheir sinensis, 1:567–568
Erythema infectiosum. *See* Fifth disease
Erythema migrans rash, 1:569, 570, 572, 573
Erythromycin
diphtheria, 1:276
necrotizing fasciitis, 2:659
nocardiosis, 2:668
nosocomial infections, 2:674
psittacosis, 2:760
rat-bite fever, 2:786
relapsing fever, 2:796, 797
scarlet fever, 2:857
trachoma, 2:968
whooping cough, 2:1068
Eschars, typhus, 2:997
Escherichia coli infection, 1:*61*
antibacterial drug issues, 1:59
antibiotic resistance, 1:62
anti-cytokine antibody syndrome, 1:53
antimicrobial soap overuse, 1:67
bacterial diseases, 1:99–100
Chipotle Mexican Grill restaurants, 2:671, 672
culture and sensitivity, 1:256
O157:H7, 1:338–341
resistant organisms, 2:800
Escherichia coli O157:H7, 1:**338–341,** *339*
animal vaccine, 1:302
bacterial diseases, 1:99–100
emerging infectious diseases, 1:311–312
food-borne disease, 1:355–356
gastroenteritis, 1:359
microbial evolution, 2:614
vaccine use for *Salmonella* infection, 2:842
Eskazole. *See* Albendazole
Esomeprazole, 1:411
Esophageal cancer, 1:411–412
Esophagus, enlargement of the, 1:173
Essential medicines, 1:270–272, 2:600–601
Estonia, 1:277, 405
Estrogen, 2:1074
Ethical issues
Asilomar Conference, 1:81–82
human research subjects, 1:344
Koch's postulates, 1:520
leprosy patients, treatment of, 1:546
polio vaccine, 2:739
self-experimentation by scientists, 1:345
Tuskegee syphilis study, 2:937–938, 939
women's reproductive rights in Latin America, 1:76
Ethiopia
African sleeping sickness, 1:*3*
child marriage, 1:15, 2:1005
cholera, 1:199
dracunculiasis, 1:283, 285
immigration, 1:474
leishmaniasis, 1:539
leprosy, 1:546
relapsing fever, 2:796
sanitation, 2:845
trachoma, 2:*968*
Ethnic cleansing, 1:263
Ethylene oxide sterilization, 2:915
Europe
AIDS history, 1:18
alveolar echinococcosis, 1:24
anellovirus, 1:30
animal importation, 1:39, 40
anisakiasis, 1:43, 45
anthrax, 1:47, 50
antimicrobial soap substances, 1:66
arthropod-borne diseases, 1:75
avian influenza, 1:88
babesiosis, 1:95, 96
biosafety level 4 laboratories, 1:421
blood supply and transfusions, 1:125
bloodborne infections transmitted through barber shops, 1:131*s*
bovine spongiform encephalopathy, 1:137, 138, 242
British beef ban, 1:138
candidiasis, 1:160
chikungunya, 1:181, 2:614
Clostridium difficile infection, 1:211, 212
colds, 1:228
cryptosporidiosis, 1:251
diphtheria, 1:277
dysentery, 1:290
extreme weather events, 1:204
glanders, 1:380
hantavirus, 1:404, 405
health care provider handwashing compliance, 2:642
hepatitis A, 1:424
hepatitis C, 1:431
hepatitis D, 1:435

H5N1, 1:496
influenza pandemic of 1918, 2:1048
legislation and international law, 1:533–534
leprosy, 1:544
lice infestation, 1:554
liver fluke infections, 1:561
Lyme disease, 1:571
malaria, 2:579
Médecins Sans Frontières, 2:602
microsporidiosis, 2:623
mosquito-borne diseases, 2:637
MRSA, 2:640
mumps, 2:647
necrotizing fasciitis, 2:659
norovirus infection, 2:670
pinworm infection, 2:705
plague, 2:711–712
Pneumocystis jirovecii pneumonia, 2:721
polio, 2:733, 734, 740
protozoan diseases, 2:755
rabies eradication, 2:778
re-emerging infectious diseases, 2:792
relapsing fever, 2:796
Rift Valley fever, 2:814
rotavirus, 2:830
SARS, 2:850
scarlet fever, 2:857
sex of animals used in research, 2:1074
smallpox, 2:891, 1020
syphilis, 2:936
taeniasis, 2:942
talaromycosis, 2:945
tapeworm infections, 2:949
tick-borne diseases, 2:957, 958
travel, 2:970
trichinellosis, 2:972, 974
tularemia, 2:990
typhus, 2:998, 999
typhus fever, 2:1048
UK beef ban, 1:241–242
vancomycin-resistant *Enterococci,* 2:1026
water-borne disease, 2:1055
West Nile virus, 2:1058, 1060
yersiniosis, 2:1097
Zika virus, 2:1101
zoonoses, 2:1106, 1107
European Centre for Disease Prevention and Control, 1:240, 2:647, 796
European Commission, 1:264
European Council, 1:264
European hares, 1:244
European Medicines Agency, 1:361, 2:893
European Nucleotide Archive, 1:363
European Parliament, 1:264
European Union
antimicrobial soap substances ban, 1:67
Biosafety level 4 facilities, 1:246
demographics and infections disease, 1:263–264
nontherapeutic antibiotic use in agriculture, 1:64, 2:1027
rubella, 2:836
trichinellosis, 2:973, 974
triclosan ban, 2:916
yersiniosis, 2:1097
Eustachian tube blockage, 1:293, 294
Euthanasia and Venezuelan equine encephalitis, 2:1035
Evang, Karl, 2:1076
Evolution
antibacterial resistance, 2:745
microbial evolution, 2:611–614
resistant organisms, 2:801, 803
Excerpt from Global Sepsis Alliance Press Release, *2:869–870*
Exclusion policies
fifth disease, 1:348*s*
hand, foot, and mouth disease, 1:398*s*
pandemic preparedness, 2:692
Executive Board, WHO, 2:899
Executive Order 13295, 1:509, 535, 2:850–851
Executive Order-Combating Antibiotic Resistant Bacteria, 2:*746*
Exhaustion, 1:122, 2:626
Exopolysaccharide coatings, 1:465
Exotic animal trade, 1:40, 2:761, 1083–1084
Expanded Program on Immunization (WHO), 1:185
Explosive diarrhea and water-borne disease, 2:1054
Exposed: scientists who risked disease for discovery, 1:**342–346**
Extended-wear contact lenses, 1:233
External ear, 2:932*s*
Extrapulmonary tuberculosis, 2:865–867, 983–984
Extreme weather
climate change, 1:204–207
leptospirosis, 1:550
protozoan diseases, 2:757
See also Natural disasters
Extremely drug-resistant tuberculosis
airborne precautions, 1:23
bacterial diseases, 1:101
emerging infectious diseases, 1:313
immigration, 1:474
notifiable diseases, 2:678
re-emerging infectious diseases, 2:791–792
tuberculosis types, 2:986
Eye and vision disorders
AIDS, 1:12
antiviral drugs, 1:72
aspergillosis, 1:85
bacterial meningitis, 2:608
bacterial sinusitis, 1:229
Baylisascaris infection, 1:105, 107
cat scratch disease, 1:161–163, 162
Chagas disease, 1:172
Chlamydia infection, 1:189, 190, 191
CMV infection, 1:214, 216
congenital Zika syndrome, 2:1101
contact lenses and *Fusarium* keratitis, 1:232–233
Crimean-Congo hemorrhagic fever, 1:244
Cryptococcus neoformans infection, 1:248
dengue and dengue hemorrhagic fever, 1:267
developing nations and drug delivery, 1:270
dracunculiasis, 1:283
eye cancer, 1:155
fifth disease, 1:347
glanders, 1:379
gonorrhea, 1:388
herpes gladiatorum, 1:442*s*
histoplasmosis, 1:451
Japanese encephalitis, 1:512
Kawasaki disease, 1:515
leprosy, 1:545
malaria, 1:50, 2:580
measles, 2:1009
microsporidiosis, 2:624*s*
opportunistic infections, 2:683
pink eye, 2:702–704
Rift Valley fever, 2:813
river blindness, 2:820–822
rubella, 2:836
shigellosis, 2:881
shingles, 2:886, 888
smallpox, 2:890
syphilis, 2:935
taeniasis, 2:943
toxoplasmosis, 2:964
trachoma, 2:967–969
trichinellosis, 2:973
viral disease, 2:1039
Zika virus, 2:1103

F

Facial issues
bile duct blockage, 1:560–561
Lassa fever, 1:526
Lyme disease, 1:569
relapsing fever, 2:795
trichinellosis, 2:973
yaws, 2:1087
Factor VIII, 1:126
Factory farming, 2:611, *612,* 750
Fainting and toxic shock, 2:961
Falciparum, 1:473
Falkland Islands, 1:242
Fallah, Mosoka P., 1:308

Falsified medical products, 1:272
Famciclovir, 1:365, 445, 2:886
Familial Creutzfeldt-Jakob disease, 2:748, 749
Familial fatal insomnia, 2:749
Famine, 2:997–1001
Famine fever. *See* Typhus
Famotidine, 1:411
Farr, William, 1:328
Fascioliasis. *See* Liver fluke infections
Fatalities. *See* Deaths
Fatigue
- African sleeping sickness, 1:5
- AIDS, 1:12
- aspergillosis, 1:85
- babesiosis, 1:95, 96
- *Baylisascaris* infection, 1:105
- blastomycosis, 1:123
- brucellosis, 1:141
- cat scratch disease, 1:162*s*
- Chagas disease, 1:172
- chickenpox, 1:176
- chikungunya, 1:182
- CMV infection, 1:214
- coccidioidomycosis, 1:218
- colds, 1:228
- cryptosporidiosis, 1:252
- cyclosporiasis, 1:259
- Ebola, 1:302
- encephalitis, 1:317
- enterovirus 71 infection, 1:325
- Epstein-Barr virus, 1:337
- helminth disease, 1:415
- hemorrhagic fevers, 1:419
- hepatitis B, 1:426
- hepatitis E, 1:437
- HIV, 1:11
- hookworm infection, 1:458
- Legionnaires' disease, 1:530
- lice infestation, 1:552
- liver fluke infections, 1:560
- Lyme disease, 1:569, 570, 573
- monkeypox, 2:628*s*
- mononucleosis, 1:223, 2:630, 631, 632
- necrotizing fasciitis, 2:659, 660
- pneumonia, 2:726
- polio, 2:736, 737
- post-treatment Lyme disease syndrome, 1:571
- protozoan diseases, 2:753
- rickettsial disease, 2:809
- sexually transmitted infections, 2:877
- syphilis, 2:935
- talaromycosis, 2:944
- tick-borne diseases, 2:956, 957
- toxoplasmosis, 2:964
- trichinellosis, 2:973
- tuberculosis, 2:983
- vector-borne disease, 2:1029
- Venezuelan equine encephalitis virus, 2:1033
- water-borne disease, 2:1054
- Zika virus, 2:1101

Favipiravir, 2:872
FBI. *See* U.S. Federal Bureau of Investigation
FDA. *See* U.S. Food and Drug Administration
"FDA Issues Final Rule on Safety and Effectiveness of Antibacterial Soaps," 1:*68–69*
Febrile seizures, 1:187
Fecal transplants, 1:211
Fecal-oral route
- alveolar echinococcosis, 1:24
- amebiasis, 1:27–28, 29
- ascariasis, 1:79
- balantidiasis, 1:102
- *Baylisascaris* infection, 1:107
- *Clostridium difficile* infection, 1:210
- cryptosporidiosis, 1:250–251
- cyclosporiasis, 1:258, 260
- dysentery, 1:289
- enterovirus 71 infection, 1:325
- *Escherichia coli* O157:H7, 1:339
- giardiasis, 1:371, 372
- hepatitis A, 1:422, 423
- hepatitis E, 1:437
- infection control and asepsis, 1:485
- norovirus infection, 2:669
- parasitic diseases, 2:694
- polio, 2:737
- rotavirus infection, 2:829
- shigellosis, 2:880–881
- viral meningitis, 2:609
- yersiniosis, 2:1096, 1097

Federal Register, 1:111*s*
Federation of American Scientists, 2:898
Female condoms, 1:14
Ferret badgers, 2:1083
Ferrets, 1:393
Fertilizers, 2:757
Fetal development and maternal infections. *See* Maternal-to-fetal/child transmission
Fever
- African sleeping sickness, 1:2, 5
- AIDS, 1:12
- anellovirus, 1:30, 32–33
- angiostrongyliasis, 1:35
- arthropod-borne diseases, 1:75
- ascariasis, 1:79
- aspergillosis, 1:85
- avian influenza, 1:89
- B virus infection, 1:92
- babesiosis, 1:95, 96
- bacterial meningitis, 2:605, 606
- blastomycosis, 1:122, 123
- brucellosis, 1:141
- burkholderia, 1:145
- Buruli ulcer, 1:148
- *Campylobacter* infection, 1:151
- cat scratch disease, 1:161–163, 162*s*
- Chagas disease, 1:172
- chickenpox, 1:175, 176
- chikungunya, 1:*180,* 181, 182
- *Chlamydia pneumoniae,* 1:194
- *Clostridium difficile* infection, 1:210
- CMV infection, 1:214
- coccidioidomycosis, 1:218
- colds, 1:228
- Crimean-Congo hemorrhagic fever, 1:244
- cryptosporidiosis, 1:251
- cyclosporiasis, 1:259
- dengue and dengue hemorrhagic fever, 1:267
- diphtheria, 1:274–275
- dracunculiasis, 1:283
- dysentery, 1:289
- ear infections, 1:293
- Eastern equine encephalitis, 1:296
- Ebola, 1:302
- encephalitis, 1:316, 317
- enterovirus 71 infection, 1:325
- Epstein-Barr virus, 1:337
- *Escherichia coli* O157:H7, 1:340
- fifth disease, 1:347
- gastroenteritis, 1:359–360
- glanders, 1:379
- gonorrhea, 1:388, 389
- hand, foot, and mouth disease, 1:397, 398
- hantavirus, 1:404, 405
- heartland virus, 2:873*s*
- helminth disease, 1:415
- hemorrhagic fevers, 1:419, 420*s*
- hepatitis A, 1:422–425
- hepatitis C, 1:430
- hepatitis E, 1:437
- herpes gladiatorum, 1:442*s*
- herpes simplex virus 2, 1:444
- histoplasmosis, 1:448
- HIV, 1:11
- influenza, 1:488, 490, 504
- Kawasaki disease, 1:515
- Lassa fever, 1:526, 528
- Legionnaires' disease, 1:530
- leptospirosis, 1:548
- lice infestation, 1:552
- listeriosis, 1:556
- liver fluke infections, 1:560
- lung flukes, 1:566
- Lyme disease, 1:569, 571, 573
- macrophage activation syndrome, 2:575–576
- malaria, 2:579, 580, 581
- Marburg hemorrhagic fever, 2:586
- measles, 2:593
- meningitis, 2:606*s*
- monkeypox, 2:626, 628*s*
- mononucleosis, 1:223, 2:630, 631, 634, 635
- mumps, 2:645
- necrotizing fasciitis, 2:659, 660
- Nipah virus infection, 2:663

nocardiosis, 2:666
opportunistic infections, 2:682
plague, 1:116, 2:715
Pneumocystis jirovecii pneumonia, 2:722
pneumonia, 2:726, 729
polio, 2:736
Powassan virus, 2:741
protozoan diseases, 2:754
psittacosis, 2:759
puerperal fever, 2:767, 768
Q fever, 2:772
rat-bite fever, 2:785, 786, 787, 788
relapsing fever, 2:795
rickettsial disease, 2:809
Rift Valley fever, 2:813
Rocky Mountain spotted fever, 2:824, 826
rotavirus infection, 2:828
RSV infection, 2:832, 834
rubella, 2:837
Salmonella infection, 2:841
SARS, 2:850
scarlet fever, 2:857
schistosomiasis, 2:860, 861
scrofula, 2:866
severe fever with thrombocytopenia syndrome, 2:871
sexually transmitted infections, 2:876, 877
shigellosis, 2:880, 881
shingles, 1:176, 2:885, 886
smallpox, 2:891
St. Louis encephalitis, 2:905
strep throat, 2:917
strongyloidiasis, 2:929
syphilis, 2:935
talaromycosis, 2:944
tetanus, 2:953
tick-borne diseases, 2:956, 957
toxic shock, 2:961, 962
toxoplasmosis, 2:964
trichinellosis, 2:973
tuberculosis, 2:983
tularemia, 2:989, 990
typhoid fever, 2:993, 995, 995*s*
typhus, 2:997, 1001
urinary tract infection, 2:1012
vaccine reactions, 2:1022
Venezuelan equine encephalitis virus, 2:1033, 1035
viral meningitis, 2:608, 610
West Nile virus, 2:1058, 1059
yellow fever, 2:1092
yersiniosis, 2:1097
Zika virus, 2:1101, 1102
Fever blisters. *See* Cold sores
Fibrosis, 1:427
Fidaxomicin, 1:211
Field kits, 2:600
Field-based biosensors, 2:783*s*
Field-level response to outbreaks. *See* Outbreaks: field-level response
Fifth disease, 1:**347–349,** *348,* 2:1039
Filariasis, 1:**350–353,** *351*
helminth disease, 1:417
tropical infectious diseases, 2:980, 981, 981*s*
Filatov's disease. *See* Mononucleosis
Filgrastim, 1:114
Filipino people and coccidioidomycosis, 1:219
Filippo, Giovanni, 1:175
Filoviruses
animal importation, 1:41
Ebola, 1:300–304
hemorrhagic fevers, 1:419, 420
viral disease, 2:1041
virus hunters, 2:1045
Filtration. *See* Air filtration; Water filtration
Fimbriae, 1:339, 2:841
Financial issues. *See* Economic and financial issues; Funding and budgets
Finger loss and typhus, 2:998
Fingernails and herpes simplex 1 virus, 1:442
Finland
group B streptococcal infection, 2:926
yersiniosis, 2:1097
Finlay, Carlos, 1:343, 2:1043, 1093–1095
First International Sanitary Conference, 1:534
First responders. *See* Emergency response
Fischetti, Vincent, 2:659k
Fish
anisakiasis, 1:43–46
botulism, 1:135
cryptosporidiosis, 1:251
liver fluke infections, 1:561, 562
marine toxins, 2:589–592
tapeworm infections, 2:948
Fitzgerald, Brenda, 1:491
Flagella, 1:371, 570–571
Flanagan, Katie, 2:1074
Flanagan, Liam, 2:660
Flank pain, 2:1012
Flat smallpox, 2:892
Flatulence, 2:754, 929, 1062
Flatworms. *See* Flukes
Flaviviruses
dengue and dengue hemorrhagic fever, 1:266–268
hemorrhagic fevers, 1:419
hepatitis C, 1:430–432
Japanese encephalitis, 1:511–514
Powassan virus, 2:741–743
St. Louis encephalitis, 2:905–907
tropical infectious diseases, 2:980
vector-borne disease, 2:1029, 1030
viral disease, 2:1041
West Nile virus, 2:1057–1061
Zika virus, 2:1022–1023, 1100–1103
Fleas
arthropod-borne diseases, 1:75
bacterial disease, 1:100
cat scratch disease, 1:162*s,* 163
climate change, 2:698
hosts and vectors, 1:461, 463
parasitic diseases, 2:694
plague, 2:712, 713, 715–719
tapeworm infections, 2:948
typhus, 2:997, 998, 999
virus hunters, 2:1046
zoonoses, 2:1106
Fleming, Alexander, 1:57, 2:676
Flesh-eating bacteria. *See* Necrotizing fasciitis
Flies
arthropod-borne diseases, 1:75
dysentery, 1:289
hosts and vectors, 1:461
river blindness, 2:820, 821, 822
shigellosis, 2:880
tularemia, 2:990
Flint, Michigan, 2:882–883
Floods
cholera, 1:200, 201
climate change, 1:205
dengue and dengue hemorrhagic fever, 1:268
leptospirosis, 1:550
plague, 2:713
protozoan diseases, 2:757
Rift Valley fever, 2:813, 814–815, 816
Florida
AIDS, 1:8
arthropod-borne diseases, 1:75
Baylisascaris infection, 1:107
chikungunya, 1:182
climate change, 1:207
Eastern equine encephalitis, 1:298*s*
globalization and infectious disease, 1:385
HPV vaccination, 1:*469*
St. Louis encephalitis, 2:906
West Nile virus, 2:1060
yellow fever, 2:1093
Zika virus, 1:169, 2:1101
Fluconazole
candidiasis, 1:159, 160
coccidioidomycosis, 1:221
Cryptococcus neoformans infection, 1:248
ringworm, 2:818
sporotrichosis, 2:902
Flucytosine, 2:945
Fluid intake. *See* Hydration and rehydration
Fluid loss. *See* Dehydration
Flukes
helminth disease, 1:415
liver flukes, 1:560–564
lung flukes, 1:565–568

schistosomiasis, 2:860–863
See also Schistosomes
Flu-like symptoms
B virus infection, 1:91–92
blastomycosis, 1:122, 123–124
coccidioidomycosis, 1:218, 219, 221
dengue and dengue hemorrhagic fever, 1:267
Ebola, 1:302
Haemophilus influenzae, 1:395
herpes simplex virus 2, 1:444
histoplasmosis, 1:448
Lyme disease, 1:571, 572
mononucleosis, 2:631
plague, 2:715
Q fever, 2:772
rabies, 2:776
rat-bite fever, 2:785
Rift Valley fever, 2:813
SARS, 2:847, 850
smallpox, 2:890
tick-borne diseases, 2:956
toxic shock, 2:961
Venezuelan equine encephalitis virus, 2:1034
viral meningitis, 2:608
Zika virus, 2:1101
FluNet, 1:503
Fluorescence tests, 2:782
Fluorescent tests, 1:149
Fluoroquinolones
Chlamydia infection, 1:189–191
gastroenteritis, 1:360
gonorrhea, 1:389
overreliance on, 1:257
pneumonia, 2:718
Q fever, 2:773
rickettsial disease, 2:811
yersiniosis, 2:1097
Flupirtine, 1:241
Flushing, skin
Crimean-Congo hemorrhagic fever, 1:244
dengue and dengue hemorrhagic fever, 1:267
hantavirus, 1:404
malaria, 2:580
marine toxins, 2:590
Fluxid. *See* Famotidine
Foaming at the mouth, 2:775, 776
Foci of diseases, 1:320
Folinic acid, 2:755
Folliculitis, 1:465, *466*
Fomites
colds, 1:229
contact precautions, 1:235
diphtheria, 1:275
enterovirus 71 infection, 1:327
fifth disease, 1:348
gastroenteritis, 1:359
hand, foot, and mouth disease, 1:398
handwashing, 1:400
hepatitis C, 1:431
impetigo, 1:480
influenza, 1:488
lice, 1:552
Marburg hemorrhagic fever, 2:585
monkeypox, 2:626, 628
mononucleosis, 2:631
MRSA prevention, 2:642–643
mumps, 2:647
norovirus infection, 2:669
pink eye, 2:703
ringworm, 2:817
RSV infection, 2:833, 834
scabies, 2:854
scarlet fever, 2:857
scrofula, 2:866
smallpox, 2:892
strep throat, 2:917, 918*s*
trachoma, 2:967
vancomycin-resistant *Enterococci,* 2:1026
viral meningitis, 2:609
"Food Additive to Blame for C. difficile Epidemic," *1:211–213*
Food additives, 1:210, 211, 212–213
Food allergies after giardiasis, 1:373
Food and Agriculture Organization, UN, 2:778
Food chain, 2:590, 638*s*, 697
Food irradiation, 1:260, 356*s*
Food labeling, 1:357
Food packaging, smart, 1:153, 558
Food production. *See* Agriculture; Livestock
Food Safety News, 1:558, 2:672
Food-borne disease and food safety, **1:354–357,** *355*
alveolar echinococcosis, 1:24, 25*f*
angiostrongyliasis, 1:35–38
anisakiasis, 1:43–46
anthrax, 1:49
ascariasis, 1:80
bacterial diseases, 1:100
balantidiasis, 1:102–103
botulism, 1:133, 135
bovine spongiform encephalopathy, 1:136
brucellosis, 1:142*s*
Campylobacter infection, 1:151–153
CDC, 1:166
Chagas disease, 1:173
cholera, 1:197–201
climate change and protozoan diseases, 2:757
Crimean-Congo hemorrhagic fever, 1:243
cryptosporidiosis, 1:250, 251, 252, 253
cyclosporiasis, 1:258–260
dysentery, 1:289, 291
Escherichia coli O157:H7, 1:338–341
gastroenteritis, 1:359
globalization, 1:384
hantavirus, 1:404
helminth disease, 1:415, 416
hepatitis A, 1:422, 423, 424, 425
hepatitis E, 1:437–439
H5N1 virus, 1:392*s*
infection control and asepsis, 1:485
leptospirosis, 1:548, 550
listeriosis, 1:556–558
liver fluke infections, 1:560–564
lung flukes, 1:565–568
marine toxins, 2:589–592
microsporidiosis, 2:622
Nipah virus infection, 2:663–664
norovirus infection, 2:669–672
parasitic diseases, 2:694, 695
pinworm infection, 2:705
prion disease, 2:749, 750
protozoan diseases, 2:754, 755
public health, 2:766
resistant organisms, 2:801
Salmonella infection, 2:840–842
sanitation, 2:845–846
SARS, 2:847
SEB intoxication, 2:1052
shellfish poisoning, 2:1054
shigellosis, 2:880–883
Staphylococcus aureus infections, 2:911, 912
taeniasis, 2:940–943
tapeworm infections, 2:948–950
toxoplasmosis, 2:964, 966
trichinellosis, 2:972–974, 973*s*
tularemia, 2:989, 990, 991
typhoid fever, 2:993
whipworm, 2:1062
yersiniosis, 2:1096–1099
zoonoses, 2:1106, 1107
Foodborne Diseases Active Surveillance Network, 2:1097, 1098
FoodNet, 2:1097, 1098
Food-service and restaurants, 1:11, 2:671
Foot and mouth disease. *See* Hand, foot, and mouth disease
Foot issues
hand, foot, and mouth disease, 1:397
Kawasaki disease, 1:515–516
rat-bite fever, 2:785
toxic shock, 2:961
Footwear and strongyloidiasis, 2:929
Fore people, 1:138*s*, 522, 523–525, 2:749
Forests. *See* Deforestation; Wooded areas and forests
Formaldehyde, 1:281
Former Soviet Union
diphtheria, 1:274, 276, 277–278
liver fluke infections, 1:561
war, 2:1050

Fort Collins, CO, 1:166
Fort Detrick, MD, 2:893, 1016
Forward to *World Malaria Report,* 2:*582–583*
Fosamprenavir, 1:13
Foscarnet, 1:215, 318
Fosfomycin, 2:1013, 1014
Fossil fuels, burning of, 1:204
Four Corners region, 1:407
Fournier, Jean Alfred, 2:657
Fournier gangrene, 2:658
Foxes
  alveolar echinococcosis, 1:24, 25, 25*f*
  leishmaniasis, 1:539
  Powassan virus, 2:741
  rabies, 2:776
  wildlife trade, 2:1083
France
  AIDS pandemic history, 1:19
  avian influenza, 1:89
  bovine spongiform encephalopathy, 1:137
  British beef ban, 1:138
  chikungunya, 1:181
  Creutzfeldt-Jakob disease, 1:242
  enterovirus 71 infection, 1:325
  influenza pandemic of 1918, 2:1048
  legislation and international law, 1:534
  lice infestation, 1:554
  plague, early history of, 2:711
  rabies eradication, 2:778
  scrofula, 2:865
  trichinellosis, 2:974
  vancomycin-resistant *Enterococci,* 2:1026
Francisella tularensis. See Tularemia
Franco, Tania, 2:1102
Frank, Anne, 2:999
French Polynesia
  angiostrongyliasis, 1:38
  arthropod-borne diseases, 1:75–76
  viral disease, 2:1042
  Zika virus, 2:1101
Frequency, disease, 1:330
Friction and handwashing, 1:401
Frieden, Tom, 2:1027
Friedrich, Richard, 1:394
Frontiers in Cellular and Infection Microbiology, 1:245–246
Frosch, Paul, 2:1043
Fruit bats, 2:*587*
  Ebola, 1:301, 304
  hemorrhagic fevers, 1:420*s*
  Marburg hemorrhagic fever, 2:586
  Nipah virus infection, 2:662–663, 664
Fulminant hepatitis E, 1:437
Fumagillin, 2:624
Fume hoods, 1:486
Fumigation. *See* Spraying programs
Funding and budgets
  African sleeping sickness research, 1:4
  AIDS prevention, 1:14
  biodefense research and development, 1:118
  bioterrorism preparedness, 2:1051*s*
  CDC, 1:164
  developing nations and drug delivery, 1:271
  Syrian refugee health outreach, 1:264–265
  UNICEF, 2:1004
  United Nations Millennium Goals, 2:1009
  vaccine development, 2:1023
  yaws research, 2:1090
  See also Economic and financial issues
Funeral customs. *See* Burial and mourning customs
Fungal disease. *See* Mycotic disease
Fungisome. *See* Amphotericin B
Furious rabies, 2:776
Fusarium keratitis, contact lenses and. *See* Contact lenses and *Fusarium* keratitis
Fusion inhibitors, 1:13

G

Gabon, 1:41, 301, 302, 304
Gain of function approach to vaccines, 1:82
Gajdusek, Carleton, 1:138*s,* 522, *523*
Galen, 1:387, 2:710
Galilei, Galileo, 2:618
Gallo, Robert, 2:806*s*
Gambia, 2:968*s,* 1074
Gambian rats, 2:627
Gametocytes, 2:580
Gamgee, John, 1:39
Gamma globulin, 1:515
Gammatorquevirus, 1:30
Ganciclovir, 1:72, 215, 318
Gangrene
  necrotizing fasciitis, 2:657, 658, 659
  plague, 2:715
  rickettsial disease, 2:810
  Rocky Mountain spotted fever, 2:825
  tetanus, 2:952
  typhus, 2:997
  war, 2:1050
Gaol fever. *See* Typhus
Gardasil
  cancer, 1:155*s*
  HPV, 1:469
  sexually transmitted infections, 2:878
  vaccines for infectious diseases that lead to cancer, 1:156
Gas, intestinal. *See* Intestinal gas
Gastric cancer. *See* Stomach cancer
Gastritis and *Helicobacter pylori,* 1:344, 409, 411
Gastroenteritis, 1:**358–361,** *360*
  Escherichia coli O157:H7, 1:338–341
  norovirus infection, 2:669–672, 670
  rotavirus infection, 1:186, 2:828–831
  viral disease, 2:1039, 1041
Gastrointestinal diseases or symptoms
  angiostrongyliasis, 1:35
  anthrax, 1:115
  bacterial diseases, 1:100
  Baylisascaris infection, 1:105–108
  Chagas disease, 1:173
  cholera, 1:197–201
  CMV infection, 1:214
  cohorted communities, 1:223, 224
  cryptosporidiosis, 1:250–253
  cyclosporiasis, 1:258–260
  dysentery, 1:289–292
  enterovirus 71 infection, 1:324–327
  Escherichia coli O157:H7, 1:338–341
  food-borne disease, 1:354–357
  gastroenteritis, 1:358–361
  hantavirus, 1:405
  Helicobacter pylori, 1:409–412
  intra-abdominal infections, 1:59
  macrophage activation syndrome, 2:575
  marine toxins, 2:591
  opportunistic infections, 2:683
  pinworm infection, 2:705
  rat-bite fever, 2:785
  Rocky Mountain spotted fever, 2:824
  rotavirus infection, 2:828–831
  Salmonella infection, 2:840–842
  schistosomiasis, 2:861
  shigellosis, 2:880–883
  sporotrichosis, 2:901
  strongyloidiasis, 2:929
  taeniasis, 2:941
  trichinellosis, 2:972, 973
  viral disease, 2:1039
  war, 2:1049
  water-borne disease, 2:1054
  whipworm, 2:1062
  yersiniosis, 2:1096–1099

Gates Foundation. *See* Bill & Melinda Gates Foundation
GAVI. *See* Global Alliance for Vaccines and Immunization
Gay men. *See* Men who have sex with men
Geese and schistosomes, 2:931
Gelsinger, Jesse, 2:808
GenBank, 1:363, 364, 2:713
Gender
  African sleeping sickness deaths, 1:4
  ascariasis, 1:80
  blastomycosis, 1:122
  brucellosis, 1:141–142
  HPV, 1:470–471
  Kawasaki disease, 1:517
  nocardiosis, 2:667
  river blindness, 2:821
  Rocky Mountain spotted fever, 2:825
  sporotrichosis, 2:903
  trichomoniasis, 2:975
  tularemia, 2:991
  women and infectious disease, 2:1071–1074
Gene sequencing
  genetic identification of microorganisms, 1:363–364
  microbial evolution, 2:613–614
  plague, 2:713–714
  re-emerging infectious disease research, 2:792
  Rocky Mountain Laboratory, 2:656
  SARS, 2:849–850
Gene therapy and retroviruses, 2:808
"General Bioterrorism and Military Health Risks" (Brundtland), 1:114–115
"General Ecological Models for Human Subsistence, Health and Poverty," 1:309
Genesee County, MO, 2:883
Genesee County Health Department, 2:883
Genetic engineering
  alpha interferon, 1:14
  Ebola vaccine, 1:304
  edible vaccines, 1:82*s*
  hepatitis B vaccine, 1:428
  Japanese encephalitis vaccine, 1:514
  kuru research, 1:524
  malaria-resistant mosquitoes, 2:638
  microbial evolution, 2:613
  smallpox, 2:898, 899
  See also Bioengineering
Genetic identification of microorganisms, 1:**362–364**
  babesiosis, 1:96, 97
  CDC, 1:340*s*
  plague, 2:713–714
  Rocky Mountain Laboratory, 2:656
  SARS, 2:849–850
  typing, 1:256–257
Genetic testing
  amebiasis, 1:29
  gonorrhea, 1:389
  HIV, 1:12–13
  relapsing fever, 2:798
  strep throat, 2:919
Genetics and genetic research
  Advanced Diagnostics Program, 2:783*s*
  anellovirus, 1:30
  antibacterial drugs, 1:57, 58
  antibiotic drug development, 2:676
  antibiotic resistance, 1:62–63
  antiviral drugs, 1:71, 72
  Asilomar Conference, 1:81–82
  biodefense research and development, 1:118–119
  Buruli ulcer, 1:150
  Campylobacter infection, 1:153
  cancer, 1:155
  cryptosporidiosis, 1:252
  Ebola, 1:302, 303, 304
  edible vaccines, 1:82*s*
  emerging infectious disease research, 1:313
  Epstein-Barr virus, 1:335
  Escherichia coli O157:H7, 1:338
  group B streptococcal infection, 2:926–927
  Helicobacter pylori infection, 1:412
  HIV, 1:454
  influenza, 1:489
  influenza pandemic of 1918, 1:496
  Kawasaki disease, 1:515
  kuru, 1:524–525
  leprosy, 1:545, 546
  microbial evolution, 2:611–614
  microbial identification techniques, 1:256–257
  MRSA, 2:641
  plague, 2:713–714
  prion disease, 2:749
  rapid diagnostic tests, 2:781, 782, 783
  re-emerging infectious disease research, 2:792
  resistant organisms, 2:801, 802*s*
  retroviruses, 2:805, 806
  Rocky Mountain Laboratory, 2:656
  RSV, 2:834
  smallpox, 2:896, 898, 899
  superbugs, 2:1027*s*
  tuberculosis vaccine research, 2:985
  USAMRIID, 2:1017
  vaccines and vaccine development, 2:1023
  vector-borne diseases, 2:1031
  Venezuelan equine encephalitis virus, 2:1035
  viral disease, 2:1037, 1038–1039
  West Nile virus, 2:1060
  women, 2:1074
  Zika virus, 2:1100
  zoonoses, 2:1107
Geneva, Switzerland, 2:604, 751, 1076
Genital candidiasis, 1:159
Genital herpes, 1:**365,** *365*
  AIDS susceptibility, 1:11
  sexually transmitted infections, 2:877
  See also Herpes simplex virus 2
Genital warts, 1:468, 469–470, 2:877–878
Genitals
  B virus infection, 1:92
  blastomycosis, 1:122
  Chlamydia infection, 1:189, 190
  filariasis, 1:350, 352
  herpes simplex 1 virus, 1:440, 441
  herpes simplex virus 2, 1:444, 446
  mycotic disease, 2:650
  syphilis, 2:934, 936
  viral disease, 2:1039
Genitourinary tract infection, 1:122
Genocide, 1:263
Gentamicin, 1:142, 2:718, 991
Geographic focality, 1:320
Geographic medicine, 1:375–377
Geographic Medicine and Health Promotion Branch, CDC, 1:385
George Institute, 2:869
Georgetown University, 1:117
Georgia (country), 1:277
Georgia (state)
  avian influenza, 1:89
  babesiosis, 1:96
  burkholderia, 1:145
  heartland virus, 2:873*s*
  illegal snails, 1:38
  influenza pandemic of 1918, 2:1048
Gerbils
  giardiasis vaccine, 1:373
  rat-bite fever, 2:785
  wildlife trade, 2:1083
Germ theory of disease, 1:**366–370**
  cholera, 1:200
  microorganisms, 2:615–616
  nosocomial infections, 2:674
  See also Koch's postulates
German measles. *See* Rubella
German Society for International Cooperation, 1:563
Germany
  anthrax, 1:48
  avian influenza, 1:89
  bovine spongiform encephalopathy, 1:137

chickenpox vaccine, 1:177
glanders, 1:381
hemorrhagic fevers, 1:420*s*
human research subjects, 1:344
leptospirosis, 1:550
Lyme disease, 1:570
Marburg hemorrhagic fever, 2:585
microscopes and microscopy, 2:619
plague, early history of, 2:711
relapsing fever, 2:796, 797–798
SARS, 2:849
war, 2:1049
yersiniosis, 2:1097
Gerstmann-Strauss-Scheinker syndrome, 2:749
"Get a Kit" program, 1:117
Get Ahead of Sepsis program (CDC), 1:168
Get Smart: Know When Antibiotics Work campaign, 2:803
Ghana
avian influenza, 1:89
Buruli ulcer, 1:149
child marriage, 2:1005
dracunculiasis, 1:283
malaria vaccine, 1:205, 2:581
trachoma, 2:968*s*
yaws, 2:1089, 1090
Ghoson, Joseph, 1:383
Giant African land snails, 1:38
Giant intestinal roundworm. *See* Ascariasis
Giard, Alfred, 1:371
Giardiasis, 1:**371–374,** *373*
opportunistic infections, 2:683
protozoan diseases, 2:754
water-borne disease, 2:1054
GIDEON, 1:**375–377,** 2:1063
"GIDEON: A World Wide Web-Based Program for Diagnosis and Informatics in Infectious Diseases," 1:*376–377*
Giemsa stain, 2:620
Giese, Jeanna, 2:778
Gigantobilharzia, 2:931
Gilbert, Charles E., 1:107–108
Gilchrist, Thomas, 1:121–122
Gilchrist's mycosis. *See* Blastomycosis
Gilead, 1:541
Gingivostomatitis, 1:92, 441
Gipson, John L., 2:634
Girls
child marriage, 1:15, 2:1005–1006
measles vaccine clinical trials, 2:1073
whipworm, 2:1064
Gland swelling or pain
CMV infection, 1:214
fifth disease, 1:347
glanders, 1:379
mononucleosis, 2:630, 634
rubella, 2:837
scarlet fever, 2:856
sexually transmitted infections, 2:877
strep throat, 2:917
tularemia, 2:990
typhus, 2:997
Glanders, 1:144, 145, 146, **378–382,** *379*
Glandular fever. *See* Mononucleosis
Glaucoma and leprosy, 1:545
GlaxoSmithKline, 1:424–425
Global Action Plan for the Prevention and Control of Pneumonia and Diarrhoea, 2:730
Global Alliance for Rabies Control, 2:778–779
Global Alliance for the Elimination of Leprosy, 1:547
Global Alliance for Vaccines and Immunization
Haemophilus influenzae, 1:396
rotavirus, 1:361, 2:831
UNICEF, 2:1005
Zika virus, 1:169
Global Burden of Disease Study, 2:756
Global Buruli Ulcer Initiative, 1:149, 150
Global Capacities Alert and Response team, WHO, 2:688
Global Coalition Against Child Pneumonia, 2:730
Global disparities in AIDS deaths, 1:14
Global Foodborne Infections Network, 2:842
Global Fund to Fight AIDS, Tuberculosis and Malaria, 1:312, 2:981*s,* 1009
Global Health Sector Strategy on STIs, 2:879
Global Health Sector Strategy on Viral Hepatitis, 1:435
Global Heart, 2:920
Global Infectious Diseases and Epidemiology Online Network. *See* GIDEON
Global Influenza Surveillance and Response System, 1:393, 496, 503
Global Leprosy Strategy, 1:547, 2:1078
Global Measles and Rubella Strategic Plan, 2:838
Global Movement for Children, 2:1003–1004, 1004–1005
Global Outbreak Alert and Response Network, 2:686, 1077
Global Polio Eradication Initiative, 1:73, 2:732–734, 734*s,* 736–737, 740, 1077–1078
Global Programme to Eliminate Lymphatic Filariasis, 1:351, 352
Global Public Health Intelligence Network, 2:1077
Global Salm-Surv program, 2:842
Global Sepsis Alliance, 2:868
Global Strategic Framework for Integrated Vector Management, 1:463
Global Task Force on Cholera Control, 1:200
Global Trachoma Mapping Project, 2:969
Global warming. *See* Climate change
Globalization, 1:**383–386**
food-borne disease, 1:260
isolation and quarantine, 1:509–510
legislation and international law, 1:535
world trade, 2:1081–1083
Globe and Mail, 2:887
Glomerulonephritis, 2:920, 921
Gloves. *See* Clothing, protective; Personal protective equipment
Glutaraldehyde, 1:281–282
Glycoproteins, 1:304, 392, 454
Goa, India, 1:199
GOARN. *See* Global Outbreak Alert and Response Network
Goats
brucellosis, 1:140
burkholderia, 1:145
Crimean-Congo hemorrhagic fever, 1:244
glanders, 1:378
Q fever, 2:771–773
Venezuelan equine encephalitis virus, 2:1033
zoonoses, 2:1106
GoFundMe, 2:660
Gold and RSV vaccine, 2:834–835
Goldhammer, Gold, 1:171–172
Gonococcal Isolate Surveillance Project, 1:389
Gonorrhea, 1:**387–390,** *388*
sexually transmitted infections, 2:877, 878, 879
urinary tract infection, 2:1013
Gorakhpus, India, 1:*315*
Gorfinkel, Iris, 2:888
Gorgas, William C., 1:322*s,* 2:1095
Gorillas, 1:304, 552, 2:1085
Gottlieb, Michael S., 1:19*s*
Gowon, Yakubu, 1:417
GPHIN. *See* Global Public Health Intelligence Network
Graham, Barney S., 2:1023
Gram, Hans Christian, 1:254, 255–256
Gram stains
culture and sensitivity, 1:255–256, 257
microscopes and microscopy, 2:619
microsporidiosis, 2:624
Gram-negative bacteria
antibacterial drugs, 1:58
antibiotic resistance, 1:62, 63
cholera, 1:197

culture and sensitivity, 1:255, 256
Escherichia coli O157:H7, 1:338
meningitis, 2:605
microscopes and microscopy, 2:619
plague, 2:715
pneumonia, 2:728
Q fever, 2:771, 1051
Salmonella infection, 2:840
typhus, 2:997
whooping cough, 2:1066
Gram-positive bacteria
antibacterial drugs, 1:58
antibiotic resistance, 1:61–62
culture and sensitive, 1:255–256
diphtheria, 1:274
group A streptococcal infections, 2:921
group B streptococcal infections, 2:925
meningitis, 2:605
microscopes and microscopy, 2:619
necrotizing fasciitis, 2:658
Staphylococcus aureus infections, 2:911
Grant, James Augustus, 1:147
Granular conjunctivitis. *See* Trachoma
Granulocyte-macrophage colony-stimulating factor, 1:53, 54
Granulocytic ehrlichiosis, 1:571
Granulomatous vasculitis, 1:123
Graunt, John, 1:328
Gray, Fred, 2:938
Great Fire of London, 2:712
Great Lakes region
blastomycosis, 1:122
Eastern equine encephalitis, 1:297
encephalitis, 1:316
mitten crabs, 1:567
Powassan virus, 2:742
Greater Involvement of People with TB, 2:987
Greece
avian influenza, 1:89
vancomycin-resistant *Enterococci,* 2:1026
Greece, ancient
animal importation, 1:39
brucellosis, 1:140
cholera, 1:199
glanders, 1:378–379
gonorrhea, 1:387
helminth disease, 1:414
influenza, 1:488
leprosy, 1:544
malaria, 2:579
mumps, 2:644
plague, 2:710
rabies, 2:775
scrofula, 2:865
tuberculosis, 2:983
Greene, Jeremy A., 2:707
Greenhouse gases, 1:204, 205, 206
Greenland, 2:974
Gregg, Norman, 2:837
Griseofulvin, 2:818
Groopman, Jerome, 1:*70*
Gross, Ludwick, 2:1000
Grote, Alexandra, 1:352
Groundhogs (woodchucks), 2:741, 777
Group A streptococcal infections. *See* Streptococcal infections, group A
Group B streptococcal infections. *See* Streptococcal infections, group B
"Growing Burden of Tuberculosis," 2:791
Growth impairment, 1:80, 2:1062, 1064
Growth promotion, antibiotic use for, 1:64, 2:745–746
Guam, 1:36
Guananto virus, 1:418
Guangdong Province, China, 2:847, 849
Guangzhou, China, 2:1083, 1084
Guardian, 2:1107
Guatemala, 1:*259*
coccidioidomycosis, 1:220
river blindness, 2:821
Venezuelan equine encephalitis virus, 2:1034
Guerin, Camille, 2:985
Guideline for Isolation Precautions, 1:235–236
"Guidelines for Prevention of Herpesvirus Simiae (B Virus) Infection in Monkey Handlers" (CDC), 1:93
Guidelines Review committee, WHO, 2:1064
Guillain-Barré syndrome
botulism compared to, 1:134
with *Campylobacter* infection, 1:151–152
Epstein-Barr virus, 1:337
Zika virus, 2:1101
Guinea
Ebola, 1:302, 304, 2:1085
Lassa fever, 1:526, 527, 527*s*
Médecins Sans Frontières, 2:601, 602
outbreaks, field-level response to, 2:688
public health, 2:765
vaccines and vaccine development, 2:1022
virus hunters, 2:1045
Guinea pigs, 2:953, 1001
Guinea worm disease. *See* Dracunculiasis
Gulf Coast states
ascariasis, 1:79
Eastern equine encephalitis, 1:296, 297
encephalitis, 1:317
marine toxins, 2:591
West Nile virus, 2:1059–1060
Gulf War, 1:261, 2:1017, 1052
Gummatous syphilis, 2:935
Gut biome. *See* Intestinal flora
Gut flora. *See* Intestinal flora
Gynecological examination, 1:390

H

H1N1, 1:313, 490, 493–498, 2:692
HAART. *See* Highly active antiretroviral therapy
H2N2, 1:500, 502
H3N2, 1:507
H5N1, 1:**391–393,** *392*
avian influenza, 1:87–88, 89–90
dangers of, 1:491, 496–497
globalization and infectious disease, 1:385
immigration, 1:474
influenza epidemiology, 1:506
isolation and quarantine, 1:509
microbial evolution, 2:614
personal protective equipment, 2:700
public health, 2:764, 766
viral disease, 2:1041
world trade, 2:1083–1084
H7N9, 1:88, 2:692
Haemogogus mosquitoes, 2:637, 980
Haemophilus influenzae, 1:**394–396**
bacterial disease vaccines, 1:101
vaccine refusal, 1:186
WHO childhood vaccination recommendations, 1:185
Hahn, James Duaine, 2:659
Haiti
AIDS, 1:8, 19, 20
Biological Weapons Convention, 1:111
burkholderia, 1:145
cholera, 1:198, 200
cyclosporiasis, 1:259
developing nations and drug delivery, 1:*271*
immigration, 1:473
malaria, 2:580
measles vaccine clinical trials, 2:1073
rotavirus vaccine, 2:*830*
Halden, Rolf U., 1:68
Halibut and anisakiasis, 1:45
Hallucinations and rabies, 1:75, 2:776
Haloacetic acids, 1:282
Hamburger disease. *See Escherichia coli* O157:H7
Hand, foot, and mouth disease, 1:39, 324–327, **397–399,** 2:1084
Hand sanitizers. *See* Alcohol-based hand sanitizers

Hands
- hand, foot, and mouth disease, 1:397
- Kawasaki disease, 1:515–516
- rat-bite fever, 2:785
- ringworm, 2:818
- toxic shock, 2:961

Handshaking, 1:402, 2:609

Handwashing, 1:**400–402,** *401, 402*
- alveolar echinococcosis prevention, 1:25
- antimicrobial soaps, 1:66, 68
- ascariasis prevention, 1:80
- bacterial disease prevention, 1:101
- balantidiasis prevention, 1:102
- *Campylobacter* infection prevention, 1:152*s*
- cat scratch disease prevention, 1:163
- *Chlamydia pneumoniae* prevention, 1:195
- *Clostridium difficile* infection prevention, 1:210, 211
- cold sores prevention, 1:226
- colds prevention, 1:230
- contact lenses and *Fusarium* keratitis prevention, 1:233
- contact precautions, 1:236
- cryptosporidiosis prevention, 1:250, 251, 252
- dysentery prevention, 1:290–291
- enterovirus 71 infection prevention, 1:327
- *Escherichia coli* O157:H7 prevention, 1:341
- food-borne disease prevention, 1:355
- gastroenteritis prevention, 1:359
- germ theory of disease, 1:366
- group A streptococcal infection prevention, 2:922
- helminth disease prevention, 1:416
- hepatitis A prevention, 1:424, 425
- hepatitis E prevention, 1:439
- impetigo prevention, 1:480, 481
- infection control and asepsis, 1:*484,* 485
- Marburg hemorrhagic fever prevention, 2:586
- measles prevention, 2:595
- MRSA prevention, 2:642
- mumps prevention, 2:646
- norovirus infection prevention, 2:670
- nosocomial infection prevention, 2:674, 675
- opportunistic infection prevention, 2:684
- pink eye prevention, 2:703
- pinworm infection prevention, 2:707
- pneumonia prevention, 2:729
- psittacosis prevention, 2:760
- puerperal fever prevention, 2:768, 769
- rat-bite fever prevention, 2:786, 788
- rotavirus infection prevention, 2:829
- RSV infection prevention, 2:833, 834
- *Salmonella* infection prevention, 2:842
- scarlet fever prevention, 2:857
- shigellosis prevention, 2:880, 882, 883
- shingles prevention, 2:887
- standard precautions, 1:486*s,* 2:908–909, 910
- strep throat prevention, 2:918*s,* 919
- taeniasis prevention, 2:942
- tapeworm infection prevention, 2:950
- toxoplasmosis prevention, 2:966
- tularemia prevention, 2:991
- vancomycin-resistant *Enterococci* prevention, 2:1026
- viral meningitis prevention, 2:610
- water-borne disease prevention, 2:1055
- whipworm prevention, 2:1062, 1063
- yersiniosis prevention, 2:1098, 1098*s*

Hanoi, Vietnam, 2:848

Hansen, Gerhard Henrik Armauer, 1:544

Hansen's disease. *See* Leprosy

Hantavirus, 1:**404–408,** *406*
- emerging infectious diseases, 1:312
- hemorrhagic fevers, 1:418, 419, 420
- USAMRIID, 2:1018

Hares
- Crimean-Congo hemorrhagic fever, 1:244
- taeniasis, 2:940
- tularemia, 2:990
- typhus, 2:998

Harvard Medical School Department of Ambulatory Care, 1:271

Haskell, County, KS, 2:1047–1048

Havana, Cuba, 2:1043

"Havana Physician Who Solved the Yellow Fever Problem Is Extolled Here and Abroad," 2:*1093–1095*

Haverhill fever. *See* Rat-bite fever

Hawaii
- angiostrongyliasis, 1:36
- burkholderia, 1:145
- dengue and dengue hemorrhagic fever, 1:266, 267
- globalization and infectious disease, 1:385
- gonorrhea, 1:389
- liver fluke infections, 1:561
- marine toxins, 2:590

Hawk eagles, 2:1083

He, Biao, 2:779

Head lice, 1:552, 553

Headache
- AIDS, 1:12
- angiostrongyliasis, 1:35
- arthropod-borne diseases, 1:75
- aspergillosis, 1:85
- B virus infection, 1:92
- bacterial meningitis, 2:605
- blastomycosis, 1:122
- burkholderia, 1:145
- cat scratch disease, 1:161–163, 162*s*
- Chagas disease, 1:172
- chickenpox, 1:176
- chikungunya, 1:181
- *Chlamydia* infection, 1:190
- coccidioidomycosis, 1:218
- Crimean-Congo hemorrhagic fever, 1:244
- cryptosporidiosis, 1:252
- dengue and dengue hemorrhagic fever, 1:267
- Eastern equine encephalitis, 1:296
- encephalitis, 1:316, 317, 318
- glanders, 1:379
- hantavirus, 1:404, 405
- helminth disease, 1:415
- hemorrhagic fevers, 1:419, 420*s*
- herpes simplex virus 2, 1:444
- influenza, 1:504
- Japanese encephalitis, 1:511, 512
- Legionnaires' disease, 1:530
- lice infestation, 1:552
- listeriosis, 1:556
- Lyme disease, 1:569, 571, 573
- macrophage activation syndrome, 2:575
- malaria, 2:580
- Marburg hemorrhagic fever, 2:586
- marine toxins, 2:590
- meningitis, 1:223, 2:606*s*
- monkeypox, 2:626, 628*s*
- mononucleosis, 2:631
- mumps, 2:645, 646
- Nipah virus infection, 2:663
- nocardiosis, 2:666
- plague, 1:116, 2:715
- pneumonia, 2:726
- polio, 2:736
- post-treatment Lyme disease syndrome, 1:572
- Powassan virus, 2:741
- protozoan diseases, 2:753
- psittacosis, 2:759
- Q fever, 2:772
- rat-bite fever, 2:785, 787
- relapsing fever, 2:795
- rickettsial disease, 2:809
- Rift Valley fever, 2:813

Rocky Mountain spotted fever, 2:824
Salmonella infection, 2:841
SARS, 2:847
scarlet fever, 2:856
schistosomiasis, 2:861
severe fever with thrombocytopenia syndrome, 2:871
sexually transmitted infections, 2:876, 877
shingles, 1:176, 2:885
St. Louis encephalitis, 2:905
strep throat, 2:917
syphilis, 2:935
taeniasis, 2:943
tick-borne diseases, 2:956, 957, 958
toxoplasmosis, 2:964
trichinellosis, 2:973
tularemia, 2:989, 990
typhoid fever, 2:993, 995, 995*s*
typhus, 2:997
vaccine reactions, 2:1022
Venezuelan equine encephalitis virus, 2:1033
viral meningitis, 2:607, 609
West Nile virus, 2:1058, 1059
yellow fever, 2:1092
Zika virus, 2:1101
Health Canada, 1:248
Health care facilities. *See* Hospitals and health care facilities
Health care workers
AIDS transmission, 1:8
anthrax, 1:48
antibiotic overuse, 1:257
antimicrobial soap use, 1:67, 68
chickenpox, 1:177
childbirth attendance, 2:768*t*, 769
Clostridium difficile infection, 1:210
contact precautions, 1:235–238, 236, *236*
Crimean-Congo hemorrhagic fever, 1:243, 244
cryptosporidiosis, 1:251
disinfection, 1:282
droplet precautions, 1:286–288
drug prices, 2:707
Ebola, 1:304
economic development, 1:308
handwashing compliance, 2:642, 910
hepatitis B, 1:427, 428*s*
hepatitis C, 1:431
herpes simplex 1, 1:442
infection control and asepsis, 1:483–487
isolation and quarantine, 1:510
Lassa fever, 1:527, 528
Médecins Sans Frontières, 2:599–602
Middle East respiratory syndrome, 1:386
monkeypox, 2:627
needlestick injuries, 1:129–130, 131
nosocomial infections, 2:*674*, 675
parasitic disease prevention, 2:696
personal protective equipment, 2:699–701
public health, 2:764*s*
SARS, 2:848
sepsis education, 2:869
standard precautions, 2:908–910
Syrian refugee health outreach, 1:264–265
travel, 2:971
tuberculosis, 2:984, 985, 986, 987–988
typhus, 2:999
Health care-associated infections. *See* Nosocomial infections
Health departments and botulism antitoxins, 1:135
Health in 2015: From MDGs to SDGs, 2:1010*s*
Health insurance, 1:432, 536
Health Insurance Portability and Accountability Act, 1:536
Health Organization, 2:1076
Health Protection Agency, UK. *See* UK Health Protection Agency
Health Protection Agency Centre for Infections, 2:858
Healthcare-associated infections. *See* Nosocomial infections
"Healthy Pets for Health People" guidelines (CDC), 1:162*s*
Healy, Melissa, 2:675
Hearing loss. *See* Deafness and hearing loss
Heart disease or symptoms
aspergillosis, 1:85
avian influenza, 1:89
bacterial meningitis, 2:604–605
brucellosis, 1:141, 142
Chagas disease, 1:171, 173
Chlamydia pneumoniae, 1:193, 195
coccidioidomycosis, 1:219
Cryptococcus neoformans infection, 1:248
diphtheria, 1:274, 275
Ebola, 1:302
enterovirus 71 infection, 1:326
group A streptococcal infections, 2:921
group B streptococcal infection, 2:926–927
hookworm infection, 1:458
impetigo, 1:482
with influenza, 1:489
Kawasaki disease, 1:515, 516, 517
Lyme disease, 1:569, 571
pneumonia risk factors, 2:626
relapsing fever, 2:795
rubella, 2:837
shingles as a risk factor for, 2:888
Staphylococcus aureus infections, 2:912
strep throat, 2:917
syphilis, 2:934, 935
tick-borne diseases, 2:958
vector-borne disease, 2:1029
viral disease, 2:1039
yellow fever, 2:1092
Heart rate abnormalities
Chagas disease, 1:173
cholera, 1:198, 201
dengue and dengue hemorrhagic fever, 1:267
diphtheria, 1:276
enterovirus 71 infection, 1:326
hookworm infection, 1:458
Lyme disease, 1:569
necrotizing fasciitis, 2:659
scarlet fever, 2:857
tetanus, 2:953
Heart valve replacement, 2:683, 773
Heartland virus, 2:872, 873*s*, 957
Heat, sterilization by, 2:914, 915
Hebard, Sara, 2:660
Heberden, William, 1:175
Hedberg, Craig, 1:558
Hedgehogs and the wildlife trade, 2:1083
Heine, Heinrich, 1:201
Helicobacter pylori, 1:**409–413,** *410*
bacterial diseases, 1:100
cancer, 1:155
Koch's postulates, 1:520–521
self-experimentation of scientists, 1:343–345
"*Helicobacter pylori* and Gastric Cancer: Factors That Modulate Disease Risk," 1:411
Hell, Stefan W., 2:620
Helminth disease, 1:**414–417,** *415, 416*
alveolar echinococcosis, 1:24–26
ascariasis, 1:78–80
climate change, 2:698
dracunculiasis, 1:283–285
hookworm infection, 1:457–460
liver fluke infections, 1:560–564
lung flukes, 1:565–568
parasitic diseases, 2:694, 695
pinworm infection, 2:705–708
river blindness, 2:820–822
sanitation, 2:845
schistosomiasis, 2:860–863
strongyloidiasis, 2:928–930
taeniasis, 2:940–943
tapeworm infections, 2:948–950
trichinellosis, 2:972–974
tropical infectious diseases, 2:980
whipworm, 2:1062–1064

Helmith disease
angiostrongyliasis, 1:35–38
filariasis, 1:350–352
Helper T cells, 1:454, 455, 478
Hemagglutinin proteins
avian influenza, 1:88
H5N1, 1:392
influenza, 1:489
influenza pandemic of 1918, 1:494
influenza pandemic of 1957, 1:500
Hematuria. *See* Bloody urine
Hemodialysis, 1:340, 341, 432*s*, 531
Hemolysis, 2:921, 925
Hemolytic anemia, 1:96
Hemolytic uremic syndrome, 1:340
Hemophagocytic lymphohistiocytosis, 2:575–576
Hemophilus bacterial disease, 1:187
Hemoptysis. *See* Coughing up blood
Hemorrhage. *See* Bleeding
Hemorrhagic fever renal syndrome, 1:404
Hemorrhagic fevers, 1:**418–421,** *419*
bioterrorism, 1:114–115
Crimean-Congo hemorrhagic fever, 1:243–246
dengue and dengue hemorrhagic fever, 1:266–268
hantavirus, 1:404–407
isolation and quarantine, 1:509
Marburg hemorrhagic fever, 2:585–587
Rift Valley fever, 2:813–816
viral disease, 2:1041
yellow fever, 2:1092
Hemorrhagic smallpox, 2:892
Henan Province, China, 2:872
Henderson Act of 1943, 2:937
Hendon, Ernest, 2:937
Hendon, North, 2:937
Henipavirus genus, 2:662
Henn, Steve, 1:554
Henry, Jim, 2:883
Henry V (English king), 1:289
HEPA filters, 1:22, 23
Hepadnaviridae, 2:1039
Hepatitis
Cryptococcus neoformans infection, 1:248
Marburg hemorrhagic fever, 2:586
psittacosis, 2:759
relapsing fever, 2:795
Hepatitis A, 1:185, **422–425,** *423*
Hepatitis B, 1:**426–429**
avian influenza, 1:156
barber shops, 1:131*s*
blood supply, 1:126, 129
bloodborne pathogens, 1:129, 130, 131
cancer, 1:154, 155
with hepatitis A, 1:423
with hepatitis D, 1:434, 435, 436
vaccines, 1:155*s*
viral disease, 2:1039
WHO childhood vaccination recommendations, 1:185
zoonoses, 2:1106
Hepatitis C, 1:**430–432,** *431*
antiviral drugs, 1:70–71
barber shops, 1:131*s*
blood supply, 1:126
bloodborne pathogens, 1:129, 130, 131
cancer, 1:155
Hepatitis D, 1:**434–436,** *435, 436*
Hepatitis E, 1:**437–439,** *438,* 438*t,* 2:1039
Hepatitis G. *See* Anellovirus
Hepatocellular cancer. *See* Liver cancer
Herbal treatment for colds, 1:230
Herd immunity, 1:187, 2:1069
Herodotus, 2:865
Herpes gladiatorum, 1:442*s*
Herpes simplex 1 virus, 1:226, **440–443**
Herpes simplex virus
antiviral drugs, 1:72
encephalitis, 1:316
sexually transmitted infections, 2:877
urinary tract infection, 2:1013
Herpes simplex virus 2, 1:365, **444–447,** *445*
Herpesviruses
B virus infection, 1:91–94
cancer, 1:155
CMV infection, 1:214–217
Epstein-Barr virus, 1:335–337
herpes simplex 1 virus, 1:440–443
mononucleosis, 2:630–635
sexually transmitted infections, 2:877
shingles, 2:885–888
viral disease, 2:1039
Herring and anisakiasis, 1:45
Herring worm, 1:43
Hewings-Martin, Yella, 1:211
HHV-8, 1:155
High-efficiency particulate air (HEPA) filters, 1:22, 23
High-level disinfection, 1:280
Highly active antiretroviral therapy, 1:13–14, 72–73, 2:722
Hignett, Katherine, 2:858
Hippocrates
brucellosis, 1:140
cholera, 1:199
diphtheria, 1:277
epidemiology, 1:328
influenza, 1:488
mumps, 2:644
tuberculosis, 2:983
weather-epidemics relationship, 1:203
Hispanic Americans and AIDS, 1:13
Histamine, 2:590, 592, 702
Histochemical tests formicrosporidiosis, 2:624
Histology, 1:149, 2:945
Histoplasmosis, 1:**448–452,** *449, 450*
History of the Peloponnesian War, 2:710
History of the Wars, 2:711
HIV, 1:**453–456**
AIDS test kit, 1:*454*
antiviral drugs, 1:72
blood supply, 1:125–126
bloodborne pathogens, 1:129, 130, 131
cancer, 1:155
candidiasis risk factors, 1:158, 159
cat scratch disease, 1:161–163
Chlamydia infection as a risk for, 1:190
climate change, 1:206
CMV infection risk factors, 1:214, 215
cohorted communities, 1:223, 224
Cryptococcus neoformans infection, 1:247–248, 249
cryptosporidiosis, 1:251, 252, 253
developing nations and drug delivery, 1:271, 272*s*
diagnosis, 1:12–13
discovery of, 2:806*s*
diseases that weaken the immune system, 2:667*s*
economic development, 1:309
emerging infectious diseases, 1:312
epidemiology, 1:331–332
extremely drug-resistant tuberculosis, 1:23
genital herpes as risk factor for, 1:365
with glanders, 1:379
gonorrhea as a risk factor for, 1:389, 390
helminth disease, 1:416
hepatitis B risk factors, 1:427
hepatitis C, 1:432, 432*s*
herpes simplex 1 virus, 1:442
herpes simplex virus 2, 1:446
histoplasmosis risk factors, 1:449, 451
immigration, 1:474
immune response, 1:478, 479
Koch's postulates, 1:521
Legionnaires' disease, 1:530
leishmaniasis, 1:541
measles, 2:595
Médecins Sans Frontières, 2:600–601
microsporidiosis, 2:623–624
mosquito-borne diseases, 2:638

mycotic disease, 2:650, 651
National Institute of Allergy and Infectious Diseases, 2:654
opportunistic infections, 2:682, 683, 684
origins of, 1:17–18
percentage of people living with HIV, 1:*7*
Pneumocystis jirovecii pneumonia, 2:721–724
re-emerging infectious diseases, 2:790–791, 792
retroviruses, 2:805, 806, 808
ringworm, 2:819
scrofula, 2:866, 867
sexually transmitted infections, 2:876–877, 878, 879
signs and symptoms, 1:11
syphilis, 2:936–937
talaromycosis, 2:946
transmission, 1:8–11
trichomoniasis, 2:977
UNICEF, 2:1006
United Nations Millennium Goals, 2:1007, 1008–1009, 1010
viral disease, 2:1038, 1041
West Nile virus, 2:1060
women, 2:1072–1073
See also AIDS
HIV fusion inhibitors, 1:13
HIV Risk Reduction Tool, 1:455*s*
Hives, 1:566
H7N9 influenza, 1:88
Hoarseness, 1:194, 229, 274
Hodgkin's lymphoma, 1:155, 337, 2:683
Hoffmann, Constanze, 1:49
Holmes, Oliver Wendell, 2:673–674, 767, 768
Homelessness
hepatitis A, 1:423, *423,* 425
lice infestation, 1:554
tuberculosis, 2:985–986
Homosexual men. *See* Men who have sex with men
Honduras, 1:205, 220
Honey, 1:135
Hong Kong
avian influenza, 1:88
ProMED, 2:752
SARS, 2:847–848, 849
scarlet fever, 2:858–859
talaromycosis, 2:945
travel, 2:970
Hong Kong International Airport, 2:*971*
Hooke, Robert, 1:366, 2:618
Hookworm infection, 1:**457–460,** *459,* 2:1106
Horby, Peter, 1:*329*
Horizontal gene transfer, 2:611, 612, 613
Hormones
iatrogenic Creutzfeldt-Jakob disease, 1:241
urinary tract infection, 2:1013
women and vaccines, 2:1074
Horn of Africa countries, 2:797, 798
Horses
burkholderia, 1:144, 145
Eastern equine encephalitis, 1:296, 297
encephalitis, 1:317
glanders, 1:378–379, 380, *380,* 381
histoplasmosis, 1:449
hosts and vectors, 1:461
leptospirosis, 1:548
rabies, 2:777
tetanus, 2:953
vector-borne disease, 2:1029
Venezuelan equine encephalitis virus, 2:1033–1035
West Nile virus, 2:1057, 1060
Hospital Donostia, 1:*236*
Hospital gangrene, 2:657
Hospital Infection Control Practices Advisory Committee, 1:235
Hospital-acquired infections. *See* Nosocomial infections
Hospitalization
airborne precautions, 1:21–23
availability of hospital beds, by country, 1:21*t*
babesiosis, 1:*95*
Campylobacter infection, 1:151
chickenpox, 1:177, 178*s*
Chlamydia pneumoniae, 1:195
coccidioidomycosis, 1:219
diphtheria, 1:276
dysentery, 1:290
Eastern equine encephalitis, 1:297
enterovirus 71 infection, 1:326
food-borne disease, 1:357
gastroenteritis, 1:358, 359–360
hepatitis A, 1:424–425
measles, 2:594
parasitic diseases, 2:695
plague, 2:718
Powassan virus, 2:742
rotavirus infection, 2:828
RSV infection, 2:832, 834
Salmonella infection, 2:841–842
Staphylococcus aureus infections, 2:912
viral meningitis, 2:607
yersiniosis, 2:1096–1099
Hospitals and health care facilities
alcohol-based hand sanitizers, 1:400
antibiotic stewardship programs, 2:746
antimicrobial soap use, 1:67, 68
Clostridium difficile infection, 1:210
contact precautions, 1:235–238
droplet precautions, 1:286–288
infection control, 2:*799*
isolation and quarantine, 1:508–510
Legionnaires' disease, 1:530, 531
norovirus infection, 2:670
resistant organisms, 2:800, 802*s*
RSV infection, 2:833
scabies, 2:853
standard precautions, 2:908–910
tuberculosis patients' rights, 2:986–988
water quality in, 1:292
Host cells
anellovirus, 1:31
antiviral drugs, 1:70–72
brucellosis, 1:140, 142
cancer, 1:154
Chlamydia infection, 1:189
Cryptococcus neoformans infection, 1:247
Ebola, 1:302
HIV, 1:12, 13
Hosts and vectors, 1:**461–464,** *462*
climate change, 2:756, 793
influenza epidemiology, 1:505
vector-borne disease, 2:1029–1032
zoonoses, 2:1106–1107
See also specific diseases
Hot dogs and listeriosis, 1:557
Hot tub rash, 1:100, **465–467,** *466*
The Hot Zone (Preston), 1:302, 304, 2:1017
Hotez, Peter J., 1:415–416
House mice, 1:405
Houseflies, 1:75, 289
Household air quality, 2:729
Households
AIDS transmission, 1:10
demographics, 1:263–264
hepatitis A, 1:423
hepatitis B, 1:427
pinworm infection, 2:706
public health, 2:764
Houston, TX, 1:207, 2:670
"How a History of Eating Human Brains Protected This Tribe from Brain Disease," 1:*523–525*
"How Charles Nicolle of the Pasteur Institute Discovered that Epidemic Typhus Is Transmitted by Lice," 2:*1000–1001*
Howard, Carter, 2:937
HPV, 1:**468–471**
avian influenza, 1:156
cancer, 1:154, 155
Chlamydia infection, effect of, 1:190
opportunistic infections, 2:683
sexually transmitted infections, 2:877–878, 879
vaccines, 1:155*s, 469*

WHO childhood vaccination recommendations, 1:185
women, 2:1073
HTLV. *See* Human T-cell leukemia virus (HTLV)
Hubei Province, China, 2:871–872
Huey, Jason Chan Meng, 2:659
Hugonnet, Stéphane, 2:688
Human encroachment into wildlife areas
Baylissacaris infection, 1:107, 304
gastroenteritis, 1:359–360
leptospirosis, 1:550
microbial evolution, 2:611
Rocky Mountain Laboratory research, 2:655
zoonoses, 2:1107
Human granulocytic ehrlichiosis, 1:571
Human growth hormone, 1:241
Human papillomavirus. *See* HPV
Human parvovirus B19, 1:347
Human rabies immunoglobulin, 2:777
Human research subjects, 2:937–938, 1071, 1073–1074. *See also* Self-experimentation by scientists
Human Rights Watch, 2:1108
Human T-cell leukemia virus (HTLV), 2:806, 806*s*
Human T-cell leukemia virus III, 1:19
Human T-lymphotrophic virus, 1:126, 155
Human Vaccines and Immunotherapies, 1:528
Humanitarian aid. *See* Developing nations and drug delivery; specific nongovernmental organizations
Hungary, 1:89, 325, 2:767–768
Hunger programs, UNICEF, 2:1006
Hunters. *See* Outdoor recreation
Hurricane Katrina, 1:201, 207, 2:670, 883
Hurricane Mitch, 1:205
Hurricanes. *See* Natural disasters
Hyalomma ticks, 1:243, 244
Hyderabad, India, 1:*395*
Hydration and rehydration
Campylobacter infection, 1:151
chikungunya, 1:182
cholera, 1:197, 198
cryptosporidiosis, 1:250, 252
dysentery, 1:290
Escherichia coli O157:H7, 1:340
gastroenteritis, 1:360
hand, foot, and mouth disease, 1:398
influenza, 1:490
mononucleosis, 2:630, 635
norovirus infection, 2:670
pneumonia, 2:729
Powassan virus, 2:742
rotavirus infection, 2:830
sanitation-related diseases, 2:845
scarlet fever, 2:857
shigellosis, 2:882
St. Louis encephalitis, 2:906
strep throat, 2:918
toxic shock, 2:961
urinary tract infection, 2:1013
viral meningitis, 2:610
water-borne disease, 2:1055
Zika virus, 2:1102
Hydrocele, 1:351
Hydrocephalus, 2:943
Hydrogen peroxide, 1:282
Hydrophobia, 2:776
Hydrosalpinx, 1:191
Hydroxychloroquine, 2:773
Hygiene
ascariasis, 1:80
bacterial disease prevention, 1:101
balantidiasis prevention, 1:103
Chlamydia infection, 1:190
cholera, 1:198–199
Clostridium difficile infection, 1:210
cohorted communities, 1:224
colds, 1:230
contact lenses and *Fusarium* keratitis, 1:233
cryptosporidiosis, 1:251
dysentery, 1:290–291, 292
enterovirus 71 infection, 1:327
Escherichia coli O157:H7 prevention, 1:341
filariasis, 1:352
food-borne disease, 1:356
gastroenteritis, 1:359
hand, foot, and mouth disease, 1:398
handwashing, 1:400–402
helminth disease, 2:1064
hepatitis A, 1:422, 424
hepatitis E, 1:439
herpes simplex 1 virus, 1:443
impetigo, 1:480, 481
leptospirosis, 1:549*s*
lice infestation, 1:553
measles prevention, 2:595
microsporidiosis, 2:624
mumps prevention, 2:646
norovirus infection prevention, 2:670
nosocomial infection prevention, 2:675
parasitic diseases, 2:696
pink eye, 2:703
pinworm infection, 2:706
pneumonia prevention, 2:729
puerperal fever, 2:768
Q fever, 2:773
ringworm, 2:818, 819
rotavirus infection, 2:829
RSV infection, 2:833, 834
Salmonella infection, 2:840, 842
sanitation, 2:845
scarlet fever, 2:857
schistosomiasis, 2:860
sepsis, 2:869
shigellosis, 2:880, 882
strep throat, 2:918*s*, 919
strongyloidiasis, 2:930
taeniasis, 2:942
tapeworm infections, 2:949, 950
toxoplasmosis prevention, 2:966
trachoma, 2:968, 969
tropical infectious diseases, 2:982
typhoid fever, 2:995
typhus, 2:998
viral meningitis prevention, 2:610
water-borne diseases, 2:1053
yersiniosis, 2:1096, 1098
Hyperendemicity
malaria, 2:579
sporotrichosis, 2:902
trachoma, 2:967
Hyperinfection, 2:928, 929
Hypermutation and leprosy, 1:545
Hypertension, 1:326, 2:729, 953
Hypertonia and congenital Zika syndrome, 2:1101
Hypervirulence, 1:212–213
Hypotension
babesiosis, 1:96
cholera, 1:201
dengue and dengue hemorrhagic fever, 1:267
hantavirus, 1:404
relapsing fever, 2:795
rickettsial disease, 2:811
toxic shock, 2:961
Hypoxia and *Pneumocystis jirovecii* pneumonia, 2:722

I

Iacono, Giovanni Lo, 1:526
Iatrogenic Creutzfeldt-Jakob disease, 1:240–241, 2:749
Ibuprofen
chikungunya, 1:182
mononucleosis, 2:634
mumps, 2:646
scarlet fever, 2:857
shingles, 2:886
strep throat, 2:918
Ice cream, 1:141, 212
ICUs. *See* Intensive care units
Idaho, 2:795, 824
Identification of microorganisms
babesiosis, 1:96, 97
bovine spongiform encephalopathy, 1:139
Campylobacter bacteria, 1:151
CDC, 1:167, 169, 340, 340*s*
cholera, 1:197
Clostridium difficile, 1:209
culture and sensitivity, 1:254–257
Cyclospora, 1:258–259

diphtheria, 1:276
Ebola, 1:41
genetic identification, 1:362–364
germ theory of disease, 1:369
GIDEON, 1:376
plague, 2:713–714
Rocky Mountain Laboratory, 2:656
SARS, 2:849–850
typing, 1:256–257
USAMRIID, 2:1017
Idoxuridine, 1:72
Iliad (Homer), 1:47
Illegal, unreported, and unregulated fishing and hunting, 2:1085
Illegal abortion, 1:76*s*, 2:1108
Illinois, 1:317, 2:873*s*
Imipenem, 1:380, 2:730
Immigration, 1:**472–475,** *473*
demographics and infectious disease, 1:261, 263, 264
Eastern equine encephalitis, 1:298
hepatitis E, 1:438
legislation and international law, 1:536–537
leishmaniasis, 1:541
leprosy, 1:544
malaria, 2:582
parasitic diseases, 2:695, 696
plague, 2:712–713
relapsing fever, 2:797–798
river blindness, 2:820, 821
schistosomiasis, 2:860, 862, 863
scrofula, 2:866
shigellosis, 2:882
smallpox, 2:890
strongyloidiasis, 2:929
taeniasis, 2:941
tapeworm infections, 2:950
tuberculosis, 2:985
typhus, 2:997–1001
war, 2:1048, 1050
world trade, 2:1082
zoonoses, 2:1106
Immune globulin
hepatitis A, 1:423, 424
monkeypox, 2:628
rabies, 2:777
RSV infection, 2:834
tetanus, 2:954
Immune response, 1:*476,* **476–479**
African sleeping sickness, 1:2
Epstein-Barr virus, 1:335
scabies, 2:852
women, 2:1074
Immune system
anti-cytokine antibody syndrome, 1:53
aspergillosis, 1:85
Buruli ulcer, 1:148
colds, 1:229
Cryptococcus neoformans infection, 1:247
diseases that weaken the immune system, 2:667*s*
Epstein-Barr virus, 1:337
fifth disease, 1:347, 349
germ theory of disease, 1:370
HIV, 1:11, 455
macrophage activation syndrome, 2:575–576
macrophages, 2:576*s*
mononucleosis, 2:632
older adults, 1:263
RSV vaccine research, 2:835
Immunity
cat scratch disease, 1:161
chickenpox, 1:175, 177
chikungunya, 1:181
diphtheria, 1:275, 276–277
Eastern equine encephalitis, 1:297
fifth disease, 1:348
hepatitis B vaccine, 1:428
histoplasmosis, 1:448, 451
influenza pandemic of 1918, 1:495
measles, 2:593
mumps, 2:644
St. Louis encephalitis, 2:905
typhus, 2:998
whooping cough vaccine, 2:1068–1069
Immunization Plus program, 2:1005
Immunocompromised individuals
airborne precautions, 1:23
amebiasis, 1:28
aspergillosis, 1:85
babesiosis, 1:96
blastomycosis, 1:122
burkholderia, 1:146
cancer, 1:155
candidiasis, 1:157, 158, 159, 160
cat scratch disease, 1:161–163, 162
chickenpox, 1:175, 177
chickenpox vaccine precautions, 1:178
climate change and malaria, 1:206
Clostridium difficile infection, 1:209
CMV infection, 1:214–215, 216
coccidioidomycosis, 1:219
cohorted communities, 1:224
cryptosporidiosis prevention, 1:253
cyclosporiasis, 1:259, 260
diseases that weaken the immune system, 2:667*s*
encephalitis, 1:317
Escherichia coli O157:H7, 1:340
fifth disease, 1:349
food-borne disease, 1:356
gastroenteritis, 1:358
group A streptococcal infections, 2:921
Haemophilus influenzae, 1:394
helminth disease, 1:416
hepatitis B, 1:426
hepatitis E, 1:437, 438
herpes simplex 1 virus, 1:441, 442, 443
herpes simplex virus 2, 1:446
histoplasmosis, 1:448, 449, 451
hot tub rash, 1:465, 466
immune response, 1:479
influenza, 1:489
Legionnaires' disease, 1:530, 531
listeriosis, 1:556
malaria, 2:580
marine toxins, 2:592
measles, 2:595
methicillin-resistant *Staphylococcus aureus,* 1:67
microsporidiosis, 2:623
monkeypox, 2:628
mononucleosis, 2:633
mumps vaccine, 2:646
mycotic disease, 2:649, 650, 651
nocardiosis, 2:666, 667, 668
norovirus infection, 2:669
nosocomial infections, 2:674
opportunistic infections, 2:682, 683, 684
Pneumocystis jirovecii pneumonia, 2:721–724
pneumonia, 2:725, 726, 729
protozoan diseases, 2:754, 755
psittacosis, 2:760
puerperal fever, 2:767
re-emerging infectious diseases, 2:792
ringworm, 2:819
rotavirus infection, 2:829–830
scabies, 2:852, 853, 854
scrofula, 2:866
sepsis, 2:868
shigellosis, 2:882
shingles, 1:177, 2:886, 887
sporotrichosis, 2:901–902
Staphylococcus aureus infections, 2:912
strongyloidiasis, 2:928, 929
superbugs, 2:1027*s*
swimmer's ear, 2:933
talaromycosis, 2:944, 945
toxoplasmosis, 2:964, 965*s*, 966
tuberculosis, 1:59, 2:984, 985, 986
urinary tract infection, 2:1013
vaccines and vaccine development, 2:1023
vancomycin-resistant *Enterococci,* 2:1026
viral meningitis, 2:607
water-borne disease, 2:1055
West Nile virus, 2:1060
women, 2:1072, 1073

Immunofluorescent microscopy, 2:620
Immunohistochemical staining, 1:244
Immunosuppressants
anti-cytokine antibody syndrome, 1:54
chickenpox vaccine precautions, 1:178
CMV infection risk factors, 1:215
fifth disease, 1:349
gastroenteritis, 1:358
macrophage activation syndrome, 2:576
Pneumocystis jirovecii pneumonia, 2:721
strongyloidiasis with, 2:929
urinary tract infection, 2:1013
water-borne disease, 2:1055
Immunotests, 2:781–782
Impax Laboratories, 2:707, 708
Imperial College London, 2:863
Impetigo, 1:**480–482,** *481*
Implanted devices
biofilms, 2:802*s*
Chagas disease, 1:173
hearing aids, 2:606
Staphylococcus aureus infections, 2:912
sterilization, 2:914
Imvamune, 2:893
"In Disaster's Wake: Tsunami Lung," 2:*730–731*
"In Soil Dwelling Bacteria, Scientists Find a New Eapon to Fight Drug-Resistant Superbugs," 2:*675–676*
Inactivated vaccines
polio vaccine, 2:733–734, 738
typhoid fever, 2:994
vaccines and vaccine development, 2:1022*s*
Incarcerated people. *See* Prisons and prisoners
Incidence and epidemiology, 1:330
Income and economic development, 1:306–307
Incontinence, 1:485, 2:825
Increased Prevalence of Anellovirus in Pediatric Patients with Fever, 1:*32–33*
India
AIDS deaths, 1:15, 20
amebiasis, 1:28
avian influenza, 1:89
bacterial meningitis, 2:606
blood supply, 1:126
burkholderia, 1:145
chikungunya, 1:180, *180,* 181
child marriage, 2:1005
cholera, 1:197, 198, 199, 201, 533
climate change, 1:205
CMV infection, 1:215
Crimean-Congo hemorrhagic fever, 1:244
cyclosporiasis, 1:259
dengue and dengue hemorrhagic fever, 1:267, *267*
diphtheria, 1:276
dysentery, 1:290
economic development, 1:308–309
encephalitis, 1:*315,* 317, 318
filariasis, 1:351
gastroenteritis, 1:358–361
glanders, 1:380
Haemophilus influenzae vaccination, 1:*395*
handwashing, 1:*401*
hookworm infection, 1:58, 457
Japanese encephalitis, 1:512, 513–514, 513*s,* 514
leishmaniasis, 1:539, 540, 541
leprosy, 1:547, 2:1078
leptospirosis, 1:*549*
microsporidiosis, 2:624*s*
mycotic disease, 2:652
Nipah virus infection, 2:663
outbreaks, field-level response to, 2:686
plague, 2:712–713
polio eradication campaign, 2:733
protozoan diseases, 2:755
rabies, 2:778
re-emerging infectious diseases, 2:791*s*
relapsing fever, 2:796
resistant organisms research, 2:803
rotavirus, 2:831
rubella, 2:839
sanitation, 2:846
SARS, 2:849
smallpox, 2:893
taeniasis, 2:942
talaromycosis, 2:945
tapeworm infections, 2:949
trade, 2:1081
tropical infectious diseases, 2:981
typhoid fever, 2:994, 995
typhus, 2:997, 999
United Nations Millennium Goals, 2:1009
vector-borne disease, 2:*1030*
Indian Journal of Medical Research, 2:839
Indian Ocean islands, 1:181, 2:999
Indiana
babesiosis, 1:96
blastomycosis, 1:123
encephalitis, 1:317
histoplasmosis, 1:451
illegal snails, 1:38
Indigenous communities
blastomycosis, 1:122
hepatitis C, 1:431
smallpox, 2:890, 893
trade, 2:1081
trichinellosis, 2:973
Indigestion. *See* Gastrointestinal diseases or symptoms
Indinavir, 1:13
Indirect contact transmission, 1:235
Indomethacin, 2:886
Indonesia
ascariasis, 1:79
cholera, 1:198
cyclosporiasis, 1:259
encephalitis, 1:317
fruit bats, 2:663
fumigation, 2:*636*
hand, foot, and mouth disease, 1:397
leprosy, 1:546
plague, 2:717
SARS, 2:848–849
smallpox, 2:897
United Nations Millennium Goals, 2:1009
water-borne diseases, 2:*1053*
women, 2:*1072*
Indoor cooking issues, 2:729
Indo-Pacific basin, 1:36
Industrial Revolution, 1:39, 204, 553
Industrialized nations. *See* Developed nations
Infanticide and leprosy, 1:546*s*
Infantile diarrhea. *See* Rotavirus infection
Infantile paralysis. *See* Polio
Infants
bacterial meningitis, 2:606
botulism, 1:135
candidiasis, 1:159
chickenpox, 1:175, 177
Chlamydia infection, 1:190
CMV infection, 1:215, 216
diphtheria, 1:277
dysentery, 1:290
ear infections, 1:295
enterovirus 71 infection, 1:324, 325, 326, 327
gastroenteritis, 1:358–361
gonorrhea, 1:389
group B streptococcal infection, 2:924, 925–926
Haemophilus influenzae, 1:395
hand, foot, and mouth disease, 1:398
hepatitis B, 1:427
hepatitis B vaccine, 1:155*s,* 428, 428*s*
herpes simplex 1 virus, 1:442, 443
herpes simplex virus 2, 1:446
hookworm infection, 1:458
infection control and asepsis, 1:485
influenza, 1:488
Lassa fever, 1:527
malaria, 2:580
measles, 2:593
norovirus infection, 2:669

nosocomial infections, 2:675
opportunistic infections, 2:683
pink eye, 2:703, 704
pneumonia, 2:727
polio eradication campaign, 2:733
Powassan virus, 2:742*s*
rotavirus infection, 2:829
RSV infection, 2:832, 833, 834
rubella, 2:837
sepsis, 2:868, 1079
Staphylococcus aureus infections, 2:912
tetanus, 2:952, 954
viral disease, 2:1041
viral meningitis, 2:607, 608, 609
whooping cough, 2:1066, 1067, 1069
yersiniosis, 2:1096, 1098
Infection and Drug Resistance, 2:1026
Infection control and asepsis, 1:**483–487,** *484,* 2:*799*
airborne precautions, 1:21–23
brucellosis, 1:141
Chagas disease, 1:173
contact precautions, 1:235–238
disinfection, 1:280–282
droplet precautions, 1:286–288
germ theory of disease, 1:369
handwashing, 1:400–401, 400–402
isolation and quarantine, 1:508–510
Lassa fever, 1:527, 528
MRSA, 2:642
nosocomial infections, 2:673, 675
overreliance on antibiotics, 1:257
personal protective equipment, 2:699–701
pneumonia, 2:729
prion disease, 2:750
public health, 2:764–765
SARS, 1:*384*
smallpox, 2:893
sports, 1:442*s*
standard precautions, 2:908–910
sterilization, 2:914–916
superbugs, 2:1027*s*
USAMRIID, 2:1016
vancomycin-resistant *Enterococci,* 2:1026, 1027, 1028
Infections in the Immunosuppressed Patient, 2:722
"Infections Reveal Inequality between the Sexes," 2:*1073–1074*
Infectious Diseases Society of America, 1:257, 2:728
Infectious waste, 1:485
Infertility
Chlamydia infection, 1:189, 191
gonorrhea, 1:387, 388, 389
mumps, 2:646
sexually transmitted infections, 2:877
Inflammation
ascariasis, 1:79
bacterial meningitis, 2:604
Chagas disease, 1:173
Clostridium difficile infection, 1:209
ear infections, 1:293
encephalitis, 1:318
group A streptococcal infections, 2:921
Helicobacter pylori, 1:409, 410–411
immune system, 1:478
influenza, 1:504
microsporidiosis, 2:624*s*
opportunistic infections, 2:683
pneumonia, 2:725
river blindness, 2:820
swimmer's ear and swimmer's itch, 2:933
viral disease, 2:1039, 1041
"Inflammation Affects Fetal Cardiac Gene Expression and May Be Linked to Adult Heart Disease," *2:926–927*
Inflammatory disease, 1:54, 572
Inflammatory mediators, 1:229
Inflammatory response, 2:854
Influenza, 1:**488–492,** *489*
antiviral drugs, 1:71–72, 73
avian influenza, 1:87–90
CDC, 1:169
cohorted communities, 1:224
colds *vs.,* 1:229, 489*t*
emerging infectious diseases, 1:313, 314
H5N1, 1:391–393
influenza pandemic of 1918, 1:493–498
influenza pandemic of 1957, 1:499–502
isolation and quarantine, 1:509
microbial evolution, 2:614
National Institute of Allergy and Infectious Diseases, 2:655
pandemic preparedness, 2:690–693
personal protective equipment, 2:700
pneumonia, 2:726
public health, 2:763–764, 764*s,* 765–766
rapid diagnostic tests, 2:783
recombinant technology, 1:82
vaccines, 1:*504,* 2:729, 1023
viral disease, 2:1041
women, 2:1074
world trade, 2:1083–1084
zoonoses, 2:1106
Influenza: tracking seasonal influences and virus mutation, 1:489, **503–507**
Influenza pandemic of 1918, 1:**493–498,** *495*
emerging infectious diseases, 1:314
influenza pandemics, 1:490, 491
public health, 2:764
war, 2:1047–1048
Influenza pandemic of 1957, 1:**499–502,** *500*
Information dissemination, public, 2:687
Informed consent and human research subjects, 1:344, 345
Infrastructure, health care
arthropod-borne disease, 1:75
blood supply, 1:125
cholera, 1:197, 198, 200, 201
climate change, 1:207
demographics, 1:261, 264
developing nations and drug delivery, 1:271
diphtheria, 1:277
disinfection, 1:281
Ebola, 2:765
economic development, 1:306
epidemiology, 1:333
field-level response to outbreaks, 2:686, 687
handwashing, 1:402
helminth disease, 1:414
hepatitis E, 1:439
Médecins Sans Frontières, 2:602
natural disasters, 2:730
pandemic preparedness, 2:690, 691, 692
protozoan diseases, 2:754
re-emerging infectious diseases, 2:792
typhoid fever, 2:995
typhus, 2:1000
virus hunters, 2:1045
war and poverty, 2:740
war and public health, 2:1050
whipworm, 2:1063
whooping cough, 2:1068
world trade, 2:1081
Inglesby, Thomas V., 1:118
Inhalational transmission
anthrax, 1:49, 50, 51, 115
blastomycosis, 1:121, 122
botulism, 1:134*s,* 135
brucellosis, 1:141
coccidioidomycosis, 1:218, 219
colds, 1:229
Cryptococcus neoformans infection, 1:247
histoplasmosis, 1:448, 449
Legionnaires' disease, 1:530
microsporidiosis, 2:622–623
mycotic disease, 2:650
nocardiosis, 2:666
plague, 2:716

psittacosis, 2:759
Q fever, 2:771, 772
rabies, 2:776
RSV infection, 2:833
rubella, 2:837
smallpox, 2:890, 891
sporotrichosis, 2:901
talaromycosis, 2:945
tuberculosis, 2:983
tularemia, 2:990, 991*s*
viral disease, 2:1041
war, 2:1050, 1051, 1052
Initiative for Vaccine Research, 1:77
Injection drug users
AIDS, 1:8, 19, 20
anthrax, 1:48, 49
bloodborne infections, 1:129, 131
hepatitis A, 1:422, 423
hepatitis B, 1:426, 427
hepatitis C, 1:430, 431, 432*s*
hepatitis D, 1:434–435
tetanus, 2:952
Injuries
inflammation, 1:318
leprosy, 1:545
tetanus, 2:952, 953
Innate immunity, 2:792
Inoculating loop, 2:915
Insect repellents and disease prevention
babesiosis, 1:97
Chagas disease, 1:173
chikungunya, 1:180, 182
Crimean-Congo hemorrhagic fever, 1:245
encephalitis, 1:318
filariasis, 1:352
Japanese encephalitis, 1:513
Lyme disease, 1:572
malaria, 2:581
plague, 2:718, 719
Powassan virus, 2:742
relapsing fever, 2:797
rickettsial disease, 2:809, 811
Rift Valley fever, 2:815
river blindness, 2:821
Rocky Mountain spotted fever, 2:826
swimmer's ear and swimmer's itch, 2:933
tick-borne disease, 2:958
tularemia, 2:989, 991
Venezuelan equine encephalitis virus, 2:1035
viral diseases, 2:1041
West Nile virus, 2:1061
Zika virus, 2:1102
Insect-borne diseases. *See* Arthropod-borne diseases
Insecticides. *See* Pesticides
Insomnia, 1:3, 2:749
Instances of the Communication of Cholera through the Medium of Polluted Water at Newburn on the Tyne, 1:*333*
Institute of Viral Preparations, Russia, 2:897
Institute Pasteur. *See* Pasteur Institute
Integrase strand transfer inhibitors (INSTIs), 1:13
Integrated Disease Surveillance and Response program, 1:169
Integrated vector management, 1:463*s*, 2:639
Intellectual disability, 1:80, 215, *216*, 2:836, 837
Intensified Smallpox Eradication Program, 2:891, 896
Intensive care units
candidiasis risk factors, 1:159
nosocomial infections, 2:675
opportunistic infections, 2:683, 684
pneumonia, 2:725, 728, 729
public health, 2:765
tetanus, 2:954
toxic shock, 2:961, 962
Interferons
anti-cytokine antibody syndrome, 1:53
antiviral drugs, 1:71
hepatitis C, 1:431–432
hepatitis D, 1:435
Intergovernmental Panel on Climate Change, 2:696
Interleukin 6, 1:53
Interleukin-1 inhibitors, 2:576
Intermediate hosts, 1:461
Intermediate leprosy, 1:545
Intermediate-level disinfection, 1:280
Internally displaced persons, 1:438, 472, 473
International adoption, 1:474–475
International Agency for the Prevention of Blindness, 2:822
International Alliance for the Control of Scabies, 2:854
International Association of National Public Health Institutes, 1:164
International Center for Research on Women, 1:73
International Centre for Diarrhoeal Diseases Research, 2:664
International Classification of Diseases, 2:787
International Code of Marketing of Breast-milk Substitutes, 2:1003
International Committee on the Taxonomy of Viruses, 1:20, 30
International Consortium on Combating Wildlife Crime, 2:1085
International cooperation
avian influenza prevention and control, 1:89–90
Buruli ulcer programs, 1:150
CDC, 1:164, 169
DNA databases, 1:363
globalization and infectious disease, 1:385
isolation and quarantine, 1:510
liver fluke infections prevention, 1:563
outbreaks, field-level response to, 2:686–687
pneumonia prevention, 2:730
International Emerging Infections Program, CDC, 1:385
International Health Division, Rockefeller Foundation, 2:1043
International Health Regulations
immigration, 1:474
legislation and international law, 1:536–537
notifiable diseases, 2:681
public health, 2:763
SARS, 2:851
World Health Organization, 2:1076
world trade, 2:1084
International law. *See* Legislation and international law
International Network for the Rational Use of Drugs, 1:271
International Network to Promote Household Water Treatment and Safe Storage, 1:29, 2:1055
International Red Cross
legislation and international law, 1:535
outbreaks, field-level response to, 2:687
tsunami lung, 2:730
International Sanitary Regulations, 2:1076
International Society for Infectious Diseases, 2:751–752
International Standards for Tuberculosis Care, 2:987
International Trachoma Initiative, 2:967
"Internationally Adopted Children--Immigration Status," 1:*474–475*
Internet resources
FluNet, 1:503
Global Public Health Intelligence Network, 2:1077
HIV Risk Reduction Tool, 1:455*s*
ProMED, 2:752
public health, 2:762
Intertrigo, 1:159
Intestinal flora
bacteria, positive role of, 1:411
Clostridium difficile infection, 1:210, 211, 212–213
Koch's postulates exceptions, 1:520*s*
puerperal fever, 2:769

Intestinal gas
cyclosporiasis, 1:259
giardiasis, 1:371
hookworm infection, 1:458
water-borne disease, 2:1054
Intestinal perforation, 1:103
Intestinal tract obstruction, 1:79, 80
Intracellular infections, 1:53
Intramuscular injections, 1:142
Intravenous antibiotics
bacterial meningitis, 2:606
glanders, 1:380
group B streptococcal infections, 2:925
leptospirosis, 1:549
Lyme disease controversies, 1:573
MRSA, 2:642
Staphylococcus aureus infections, 2:913
tsunami lung, 2:730
vancomycin-resistant *Enterococci*, 2:1027
Intravenous catheters
biofilms, 2:802*s*
candidiasis risk factors, 1:158–159
nosocomial infection prevention, 2:675
Intravenous corticosteroids, 1:318
Intravenous fluids
Campylobacter infection, 1:151
cholera, 1:198
dysentery, 1:290
Powassan virus, 2:742
rotavirus infection, 2:830
St. Louis encephalitis, 2:906
Intravenous immune globulin, 2:954
Introduced diseases and endemicity development, 1:321
Inuits, 2:973
Invasive infections
aspergillosis, 1:53
candidiasis, 1:158–159, 159–160
group A streptococcal infections, 2:920, 922
group B streptococcal infections, 2:925
Invasive species as vectors, 1:385
Iodine, 1:281
Iodoquinol, 1:103
Iowa, 1:317
IR3535, 2:907, 1035*s*
Iran
avian influenza, 1:89
balantidiasis, 1:103
leishmaniasis, 1:539
microsporidiosis, 2:624*s*
Pneumocystis jirovecii pneumonia, 2:721
trachoma, 2:968*s*
Iraq
avian influenza, 1:88
demographics, 1:261
leishmaniasis, 1:541
war, 2:1050, 1052
Iraq War, 1:59, 2:1048–1049
Ireland, 1:137, 2:998
Iron deficiency. *See* Anemia
Iron lungs, 2:*738*
Iron supplementation and whipworm, 2:1063
Irradiation, food, 1:260, 356*s*
Irrigation and encephalitis, 1:317
Irritability
ear infections, 1:293
enterovirus 71 infection, 1:325
macrophage activation syndrome, 2:575
pinworm infection, 2:705
protozoan diseases, 2:753
viral meningitis, 2:608
Irritable bowel syndrome, 1:152, 371
Ishaq, Sauid, 1:411
Island nations and climate change, 2:757
Isodid ticks, 1:243
Isolation and quarantine, 1:**508–510,** *509*
animal importation, 1:40
contact precautions, 1:237
diphtheria, 1:276
extremely drug-resistant tuberculosis, 2:986
glanders, 1:380
globalization and infectious disease, 1:385
hemorrhagic fevers prevention, 1:420
immigration, 1:474
imported animals, 2:778
infection control and asepsis, 1:484
influenza pandemic of 1957, 1:501
Lassa fever, 1:527
legislation and international law, 1:533, 535, 536
leprosy, 1:544, 546, 547
pandemic preparedness, 2:692
plague, 2:712, 718
public health, 2:764
Rift Valley fever, 2:816
SARS, 2:849, 850–851
smallpox, 2:893
typhoid fever, 2:995*s*
USAMRIID, 2:1016
vancomycin-resistant *Enterococci*, 2:1027
Israel
avian influenza, 1:89
chickenpox vaccine, 1:177
zoonoses, 2:1106
Italy
avian influenza, 1:89, 491
bloodborne infections transmitted through barber shops, 1:131*s*
chickenpox vaccine, 1:177
chikungunya, 1:*180*
immigration, 1:474
lice infestation, 1:554
malaria, 2:579
plague, early history of, 2:711
quarantine, 1:508, 533
relapsing fever, 2:796, 797
Itching
African sleeping sickness, 1:5
B virus infection, 1:92
chickenpox, 1:176
helminth disease, 1:415
herpes simplex virus 2, 1:444
hookworm infection, 1:458
lice infestation, 1:552
marine toxins, 2:591
pinworm infection, 2:705
river blindness, 2:820
scabies, 2:852
schistosomiasis, 2:861
sexually transmitted infections, 2:878
shingles, 2:886, 887
smallpox, 2:890
swimmer's ear and swimmer's itch, 2:931, 932, 933
trichinellosis, 2:973
trichomoniasis, 2:976
vaccine reactions, 2:1022
yaws, 2:1087
Itraconazole
aspergillosis, 1:85
blastomycosis, 1:122
coccidioidomycosis, 1:221
ringworm, 2:818
sporotrichosis, 2:902
talaromycosis, 2:945
Ivanovski, Dmitri, 2:1043
Ivermectin
developing nations and drug delivery, 1:270, 272
lice infestation, 1:553
river blindness, 2:820, 821, *821*, 822
scabies, 2:854
strongyloidiasis, 2:929, 930
tropical infectious diseases, 2:981
Ivins, Bruce, 1:48, 2:1017
Ivory Coast. *See* Cote d'Ivoire
IXIARO vaccine, 1:318
Ixodes ticks, 2:*871*
babesiosis, 1:95
Lyme disease, 1:569, 572
Powassan virus, 2:741
tick-borne diseases, 2:957, 958

J

Jackals, 1:539, 2:776
Jail fever. *See* Typhus
Jakarta, Indonesia, 1:198, 2:*1053, 1072*
Jamaica, 1:472
Janssen, Hans, 2:618

Janssen, Zacharias, 2:618
Japan
alveolar echinococcosis, 1:24
anisakiasis, 1:*43,* 45
anthrax, 1:47, 50
antibiotic resistance, 1:62
antimicrobial soaps, 1:67
Aum Shinrikyo attack, 1:304
bacterial meningitis, 2:604
bloodborne infections transmitted through barber shops, 1:131*s*
burkholderia, 1:146*s*
chickenpox vaccine, 1:177
encephalitis, 1:318
glanders, 1:381
hand, foot, and mouth disease, 1:397
hepatitis D, 1:434
hepatitis E, 1:438
hookworm infection, 1:58
human research subjects, 1:344
influenza epidemiology, 1:506
Japanese encephalitis, 1:511–512, 513–514
Kawasaki disease, 1:515
leprosy, 1:546*s*
lung flukes, 1:566
MRSA, 2:640
ProMED, 2:752
retroviruses, 2:806
severe fever with thrombocytopenia syndrome, 2:872
smallpox, 2:893
taeniasis, 2:942
talaromycosis, 2:945
tick-borne diseases, 2:957
triclosan, 2:916
tularemia, 2:989
whipworm, 2:1063
Japanese descent and Kawasaki disease, 1:517
Japanese encephalitis, 1:77, 318, **511–514,** *512*
Jaundice
hepatitis A, 1:422–425
hepatitis B, 1:426
hepatitis C, 1:430
hepatitis D, 1:434
hepatitis E, 1:437
leptospirosis, 1:548
malaria, 2:580
Marburg hemorrhagic fever, 2:586
mononucleosis, 2:631
protozoan diseases, 2:753
relapsing fever, 2:796
toxoplasmosis, 2:964
yellow fever, 2:1092
Java, 1:36
Jefferson, David, 1:*297*
Jenner, Edward
germ theory of disease, 1:366
smallpox, 2:891, 896
smallpox vaccine, 1:184
vaccines, 2:1020
Jewish persecution, 2:712
Jimmy and Rosalyn Carter Humanitarian Award, 2:1079
Jirovec, Otto, 2:722
Jock itch, 2:650, 817
John Cunningham virus, 2:683
Johns Hopkins University, 1:117
Johnson, Karl, 2:1045
Joint Biological Agent Identification and Detection System, 2:1018
Joint Monitoring Programme for Water Supply, Sanitation and Hygiene, 2:1079
Joint United Kingdom Blood Transfusion and Tissue Transplantation Services Professional Committee, 1:126
Joint United Nations Programme on HIV and AIDS. *See* UNAIDS
Joints and joint pain
African sleeping sickness, 1:5
blastomycosis, 1:122
cat scratch disease, 1:161–163
chikungunya, 1:*180,* 181, 182
coccidioidomycosis, 1:218, 219
congenital Zika syndrome, 2:1101
cryptosporidiosis, 1:252
dengue and dengue hemorrhagic fever, 1:267
fifth disease, 1:347, 348
gonorrhea, 1:388
group A streptococcal infections, 2:921
group B streptococcal infections, 2:925
Haemophilus influenzae, 1:395
hepatitis B, 1:426
hepatitis D, 1:434
Lyme disease, 1:569, 571
rat-bite fever, 2:785, 787, 788
relapsing fever, 2:795
Rocky Mountain spotted fever, 2:824
schistosomiasis, 2:861
sporotrichosis, 2:901
tick-borne diseases, 2:958
trichinellosis, 2:973
tularemia, 2:989, 990
vector-borne disease, 2:1029
yersiniosis, 2:1097
Zika virus, 2:1101
Jones, Joseph, 2:657
Jordan, 1:89, 541
Journal of Clinical Investigation, 1:415–416, 2:1023
Journal of Experimental Medicine, 1:478*s*
Journal of Family Practice, 1:491
Journal of General Virology, 1:31
Journal of Infectious Diseases
chickenpox vaccine, 1:179
influenza pandemic of 1957, 1:499
National Institute of Allergy and Infectious Diseases, 2:655
women and infectious disease, 2:1071
Zika virus vaccine development, 2:1022–1023
Journal of the American Medical Association, 2:739
Journal of Virology, 1:325, 2:779
Journal of Virus Eradication, 1:217
Journals, CDC, 1:168
June, Carl H., 1:479
Jungle fever, 2:1046
Junin virus, 1:418
Juquitiba virus, 1:406
Justice, patients' right to, 2:987
Justinian (Roman emperor), 2:710
Justinian plague, 2:710–711, 714, 716

K

Kabul, Afghanistan, 1:*291, 539*
Kalazar. *See* Visceral leishmaniasis
Kaliningrad, Russia, 1:277
Kampala, Uganda, 1:147
Kampuchea, 1:561
Kandahar, Afghanistan, 1:278
Kansas, 2:795, 873*s*
Kaplan, Sarah, 1:523
Kaposi's sarcoma
AIDS, 1:8, 12, 18, 19
antiviral drugs, 1:73
cancer, 1:155
opportunistic infections, 2:683
sexually transmitted infections, 2:877
viral disease, 2:1039
Katayama fever, 2:861
Katz, Rebecca, 2:1084
Kawasaki, Tomisaku, 1:515
Kawasaki disease, 1:**515–518,** *516,* 517*t,* 2:575
Kaya, Rolland, 1:5
Kazakhstan, 1:89, 277
Kennedy, Cheryl, 2:707
Kentucky
babesiosis, 1:96
heartland virus, 2:873*s*
hepatitis B, 1:428
histoplasmosis, 1:449
impetigo, 1:480
Kenya
African sleeping sickness, 1:3
leishmaniasis, 1:539
malaria vaccine, 1:205, 2:581
plague, 2:716
re-emerging infectious diseases, 2:790
Rift Valley fever, 2:813, 815, 816
Kerala, India, 1:*180*
Keratitis, 1:232–233, 442*s*
Keratoconjunctivitis, 2:624*s,* 1039
Kerions, 2:817

Kern County, CA, 1:221
Ketoconazole, 1:221, 2:818, 945
Key, George, 2:937
"The Key to Keeping Lice at Bay? A Lot of Hot Air," 1:*554*
Khabarovsk, Russia, 2:*609,* 610
Khon Kaen University, 1:563
Khutu, Diana, 1:122
Kid Power, UNICEF, 2:1004
Kidney dialysis, 1:340, 341, 432*s,* 531
Kidney disease or symptoms
  babesiosis, 1:95, 96–97
  blastomycosis, 1:122
  cholera, 1:198
  dysentery, 1:289
  Escherichia coli O157:H7, 1:338, 339, 340
  food-borne disease, 1:354, 356
  glanders, 1:379
  group A streptococcal infections, 2:921
  hantavirus, 1:404
  herpes simplex 1 virus, 1:442
  impetigo, 1:482
  Legionnaires' disease, 1:530, 531
  leptospirosis, 1:548
  malaria, 2:580
  nocardiosis, 2:666
  protozoan diseases, 2:753
  rickettsial disease, 2:810
  Rocky Mountain spotted fever, 2:824
  scabies, 2:853
  strep throat, 2:917
  tuberculosis risk factors, 2:984
  tularemia, 2:990
  typhus, 2:998
  urinary tract infection, 2:1012, 1013, 1014
  viral disease, 2:1039
  yellow fever, 2:1092
Kidney transplantation, 1:341
Kilbourne, Frederick L., 1:95
King, Charles H., 2:863
The King's Evil. *See* Scrofula
Kinshasa, Congo, 1:17–18
Kinshasa, Democratic Republic of the Congo, 2:995
Kinyoun, Joseph J., 2:653–654
Kiragu, Andrew, 2:597
Kirby-Bauer disc diffusion susceptibility test, 1:256
Kisangani, Democratic Republic of Congo, 1:243
Kissing bugs, 1:172
Kissing disease. *See* Mononucleosis
Kissinger, Patricia, 2:976
Klasing, Amanda, 2:1108
Klebsiella infection, 1:62
Klein, Sabra, 2:1074
Koch, Robert, 1:*254, 368, 520*
  anthrax, 1:47
  culture and sensitivity techniques, 1:254–255
  germ theory, 1:200, 367
  Koch's postulates, 1:369*s,* 519–521
  microorganisms, 2:615–616
Koch's postulates, 1:254–255, **519–521**
KOH test, 1:122
Kolkata, India, 1:198
Koltsovo, Russia, 1:168, 2:1051
Koplik spots, 2:593, 594
Korea
  emerging infectious diseases, 1:312
  encephalitis, 1:318
  hemorrhagic fevers, 1:419, 420
  liver fluke infections, 1:562
  typhus, 2:998
Krishnaswami, C. S., 1:379
Kruse, Walter M., 1:228
Kunimoto, Mamoru, 1:546*s*
Kunming, China, 1:*384*
Kurds, 1:261
Kuru, 1:138*s,* 241, **522–525,** 2:749
Kuwait, 1:89, 2:652
Kwakye-Maclean, Cynthia, 2:1090
Kwan Sui-Chu, 2:848, 970–971
KwaZulu-Natal Province, South Africa, 2:791
Kwok, Robert, 1:278
Kyasanur Forest disease, 1:419

L

La Crosse encephalitis, 1:317, 2:1106
Labeling, food, 1:357
Labor and employment issues
  dracunculiasis, 1:284–285
  economic development, 1:307
  plague, 2:712
  tuberculosis patients' rights, 2:988
Laboratories and laboratory workers
  B virus infection, 1:91–92, 93
  brucellosis, 1:142
  Chagas disease, 1:172
  culture and sensitivity, 1:254–257
  glanders, 1:380
  hemorrhagic fevers, 1:420*s*
  infection control and asepsis, 1:486
  monkeypox, 2:627
  typhus, 2:1001
Laboratory of Hygiene, 2:653–654
Lactobacillus, 1:211, 354
Lafferty, Kevin D., 2:697, 698
Laguna Negra virus, 1:406
Lake Chad basin countries, 1:473
Lambeth Company, 1:329
Lancefield, Rebecca, 2:920–921
Lancefield groups, 2:920–921
Lancet
  Ebola vaccine, 2:1022
  MMR vaccine, 2:1021
  pinworm infection, 2:706
  river blindness, 2:821
  undernutrition, 1:205
  yellow fever, 2:1095
Lancet Global Health, 2:814, 922
Lancet Infectious Diseases
  scarlet fever, 2:858
  schistosomiasis, 2:863
  whooping cough, 2:1067
Land use issues, 1:451
Landsteiner, Karl, 2:736
Lansoprazole, 1:411
Laos
  burkholderia, 1:145
  glanders, 1:380
  liver fluke infections, 1:561
  lung flukes, 1:566
  trachoma, 2:968*s*
  trichinellosis, 2:974
"The Largest Q Fever Outbreak Ever Reported," 2:*773*
Larvae
  dracunculiasis, 1:283, 284
  filariasis, 1:350, 351*s*
  hookworm infection, 1:457
  lung flukes, 1:565–566
  Lyme disease, 1:571
  parasitic diseases, 2:695
  pinworm infection, 2:705
  strongyloidiasis, 2:928
  swimmer's ear and swimmer's itch, 2:931
  taeniasis, 2:940–943
  tapeworm infections, 2:949
  trichinellosis, 2:972, 973, 974
Larvicides, 2:822
Laryngitis, 1:194
Lasker Award, 2:601–602
Lassa fever, 1:**526–528,** *527*
  globalization, 1:383
  hemorrhagic fevers, 1:418
  USAMRIID, 2:1016
Latency
  Epstein-Barr virus, 1:335, 337
  sexually transmitted infections, 2:877
  syphilis, 2:935
  tuberculosis, 2:983
  yaws, 2:1087, 1089–1090
  See also Dormancy
Latin America
  amebiasis, 1:28
  arthropod-borne diseases, 1:76*s*
  avian influenza, 1:156
  candidiasis, 1:160
  Chagas disease, 1:171, 172, 173
  cholera, 1:199, 201
  climate change, 1:206
  dengue and dengue hemorrhagic fever, 1:266, 267
  developing nations and drug delivery, 1:271
  diphtheria, 1:276
  environmental health risks, 2:1077

gastroenteritis, 1:358–361
hepatitis E, 1:438
histoplasmosis, 1:448
maternal mortality, 2:769
mosquito-borne diseases, 2:637
parasitic diseases, 2:695
plague, 2:715, 716, 717
rabies, 2:777
sanitation, 2:844
taeniasis, 2:942
tapeworm infections, 2:949
travel, 2:970
trichinellosis, 2:973
tropical infectious diseases, 2:981
United Nations Millennium Goals, 2:1009
yaws, 2:1087, 1088
Latvia, 1:277
Lavage, 1:54
Lawa Lake Project, 1:563–564
Lawsuits, 1:510
Lazear, Jesse, 1:342–343, 344, 2:1043, 1094, 1095
League of Nations, 2:737, 1076
Leahy, Patrick, 1:48
Learning disabilities and hookworm infection, 1:459
Lebanon, 1:541
Lechiguanas virus, 1:406
Leeuwenhoek, Antoni van, 2:*615*
germ theory of disease, 1:366
giardiasis, 1:371
microorganisms, 2:615
microscopes and microscopy, 2:618
Leg pain, 2:787, 935
Legionnaires' disease, 1:169, *529*, **529–532**
Legislation and international law, 1:**533–537**
Biological Weapons Convention, 1:47, 109–111
bioterrorism preparedness, 2:1051*s*
Chengdu Declaration for Action, 2:943
Convention on the Rights of the Child, 2:1003
Declaration of Helsinki, 1:344, 2:937
Declaration of the Rights of the Child, 2:1003
disinfections, 1:282
isolation and quarantine, 2:986
Paris Climate Agreement, 1:206
Public Health Service Act, 1:508
smallpox, 2:893–894
trichinellosis, 2:974
United Nations Convention on the Rights of the Child, 2:1004
USA PATRIOT Act, 1:111*s*
Vaccination Act, UK, 2:891
Vaccination Assistance Act, 1:185
Leiden Medical Center, 1:212
Leidy, Joseph, 2:972
Leishmaniasis, 1:**538–542,** *539, 540*
parasitic diseases, 2:695
protozoan diseases, 2:754, 755
tropical infectious diseases, 2:980, 981
Lemming fever. *See* Tularemia
Lenze, Paul E., Jr., 1:264
Leopards and the wildlife trade, 2:1083
Lepromatous leprosy, 1:545–546
Leprosy, 1:**543–547,** *544*
Koch's postulates exceptions, 1:520*s*
tropical infectious diseases, 2:980, 981, 981*s*
World Health Organization, 2:1078
Leprosy Prevention Law (Japan), 1:546*s*
Leptospirosis, 1:205, **548–551,** *549,* 2:1106
Lesions
anthrax, 1:*48*, 49
B virus infection, 1:92
blastomycosis, 1:122, 123
Buruli ulcer, 1:147–150
dracunculiasis, 1:283
glanders, 1:379
gonorrhea, 1:388
hand, foot, and mouth disease, 1:397
herpes simplex virus 2, 1:444
histoplasmosis, 1:449
impetigo, 1:480, *481*
leishmaniasis, 1:538, 539, *539,* 539–540, 541
leprosy, 1:543, 545
leptospirosis, 1:549*s*
nocardiosis, 2:666
protozoan diseases, 2:754
ringworm, 2:817, 818
scrofula, 2:865, 866
sexually transmitted infections, 2:877
smallpox, 2:891, 892
sporotrichosis, 2:901, 902
syphilis, 2:877, 934
talaromycosis, 2:944–945
yaws, 2:1087, 1089, 1090
Lesotho, 2:792
Less developed nations. *See* Developing nations
Lethargy, 2:575, 666
"Letter: Louseborne Relapsing Fever in Young Migrants, Sicily, Italy, July-September 2015," 2:*797–798*
Lettuce and cyclosporiasis outbreaks, 1:258
Leucovorin. *See* Folinic acid
Leukemia, 2:929, 1041
Leukocytosis, 2:944
Leukopenia, 1:267
Levine, Bruce L., 1:479
Levofloxacin
Legionnaires' disease, 1:531
plague, 2:718
pneumonia, 2:718
typhus, 2:1000
Lewis, Kim, 2:676
Liberia
Ebola, 1:302, 2:1085
field-level response to Ebola outbreak, 2:*685*
Lassa fever, 1:526, 527, 527*s*
Médecins Sans Frontières, 2:601
public health, 2:765
Libya, 2:797–798
Lice infestation, 1:**552–555,** *553.* *See also* Louse-borne diseases
Life cycle
lung flukes, 1:*566*
protozoa, 2:757
strongyloidiasis, 2:928
tapeworms, 2:948, *949*
toxoplasmosis, 2:964
whipworm, 2:1062
Life expectancy, 2:1010*s,* 1079
Life sciences and bioterrorism, 1:118
Lifelong immunity
chickenpox, 1:177
endemic typhus, 2:998
fifth disease, 1:348
hepatitis B vaccine, 1:428
measles, 2:593
mumps, 2:644
St. Louis encephalitis, 2:905
Lifetime prevalence, 1:330
Ligase change reaction, 1:364
Light field microscopy, 2:620
Light microscopes, 2:618–619
Light sensitivity. *See* Photosensitivity
Light therapy. *See* Phototherapy
Limb issues
Buruli ulcer, 1:148
fetal development and maternal chickenpox, 1:177
malaria, 2:580
typhus, 2:997, 998
Limbic encephalitis, 1:316
Limmathurotsakul, Direk, 1:381
Lindane shampoo, 1:553
Linens. *See* Bedding
Linezolid, 2:1027
Lipopolysaccharides, 2:841
Liposomal amphotericin B, 1:540, 541, 2:755
Liposome preparations, 1:248
Lister, Joseph
airborne precautions, 1:21
antibacterial drugs, 1:56
contact precautions, 1:235
disinfection, 1:280
germ theory of disease, 1:367
infection control, 1:400, 484
Listeriosis, 1:356, **556–558,** *557*
Lithuania
diphtheria, 1:277
international adoption, 1:475

plague, 2:712
smallpox, 2:890
Little Ice Age, 2:711
Liu Jianlun, 2:847, 970
Live virus vaccines. *See* Attenuated vaccines
Liver cancer
avian influenza, 1:156
cancer, 1:154, 155, 155*s*
hepatitis B, 1:426, 427, 428
hepatitis C, 1:432
hepatitis D, 1:434
viral disease, 2:1039
Liver disease or symptoms
amebiasis, 1:27
ascariasis, 1:79
avian influenza, 1:89, 156
babesiosis, 1:95, 96
Baylisascaris infection, 1:105
brucellosis, 1:141
cat scratch disease, 1:161–163
Cryptococcus neoformans infection, 1:248
dysentery, 1:289, 290
glanders, 1:379
helminth disease, 1:415
hepatitis A, 1:422–425
hepatitis B, 1:426–428, 427, 428
hepatitis C, 1:430–432, 431
hepatitis D, 1:434–436
hepatitis E, 1:437–439
leishmaniasis, 1:538
liver fluke infections, 1:560
macrophage activation syndrome, 2:575–576
malaria, 2:580
Marburg hemorrhagic fever, 2:586
mononucleosis, 2:631, 634
nocardiosis, 2:666
protozoan diseases, 2:754, 755
psittacosis, 2:759
relapsing fever, 2:795, 796
rickettsial disease, 2:810
rubella, 2:837
schistosomiasis, 2:861
strongyloidiasis, 2:929
talaromycosis, 2:944
tularemia, 2:989, 990
viral disease, 2:1039
water-borne disease, 2:1054
yellow fever, 2:1092
Liver failure
CMV infection, 1:216
hepatitis D, 1:435
leptospirosis, 1:548
Marburg hemorrhagic fever, 2:586
talaromycosis, 2:945
Liver fluke infections, 1:*560*, **560–564**
Liver tissue test for brucellosis, 1:142
Liver transplantation, 1:428, 435
Liverpool, England, 2:795
Liverpool School of Tropical Medicine, 2:1031
Livestock
animal importation, 1:39, 40, *40*
anthrax, 1:47, 50
antibiotic resistance, 1:63, 64
antibiotics, 2:1027–1028
avian influenza, 1:88–89
balantidiasis, 1:102, 103
bovine spongiform encephalopathy, 1:136–139, 241–242
brucellosis, 1:140–142, 141–142
burkholderia, 1:142, 145, 146
Campylobacter infection, 1:152–153
Crimean-Congo hemorrhagic fever, 1:243, 244, 245
cryptosporidiosis, 1:251
deworming, 2:950
Escherichia coli O157:H7, 1:338, 339, 340–341
food-borne disease, 1:355, 356
hemorrhagic fevers, 1:419
histoplasmosis, 1:449
H5N1 virus, 1:392*s*, 393
hosts and vectors, 1:*462*
leptospirosis, 1:548, 549
listeriosis, 1:556
liver fluke infections, 1:561, 562
microbial evolution, 2:611, *612*, 614
Nipah virus infection, 2:662, 663–664
President's Initiative on Combating Antibiotic Resistance, 2:745–746
prion disease, 2:748, 749, 750
protozoan diseases, 2:754
psittacosis, 2:760
Q fever, 2:771–773, *772*, 773
resistant organisms, 2:801, 802, 803
Rift Valley fever, 2:813, 815, 816
Salmonella infection, 2:841
Staphylococcus aureus infections, 2:912
taeniasis, 2:940, 941, 942
tapeworm infections, 2:948
toxoplasmosis, 2:964
transmissible spongiform encephalopathies, 1:523
trichinellosis, 2:974
Venezuelan equine encephalitis virus, 2:1033
war, 2:1051
zoonoses, 2:1106
Lo, Nathan C., 2:863
Loa loa, 1:351*s*, 2:821
Lobsters, 2:591
Lockjaw. *See* Tetanus
Loeffler, Friedrich, 2:1043
Logging, 2:664
London, England
epidemiology, 1:328, 329
On the Mode of Communication of Cholera (Snow), 1:333
plague, 2:712
sanitation, 2:844
typhus, 2:998
London School, 2:1095
Lone Star ticks, 2:873*s*
Loney, Sydney, 1:123
Long-term care facilities. *See* Nursing homes and long-term care facilities
Lopinavir, 1:13
Los Angeles, CA
AIDS pandemic history, 1:18, 19*s*
hepatitis A, 1:424
mitten crabs, 1:567
plague, 2:717
Los Angeles Times, 1:491, 2:675
Louis XVI, 2:865
Louisiana
dengue, 1:266
Hurricane Katrina, 1:201, 207
leprosy treatment center, 1:545
St. Louis encephalitis, 2:906
Louisville, KY, 1:480
Louse-borne diseases, 2:*796*
parasitic diseases, 2:694
relapsing fever, 2:795, 796–797, *797–798*
sexually transmitted infections, 2:878
typhus, 2:997, 998, 999, 1000–1001
war, 2:1048
See also Lice infestation
LouseBuster, 1:554
Low birth weight
candidiasis risk factors, 1:159
malaria, 2:581
pneumonia risk factors, 2:727
urinary tract infection, 2:1013
Low body temperature and relapsing fever, 2:795
Low body weight as tuberculosis risk factor, 2:984
Low socioeconomic status. *See* Socioeconomic status
Low-level disinfection, 1:280
Lu Han, Kang Li, 1:327
Lubombo Spatial Development Initiative, 1:206
Lumbar puncture. *See* Cerebrospinal fluid tests
Lumsden, W. H. R., 1:181
Lung biopsy, 2:667
Lung disease or symptoms
anthrax, 1:47
anti-cytokine antibody syndrome, 1:53, 54
ascariasis, 1:79
aspergillosis, 1:84–86
bacterial diseases, 1:100
blastomycosis, 1:121–124
botulism, 1:135
burkholderia, 1:144, 146

cat scratch disease, 1:161–163
coccidioidomycosis, 1:221
cryptosporidiosis, 1:251
glanders, 1:379
hantavirus, 1:404
helminth disease, 1:415
histoplasmosis, 1:448–449, *450*
hookworm infection, 1:458
hot tub rash, 1:465, 466–467
with influenza, 1:489
Legionnaires' disease, 1:529–531
lung flukes, 1:565–568
microsporidiosis, 2:623
with MRSA, 2:642
mycotic disease, 2:650
nocardiosis, 2:666, 667
Pneumocystis jirovecii pneumonia, 2:721–724
pneumonia, 2:626, 725–731, 726
RSV infection, 2:832–835
SEB intoxication, 2:1052
sporotrichosis, 2:901, 902
strongyloidiasis, 2:929
talaromycosis, 2:944
tuberculosis, 2:983–988
tularemia, 2:989, 990
water-borne disease, 2:1054
Lung flukes, 1:*565,* **565–568,** *566*
Lunkov, Nikolai, 1:*110*
Luzon, Philippines, 1:*351*
Lyme, CT, 1:570
Lyme disease, 1:**569–574**
blastomycosis *vs.,* 1:121
climate change, 1:206, 2:698
Rocky Mountain Laboratory, 2:656
tick-borne diseases, 2:956–957, 958
vector-borne disease, 2:1029
zoonoses, 2:1107
LYMErix, 1:572
Lymph gland swelling or pain. *See* Gland swelling or pain
Lymph node biopsy, 2:756, 945
Lymph node swelling or pain
African sleeping sickness, 1:2
AIDS, 1:19
brucellosis, 1:141
cat scratch disease, 1:161–163, 162, 162*s*
dengue and dengue hemorrhagic fever, 1:267
filariasis, 1:350
herpes gladiatorum, 1:442*s*
herpes simplex virus 2, 1:444
HIV, 1:11
Kawasaki disease, 1:515
Lyme disease, 1:569
macrophage activation syndrome, 2:575–576
monkeypox, 2:628*s*
mononucleosis, 2:630, 631, 634
nocardiosis, 2:666
plague, 1:116, 2:715
scrofula, 2:866
sexually transmitted infections, 2:877
swimmer's ear and swimmer's itch, 2:932
talaromycosis, 2:944
toxoplasmosis, 2:964
West Nile virus, 2:1059
yaws, 2:1087
Lymphatic filariasis. *See* Filariasis
Lymphatic system
blastomycosis, 1:122
immune response, 1:477–478
sporotrichosis, 2:901
tularemia, 2:989
Lymphedema, 1:350, 351, 352, 478
Lymphocytes, 2:634
Lymphocytic choriomeningitis, 2:1041
Lymphogranuloma venereum, 1:190
Lymphoma
AIDS, 1:12
cancer, 1:155
Helicobacter pylori, 1:411
strongyloidiasis with, 2:929
Lymphopenia and avian influenza, 1:89
Lysol, 1:281
Lyssavirus. See Rabies

M

M proteins, 2:921
Mabey, David, 2:1089
Macaque monkeys, 1:*91,* 91–94, 2:581, 926–927
Macedonia, 2:579
Machupo virus, 1:418
Mackerel, 1:45
Macrolides, 1:189–191
Macrophage activation syndrome, 2:**575–577**
Macrophages and the immune system, 2:576*s*
Macrotube dilution susceptibility test, 1:256
Mad cow disease. *See* Bovine spongiform encephalopathy
Madagascar
angiostrongyliasis, 1:36
arthropod-borne diseases, 1:75
influenza, 1:491
leprosy, 1:546, 2:1078
plague, 1:13, 2:715, *717,* 717–718
Madeira Islands, 1:267
Magnetic resonance imaging, 2:667
Mahajan, Vikram K., 2:902
Maharashtra, India, 2:839
Mahler, Halfdan T., 1:220
Maine, 1:571
Major histocompatibility complex, 1:476
Malacidin, 2:675–676
Malaise
hemorrhagic fevers, 1:420*s*
hepatitis A, 1:422
hepatitis B, 1:426
hepatitis D, 1:434
hepatitis E, 1:437
herpes gladiatorum, 1:442*s*
mumps, 2:645
SARS, 2:847
sexually transmitted infections, 2:877
shigellosis, 2:883
typhoid fever, 2:995*s*
vaccine reactions, 2:1022
Malaria, 2:*578,* **578–584**
arthropod-borne diseases, 1:75, 77
babesiosis *vs.,* 1:96
CDC, 1:165
climate change, 1:204, 207
DDT, 2:1045
dengue and dengue hemorrhagic fever *vs.,* 1:266
economic development, 1:309
emerging infectious diseases, 1:312–313
endemicity, 1:321, 322, 322*s*
hosts and vectors, 1:461, 462
immigration, 1:472, 473
infection control and asepsis, 1:486
Médecins Sans Frontières, 1:5, 2:601
mosquito-borne diseases, 2:637, 638
opportunistic infections, 2:684
parasitic diseases, 2:695, 696
protozoan diseases, 2:753, 755, 756
re-emerging infectious diseases, 2:790–791, 791*s*
resistant organisms, 2:802
travel, 2:971
treated bed nets and the lifespan of mosquitoes, 2:1031–1032
tropical infectious diseases, 2:979–980, 981, 982
UNICEF, 2:1005
United Nations Millennium Goals, 2:1008, 1009, 1010
vector-borne disease, 2:1029, 1030–1031
women, 2:1072
zoonoses, 2:1105, 1107
Malarone. *See* Atovaquone; Proguanil
Malathion, 1:553, 2:853
Malawi
African sleeping sickness, 1:3
AIDS, 1:8
child marriage laws, 1:15
malaria vaccine, 1:205, 2:581
plague, 2:716

re-emerging infectious diseases, 2:790
typhoid fever, 2:996
Malawista, Stephen E., 1:570
Malaysia
avian influenza, 1:88, 89
burkholderia, 1:145
enterovirus 71 infection, 1:325, 326
glanders, 1:380
hand, foot, and mouth disease, 1:397, 398
Nipah virus infection, 2:662, 663, 664
Males, Michelle, 1:*339*
Mali, 1:1, 169, 2:688
Mallon, Mary ("Typhoid Mary"), 2:993, 995*s*
Malnutrition
ascariasis, 1:79, 80
candidiasis risk factors, 1:158
climate change, 1:205
cryptosporidiosis-related death risk factors, 1:253
diphtheria, 1:277
dracunculiasis, 1:285
filariasis, 1:352
helminth disease, 1:417
hookworm infection, 1:458
opportunistic infections, 2:682, 683, 684
Pneumocystis jirovecii pneumonia, 2:721
protozoan diseases, 2:755
typhus, 2:998, 999
Vitamin A Global Initiative, 2:1005
war, 2:1050
whooping cough, 2:1068
women, 2:1072
Malta fever. *See* Brucellosis
Mammals
acariasis, 1:78
anellovirus, 1:30
anisakias and marine mammals, 1:43, *44,* 45
blastomycosis, 1:121
Crimean-Congo hemorrhagic fever, 1:244
Eastern equine encephalitis, 1:296
Ebola, 1:303
giardiasis, 1:371, 372
influenza, 1:494
monkeypox, 2:626
Pneumocystis jirovecii, 2:721
Powassan virus, 2:741
prions, 1:524
rabies, 2:775, *776–777*
rickettsial disease, 2:809, 810
schistosomes, 2:931
sporotrichosis, 2:903
trichinellosis, 2:973
virus hunters, 2:1046
world trade in, 2:1083, 1084
Manchuria, 1:13
Manitoba, Canada, 1:25
Mano River Union Lassa Fever Network, 1:527*s*
Manson, Patrick, 1:343, 2:637
Mansonella infection. *See* Filariasis
Maporal virus, 1:406
Maps
antibiotic prescriptions, 1:*57*
Buruli ulcer distribution, 1:*149*
Chagas disease endemicity, 1:*172*
chikungunya, 1:*181*
CMV infection, 1:*215*
coccidioidomycosis, 1:*220*
Crimean-Congo hemorrhagic fever, 1:*245*
dengue and dengue hemorrhagic fever, 1:*268*
DTP vaccines, 2:*952*
emerging infectious diseases, 1:*311*
enterovirus 71 infection, 1:*325*
glanders, 1:*379*
hantavirus, 1:*406*
hepatitis D, 1:*436*
histoplasmosis, 1:*449*
leishmaniasis, 1:*540*
MRSA, 2:*641*
plague, 2:*718*
Rift Valley fever, 2:*814*
river blindness, 2:*822*
Rocky Mountain spotted fever, 2:*825*
rotavirus infection, 2:*829*
Salmonella infection, 2:*841*
schistosomiasis, 2:*862*
sporotrichosis, 2:*902*
strongyloidiasis, 2:*930*
taeniasis, 2:*942*
West Nile virus, 2:*1059*
Marburg hemorrhagic fever, 2:**585–587,** 586*t*
animal importation, 1:41
hemorrhagic fevers, 1:419, 420, 420*s*
National Institute of Allergy and Infectious Diseases, 2:655
USAMRIID, 2:1018
viral disease, 2:1041
Marchbein, Deane, 2:602
Marcus Aurelius, 2:710
Marginalized groups, 2:600
Marine mammals and anisakiasis, 1:43, 45
Marine microorganisms, 2:591*s*
Marine toxins, 2:*589,* **589–592**
Marler, Bill, 2:671, 672
Marlow, Jeffrey, 2:1046
Mars *Odyssey,* 2:916
Marshall, Barry, 1:343–344, 409, 411, 412*s,* 520–521
Marshall, J. Robin, 1:345
Marston, Barbara J., 2:765
Martinique, 2:1042
Maryland, 1:298*s,* 571
Masks. *See* Personal protective equipment
Mass migration
demographics and infectious disease, 1:261, 263, 264
river blindness, 2:820
typhus, 2:997, 1000
Mass spectrometry, 1:117
Mass vaccination
cholera, 1:199, 200
diphtheria, 1:274, 275, 277–278
measles, 2:594, 595
mumps, 2:645–646
polio, 2:732–734, 740
public health, 2:763
rubella, 2:839
smallpox, 2:897
vaccines and vaccine development, 2:1022, 1023
vs. ring vaccination, 1:115
Massachusetts
babesiosis, 1:96
Lyme disease, 1:571
norovirus infection, 2:671
Powassan virus, 2:742, 742*s*
public health, 2:765–766
Massachusetts General Hospital, 2:730
Mastitis, 2:912
Mastoiditis, 2:857
Mastomys rats, 1:526, 527
Maternal age as pneumonia risk factor, 2:727
Maternal health and the United Nations Millennium Goals, 2:1007
Maternal mortality
group A streptococcal infections, 2:922
Médecins Sans Frontières, 2:602
puerperal fever, 2:767–769
United Nations Millennium Goals, 2:769, 1007
Maternal-to-fetal/child transmission
African seeping sickness, 1:2
AIDS, 1:8, 12–13, 15, 20
antiviral drugs for prevention of, 1:72
Chagas disease, 1:172, 173
chickenpox, 1:177
chikungunya, 1:181
Chlamydia infection, 1:190
CMV infection, 1:214, 215, 216
genital herpes, 1:365
gonorrhea, 1:388
group B streptococcal infection, 2:926–927
group B streptococcal infections, 2:924–927
hepatitis B, 1:426, 427
hepatitis D, 1:434
hepatitis E, 1:437
herpes simplex 1 virus, 1:441, 443
herpes simplex virus 2, 1:445, 446*s*

listeriosis, 1:556
malaria, 2:581
measles, 2:594
mosquito-borne diseases, 2:637
pink eye, 2:702
protozoan diseases, 2:754, 756
rubella, 2:836, 837
scrofula, 2:866
sexually transmitted infections, 2:877
syphilis, 2:936
toxoplasmosis, 2:965–966
trichomoniasis, 2:977
Venezuelan equine encephalitis virus, 2:1035
viral disease, 2:1042
West Nile virus, 2:1060
women, 2:1072
Zika virus, 2:687, 1101
Mathematical demographic models, 1:261–262, 263
Mather, Thomas, 2:958
Mavyret, 1:432
Mayo Clinic, 1:230, 517*s*, 2:954
McCallum, Peter, 1:147
McElvania TeKippe, Erin, 1:32
McGeer, Allison, 2:888
McGuireWoods, 2:671
McMullan, Laura K., 2:873
MDGs. *See* United Nations Millennium Goals
Measles, 2:**593–598,** *594*
childhood vaccination, 1:187
climate change, 1:205
deaths due to, 1:186
endemicity, 1:320–321
globalization, 1:384
infection control and asepsis, 1:487
opportunistic infections, 2:684
United Nations Millennium Goals, 2:1009
vaccination and elimination of, 1:185
vaccine refusal, 1:186
viral disease, 2:1041
viral meningitis, 2:610
WHO childhood vaccination recommendations, 1:185
zoonoses, 2:1106
Measles and Rubella Initiative, 2:595
Meat
AIDS, origins of, 1:17, 18
animal importation, 1:39, 40
anthrax, 1:49
bovine spongiform encephalopathy, 1:136, 137, 138, 139
brucellosis, 1:142*s*
Campylobacter infection, 1:152, 152*s*, 153
Creutzfeldt-Jakob disease, 1:239, 240, 241–242
drug-resistant bacteria, 1:64
Ebola, 1:304
Escherichia coli O157:H7, 1:340, 341
food-borne disease, 1:355, 356, 357
gastroenteritis, 1:359
germ theory research, 1:366
helminth disease, 1:415, 416
hepatitis E, 1:437, 438, 439
H5N1, 1:392*s*
kuru, 1:524
listeriosis, 1:556, 557–558
liver flukes, 1:562
norovirus infection, 2:669
parasitic diseases, 2:694, 695
prion disease, 2:748, 749, 750
protozoan diseases, 2:754
resistant organisms, 2:801
Salmonella infection, 2:841, 842
taeniasis, 2:940–943, 942
tapeworm infections, 2:948, 950
toxoplasmosis, 2:964, 965*s*, 966
trehalose, 1:212
trichinellosis, 2:972, 973–974, 973*s*, 974
tularemia, 2:991
world trade, 2:1083–1084, 1085
yersiniosis, 2:1096, 1097–1098, 1098*s*
zoonoses, 2:1107
Mebendazole
costs, 2:707, 708
hookworm infection, 1:58
liver fluke infections, 1:562
pinworm infection, 2:706
toxocariasis, 1:80*s*
trichinellosis, 2:974
whipworm, 2:1062, 1063, 1064
Mechanical ventilation
Legionnaires' disease, 1:531
pneumonia, 2:725, 729
RSV infection, 2:834
West Nile virus, 2:1059
Médecins Sans Frontières, 2:**599–603,** *600*
African sleeping sickness, 1:1, 5
developing nations and drug delivery, 1:270, 271
diphtheria, 1:278
epidemiology, 1:332
isolation and quarantine, 1:510
legislation and international law, 1:535
outbreaks, field-level response to, 2:686, 687, 688
plague, 2:717
typhoid fever, 2:995
Media response to AIDS, 1:*17*
Medical equipment
contact precautions, 1:236–237
standard precautions, 2:909, 910
sterilization, 2:914
Medical information, patients' right to, 2:987
Medical Journal of Australia, 2:730
Medical Mycology, 2:903
The Medical Record, 2:1094, 1095
Medication stockpiling. *See* Stockpiling, drug
Medication-related adverse events. *See* Adverse effects
Medicine, 2:1000
Mediterranean countries
brucellosis, 1:141
dengue and dengue hemorrhagic fever, 1:267
hookworm infection, 1:58
tapeworm infections, 2:949
typhus, 2:997, 999
Zika virus, 2:1102
Mefloquine, 2:581
Meister, Joseph, 2:778
Melarsoprol, 1:3, 4
Melioidosis. *See* Glanders
Memory loss
encephalitis, 1:316
HIV symptoms, 1:11
marine toxins, 2:591, 592
picornaviruses, 1:230
Powassan virus, 2:741
syphilis, 2:935
toxic shock, 2:961
Men
Chlamydia infection, 1:189, 190, 191
filariasis, 1:351, 352
HPV, 1:470–471
leptospirosis, 1:550
mumps, 2:646
protozoan diseases, 2:754
sexually transmitted infections, 2:877, 878
trichomoniasis, 2:975, 976
Tuskegee syphilis study, 2:937–938
urinary tract infection, 2:1013
Men who have sex with men
AIDS pandemic history, 1:19, 20
cancer, 1:155
Chlamydia infection, 1:190
giardiasis, 1:371*s*
gonorrhea risk factors, 1:389
hepatitis A, 1:423, 425
hepatitis B, 1:427
hepatitis C, 1:431
hepatitis D, 1:435
Pneumocystis jirovecii pneumonia, 2:721
shigellosis, 2:882
syphilis, 2:936–937
Mengele, Josef, 1:344
Meningitis
angiostrongyliasis, 1:35, 36
anti-cytokine antibody syndrome, 1:53
aspergillosis, 1:85
bacterial sinusitis, 1:229

blastomycosis, 1:123
childhood vaccination, 1:187
coccidioidomycosis, 1:218, 219, 221
cohorted communities, 1:223–224, 224*s,* 225
Cryptococcus neoformans infection, 1:247–248
enterovirus 71 infection, 1:326
food-borne disease, 1:356
gonorrhea, 1:388
group B streptococcal infections, 2:924, 925
Haemophilus influenzae, 1:394, 395, 396
hand, foot, and mouth disease, 1:397, 398–399
herpes simplex virus 2, 1:444
Kawasaki disease, 1:517
leptospirosis, 1:548
mycotic disease, 2:651
polio, 2:736
Powassan virus, 2:741–743
rat-bite fever, 2:786
relapsing fever, 2:795
scarlet fever, 2:857
shingles, 2:888
sporotrichosis, 2:901–902
Staphylococcus aureus infections, 2:912
taeniasis, 2:943
vancomycin-resistant *Enterococci,* 2:1025
viral disease, 2:1039
West Nile virus, 2:1057, 1059, 1060, 1061
WHO childhood vaccination recommendations, 1:185
Meningitis, bacterial, 2:**604–606**
cohorted communities, 1:223–224
encephalitis with, 1:315
Haemophilus influenzae, 1:394, 395, 396
viral meningitis *vs.,* 2:608, 609, 610
Meningitis, viral, 1:326, 2:605, **607–610,** 607*t*
Meningitis B vaccine for gonorrhea, 1:389
Meningitis Research Foundation, 2:607, 610
Meningoencephalitis, 2:813
Mensch, Judith, 1:570
Menstruation, 1:230*s,* 388
Mental development and hookworm infection, 1:58, 459
Mental health facilities, 1:290
Mental retardation. *See* Intellectual disability
Mental status changes
bacterial meningitis, 2:604
cat scratch disease, 1:162
dengue and dengue hemorrhagic fever, 1:267
Legionnaires' disease, 1:530
macrophage activation syndrome, 2:575
necrotizing fasciitis, 2:659
relapsing fever, 2:796
typhoid fever, 2:993
MeNZB vaccine for gonorrhea, 1:389
Mepacrine, 2:579
Merck & Co., 1:270, 272, 424, 2:822
Merck Manual Professional Edition, 2:728
Mercury in vaccines, 1:186, 187, 2:838*s,* 1021–1022
Mercy (ship), 2:730
Meropenem, 1:380, 2:802*s*
Mesopotamia, 1:39, 47
Mesothelioma, 1:155
Messenger ribonucleic acid (mRNA), 1:72
Methenamine hippurate, 2:1014
Methicillin resistance, 1:62, 2:802
Methicillin-resistant *Staphylococcus aureus. See* MRSA
Methylprednisolone, 2:576
Metrifonate, 2:862
Metrol Health Medical Center, 1:470
Metronidazole
balantidiasis, 1:103
Clostridium difficile infection, 1:211
dysentery, 1:290
giardiasis, 1:373
Helicobacter pylori, 1:411
protozoan diseases, 2:755
tetanus, 2:954
trichomoniasis, 2:976
tsunami lung, 2:730
Metropole Hotel, 2:847, 970
Mexico
brucellosis, 1:141
burkholderia, 1:145
Chagas disease, 1:171, 173
coccidioidomycosis, 1:218, 220
cyclosporiasis, 1:258, 259
encephalitis, 1:317
food-borne disease, 1:355
hantavirus, 1:406
hepatitis E, 1:438
measles, 2:595, 597
mycotic disease, 2:651
parasitic diseases, 2:695
protozoan diseases, 2:755
river blindness, 2:821
Rocky Mountain spotted fever, 2:825
Salmonella infection, 2:842
trachoma, 2:968*s*
trichinellosis, 2:974
typhus, 2:999
Venezuelan equine encephalitis virus, 2:1034
Mexico City, 2:656, 809
Meyaard, Linde, 2:1074
Miami-Dade County, FL, 1:169
Miasmas, 2:712
Mice
babesiosis, 1:97
Baylisascaris infection, 1:107
Creutzfeldt-Jakob disease, 1:241
disinfection byproducts, effects of, 1:282
hantavirus, 1:405–406, 407, *407*
influenza virus particles, 1:495
kuru, 1:524
Lyme disease, 1:571
pigmentation research, 1:478*s*
Powassan virus, 2:741
rabies vaccine research, 2:779
rat-bite fever, 2:785
toxic shock research, 2:963
typhus, 2:998
virus hunters, 2:1046
Michael, Grace, 2:1090
Michigan, 1:298*s,* 424–425
"Michigan Hit Hard by Deadly Hepatitis A Outbreak," 1:*424–425*
Miconazole, 2:818, 945
Microarray technology, 1:364
Microbes. *See* Microorganisms
Microbes and Infection, 2:1000
Microbial evolution, 2:**611–614**
climate change, 1:203, 205
HIV, 1:454
leprosy, 1:547
nosocomial infections, 2:673
President's Initiative on Combating Antibiotic Resistance, 2:745
resistant organisms, 2:799–803
smallpox, 2:890
viral disease, 2:1041
Microbicides, 1:14, 2:1073
Microbiology
culture and sensitivity, 1:254–257
marine microorganisms, 2:591*s*
microorganisms, 2:615–617
microscopy, 2:618–620
Microbiology tests, 2:728
Microcephaly, 1:*312,* 2:*1100*
congenital Zika syndrome, 2:1101
mosquito-borne diseases, 2:637
Zika virus, 1:76*s,* 2:687, 1101, 1103, 1107, 1108
Microfilariae and river blindness, 2:820
Micronesia
angiostrongyliasis, 1:36
arthropod-borne diseases, 1:75
climate change and protozoan diseases, 2:757
Zika virus, 2:1101, 1102
Microorganisms, 2:**615–617**
climate change, 1:204
culture and sensitivity, 1:254–257
disinfection, 1:280–282

genetic identification of, 1:362–364
handwashing, 1:282
Koch's postulates, 1:369, 519–521
marine microorganisms, 2:591, 592
microbial evolution, 2:611–614
microscopes and microscopy, 2:618–620
microscopy, 2:618–620
personal protective equipment, 2:699, 700
rapid diagnostic tests, 2:781–783
resistant organisms, 2:799–803
standard precautions, 2:909–910
sterilization, 2:914–916
triclosan exposure, 1:67
USAMRIID, 2:1015–1018
See also specific microorganisms and diseases
Microscopes and microscopy, 2:**618–621,** *619*
Crimean-Congo hemorrhagic fever, 1:244
microorganism identification, 1:363
trichomoniasis, 2:976
virus hunters, 2:1045
MicroSEQ, 1:364
Microsporidiosis, 2:**622–625,** *623,* 683
Microtube dilution test, 1:256
Mid-Atlantic states, 1:107, 449
Middle Ages, 1:544, 2:711–712, 716
Middle America Research Unit, 2:1045
Middle East
arthropod-borne diseases, 1:75
avian influenza, 1:88
bloodborne infections transmitted through barber shops, 1:131*s*
brucellosis, 1:141
burkholderia, 1:142, 145
demographics, 1:263
dysentery, 1:290
encephalitis, 1:317
glanders, 1:380
leprosy, 1:544
liver fluke infections, 1:561
malaria, 2:579
protozoan diseases, 2:755
re-emerging infectious diseases, 2:792
river blindness, 2:821
schistosomiasis, 2:861
taeniasis, 2:942
West Nile virus, 2:1057, 1060
Middle East, ancient, 1:414, 2:710
Middle East respiratory syndrome, 1:386
Middle-African hedgehogs, 1:244
Midwestern United States
Baylisascaris infection, 1:107
blastomycosis, 1:122
encephalitis, 1:317
Powassan virus, 2:742
St. Louis encephalitis, 2:906
Migration. *See* Immigration
Migratory polyarthritis, 1:388
Military
anthrax vaccines, 1:50
antibiotic resistance, 1:59
brucellosis, 1:142
CDC origins, 1:165
diphtheria, 1:277
dysentery, 1:290
influenza pandemic of 1918, 2:1047–1048
leishmaniasis, 1:540, 541
leptospirosis, 1:549
SARS, 2:851
strongyloidiasis, 2:929
typhus, 2:998
USAMRIID, 2:1017
yellow fever research, 1:342–343
See also War
Milk
brucellosis, 1:140, 141
pasteurization, 1:356
Q fever, 2:773
rat-bite fever, 2:786
scrofula, 2:866
tuberculosis, 2:983
yersiniosis, 2:1096, 1098
Millennium Declaration, 2:1006
Millennium Development Goals. *See* United Nations Millennium Goals
Millennium Development Goals Report 2015, 2:1006
Millennium Fund, 2:790
Miller, Laurie C., 1:474
Miltefosine, 1:540, 2:755
Milwaukee, WI, 1:250, 252, 2:1054
Minghui, Ren, 1:321
Minikel, Eric, 1:525
Minimal inhibitory concentration, 1:256
Ministry of Health and Family Welfare, India, 1:308
Mink, 1:136
Minnesota
alveolar echinococcosis, 1:25
babesiosis, 1:96
Center for Disease Research and Policy, 1:491
Lyme disease, 1:571
measles outbreak, 2:596–598
Minocycline, 2:642, 668, 913
Minoia, Francesca, 2:575
Mintezol. *See* Thiabendazole
Miracidia, 1:415, 565–566
Mirazimi, Ali, 1:245
Miscarriage
chickenpox, 1:177
genital herpes, 1:365
hepatitis E, 1:437
listeriosis, 1:556
malaria, 2:581
measles, 2:594
mumps, 2:646
Rift Valley fever, 2:814
rubella, 2:837
syphilis, 2:936
"Misdiagnosed Sepsis Now a Global Health Priority for World Health Organization," 2:*869–870*
Misdiagnosis
babesiosis, 1:96
blastomycosis, 1:121
dengue and dengue hemorrhagic fever, 1:266
Lyme disease, 1:573
Nipah virus infection, 2:664
psittacosis, 2:760
Misinformation and outbreaks, 2:687
Mississippi, 2:906
Mississippi River basin
blastomycosis, 1:122
encephalitis, 1:317
histoplasmosis, 1:448
lung flukes, 1:567
Mississippi River Valley disease. *See* Histoplasmosis
Missouri
babesiosis, 1:96
heartland virus, 2:873*s*
histoplasmosis, 1:449
lung flukes, 1:567
St. Louis encephalitis, 2:905
Mites
hosts and vectors, 1:461
scabies, 2:852
typhus, 2:997, 998, 999
virus hunters, 2:1046
Mitigation of climate change, 1:206
Mitten crabs, 1:567–568
MMR vaccine
measles, 2:595–598, 595*s*
meningitis, 2:607
mumps, 2:647
research, 2:838*s*
rubella, 2:838, 839
vaccines and vaccine development, 2:1021, 1022*s*
viral meningitis, 2:610
MMRV vaccine, 2:838
Model Food Code, 1:153
Model List of Essential Medicines, 1:270
Model State Emergency Health Powers Act, 1:117, 535–536
Modeling, computer. *See* Computer modeling
Modified measles, 2:593–594
Modified smallpox, 2:892
Modified vaccinia Ankara, 2:791
Moerner, Tilliam E., 2:620
MoistureLoc, 1:232
Mold and antibiotics, 1:57
Moldova, 1:277
Molecular biology
amebiasis tests, 1:29

antiviral drugs, 1:71
Asilomar Conference, 1:81–82
genetic identification of microorganisms, 1:362–364
germ theory of disease, 1:369
kuru research, 1:524–525
microbial identification techniques, 1:256–257
plague, 2:713–714
RSV infection, 2:833–834
Molecular tests
rapid diagnostic tests, 2:781, 782, 783
relapsing fever, 2:797
Moles, 1:258
Mongolia, 1:13, 89
Monitoring. *See* Surveillance
Monkey B virus. *See* B virus infection
Monkeypox, 2:**626–629,** *627*
animal importation, 2:1084
globalization and infectious disease, 1:384, 385
viral disease, 2:1039
Monkeys
animal importation, 1:41
B virus infection, 1:91–94
cat scratch disease, 1:163
dengue and dengue hemorrhagic fever, 1:266
Ebola, 1:303, 2:1022, 1085
group B streptococcal infection, 2:926–927
hemorrhagic fevers, 1:420*s*
malaria, 2:581
Marburg hemorrhagic fever, 2:585
monkeypox, 2:626
SARS research, 2:850
virus hunters, 2:1046
zoonoses, 2:1106
Mono. *See* Mononucleosis
"Mono: Tough for Teens and Twenty-Somethings," 2:*633–635*
Monongahela virus, 1:406
Mononucleosis, 2:*630,* **630–635**
CMV infection, 1:214
Epstein-Barr virus, 1:335, 337
viral disease, 2:1039
Monovalent vaccines, 2:734
Monroe, Christopher, 2:937
Monrovia, Liberia, 2:601
Monsoons, 1:200, 205, 513*s*
Montana
brucellosis, 1:143
Q fever, 2:771
relapsing fever, 2:795
Rocky Mountain Laboratory, 2:655–656
Montenegro, 2:1050
Montpellier, France, 1:181
Montreal, Quebec, Canada, 1:474
Montresor, Antonio, 2:1064
Mood swings, 1:244
Morabito, Kaitlyn M., 2:1023
Morbidity and Mortality Weekly Report
Baylisascaris infection, 1:107
CDC journals, 1:168
coccidioidomycosis, 1:220
notifiable diseases, 2:679
Morbidity rates, 1:306, 329
Morbillivirus. See Rinderpest
Morgantown, WV, 1:166
Morocco, 1:259, 2:778, 968*s*
Mortality. *See* Deaths
Morton, Richard, 1:175
Moscow, Russia, 1:277, 2:897
Mosquirix. *See* RTS,S/AS01 vaccine
Mosquito netting. *See* Netting, bed
Mosquito-borne diseases, 2:**636–639,** *1105*
arthropod-borne diseases, 1:75
Buruli ulcer, 1:148
chikungunya, 1:180
climate change, 1:204, 205–206, 207
dengue and dengue hemorrhagic fever, 1:266–268
Eastern equine encephalitis, 1:296–298, 298*s*
encephalitis, 1:316, 317, 318
endemicity, 1:321
filariasis, 1:350–352
fumigation for prevention of, 2:*636*
globalization and infectious disease, 1:385
hemorrhagic fevers, 1:419
hosts and vectors, 1:461
immigration, 1:473
infection control and asepsis, 1:486
Japanese encephalitis, 1:511–514
malaria, 2:578–583
outbreaks, field-level response to, 2:687
parasitic diseases, 2:694
protozoan diseases, 2:753
re-emerging infectious diseases, 2:790–791, 791*s*, 792
Rift Valley fever, 2:813–816
St. Louis encephalitis, 2:905–907, *906*
tropical infectious diseases, 2:*979,* 979–980
tularemia, 2:990
United Nations Millennium Goals, 2:1009
vector-borne disease, 2:1029, 1030–1031
Venezuelan equine encephalitis virus, 2:1033–1035
viral disease, 2:1042
viral meningitis, 2:609
virus hunters, 2:1043–1044, 1045, 1046
West Nile virus, 2:1057–1061
yellow fever, 1:345–346, 2:1092–1095
Zika virus, 2:1100–1103
zoonoses, 2:1105, 1106, 1107–1108
Moss, Frederick, 2:937, 939
Mother-to-child infection. *See* Maternal-to-fetal/child transmission
Motor issues. *See* Movement issues
Mountain, Joseph Walter, 1:165
Mourning customs. *See* Burial and mourning customs
Mouth symptoms
B virus infection, 1:92
enterovirus 71 infection, 1:325
hand, foot, and mouth disease, 1:397
herpes simplex 1 virus, 1:440, 441
histoplasmosis, 1:449
Kawasaki disease, 1:515
marine toxins, 2:590, 591
talaromycosis, 2:945
tularemia, 2:990
viral disease, 2:1039
Movement issues
African sleeping sickness, 1:3
Baylisascaris infection, 1:105, 107
Buruli ulcer, 1:148
Creutzfeldt-Jakob disease, 1:240
Japanese encephalitis, 1:512
malaria, 2:580
nocardiosis, 2:666
opportunistic infections, 2:683
prion disease, 2:749, 750
protozoan diseases, 2:753
Rocky Mountain spotted fever, 2:825
Zika virus, 2:1103
Moxifloxacine, 2:773
Mozambique
child marriage, 2:1005
cholera, 1:200
leprosy, 1:546, 2:1078
malaria, 1:206
outbreaks, field-level response to, 2:686–687
plague, 2:716
re-emerging infectious diseases, 2:792
MR vaccine, 2:646
MRSA, 2:**640–643,** *641, 642*
antibacterial drug issues, 1:59
antibiotic resistance, 1:62, 63–64
antimicrobial soap use for prevention of, 1:67
bacterial diseases, 1:100
contact precautions, 1:237
demographics, 1:263
infection control and asepsis, 1:485
isolation and quarantine, 1:509
nosocomial infections, 2:674–675
President's Initiative on Combating Antibiotic Resistance, 2:746

research, 2:675–676
resistant organisms, 2:801, 802*s*
Staphylococcus aureus infections, 2:912–913
vancomycin, 2:1025
with vancomycin-resistant *Enterococci,* 2:1026
Mucocutaneous leishmaniasis, 1:539, 540, 2:755
Mucosa-associated lymphoid tissue lymphoma, 1:155
Mucosal bleeding, 1:526, 2:575
Mucus membranes and leprosy, 1:545
Mules
burkholderia, 1:144
glanders, 1:378, 381
transmissible spongiform encephalopathies, 1:136
Venezuelan equine encephalitis virus, 2:1035
Mullis, Kary, 2:616*s*, 782
Multibacillary leprosy, 1:546–547
Multidrug resistance
bacterial diseases, 1:62
drug development research, 2:675–676
isolation and quarantine, 1:509
plague, 2:716–717, 718
pneumonia, 2:729
resistant organisms, 2:799, 801
Salmonella infection, 2:842
sexually transmitted infections, 2:878–879
tuberculosis, 2:985
typhoid fever, 2:994, 996
urinary tract infection, 2:1013, 1014
Multidrug resistant *Acinetobacter baumannii,* 1:59
Multidrug therapy for leprosy, 1:545, 546–547, 2:1078
Multidrug-resistant tuberculosis
bacterial diseases, 1:101
economic development, 1:308
genetic identification of microorganisms, 1:363
re-emerging infectious diseases, 2:791
Multimammate rats, 1:244
Multiple organ failure
macrophage activation syndrome, 2:575–576
sepsis, 2:868
toxic shock, 2:961, 962
tularemia, 2:990
Multiple sclerosis, 1:195, 337, 2:808
Multiplex PCR, 1:364
Mumbai, India, 1:*74*
Mumps, 2:*644,* **644–648**
meningitis, 2:607
vaccination and elimination of, 1:185
viral meningitis, 2:609, 610
Mupirocin, 2:674
Murine typhus. *See* Endemic typhus
Murray, Polly, 1:570
Muscle aches or pain. *See* Myalgia
Muscle biopsy, 2:974
Muscle inflammation and microsporidiosis, 2:624*s*
Muscle spasms
Japanese encephalitis, 1:512
rabies, 2:776
tetanus, 2:953, 954
West Nile virus, 2:1059
Muscle tremors. *See* Tremors
Muskrats, 1:405
Mussels, 2:591
Mutation
avian influenza, 1:88
influenza, 1:503–507
microbial evolution, 2:611, 612–613
Myalgia
avian influenza, 1:89
B virus infection, 1:92
babesiosis, 1:95, 96
blastomycosis, 1:122
brucellosis, 1:141
Crimean-Congo hemorrhagic fever, 1:244
cyclosporiasis, 1:259
dengue and dengue hemorrhagic fever, 1:267
Ebola, 1:302
glanders, 1:379
helminth disease, 1:415
hemorrhagic fevers, 1:419, 420*s*
influenza, 1:488, 504
Japanese encephalitis, 1:512
Legionnaires' disease, 1:530
marine toxins, 2:591
monkeypox, 2:626, 628*s*
mononucleosis, 2:631, 634
pneumonia, 2:726
polio, 2:737
protozoan diseases, 2:753
rat-bite fever, 2:787
relapsing fever, 2:795
Rift Valley fever, 2:813
Rocky Mountain spotted fever, 2:824
schistosomiasis, 2:861
tick-borne diseases, 2:956
toxoplasmosis, 2:964
trichinellosis, 2:973
tularemia, 2:989, 990
typhoid fever, 2:993
Venezuelan equine encephalitis virus, 2:1033
West Nile virus, 2:1058
Zika virus, 2:1101
Myanmar
avian influenza, 1:89
burkholderia, 1:145
demographics, 1:261
glanders, 1:379
Japanese encephalitis, 1:514
leprosy, 1:546
malaria, 2:579
plague, 2:717
trachoma, 2:968*s*
Mycobacteria
anti-cytokine antibody syndrome, 1:53–54
Buruli ulcer, 1:147–150
leprosy, 1:543
Mycobacterium leprae. See Leprosy
Mycobacterium tuberculosis. See Tuberculosis
Mycobacterium ulcerannus. See Buruli ulcer
Mycolactone toxins, 1:149
Mycoplasma pneumonia, 2:726
Mycotic disease, 2:**649–652,** *650*
aspergillosis, 1:84–86
blastomycosis, 1:121–124
candidiasis, 1:157–160
coccidioidomycosis, 1:218–222
contact lenses and *Fusarium* keratitis, 1:232–233
Cryptococcus neoformans infection, 1:247–249
droplet precautions, 1:286
histoplasmosis, 1:448–451
HIV, 1:11
microorganisms, 2:616
microsporidiosis, 2:622–624
nosocomial infections, 2:675
opportunistic infections, 2:682, 683
Pneumocystis jirovecii pneumonia, 2:721–724
pneumonia, 2:725
ringworm, 2:817–819
sporotrichosis, 2:901–903
talaromycosis, 2:944–946
Mycotic Diseases Branch, CDC, 2:651
Myelitis, 1:315
Myocarditis
Cryptococcus neoformans infection, 1:248
diphtheria, 1:275
enterovirus 71 infection, 1:326
relapsing fever, 2:795
viral disease, 2:1039
Myriapods, 1:258
Myringotomy, 1:294

N

N, N-diethyl-meta-toluamide. *See* DEET
N-95 respirators, 1:*22,* 23
NAACP, 2:937
Nacht, Sheri, 1:554
Nägeli, Karl Wilhelm von, 2:622
Nails and mycotic infections, 1:159, 2:817
Nairovirus. See Crimean-Congo hemorrhagic fever

Namibia, 2:716
Nanoparticles, 2:834–835
Nantucket, MA, 1:95
Nantucket fever. *See* Babesiosis
Napoleon, 2:998, 1048
Naproxen, 1:182, 2:646, 886
Narrow-spectrum antibiotics, 1:57
NASA, 2:916*s*
Nasal discharge, 1:274–275, 504
Nasal inflammation, 1:504
Nashville, TN, 1:195
Nasogastric intubation and pneumonia, 2:729
Nasogastric suction for anisakiasis, 1:45
Nasopharyngeal carcinoma, 1:155, 337
Natal multimammate rats, 1:526
Natamycin, 1:232
National Academy of Sciences, 1:51
National Action Plan for Combating Antibiotic-Resistant Bacteria, 2:744
National Aeronautics and Space Administration (NASA), 2:916*s*
National Antimicrobial Resistance Monitoring System, 2:746
National Association for the Advancement of Colored People (NAACP), 2:937
National Biocontainment Laboratories, 2:792
National Biodefense Strategy, 2:1015
National Bioethics Advisory Commission, 2:939
National Blood Service, UK, 2:1060
National Botulism Surveillance System, 1:134
National Campaign for Appropriate Antibiotic Use in the Community, 2:803
National Cancer Institute, 1:19, 2:806
National Center for Biotechnology Information, 1:78, 363, 2:660, 962*s*
National Center for Chronic Disease Prevention, 1:168
National Center for Emerging and Zoonotic Infectious Diseases, CDC, 2:792–793
National Center for HIV/AIDS, Viral Hepatitis, STD, and TB Prevention, 2:965*s*
National Center for Infectious Diseases, 1:348*s*
National Committee on Clinical Laboratory Standards, 1:256
National Congenital Rubella Registry, 2:837–838
National Electronic Disease Surveillance system, 1:536
National Electronic Telecommunications System for Surveillance, 2:679
National Foundation for Infantile Paralysis, 2:739*s*
National Foundation for Infectious Diseases, 2:1079
National Hockey League, 2:647
National Hospital of Pediatrics, Vietnam, 1:*329*
National Immigration Agency, Taiwan, 1:474
National Immunization Program, 2:838
National Influenza Centres, 1:503
National Institute for Infectious Diseases (Japan), 1:506
National Institute for Medical Research (UK), 1:506
National Institute for Occupational Safety and Health, 1:23, 167, 451
National Institute for Viral Disease Control and Prevention (China), 1:506
National Institute of Allergy and Infectious Diseases, 2:**653–656**
  biodefense research and development, 1:118
  colds, 1:230*s*
  glanders, 1:378, 381
  re-emerging infectious diseases, 2:790
  resistant organisms, 2:802
  vaccines and vaccine development, 2:1022
National Institute of Neurological Disorders and Stroke, 1:317
National Institutes of Health
  Asilomar Conference guidelines, 1:82
  Biomedical Advanced Research and Development Authority, 1:114
  chikungunya vaccine research, 1:182
  coccidioidomycosis, 1:219
  GenBank, 1:363
  influenza pandemic of 1957, 1:501
  National Institute of Allergy and Infectious Diseases, 2:654
  Pneumocystis jirovecii pneumonia, 2:723
  ringworm, 2:818
  smallpox, 2:894, 898
  Task Force on Antimicrobial Resistance, 1:256*s*
  trachoma, 2:968
  virus hunters, 2:1045
  women and infectious disease, 2:1074
National Library of Medicine, 2:962*s,* 968, 999
National Microbiological Institute, 2:654
National Microbiology Laboratory, 1:304
National newspaper, 1:528
National Nosocomial Infection Surveillance System, 2:1026
National Notifiable Diseases Surveillance System
  babesiosis, 1:97
  brucellosis, 1:141
  notifiable diseases, 2:679
  plague, 2:718
  tetanus, 2:954
National Oceanographic and Atmospheric Administration, 2:592
National Parasite Collection, 2:697
National Pediculosis Association, 1:553, 554
National Science Advisory Board for Biosecurity, 1:496
National Strategy for Pandemic Influenza Implementation Plan, 2:691
Native Americans
  blastomycosis, 1:122
  smallpox, 2:890, 893
  trade, 2:1081
Natural disasters
  cholera, 1:198, 200, 201
  demographics, 1:263
  dengue and dengue hemorrhagic fever, 1:268
  endemicity, 1:322
  shigellosis, 2:882
  tsunami lung, 2:730–731
  typhoid fever, 2:995
  typhus, 2:998
  See also Extreme weather
Natural immunity, 1:12
Nature
  anthrax, 1:49
  Clostridium difficile infection, 1:211, 212
  Ebola, 1:303
  giardiasis vaccine, 1:373
  influenza virus particles, 1:495
  kuru, 1:524–525
  vaccine safety, 1:278
Nature Communications, 1:545
Nature Ecology & Evolution, 1:309
Nausea
  AIDS, 1:12
  angiostrongyliasis, 1:35
  anisakiasis, 1:45
  ascariasis, 1:79
  B virus infection, 1:92
  Baylisascaris infection, 1:105
  botulism, 1:133
  Campylobacter infection, 1:151
  candidiasis, 1:159
  chikungunya, 1:*180,* 181
  Clostridium difficile infection, 1:210
  cryptosporidiosis, 1:251
  dysentery, 1:289
  encephalitis, 1:316
  Escherichia coli O157:H7, 1:340
  food-borne disease, 1:354
  giardiasis, 1:371

hand, foot, and mouth disease, 1:397
hantavirus, 1:404
heartland virus, 2:873*s*
hemorrhagic fevers, 1:419
hepatitis A, 1:422
hepatitis B, 1:426
hepatitis C, 1:430
hepatitis D, 1:434
hepatitis E, 1:437
influenza, 1:488
Legionnaires' disease, 1:530
listeriosis, 1:556
liver fluke infections, 1:560
malaria, 2:580
marine toxins, 2:591
Nipah virus infection, 2:663
nocardiosis, 2:666
protozoan diseases, 2:754
Q fever, 2:772
rat-bite fever, 2:785
relapsing fever, 2:795
Rocky Mountain spotted fever, 2:824
Salmonella infection, 2:841
schistosomiasis, 2:861
shigellosis, 2:880, 881
tapeworm infections, 2:948
trichinellosis, 2:972
tularemia, 2:989
viral meningitis, 2:608
water-borne disease, 2:1054
West Nile virus, 2:1058
whipworm, 2:1062
yellow fever, 2:1092
Neale, James R., 2:671
Nebraska, 1:317
Neck pain
bacterial meningitis, 2:605
Crimean-Congo hemorrhagic fever, 1:244
hemorrhagic fevers, 1:419
Lyme disease, 1:569
Neck stiffness
angiostrongyliasis, 1:35
enterovirus 71 infection, 1:326
Haemophilus influenzae, 1:395
hemorrhagic fevers, 1:419
histoplasmosis, 1:449
Japanese encephalitis, 1:512
meningitis, 1:223, 2:606*s*
mumps, 2:645
polio, 2:736
relapsing fever, 2:795
St. Louis encephalitis, 2:905
tick-borne diseases, 2:958
viral meningitis, 2:607
West Nile virus, 2:1059
Necrotizing enterocolitis, 1:159
Necrotizing fasciitis, 2:*657*, **657–661**
bacterial diseases, 1:101
group A streptococcal infections, 2:920
MRSA, 2:640
Needles and disease transmission
AIDS, 1:8
bloodborne pathogens, 1:129, 131
hepatitis B, 1:426
hepatitis C, 1:431
Marburg hemorrhagic fever, 2:587
Negative pressure rooms, 1:22, 23
Neglected diseases
globalization and infectious disease, 1:385
scabies, 2:854
toxocariasis, 1:80*s*
tropical infectious diseases, 2:979, 980, 981*s*, 982
yaws, 2:1090
Neglected Tropical Diseases Department WHO, 2:1064
Neisser, Albert, 1:387, 544
Neisseria meningitides, 1:223, 2:605
Nelfinavir, 1:13
Nelson, Christina, 1:573
Nematode infections. *See* Roundworm infections
Nemours Foundation, 2:932
Neonatal gonorrhea, 1:388
Neonatal infants. *See* Newborns
Neonatal transmission. *See* Maternal-to-fetal/child transmission
Nepal
bacterial meningitis, 2:606
child marriage, 2:1005
cyclosporiasis, 1:259
immigration, 1:473
Japanese encephalitis, 1:513*s*, 514
leishmaniasis, 1:540, 541
leprosy, 1:546, 2:1078
re-emerging infectious diseases, 2:791*s*
rotavirus, 2:831
Nephritis, 2:1039
Nephropathia epidemica, 1:405
Nephrotic syndrome, 2:580
Nerve damage or pain
Buruli ulcer, 1:147
diphtheria, 1:275
Escherichia coli O157:H7, 1:340
leprosy, 1:543, 545–546
shingles, 2:885, 886
Nervous system. *See* Neurological disease or symptoms
Nervousness and pinworm infection, 2:705
Netherlands
anisakiasis, 1:45
avian influenza, 1:89, 491
enterovirus 71 infection, 1:325
immigration, 1:474
lice infestation, 1:554
Q fever, 2:772, 773
relapsing fever, 2:796, 797–798
smallpox research, opposition to, 2:899
vancomycin-resistant *Enterococci,* 2:1027
Netherlands Journal of Medicine, 2:773
Netting, bed
chikungunya, 1:180, 182
filariasis, 1:352
hosts and vectors, 1:462
infection control, 1:486
Japanese encephalitis, 1:513
leishmaniasis, 1:540
malaria, 2:581, 582, 583
mosquito-borne disease, 2:638, 639
parasitic disease, 2:*694*
Rift Valley fever, 2:815
treated bed nets and the life span of mosquitoes, 2:1031–1032
tropical infectious diseases, 2:982
United Nations Millennium Goals, 2:1009
vector-borne disease, 2:1031
West Nile virus, 2:1059
yellow fever, 2:1093
Neupogen. *See* Filgrastim
Neuraminidase inhibitors, 1:490
Neuraminidase proteins
avian influenza, 1:88
H5N1, 1:392
influenza, 1:489
influenza pandemic of 1918, 1:494
influenza pandemic of 1957, 1:500
Neurocysticercosis, 2:949, 950
Neurological disease or symptoms
African sleeping sickness, 1:2, 4, 5
ascariasis, 1:79
B virus infection, 1:91, 92
bacterial meningitis, 2:608
Baylisascaris infection, 1:105
Chlamydia pneumoniae, 1:193, 195
CMV infection, 1:214
coccidioidomycosis, 1:218
Creutzfeldt-Jakob disease, 1:240
Cryptococcus neoformans infection, 1:249
diphtheria, 1:274
Eastern equine encephalitis, 1:296–298, 297, 298
encephalitis, 1:316
enterovirus 71 infection, 1:324–327
glanders, 1:379
helminth disease, 1:415
herpes simplex 1 virus, 1:443
Japanese encephalitis, 1:512, 513
Lassa fever, 1:526, 527
Lyme disease, 1:573
macrophage activation syndrome, 2:575
malaria, 2:580
microsporidiosis, 2:624*s*

mosquito-borne diseases, 2:637
mumps, 2:645
Nipah virus infection, 2:664
nocardiosis, 2:666
opportunistic infections, 2:683
picornaviruses, 1:230
prion disease, 2:748–750
protozoan diseases, 2:753
psittacosis, 2:759
rabies, 2:775–779, 776
relapsing fever, 2:795, 796
sexually transmitted infections, 2:877
sporotrichosis, 2:901, 902
strongyloidiasis, 2:929
syphilis, 2:935, 936
taeniasis, 2:942–943
tapeworm infections, 2:949, 950
tetanus, 2:952–955
tropical infectious diseases, 2:980
tsunami lung, 2:730
West Nile virus, 1:206
See also Brain disease or symptoms
Neurosyphilis, 2:935
Neurotoxins, 1:133–135, 2:591, 952
Neutrophils, 1:410, 478
Nevada, 1:220, 2:795
Nevirapine, 1:13
New African magazine, 2:1079
New Caledonia, 1:36
New England Journal of Medicine
abortion in Brazil, 2:1108
anti-cytokine antibody syndrome, 1:53
Chlamydia pneumoniae, 1:195
clinical trials, 1:331
drug-resistant bacteria in meat, 1:64
Koch's postulates, 1:521
rotavirus vaccine, 1:81
tsunami lung, 2:730
New Guinea, 1:138*s,* 522, 2:579, 749
New Hampshire, 1:571
New Jersey
babesiosis, 1:96
Eastern equine encephalitis, 1:298*s*
Lyme disease, 1:571
Powassan virus, 2:742
New Mexico
coccidioidomycosis, 1:220
hantavirus, 1:407
plague, 2:717
relapsing fever, 2:795
smallpox, 2:896
West Nile virus, 2:1060
New Orleans, LA
angiostrongyliasis, 1:36
dengue and dengue hemorrhagic fever, 1:266
Hurricane Katrina, 1:201, 207
St. Louis encephalitis, 2:906
New World leishmaniasis, 2:755
New York
AIDS pandemic history, 1:18, 19*s*
burkholderia, 1:142
Eastern equine encephalitis, 1:298*s*
encephalitis, 1:317
globalization and infectious disease, 1:385
illegal snails, 1:38
Lyme disease, 1:571
mosquito-borne diseases, 2:637
mycotic disease, 2:652
Powassan virus, 2:742
typhoid fever, 2:995*s*
yellow fever, 2:1092
New York City, NY, 1:474, 2:1058
New York Post, 1:48
New York Times
"Chipotle Is Subpoened in Criminal Inquiry over Norovirus Outbreak," 2:671
drug development, 1:63
Ebola vaccine, 2:1022
polio vaccine, 2:739
"A Zika Tale in a Favela," 2:1102–1103
New York-1 virus, 1:406
New Yorker, 1:412*s*
New Zealand, 1:424, 2:949
Newborns
bacterial meningitis, 2:606
candidiasis, 1:159
chickenpox, 1:175, 177
Chlamydia infection, 1:190
CMV infection, 1:215, 216
enterovirus 71 infection, 1:326
gastroenteritis, 1:358–361
gonorrhea, 1:389
group B streptococcal infection, 2:924, 925–926
herpes simplex 1 virus, 1:443
herpes simplex virus 2, 1:446
hookworm infection, 1:458
pink eye, 2:704
RSV infection, 2:832
rubella, 2:837
tetanus, 2:952, 954
Nexium. *See* Esomeprazole
NGOs. *See* Nongovernmental organizations
Nicaragua, 1:550, 2:*727*
Nicks, Bobbie, 2:883
Niclocide. *See* Niclosamide
Niclosamide, 2:942, 950
Nicolle, Charles, 2:1000–1001
Nifurtimox
Chagas disease, 1:171, 173
parasitic diseases, 2:695
protozoan diseases, 2:756
tropical infectious diseases, 2:981
Niger
avian influenza, 1:89
child marriage, 2:1005
Rift Valley fever, 2:816
smallpox vaccination, 2:*896*
Nigeria
ascariasis, 1:79
avian influenza, 1:89
cholera, 1:200
dengue and dengue hemorrhagic fever, 1:266
dracunculiasis, 1:283
Ebola, 1:169
emerging infectious diseases, 1:314
immigration, 1:473
Lassa fever, 1:526, 527, 528
leprosy, 1:546
monkeypox, 2:628
outbreaks, field-level response to, 2:688
polio, 1:184, 487, 2:733, 734, 734*s*
rotavirus, 2:829, 831
United Nations Millennium Goals, 2:1009
yellow fever, 2:1092–1095
Zika virus, 2:1101
Night sweats, 1:122, 2:666, 877
Nightingale, Florence, 1:400
NIH. *See* National Institutes of Health
Nikaido, Hiroshi, 2:801
Nikkomycin Z, 1:221
Nile River Valley, 2:713
Nine-banded armadillos, 1:545
"1957 Flu Pandemic," 1:*501–502*
"Nipah: Fearsome Virus That Caught the Medical and Scientific World Off-Guard," 2:*664*
Nipah virus infection, 2:*662,* **662–665**
Nippon Foundation, 2:1078
Nishizawa, T., 1:30
Nitazoxanide, 1:252, 373
Nitzchia pungens, 2:591
Nixon, Richard, 1:142, 2:893, 1016
Nizatidine, 1:411
Nobel Prize
Betzig, Eric, 2:620
Enders, John F., 2:736, 739
Gajdusek, Carleton, 1:138*s*
Hell, Stefan W., 2:620
Koch, Robert, 1:47, 369*s,* 519
Marshall, Barry, 1:344, 411, 521
Médecins Sans Frontières, 2:599
Moerner, William E., 2:620
Mullis, Kary, 2:616*s,* 782
Nicolle, Charles, 2:1001
Pasteur Institute, 2:778
Prusiner, Stanley, 1:242, 2:750
Robbins, Frederick, 2:736, 739
Rous, Peyton, 1:154
UNICEF, 2:1003
Warren, J. Robin, 1:344, 411
Weller, Thomas, 2:736, 739

Nocardiosis, 1:53, 2:**666–668,** *667,* 730
Nodules, 2:901, 944, 1087
Nomads and African sleeping sickness, 1:5
Non-*albicans* candidiasis, 1:158
Nongovernmental organizations
isolation and quarantine, 1:510
legislation and international law, 1:533, 535
outbreaks, field-level response to, 2:686
See also specific organizations
Non-Hodgkin lymphoma, 1:155, 2:683
Non-native species, 1:567–568
Non-nucleoside reverse transcriptase inhibitors, 1:13
Nonself *vs.* self and the immune system, 1:476–477
Nonsteroidal anti-inflammatory drugs
hand, foot, and mouth disease, 1:398
mononucleosis, 2:632
shingles, 2:886
Zika virus cautions, 2:1102
Nontherapeutic use of antibiotics, 1:64, 2:745–746, 1027–1028
Nontuberculous mycobacterial disease, 1:53
Norovirus infection, 2:**669–672,** *670*
food-borne disease, 1:355
gastroenteritis, 1:358, 359
war, 2:1049
North Africa, 1:244, 2:579, 716
North America
AIDS, 1:14, 18
alveolar echinococcosis, 1:24
anellovirus, 1:30
arthropod-borne diseases, 1:75
blastomycosis, 1:121, 122, 123
bovine spongiform encephalopathy, 1:137, 242
brucellosis, 1:142, 143
chikungunya, 2:614
cholera, 1:199
climate change, 1:206
cryptosporidiosis, 1:251
cyclosporiasis, 1:258
Eastern equine encephalitis, 1:296, 297
extremely drug-resistant tuberculosis, 1:23
helminth disease, 1:415
hepatitis A, 1:424
histoplasmosis, 1:448
infection control and asepsis, 1:486
leishmaniasis, 1:540
leprosy, 1:544
marine toxins, 2:589
Médecins Sans Frontières, 2:602
mitten crabs, 1:568
MRSA, 2:640
necrotizing fasciitis, 2:659
pinworm infection, 2:706
plague, 2:717
polio, 2:737
Powassan virus, 2:741
protozoan diseases, 2:755
public health, 2:764–765
rat-bite fever, 2:786
rickettsial disease, 2:809
smallpox, 2:890
St. Louis encephalitis, 2:906
tapeworm infections, 2:949
tick-borne diseases, 2:957, 958
tularemia, 2:990
typhoid fever, 2:995*s*
Venezuelan equine encephalitis virus, 2:1033
water-borne disease, 2:1054, 1055
West Nile virus, 2:1057–1058, 1060
yellow fever, 2:1093
Zika virus, 1:169
zoonoses, 2:1106, 1107
North American blastomycosis. *See* Blastomycosis
North Asian tick typhus, 2:810, 997
North Carolina, 1:297, 2:825
North Korea
anthrax, 1:47, 50, 51
lung flukes, 1:566
severe fever with thrombocytopenia syndrome, 2:872
North Queensland, Australia, 2:999
North Sea and anisakiasis, 1:43
North-central United States, 1:571
Northeastern Africa, 2:999
Northeastern Asia, 1:513
Northeastern United States
babesiosis, 1:95, 96
Baylisascaris infection, 1:107
encephalitis, 1:316
Lyme disease, 1:571, 572
Powassan virus, 2:741–743, 742, 742*s*
West Nile virus, 2:1058
Zika virus, 2:1102
Northeastern University, 2:676
Northern Africa, 2:769, 797
Northern Asia, 2:957
Northern Australia, 2:1102
Northern Europe, 1:434
Northern hemisphere
influenza, 1:496, 506
tapeworm infections, 2:949
tick-borne diseases, 2:958
Northern United States, 1:172, 2:742*s*
Northwestern United States, 1:248, 2:715, 717
Norwalk, OH, 2:669
Norwalk viruses, 1:224, 2:1039
Norway, 1:325, 2:1068
Norwegian scabies, 2:852–853
Nose swabs and viral meningitis, 2:609
Nosebleeds, 1:244
Nosocomial infections, 2:**673–677**
antibacterial drug issues, 1:59
antibiotic resistance, 1:62
candidiasis, 1:157, 158–159, 160
Clostridium difficile infection, 1:210, 211, 213
contact precautions, 1:237
hemorrhagic fevers, 1:419
hepatitis C, 1:430
infection control and asepsis, 1:483–487
invasive devices-associated and surgical site infections, 1:257
MRSA, 1:263, 2:640, 641, *641,* 643
mycotic disease, 2:651–652
nocardiosis, 2:666
opportunistic infections, 2:683
pneumonia, 2:726–727, 728, 729
prevention, 2:*674*
prion disease, 2:750
public health, 2:765
puerperal fever, 2:767–769
sepsis, 2:869
Staphylococcus aureus infections, 2:912, 913
urinary tract infection, 2:1013
vancomycin-resistant *Enterococci,* 2:1025–1028
"Notes from the Field: Fatal Rat-Bite Fever in a Child-San Diego County, California," 2:*787–788*
Notifiable diseases, 2:**678–681,** *679,* 680*s*
babesiosis, 1:97
brucellosis, 1:141, 142
chikungunya, 1:182
epidemiology, 1:332
legislation and international law, 1:536
Lyme disease, 2:958
mumps, 2:646
plague, 2:718
public health, 2:762–763
Q fever, 2:773
rabies, 2:777
sexually transmitted infections, 2:878
tetanus, 2:954
tularemia, 2:991
Nova Scotia, 1:406
Novartis, 1:547, 2:1078
Novobiocin, 1:380
Novosibirsk, Russia, 2:894, 1051
NPR
benznidazole, 1:173–174
Crimean-Congo hemorrhagic fever, 1:244
HPV vaccine, 1:470
lice treatment, 1:554
Médicins Sans Frontières, 2:601

whooping cough vaccine, 2:1068–1069
NSAIDs. *See* Nonsteroidal anti-inflammatory drugs
Nucleic acid tests
blood supply, 1:126
Chlamydia infection, 1:191, 191*s*
gonorrhea, 1:389
rapid diagnostic tests, 2:782
trichomoniasis, 2:976
Nucleoside reverse transcriptase inhibitors, 1:13
Numbness
B virus infection, 1:92
marine toxins, 2:591
shingles, 2:886
toxoplasmosis, 2:964
Nunn, Lois, 1:411
Nuremberg Code, 1:344
Nurses. *See* Health care workers
Nursing homes and long-term care facilities
Chlamydia pneumoniae, 1:195
Clostridium difficile infection, 1:210, 211, 213
cohorted communities, 1:223, 224
gastroenteritis, 1:358
hepatitis A, 1:423
norovirus infection, 2:670
pneumonia, 2:727
RSV infection, 2:833
scabies, 2:853
strongyloidiasis, 2:930
vancomycin-resistant *Enterococci,* 2:1027
Nutraceuticals, 2:591*s*
Nutrition, 1:307, 427. *See also* Malnutrition
Nuurali, Siman, 2:596
Nystatin, 1:159

O

Oaxaca, Mexico, 1:406
Obama, Barack, 1:509, 2:744–747, *745,* 851
Occupational risk
alveolar echinococcosis, 1:25
B virus infection, 1:91–92, 93
Baylisascaris infection, 1:107
bioterrorism preparedness, 2:1051*s*
bloodborne pathogens, 1:129–130
brucellosis, 1:141, 142
cat scratch disease, 1:163
Chagas disease, 1:172
Crimean-Congo hemorrhagic fever, 1:244
cryptosporidiosis, 1:251
hepatitis B, 1:426, 428*s*
hepatitis C, 1:431
hepatitis D, 1:435
herpes simplex 1, 1:442
histoplasmosis, 1:451
H5N1 virus, 1:392*s*
Lassa fever, 1:527, 528
Legionnaires' disease, 1:531
leptospirosis, 1:549
monkeypox, 2:627
mycotic disease, 2:651
needlestick injuries, 1:131
Nipah virus infection, 2:663–664
nosocomial infections, 2:675
plague, 2:717
protozoan diseases, 2:754
psittacosis, 2:759
Q fever, 2:771
rabies, 2:777
Rift Valley fever, 2:814
SARS, 2:971
sporotrichosis, 2:903
tuberculosis, 2:984, 985
typhus, 2:999, 1001
Venezuelan equine encephalitis virus, 2:1035
Occupational Safety and Health Administration, US, 1:129, 131, 2:701
Occupational therapy for polio, 2:738
Oceania, 1:30, 2:769, 1088
O'Connor, Daniel Basil, 2:739
Ocular histoplasmosis, 1:451
Odds ratio and epidemiology, 1:330
O'Driscoll, Tristan, 2:1026, 1027
Office for State, Tribal, Local, and Territorial Support, 1:167
Office of Criminal Investigations, FDA, 2:671
Office of Infectious Diseases, 1:168
Office of Laboratory Security, Public Health Agency of Canada, 1:80
Office of Malaria Control in War Areas, 1:165
Office of Noncommunicable Diseases, Injury, and Environmental Health, 1:168
Office of Public Health Preparedness and Response, 1:167
Office of Public Health Scientific Services, 1:168
Office of Technology Assessment, US, 1:111
Office of the Surgeon General of the Army, US. *See* U.S. Surgeons General
O157:H7 *Escherichia coli. See Escherichia coli* O157:H7
Ohio
encephalitis, 1:317
histoplasmosis, 1:449
influenza pandemic of 1957, 1:501–502
measles, 1:487, 2:594
norovirus infection, 2:669, 671
Ohio River valley, 1:122, 448
Ohio River Valley fever. *See* Histoplasmosis
Oil of lemon eucalyptus, 2:907, 1061
Ointment, antibiotic. *See* Topical medications
Okello, Anna L., 2:942
Oklahoma, 2:873*s*
Old World hantaviruses, 1:404–405, 407
Old World leishmaniasis, 2:755
Older adults and the elderly
avian influenza, 1:89
babesiosis, 1:96
bacterial meningitis, 2:606
candidiasis, 1:158, 159, 160
Clostridium difficile infection, 1:209, 210, 211, 212, 213
coccidioidomycosis, 1:219
cohorted communities, 1:223, 224
cryptosporidiosis, 1:252
demographics, 1:261, 263
Escherichia coli O157:H7, 1:340
food-borne disease, 1:356
gastroenteritis, 1:358
group B streptococcal infections, 2:925, 926
histoplasmosis, 1:449
infection control and asepsis, 1:485, 487
influenza, 1:489, 490–491
influenza pandemic of 1957, 1:499, 501
Japanese encephalitis, 1:513
listeriosis, 1:556
marine toxins, 2:592
norovirus infection, 2:669
opportunistic infections, 2:683
pension payments, 1:307
pneumonia, 2:726, 727, 729
psittacosis, 2:760
rickettsial disease, 2:811
RSV infection, 2:832, 833, 834
sanitation-related diseases, 2:844
scabies, 2:852
sepsis, 2:868, 869
severe fever with thrombocytopenia syndrome, 2:872
shingles, 1:177, 2:885, 886, 887
St. Louis encephalitis, 2:906
tetanus, 2:954
toxoplasmosis, 2:966
tuberculosis, 2:984
typhus, 2:998
urinary tract infection, 2:1014
viral disease, 2:1041
Oldstone, Michael B. A., 2:1043
Oligonucleotides, 1:72
Olympic Games, 2:1029, 1030, 1042, 1102
Oman, 2:968*s*
Omeprazole, 1:411
Omsk hemorrhagic fever, 1:419

On the Mode of Communication of Cholera (Snow), 1:333
"On the Mode of Communication of Cholera" (Snow), 1:200
Onchocerca volvulus. See Filariasis
Onchocerciasis. *See* River blindness
Onchocerciasis Control Program, 2:822
Ongula, Timish, 2:1089
Online resources. *See* Internet resources
ONRAB rabies vaccine, 2:779
Ontario, Canada
  blastomycosis, 1:122
  Escherichia coli O157:H7, 1:339, *339*
  hantavirus, 1:406
  shingles vaccines, 2:888
  West Nile virus, 2:1060
Oocysts, 1:259–260, 2:757, 964
Oophoritis, 2:645, 646
Open defecation, 2:844, 845, 846, 846*s*, 881
Operation Sea Spray, 2:1014*s*
Ophüls, William, 1:218
Opioids, 1:428, 2:886, 887
Opisthorciasis. *See* Liver fluke infections
Opossums, 1:148, 2:973, 998, 999
Opportunistic infections, 2:**682–684,** 682*t*
  AIDS, 1:8, 12, 14, 18–19
  anti-cytokine antibody syndrome, 1:53, 54
  bacterial diseases, 1:100
  Haemophilus influenzae, 1:394
  hot tub rash, 1:466
  Legionnaires' disease, 1:530
  microorganisms, 2:616–617
  microsporidiosis, 2:622, 623–624
  mycotic disease, 2:649, 651
  Pneumocystis jirovecii pneumonia, 2:721–724
  Staphylococcus aureus infections, 2:911
  talaromycosis, 2:944–946
  viral disease, 2:1038
Oracular syphilis, 2:935
Oral cancer, 1:470–471
Oral Cancer Foundation, 1:471
Oral candidiasis, 1:158, *158*
Oral contraceptives, 1:517
Oral hydration therapy. *See* Hydration and rehydration
Oral papillomas, 1:468
Oral rehydration therapy. *See* Hydration and rehydration
Oral sex
  AIDS, 1:8, 9, 11
  herpes simplex 1 virus, 1:441, 443
  herpes simplex virus 2, 1:445, 446
  HPV, 1:469, 470, 471, 2:878
  syphilis, 2:936
  trichomoniasis, 2:975
Oral vaccines
  polio vaccine, 2:733, 734, 738
  rabies vaccine, 2:779
  typhoid fever vaccine, 2:994
Oran virus, 1:406
Orange County, CA, 1:567, 2:595
Orchitis and mumps, 2:645, 646
Ordinary smallpox, 2:891
Oregon, 1:187, 2:672, 717
Organ damage
  brucellosis, 1:141
  Chagas disease, 1:173
  helminth disease, 1:416
  impetigo, 1:482
  rickettsial disease, 2:810
  schistosomiasis, 2:860
Organ failure
  Clostridium difficile infection, 1:209, 212
  glanders, 1:379
  hemorrhagic fevers, 1:420
  macrophage activation syndrome, 2:575–576
  Marburg hemorrhagic fever, 2:586
  necrotizing fasciitis, 2:659
  sepsis, 2:868
  toxic shock, 2:961, 962
  tularemia, 2:990
  typhus, 2:998
Organ transplantation
  aspergillosis, 1:85, 86, 86*s*
  cancer, 1:155
  candidiasis risk factors, 1:158
  Chagas disease, 1:172, 173
  CMV infection risk factors, 1:214–215, 215–216
  coccidioidomycosis risk factors, 1:220
  Escherichia coli O157:H7, 1:341
  hepatitis B, 1:428
  hepatitis D, 1:435
  herpes simplex 1 virus risk factors, 1:442
  histoplasmosis risk factors, 1:449
  malaria, 2:580
  microsporidiosis, 2:624*s*
  nocardiosis, 2:666
  opportunistic infections, 2:682, 684
  Pneumocystis jirovecii pneumonia, 2:721
  rabies, 2:777
  rickettsial disease, 2:810
  strongyloidiasis, 2:928, 929
  tuberculosis, 2:984
  vancomycin-resistant *Enterococci,* 2:1026
  water-borne disease, 2:1055
  West Nile virus, 1:317
Organisation Mondiale de la Santé Animale. *See* World Organization for Animal Health
Organized crime, 2:1085
Organizing, patients' right to, 2:987–988
Oriental rat flea, 2:715
Orientalis plague biotype, 2:713–714
Oritavancin, 2:1027
Orlovskaya, Russia, 1:277
Oropharyngeal cancer, 1:155*s*, 470–471, 2:1039
Orthomyxoviruses, 2:1041
Orthopoxvirus. See Monkeypox; Smallpox
Oseltamivir
  antiviral drugs, 1:73
  avian influenza, 1:89
  H5N1 virus, 1:393
  influenza, 1:490, 491, 505, 506
Osler, William, 2:1095
Oster, William, 2:729
Ostriches, 1:244
Otitis media. *See* Ear infections
O'Toole, Tara, 1:118
Outbreak (motion picture), 1:302, 304, 2:1017
Outbreaks
  CDC, 1:169
  climate change, 1:205, 206–207
  cohorted communities, 1:224, 225
  demographics, 1:261–265
  emerging infectious diseases, 1:311–314
  GIDEON, 1:375
  pandemic preparedness, 2:690–693
  personal protective equipment, 2:701
  public health, 2:762, 764–765
  travel, 2:970–971
  USAMRIID, 2:1017
  vaccines and vaccine development, 2:1022, 1023
  vector-borne disease, 2:1030
  virus hunters, 2:1045, 1046
  World Health Organization, 2:1077, 1078
  See also Specific diseases and disease types
Outbreaks: field-level response, 2:*685,* **685–689**
  Médecins Sans Frontières, 2:601–602
  ProMed, 2:751–752
  rapid diagnostic tests, 2:783
Outdoor recreation
  alveolar echinococcosis, 1:25
  Baylisascaris infection, 1:107
  giardiasis, 1:371*s,* 372
  leptospirosis, 1:548, 549, 550
  Lyme disease, 1:572
  plague, 2:717

relapsing fever, 2:797
tularemia, 2:990
Outpatient health care settings, 1:210
Ovaries and blastomycosis, 1:122
Overcrowding. *See* Crowded conditions
Over-the-counter medications
colds, 1:230
encephalitis, 1:318
fifth disease, 1:348
gastroenteritis, 1:360
Helicobacter pylori, 1:411
influenza pandemic preparedness, 2:766
lice infestation, 1:553
pinworm, 2:707–708
swimmer's ear and swimmer's itch, 2:933
Overuse of antibiotics
Clostridium difficile infection, 1:210
infections for which cultures are not possible, 1:256
resistant organisms, 1:83, 2:799
Ovex. *See* Anthelmintic drugs; Mebendazole
Oxacillin-resistant *Staphylococcus aureus. See* MRSA
Oxamniquine, 2:862
Oxford-Emergent Tuberculosis Consortium, 2:791
Oxycodone, 2:886
Oysters, 2:591
Ozone water treatment, 2:915, 1055

P

Pacemakers. *See* Implanted devices
Pacific Island descent and Kawasaki disease, 1:515, 517
Pacific Islands
angiostrongyliasis, 1:36
encephalitis, 1:318
fruit bats, 2:663
mosquito-borne diseases, 2:637
tropical infectious diseases, 2:981
yaws, 2:1089
Zika virus, 1:169, 2:1100, 1102
Pacific Northwest. *See* Northwestern United States
Packaging, smart, 1:153, 558
PACRG gene, 1:546
Pafuramidine maleate, 1:4
Paget, James, 2:972
Pain
B virus infection, 1:92
candidiasis, 1:159
Creutzfeldt-Jakob disease, 1:240
diphtheria, 1:275
dracunculiasis, 1:284
hand, foot, and mouth disease, 1:398
hemorrhagic fevers, 1:419
herpes simplex 1 virus, 1:442
herpes simplex virus 2, 1:444
leprosy and loss of pain sensation, 1:545
Lyme disease, 1:573
necrotizing fasciitis, 2:659
polio, 2:736
prion disease, 2:749
shingles, 2:885, 886–887
swimmer's ear and swimmer's itch, 2:932
vaccine reactions, 2:1022
yaws, 2:1087
Pakistan, 1:*185,* 2:*733*
avian influenza, 1:89
bacterial meningitis, 2:606
bloodborne infections transmitted through barber shops, 1:131*s*
cyclosporiasis, 1:259
dengue fever patient, 1:*204*
outbreaks, field-level response to, 2:686
polio, 1:184, 2:733, 734, 734*s*, 737, 740
rotavirus, 1:361, 2:829
United Nations Millennium Goals, 2:1009
Palivizumab, 2:834
Palliative care. *See* Comfort care
Pallor and malaria, 2:580
Palombo, Heidi, 2:634
Palpitations. *See* Heart rate abnormalities
Paltrow, Gwynneth, 2:664
Pan American Health Organization, 1:182, 361, 2:738
Panagiotakopulu, Eva, 2:713
Panama
burkholderia, 1:145
hantavirus, 1:405
Rocky Mountain spotted fever, 2:825
viral disease, 2:1042
Panama Canal
arthropod-borne diseases, 1:75
endemicity, 1:322*s*
histoplasmosis, 1:448
vector-borne disease, 2:1030
virus hunters, 2:1043
yellow fever, 2:1092
Pancreas disease or symptoms
Escherichia coli O157:H7, 1:340
Marburg hemorrhagic fever, 2:586
mumps, 2:645
taeniasis, 2:942
Pandemic Intervals Framework, 2:764*s*
Pandemic preparedness, 2:**690–693,** *691*
Pandemics
AIDS, 1:17–20
CDC, 1:169
cholera, 1:199
dengue and dengue hemorrhagic fever, 1:266
emerging infectious diseases, 1:314
influenza, 1:488, 490, 491
influenza epidemiology, 1:504, 505
influenza pandemic of 1918, 1:493–498
influenza pandemic of 1957, 1:499–502
legislation and international law, 1:534
plague, 2:712–713, 716–717
public health, 2:763–764, 764*s*, 765–766
scarlet fever, 2:857
vaccine development, 2:1023
viral disease, 2:1041
war, 2:1047–1048
zoonoses, 2:1105
Pan-drug resistance, 2:801
Pantoprazole, 1:411
Pan-tropism, 1:31
Pap tests, 1:469, 470, 2:976, 1073
Papa, Anna, 1:245
Papayas, 1:355, 2:842
Papillomas, HPV, 1:468, 469–470
Papovaviruses, 2:1039
Papua New Guinea, 1:103, 241, 2:999
"Papua New Guinea Struggles to Eradicate Yaws Disease," 2:*1088–1090*
Papules and yaws, 2:1087
Paracetamol, 1:182, 2:857
Paragonimus. *See* Lung flukes
Paraguay, 1:220, 406
Parakeets and aspergillosis, 1:86
Paralysis
bacterial meningitis, 2:604
botulism, 1:133, 135
diphtheria, 1:275
encephalitis, 1:316
enterovirus 71 infection, 1:325
food-borne disease, 1:354
Japanese encephalitis, 1:511, 512, 513
leprosy, 1:546
marine toxins, 2:591
opportunistic infections, 2:683
polio, 2:736
rabies, 2:776
Rocky Mountain spotted fever, 2:824–825
schistosomiasis, 2:861
St. Louis encephalitis, 2:905
syphilis, 2:934, 935
tick-borne diseases, 2:957, 958
tsunami lung, 2:730
West Nile virus, 2:1059

Paralytic shellfish poisoning, 2:591
Paramyxoviruses, 2:644, 662
Paraneoplastic limbic encephalitis, 1:316
Parasitic diseases, 2:**694–698,** *696*
amebiasis, 1:27–29
angiostrongyliasis, 1:35–38
anisakiasis, 1:43–46
ascariasis, 1:78–80
babesiosis, 1:95–97
balantidiasis, 1:102–103
cancer, 1:155
Chagas disease, 1:171–174
climate change, 1:204, 205
cryptosporidiosis, 1:250–253
dracunculiasis, 1:283–285
dysentery, 1:289, 290
eradication, 1:284*s*
filariasis, 1:350–352
giardiasis, 1:371–374
helminth disease, 1:414–417
hookworm infection, 1:457–460
leishmaniasis, 1:538–541
lice infestation, 1:552–554
liver fluke infections, 1:560–564
lung flukes, 1:565–568
malaria, 2:578–583
microsporidiosis, 2:622–624
mosquito-borne diseases, 2:638
pinworm infection, 2:705–708
prevention, 2:*694*
protozoan diseases, 2:753–757
resistant organisms, 2:800–801, 802
rickettsial disease, 2:809–812
river blindness, 2:820–822
schistosomiasis, 2:860–863
strongyloidiasis, 2:928–930
swimmer's ear and swimmer's itch, 2:931–933
taeniasis, 2:940–943
tapeworm infections, 2:948–950
toxoplasmosis, 2:964–966
trichinellosis, 2:972–974
trichomoniasis, 2:975, 976
tropical infectious diseases, 2:979–980
water-borne disease, 2:1054
whipworm, 2:1062–1064
World Health Organization, 2:1078
zoonoses, 2:1106
Paratyphoid fever, 2:993
Parents' refusal to vaccinate their children. *See* Refusal to vaccinate children
Paris, France, 1:534
Paris Climate Agreement, 1:206
PARK2 gene, 1:546
Parkinson's disease, 1:524, 525
Parkinsons-like symptoms, 1:3
Parodi, Allesandro, 2:576
Parotitis and mumps, 2:644, *644,* 645
Parrots and aspergillosis, 1:86
Partner notification. *See* Sexual contact notification
Partners for Parasite Control, 1:459, 460
Parvoviruses, 1:347, 348, 2:1039
Pasco, WA, 1:558
Passerine birds, 1:296, 297
Passive case findings, 2:763
Pasternack, Mark, 2:730
Pasteur, Louis
anthrax, 1:50
bacteriology, 1:519
culture and sensitivity techniques, 1:254
germ theory, 1:200, 280, 367, 2:674
microorganisms, 2:615
pasteurization, 1:356
puerperal fever, 2:767
rabies vaccine, 2:777, 778
vaccines, 2:1021
Pasteur Institute, 1:19, 2:717, 778, *815,* 1000–1001
Pasteurization, 1:356, 2:615. *See also* Unpasteurized dairy products
Pasupathy, Shanker, 2:659
PATH, 2:830
Pathogenesis and anellovirus, 1:32
Pathogens. *See* Microorganisms; specific pathogens
Patient education and sexually transmitted infections, 2:878
Patient isolation. *See* Isolation and quarantine
Patient records, 1:286
Patient transport, 1:236
Patient-care equipment. *See* Medical equipment
"The Patients' Charter for Tuberculosis Care," 2:*986–988*
Patients' rights, 2:986–988
Patriot Act, 1:111*s*
Paucibacillary leprosy, 1:546
Paula Souza, Geraldo de, 2:1076
PCR tests. *See* Polymerase chain reaction tests
Peacock, Sharon J., 1:381
Peanut butter, 1:340
Peasants' Revolt, 2:712
Pedestals, 1:339
Pediatric Infectious Diseases Society, 2:728, 921
Pediatrics, 1:179, 186–187, 2:1069
Pediculosis. *See* Lice infestation
Peek, Richard M., Jr., 1:411
Peloponnesian War, 1:290
Pelvic inflammatory disease
Chlamydia infection, 1:189–190, 191
gonorrhea, 1:388–389
HIV symptoms, 1:11
pinworm infection, 2:707
sexually transmitted infections, 2:877
trichomoniasis, 2:976
Pelvic pain, 1:389, 2:646, 877
Penicillin
anthrax, 1:115
antibacterial drugs, 1:57–58
antibiotic resistance, 1:61
culture and sensitivity, 1:256
diphtheria, 1:276
gonorrhea, 1:389
group A streptococcal infections, 2:922
group B streptococcal infections, 2:925
necrotizing fasciitis, 2:659
relapsing fever, 2:796
resistant organisms, 2:800, 801
scarlet fever, 2:857, 858
Staphylococcus aureus infections, 2:913
strep throat, 2:918
syphilis, 2:934, 936
Tuskegee syphilis study, 2:937
war, 2:1049–1050
yaws, 2:1003, 1088
Penicillin G, 1:549, 2:786
Penicillin V, 2:786
Penicillin-resistant *Staphylococcus aureus,* 1:59, 2:640, 800
Penicillin-resistant *Streptococcus* pneumonia, 2:729
Penicillins
antibacterial resistance, 2:676
MRSA, 1:59, 2:640, 800
rat-bite fever, 2:786
syphilis, 2:936
Penicillium marneffei. See Talaromycosis
Penile cancer, 1:155*s*, 468
Penile discharge, 1:189, 2:877, 878
Penis rash and candidiasis, 1:159
Penn State University, 2:1032
Pennsylvania
Baylisascaris infection, 1:105
Chagas disease, 1:172
chickenpox, 1:179
cyclosporiasis, 1:258
illegal snails, 1:38
Lyme disease, 1:571
Powassan virus, 2:742
relapsing fever, 2:795
rubella, 2:837
Pension payments, 1:307
Pentamidine, 1:3, 4, 5, 2:755
Pentavalent antimonials, 1:540, 2:755
Pentosan polysulphate, 1:241
Pepcid. *See* Famotidine
Peptic ulcers and *Helicobacter pylori* infection, 1:343–344, 409
Peptidoglycans, 1:58, 63
Pepto-Bismol. *See* Bismuth subsalicylates
Peramivir, 1:89, 490, 505
Pereira, Miriam, 2:1108
Perforated colon and amebiasis, 1:27
Pericarditis and viral disease, 2:1039

Period of communicability, 1:331
Period of prevalence, 1:330
Peripheral nerve involvement. *See* Nerve damage or pain
Peritonitis, 1:79, 210, 2:929
Permethrin
lice infestation, 1:553
malaria prevention, 2:581
scabies, 2:853
tick-borne disease prevention, 2:958
typhus prevention, 2:1000
Venezuelan equine encephalitis virus prevention, 2:1035*s*
Personal protective equipment, 2:*674*, **699–701**, *848*
bloodborne pathogens, 1:131
colds, 1:230
contact precautions, 1:235, 236
droplet precautions, 1:287
Ebola, 1:304
epidemiology, 1:331
infection control and asepsis, 1:484–485
Lassa fever, 1:528
leptospirosis, 1:549
Marburg hemorrhagic fever, 2:586
psittacosis, 2:759, 760
public health, 2:764
Q fever, 2:773
slaughtering process, 1:90
smallpox, 2:893
standard precautions, 2:909
vancomycin-resistant *Enterococci* prevention, 2:1026
viral disease prevention, 2:1041
See also Clothing, protective
Personality changes, 1:316, 2:753, 935
Personal-service workers and AIDS prevention, 1:11
Person-to-person transmission
amebiasis, 1:27–28
avian influenza, 1:89
bacterial meningitis, 2:605
brucellosis, 1:141, 142*s*
Chlamydia infection, 1:190
colds, 1:229
contact precautions, 1:237
Ebola, 1:301, 303
elbow bump greeting, 1:402
enterovirus 71 infection, 1:325
Epstein-Barr virus, 1:335
fifth disease, 1:348, 348*s*
glanders, 1:379
group A streptococcal infections, 2:921
Haemophilus influenzae, 1:395
hand, foot, and mouth disease, 1:398–399
hemorrhagic fevers, 1:419
hepatitis A, 1:424–425
impetigo, 1:480, 481–482
influenza, 1:488–489
influenza pandemic of 1918, 1:495
influenza pandemic of 1957, 1:500
lice infestation, 1:553
malaria, 2:580
Marburg hemorrhagic fever, 2:587
measles, 2:594
microbial evolution, 2:614
microsporidiosis, 2:623
mononucleosis, 2:631
Nipah virus infection, 2:663, 664
personal protective equipment, 2:700
plague, 2:716
rabies, 2:777
rickettsial disease, 2:810
ringworm, 2:817
rotavirus infection, 2:828
scabies, 2:852
scrofula, 2:866
shigellosis, 2:880, 883
smallpox, 2:892
Staphylococcus aureus infections, 2:912
strep throat, 2:917–918, 918*s*
strongyloidiasis, 2:930
vancomycin-resistant *Enterococci,* 2:1026
viral meningitis, 2:609
Perth, Australia, 1:326
Pertussis. *See* Whooping cough
Peru
burkholderia, 1:145
cholera, 1:199
cyclosporiasis, 1:258, 259
encephalitis, 1:317
hantavirus, 1:406
leishmaniasis, 1:539
plague, 2:715
sporotrichosis, 2:902, 903
Venezuelan equine encephalitis virus, 2:1034
Peshawar, Pakistan, 1:*204*
Pesticide Environmental Stewardship Program, 2:639
Pesticide resistance, 1:76, 463, 2:792
Pesticides and disease prevention
arthropod-borne diseases, 1:75
burkholderia, environmental benefits of, 1:146
DDT, 2:1045
dracunculiasis, 1:284
Eastern equine encephalitis, 1:298
hemorrhagic fevers, 1:420
infection control and asepsis, 1:486
malaria, 1:321, 2:579, 581, 583
mosquito-borne diseases, 2:638–639, 638*s*
parasitic diseases, 2:696
plague, 2:719
rickettsial diseases, 2:811
Rocky Mountain spotted fever, 2:826
treated bed nets and the lifespan of mosquitoes, 2:1031–1032
tropical infectious diseases, 2:*979,* 982
typhus, 2:1000
vector control, 1:462
vector resistance, 1:463
vector-borne diseases, 2:1030
Venezuelan equine encephalitis virus, 2:1035, 1035*s*
West Nile virus, 2:*1058,* 1061
yellow fever, 2:1093
Zika virus, 2:1102
zoonoses, 2:1107
Petechiae, 1:267, 404
Petri, Richard Julius, 1:255
Pets
alveolar echinococcosis, 1:24, 25, 25*f*
animal importation, 1:40
Campylobacter infection, 1:152*s*
cat scratch disease, 1:161–163
cryptosporidiosis, 1:251
giardiasis, 1:372
giardiasis vaccine, 1:373
histoplasmosis, 1:449
parasitic diseases, 2:695
plague, 2:716, 717, 718, 719
protozoan diseases, 2:754
psittacosis, 2:759–761
rabies, 2:775, 776–777, 778
rabies vaccination, 2:777–778
raccoons as, 1:108
rat-bite fever, 2:785, 787–788
ringworm, 2:818, 819
sporotrichosis, 2:903
tapeworm infections, 2:948
tick-borne diseases, 2:958, 959
toxocariasis, 1:80*s*
toxoplasmosis, 2:964, 965*s*
typhus, 2:998
West Nile virus, 2:1060
wildlife trade, 2:1083
zoonoses, 2:1106
Petting zoos, 1:339
Pew Charitable Trust, 1:263
Pfeiffer, Johannes, 1:394
Pfeiffer's disease. *See* Mononucleosis
Pfizer, 2:925, 969, 1089, 1090
Phage therapy, 1:63, 2:642, 803, 913
Phagocytosis, 2:575, 576*s*
Pharmaceutical companies
African sleeping sickness programs, 1:1
anthelmintic drug costs, 2:707–708
antibiotic resistance, 1:59, 63
antibiotics development, 2:803
developing nations and drug delivery, 1:270–272

group B streptococcal infection vaccines, 2:925
hepatitis A vaccine, 1:424
leprosy drug donations, 2:1078
leprosy drugs, 1:547
Médecins Sans Frontières, 2:600–601
river blindness drugs, 2:822
trachoma, antibiotics for, 2:969
yaws drugs, 2:1089, 1090
Pharmacy Times, 1:432
Pharyngitis
avian influenza, 1:89
cat scratch disease, 1:161–163
Chlamydia infection, 1:190
Chlamydia pneumoniae, 1:194
CMV infection, 1:214
colds, 1:228
dengue and dengue hemorrhagic fever, 1:267
Eastern equine encephalitis, 1:296
fifth disease, 1:347
group A streptococcal infections, 2:922, 922*s*
hand, foot, and mouth disease, 1:397
influenza, 1:488, 504
measles, 2:593
mononucleosis, 1:223, 2:630, 631
scarlet fever, 2:856, 857
sexually transmitted infections, 2:876
strep throat, 2:917–919
tularemia, 2:990
Venezuelan equine encephalitis virus, 2:1033
PHEIC. *See* Potential public health emergencies of international concern
Phenol ring structure, 1:67
Phenols, 1:281
Philadelphia, PA
Legionnaire's disease, 1:169, 529–530, 531
relapsing fever, 2:795
yellow fever, 2:1092
Philippines
angiostrongyliasis, 1:36
avian influenza, 1:89
balantidiasis, 1:103
chikungunya, 1:180, 181
Ebola, 1:303
filariasis, 1:*351*
fruit bats, 2:663
hemorrhagic fevers, 1:420*s*
leprosy, 1:546
lung flukes, 1:566
measles, 2:594, *594*
rabies, 2:779
SARS, 2:848–849
taeniasis, 2:942
typhoid fever, 2:*994*
UK beef imports, 1:139
Phillips, Dom, 2:1107
Philosophical Transactions of the Royal Society B, 1:479
Phitsanulok, Thailand, 1:514
Phlebovirus infection, 2:872, 873*s*
Photocoagulation laser eye surgery, 1:451
Photon-tunneling microscopy, 2:620
Photosensitivity
bacterial meningitis, 2:605
Crimean-Congo hemorrhagic fever, 1:244
glanders, 1:379
leprosy, 1:545
mononucleosis, 2:634
pink eye, 2:702
trachoma, 2:967
typhus, 2:997
viral meningitis, 2:607, 608
Phototherapy, 2:706–707
Physical development and hookworm infection, 1:58, 459
Physical therapy, 1:297, 2:738
Physicians. *See* Health care workers
Picard, André, 2:887
Picardeau, Mathieu, 1:549
Picaridin, 2:907, 1035*s*
Pickled herring and anisakiasis, 1:45
Picornaviruses, 1:230, 324–327, 2:1039
Piening, Turid, 1:5
Pigeon lice, 1:554
Pigs
anellovirus, 1:31
balantidiasis, 1:103
brucellosis, 1:140, 142
Campylobacter infection, 1:152
encephalitis, 1:318
H5N1 virus, 1:391–393
influenza, 1:488, 490, 491, 505
Japanese encephalitis, 1:512
leptospirosis, 1:548
liver fluke infections, 1:562
Nipah virus infection, 2:662, 663–664
protozoan diseases, 2:754
ringworm, 2:817
taeniasis, 2:940, 941
trichinellosis, 2:974
Venezuelan equine encephalitis virus, 2:1033
zoonoses, 2:1106
Pink eye, 2:**702–704,** *703*
Pin-Rid. *See* Pyrantel pamoate
Pinworm infection, 1:415, 2:**705–708,** *706*
"Pinworm Treatments Are an Expensive Drug Mistake You Don't Need to Make," 2:*707–708*
Pin-X. *See* Pyrantel pamoate
Pinyon mice, 1:406
Piperacillin-tazobactam, 2:1027
Piperazine, 1:80, 2:706
Plague, 2:*718*
arthropod-borne diseases, 1:75
bacterial diseases, 1:99, 100
bioterrorism, 1:114, 116
endemicity, 1:322*s*
immigration, 1:472, 474
isolation and quarantine, 1:509, 533
personal protective equipment, 2:699
policies regarding, 1:533
quarantine, 1:508
travel, 2:970
USAMRIID, 2:1018
vector-borne disease, 2:1029
war, 2:1050–1051
zoonoses, 2:1106
Plague, early history, 2:*709,* **709–714**
Plague, modern history, 2:**715–720,** *717*
Plague of the Philistines, 2:710
Plants, 1:57, 385
Plaques, atherosclerotic, 1:195
Plasmapheresis, 1:54
Plasmid-mediated transfer, 1:62–63
Plasmids, 2:612
Plasmodia. See Malaria
Platelet count, 1:267, 2:872
Pleomorphic bacteria, 1:394
Pleural effusion, 2:726
Pliny the Elder, 2:618
PLOS Neglected Tropical Diseases
dengue, 1:266
economic development, 1:308
Lassa fever, 1:526
leptospirosis, 1:549, 550
river blindness, 2:822
schistosomiasis, 2:863
strongyloidiasis, 2:930
PLOS One, 1:30–31, 2:712
PLOS Pathogens, 2:1049
Plot, Robert, 1:203–204
Pneumococcus. *See Streptococcus pneumoniae*
Pneumocystis carinii pneumonia. *See Pneumocystis jirovecii* pneumonia
Pneumocystis jirovecii pneumonia, 2:**721–724,** 721*s*
AIDS, 1:8, 18, 19*s*
opportunistic infections, 2:682
prevention, 2:*723*
Pneumonia, 2:**725–731,** *727*
AIDS, 1:8, 18, 19*s*
bacterial disease vaccines, 1:101
cat scratch disease, 1:162
chickenpox, 1:176
Chlamydia infection, 1:190
Chlamydia pneumoniae, 1:193–195
CMV infection, 1:214
cohorted communities, 1:223, 224
glanders, 1:379
group B streptococcal infections, 2:924, 925

Haemophilus influenzae, 1:395, 396
influenza, 1:488, 505
Legionnaires' disease, 1:529, 530
measles, 2:593
microorganisms, 2:616
nosocomial infections, 2:674
Operation Sea Spray, 2:1014*s*
opportunistic infections, 2:682
overreliance on fluoroquinolones, 1:257
Pneumocystis jirovecii pneumonia, 2:721–724, 725–726
polio, 2:737
prevention, 2:*723*
psittacosis, 2:759
Q fever, 2:772, 773
rat-bite fever, 2:786
relapsing fever, 2:795
RSV infection, 2:832, 834
SARS, 2:847, 850
scarlet fever, 2:857
Staphylococcus aureus infections, 2:912
substandard and falsified medical products, 1:272
tularemia, 2:990
war, 2:1047
whooping cough, 2:1067
Pneumonic plague, 1:116, 2:712, 717, 1029
Pneumonitis and ascariasis, 1:79
Poaching, animal, 1:304, 2:1085
Pockmarks, 2:890
Point prevalence, 1:330
Poison, rat, 2:787
Poland, 1:89, 396, 2:712
Polar bear meat, 2:974
Polio, 2:**736–740**
CDC, 1:169
childhood vaccination, 1:186
emerging infectious diseases, 1:314
eradication, 1:184
immigration, 1:473
polio eradication campaign, 2:732–735
vaccines, 1:185, 2:1021, *1021*
viral disease, 2:1039
war, 2:1049
World Health Organization, 2:1077–1078
Polio eradication campaign, 1:487, 2:**732–735**, *733*, 736–738, 740
Polio-like symptoms, 1:326
Poliomyelitis. *See* Polio
Politics and immigration, 1:474
Pollard, Charlie, 2:937
Pollution, water. *See* Water pollution
Polyarthritis and gonorrhea, 1:388
Polyendocrinopathy, 1:53
Polymerase chain reaction tests
babesiosis, 1:96, 97
babesiosis diagnosis, 1:95
Buruli ulcer, 1:149
cat scratch disease, 1:162
Crimean-Congo hemorrhagic fever, 1:244
cyclosporiasis, 1:260
encephalitis, 1:318
enterovirus 71 infection, 1:326
genetic identification of microorganisms, 1:363
microorganisms, 2:616*s*
plague, 2:713–714
rapid diagnostic tests, 2:782
rat-bite fever, 2:787
relapsing fever, 2:798
SARS, 2:850
trachoma, 2:969
viral meningitis, 2:609
Zika virus, 2:1102
Polymicrobial disease, 2:658
Polynesia, 1:36, 2:1102
Pontiac fever, 1:529, 530, 531
Popper, Erwin, 2:736
Popular Science, 1:417
Population, 1:331, 2:710, 711. *See also* Immigration
Porcupines, 2:1085
Pork. *See* Meat
Porpoises and anisakiasis, 1:45
Portugal
babesiosis, 1:96
bovine spongiform encephalopathy, 1:137
dengue and dengue hemorrhagic fever, 1:267
vancomycin-resistant *Enterococci,* 2:1026
Posaconazole, 2:945–946
Possums, 1:148, 2:973, 998, 999
Postexposure prophylaxis
bioterrorism, 1:114, 116
rabies, 2:777, 778
war, 2:1050
Postherpetic neuralgia, 1:176, 177, 2:885, 886–887, 888
Postinfection issues
encephalitis, 1:315–316
giardiasis, 1:371, 373
polio, 2:737
streptococcal glomerulonephritis, 2:921
Post-kala-azar dermal leishmaniasis, 1:538–539
Postmenopausal women, 2:1013
Posttransfusion hepatitis. *See* Hepatitis B
Post-treatment Lyme disease syndrome, 1:569, 571–572, 572–574
Potential public health emergencies of international concern, 2:1084
Potera, Carol, 2:730
Poultry
antibiotic resistance, 1:63, 64
avian influenza, 1:88–89, 90
bacterial disease, 1:100
Campylobacter infection, 1:152–153
Ebola, 1:304
emerging infectious diseases, 1:311
food-borne diseases, 1:355, 357, 401, 485
histoplasmosis, 1:449
H5N1, 1:391, 392, 392*s*
listeriosis, 1:557, 558
microbial evolution, 2:614
overcrowding, 2:*612*
psittacosis, 2:759, 760
resistant organisms, 2:803
Salmonella infection, 2:841, 842
viral disease, 2:1041
world trade, 2:1083–1084
zoonoses, 2:1106
Poverty and low socioeconomic status
Chagas disease, 1:173
diphtheria, 1:277
economic development, 1:306, 308, 309
filariasis, 1:351
gonorrhea risk factors, 1:389
helminth disease, 1:415
hepatitis A, 1:423
hookworm infection, 1:457
leishmaniasis, 1:538, 539
maternal mortality, 2:769
river blindness, 2:822
St. Louis encephalitis, 2:906
Sustainable Development Goals, 2:1010*s*
trachoma, 2:968
tropical infectious diseases, 2:979
tuberculosis, 2:985–986
UNICEF, 2:1006
water-borne disease, 2:1055
yaws, 2:1087
Zika virus, 2:1103
zoonoses, 2:1107–1108
"'Poverty Favours the Mosquito' Experts Warn Zika Virus Could Return to Brazil'", 2:*1107–1108*
Powassan virus, 1:316, 2:**741–743**, *742*, 957
Poxviruses, 2:1039. *See also* specific diseases
Prague, Czech Republic, 1:474
Prairie dogs, 2:627, 715
Praziquantel
liver fluke infections, 1:562
lung flukes, 1:567
schistosomiasis, 2:860, 862, 863
taeniasis, 2:942
tapeworm infections, 2:948, 950
Precautions. *See* Airborne precautions; Contact precautions; Droplet precautions; Standard precautions
PREDICT, 2:1046
Prednisolone, 2:576
Pre-exposure rabies vaccines, 2:777

Pregnancy
candidiasis risk factors, 1:158, 159
chickenpox, 1:175, 177
chickenpox vaccine precautions, 1:178
Chlamydia infection screening, 1:191
cholera, 1:198
Clostridium difficile infection, 1:211
CMV infection, 1:216
coccidioidomycosis risk factors, 1:219–220
dysentery, 1:290
Ebola, 1:303*s*
emerging infectious diseases, 1:312
fifth disease, 1:348
food-borne disease, 1:356
gonorrhea, 1:388
group B streptococcal infection, 2:926
hepatitis E, 1:437
herpes simplex virus 2, 1:445, 446*s*
HIV testing, 1:13
hookworm infection, 1:458
Kawasaki disease, 1:517
Lassa fever, 1:527
listeriosis, 1:556, *557,* 558
malaria, 2:580, 581
measles, 2:594
mumps vaccine, 2:646
mycotic disease, 2:650
parasitic diseases, 2:695
protozoan disease prevention, 2:755
Rift Valley fever, 2:814
rubella, 2:838
toxoplasmosis, 2:965–966
United Nations Millennium Goals, 2:1007–1008
urinary tract infection, 2:1013
viral disease, 2:1039, 1042
women, 2:1072, 1073
Zika virus, 1:76*s,* 2:1102
Premature birth
group B streptococcal infections, 2:925, 926
listeriosis, 1:556
maternal chickenpox, 1:177
measles, 2:594
syphilis, 2:936
urinary tract infection, 2:1013
whooping cough, 2:1066
Prenatal care, 1:216, 2:1007–1008
Preparedness
bioterrorism, 1:114, 116, 117–118, 2:700*s*
CDC, 1:169
emergency preparedness kits, 2:766
pandemic preparedness, 2:690–693
plague, 2:717–718, 719
public health, 2:765–766
USAMRIID, 2:1017
"President William Jefferson Clinton's Apology on Behalf of the United States of America," 2:*937–938*
President's Council of Advisors on Science and technology, 2:*745*
President's Initiative on Combating Antibiotic Resistance, 2:*745*
President's (Obama Administration) Initiative on Combating Antibiotic Resistance, 2:7**44–748**
Preston, Richard, 1:302, 2:1017
Presumptive therapy for pneumonia, 2:728
Preterm birth. *See* Premature birth
Prevacid. *See* Lansoprazole
Prevalence and epidemiology, 1:330, 331
Prevention
African sleeping sickness, 1:4–5
AIDS, 1:10, 11, 20
airborne precautions, 1:21–23
alveolar echinococcosis, 1:25*f*
anisakiasis, 1:45
anthrax, 1:50
ascariasis, 1:80
avian influenza, 1:90
babesiosis, 1:97
balantidiasis, 1:103
bloodborne infections, 1:131
bovine spongiform encephalopathy, 1:138
burkholderia, 1:145–146
Campylobacter infection, 1:152*s,* 153
Chagas disease, 1:173
chikungunya, 1:*180,* 182
Chlamydia infection, 1:191
cholera, 1:198–199, 200
cohorted communities, 1:225
contact precautions, 1:235–238
Creutzfeldt-Jakob disease, 1:241
cryptosporidiosis, 1:252, *252–253,* 252*s*
cyclosporiasis, 1:260
diphtheria, 1:278
dracunculiasis, 1:284
enterovirus 71 infection, 1:326–327
filariasis, 1:350
food-borne disease, 1:356–357
handwashing, 1:400–402
hantavirus, 1:407
helminth disease, 1:416
hemorrhagic fevers, 1:420
hepatitis B, 1:428
histoplasmosis, 1:451
HIV, 1:455*s*
hosts and vectors, 1:462
impetigo, 1:480
kuru, 1:523
Lassa fever, 1:527, *527,* 527*s*
Legionnaires' disease, 1:531
leishmaniasis, 1:541
leptospirosis, 1:549*s,* 550
liver fluke infections, 1:562–564
malaria, 2:581, 582–583
marine toxin-related illnesses, 2:592
measles, 2:595
microsporidiosis, 2:624
mosquito-borne diseases, 2:638–639
norovirus infection, 2:670
nosocomial infections, 2:673, *674,* 675
opportunistic infections, 2:684
parasitic diseases, 2:696
pinworm infection, 2:706–707
plague, 2:719
Pneumocystis jirovecii pneumonia, 2:*723*
pneumonia, 2:729–730
polio, 2:738
Powassan virus, 2:742
protozoan diseases, 2:755
Q fever, 2:773
rat-bite fever, 2:787, 788
relapsing fever, 2:797
rickettsial disease, 2:809, 811
Rift Valley fever, 2:815
scabies, 2:854*s*
St. Louis encephalitis, 2:906–907
syphilis, 2:936
taeniasis, 2:942
tapeworm infections, 2:950
tick bites, 2:958
toxoplasmosis, 2:965*s,* 966
tropical infectious diseases, 2:981, 981*s,* 982
tularemia, 2:989, 991
typhus, 2:1000
vancomycin-resistant *Enterococci,* 2:1027
vector-borne disease, 2:1030–1031
Venezuelan equine encephalitis virus, 2:1035*s*
viral disease, 2:1041
water-borne disease, 2:1054, 1055–1056
water-borne illness, 1:466*s*
West Nile virus, 2:*1058,* 1059, 1061
whipworm, 2:1062, 1063
yellow fever, 1:345–346
zoonoses, 2:1107
Prevention of Mother-to-Child Transmission program, 1:20
"The Prevention of Yellow Fever," 1:*345–346*
Prilosec. *See* Omeprazole
Primaquine, 2:581
Primary encephalitis, 1:315
Primary hosts, 1:461
Primates
AIDS, origins of, 1:17–18

anellovirus, 1:31
animal importation, 1:40, 41
B virus infection, 1:91–94
balantidiasis, 1:103
cat scratch disease, 1:163
colds, 1:228
dengue and dengue hemorrhagic fever, 1:266
Ebola, 1:303, 304, 2:1022, 1085
group B streptococcal infection, 2:926–927
hemorrhagic fevers, 1:420*s*
histoplasmosis, 1:449
lice infestation, 1:552
malaria, 2:581
typhus research, 2:1001
Venezuelan equine encephalitis virus, 2:1035
world trade, 2:1083
zoonoses, 2:1106
Prince Edward Island, Canada, 2:592
Prince of Wales Hospital, 2:848
Princeton University, 1:307
Prion Clinic, 1:241
Prion disease, 2:*748*, **748–750,** 749*s*
animal importation, 1:40
blood supply, 1:126–127
bovine spongiform encephalopathy, 1:136–139
Creutzfeldt-Jakob disease, 1:239–242
kuru, 1:522–525
standard precautions, 2:910
sterilization, 2:915
zoonoses, 2:1107
Pripsen. *See* Anthelmintic drugs
Prisoners of war, 2:1048
Prisons and prisoners
Chlamydia pneumoniae, 1:195
cohorted communities, 1:223, 224
dysentery, 1:290
hepatitis A, 1:423
hepatitis C, 1:431
scabies, 2:853
trichomoniasis, 2:976
typhus, 2:999
Privacy issues
legislation and international law, 1:536
notifiable diseases databases, 2:681
parents refusing to vaccinate their children, 1:187
tuberculosis patients' right to, 2:987
Probability and epidemiology, 1:330
Procaine, 2:786
Proceedings of the National Academy of Sciences, 2:791*s,* 1031
Procopius of Caesarea, 2:710–711
Prodrome, smallpox, 2:891
Produce, 1:258, 558
Proglottids, 2:941, 942, 948
Program for Appropriate Technology in Health (PATH), 1:156
Program for Monitoring Emerging Diseases. *See* ProMED
Program for the Elimination of Neglected Diseases in Africa, 1:270, 2:822
Programme for the Surveillance and Control of Leishmaniasis, 1:541
Progress on Drinking Water, Sanitation and Hygiene 2017, 2:1079
Progressive multifocal leukoencephalopathy, 2:683, 1039
Proguanil, 2:581
Project Bioshield, 1:51, 114, 2:654
Project HOPE, 2:730
ProMED, 2:**751–752**
Promin, 1:545
Prophylaxis
avian influenza, 1:90
bioterrorism, 1:114
Chlamydia pneumoniae prevention, 1:195
CMV infection, 1:215–216, 216–217
malaria, 2:581
opportunistic infections, 2:683
plague, 2:718
Pneumocystis jirovecii pneumonia, 2:721
public health, 2:763
typhus, 2:1000
Prostate issues, 1:122, 2:976, 1013
Prosthetic heart valves, 2:683, 773
Prostitutes. *See* Sex workers
Prostration, 1:504
Protease inhibitors, 1:13
Protective aspects of certain diseases, 1:373, 411–412
Protective equipment, personal. *See* Personal protective equipment
Protein deficiency and hookworm infection, 1:458
Protein in the urine. *See* Proteinuria
Proteins
avian influenza, 1:88
Creutzfeldt-Jakob disease, 1:240, 242
Ebola, 1:302
Escherichia coli O157:H7, 1:339
H5N1, 1:392
immune response, 1:476–477
influenza, 1:489, 494, 500
kuru, 1:522–523
prion disease, 2:748
viral disease, 2:1039
women, 2:1074
zoonoses, 2:1107
Proteinuria, 1:526
Proton pump inhibitors, 1:411
Protonix. *See* Pantoprazole
Protozoan diseases, 2:**753–758,** *755*
balantidiasis, 1:102–103
cyclosporiasis, 1:258–260
dysentery, 1:289, 290
emerging infectious diseases, 1:312
gastroenteritis, 1:359–360
giardiasis, 1:371–373
hosts and vectors, 1:461
leishmaniasis, 1:538–541
microorganisms, 2:616
opportunistic infections, 2:682–683
parasitic diseases, 2:694
sexually transmitted infections, 2:878
tick-borne diseases, 2:957, 958
toxoplasmosis, 2:964–966
tropical infectious diseases, 2:980
vector-borne disease, 2:1030–1031
Pruritis. *See* Itching
Prusiner, Stanley, 1:242, 2:750
Pseudomembranes and diphtheria, 1:274–275, 276
Pseudomonas aeruginosa dermatitis. *See* Hot tub rash
Pseudoterranova decipiens, 1:43
Psittacosis, 2:**759–760**
Psorphora mosquitoes, 2:1033
Psychiatric symptoms
Creutzfeldt-Jakob disease, 1:240
Japanese encephalitis, 1:512
prion disease, 2:749
Psychosocial issues, 1:113–114, 446
Pteropodidae, 1:301, 2:662–663
Pubic lice, 1:552, 2:878
Public awareness and education
AIDS prevention, 1:15
balantidiasis prevention, 1:103
bioterrorism preparedness, 1:117–118
Chlamydia infection prevention, 1:191
coccidioidomycosis, 1:221
developing nations and drug delivery, 1:271
Ebola, 1:304
eradication of dracunculiasis, 1:284*s*
helminth disease, 1:417, 2:1064
histoplasmosis, 1:451
liver fluke infections, 1:563
Marburg hemorrhagic fever, 2:587
Rocky Mountain spotted fever, 2:826
sepsis, 2:869
syphilis, 2:936
Syrian refugees, 1:265
Task Force on Antimicrobial Resistance, 1:256*s*
toxic shock, 2:963
United Nations Millennium Goals, 2:1010
yersiniosis, 2:1098
Public health, 2:**762–766**
arthropod-borne diseases, 1:75
bacteria identification, 1:340*s*

bioterrorism, 1:114, 116, 2:1051*s*
CDC, 1:164–169
cholera prevention, 1:200
cohorted communities, 1:223–225
economic development, 1:306–309
endemic disease, 1:322*s*
epidemiology, 1:328–333
GIDEON, 1:375–377
influenza, 1:491, 503–507
isolation and quarantine, 1:508–510
legislation and international law, 1:533–537
liver fluke infections prevention, 1:562–564
mosquito-borne diseases, 2:637
outbreaks, field-level response to, 2:685–688
pandemic preparedness, 2:690–693
President's Initiative on Combating Antibiotic Resistance, 2:744–746
resistant organisms, 2:802
Rocky Mountain Laboratory research, 2:655–656
SARS, 2:850–851
taeniasis, 2:943
tuberculosis patients' responsibilities, 2:988
United Nations Millennium Goals, 2:1008–1010
vaccines and vaccine development, 2:1020
war, 2:1049
World Health Organization, 2:1076–1080
zoonoses, 2:1107–1108
Public Health Agency of Canada, 1:80
Public Health Emergency of International Concern, 2:687
Public Health England, 2:765, 858
Public Health Reports, 2:1047
Public Health Service Act, 1:508
Public information dissemination, 2:687
Public Service Act, 1:510*s*
Puerperal fever, 1:366, 2:673–674, **767–770,** 921–922
Puerto Rico
angiostrongyliasis, 1:36
chikungunya, 1:182
climate change, 1:207
cyclosporiasis, 1:259
dengue and dengue hemorrhagic fever, 1:267
marine toxins, 2:590
yellow fever, 2:1095
Pulmonary alveolar proteinosis, 1:53, 54, 2:667
Pulmonary anthrax, 1:49
Pulmonary edema, 1:405
Pulmonary histoplasmosis, 1:448–449
Pulmonary sporotrichosis, 2:901, 902
Pulmonary tuberculosis, 1:566
Puncture wounds, 2:659, 666, 953
Purdue University, 1:117
Pus, 1:293, 380
Pustules
scabies, 2:852
shingles, 2:888
smallpox, 2:890, 1020
Puumala virus, 1:404
Puvanendran, Rukshini, 2:659
Pyelonephritis, 2:1012, 1014
Pygmy rice rats, 1:405, 406
Pyrantel pamoate, 1:80, 2:706
Pyrethrins, 1:553, 2:638
Pyrethroids, 2:638
Pyrithramine, 2:755
Pyrocide, 2:*1058*

Q

Q fever, 2:**771–774**
rickettsial disease, 2:810
tick-borne diseases, 2:957
war, 2:1051
QT interval, 2:796
QuantiFERON-TB (QFT) Gold test, 2:984
Quarantine. *See* Isolation and quarantine
Quaternary ammonium, 1:282
Quebec, Canada, 1:486, 2:1060
Queensland tick typhus, 2:810
Quinine
babesiosis, 1:97
malaria, 2:579
mosquito-borne diseases, 2:638
tick-borne diseases, 2:958
Quinolone antibiotics, 1:58, 2:933
Quinupristin/dalfopristin, 2:1027

R

Rabbit fever. *See* Tularemia
Rabbits
Baylisascaris infection, 1:107
plague, 2:715
taeniasis, 2:940
tularemia, 2:990, 991
wildlife trade, 2:1083
Rabeprazole, 1:411
Rabies, 1:41–42, 2:*775,* **775–780,** 1106, 1107
Raccoons
Baylisascaris, 1:105–108
histoplasmosis, 1:449
lung flukes, 1:567
Powassan virus, 2:741
rabies, 2:776
typhus, 2:998
Race/ethnicity
AIDS, 1:13
blastomycosis, 1:122
coccidioidomycosis, 1:219
Kawasaki disease, 1:515, 517
Rocky Mountain spotted fever, 2:825
syphilis, 2:936
trichomoniasis, 2:976
Rain forest anthrax, 1:49
Rain forests, 1:1, 2:664
Rain forests and monkeypox, 2:626, 627
Rainfall
climate change, 1:205–206, 206–207
hantavirus, 1:407
Rift Valley fever, 2:813, 814–815
Rajagopal, Lakshmi, 2:927
Rajchman, Ludwik Witold, 2:1003
Random microbial evolution, 2:611, 613, 614
Random vaccination, 1:263–264
Randomized selection of research subjects, 1:331–332
Ranitidine, 1:411
Ranson, Hilary, 2:1031, 1032
Rapid diagnostic tests, 2:**781–784,** *782*
African sleeping sickness, 1:5
AIDS, 1:12
dengue and dengue hemorrhagic fever, 1:267–268
influenza, 1:490
leishmaniasis, 1:540–541
strep throat, 2:919
RAPIDS, 2:638
Rapivab. *See* Peramivir
Rarotonga, 1:36
Rash
African sleeping sickness, 1:2
avian influenza, 1:89
bacterial meningitis, 2:605
blastomycosis, 1:122
candidiasis, 1:159
cat scratch disease, 1:161–163
Chagas disease, 1:172
chickenpox, 1:175, 176
chikungunya, 1:181
Crimean-Congo hemorrhagic fever, 1:244
dengue and dengue hemorrhagic fever, 1:267
enterovirus 71 infection, 1:325, 326
fifth disease, 1:347, *348,* 349
gonorrhea, 1:388
hand, foot, and mouth disease, 1:397
hantavirus, 1:404
helminth disease, 1:415
HIV, 1:11

hookworm infection, 1:458
hot tub rash, 1:465–467
Kawasaki disease, 1:515
lice infestation, 1:552
liver fluke infections, 1:560
Lyme disease, 1:569, 570, 571, 572, 573
Marburg hemorrhagic fever, 2:586
marine toxins, 2:590
measles, 2:593, 594, *594*
meningitis, 2:606*s*
monkeypox, 2:626, 628*s*
mononucleosis, 2:631
mycotic disease, 2:650
nocardiosis, 2:666
rat-bite fever, 2:785, 787, 788
relapsing fever, 2:795
rickettsial disease, 2:809, 810, 811
Rocky Mountain spotted fever, 2:824
rubella, 2:837
scabies, 2:853
scarlet fever, 2:856
sexually transmitted infections, 2:877
shingles, 1:176, 2:885, 886
smallpox, 2:891, 1020
swimmer's ear and swimmer's itch, 2:931
syphilis, 2:934–935
tick-borne diseases, 2:956–957
toxic shock, 2:961, 962
trichinellosis, 2:973
typhoid fever, 2:993
typhus, 2:997
viral disease, 2:1039
viral meningitis, 2:608
West Nile virus, 2:1059
yersiniosis, 2:1097
Zika virus, 2:1101
Raspberries, 1:*259*
cyclosporiasis, 1:258
Rat lungworm. *See* Angiostrongyliasis
Rat-bite fever, 2:**785–788,** *786,* 1106
Rats
angiostrongyliasis, 1:35–38, 36
climate change, 1:204
Crimean-Congo hemorrhagic fever, 1:244
hantavirus, 1:405
hosts and vectors, 1:461
Lassa fever, 1:526, 527, 528
leptospirosis, 1:550
monkeypox, 2:627
nosocomial infections, 2:675–676
plague, 2:712, 713, 715, 717, 719
rabies, 2:777
talaromycosis, 2:944, 945, *945*
tetanus, 2:953
toxic shock research, 2:963
trichinellosis, 2:973
typhus, 2:997, 998, 999
vector-borne disease, 2:1029
wildlife trade, 2:1083
zoonoses, 2:1106
Ravelli, Angello, 2:576
Ravuconazole, 2:945–946
Razor shaving, 1:131*s*
Reactivation
CMV infection, 1:214
fifth disease, 1:347
herpes simplex 1 virus, 1:226, 316, 441, 442
herpes simplex virus 2, 1:446
histoplasmosis, 1:451
tuberculosis, 1:224
Varicella zoster, 1:53, 175, 176
See also Relapse and recurrence
Read, Andrew, 2:1032
Reassortment and influenza, 1:494, 496, 500, 501, 505
Recalls, food, 1:135, 557, 558
Recife, Brazil, 1:*312,* 2:*845, 1100*
Recombinant DNA technology, 1:81–82, 2:985
Recombinant vesicular stomatitis virus-Zaire Ebola virus vaccine, 1:304
Recombivax HB, 1:155*s*
Recommendations for Counteracting Disease Spread through Migration, 1:*264–265*
"Recommendations for Prevention of and Therapy for Exposure to B Virus," 1:93
Reconstructive surgery and leishmaniasis, 1:540
Rectal prolapse and whipworm, 2:1062
Recurrence. *See* Relapse and recurrence
Red Book, 1:475
Red Cross
blood supply, 1:126, 127
diphtheria, 1:278
legislation and international law, 1:535
Measles and Rubella Initiative, 2:595
outbreaks, field-level response to, 2:687
parasitic disease screening, 2:695
tsunami lung, 2:730
Red tides, 2:591
Red-backed vole, 1:405
Redi, Francisco, 1:366
Red-meat allergies, 2:956, 957
Reed, Walter, 1:*343*
virus hunters, 2:1043
yellow fever, 2:1094, 1095
Yellow Fever Commission, 1:342, 344, 345
Re-emerging infectious diseases, 2:**789–794**
bacterial diseases, 1:101
chikungunya, 1:*180*
climate change, 1:206
demographics, 1:263
diphtheria, 1:274, 277
dysentery, 1:290
economic development, 1:308
epidemiology, 1:332
glanders, 1:381
immigration, 1:473
infection control and asepsis, 1:486
parasitic diseases, 2:756–757
trichinellosis, 2:972
tuberculosis, 1:59
zoonoses, 2:1107
See also Emerging infectious diseases
Reese's Pinworm Medicine, 2:707
Refugees
African sleeping sickness, 1:5
cholera, 1:200
demographics, 1:261, 263–264
hepatitis E, 1:438
immigration, 1:472, 473, 474
leishmaniasis, 1:541
lice infestation, 1:554
Médecins Sans Frontières, 2:600
relapsing fever, 2:796, 797–798
schistosomiasis, 2:860, 862, 863
smallpox, 2:*892*
typhus, 2:999
war, 2:1048, 1050
world trade, 2:1082
zoonoses, 2:1106
Refusal to vaccinate children
diphtheria, 1:276–277, 278
infection control and asepsis, 1:487
measles, 2:595–598
risk for communities, 1:186–187
vaccines and vaccine development, 2:1021
Regional B Biocontainment Laboratories, 2:792
Regulations. *See* Legislation and international law
Rehabilitation
polio, 2:738
tuberculosis patients' rights, 2:988
Rehydration. *See* Hydration and rehydration
Reinfection, 1:190, 210, 211
Reingold, Art, 2:1069
Reiter's syndrome, 2:841
Relapse and recurrence
blastomycosis, 1:122
coccidioidomycosis, 1:221
cryptosporidiosis, 1:251
cyclosporiasis, 1:259
herpes simplex virus 2, 1:444
leishmaniasis, 1:541

malaria, 2:580
mononucleosis, 2:633
pink eye, 2:703
yaws, 2:1087
See also Reactivation
Relapsing fever, 1:552, 554, 2:**795–798,** *796,* 957
Relative risk of disease, 1:330
Relenza. *See* Zanamivir
Religion, 1:187, 2:712, 1021
Rely superabsorbent tampons, 2:962
Renaissance, 2:712
Renal disease. *See* Kidney disease or symptoms
ReNu, 1:232
Reoviruses, 2:1039, 1041
Replication
AIDS, 1:13
anellovirus, 1:31–32, 33
antiviral drugs, 1:72
cancer, 1:154
climate change, effect of, 1:207
CMV infection, 1:217
encephalitis, 1:318
HIV, 1:444, 454, 455
influenza, 1:490, 494
Marburg hemorrhagic fever, 2:586
microbial evolution, 2:613
retroviruses, 2:805, 808
viral disease, 2:1037, 1039, *1040*
Reporting
blastomycosis, 1:123
cholera, 1:198
coccidioidomycosis, 1:218
cryptosporidiosis, 1:251
epidemiology, 1:332
influenza, 1:506
isolation and quarantine, 1:510
legislation and international law, 1:535, 536
notifiable diseases, 2:678–681
plague, 2:718
ProMED, 2:751–752
public health, 2:762–763
rabies, 2:777
SARS, 2:851
scarlet fever, 2:858
sexually transmitted infections, 2:878
tropical infectious diseases, 2:981
women and infectious diseases, 2:1072
Reproductive rights. *See* Abortion; Contraception
Reproductive system infections
Chlamydia infection, 1:189–190, 191
disinfection byproducts, effects of, 1:282
gonorrhea, 1:389–390
sanitation, 2:844
Reptiles, 1:40, 371, 2:1083
Research
ADHD medications and sexually transmitted infections, 2:977
Advanced Diagnostics Program, 2:783*s*
African sleeping sickness, 1:4
AIDS, 1:12, 14, 20
amebiasis, 1:29
anellovirus, 1:32–33
animal importation, 1:40
antibiotic resistance, 1:59, 63
antiviral drugs, 1:72, 73
arthropod-borne diseases, 1:77
Asilomar Conference, 1:81–82, 81–83
avian influenza, 1:155
B virus, 1:93
biodefense research and development, 1:118–119
biological warfare research, 2:1015–1018
Buruli ulcer, 1:149, 150
Campylobacter infection, 1:153
CDC, 1:167–168, 169
climate change, 1:205
climate change and parasites, 2:697–698
climate change and re-emerging infectious diseases, 2:793
CMV infection, 1:214, 217
coccidioidomycosis, 1:221
colds, 1:230
ear infections, 1:295
Ebola, 1:302, 303–304, 419, 2:602
edible vaccines, 1:82*s*
emerging infectious diseases, 1:313
epidemiology, 1:330, 331–332
Escherichia coli O157:H7, 1:340–341
Fusarium keratitis, 1:232–233
genital herpes, 1:365
germ theory of disease, 1:369
giardiasis, 1:373
gonorrhea, 1:389
group A streptococcal infection, 2:922
group B streptococcal infection, 2:925, 926–927
Health Insurance Portability and Accountability Act, 1:536
Helicobacter pylori, 1:409, 412
hepatitis D, 1:435
herpes simplex virus 2, 1:445, 446
HIV, 1:130, 455
H5N1, 1:393, 2:614
immune system and tattoos, 1:478*s*
influenza drugs, 1:505
Japanese encephalitis, 1:513, 514
Kawasaki disease, 1:517–518
Koch's postulates, 1:519–521
Lassa fever, 1:528
leishmaniasis, 1:540
leprosy, 1:545
lice infestation, 1:554
listeriosis, 1:558
malaria, 2:579, 581–582
marine toxin-related illnesses, 2:592
Médecins Sans Frontières, 2:600
microbial evolution, 2:614
microsporidiosis, 2:624
MMR vaccine and autism, 2:838*s*
mosquito-borne diseases, 2:638, *815*
MRSA, 2:642, 643
mycotic disease, 2:652
National Institute of Allergy and Infectious Diseases, 2:654
Nipah virus infection, 2:663
norovirus infection, 2:671
nosocomial infections, 2:675–676
Operation Sea Spray, 2:1014*s*
opportunistic infections, 2:684
outbreaks, field-level response to, 2:687
parasitic diseases, 2:695–696
pink eye, 2:704
plague, 2:713–714, 718, 719
pneumonia, 2:729
polio, 2:739*s*
prion disease, 2:750
Project Bioshield, 1:114
Q fever, 2:773
rabies, 2:778, 779
rapid diagnostic tests, 2:783
re-emerging infectious diseases, 2:791, 792
resistant organisms, 2:803
retroviruses, 2:808
rickettsial disease, 2:811
Rift Valley fever, 2:813, 815
Rocky Mountain Laboratory, 2:655–656
rotavirus, 2:830, 831
RSV, 2:834–835
Salmonella, 2:842
schistosomiasis, 2:863
self-experimentation of scientists, 1:342–346
sepsis, 2:869
sexually transmitted infections, 2:879
shigellosis, 2:882
shingles, 2:888
smallpox, 2:898, 899
St. Louis encephalitis, 2:907
Staphylococcus aureus infections, 2:913
sterilization, 2:915, 916*s*
talaromycosis, 2:946
toxic shock, 2:963
treated bed nets and the lifespan of mosquitoes, 2:1031–1032
tropical infectious diseases, 2:981–982

tuberculosis, 2:983, 985
tularemia, 2:991
Tuskegee syphilis study, 2:937–938
typhoid fever, 2:996
typhus, 2:999–1000, 1001
vaccines and vaccine development, 2:1020–1023
vancomycin-resistant *Enterococci,* 2:1026, 1027
Venezuelan equine encephalitis virus, 2:1033–1035
viral meningitis, 2:610
virus hunters, 2:1043–1046
West Nile virus, 2:1058
women, 2:1071, 1073–1074
worm therapy, 1:417
yaws, 2:1090
yellow fever, 2:1093–1095
Research and Markets, 1:135
Research laboratories. *See* Laboratories and laboratory workers
Reservoirs. *See* Hosts and vectors; specific diseases
"Residents of Flint, Mich., Are Still Afraid of the City's Water," 2:*882–883*
Resistance, vector, 1:463
Resistant organisms, 2:*799,* **799–804**
arthropod-borne diseases, 1:76
disinfection, 1:281, 282
germ theory of disease, 1:369–370
microbial evolution, 2:611–614
microorganisms, 2:617
re-emerging infectious diseases, 2:790, 792
sterilization, 2:915–916
Task Force on Antimicrobial Resistance, 1:256*s*
See also Antibiotic resistance; Drug resistance
Resolution on Sepsis, WHO, 2:869–870
Respirators, 1:*22,* 23, 2:700
Respiratory diphtheria, 1:274–275
Respiratory syncytial virus infection. *See* RSV infection
Respiratory system disease or symptoms
B virus infection, 1:92
burkholderia, 1:145
Chlamydia pneumoniae, 1:193–195
climate change, 1:205
colds, 1:228–230
diphtheria, 1:274–275
ear infections, 1:293
glanders, 1:379
group A streptococcal infections, 2:921
Haemophilus influenzae, 1:394–396
malaria, 2:580
Middle East respiratory syndrome, 1:386
necrotizing fasciitis, 2:659
Nipah virus infection, 2:662, 663
nosocomial infections, 2:674
opportunistic infections, 2:684
personal protective equipment, 2:700
pneumonia, 2:729
polio, 2:736–737
Powassan virus, 2:742
protozoan diseases, 2:753
psittacosis, 2:760
rabies, 2:776
resistant organisms, 2:803
Rocky Mountain spotted fever, 2:824
RSV infection, 2:832–835
SARS, 2:847–851
St. Louis encephalitis, 2:906
tularemia, 2:990
Responsibilities, patient, 2:988
Rest
chikungunya, 1:182
encephalitis, 1:318
hepatitis B, 1:427
influenza, 1:490
mononucleosis, 2:630, 632, 635
nocardiosis, 2:668
pneumonia, 2:729
scarlet fever, 2:857
strep throat, 2:918
viral meningitis, 2:610
Zika virus, 2:1102
Restaurants and food-borne diseases, 1:11, 2:671–672
Reston, VA, 1:41, 302, 303, 2:1017
Reston ebolavirus, 2:1017
Restriction enzymes, 1:81
Retinitis, 1:214
Retinochoroiditis, 2:964
Retroorbital pain, 1:267
Retroviral gene therapy, 2:806
Retroviruses, 2:*805,* **805–808**
cancer, 1:155
HIV, 1:453–456
viral disease, 2:1041
Réunion Island, 1:181
Reuters, 1:558
Reverse transcriptase, 2:806, 1041
Reverse transcriptase polymerase chain reaction, 1:364
Rex, David, 1:501–502
Reye syndrome, 2:632, 634
Rhabdovirus group and rabies, 2:776
Rhesus monkeys and SARS research, 2:850
Rheumatic diseases and macrophage activation syndrome, 2:575–576
Rheumatic fever, 2:857, 917, 920, 921
Rhinitis. *See* Colds
Rhode Island, 1:96, 571
Ribasphere. *See* Ribavirin
Ribavirin
antiviral drugs, 1:71
Crimean-Congo hemorrhagic fever, 1:245
hantavirus, 1:407
hepatitis C, 1:431, 432
Lassa fever, 1:528
measles, 2:595
Nipah virus infection, 2:663
rabies, 2:778
RSV infection, 2:834
Ribosomes and antibiotics, 1:58
Rice production and encephalitis, 1:318
Rice rats, 1:405
"Rice-water stool," 1:197, 198, 201
Ricin toxin, 2:1018
Ricketts, 2:809
Ricketts, Howard Taylor, 2:656, 809, 824, 997
Rickettsial disease, 2:**809–812,** *810,* 810*t*
Rocky Mountain spotted fever, 2:824–826
tick-borne diseases, 2:957
typhus, 2:997–1001
Rifampicin
brucellosis, 1:142
Buruli ulcer, 1:149
leprosy, 1:545, 546, 2:1078
Q fever, 2:773
re-emerging infectious diseases, 2:791
tropical infectious diseases, 2:981
typhus, 2:1000
Rifampin. *See* Rifampicin
Rift Valley fever, 1:418, 419, 2:**813–816,** *814, 815*
Rights and responsibilities of tuberculosis patients, 2:986–988
Rigors and rat-bite fever, 2:787
Rimantadine, 1:393, 490, 505
Rinderpest, 1:40
Ring vaccination, 1:115, 2:1022
Ringworm, 1:42, 2:**817–819,** *818,* 819*t*
Rio de Janeiro, Brazil, 2:902, 903, 1029, 1030, 1042
Rio Grande do Norte, Brazil, 2:1101
Rio Mamore virus, 1:406
Risk assessment and epidemiology, 1:329–330
Risk Management and Healthcare Policy, 2:942
Risks, vaccination, 1:187
Risky sexual behaviors and ADHD medications, 2:977
Ritonavir, 1:13
Rituximab, 1:54
River blindness, 2:**820–822,** *821, 822*
developing nations and drug delivery, 1:270

helminth disease, 1:417
tropical infectious diseases, 2:981*s*
Rizzetto, Mario, 1:434
RNA
Ebola, 1:302, 303
influenza pandemic of 1918, 1:496
Venezuelan equine encephalitis virus, 2:1033
viral disease, 2:1039
Zika virus, 2:1102
RNA viruses
gastroenteritis, 1:358, *360*
genetic identification of microorganisms, 1:364
hemorrhagic fevers, 1:418–419
hepatitis A, 1:422–425
hepatitis C, 1:430–432
hepatitis D, 1:434–436
hepatitis E, 1:437–439
HIV, 1:453–456
Japanese encephalitis, 1:511–514
Marburg hemorrhagic fever, 2:585–587
measles, 2:593–598
mumps, 2:644–647
rabies, 2:775–779
retroviruses, 2:805–808
RSV infection, 2:832–835
rubella, 2:836–839
viral disease, 2:1039
Robbins, Frederick, 2:736, 739
Robicheau, Joan, 2:887–888
Robinson, Marion, 1:181
Rockefeller Foundation, 2:1043, 1045
Rockefeller University, 2:676
Rockfish and anisakiasis, 1:45
Rocky Mountain Laboratory, 2:654, 655–656
Rocky Mountain spotted fever, 2:*810*, **824–827**, *825, 826*
National Institute of Allergy and Infectious Diseases, 2:656
rickettsial disease, 2:809, 810, 811
tick-borne diseases, 2:956–957
typhus, 2:997, 999
Rocky Mountain wood ticks, 2:824
Rocky Mountains region, 1:134
Rodents
alveolar echinococcosis, 1:25, 25*f*, 26
anellovirus, 1:31
angiostrongyliasis, 1:35
animal importation, 2:1084
babesiosis, 1:97
balantidiasis, 1:103
climate change, 1:204
Crimean-Congo hemorrhagic fever, 1:244
cyclosporiasis, 1:258
globalization, 1:384
hantavirus, 1:404–407
hemorrhagic fevers, 1:418, 419, 420
Lassa fever, 1:526–528, 527, 528
leishmaniasis, 1:539, 540
leptospirosis, 1:548, 550
monkeypox, 2:626, 627
plague, 2:712, 713, 715, 717, 719
Powassan virus, 2:741
rabies, 2:777
rat-bite fever, 2:785–788, 787
relapsing fever, 2:795
smallpox, 2:890
talaromycosis, 2:944, 945
tapeworm infections, 2:948
tetanus, 2:953
toxic shock research, 2:963
toxoplasmosis, 2:964
tularemia, 2:990
typhus, 2:997, 998, 999
vector-borne disease, 2:1029
Venezuelan equine encephalitis virus, 2:1033, 1035
virus hunters, 2:1045, 1046
Rohingya people, 1:261, 2:*892*
Roll Back Malaria program, 2:1005
Roma persecution, 2:712
Roman Empire, late, 2:710–711
Romaña, Cecilio, 1:172
Romania, 1:89, 2:973, 974
Rome, ancient
animal importation, 1:39
leprosy, 1:544
lice infestation, 1:552–553
plague, 2:710
Roosevelt, Franklin D., 2:737
Rose gardener's disease. *See* Sporotrichosis
Ross, Ronald, 1:343
Rossbach, Michael Joseph, 2:920
Rotary International, 2:732, 740, 1077
Rotavirus infection, 2:**828–831**, *829, 830*
childhood vaccinations, 1:186
cohorted communities, 1:224
gastroenteritis, 1:358–359, 361
viral disease, 2:1041
WHO childhood vaccination recommendations, 1:185
Rotavirus Vaccination Program, 1:361, 2:830
Roundworm infections, 1:*78, 415*
angiostrongyliasis, 1:35–38
animal importation, 1:42
anisakiasis, 1:43–46
ascariasis, 1:78–80
dracunculiasis, 1:283–285
filariasis, 1:350–352
helminth disease, 1:414–415
hookworm infection, 1:457–460
parasitic diseases, 2:695
pinworm infection, 2:705–708
strongyloidiasis, 2:928–930
toxocariasis, 1:80*s*
trichinellosis, 2:972–974
Rous, Peyton, 1:154
Rous sarcoma virus, 2:806
Rousseff, Dilma, 2:1108
Roux, Emile, 2:1001
Roxithromycin, 2:1000
Royal Academy of Havana, 2:1094
Royal Caribbean, 2:670
Royalty as healers, 2:865, *866*
RSV infection, 2:**832–835,** *833*
RTS,S vaccine, 2:791
RTS,S/AS01 vaccine, 2:581–582
Rubella, 1:185, 2:*836,* **836–839,** 1041
Rubeola. *See* Measles
Ruminants and taeniasis, 2:940, 941
Runny nose
avian influenza, 1:89
Chlamydia pneumoniae, 1:194
colds, 1:228
ear infections, 1:293
RSV infection, 2:832
Rupp, Nicholas, 1:425
Rural areas
Chagas disease, 1:173
demographics, 1:262
dracunculiasis, 1:283
Ebola, 1:303, 304
economic development, 1:307, 309
Japanese encephalitis, 1:513
leishmaniasis, 1:539, 540, 541
liver fluke infections, 1:563
maternal mortality, 2:769
monkeypox, 2:627
rabies, 2:775
rapid diagnostic tests, 2:783
sanitation, 2:846*s*
schistosomiasis, 2:861, 863
yaws, 2:1087
yellow fever, 2:1093
Russell, Josiah C., 2:711
Russia
alveolar echinococcosis, 1:24
anthrax, 1:48
avian influenza, 1:89
Biological Weapons Convention, 1:110
Crimean-Congo hemorrhagic fever, 1:243
diphtheria, 1:187, 277
encephalitis, 1:317
H5N1, 1:496
international adoption, 1:475
lice infestation, 1:554
liver fluke infections, 1:561
Powassan virus, 2:741–743, 742
protozoan diseases, 2:755
smallpox, 2:890, 892, 894, 896, 897, 898
tick-borne diseases, 2:957
typhus, 2:998, 999
viral meningitis, 2:*609,* 610
war, 2:1048, 1051

rVSV-ZEBOV vaccine, 2:1022
Rwanda
AIDS pandemic history, 1:18
cholera, 1:200, 201
re-emerging infectious diseases, 2:790

S

Saaremaa virus, 1:405
Sabia virus, 1:418
Sabin, Albert, 1:184, 2:738, 739*s*
Sabin, Florence, 1:*535,* 536*s*
Sabin Health Laws, 1:536*s*
Sabin Vaccine Institute, 2:863
Saccharomyces boulardii, 1:211
Sacramento County, CA, 1:221
"Safe Management of Patients with Ebola Virus Disease in U.S. Hospitals," 1:*237–238*
SAFE strategy, 2:968–969, 968*s*
Safe Water Program, CDC, 2:1055
Safer sex practices
AIDS, 1:11, 14, 15
gonorrhea, 1:390
sexually transmitted infections, 2:878
syphilis, 2:936
Safety and the Asilomar Conference guidelines, 1:81–82
Saipan, 1:36
Salad, bagged, 1:558
Salah, Suaado, 2:596, 598
Salerno, Italy, 1:*473*
Salivary glands, 2:776, 932
Salk, Jonas, 1:184, 2:738, 739*s,* *1021*
Salmon, Daniel, 2:840
Salmon and anisakiasis, 1:45
Salmonella infection, 2:**840–843,** *841*
animal importation, 1:40
anti-cytokine antibody syndrome, 1:53
food-borne disease, 1:355
zoonoses, 2:1106
Salmonella typhi. See Typhoid fever
Salmonellosis. *See Salmonella* infection
Salpingitis, 1:388, 2:707, 877
Salt Lake County, UT, 1:425
Samples, virus. *See* Virus sharing
San Diego, CA, 1:*423,* 2:787–788
San Francisco, CA
AIDS pandemic history, 1:19*s*
coccidioidomycosis, 1:218
mitten crabs, 1:567
shigellosis, 2:882
San Joaquin, Bolivia, 2:1045
San Joaquin Valley, CA, 1:220, 221
Sanatoriums, tuberculosis, 2:984
Sandflies, 1:538, 539, 540, 541, 2:980
Sandia National Laboratories, 2:899
Sanitation, 1:198*t,* 2:**844–846,** *845*
amebiasis, 1:28, 29
ascariasis, 1:80
balantidiasis, 1:102, 103
cholera, 1:197, 198, 200, 201
climate change, 1:205, 207
cryptosporidiosis, 1:250
demographics, 1:261
dengue and dengue hemorrhagic fever, 1:268
diphtheria, 1:275, 277
dysentery, 1:289, 290, 291, 292
economic development, 1:307
endemicity, 1:322, 322*s*
group A streptococcal infections, 2:921
helminth disease, 1:415, 416, 417, 2:1064
hepatitis A, 1:424
hepatitis E, 1:437, 438, 439
hookworm infection, 1:458
hosts and vectors, 1:463
immigration, 1:473
legislation s, 1:534, 535
leishmaniasis, 1:539, 541
leptospirosis, 1:550
liver fluke infection prevention, 1:562
mosquito-borne diseases, 2:638
mycotic disease, 2:651
parasitic diseases, 2:696
pinworm infection prevention, 2:707
plague, 2:717, 719
protozoan diseases, 2:754, 755
puerperal fever, 2:768
re-emerging infectious diseases, 2:793
schistosomiasis, 2:860, 862
sepsis, 2:869
shigellosis, 2:880, 881, 882
strongyloidiasis, 2:930
tapeworm infections, 2:948, 949, 950
trachoma, 2:967, 969
tropical infectious diseases, 2:979, 982
typhoid fever, 2:995
UNICEF, 2:1006
war, 2:1049
water-borne diseases, 2:1053–1056
whipworm, 2:1062, 1063
World Health Organization, 2:1078–1079
yaws, 2:1087
Yemen, 1:*199*
Zika virus, 2:1107–1108
Sanitizers, alcohol-based. *See* Alcohol-based hand sanitizers
Sanofi Pasteur, 1:268
Santosham, Mathuram, 2:831
Saquinivir, 1:13
Sarawak, 1:36
Sarcoptes scabei infection. *See* Scabies
Sarin gas attacks, 1:304
SARS, 2:*679,* **847–851,** *848*
cohorted communities, 1:225
globalization and infectious disease, 1:385
infection control, 1:*384*
isolation and quarantine, 1:509
nosocomial infections, 2:675
notifiable diseases, 2:678
public health, 2:763, 764–765, 766
travel, 2:970–971
viral disease, 2:1041
world trade, 2:1083, 1084
Sashimi and anisakiasis, 1:45
Satcher, David, 2:937
Saudi Arabia
avian influenza, 1:89
relapsing fever, 2:796
Rift Valley fever, 2:814, 816
Scabicides, 2:853
Scabies, 2:**852–855,** *853,* 878
Scalded skin syndrome, 2:912
Scallops, 1:423, 2:591
Scalp ringworm, 2:817, 818
Scandinavia, 1:570, 2:737, 857
Scanning electron microscopes, 2:620
Scarlatina, 2:856
Scarlet fever, 2:**856–859,** *857,* 917, 921
"Scarlet Fever: A Sudden and Dramatic Outbreak Has Been Recorded in England and Scientists Can't Explain Why," 2:*858–859*
Scarring, 2:886, 890, 967, 968, 969
Schenck, Benjamin Robinson, 2:901
Schenck's disease. *See* Sporotrichosis
Schistosomes, 1:415, 2:860–863, 931–933
Schistosomiasis, 2:**860–864,** *861,* *862*
cancer, 1:155
helminth disease, 1:415, 417
hosts and vectors, 1:461
sanitation, 2:845
Schistosomiasis Control Initiative, 2:863
Schlafly, Phyllis, 1:187
Schleiss, Mark R., 1:217
Schneider, Stephen, 1:205
Schonlein, Johann Lukas, 2:983
School immunization laws, 1:185
Schools
Chlamydia pneumoniae, 1:195
histoplasmosis, 1:451
lice infestation, 1:553
See also Cohorted communities
Schottmuller, Hugo, 2:925
Schuchat, Anne, 1:*166*
Science, 2:791*s*
Science Daily, 1:206
Scientific American, 2:1046
Scientific Reports, 1:327

Scientists, self-experimentation by. *See* Self-experimentation by scientists
Scollard, David M., 1:545
Scombrotoxic fish poisoning, 2:590
Scotland, 1:89
Scrapie, 1:136, 138*s*
Scratches. *See* Bites and scratches
Screening
  African sleeping sickness, 1:5
  AIDS, 1:8
  blood supply, 1:125, 126, 127
  Chlamydia infection, 1:191
  CMV infection, 1:216
  cohorted communities, 1:224–225
  Eastern equine encephalitis, 1:297
  epidemiology, 1:331
  eradication, 1:284*s*
  gonorrhea, 1:389, 390
  group B streptococcal infection, 2:926
  hepatitis B, 1:426
  hepatitis C, 1:431
  HIV, 1:12
  HPV, 1:470
  public health, 2:764
  strongyloidiasis, 2:928
  Syrian refugees, 1:264
Scripps Research, 1:12
Scrofula, 2:**865–867**
Scrub typhus, 1:418, 2:810–811, 997, 998, 999, 1000
SDGs. *See* Sustainable Development Goals (SDGs)
Seafood
  angiostrongyliasis, 1:35
  anisakiasis, 1:43–46
  botulism, 1:135
  Campylobacter infection, 1:152
  cryptosporidiosis, 1:251
  gastroenteritis, 1:359
  hepatitis A, 1:423
  liver fluke infections, 1:561, 562
  lung flukes, 1:565–568
  marine toxins, 2:589–592
  tapeworm infections, 2:948
  water-borne diseases, 2:1054
Seal worm, 1:43
Seals and Sea lions, 1:31, 45
Seasonality
  cat scratch disease, 1:163
  chickenpox, 1:177
  cholera, 1:200
  climate change and re-emerging infectious diseases, 2:791*s*
  cyclosporiasis, 1:259
  demographics, 1:263
  dracunculiasis, 1:284–285
  dysentery, 1:290
  Eastern equine encephalitis, 1:296, 298*s*
  fifth disease, 1:348
  hosts and vectors, breeding seasons of, 1:463
  impetigo, 1:480
  influenza, 1:489, 503–507
  Japanese encephalitis, 1:513
  Kawasaki disease, 1:517
  Lassa fever, 1:527
  Lyme disease, 1:572
  mumps, 2:645
  plague, 2:713
  pneumonia, 2:726
  polio, 2:736
  Powassan virus, 2:742
  re-emerging infectious diseases, 2:792
  Rocky Mountain spotted fever, 2:825
  rotavirus infection, 2:828
  RSV infection, 2:833
  rubella, 2:837
  severe fever with thrombocytopenia syndrome, 2:872
  strep throat, 2:918
  swimmer's ear and swimmer's itch, 2:932
  tick-borne diseases, 2:956, 958
  tularemia, 2:990–991
  typhus, 2:999
  viral meningitis, 2:609, 610
  West Nile virus, 2:1059
  whooping cough, 2:1067
  yersiniosis, 2:1096–1099
Seattle Children's Research Institute, 2:927
SEB intoxication, 2:1052
Secondary encephalitis, 1:315–316
Secondary infections
  Eastern equine encephalitis, 1:297
  Ebola, 1:303
  influenza, 1:488, 490
  influenza pandemic of 1957, 1:501
  Japanese encephalitis, 1:512
  measles, 2:595
  mononucleosis, 2:632
  SARS, 2:848
  tropical infectious diseases, 2:980
Secondary syphilis, 2:877
Securities and Exchange Commission, US, 2:671
Security and patients' rights, 2:988
Segretain, Gabriel, 2:944
Seizures
  AIDS, 1:12
  B virus infection, 1:92
  cholera, 1:198
  CMV infection, 1:216
  Eastern equine encephalitis, 1:296
  encephalitis, 1:316, 317, 318
  enterovirus 71 infection, 1:326
  helminth disease, 1:415
  hemorrhagic fevers, 1:420
  Japanese encephalitis, 1:511, 512, 513
  lung flukes, 1:567
  macrophage activation syndrome, 2:575
  malaria, 2:580
  meningitis, 2:606*s*
  nocardiosis, 2:666
  Powassan virus, 2:741
  protozoan diseases, 2:753
  rabies, 1:75, 2:776
  relapsing fever, 2:795
  scarlet fever, 2:857
  schistosomiasis, 2:861
  shigellosis, 2:882
  St. Louis encephalitis, 2:905
  syphilis, 2:935
  taeniasis, 2:943
  toxoplasmosis, 2:964
  tropical infectious diseases, 2:980
  vaccine reactions, 2:1022
  West Nile virus, 2:1059
  whooping cough, 2:1066
  Zika virus, 2:1103
Select Agent Program, CDC, 1:111*s*
Selective pressures and microbial evolution, 1:62, 313–314, 2:611–612, 803
Selective surveillance, 1:86*s*
Selenium sulfide, 2:818
Self *vs.* nonself and the immune system, 1:476–477
Self-experimentation by scientists
  Helicobacter pylori, 1:409
  Koch's postulates, 1:520–521
  lice infestation research, 1:554
  virus hunters, 2:1046
  yellow fever, 1:342–346, 2:1093–1095
Self-isolation and SARS, 2:848
Semmelweis, Ignaz, 1:366, 400, 2:674, 767–768, *768*
Seneca, 2:618
Senegal
  AIDS, 1:15
  measles vaccine clinical trials, 2:1073
  outbreaks, field-level response to, 2:688
  resistant organisms, 2:802
  rubella vaccine, 2:*836*
Senegal River Project, 2:815
Sensation loss and leprosy, 1:54, 543
Sensitivity. *See* Culture and sensitivity
Seoul virus, 1:405, 406, 407
Separate rooms and droplet precautions, 1:286–287
Sepsis, 2:**868–870**
  broad-spectrum antibiotics, 1:257
  CDC, 1:168
  dysentery, 1:289
  enterovirus 71 infection, 1:326
  group B streptococcal infection, 2:926

group B streptococcal infections, 2:924, 925
infection control and asepsis, 1:485
listeriosis, 1:556
puerperal fever, 2:769
scabies, 2:853
urinary tract infection, 2:1014
World Health Organization, 2:1079
Septic scarlet fever, 2:857
Septic shock, 1:379, 388
Septicemia
bacterial meningitis, 2:604
Clostridium difficile infection, 1:210
glanders, 1:379
meningitis, 2:606*s*
Staphylococcus aureus infections, 2:912
toxic shock, 2:961–963
Septicemic plague, 2:711–712
Serbia
avian influenza, 1:89
trichinellosis, 2:974
typhus, 2:998–999
war, 2:1048, 1050
Serological tests. *See* Blood tests
Serotypes
cholera, 1:197, 199
dengue virus, 1:268
Salmonella, 2:840, 842
Serpa, Cleane, 2:1108
Serratia marcescens, 2:1014*s*
Serum hepatitis. *See* Hepatitis B
7-Eleven, 1:425
Severe acute respiratory syndrome. *See* SARS
Severe fever with thrombocytopenia syndrome, 2:**871–873**
Sewer systems. *See* Sanitation
Sex workers
AIDS prevention, 1:15
hepatitis D, 1:435
women, 2:1073
Sexual abuse and trichomoniasis, 2:977
Sexual behavior, 2:977, 1009
Sexual contact notification and testing
Chlamydia infection, 1:191
herpes simplex virus 2, 1:446*s*
sexually transmitted infections, 2:878
syphilis, 2:936
Sexually transmitted infections, 2:**875–879**
brucellosis, 1:141, 142*s*
Chlamydia infection, 1:189, 190, 191
cohorted communities, 1:224
dysentery, 1:292
Ebola prevention, 1:303*s*
Epstein-Barr virus, 1:335
genital herpes, 1:365
gonorrhea, 1:387–390
hepatitis A, 1:422, 423
hepatitis B, 1:426, 427
hepatitis B vaccine, 1:428*s*
herpes simplex 1 virus, 1:441, 443
herpes simplex virus 2, 1:444–446, 445, 446
HPV, 1:468–470
lice, 1:552
microsporidiosis, 2:623
mosquito-borne diseases, 2:637
protozoan diseases, 2:754, 756
scabies, 2:852
shigellosis, 2:880
syphilis, 2:934–939
testing, 2:*876*
trichomoniasis, 2:975–977
United Nations Millennium Goals, 2:1009
urinary tract infection, 2:1012–1013
viral disease, 2:1041
women, 2:1071, 1073
Zika virus, 2:1108
See also AIDS; HIV
Shalala, Donna, 2:938
Shapin, Steven, 1:200
Sharing, virus. *See* Virus sharing
Sharp, Joshua, 1:12
Sharps. *See* Needles and disease transmission
Shear, Neil, 1:123
Sheep
anthrax, 1:47
brucellosis, 1:140
burkholderia, 1:145
Crimean-Congo hemorrhagic fever, 1:244
cryptosporidiosis, 1:251
glanders, 1:378
hemorrhagic fevers, 1:419
liver fluke infections, 1:561, 562
lung flukes, 1:567
Q fever, 2:771–773
Rift Valley fever, 2:814, 815
scrapie, 1:136, 138*s*
taeniasis, 2:940, 941
tetanus, 2:953
toxoplasmosis, 2:964
Venezuelan equine encephalitis virus, 2:1033
zoonoses, 2:1106
Sheep pox, 1:39
Shellfish. *See* Seafood
Shiga, Kiyoshi, 1:289–290, 2:880
Shigella infection. *See* Shigellosis
Shigellosis, 2:**880–884,** *881*
bacterial diseases, 1:100
dysentery, 1:289–290, 291
food-borne disease, 1:355
Shingles, 1:11, 2:**885–889,** *886*
anti-cytokine antibody syndrome, 1:53
antiviral drugs, 1:72
chickenpox, 1:175, 176, 177, 178
chickenpox vaccine, 1:179
viral disease, 2:1039
Shingrix, 1:177, 2:887, 888
Shining Mountain, 1:186–187
Ship fever. *See* Typhus
Ship travel. *See* Cruise ships
Shivering, 2:580, 753, 795
Shock
cholera, 1:198, 201
Ebola, 1:302
food-borne disease, 1:355
glanders, 1:379
gonorrhea, 1:388
hantavirus, 1:404
necrotizing fasciitis, 2:659
toxic shock, 1:169, 2:912, 920, 961–963
Shonka, Nicole, 2:722
Shope, Robert, 2:1045–1046
Short, Erica E., 2:756
Shortness of breath
AIDS, 1:12
avian influenza, 1:89
blastomycosis, 1:122
SARS, 2:850
strongyloidiasis, 2:929
Short-tailed cane mice, 1:405
Shunts, 1:221
Sicily, 2:711, 797–798
"Sick City," 1:*200–201*
Side effects
antiviral drugs, 1:73
Cryptococcus neoformans infection drugs, 1:248
ivermectin, 2:821
See also Adverse effects
Sierra Leone
child marriage, 2:1005
Ebola, 1:302, 2:1085
epidemiology, 1:332
hemorrhagic fevers, 1:*419*
Lassa fever, 1:526, 527, 527*s*
Médecins Sans Frontières, 2:601, 602
public health, 2:765
Sightsavers, 2:969
Silbereld, Ellen K., 1:64
Silent Spring (Carson), 2:638*s*
Siliguri, India, 1:*267*
Simi Valley, CA, 2:671
Simian immunodeficiency virus (SIV), 1:17–18
Simmons, Fred, 2:937
Simond, Paul-Louis, 2:716
Simulation models. *See* Computer modeling
Sin Nombre virus, 1:406, 407, 419
Singapore
British beef ban, 1:138
enterovirus 71 infection, 1:326
glanders, 1:380
hand, foot, and mouth disease, 1:397, 398

Nipah virus infection, 1:64, 2:662
SARS, 2:848–849, 851
Singer, Mervyn, 2:868
Singh, Maya, 1:*401*
Sinus infection, 1:85, 2:917
Sinusitis, 1:190, 256
Sircar, Anita D., 1:107
Skin biopsy, 1:122, 2:945
Skin diseases or symptoms
B virus infection, 1:92
Baylisascaris infection, 1:105
blastomycosis, 1:122
Buruli ulcer, 1:147–150, 148
cholera, 1:201
coccidioidomycosis, 1:218
dengue and dengue hemorrhagic fever, 1:267
diphtheria, 1:275
gonorrhea, 1:388
histoplasmosis, 1:449
hot tub rash, 1:465–467
HPV, 1:468
impetigo, 1:480–482
leishmaniasis, 1:538, 539–540, 541
leprosy, 1:543, 545
macrophage activation syndrome, 2:575
mycotic disease, 2:649, 650
necrotizing fasciitis, 2:659
nocardiosis, 2:666
pinworm infection, 2:705
ringworm, 2:817
river blindness, 2:820, 821
scabies, 2:852–855
shingles, 2:886
sporotrichosis, 2:901–903
Staphylococcus aureus infections, 2:912, *912*
strongyloidiasis, 2:929
swimmer's itch, 2:931–933
talaromycosis, 2:944–945
tularemia, 2:990
viral disease, 2:1039
yaws, 2:1087, 1089, 1090
Skin tests, 1:85, 2:984
Skinner, Ginger, 2:707
Skunks
hosts and vectors, 1:461
lung flukes, 1:567
Powassan virus, 2:741
rabies, 2:776
typhus, 2:998
Slapped cheek syndrome. *See* Fifth disease
Slash-and-burn logging, 2:664
Slaughter and slaughterhouses
avian influenza, 1:90
bacterial disease, 1:100
bovine spongiform encephalopathy, 1:138, 139, 241
brucellosis, 1:141
Campylobacter, 1:152
Creutzfeldt-Jakob disease, 1:241
Crimean-Congo hemorrhagic fever, 1:244
Escherichia coli O157:H7, 1:339, 341
food-borne disease, 1:355, 356
hemorrhagic fevers, 1:419
H5N1, 1:*392s*
influenza, 1:501
Nipah virus infection, 2:662, 664
prion diseases, 2:750
Q fever, 2:771
Rift Valley fever, 2:814
Salmonella, 2:841
taeniasis, 2:942
trichinellosis, 2:973
yersiniosis, 2:1098
zoonoses, 2:1107
See also Culling, animal
Slavic countries, 2:942
Sleep issues, 1:1–5, 3, 2:705, 749
Sleepiness
African sleeping sickness, 1:1–5
enterovirus 71 infection, 1:325, 326
Nipah virus infection, 2:663
viral meningitis, 2:608
Sleeping sickness. *See* African sleeping sickness
Slim disease, 1:18, 19
Sloths, 2:1046
Slovakia, 1:89
Slovenia, 1:89, 2:849, 1042
Slugs, 1:35, 36
Smallpox, 2:**890–895,** *892*
bioterrorism, 1:114–115
chickenpox compared to, 1:175
eradication and storage, 1:168, 184–185, 187, 2:896–899
germ theory of disease, 1:366
isolation and quarantine, 1:509
monkeypox compared to, 2:626
plague, 2:710
vaccine, 2:*896,* 1020–1021, 1022, 1023
viral disease, 2:1039
war, 2:1051
World Health Organization, 2:738–739, 1077
world trade, 2:1081
zoonoses, 2:1106
Smallpox eradication and storage, 2:738–739, 891, 893, **896–900,** *898,* 1077
Smart packaging, 1:153, 558
SmartGene, 1:364
Smell, sense of, 1:228–229
Smith, Bradley T., 1:118
Smith, Hamilton, 1:81
Smith, Theobald, 1:95, 2:840, *842*
Smithsonian Institution, 2:697
Smoking, 1:167
Smyth, Jamie, 2:1088
Snails, 1:*36*
angiostrongyliasis, 1:35, 36
hosts and vectors, 1:461
liver fluke infections, 1:562
lung flukes, 1:565–568
schistosomiasis, 2:860, 861, 862
swimmer's ear and swimmer's itch, 2:931–932, 933
Snake River Valley, 2:824
Snakes, 1:258, 2:1083
Sneezing, 1:*287*
chickenpox, 1:176
Chlamydia infection, 1:190
Chlamydia pneumoniae, 1:193
colds, 1:228, 229, 230
diphtheria, 1:275
encephalitis, 1:317
enterovirus 71 infection, 1:327
group A streptococcal infections, 2:921
measles, 2:593, 594
mumps, 2:645
necrotizing fasciitis, 2:659
RSV infection, 2:833
rubella, 2:837
scarlet fever, 2:857
strep throat, 2:917, 918*s*
viral meningitis, 2:609
Snow, John
cholera, 1:200
epidemiology, 1:329
germ theory of disease, 1:366–367
legislation and international law, 1:534
On the Mode of Communication of Cholera (Snow), 1:333
outbreaks, field-level response to, 2:685–686
sanitation, 2:844
Snow peas and cyclosporiasis, 1:258
Snyder, Rick, 2:883
Social distancing and public health, 2:692, 766
Social issues
AIDS, 1:20
dracunculiasis, 1:284–285
economic development, 1:308
filariasis, 1:350, 352
herpes simplex virus 2, 1:446
leishmaniasis, 1:541
leprosy, 1:544, 546*s,* 547
maternal mortality, 2:769
mononucleosis, 2:632
plague, 2:712
vector-borne disease, 2:1031
Zika virus, 1:76*s*
Social justice, 1:308, 309
Socioeconomic status
Chagas disease, 1:173
diphtheria, 1:277
economic development, 1:306, 308, 309
filariasis, 1:351
gonorrhea risk factors, 1:389
helminth disease, 1:415
hepatitis A, 1:423

herpes simplex 1 virus, 1:442
hookworm infection, 1:457
leishmaniasis, 1:538, 539
maternal mortality, 2:769
mononucleosis, 2:632
river blindness, 2:821, 822
St. Louis encephalitis, 2:906
Sustainable Development Goals, 2:1010*s*
trachoma, 2:968
tropical infectious diseases, 2:979
tuberculosis, 2:985–986
UNICEF, 2:1006
water-borne disease, 2:1055
yaws, 2:1087
Zika virus, 2:1103
zoonoses, 2:1107–1108
Sodium hypochlorite, 1:281, 282
Sodoku. *See* Rat-bite fever
Sofosbuvir, 1:432
Software, 1:375–377
Soil
anthrax, 1:47
antibiotic drug development, 2:675–676
ascariasis, 1:79, 80
brucellosis, 1:141
coccidioidomycosis, 1:218, 219, 221
glanders, 1:379
helminth disease, 1:415, 416
histoplasmosis, 1:448, 449
hookworm infection, 1:457, 458
leptospirosis, 1:548, 550
mycotic disease, 2:650, 651
necrotizing fasciitis, 2:660
nocardiosis, 2:666
strongyloidiasis, 2:928, 929
taeniasis, 2:941
talaromycosis, 2:945
tetanus, 2:953
tularemia, 2:990
whipworm, 2:1062, 1063
Soldiers. *See* Military
Solid fueled indoor cooking, 2:729
Solomon Islands, 2:1089
Solution-phase hybridization, 1:363–364
Somali immigrants, 2:596–598
Somalia
Biological Weapons Convention, 1:111
immigration, 1:474
leishmaniasis, 1:539
relapsing fever, 2:797–798
Rift Valley fever, 2:815
smallpox, 2:896, 897
Sore throat. *See* Pharyngitis
Sorensen, Cecilia, 1:207
Sores. *See* Lesions
South Africa
antiviral drugs, 1:73
British beef ban, 1:138
CMV infection, 1:215
Crimean-Congo hemorrhagic fever, 1:244
Ebola, 1:302
economic development, 1:307
extremely drug-resistant tuberculosis, 1:23
microsporidiosis, 2:624*s*
plague, 2:716
rabies, 2:778, 779
re-emerging infectious diseases, 2:791–792
rotavirus, 2:831
smallpox research, opposition to, 2:899
typhus, 2:998
South America
AIDS, 1:15, 18
anellovirus, 1:30
anisakiasis, 1:45
anthrax, 1:49
arthropod-borne diseases, 1:75
babesiosis, 1:96
blastomycosis, 1:122
brucellosis, 1:141
burkholderia, 1:142
Buruli ulcer, 1:147–150
Chagas disease, 1:171, 173, 174
chikungunya, 2:614
coccidioidomycosis, 1:220
dysentery, 1:290
Eastern equine encephalitis, 1:296, 297
encephalitis, 1:317
extremely drug-resistant tuberculosis, 1:23
filariasis, 1:351
glanders, 1:380
Haemophilus influenzae, 1:396
hantavirus, 1:404
hepatitis D, 1:434, 435
histoplasmosis, 1:449
immigration, 1:474
leishmaniasis, 1:539
leprosy, 1:544
lung flukes, 1:566
malaria, 2:580, 581
mosquito-borne diseases, 2:637
mycotic disease, 2:651, 652
outbreaks, field-level response to, 2:687
protozoan diseases, 2:755
relapsing fever, 2:796
resistant organisms, 2:800
river blindness, 2:821
Rocky Mountain spotted fever, 2:825
schistosomiasis, 2:862
scrofula, 2:867
smallpox, 2:890
St. Louis encephalitis, 2:906
taeniasis, 2:943
tapeworm infections, 2:949
travel, 2:970
tropical infectious diseases, 2:981
typhoid fever, 2:994
typhus, 2:998, 999
vector-borne disease, 2:1030
Venezuelan equine encephalitis virus, 2:1033, 1034, 1035
virus hunters, 2:1043
water-borne disease, 2:1055
whipworm, 2:1063
yellow fever, 2:1092
Zika virus, 1:169, 462, 2:1102
South Asia
AIDS deaths, 1:15
arthropod-borne diseases, 1:77
cholera, 1:198
hepatitis E, 1:437
pneumonia, 2:727
smallpox, 2:1077
taeniasis, 2:942
South Korea
British beef ban, 1:138
filariasis eradication, 1:350, 352
Kawasaki disease, 1:515
liver fluke infections, 1:561
severe fever with thrombocytopenia syndrome, 2:872
South Pacific
burkholderia, 1:145
glanders, 1:380
marine toxins, 2:590
South Sudan
dracunculiasis, 1:285
leishmaniasis, 1:539
parasitic disease prevention, 2:*694*
South Vietnam, 2:1051
South-central United States, 2:811
Southeast Asia
amebiasis, 1:28
angiostrongyliasis, 1:36
ascariasis, 1:79
burkholderia, 1:145
Buruli ulcer, 1:147–150
chikungunya, 1:180, 181
cholera, 1:533
cyclosporiasis, 1:259
dengue and dengue hemorrhagic fever, 1:267
diphtheria, 1:276
dysentery, 1:290
enterovirus 71 infection, 1:326
filariasis, 1:351
glanders, 1:378, 380
Japanese encephalitis, 1:511, 513
leishmaniasis, 1:541
malaria, 2:580, 581
maternal mortality, 2:769
mosquito-borne diseases, 2:637
nosocomial infections, 2:675
Pacific countries, 1:147–150
plague, 2:712–713, 715, 716, 719
polio, 2:734, 740
protozoan diseases, 2:755
rabies, 2:779
rubella, 2:838
SARS, 2:848–849
schistosomiasis, 2:861

syphilis, 2:936
taeniasis, 2:942
talaromycosis, 2:944, 945, 946
trichinellosis, 2:973
tropical infectious diseases, 2:981
typhus, 2:997, 999
whipworm, 2:1063
wildlife trade, 2:1083
Zika virus, 2:1102
Southeastern United States
blastomycosis, 1:122
histoplasmosis, 1:449
marine toxins, 2:591
rickettsial disease, 2:811
strongyloidiasis, 2:929
whipworm, 2:1063
Southern Africa
developing nations and drug delivery, 1:272*s*
dysentery, 1:290
re-emerging infectious diseases, 2:791*s*
Rift Valley fever, 2:814
United Nations Millennium Goals, 2:1009
Southern Asia, 2:769
Southern Atlantic states, 2:825
Southern blot analysis, 1:363
Southern Brazil, 2:791*s*
Southern California, 1:424–425, 2:999
Southern China, 1:457, 2:861
Southern Europe, 1:434, 2:942
Southern flying squirrels, 2:999
Southern hemisphere, 1:496, 506, 2:958
Southern tick-associated rash illness, 2:956–957
Southern United States
blastomycosis, 1:122
Chagas disease, 1:172, 173
strongyloidiasis, 2:928
Southwark and Vauxhall, 1:329
Southwestern Asia, 1:50
Southwestern United States
coccidioidomycosis, 1:218–219, 221
hantavirus, 1:406, 407
plague, 2:715, 716, 717, 719
relapsing fever, 2:796
Soviet Union
anthrax, 1:47, 48
biological weapons, 1:109–110
childhood-associated infectious disease eradication, 1:184–185
glanders, 1:381
smallpox, 2:893–894
war, 2:1051
See also Former Soviet Union
Soviet-Afghan War, 1:381
Spain
anisakiasis, 1:45
avian influenza, 1:89
babesiosis, 1:96
chickenpox vaccine, 1:177
diphtheria, 1:277
Ebola, 2:601
relapsing fever, 2:796
SARS, 2:849
trichinellosis, 2:974
Spanish flu. *See* Influenza pandemic of 1918
Spas. *See* Hot tub rash
Spasms. *See* Muscle spasms
Speaker, Andrew, 1:474
Special Pathogens Branch, CDC, 1:168
Special Program for Research and Training in Tropical Diseases, 1:4
Specificity, test, 1:331
Specter, Michael, 1:412*s*
Spectroscopy, 1:117
Speech issues, 1:133, 2:741, 753
Speelman, P., 2:773
Spencer, Charles A., 2:618–619
Sphagnum moss, 2:903
Spiers, Ronald, 1:*110*
Spinal cord
bacterial meningitis, 2:604, 605
helminth disease, 1:415
schistosomiasis, 2:861
Spinal cord injuries, 2:1014
Spinal polio, 2:736
Spinal tap. *See* Cerebrospinal fluid tests
Spirillum minus. See Rat-bite fever
Spirochetes
Lyme disease, 1:570–571
relapsing fever, 2:797
syphilis, 2:934
yaws, 2:1087
Spironolactone, 1:72
Spleen symptoms
ascariasis, 1:79
babesiosis, 1:96
brucellosis, 1:141
cat scratch disease, 1:161–163
dysentery, 1:289
glanders, 1:379
leishmaniasis, 1:538, 540
macrophage activation syndrome, 2:575–576
malaria, 2:580
mononucleosis, 2:631, 632, 634
protozoan diseases, 2:754
rickettsial disease, 2:810
rubella, 2:837
schistosomiasis, 2:861
talaromycosis, 2:944
tularemia, 2:990
Spontaneous antibiotic resistance, 1:62
Spontaneous bovine spongiform encephalopathy, 1:139
Sporadic Creutzfeldt-Jakob disease, 1:240, 2:749
Spores
anthrax, 1:47, 49, 51, 115
bacterial diseases, 1:100
blastomycosis, 1:122
botulism, 1:133–134, 135
Clostridium difficile infection, 1:209, 210
coccidioidomycosis, 1:218, 221
Cryptococcus neoformans infection, 1:247–248
disinfection, ineffectiveness of, 1:280
food-borne disease, 1:354, 356
histoplasmosis, 1:448, 449, 451
microsporidiosis, 2:622–623, 624
mycotic disease, 2:649, 650, 651
sterilization, 2:915, 916*s*
talaromycosis, 2:945
war, 2:1050
Sporothrix schenckii. See Sporotrichosis
Sporotrichosis, 2:651, **901–904,** *902, 903*
Sports and athletes
herpes simplex 1, 1:442*s*
mononucleosis, 2:634
scabies prevention, 2:854*s*
See also Athletic facilities
Spotted fevers
Rocky Mountain spotted fever, 2:656, 809, 810, 811, 824–826
tick-borne diseases, 2:956–957
typhus, 2:997, 998
Spraying programs
climate change, 1:206
Eastern equine encephalitis, 1:298
endemic diseases, 1:321
hemorrhagic fevers, 1:420
hosts and vectors, 1:462
infection control, 1:486
malaria, 2:583
mosquito-borne diseases, 2:*636,* 638
river blindness, 2:822
vector-borne disease, 2:1030
West Nile virus, 2:1061
yellow fever, 2:1093
zoonoses, 2:1107
Sputum tests
aspergillosis, 1:85
blastomycosis, 1:122
burkholderia, 1:145–146
coccidioidomycosis, 1:220
glanders, 1:380
tuberculosis, 2:984
Squid and anisakiasis, 1:45
Squirrels
Baylisascaris infection, 1:107
encephalitis, 1:317
plague, 2:715
Powassan virus, 2:741
rat-bite fever, 2:785
taeniasis, 2:940
tularemia, 2:990
typhus, 2:999
West Nile virus, 2:1060
wildlife trade, 2:1083

Sri Lanka, 1:318, 546, 2:999
ST-246, 2:892
St. Lawrence River valley, 1:448
St. Louis encephalitis, 1:317, 418, 2:**905–907,** *907*
St. Martin, 1:182
St. Petersburg, Russia, 1:277
Stage 1 and Stage 2 Disinfectants and Disinfection Byproducts Rules (EPA), 1:282
Stager, Margaret, 1:470
Staining
- aspergillosis, 1:85
- bacterial meningitis, 2:605
- culture and sensitivity, 1:255–256, 257
- microscopes and microscopy, 2:618, 619–620
- microsporidiosis, 2:624

Standard precautions, 2:**908–910,** *909*
- Ebola prevention, 1:237
- infection control and asepsis, 1:484, 486*s*
- Lassa fever, 1:527
- Marburg hemorrhagic fever prevention, 2:586
- nosocomial infection prevention, 2:675

Stanford University Hospital, 2:1014*s*
Staph infections. *See Staphylococcus aureus* infections
Staphylococcal enterotoxin B, 2:1018, 1052
Staphylococcus aureus infections, 2:*911,* **911–913,** *962*
- antibacterial drug issues, 1:59
- antibiotic resistance, 1:61–62
- anti-cytokine antibody syndrome, 1:53
- antimicrobial soap use, 1:66
- CDC, 1:169
- impetigo, 1:480, 481
- infection control and asepsis, 1:487
- influenza, 1:488–489
- nosocomial infections, 2:674–675
- pneumonia, 2:729
- resistant organisms, 2:800, 801, 802
- SEB intoxication, 2:1052
- toxic shock, 2:961–963
- USAMRIID, 2:1018
- *See also* MRSA

State of Palestine, 1:111
State of the World's Children 2016, 2:1006
State Research Center of Virology and Biotechnology, Russia, 1:168, 2:894, 897
States
- babesiosis, 1:97
- bioterrorism, 1:117
- botulism antitoxin, 1:135
- Model State Emergency Health Powers Act, 1:535–536

Statistics and epidemiology, 1:328, 329
Stavudine, 1:13
STDs. *See* Sexually transmitted infections
Steele, Duncan, 2:831
Steere, Allan C., 1:570
Stegomyia calopus, 2:1094
Steiner, Rudolf, 1:187
Stem cell transplantation, 1:86*s*
Sterile male mosquitoes, 1:462, 486, 2:1031, 1093
Sterilization (disinfection), 2:**914–916,** *915*
- nosocomial infection prevention, 2:675
- puerperal fever prevention, 2:769
- *vs.* disinfection, 1:280
- *See also* Disinfection

Sterilization (reproductive), 1:546*s*
Sterling, VA, 2:671
Sterne, Max, 1:50
Steroid use as candidiasis risk factor, 1:159
Stewart, William, 1:61
Stiff neck. *See* Neck stiffness
Stigmatization. *See* Social issues
Stillbirth
- group B streptococcal infections, 2:925
- hepatitis E, 1:437
- listeriosis, 1:556
- Venezuelan equine encephalitis virus, 2:1035

Still's disease, 2:575
Stinchfield, Patsy, 2:598
Stinear, Tim, 1:150
STIs. *See* Sexually transmitted infections
Stockpiling, drug
- anthrax vaccines, 1:51
- antiviral drugs, 1:496, 505
- bioterrorism, 1:114, 115, 116, 2:700*s*
- H5N1 vaccine, 1:497
- pandemic preparedness, 2:691–692
- plague antibiotics, 2:719
- public health, 2:763–764
- smallpox drugs, 2:892, 899
- tularemia drugs, 2:991*s*
- USAMRIID, 2:1016

Stomach cancer
- cancer, 1:155
- Epstein-Barr virus, 1:337
- *Helicobacter pylori,* 1:409, 411

Stomach cramps. *See* Abdominal cramps
Stomach pain. *See* Abdominal pain
Stomach symptoms. *See* Gastrointestinal diseases or symptoms
Stomach ulcers, 1:343–344, 409
Stomatitis, 1:92
Stool abnormalities and protozoan diseases, 2:754
Stool pills, 1:*209*
Stool tests
- ascariasis, 1:79
- cyclosporiasis, 1:259–260
- dysentery, 1:290
- giardiasis, 1:372
- lung flukes, 1:567
- protozoan diseases, 2:755
- *Salmonella* infection, 2:842
- strongyloidiasis, 2:929
- trichinellosis, 2:974
- typhoid fever, 2:993
- viral meningitis, 2:609
- whipworm, 2:1063

Storage, smallpox. *See* Smallpox eradication and storage
Strabismus, 1:135
Strategic Advisory Group of Experts on Immunization, 2:779
Strategic Framework, CDC, 1:166
Strategic National Stockpile, 1:114, 2:893, 899
Stratford Hotel, 1:529–530
Strawberries and hepatitis A, 1:423
Strawberry tongue, 1:515
Strep throat, 2:**917–919,** *918,* 922, 922*s*
Streptobacillus moniliformis. See Rat-bite fever
Streptococcal infections
- anti-cytokine antibody syndrome, 1:53
- antimicrobial soap use, 1:66
- group B streptococcal infections, 2:924–927
- impetigo, 1:480, 481, 482
- pneumonia, 2:728–729
- puerperal fever, 2:767
- scabies, 2:853

Streptococcal infections, group A, 2:**920–923,** *921*
- group B streptococcal infections compared to, 2:925
- with influenza, 1:488
- meningococcus, 2:606
- necrotizing fasciitis, 2:658
- prevention, 1:481*s*
- puerperal fever, 2:767
- scarlet fever, 2:856
- strep throat, 2:917–919
- toxic shock, 2:961, 963

Streptococcal infections, group B, 2:*924,* **924–927**
Streptococcus pneumoniae
- bacterial meningitis, 2:606
- influenza, 1:505
- meningitis, 2:606
- vaccines, 1:186, 2:729
- WHO childhood vaccination recommendations, 1:185

Streptococcus pyogenes
group A streptococcal infections, 2:920–922
nosocomial infections, 2:673
scarlet fever, 2:856
strep throat, 2:917–919
toxic shock, 2:961, 963
Streptomycin
brucellosis, 1:142
Buruli ulcer, 1:149
plague, 2:718
tularemia, 2:991
Stress
colds, 1:230*s*
economic development, 1:307
herpes simplex 1 virus, 1:441, 443
mycotic disease, 2:650
Striated muscles and lung flukes, 1:566
Strip diagnostic tests, 2:783
Striped field mice, 1:405
Strokes, 1:195, 2:888
Strongyloidiasis, 2:**928–930,** *929, 930*
Stuffy nose, 1:228, 293
Stunted growth and sanitation, 2:844
Stupor
Japanese encephalitis, 1:512
malaria, 2:580
St. Louis encephalitis, 2:905
Subacute sclerosing panencephalitis, 2:594
Subcutaneous mycotic infection, 2:649, 650
Sub-Saharan Africa
African sleeping sickness, 1:5
anthrax, 1:49
antiviral drugs, 1:72–73
avian influenza, 1:156
bacterial meningitis, 2:605
cryptosporidiosis prevention, 1:253
dracunculiasis, 1:283
emerging infectious disease, 1:313
Haemophilus influenzae, 1:396
hepatitis B, 1:427
immigration, 1:473
malaria, 2:578, 580, 581, 582–583
maternal mortality, 2:769
nosocomial infections, 2:675
pneumonia, 2:727
protozoan diseases, 2:755
re-emerging infectious diseases, 2:790, 791, 792
sanitation, 2:844, 845
schistosomiasis, 2:863
scrofula, 2:867
tropical infectious diseases, 2:979, 981
UNICEF, 2:1005
United Nations Millennium Goals, 2:1008, 1009
viral disease, 2:1041
women, 2:1073
Substance abuse. *See* Drug abuse; Injection drug users
Substandard and falsified medical products, 1:272
Subtropics
ascariasis, 1:78
climate change and parasitic diseases, 2:756
dysentery, 1:290
Japanese encephalitis, 1:513
leishmaniasis, 1:538, 539
lung flukes, 1:565
malaria, 2:578, 580
parasitic diseases, 2:695
ringworm, 2:818
sporotrichosis, 2:902
strongyloidiasis with, 2:929
Sudan
African sleeping sickness, 1:3
avian influenza, 1:89
cholera, 1:199, 200, 201
demographics, 1:261
dracunculiasis, 1:283
Ebola, 1:41, 302
hemorrhagic fevers, 1:420, 420*s*
leishmaniasis, 1:539
outbreaks, field-level response to, 2:686
relapsing fever, 2:796
Rift Valley fever, 2:815
Sudden infant death syndrome, 1:278
Suffocation and diphtheria, 1:274, 275
Sulfadiazine, 1:380, 2:668, 755
Sulfamethoxazole. *See* Trimethoprim-sulfamethoxazole
Sulfonamide drugs, 2:668
Sulfone drugs, 1:545
Sumatra, 2:730
Summary of Notifiable Infectious Diseases, 2:679
Sun, Lena H., 1:572, 2:596
Sunlight exposure and herpes simplex 1 virus, 1:443
Sunshine Project, 2:899
Superabsorbent tampons, 2:962
Superbugs, 1:434, 435, 2:1027*s*
Superficial mycotic infection, 2:649
Superresolution microscopy, 2:620
Superspreaders and SARS, 2:847
Supplemental oxygen therapy, 2:834
Supportive treatment
cyclosporiasis, 1:260
Eastern equine encephalitis, 1:297
Escherichia coli O157:H7, 1:340
Japanese encephalitis, 1:513
Lassa fever, 1:528
Nipah virus infection, 2:663
Powassan virus, 2:742
trichinellosis, 2:974
zoonoses, 2:1107
Suramin, 1:3, 4
Surgeons General, U.S. *See* U.S. Surgeons General
Surgery
anisakiasis, 1:45
aspergillosis, 1:85
Baylisascaris infection, 1:107
Buruli ulcer, 1:149
Chagas disease, 1:173
Chlamydia infection, 1:191
coccidioidomycosis, 1:221
contact precautions, 1:236, *236, 237*
diphtheria, 1:276
ear infections, 1:294
filariasis, 1:352
group A streptococcal infections, 2:921
HPV, 1:470
leishmaniasis, 1:540
lung flukes, 1:567
necrotizing fasciitis, 2:657, 659
ocular histoplasmosis, 1:451
personal protective equipment, 2:699, 701
scrofula, 2:866
sporotrichosis, 2:902
strep throat, 2:919
toxic shock, 2:961
trachoma, 2:969
Surgical instruments
nosocomial infection prevention, 2:675
prion disease, 2:750
standard precautions, 2:910
sterilization, 2:914
Surgical scrubbing, 1:281
Surgical site infections, 1:257
Surveillance
African sleeping sickness, 1:4–5
aspergillosis, 1:86*s*
bioterrorism, 1:115, 117
botulism, 1:134
Campylobacter infection, 1:153
CDC, 1:167, 168–169
cholera, 1:198, 199, 200
emerging infectious diseases, 1:313
encephalitis, 1:319
epidemiology, 1:332
globalization, 1:385
gonorrhea, 1:389
H5N1, 1:393
influenza, 1:496, 503, 505, 506
leishmaniasis, 1:541
leptospirosis, 1:549
liver fluke infections, 1:563–564
National Institute of Allergy and Infectious Diseases, 2:655
nosocomial infections, 2:674
notifiable diseases, 2:678–681, 680*s*
plague, 2:718, 719

polio eradication campaign, 2:733, 734
public health, 2:762, 764, 765
Salmonella infection, 2:842
SARS, 2:851
smallpox, 2:897
trachoma, 2:968*s*
vancomycin-resistant *Enterococci,* 2:1026, 1027
Venezuelan equine encephalitis virus, 2:1035
water-borne disease, 2:1055
World Health Organization, 2:1077
Susceptibility to disease and world trade, 2:1082
Sushi and anisakiasis, 1:45
Sustainable Development Goals (SDGs), 1:352, 2:1006, 1010*s,* 1079
SV40, 1:155
Sverdlovsk, Russia, 1:48
Swallowing problems
AIDS, 1:12
botulism, 1:133
candidiasis, 1:159
strep throat, 2:917
tetanus, 2:953
Swamps, 1:297, 298, 298*s*
Swaziland, 1:206, 2:792
Sweating
babesiosis, 1:96
glanders, 1:379
HIV, 1:11
malaria, 2:580
marine toxins, 2:590, 591
pneumonia, 2:726
protozoan diseases, 2:753
relapsing fever, 2:795
Salmonella infection, 2:841
scrofula, 2:866
tetanus, 2:953
typhus, 2:997
Sweden
avian influenza, 1:89
babesiosis, 1:96
group B streptococcal infection, 2:926
pertussis, 1:187
public health, 2:763
Swedish International Development Cooperation Agency, 2:846
Sween District, Uganda, 2:587
Swelling
dracunculiasis, 1:284
Kawasaki disease, 1:515
leprosy, 1:543
necrotizing fasciitis, 2:659
strongyloidiasis, 2:929
swimmer's ear and swimmer's itch, 2:933
vaccine reactions, 2:1022
See also Gland swelling or pain; Lymph node swelling or pain
Swimmer's ear and swimmer's itch, 1:294*s,* 2:**931–933,** *932*
Swimming
cryptosporidiosis, 1:251, 252, 253
helminth disease prevention, 1:416
hookworm infection, 1:458
hot tub rash, 1:465
Legionnaires' disease, 1:531
sanitation, 2:846
schistosomiasis, 2:862
shigellosis, 2:883
swimmer's ear and swimmer's itch, 2:931, 932, 933
viral meningitis, 2:610
water-borne disease, 2:1055
Swine. *See* Pigs
Swine fever and world trade, 2:1084
Swine flu. *See* H1N1
Switzerland
avian influenza, 1:89
babesiosis, 1:96
bacterial meningitis, 2:604
Biosafety level 4 facilities, 1:246
lice infestation, 1:554
ProMED, 2:751
rabies eradication, 2:778
relapsing fever, 2:797–798
Swollen glands. *See* Gland swelling or pain
Sylvatic rabies, 2:777
Symphony Health, 2:707
Synthetic vaccines, 2:1022*s,* 1023
Syphilis, 2:**934–939,** *935*
AIDS susceptibility, 1:11
antibacterial drugs, 1:57
sexually transmitted infections, 2:877, 878, 879
spirochetes, 1:571
travel, 2:970
Syria, 1:111, 539, 541
Syria, ancient, 1:277
Syrian refugees, 1:263–264
Systemic infection
juvenile idiopathic arthritis, 2:575
mycotic infections, 2:649
nocardiosis, 2:666
talaromycosis, 2:944–945
Systemic lupus erythematosus, 2:575, 576
Systrom, David, 2:730
Sze, Szeming, 2:1076

T

T cells
AIDS, 1:8, 12
HIV, 1:454, 455, 2:790
immune response, 1:478, 479
Pneumocystis jirovecii pneumonia, 2:723–724
Tabes dorsalis, 2:935
Taenia infection. *See* Taeniasis
Taeniasis, 2:*940,* **940–943,** 980
Tagamet. *See* Cimetidine
Tahiti, 1:36
Taipei, Taiwan, 1:435
Taiwan
ADHD medications and sexually transmitted infections, 2:977
angiostrongyliasis, 1:36, 38
chickenpox vaccine, 1:177
Chlamydia pneumoniae, 1:193
encephalitis, 1:318
enterovirus 71 infection, 1:325, 326
hand, foot, and mouth disease, 1:397, 398
hepatitis D, 1:435
hepatitis E, 1:438
immigration, 1:474
lung flukes, 1:565–568
Taiwan National Health Insurance Research Database, 2:977
Tajikistan, 1:277
Talaromyces marneffei. See Talaromycosis
Talaromycosis, 2:**944–947,** *946*
Taliban, 2:734, 734*s*
Tamiflu. *See* Oseltamivir
Tampons and toxic shock, 2:961–963
Tanzania
African sleeping sickness, 1:3
AIDS pandemic history, 1:18
Biological Weapons Convention, 1:111
leprosy, 1:546, 2:1078
outbreaks, field-level response to, 2:686
plague, 2:716
rabies, 2:779
Rift Valley fever, 2:815, 816
Zika virus, 2:1101
Tape tests, 2:706
Tapeworm infections, 1:*25,* 2:**948–951,** *949, 950*
alveolar echinococcosis, 1:24, 25
climate change, 2:698
helminth disease, 1:415
parasitic diseases, 2:695
taeniasis, 2:940–943
tropical infectious diseases, 2:980
Task Force on Antimicrobial Resistance, 1:256*s*
Taste and colds, 1:229
Tattooing, 1:11, 432, 478*s,* 2:952
TB/IV Clinical Manual, 2:867
Tdap vaccine, 1:276, 277, 2:*1067,* 1068–1069
Tearing, eye, 2:702, 703*s,* 967
Technology
Asilomar Conference, 1:81–82
biodefense research and development, 1:118–119

bioengineered edible vaccines, 1:82*s*
bioterrorism identification technology, 1:117
Campylobacter infection prevention, 1:153
cooking technology and pneumonia prevention, 2:729
economic development, 1:309
genetic identification of microorganisms, 1:362–364
listeriosis prevention, 1:558
retroviruses, 2:808
RSV vaccine development, 2:834
smart packaging, 1:153, 558
Tecovirimat, 1:115, 2:892
Tedizolid, 2:1027
Telaprevir, 1:432
Telavancin, 2:1027
Telithromycin, 2:1000
Temer, Michel, 2:1108
Temperate climates
chickenpox, 1:177
diphtheria, 1:275
pinworm infection, 2:706
strongyloidiasis with, 2:929
swimmer's ear and swimmer's itch, 2:932
vector-borne disease, 2:1030
Temperature cycling, 1:2
Tendon pain, 1:388, 569
Tenesmus, 2:883
Tennessee, 1:428, 449, 2:873*s*
Tenofovir alafenamide, 1:13
Tenofovir disoproxil fumarate, 1:13
Tenosynovitis, 1:388
Terbinafine, 2:818
Terrorism. *See* Bioterrorism
Testes
blastomycosis, 1:122
gonorrhea, 1:388
leprosy, 1:545
Tetanospasmin, 2:952
Tetanus, **2:952–955,** *953*
bacterial disease vaccines, 1:101
unvaccinated children, 1:186
vaccines, 1:184, 185, 2:1022*s*
war, 2:1049
WHO childhood vaccination recommendations, 1:185
Tetracycline
anthrax, 1:115
balantidiasis, 1:103
Chlamydia infection, 1:189–191
glanders, 1:380
Helicobacter pylori, 1:411
nosocomial infections, 2:674
plague, 2:718
psittacosis, 2:759, 760
rat-bite fever, 2:786
relapsing fever, 2:796, 797
rickettsial disease, 2:811
syphilis, 2:936
trachoma, 2:968
typhus, 2:999
Texas
animal importation, 1:40
chikungunya, 1:182
coccidioidomycosis, 1:220
dengue and dengue hemorrhagic fever, 1:266, 267
encephalitis, 1:317
globalization and infectious disease, 1:385
histoplasmosis, 1:449
isolation and quarantine, 1:510
norovirus infection, 2:670
relapsing fever, 2:795
smallpox, 2:896
typhus, 2:999
Venezuelan equine encephalitis virus, 2:1034
West Nile virus, 2:1059, 1060
Thailand
AIDS deaths, 1:15
angiostrongyliasis, 1:36
avian influenza, 1:88
burkholderia, 1:144, 145
cholera, 1:197
glanders, 1:380, 381
Haemophilus influenzae, 1:396
hantavirus, 1:405
HIV vaccine research, 2:654
Japanese encephalitis, 1:514
leishmaniasis, 1:540
liver fluke infections, 1:561, 562
lung flukes, 1:566
SARS, 2:848–849
talaromycosis, 2:945
tick-borne diseases, 2:957
wildlife trade, 2:1083
"Thailand Uses Integrated Ecosystems Health Approach to Beat Cancer-Causing Disease," 1:*562–564*
Thailand virus, 1:405
Thalamus and prion disease, 2:749
Therapeutic vaccines and AIDS research, 1:20
Thiabendazole, 1:80
Thimerosal, 2:838*s,* 1021–1022
Third World Network, 2:899
"'This Is a Game-changer': New Shingles Vaccine Dramatically Improves Protection," 2:*887–888*
"This Man Thought He Had the Flu. Months Later, He Could Barely Eat or Talk," 1:*123–124*
"This Vaccine Can Prevent Cancer, But Many Teenagers Still Don't Get It," 1:*470–471*
Thomas, Bolaji N., 2:756
Thomas, Lian Francesca, 2:942
Thompson, Sara, 2:1084
Thorny-headed worms, 2:698
3TC and AIDS, 1:13
Throat cancer, 1:468
Throat redness, 1:244
Throat soreness. *See* Pharyngitis
Throat spasms and rabies, 1:75, 2:776
Throat swabs, 2:609, 917
Thrombocytopenia, 2:871–873
Thrombocytopenic purpura, 1:340
Thrombosis, 2:997
Thrush. *See* Candidiasis
Thucydides, 2:710
Tiabendazole, 2:974
Tick removal
babesiosis, 1:97
Lyme disease, 1:572
rocky Mountain spotted fever prevention, 2:826
tick-borne diseases, 2:957, 958
Tick-borne diseases, 1:*570,* **2:956–960,** *957*
animal importation, 2:1084
babesiosis, 1:95–97
climate change, 2:698
Crimean-Congo hemorrhagic fever, 1:243–246
encephalitis, 1:316, 317
heartland virus, 2:873*s*
hemorrhagic fevers, 1:419
hosts and vectors, 1:461
Lyme disease, 1:569–574
parasitic diseases, 2:694
Powassan virus, 2:741–743
Q fever, 2:771
relapsing fever, 2:795, 797
rickettsial disease, 2:809–812
Rocky Mountain spotted fever, 2:824–826
severe fever with thrombocytopenia syndrome, 2:871–873
tularemia, 2:990
typhus, 2:997–1001, 999
vector-borne disease, 2:1029
viral meningitis, 2:609
virus hunters, 2:1046
zoonoses, 2:1107
Tick-borne encephalitis, 2:957, *957,* 958
Tigecycline, 2:1027
Tinea, 2:650, 817–819
Tingling sensation, 1:92, 2:886, 932
Tinidazole
giardiasis, 1:373
Helicobacter pylori, 1:411
protozoan diseases, 2:755
trichomoniasis, 2:976
Tips From Former Smokers campaign, 1:167
Tiredness. *See* Fatigue
Tissue tests
blastomycosis, 1:122
Buruli ulcer, 1:149
coccidioidomycosis, 1:220
herpes simplex virus 2, 1:445
TLR7 protein, 2:1074
Toe loss and typhus, 2:998
Togaviruses, 2:836, 1041. *See also* Chikungunya
Togo, 1:149

Tokyo, Japan, 2:752
Toledo, OH, 2:671
Tolerance, DDT, 1:321
Tongue issues, 1:515, 2:856
Tonsillectomy, 2:919
Tonsillitis, 1:12, 2:631, 634, 917
Toothpastes, 1:68, 2:916
Topical medications
  eye drops, 2:703, 704
  hot tub rash, 1:466
  impetigo, 1:481
  lice infestation, 1:553
  pink eye, 2:702, 703, 704
  ringworm, 2:818
  scabies, 2:853–854
  swimmer's ear and swimmer's itch, 2:933
  trachoma, 2:968–969
TORCH test, 1:442
Torgerson, Paul R., 1:550
Toronto, Ontario, 2:764–765, 1060
Toronto Public Health, 2:764–765
Torque teno virus. *See* Anellovirus
Total community treatment, 2:1089–1090
Touré, Amadou Toumani, 1:417
Towards Universal Access, 2:1010
Toxic megacolon, 1:212
Toxic scarlet fever, 2:857
Toxic shock, 2:**961–963,** *962*
  CDC, 1:169
  group A streptococcal infections, 2:920
  Staphylococcus aureus infections, 2:912
Toxins
  bacterial diseases, 1:100
  botulism, 1:133–135
  climate change, 1:205
  Clostridium difficile infection, 1:209
  diphtheria, 1:274, 275, 276
  Escherichia coli O157:H7, 1:338, 339
  marine toxins, 2:589–592
  necrotizing fasciitis, 2:657
  parasitic diseases, 2:696
  plague, 2:716
  Salmonella infection, 2:841
  talaromycosis, 2:945
  tetanus, 2:952, 954
  tick-borne diseases, 2:957
  toxic shock, 2:961–963
  vaccines and vaccine development, 2:1022*s*
  whooping cough, 2:1066, 1069
Toxocariasis, 1:80*s*
Toxoid vaccines, 2:952, 1022*s*
Toxoplasma infection. *See* Toxoplasmosis
Toxoplasmosis, 2:**964–966,** *965*
  opportunistic infections, 2:682–683
  parasitic diseases, 2:695
  protozoan diseases, 2:754, 755, 756
TPOXX, 2:892
Tracheostomy, 1:276
Trachoma, 2:**967–969,** *968*
  Chlamydia infection, 1:189, 190, *190,* 191
  tropical infectious diseases, 2:981*s*
Tracing, contact. *See* Contact tracing
Trade. *See* World trade
Trade agreements, 1:534–535
"Trafficking Wildlife and Transmitting Disease: Bold Threats in an Era of Ebola," 2:*1084–1085*
Transactions of the Royal Society of Tropical Medicine and Hygiene, 2:999–1000
Transfusions. *See* Blood supply
Transgender women, 2:1074
Transgenic crop vaccines, 1:82*s*
Translational inhibition, 1:57
Transmissible mink encephalopathy, 1:136
Transmissible spongiform encephalopathies
  bovine spongiform encephalopathy, 1:136–139
  Creutzfeldt-Jakob disease, 1:239–242
  kuru, 1:522–525
  prion disease, 2:748–750
Transmission electron microscopes, 2:620
Transplantation, corneal, 1:232
Transplantation, organ. *See* Organ transplantation
Transport, patient, 1:236
Trap-and-slaughter campaigns, 1:143
Travel, 2:**970–971,** *971*
  African sleeping sickness, 1:3
  amebiasis, 1:28
  angiostrongyliasis, 1:36
  arthropod-borne diseases, 1:74, 75
  ascariasis, 1:79
  brucellosis, 1:142*s*
  burkholderia, 1:145
  CDC notices, 1:386
  Crimean-Congo hemorrhagic fever, 1:244
  cryptosporidiosis, 1:251
  cyclosporiasis, 1:258
  dengue and dengue hemorrhagic fever, 1:268
  dysentery, 1:289, 290, *291,* 292
  epidemiology, 1:332
  giardiasis, 1:371*s*
  globalization, 1:383–386
  hepatitis A, 1:422, 423, 424
  hepatitis B, 1:428*s*
  hepatitis E, 1:437, 439
  influenza, 1:505–506
  influenza pandemic of 1918, 1:495
  Japanese encephalitis, 1:512, 513–514
  Lassa fever, 1:528
  legislation and international law, 1:536
  leishmaniasis, 1:540
  leptospirosis, 1:550
  malaria, 2:579, 580, 581, 582
  measles, 2:594
  microsporidiosis, 2:623
  mosquito-borne diseases, 2:639
  plague, 2:710, 718
  polio, 2:738
  ProMED, 2:752
  protozoan diseases, 2:755
  public health, 2:763, 764
  rabies vaccine, 2:777
  relapsing fever, 2:796, 797
  rickettsial disease, 2:811
  Rift Valley fever, 2:814, 816
  sanitation, 2:845–846
  SARS, 2:848–849, 849*s,* 850, 851
  schistosomiasis, 2:860, 862
  shigellosis, 2:882
  spread of disease, 1:472
  talaromycosis, 2:945
  tapeworm infections, 2:950
  trichinellosis, 2:974
  tuberculosis, 2:986
  typhoid fever, 2:993, 994, 995
  typhus, 2:999, 1000
  war, 2:1048
  wildlife, 2:1085
  world trade, 2:1081, 1082–1083
  Zika virus, 2:1101, 1102
  zoonoses, 2:1106
Travel restrictions and public health, 2:763
"Traveling the Extra Mile to Treat Sleeping Sickness in the DRC," 1:*5*
"Treated Bed Nets Shorten the Lifespan Even of Mosquitos That Evolved Resistance," 2:*1031–1032*
Treaties. *See* Legislation and international law
"Treating ADHD with Medication May lower the Risk of Sexually Transmitted Infections," 2:*977*
Tree porcupines, 2:1046
Trehalose, 1:210, 211, 212–213
Trematodes. *See* Flukes
Tremors
  encephalitis, 1:317
  Japanese encephalitis, 1:512
  Lassa fever, 1:527
  St. Louis encephalitis, 2:905
  syphilis, 2:935
Trench fever, 1:552
Treponema pallidum. See Syphilis
Treponema pertenue. See Yaws
Triatoma infestans, 1:172
Trichinellosis, 2:**972–974,** *973,* 1106, 1107
Trichobilharzia, 2:931

Trichomoniasis, 2:**975–978,** *976*
  parasitic diseases, 2:695
  protozoan diseases, 2:754, 756
  sexually transmitted infections, 2:878
Trichophyton interdigitale, 2:650
Trick-or-Treat for UNICEF, 2:1004
Triclabendazole, 1:562, 567
Triclocarban, 1:66, 67, 69
Triclosan, 1:66, 67–68, 69, 2:915–916
Trifluridine, 1:72
Trihalomethanes, 1:282
Trimethoprim-sulfamethoxazole
  brucellosis, 1:142
  cyclosporiasis, 1:260
  glanders, 1:380
  MRSA, 2:642
  nocardiosis, 2:668
  Q fever, 2:773
  Staphylococcus aureus infections, 2:913
  typhoid fever, 2:994
  war, 2:1049
  yersiniosis, 2:1097
Trophozoites, 1:27, 371, 372, 2:754
Tropical infectious diseases, 2:*979,* **979–982**
  deworming and the prevention of, 2:1064
  economic development, 1:308
  scabies, 2:854
  UNICEF, 2:1003
  vector-borne disease, 2:1030, 1031
  yaws, 2:1090
Tropics
  African sleeping sickness, 1:1
  ascariasis, 1:78, 79, 80
  burkholderia, 1:145
  chickenpox, 1:177
  climate change and parasitic diseases, 2:756
  diphtheria, 1:275
  dysentery, 1:290
  filariasis, 1:351
  Japanese encephalitis, 1:513
  leishmaniasis, 1:538, 539
  leptospirosis, 1:548, 549, 550
  lung flukes, 1:565
  malaria, 2:578, 579, 580, 581
  monkeypox, 2:626, 627
  parasitic diseases, 2:695
  pinworm infection, 2:706
  protozoan diseases, 2:755
  ringworm, 2:818
  scabies, 2:853
  sporotrichosis, 2:902
  strongyloidiasis with, 2:929
  whipworm, 2:1062, 1063
  yaws, 2:1088
  yellow fever, 2:1093
Trypanosoma brucei infections. *See* African sleeping sickness
Trypanosoma cruzi infections. *See* Chagas disease
Tsergouli, Katerina, 1:245
Tsetse flies, 1:1, 2, 3, 2:753, 980
Tsioka, Katerina, 1:245
Tsunami lung, 2:730–731
Tuberculoid leprosy, 1:545
Tuberculosis, 1:*99,* 2:**983–988,** *984*
  airborne precautions, 1:21
  anti-cytokine antibody syndrome, 1:53
  bacterial disease vaccines, 1:101
  cohorted communities, 1:223, 224
  disinfection, 1:280
  economic development, 1:308–309
  emerging infectious diseases, 1:311, 313
  epidemiology, 1:330
  genetic identification of microorganisms, 1:363
  immigration, 1:473–474
  infection control and asepsis, 1:485
  isolation and quarantine, 1:509
  lung flukes *vs.,* 1:566
  Médecins Sans Frontières, 2:601
  microbial evolution, 2:614
  opportunistic infections, 2:682
  personal protective equipment, 2:700
  protozoan diseases, 2:755
  re-emerging infectious diseases, 2:791–792
  scrofula, 2:865–867
  talaromycosis *vs.,* 2:945
  United Nations Millennium Goals, 2:1008, 1009, 1010
  WHO childhood vaccination recommendations, 1:185
  women, 2:1072–1073, 1074
  zoonoses, 2:1106
Tugela Ferry, South Africa, 2:792
Tulare County, Ca, 2:989–990
Tularemia, 2:*989,* **989–992**
  bioterrorism, 1:114–115
  tick-borne diseases, 2:957
  war, 2:1051
Tuna and anisakiasis, 1:45
Tunis, 2:1001
Turkey
  avian influenza, 1:88
  bloodborne infections, 1:131*s*
  chickenpox vaccine, 1:177
  Crimean-Congo hemorrhagic fever, 1:244, 245
  leishmaniasis, 1:541
Turkmenistan, 1:277
Tuskegee syphilis study, 2:937–938
Type A botulism toxin, 1:134
Type B botulism toxin, 1:134
Type E botulism toxin, 1:134
Typhoid fever, 2:**993–996,** *994*
  bacterial disease vaccines, 1:101
  sanitation, 2:844
  typhus *vs.,* 2:997
  WHO childhood vaccination recommendations, 1:185
Typhoid Mary. *See* Mallon, Mary
Typhoid psychosis, 2:993
Typhoon Nina, 2:757
Typhus, 2:**997–1002**
  lice infestation, 1:552, 554
  relapsing fever, 2:796
  rickettsial disease, 2:809, 810, 811
  sanitation, 2:844
  World War I, 2:1048

U

Uganda
  African sleeping sickness, 1:3
  AIDS, 1:15, 18, 19
  Buruli ulcer, 1:147
  cancer viruses, 1:154
  child marriage, 2:1005
  Ebola, 1:302
  emerging infectious diseases, 1:312
  hemorrhagic fevers, 1:420*s*
  Marburg hemorrhagic fever, 2:585, 587
  mosquito-borne diseases, 2:637, 638
  outbreaks, field-level response to, 2:686
  pediatric AIDS, 1:20
  plague, 2:716
  typhoid fever, 2:995
  Zika virus, 2:1101
Uige, Angola, 2:586–587
UK Agricultural and Horticultural Development Board, 1:139
UK Department of Health, 1:126
UK Department of International Development, 1:332–333
UK Food Standards Agency, 1:138, 139
UK Health Protection Agency
  Creutzfeldt-Jakob disease, 1:241
  outbreaks, field-level response to, 2:687
  scarlet fever, 2:857–858
  sexually transmitted infections, 2:878
UK Meat and Livestock Commission, 1:138
UK Medical Research Council, 1:241, 242
Ukraine, 1:89, 277
Ulcers
  diphtheria, 1:275
  enterovirus 71 infection, 1:325, 327
  Fusarium keratitis, 1:233

hand, foot, and mouth disease, 1:397
Helicobacter pylori, 1:343–344, 409
leprosy, 1:543
mycotic disease, 2:650
trachoma, 2:968
viral disease, 2:1039
Ultraviolet light, 1:281, 2:1055
UNAIDS
AIDS history, 1:17, 20
antiviral drugs, 1:73
developing nations and drug delivery, 1:272*s*
HIV, 1:453
leishmaniasis, 1:541
United Nations Millennium Goals, 2:1009, 1010
Unconsciousness
cholera, 1:198
encephalitis, 1:317
meningitis, 2:606*s*
rabies, 2:776
relapsing fever, 2:795
Undecylenic acid, 2:818
Undernutrition. *See* Malnutrition
Underreporting. *See* Reporting
UNICEF, 2:**1003–1006,** *1005*
African sleeping sickness, 1:4
cholera, 1:198
diphtheria, 1:277
emerging infectious disease, 1:313
gastroenteritis, 1:361
Global Polio Eradication Initiative, 2:732, 740, 1077
helminth disease, 1:417
Joint Monitoring Programme for Water Supply, Sanitation and Hygiene, 2:1079
measles, 2:595
outbreaks, field-level response to, 2:687
pneumonia, 2:730
polio eradication campaign, 2:734
sanitation, 2:846
smallpox eradication, 1:185
Union of Concerned Scientists, 1:64
United Against Rabies campaign, 2:779
United Arab Emirates, 2:*691,* 872
United Kingdom
animal importation, 1:40
anthrax, 1:47–48, 50
avian influenza, 1:89
biosafety level 4 laboratories, 1:421
blood supply, 1:126, 127
bovine spongiform encephalopathy, 1:136, 137, 138–139
chickenpox vaccine, 1:177–178
cholera, 1:199, 200
Clostridium difficile infection, 1:211
Creutzfeldt-Jakob disease, 1:239, 241, 242
diphtheria, 1:275, 277
dysentery, 1:290
Ebola, 1:302
enterovirus 71 infection, 1:325
epidemiology, 1:328–329, 332–333
Escherichia coli O157:H7, 1:338
globalization, 1:384
group B streptococcal infection, 2:926
Haemophilus influenzae, 1:396
hand, foot, and mouth disease, 1:397
immigration, 1:473–474
influenza epidemiology, 1:506
isolation and quarantine, 1:533
Meningitis Research Foundation, 2:610
methicillin-resistant *Staphylococcus aureus,* 1:485
MRSA, 2:640
mycotic disease, 2:652
notifiable diseases, 2:678, 681
outbreaks, field-level response to, 2:687
pink eye, 2:704
plague, early history of, 2:711
polio, 2:737
prion disease, 2:748, 749, 750
relapsing fever, 2:795
sanitation, 2:844
SARS, 2:849
scarlet fever, 2:857–859
scrofula, 2:865
smallpox, 2:891
tuberculosis research, 2:983
typhoid fever, 2:994
typhus, 2:998
vaccines, 2:1021
vancomycin-resistant *Enterococci,* 2:1026
variant Creutzfeldt-Jakob disease, 1:523
war, 2:1049
West Nile virus, 2:1060
whooping cough vaccine, 2:1068
United Nations
AIDS, 1:17
Biological Weapons Convention, 1:110–111
bushmeat, 1:304
cholera, 1:198
filariasis, 1:352
hemorrhagic fevers, 1:420–421
internally displaced persons, 1:472
legislation and international law, 1:533, 534–535, 536
Médecins Sans Frontières, 2:601
sanitation, 2:846
sepsis in member states, 2:868
water-borne disease, 2:1055
See also UNAIDS; UNICEF; World Health Organization
United Nations Children's Fund. *See* UNICEF
United Nations Conference on International Organization, 2:1076
United Nations Convention on the Rights of the Child, 2:1004
United Nations Development Group, 2:1003
United Nations Development Program, 1:4, 2:1005
United Nations General Assembly, 2:1003, 1004
United Nations High Commissioner for Refugees, 1:263
United Nations International Decade for Action, 2:1055
United Nations Millennium Goals, 2:**1007–1011**
filariasis, 1:352
maternal mortality, 2:769
UNICEF, 2:1004, 1006
World Health Organization, 2:1079
United Nations Millennium Summit, 2:1006
United Nations Mission for Ebola Emergency Response, 2:687
United Nations Population Fund, 2:1073
United Nations Secretariat Building, 2:*1008*
United Nations Security Council, 2:601
United States
African sleeping sickness, 1:3
AIDS, 1:13, 18–19
airborne precautions, 1:21
alveolar echinococcosis, 1:24
amebiasis, 1:28
angiostrongyliasis, 1:36, 38
animal importation, 1:40
anisakiasis, 1:45
anthrax, 1:47–48, 50, 51
antimicrobial soap substance bans, 1:66
arthropod-borne diseases, 1:75
ascariasis, 1:79
aspergillosis, 1:85, 86*s*
avian influenza, 1:156
babesiosis, 1:95, *95,* 96, 97
Baylisascaris infection, 1:107
biological weapons, 1:109
biosafety level 4 facilities, 1:246, 421
bioterrorism, 1:113–114
blastomycosis, 1:123
blood supply, 1:125, 126, 127
botulism, 1:134
bovine spongiform encephalopathy, 1:137
brucellosis, 1:141
burkholderia, 1:145

Campylobacter infection, 1:151
candidiasis, 1:160
CDC, 1:164–169
Chagas disease, 1:172, 173
chickenpox, 1:176, 177, 178–179, 178*s*
chikungunya, 1:182
childhood-associated infectious diseases, immunization impacts, 1:185
Chlamydia infection, 1:190
Chlamydia pneumoniae, 1:193
Clostridium difficile infection, 1:210, 211, 212
CMV infection, 1:215
coccidioidomycosis, 1:218–219
colds, 1:230
contact lenses and *Fusarium* keratitis, 1:233
contact precautions, 1:237
Creutzfeldt-Jakob disease, 1:241
Cryptococcus neoformans infection, 1:248
cryptosporidiosis, 1:250, 251, 252
cyclosporiasis, 1:258, 259
dengue and dengue hemorrhagic fever, 1:266, 267
diphtheria, 1:275, 277
dysentery, 1:290
ear infections, 1:294
Eastern equine encephalitis, 1:296, 297, 298
Ebola, 2:601
emerging infectious diseases, 1:312
encephalitis, 1:316–317, 318, 319
endemicity, 1:320
enterovirus 71 infection, 1:325
epidemiology, 1:330, 331
Epstein-Barr virus, 1:335, 336
Escherichia coli O157:H7, 1:339, 340
fake vaccination program, 2:734*s*
food-borne diseases, 1:354, 355, 357
gastroenteritis, 1:358
genetic identification of microorganisms, 1:364
giardiasis, 1:372
glanders, 1:378, 380, *380,* 381
globalization and infectious disease, 1:385
gonorrhea, 1:388–389
group B streptococcal infection, 2:925–926
Haemophilus influenzae, 1:395
hantavirus, 1:404, 405, *406*
health care provider handwashing compliance, 2:642
heartland virus, 2:872
hemorrhagic fevers, 1:420*s*
hepatitis A, 1:423
hepatitis B, 1:427, 428
hepatitis C, 1:431, 432
hepatitis D, 1:434, 435–436
herpes simplex virus 2, 1:445
highly active antiretroviral therapy (HAART), 1:13–14
histoplasmosis, 1:448, 449, 451
hosts and vectors, 1:462
immigration, 1:472, 473–474
influenza, 1:490, 491
influenza epidemiology, 1:503, 504–505
influenza pandemic of 1918, 1:493
influenza pandemic of 1957, 1:499
isolation and quarantine, 1:508, 509, 510*s*
Japanese encephalitis, 1:513
Kawasaki disease, 1:517
Lassa fever, 1:527
Legionnaires' disease, 1:529–530
legislation and international law, 1:535–536
lice infestation, 1:554
listeriosis, 1:556, 558
lung flukes, 1:567
Lyme disease, 1:570, 571
marine microorganisms, 2:591*s*
marine toxins, 2:589, 591, 592
measles, 1:487, 2:594
methicillin-resistant *Staphylococcus aureus,* 1:485
microsporidiosis, 2:624*s*
monkeypox, 2:627, 628
mononucleosis, 2:631–632
mosquito-borne diseases, 2:637, 638*s*
MRSA, 2:640, 641
mumps, 2:644, 645, 646, 647
mycotic disease, 2:651, 652
necrotizing fasciitis, 2:659
norovirus infection, 2:670
nosocomial infections, 1:483, 487, 2:675
notifiable diseases, 2:678–681
outbreaks, field-level response to, 2:687
pandemic preparedness, 2:691–693
parasitic diseases, 2:695
Paris climate agreement, 1:206
personal protective equipment, 2:701
pinworm infection, 2:705, 706
plague, 2:715–716, *718*
Pneumocystis jirovecii pneumonia, 2:721
pneumonia, 2:725, 727, 729
polio, 2:732, 737
Powassan virus, 2:741–743, 742, 742*s,* 743
premature births, 2:926
protozoan diseases, 2:755, 756
psittacosis, 2:759
Q fever, 2:772
rabies, 2:777, 778, 779
re-emerging infectious diseases, 2:790, 791, 792
relapsing fever, 2:795, 796, 797
resistant organisms, 2:803
retroviruses, 2:806
rickettsial disease, 2:811
Rocky Mountain spotted fever, 2:824, 825, 826
rotavirus infection, 2:829
RSV infection, 2:834
rubella, 2:836, 837, 839
Salmonella infection, 2:842
SARS, 2:849, 850
scarlet fever, 2:857
scrofula, 2:866
sepsis, 2:868
sexually transmitted infections, 2:877*s,* 878–879
shigellosis, 2:882, 883
shingles, 2:885, 886
smallpox, 2:890, 891, 892, 893–894
smallpox eradication and storage, 2:896, 897–898
smallpox research, 2:899
smallpox vaccine stockpile, 1:115
St. Louis encephalitis, 2:905–907, 906, *907*
Staphylococcus aureus infections, 2:912
strep throat, 2:918
strongyloidiasis, 2:928, 929
swimmer's ear and swimmer's itch, 2:931
syphilis, 2:936
taeniasis, 2:942
talaromycosis, 2:945
tapeworm infections, 2:949
tetanus, 2:953
tick-borne diseases, 2:957, 958
toxic shock, 2:962*s*
toxoplasmosis, 2:966
travel, 2:970, 971
trichinellosis, 2:974
trichomoniasis, 2:975, 976
triclosan, 2:916
tuberculosis, 2:984, 985–986
tularemia, 2:989, 991
typhoid fever, 2:993
typhus, 2:997, 999
UNICEF, 2:1004
vaccine refusal, 1:186
vancomycin-resistant *Enterococci,* 2:1026, 1027
Venezuelan equine encephalitis virus, 2:1034
viral disease, 2:1042
viral meningitis, 2:607, 609
war, 2:1051
water-borne diseases, 2:1053, 1054, 1055
West Nile virus, 2:1058, *1059,* 1059–1060
whipworm, 2:1063

whooping cough, 2:1066, 1067, 1068
women, 2:1073
yellow fever, 2:1092
yersiniosis, 2:1096–1099, 1097, 1098
Zika virus, 2:1101, 1102
zoonoses, 2:1106
United States Agency for International Development, 1:563
United States Army Medical Research Institute of Infectious Diseases. *See* USAMRIID
Universal health coverage, 2:1079
Universal precautions, 2:908
University of Arizona, 1:221
University of Birmingham, 2:983
University of California, Berkeley, 2:697
University of Georgia, 1:12
University of Minnesota, 2:597
University of North Carolina, 1:4
University of Oklahoma, 1:212
University of Oregon, 1:212
University of Pennsylvania, 1:445
University of Texas, 1:455
University of Thailand, 1:563
University of Washington School of Medicine, 2:926–927
Unpasteurized dairy products
brucellosis, 1:140, 141, 142*s*
Campylobacter infection, 1:152*s*
listeriosis, 1:557
rat-bite fever, 2:786
scrofula, 2:866
tuberculosis, 2:983
yersiniosis, 2:1098
Unsafe abortion, 2:1108
Upper respiratory infections. *See* Respiratory system disease or symptoms
Ural Mountains, 1:48
Urban areas
dengue and dengue hemorrhagic fever, 1:268
leishmaniasis, 1:541
re-emerging infectious diseases, 2:793
tuberculosis, 2:986
water-borne disease, 2:1054
yellow fever, 2:1092
zoonoses, 2:1107
Urban rabies, 2:777
Urban transmission, Zika virus, 2:1101
Urbani, Carlo, 2:848, 849
Urethral discharge, 1:387–388
Urethral swabs, 1:191*s*
Urethritis
Chlamydia infection, 1:189, 191
gonorrhea, 1:387
protozoan diseases, 2:754
sexually transmitted infections, 2:878
urinary tract infection, 2:1012
viral disease, 2:1039
Urinary catheters. *See* Catheters
Urinary incontinence. *See* Incontinence
Urinary tract infection, 2:**1012–1014,** *1013*
antibiotic resistance, 1:59
blastomycosis, 1:122
herpes simplex virus 2, 1:444
nosocomial infections, 1:257
polio, 2:737
schistosomiasis, 2:861, 862
trichomoniasis, 2:975–977
vancomycin-resistant *Enterococci,* 2:1025
Urination issues
Chlamydia infection, 1:189
gonorrhea, 1:387
herpes simplex virus 2, 1:444
Legionnaires' disease, 1:530
sexually transmitted infections, 2:877
shigellosis, 2:881
trichomoniasis, 2:976
urinary tract infection, 2:1012
Urine tests
blastomycosis, 1:122
glanders, 1:380
viral meningitis, 2:609
Uruguay, 1:177
U.S. Agency for International Development, 1:253, 2:1046
U.S. Air Force, 2:1049
U.S. Animal and Plant Health Inspection Service, 2:779
U.S. Arms Control Association, 1:111
U.S. Army
influenza pandemic of 1918, 2:1047–1048
Operation Sea Spray, 2:1014*s*
smallpox, 2:893
virus hunters, 2:1043–1044
Yellow Fever Commission, 2:1092, 1095
U.S. Army Medical Research and Development Command, 2:1016
U.S. Army Medical Research Institute of Chemical Diseases, 2:1018
U.S. Army Medical Research Institute of Infectious Diseases. *See* USAMRIID
U.S. Biomedical Advanced Research and Development, 2:893
U.S. Centers for Disease Control and Prevention. *See* CDC
U.S. Central Intelligence Agency, 1:116
U.S. Congress
CDC, 1:166
disease reporting, 1:385, 2:678
Project Bioshield, 1:114
smallpox virus, 2:899
U.S. Council of State and Territorial Epidemiologists, 2:679
U.S. Department of Agriculture
animal importation, 1:39, 40
biological weapons, 1:111*s*
bovine spongiform encephalopathy, 1:139
Eastern equine encephalitis-carrying mosquitoes, 1:298*s*
food-borne disease and food safety, 1:357
globalization and infectious disease, 1:385
listeriosis, 1:557
Salmonella infection, 2:842
snails, seizure of, 1:38
Task Force on Antimicrobial Resistance, 1:256*s*
world trade, 2:1084
yersiniosis, 2:1097, 1098, 1098*s*
U.S. Department of Defense
Advanced Diagnostics Program, 2:783*s*
anthrax, 1:49
antibiotic resistance, 1:59
biological warfare research, 2:1015–1018
Biomedical Advanced Research and Development Authority, 1:114
leishmaniasis, 1:541
Task Force on Antimicrobial Resistance, 1:256*s*
war and infectious disease, 2:1052
U.S. Department of Health and Human Services, 1:111*s*
anthrax vaccine stockpile, 1:51
Biomedical Advanced Research and Development Authority, 1:114
bioterrorism, 1:114
National Institute of Allergy and Infectious Diseases, 2:653
pandemic preparedness, 2:692
Tuskegee syphilis study, 2:938
See also CDC
U.S. Department of Homeland Security, 1:114
U.S. Department of Justice, 2:1017
U.S. Department of State, 1:111
U.S. Department of Veterans Affairs, 1:256*s*
U.S. Federal Bureau of Investigation
anthrax attacks, 1:48, 2:1017
bioterrorism, 1:113
smallpox specimens, 2:894
U.S. Food and Drug Administration
AIDS, 1:11, 19–20
albendazole, 1:45
antibiotic use in livestock, 1:64, 2:746
antimicrobial soaps, 1:66, 67, 68–69
avian influenza, 1:89

Biomedical Advanced Research and Development Authority, 1:114
botulism recalls, 1:135
Campylobacter infection, 1:153
Chagas disease drugs, 1:171, 173–174
Chipotle subpoena, 2:671
cholera vaccine, 1:199
cryptosporidiosis, 1:251, 252
enrofloxacin, 2:803
food-borne disease and food safety, 1:356*s*, 357
gene therapy trials, 2:808
hepatitis C drugs, 1:432
H5N1 vaccine, 1:497
immune response, 1:479
leishmaniasis drugs, 1:540
listeriosis, 1:557, 558
plague drugs, 1:116, 2:718
protozoan diseases drugs, 2:755
rabies vaccine, 2:777
rotavirus vaccine, 1:361, 2:830
shingles, 1:177, 2:887
smallpox, 2:892, 893, 894, 898
trehalose, 1:212
triclosan ban, 2:916
yersiniosis, 2:1098
U.S. Food Safety and Inspection Service, 1:558
U.S. Government Accountability Office, 2:1074
U.S. Health Resources and Services Administration, 1:256*s*
U.S. Homeland Security Council, 2:691
U.S. National Vital Statistics, 2:727
U.S. Navy, 2:730
U.S. Navy Preventive Medicine Department, 2:1048–1049
U.S. Postal Service, 1:116, 2:1017
U.S. President's Emergency Plan for AIDS Relief, 2:981*s*
U.S. President's Malaria Initiative, 2:1009
U.S. Public Health Service
influenza epidemiology, 1:507
leprosy, 1:544–545
Tuskegee syphilis study, 2:937–938
war, 2:1047
U.S. Public Health Service Act, 2:986
U.S. Surgeons General
SARS, 2:850
Tuskegee syphilis study, 2:937
USAMRIID, 2:1016
U.S. 21st Century Cures Act, 2:803
U.S. Veterans Health Administration, 1:116
U.S. Virgin Islands, 1:267
USA PATRIOT Act, 1:111*s*
USAID, 1:563
USAMRICD. *See* U.S. Army Medical Research Institute of Chemical Diseases
USAMRIID, 2:*1015*, **1015–1019**
Utah
coccidioidomycosis, 1:220
hantavirus, 1:407
hepatitis A, 1:424–425
relapsing fever, 2:795
Uttar Pradesh, India, 1:513*s*
Uzbekistan, 1:277

V

Vaccination Act, UK, 2:891
Vaccination Assistance Act, 1:185
Vaccine Alliance. *See* Global Alliance for Vaccines and Immunization
Vaccine Safety Council, 2:597
Vaccines, animal, 1:*297*
anthrax, 1:47, 50
brucellosis, 1:140, 141, 142
Eastern equine encephalitis, 1:297
Escherichia coli O157:H7, 1:302, 340–341
giardiasis, 1:373
liver fluke infections, 1:562
parasitic diseases, 2:695
Q fever, 2:773
rabies, 2:777–778, 779
Rift Valley fever, 2:815
Venezuelan equine encephalitis virus, 2:1035
war, 2:1051
West Nile virus, 2:1060
Vaccines and vaccine development, 2:**1020–1024**, *1021*
AIDS, 1:*9*, 20
anthrax, 1:50, 115
arthropod-borne diseases, 1:77
avian influenza, 1:89, 90, 156
B virus, 1:93
bacterial diseases, 1:101
bacterial meningitis, 2:606
bioengineered edible vaccines, 1:82*s*
bioterrorism, 1:115, 116
Buruli ulcer, 1:149
cancer, 1:154, 155, 155*s*
CDC, 1:167, 169
chickenpox, 1:175, *176*, 178–179, 178*s*
chikungunya, 1:182
childhood-associated infectious diseases, 1:184–187
Chlamydia infection, 1:191
cholera, 1:199, 200
CMV infection, 1:214, 216, 217
cohorted communities, 1:224*s*, 225
Crimean-Congo hemorrhagic fever, 1:245
demographics, 1:263–264
dengue and dengue hemorrhagic fever, 1:268
diphtheria, 1:274, *275*, 276, 278
DTP vaccines, 2:*952*
ear infections, 1:295
Ebola, 1:302, 303–304, 419, 2:602
emerging infectious diseases, 1:314
encephalitis, 1:318
endemic diseases, 1:320–321
enterovirus 71 infection, 1:326
Escherichia coli O157:H7, 1:341
gastroenteritis, 1:359, 361
genital herpes, 1:365
GIDEON, 1:375
globalization and infectious disease, 1:385
gonorrhea, 1:389
group A streptococcal infections, 2:922
group B streptococcal infection, 2:925
Haemophilus influenzae, 1:394, *395*, 396
Helicobacter pylori, 1:412
hemorrhagic fevers, 1:420
hepatitis A, 1:423, *423*, 424–425
hepatitis B, 1:426, *427*, 428, 428*s*
hepatitis D, 1:435
hepatitis E, 1:437, 438
herpes simplex virus 2, 1:445
HIV, 1:130
H5N1, 1:497
HPV, 1:468, 469, *469*, 470–471
immigration, 1:474
infection control and asepsis, 1:487
influenza, 1:490–491, 496, 501, 504–505, 506
internationally adopted children, 1:475
Japanese encephalitis, 1:511–512, *512*, 513, 514
Lassa fever, 1:528
legislation and international law, 1:536–537
leishmaniasis, 1:540
leptospirosis, 1:548
Lyme disease, 1:572
malaria, 1:205, 2:579, 581
measles, 2:593, 595–598
microorganisms, 2:617
MMR vaccine, 2:838*s*
mosquito-borne diseases, 2:638, 639
MRSA, 2:643
mumps, 2:644, 645–646, 646–647
National Institute of Allergy and Infectious Diseases, 2:654
norovirus infection, 2:671
outbreaks, field-level response to, 2:687

pandemic preparedness, 2:691–692
parasitic diseases, 2:695–696
plague, 2:719
pneumonia, 2:729
polio, 1:*185,* 2:732–734, 737, 738, 740
public health, 2:763, 765
Q fever, 2:772, 773
rabies, 2:775, *775,* 777, 779
recombinant technology, 1:82
re-emerging infectious diseases, 2:791, 792
rickettsial disease, 2:811
Rift Valley fever, 2:813
Rocky Mountain Laboratory, 2:656
rotavirus, 2:828, 829, *830,* 831
RSV, 2:834–835
rubella, 2:836, *836,* 837–838, 839
Salmonella, 2:842
schistosomiasis, 2:863
sepsis, 2:869
sexually transmitted infections, 2:878, 879
shingles, 1:177, 2:885, 887–888
smallpox, 2:891, 893, 894, 897, 898, 899
smallpox vaccine for monkeypox prevention, 2:627–628, 628*s*
Tdap vaccine, 2:*1067*
tetanus, 2:953, 954
tick-borne diseases, 2:957, 958
tropical infectious diseases, 2:981, 982
tuberculosis, 2:985
tularemia, 2:991
typhoid fever, 2:993, 994–995, 996
UNICEF, 2:*1005,* 1006
USAMRIID, 2:1017, 1018
vector-borne disease, 2:1031
Venezuelan equine encephalitis virus, 2:1034, 1035
viral diseases, 1:71–72, 2:1041
viral meningitis prevention, 2:610
war, 2:1049, 1050–1051, 1052
whooping cough, 2:1066, 1067–1068, 1068–1069
women, 2:1073–1074
World Health Organization, 2:1076, 1077–1078
yellow fever, 2:1092
Vaccinia immune globulin medications, 2:628
Vaccinia virus, 2:897, 1039
Vaginal bleeding, abnormal, 2:877
Vaginal cancer, 1:155*s,* 468
Vaginal candidiasis, 1:159
Vaginal discharge
Chlamydia infection, 1:189
gonorrhea, 1:388
protozoan diseases, 2:754
puerperal fever, 2:767
sexually transmitted infections, 2:877
Vaginitis, 2:707, 754
Valacyclovir
genital herpes, 1:365
herpes simplex virus 2, 1:445, 446*s*
shingles, 2:886
Valganciclovir, 1:215
Valley fever. *See* Coccidioidomycosis
Valproate, 1:241, 2:750
Van Der Linden, Vanessa, 1:*312*
Van Tieghem, Edouard Leon, 1:121
Vancomycin
antibiotic resistance, 1:62
Clostridium difficile infection, 1:211
MRSA, 2:642
tsunami lung, 2:730
Vancomycin intermediate-resistant *Staphlyococcus aureus,* 2:643
Vancomycin-resistant *Enterococci,* 1:100, 487, 509, 2:**1025–1028,** *1026*
Vancomycin-resistant *Staphylococcus aureus,* 1:237, 2:642
Vancouver, George, 2:589
Vancouver Island, Canada, 1:248
Vanuatu, 2:1089
Variant Creutzfeldt-Jakob disease
animal importation, 1:40
blood supply, 1:126–127
bovine spongiform encephalopathy, 1:136, 139
BSE inquiry, 1:138*s*
Creutzfeldt-Jakob disease types, 1:239–242
kuru, 1:524
prion disease, 2:749, 750
Varicella. *See* Chickenpox
Varicella zoster virus. *See* Shingles
Varicella-zoster immune globulin (VZIG), 1:178
Variola virus. *See* Smallpox
Variolation, 2:710, 891, 1020
Vascular bleeding and hantavirus, 1:404
VaxGen Inc., 1:51
Vector resistance, 1:463
Vector-borne disease, 1:204, 205–206, 2:**1029–1032,** *1030. See also* Arthropod-borne diseases; Hosts and vectors
Vegetables and food-borne disease, 1:556, 557, 558, 562
Venereal diseases. *See* Sexually transmitted infections
Venezuela
coccidioidomycosis, 1:220
encephalitis, 1:317
hantavirus, 1:405, 406
river blindness, 2:821
Venezuelan equine encephalitis virus, 2:1034, 1035
Venezuelan equine encephalitis virus, 1:317, 2:**1033–1036,** *1034*
Venezuelan hemorrhagic fever, 1:418
Venice, Italy, 1:508
Ventilation systems and infection control, 1:486
Ventilator-associated pneumonia, 1:257, 2:674
Ventura County Environmental Health Division, 2:671
Vermifuges. *See* Anthelmintic drugs
Vermont, 1:123, 571
Vermox. *See* Anthelmintic drugs; Mebendazole
Verotoxins, 1:338
Vertigo and African sleeping sickness, 1:5
Vesicular stomatitis viruses, 1:304
Vesper mice, 1:406
Veterinarians
alveolar echinococcosis, 1:25
B virus infection, 1:91–92
Baylisascaris infection, 1:107
brucellosis, 1:141
cat scratch disease, 1:163
Crimean-Congo hemorrhagic fever, 1:244
leptospirosis, 1:549
monkeypox, 2:627
plague, 2:717
psittacosis, 2:759
Q fever, 2:771, 773
Rift Valley fever, 2:814
sporotrichosis, 2:903
Veterinary vaccines. *See* Vaccines, animal
Vibrio cholerae, 1:197
Vical, 1:216
Victoria, Australia, 1:147, 150
Victorian Infectious Diseases Reference Laboratory (Australia), 1:506
Vienna General Hospital, 2:674
Vietnam
avian influenza, 1:88
burkholderia, 1:144, 145
epidemiology, 1:*329*
Japanese encephalitis, 1:512, 513–514
liver fluke infections, 1:562
lung flukes, 1:566
plague, 2:717
SARS, 2:848
talaromycosis, 2:945
Vietnam War, 2:1050–1051
Violence against polio eradication campaign workers, 2:734, 734*s*
Vipers, 1:258
Viral disease, 2:**1037–1042,** *1038, 1040*
antibiotic resistance, 1:63
anti-cytokine antibody syndrome, 1:54
antiviral drugs, 1:70–73

biodefense research and development, 1:119
cancer, 1:154–156
CDC, 1:169
climate change, 1:206–207
CMV infection, 1:214–217
cohorted communities, 1:224
cold sores, 1:226
colds, 1:228–230
droplet precautions, 1:286, 287–288
Ebola, 1:300–304
encephalitis, 1:315–319
enterovirus 71 infection, 1:324–327
Epstein-Barr virus, 1:335–337
fifth disease, 1:347–349
gastroenteritis, 1:358–359, *360*, 361
genetic identification of microorganisms, 1:364
genital herpes, 1:365
hand, foot, and mouth disease, 1:397–399
heartland virus, 2:873*s*
hemorrhagic fevers, 1:418–421
hepatitis A, 1:422–425
hepatitis B, 1:426–428
hepatitis C, 1:430–432
hepatitis D, 1:434–436
hepatitis E, 1:437–439
herpes simplex 1 virus, 1:440–443
herpes simplex virus 2, 1:444–446
HIV, 1:453–456
H5N1, 1:391–393
HPV, 1:468–470
influenza, 1:488–491, 503–507
influenza pandemic of 1918, 1:493–498
influenza pandemic of 1957, 1:499–502
Japanese encephalitis, 1:511–514
Lassa fever, 1:526–528
Marburg hemorrhagic fever, 2:585–587
measles, 2:593–598
meningitis, 1:326, 2:605, 607–610
microbial evolution, 2:614
microorganisms, 2:616
microscopes and microscopy, 2:619
Middle East respiratory syndrome, 1:386
monkeypox, 2:626–628
mononucleosis, 2:630–635
mumps, 2:644–647
Nipah virus infection, 2:662–664
norovirus infection, 2:669–672
opportunistic infections, 2:683
pneumonia, 2:725, 726
polio, 2:732–734, 736–740
Powassan virus, 2:741–743
re-emerging infectious diseases, 2:792
retroviruses, 2:805–808
Rift Valley fever, 2:813–816
rotavirus infection, 2:828–831
RSV infection, 2:832–835
rubella, 2:836–839
SARS, 2:847–851
severe fever with thrombocytopenia syndrome, 2:871–873
sexually transmitted infections, 2:876–877, 878, 879
shingles, 2:885–888
smallpox, 2:890–894
St. Louis encephalitis, 2:905–907
tick-borne diseases, 2:957, 958
urinary tract infection, 2:1013
vector-borne disease, 2:1029
Venezuelan equine encephalitis virus, 2:1033–1035
West Nile virus, 2:1057–1061
yellow fever, 2:1092–1095
Zika virus, 2:1100–1103
zoonoses, 2:1106
Viral hemorrhagic fevers. *See* Hemorrhagic fevers
Viral load, 1:8, 206, 2:741
Viral samples. *See* Virus sharing
Viral shedding, 1:441, 443, 444
Virazole. *See* Ribavirin
Virgin Islands, 1:182, 266, 267, 2:590
Virginia, 1:303, 571, 2:671, 742
Virions, 2:1038–1039
Virology, 2:1043–1046
Virulence
Clostridium difficile infection, 1:212–213
Salmonella infection, 2:841
scarlet fever, 2:856
Virus hunters, 2:**1043–1046,** *1044*
Virus sharing, 1:89–90, 385
Viruses, Plagues, and History, 2:1043
Viruslike particles, 1:182
Visceral leishmaniasis, 1:538–541, 2:754, 755, 756, 980
VISION 2020, 2:822
Vision disorders. *See* Eye and vision disorders
Vital Signs (CDC), 1:167
Vitamin A, 2:595
Vitamin A Global Initiative, 2:1005
Vitamin C, 1:230
Vlasits, Anna, 2:1031
Voles, 1:405
Voluntary isolation and quarantine, 1:508, 2:850
Vomit tests, 1:79
Vomiting
AIDS, 1:12
amebiasis, 1:27
angiostrongyliasis, 1:35
anisakiasis, 1:45
ascariasis, 1:79
B virus infection, 1:92
bacterial diseases, 1:100
Campylobacter infection, 1:151
candidiasis, 1:159
Chagas disease, 1:172
chikungunya, 1:*180,* 181
cholera, 1:197, 198, 201
Clostridium difficile infection, 1:210
Crimean-Congo hemorrhagic fever, 1:244
cryptosporidiosis, 1:250, 251
dysentery, 1:289
Ebola, 1:302
encephalitis, 1:317
enterovirus 71 infection, 1:326
Escherichia coli O157:H7, 1:340
food-borne disease, 1:354
gastroenteritis, 1:358–361, 359–360
hantavirus, 1:404
hemorrhagic fevers, 1:419, 420*s*
hepatitis E, 1:437
Japanese encephalitis, 1:512
Lassa fever, 1:526
Legionnaires' disease, 1:530
leptospirosis, 1:548
listeriosis, 1:556
Marburg hemorrhagic fever, 2:586
marine toxins, 2:590
meningitis, 2:606*s*
necrotizing fasciitis, 2:660
norovirus infection, 2:669, 670
pinworm infection, 2:705
polio, 2:736
Powassan virus, 2:741
Q fever, 2:772
rat-bite fever, 2:785, 787
relapsing fever, 2:795
Rocky Mountain spotted fever, 2:824
rotavirus infection, 2:828
Salmonella infection, 2:841
scarlet fever, 2:856
severe fever with thrombocytopenia syndrome, 2:871
taeniasis, 2:943
toxic shock, 2:961
trichinellosis, 2:972
typhus, 2:997
viral meningitis, 2:608
water-borne disease, 2:1054
West Nile virus, 2:1058–1059
yellow fever, 2:1092
Voriconazole, 1:85, 159, 2:946
Vulvar cancer, 1:155*s*, 468
Vulvovaginal candidiasis, 1:158
Vulvovaginal swabs, 1:191*s*

W

Wakefield, Andrew, 2:596, 1021
Waksman, Selman, 1:57
Wales, 2:857, 994

A Walk Across Africa (Grant), 1:147
Walker, Mark J., 2:858
Walker, Polly, 1:64
Walkerton, Ontario, Canada, 1:339
Walking Palms Global Initiative, 1:207
Walking pneumonia, 2:726
Walruses, 2:973
Walton, David, 2:659
War, 2:**1047–1052,** *1049*
  battlefield medicine, 2:1018
  cholera, 1:198, 200
  demographics, 1:261, 263
  dysentery, 1:290
  helminth disease, 1:416
  legislation and international law, 1:535
  leishmaniasis, 1:541
  leptospirosis, 1:550
  lice infestation, 1:554
  malaria, 2:581
  Médecins Sans Frontières, 2:600
  plague, 2:711
  polio eradication campaign, 2:734, 734*s*
  smallpox, 2:890
  typhoid fever, 2:995
  typhus, 2:997–1001, 998, 999, 1000
  Yemen, 1:*199*
  See also Biological weapons; Military; specific wars
Warren, Charles Henry, 2:995*s*
Warren, J. Robin, 1:343–344, 409, 411, 412*s*
Warren, Stafford, 1:344
Warts
  HPV, 1:468, 469–470
  sexually transmitted infections, 2:877–878
  viral disease, 2:1039
Washington
  animal importation, 1:40
  babesiosis, 1:96
  bovine spongiform encephalopathy, 1:139
  Chlamydia pneumoniae, 1:193
  coccidioidomycosis, 1:220
  Escherichia coli infection, 2:672
  listeriosis outbreak, 1:558
  relapsing fever, 2:795
  whooping cough, 2:1069
Washington Post, 1:524, 572, 2:596, 882, 961
Wasser, Lauren, 2:963
Wastewater, triclosan in, 1:68
Wasting and tuberculosis, 2:983
Water filtration
  cryptosporidiosis, 1:252*s*, 253
  dracunculiasis, 1:284, 284*s*, 285
  giardiasis, 1:372
  schistosomiasis, 2:862
  shigellosis, 2:883
  water-borne disease, 2:1054, 1055
Water fleas, 1:283, 463
Water pollution, 2:933, 1055, 1055*s*
Water treatment
  cryptosporidiosis, 1:252
  germ theory of disease, 1:369
  water-borne diseases, 2:1054, 1055, 1055*s*
Water-borne diseases, 2:*1053,* **1053–1056**
  amebiasis, 1:28–29
  ascariasis, 1:79
  bacterial diseases, 1:100, 101
  balantidiasis, 1:102, 103
  Buruli ulcers, 1:147–148
  Campylobacter infection, 1:151–153
  cholera, 1:197–201, 198–199, 200
  climate change, 1:204, 205, 207
  cryptosporidiosis, 1:250–253
  demographics, 1:261
  dengue and dengue hemorrhagic fever, 1:268
  disinfection, 1:281, 282
  dracunculiasis, 1:283–285
  dysentery, 1:289–292
  economic development, 1:307
  emerging infectious diseases, 1:312, 314
  epidemiology, 1:329, 333
  Escherichia coli O157:H7, 1:338–341
  gastroenteritis, 1:359–360
  germ theory, 1:366–367
  giardiasis, 1:371–374
  glanders, 1:379, 381
  helminth disease, 1:415, 416, 417, 2:1064
  hepatitis A, 1:422, 423
  hepatitis E, 1:437–439
  hosts and vectors, 1:463
  hot tub rash, 1:465–467
  Legionnaires' disease, 1:529–531
  legislation s, 1:534
  leptospirosis, 1:548–550, 549*s*
  liver fluke infections, 1:560, 562
  microsporidiosis, 2:622–624
  parasitic diseases, 2:694, 696
  prevention, 1:466*s*
  protozoan diseases, 2:754, 755, 757
  public health, 2:766
  rat-bite fever, 2:786
  resistant organisms, 2:801
  rotavirus infection, 2:828–831
  Salmonella infection, 2:840–842
  sanitation, 2:845, 846
  schistosomiasis, 2:860–863
  sepsis, 2:869
  shigellosis, 2:880–883
  sterilization, 2:915
  swimmer's ear and swimmer's itch, 2:931–933
  tapeworm infections, 2:950
  toxoplasmosis, 2:964
  tularemia, 2:989, 990, 991
  typhoid fever, 2:993, 995
  war, 2:1049
  World Health Organization, 2:1078–1079
  yersiniosis, 2:1096, 1098
  See also Sanitation
Waterfowl and schistosomes, 2:931
Watery diarrhea
  avian influenza, 1:89
  cholera, 1:201
  Clostridium difficile infection, 1:210
  Escherichia coli O157:H7, 1:340
  rotavirus infection, 2:828–829
  Salmonella infection, 2:841
Weakness
  alveolar echinococcosis, 1:24
  arthropod-borne diseases, 1:75
  brucellosis, 1:141
  cat scratch disease, 1:161–163
  enterovirus 71 infection, 1:326
  hookworm infection, 1:458
  marine toxins, 2:591
  mononucleosis, 2:631
  necrotizing fasciitis, 2:659
  Nipah virus infection, 2:663
  plague, 2:715
  polio, 2:737
  Powassan virus, 2:741
  rat-bite fever, 2:787
  relapsing fever, 2:795
  Rift Valley fever, 2:813
  Salmonella infection, 2:841
  schistosomiasis, 2:861
  tularemia, 2:990
  typhoid fever, 2:993
Wealth and economic development, 1:307
Weapons, biological. *See* Biological weapons
Weasels, 2:785
Weather
  climate change and parasitic diseases, 2:756, 757
  colds, 1:229–230, 230*s*
  leptospirosis, 1:550
  protozoan diseases, 2:757
  Rift Valley fever, 2:813
  RSV infection, 2:833
  See also Floods; Natural disasters
Weather and climate change, 1:203–207
Websites. *See* Internet resources
Wehlie, Tahlil, 2:598
Weight loss
  AIDS, 1:12
  alveolar echinococcosis, 1:24
  aspergillosis, 1:85
  balantidiasis, 1:102
  blastomycosis, 1:122
  burkholderia, 1:145
  cryptosporidiosis, 1:251
  cyclosporiasis, 1:259
  dysentery, 1:289

giardiasis, 1:371
herpes gladiatorum, 1:442*s*
HIV, 1:11
hookworm infection, 1:458
Marburg hemorrhagic fever, 2:586
microsporidiosis, 2:623
opportunistic infections, 2:683
protozoan diseases, 2:753, 754
Q fever, 2:772
Rift Valley fever, 2:813
schistosomiasis, 2:861
scrofula, 2:866
sexually transmitted infections, 2:877
syphilis, 2:935
taeniasis, 2:941
talaromycosis, 2:944
tuberculosis, 2:983
water-borne disease, 2:1054
whipworm, 2:1062
Weil, Adolf, 1:548
Weingarten, Rebecca A., 2:1027
Well water, 1:339
Wellcome Trust Sanger Institute, 1:212
Weller, Thomas, 2:736, 739
West Africa
cholera, 1:201
Ebola, 1:114, 2:1022
economic development, 1:308
globalization and infectious disease, 1:385
hepatitis E, 1:438
Lassa fever, 1:526, 527
leprosy, 1:544
Médecins Sans Frontières, 2:599, 602
monkeypox, 2:626, 627, 628
outbreaks, field-level response to, 2:687
plague, 2:716
public health, 2:765
Rift Valley fever, 2:815
river blindness, 2:820, 821, 822
USAMRIID, 2:1017
yellow fever, 2:1092
West African trypanosomiasis. *See* African sleeping sickness
West Asia, 2:792, 1057
West Coast, United States, 1:107
West Nile virus, 2:**1057–1061,** *1058, 1059*
arthropod-borne diseases, 1:77
blood supply, 1:126
climate change, 1:206
demographics, 1:263
encephalitis, 1:317, 319
globalization and infectious disease, 1:385
hosts and vectors, 1:463
mosquito-borne diseases, 2:637
re-emerging infectious diseases, 2:792
St. Louis encephalitis, relation to, 2:906
travel, 2:970
vector-borne disease, 2:1030
viral disease, 2:1041
zoonoses, 2:1106, 1107
West Virginia, 1:428, 449
Western Africa, 1:266, 290
Western equine encephalitis, 1:317, 2:1029, 1033
Western Europe
AIDS deaths, 1:14
avian influenza, 1:156
Crimean-Congo hemorrhagic fever, 1:244
diphtheria, 1:275, 277
endemicity, 1:320
epidemiology, 1:331
helminth disease, 1:415
scarlet fever, 2:857
whipworm, 2:1063
Western Hemisphere
chikungunya, 1:181
cholera, 1:199
coccidioidomycosis, 1:218, 220
mosquito-borne diseases, 2:637
polio eradication, 1:187
Zika virus, 2:687
Western Pacific countries
dengue and dengue hemorrhagic fever, 1:267
hepatitis B, 1:427
Japanese encephalitis, 1:511
malaria, 2:580, 581
polio, 2:733, 734, 740
Western United States
botulism, 1:134
encephalitis, 1:317
relapsing fever, 2:795, 796, 797
St. Louis encephalitis, 2:906
Wetlands and Eastern equine encephalitis, 1:298
Whales, 1:45, 2:973
"What If Cipro Stopped Working?", 1:*64*
"What You Know about Ticks May Be Just Wrong Enough!", 2:*958–959*
Wheezing
ascariasis, 1:79
aspergillosis, 1:85
dracunculiasis, 1:283
RSV infection, 2:832
strongyloidiasis, 2:929
Whidbee, Delano, 2:883
Whipworm, 2:**1062–1065,** *1063*
White, Ryan, 1:*129*
White blood cells
immune response, 1:478
lung flukes, 1:567
macrophage activation syndrome, 2:575–576
severe fever with thrombocytopenia syndrome, 2:872
White-footed mice, 1:406, 2:741
Whitmore, Alfred, 1:379
Whitmore's disease. *See* Glanders
WHO. *See* World Health Organization (WHO)
"WHO Guide to Identifying the Economic Consequences of Disease and Injury," 1:309
"WHO Recommends Large-Scale Deworming to Improve Children's Health and Nutrition," 2:*1064*
Whooping cough, 2:**1066–1070**
bacterial disease vaccines, 1:101
childhood vaccination, 1:187
unvaccinated children, 1:186
vaccine refusal, 1:186
WHO childhood vaccination recommendations, 1:185
"Whooping Cough Vaccine's Protection Fades Quickly," 2:*1068–1069*
Wild animals
alveolar echinococcosis, 1:25
anellovirus, 1:31
Baylisascaris infection, 1:108
brucellosis, 1:141
Chagas disease, 1:173
Crimean-Congo hemorrhagic fever, 1:243, 244
hemorrhagic fevers, 1:418–419
histoplasmosis, 1:449
leptospirosis, 1:548
liver fluke infections, 1:560
lung flukes, 1:565
microsporidiosis, 2:622
as pets, 1:107
psittacosis, 2:759
rabies, 2:777, 778, 779
SARS, 2:849
world trade in, 2:1081, 1083–1085
Wild boars, 1:31, 2:973, 1083
Wild game meat, 2:973, 973*s*, 974
Wildlife areas, human encroachment into. *See* Human encroachment into wildlife areas
Wilson, Keith T., 1:411
Wiltshire, UK, 2:857
Winnipeg, Manitoba, Canada, 1:304
Winslet, Kate, 2:664
Winter diarrhea. *See* Rotavirus infection
Wisconsin
blastomycosis, 1:122
encephalitis, 1:317
Lyme disease, 1:571
Powassan virus, 2:742, 742*s*
water-borne disease, 2:1054
Wolbachia, 1:462, 2:1093
Wolves, 2:697, 776, 777
Women, 2:**1071–1075,** *1072*
Brazil, 2:1108
Chlamydia infection, 1:189–190, 191, 191*s*
gonorrhea, 1:389–390

HPV, 1:468–469
kuru, 1:522, 523
mumps, 2:646
protozoan diseases, 2:754
rubella, 2:838
sexually transmitted infections, 2:877, 878
toxic shock, 2:961, 962–963
trachoma, 2:967, 969
trichomoniasis, 2:975, 976, 977
urinary tract infection, 2:1012–1013
vulvovaginal candidiasis, 1:158
Zika virus, 1:76*s*
Wood, Leonard, 2:1094
Wood Buffalo National Park, 1:142
Wood lamp, 2:818
Wood rats, 2:715
Wood ticks, 2:824
Woodchucks, 2:741, 777
Woodcock, Janet, 1:68
Wooded areas and forests
blastomycosis, 1:122
Lyme disease, 1:572
Powassan virus, 2:742
relapsing fever, 2:797
rickettsial disease, 2:811
river blindness, 2:820
Rocky Mountain spotted fever, 2:825, 826
tick-borne diseases, 1:206, 2:958
virus hunters, 2:1045, 1046
yaws, 2:1088
Zika virus, 2:1101
See also Deforestation
Woodruff, Robert, 1:166
Woods, Robert, 1:12
Woods Hold Oceanographic Institution, 2:592
Wooster, OH, 1:501
Workdays lost, 1:230
World Bank
African sleeping sickness, 1:4
cryptosporidiosis prevention, 1:253
Global Fund to Fight AIDS, Tuberculosis and Malaria, 2:1009
legislation and international law, 1:533
sanitation, 2:846
"Trafficking Wildlife and Transmitting Disease: Bold Threats in an Era of Ebola," 2:1084–1085
UNICEF, work with, 2:1005
wildlife crime, 2:1085
Zika virus, 2:1102
World Care Council, 2:986–988
World Economic Forum, 1:115
World Health Assembly
Buruli ulcer, 1:149
childhood-associated infectious disease eradication, 1:184–185
filariasis, 1:352
hepatitis D, 1:435
legislation and international law, 1:537
leprosy, 1:547
schistosomiasis, 2:863
sepsis, 2:868
smallpox, 2:898
United Nations Millennium Goals, 2:1009
World Health Organization, 2:1076
World Health Organization (WHO), 2:**1076–1080,** *1078*
African sleeping sickness, 1:1, 3, 4
AIDS, 1:8, 13, 20
alveolar echinococcosis prevention, 1:25
amebiasis prevention, 1:29
animal importation, 2:1084
antibiotics, distribution of, 1:58
antimicrobial resistance, 2:745
arthropod-borne diseases, 1:75, 77
ascariasis, 1:78
avian influenza, 1:87, 88, 89–90, 156
bioterrorism, 1:114–115
blood supply, 1:126, 127
Brazil's sanitation situation, 2:1108
Buruli ulcer, 1:148, *149*
CDC, partnership with, 1:169
Chagas disease, 1:173
chickenpox, 1:177
chikungunya, 1:*180*
childhood-associated infectious disease eradication, 1:184–185
Chlamydia infection, 1:189, 191
cholera, 1:198, 199, 200, 201
climate change, 1:205
Crimean-Congo hemorrhagic fever, 1:243, 245
cryptosporidiosis prevention, 1:252–253
DDT use, 1:77
Declaration of Helsinki, 2:937
dementia, 1:525
dengue and dengue hemorrhagic fever, 1:267
developing nations and drug delivery, 1:270, 271
deworming recommendations, 2:1064
diphtheria, 1:276, 277, 278
dracunculiasis, 1:285
dysentery, 1:291, 292
Ebola, 1:301, 303, 303*s,* 2:602
economic development, 1:306–309, 307
elbow bump greeting, 1:402
emerging infectious diseases, 1:312–313, 314
encephalitis, 1:318
endemicity, 1:321
epidemiology, 1:332
extremely drug-resistant tuberculosis, 1:23
filariasis, 1:351
food irradiation for cyclosporiasis prevention, 1:260
food-borne disease and food safety, 1:356, 357
gastroenteritis, 1:361
germ theory of disease, 1:369
Global Polio Eradication Initiative, 1:73, 2:736, 737, 738, 740
globalization and infectious disease, 1:385
Gonococcal Antimicrobial Surveillance Programme, 1:389*s*
gonorrhea, 1:389, 390
group A streptococcal infections, 2:920
Haemophilus influenzae, 1:394, 395, 396
handwashing, 1:402
helminth disease, 1:416, 417
hepatitis A, 1:423
hepatitis C, 1:431
hepatitis D, 1:434, 435
hepatitis E, 1:437
herpes simplex 1 virus, 1:442
herpes simplex virus 2, 1:445
HIV prevalence, 1:224
H5N1, 1:391, 392*s,* 393, 2:614
hookworm infection, 1:457, 458, 459, 460
HPV, 1:469
immigration, 1:472, 473, 474
influenza, 1:490, 491
influenza epidemiology, 1:503, 506
influenza pandemics, 1:496, 500, 501
integrated vector management, 1:463*s*
isolation and quarantine, 1:510
Japanese encephalitis, 1:512, 514
Lassa fever, 1:526, 527*s*
legislation and international law, 1:534–535, 536–537
leishmaniasis, 1:538, 539, 541
leprosy, 1:543, 545, 547
leptospirosis, 1:548, 549*s*
liver fluke infections, 1:562, 563
malaria, 1:462, 2:580, 582–583
Marburg hemorrhagic fever, 2:585, 586, 587
measles, 2:593, 594, 595
Médecins Sans Frontières, 2:601
microsporidiosis, 2:624
monkeypox, 2:627
mosquito netting campaign, 1:486, 2:1093
mosquito-borne diseases, 2:637
nosocomial infections, 2:675
notifiable diseases, 2:681
outbreaks, field-level response to, 2:685, 687, 688

pandemic preparedness, 2:690–691
parasitic diseases, 2:695, 696
plague, 2:715, 717, 718
pneumonia, 2:727, 729–730
polio eradication, 1:487, 2:732, 733, 734, 734*s*
prion diseases, 2:910, 915
ProMED, 2:751, 752
protozoan diseases, 2:755
public health, 2:763, 765
rabies, 2:775, 777, 778, 779
rapid diagnostic tests, 2:783
re-emerging infectious diseases, 2:789, 791
resistant organisms, 2:801, 802–803
Rift Valley fever, 2:814, 816
river blindness, 2:821, 822
rotavirus, 2:829, 830, 831
rubella, 2:838
Salmonella infection, 2:841, 842
sanitation, 2:845, 846*s*
SARS, 2:848–849, 849*s*
scabies, 2:854
schistosomiasis, 2:860, 863
scrofula, 2:867
sepsis, 2:868–870
sexually transmitted infections, 2:878, 879
smallpox, 2:891, 894, 896–899
syphilis, 2:935, 936
taeniasis, 2:943
talaromycosis, 2:946
tetanus, 2:954
trachoma, 2:967, 968–969, 968*s*
trichomoniasis, 2:975
tropical infectious diseases, 2:979, 980, 981, 981*s*, 982
tuberculosis, 1:101, 2:984, 986
tularemia, 2:991
typhoid fever, 2:994–995, 996
typhus, 2:999, 1000
UNICEF, work with, 2:1005
United Nations Millennium Goals, 2:1009, 1010
unvaccinated children, 1:186
vector-borne disease, 2:1029, 1030, 1031
viral disease, 2:1041, 1042
war, 2:1051
water-borne diseases, 2:1053–1056
West Nile virus, 2:1058, 1059
whipworm, 2:1064
whooping cough, 2:1068
women and infectious disease, 2:1071–1072, 1073
world trade, 2:1083, 1084
yaws, 2:1088, 1089, 1090
yellow fever, 2:1092–1095
zoonoses, 2:1105, 1107

"World Malaria Report," 2:*582–583*, 981
World Organization for Animal Health, 1:137, 2:778
World Pneumonia Day, 2:729–730
World Summit for Children, 2:1003
World Toilet Day, 2:846
World Tourism Organization, 1:383
World trade, 2:**1081–1086**
cholera, 1:199, 200, 201
economic development, 1:308
globalization, 1:383, 384, 385
legislation and international law, 1:533, 534–535, 536
leprosy, 1:544
plague, 2:710, 711, 718
zoonoses, 2:1106
World Trade Organization, 1:533
World Vision International, 1:486, 2:1031, 1093
World War I
anthrax, 1:50
burkholderia, 1:146*s*
emerging infectious diseases, 1:314
influenza pandemic of 1918, 1:490, 493, 495
malaria, 2:579
relapsing fever, 2:796
syphilis, 2:936
tuberculosis, 2:985
typhus, 2:998–999
war, 2:1047–1048
World War II
anthrax, 1:50
CDC, origins of the, 1:165
glanders, 1:381
human research subjects, 1:344
malaria, 2:579
Pneumocystis jirovecii pneumonia, 2:721
relapsing fever, 2:796
smallpox, 2:893
tularemia, 2:991
typhus, 2:999
war, 2:1049–1050
World Wildlife Fund, 1:304
Worldwide Facial Injectables Market Drivers, Opportunities, Trends, and Forecasts (Research and Markets), 1:135
Worm therapy, 1:417
Worming. *See* Deworming
Wounds
B virus infection, 1:93
botulism, 1:133
brucellosis, 1:140–141
cat scratch disease, 1:161–163, 162*s*
group A streptococcal infections, 2:921
impetigo, 1:480, 481
necrotizing fasciitis, 2:659, 660
rat-bite fever, 2:785
Staphylococcus aureus infections, 2:911, 912
tetanus, 2:952, 953, 954
tsunami lung, 2:730
war, 2:1049–1050
Wroblewski, Lydia E., 1:411
Wuchereria bancrofti. See Filariasis

X

XDR-TB. *See* Extremely drug-resistant tuberculosis
X-rays
anisakiasis, 1:45
aspergillosis, 1:85
avian influenza, 1:89
blastomycosis, 1:122
coccidioidomycosis, 1:220, 221
Legionnaires' disease, 1:531
lung flukes, 1:567
nocardiosis, 2:667
pneumonia, 2:726
tuberculosis, 2:983, 984

Y

Yale Arbovirus Research Unit, 2:1046
Yambuku, Zaire, 2:1045
Yap, Micronesia, 2:1101, 1102
Yaws, 2:**1087–1091,** *1088*
tropical infectious diseases, 2:980, 981
UNICEF, 2:1003
Yaws Eradication Strategy, 2:1088
Yeasts. *See* Mycotic disease
Yekaterinburg, Russia, 1:48
Yellow fever, 2:**1092–1095,** *1093*
arthropod-borne diseases, 1:75
CDC, 1:169
endemicity, 1:322*s*
hemorrhagic fevers, 1:419, 420
immigration, 1:474
mosquito-borne diseases, 2:637
prevention of, 1:345–346
quarantine, 1:508
research, 1:342–343
Rocky Mountain Laboratory, 2:656
self-experimentation of scientists, 1:344
travel, 2:971
tropical infectious diseases, 2:981
vector-borne disease, 2:1030, 1031
virus hunters, 2:1043, 1045
WHO childhood vaccination recommendations, 1:185
Yellow Fever Commission, 1:342–343, 344, 2:1043–1044, 1045, 1092, 1095
Yellow pygmy rice rats, 1:405

Yemen, 1:*199*
child marriage, 2:1005
cholera, 1:198
Médecins Sans Frontières, 2:*600*
Rift Valley fever, 2:814, 816
river blindness, 2:821
war, 2:1049
water-borne disease, 2:1054–1055
Yerkes National Primate Research Center, 1:91–92
Yersin, Alexandre-Emile-John, 2:715, 716
Yersinia pestis
arthropod-borne diseases, 1:75
bacterial diseases, 1:99, 100
bioterrorism, 1:116
plague, early history, 2:709
plague, modern history of, 2:715, 719
vector-borne disease, 2:1029
zoonoses, 2:1106
"*Yersinia pestis* Orientalis in Remains of Ancient Plague Patients," 2:*713–714*
Yersiniosis, 2:**1096–1099,** *1097*
Yolo County, CA, 2:670
Young adults
Chlamydia infection, 1:191
cohorted communities, 1:224*s*
Creutzfeldt-Jakob disease, 1:240
diphtheria vaccine, 1:276
Epstein-Barr virus, 1:335, 337
gonorrhea, 1:389
hepatitis B vaccine, 1:428
influenza, 1:490, 495
Lassa fever, 1:527
leptospirosis, 1:550
mononucleosis, 2:630, 631, 633–635
mumps, 2:647
pneumonia, 2:726
rickettsial disease, 2:811
toxic shock, 2:961
tuberculosis, 2:985

Z

Zaire
African sleeping sickness, 1:3
AIDS pandemic history, 1:18
Ebola, 1:41
hemorrhagic fevers, 1:420
virus hunters, 2:1045
See also Democratic Republic of the Congo
Zalcitabine, 1:13
Zambia
AIDS pandemic history, 1:18
child marriage, 1:15, 2:1005
mosquito-borne diseases, 2:638
Zanamivir, 1:89, 393, 490, 496, 505
Zantac. *See* Ranitidine
Zentel. *See* Albendazole
Zhadanov, Victor, 1:184–185
Zhongshan Hospital, 2:970
Zidovudine, 1:72
Ziehl-Neelsen stain, 1:149, 2:619–620
"A Zika Tale in a Favela," 2:*1102–1103*
Zika virus, 1:*312,* 2:*1100,* **1100–1103**
arthropod-borne diseases, 1:75–76, 76*s*, 77
CDC, 1:166, 169
climate change, 1:206–207
endemicity, 1:321
hosts and vectors, 1:462, 463
infection control and asepsis, 1:486
Koch's postulates, 1:521
microbial evolution, 2:614
mosquito-borne diseases, 2:637
notifiable diseases, 2:681
outbreaks, field-level response to, 2:687
Rocky Mountain Laboratory, 2:655
vaccines and vaccine development, 2:1022–1023
vector-borne disease, 2:1029
viral disease, 2:1042
Zimbabwe
African sleeping sickness, 1:3
Marburg hemorrhagic fever, 2:585
plague, 2:716
re-emerging infectious diseases, 2:792
Zimmer, Carl, 2:697
Zinc gluconate, 1:230
Zoo staff, 1:163
Zoonoses, 2:*1105,* **1105–1109**
animal importation, 1:39–42
arenaviruses, 1:418
avian influenza, 1:87–90
balantidiasis, 1:102–103
Baylisascaris infection, 1:105–108
bovine spongiform encephalopathy, 1:136–139
brucellosis, 1:140–142
burkholderia, 1:144–146
Buruli ulcer, 1:148
Campylobacter infection, 1:152
cat scratch disease, 1:161–163
Ebola, 1:303, 2:1085
emerging infectious diseases, 1:311–314
glanders, 1:381
globalization, 1:384, 385
H5N1 virus, 1:391–393
Lassa fever, 1:526–528
leptospirosis, 1:548–550
liver fluke infections, 1:560–564
monkeypox, 2:626–628
Nipah virus infection, 2:662–664
plague, 2:715–719
psittacosis, 2:759–760
Q fever, 2:771–773
rabies, 2:775–779
rat-bite fever, 2:785–788
relapsing fever, 2:795–798
toxoplasmosis, 2:964–966
tularemia, 2:989–991
virus hunters, 2:1043–1046
world trade, 2:1084
Zostavax, 1:177, 2:887, 888
Zoster. *See* Shingles